Essentials of
Exercise
Physiology
SECOND EDITION

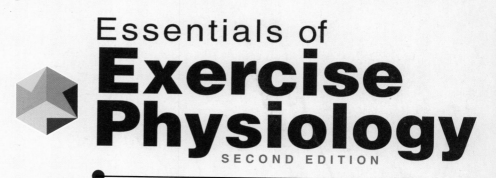

Essentials of
Exercise
Physiology

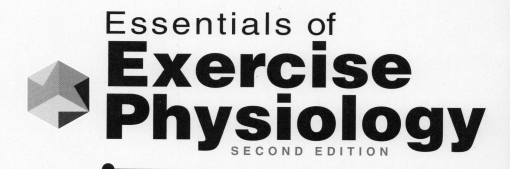

SECOND EDITION

William D. McArdle
Professor Emeritus
Department of Family, Nutrition, and Exercise Science
Queens College of the City University of New York
Flushing, New York

Frank I. Katch
Professor
Department of Exercise Science
University of Massachusetts
Amherst, Massachusetts

Victor L. Katch
Professor
Department of Movement Science
Division of Kinesiology
Associate Professor, Pediatrics
School of Medicine
University of Michigan
Ann Arbor, Michigan

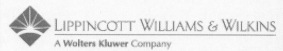

LIPPINCOTT WILLIAMS & WILKINS
A **Wolters Kluwer** Company
Philadelphia · Baltimore · New York · London
Buenos Aires · Hong Kong · Sydney · Tokyo

Editor: Eric Johnson
Managing Editor: Karen Gulliver
Marketing Manager: Christine Kushner
Design Coordinator: Doug Smock

Printed in the United States of America

ISBN: 0-683-30507-7

To purchase additional copies of this book, call our customer service department at (800) 638-3030 or fax orders to (301) 824-7390. International customers should call (301) 714-2324.

00 01 02 03 04
1 2 3 4 5 6 7 8 9 10

To those who provide great meaning to my life: Kathleen, Theresa, Amy, Kevin, Jennifer, Christian, Liam, and Nicole

—BILL MCARDLE

To my beautiful wife Kerry and our great children, David, Kevin, and Ellen

—FRANK I. KATCH

To Heather, Erika, Leslie, and Jesse. You light up my life

—VICTOR L. KATCH

Preface

Introduction

Our goals in the first edition of *Essentials of Exercise Physiology* were to reveal the exciting nature of the science behind exercise physiology and share our passion for the field with others. Our goals for this second edition of *Essentials of Exercise Physiology* remain the same. We have updated almost every section to include and reflect the numerous advances in the field over the past five years. This includes integrating new scientific findings with practical applications to enhance understanding in the field. This has not been an easy task, as exercise physiology has exponentially expanded its knowledge base through the efforts of researchers from many different and new disciplines. A complete understanding of the practical applications of exercise physiology to diverse populations has become a *de facto* requirement for employment in the health-related sciences; we believe this new edition to be the ideal book to help students bridge the gap between theory and practice. Below, we highlight the many new features and advantages of the second edition of *Essentials of Exercise Physiology*.

Organized to Facilitate Student Learning

The second edition of *Essentials of Exercise Physiology* has undergone changes in response to constructive advice from professors and students worldwide about how to improve the teaching and learning of exercise physiology. However, we have maintained the core emphasis of the text—a focus on understanding the interrelationships among energy intake, energy production during exercise, and physiologic systems that support physical activity and training responsiveness.

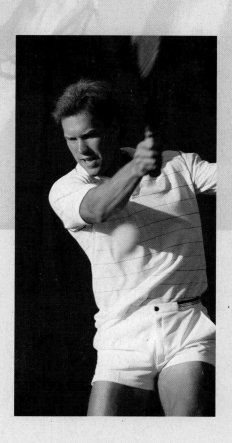

- **Section I:** *Introduction to Exercise Physiology* introduces the historical roots of exercise physiology and delves into the basics of the scientific method, with emphasis on how theories, laws, and facts interrelate to create new knowledge.

- **Section II:** *Nutrition and Energy Transfer*, composed of eight chapters, emphasizes the interrelationship between optimal nutrition and energy metabolism, and how energy transfers from stored nutrients to muscle cells to produce movement during diverse forms of physical activity.

- **Section III:** *The Physiologic Support Systems* contains four chapters that review the fundamental physiologic support systems—pulmonary, circulatory, neuromuscular, and hormonal—and their interactive contributions to energy transfer in exercise and adaptation to training.

- **Section IV:** *Exercise Training and Adaptation in Functional Capacity* describes the application of the scientific principles of exercise training, including the functional and structural adaptation responses to chronic exercise overload.

- **Section V:** *Factors Affecting Physiological Function, Energy Transfer, and Exercise Performance* has two chapters that focus on the effects of environmental challenges and ergogenic substances on energy transfer and human exercise performance.

- **Section VI:** *Optimizing Body Composition, Aging, and Health-Related Exercise Benefits* features the health-related aspects of regular physical activity, with four chapters devoted to body composition assessment and the important role exercise plays in weight control, successful aging, overall good health, and rehabilitation from disease. In new Chapter 21, we discuss the emerging role of the clinical exercise physiologist in the health-related professions.

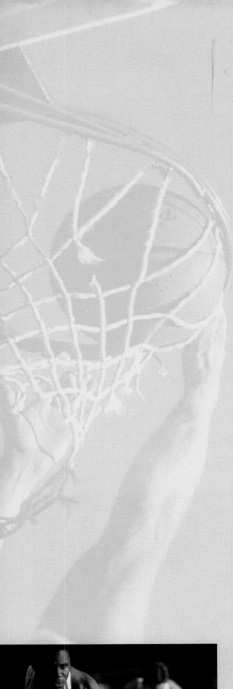

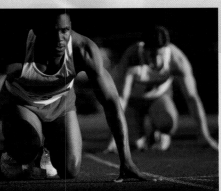

New to the Second Edition

The following points highlight new and expanded content of the second edition of *Essentials of Exercise Physiology*:

- **A new Chapter 1, Origins of Exercise Physiology: Foundations for the Field of Study,** provides an overview of the history of exercise physiology. For the first time in any of our texts, we also introduce basic scientific inquiry related to exercise physiology, and illustrate how to discern good exercise physiology research, explain how different scientific laws and theories develop, illustrate the differences among theoretical, empirical, basic, and applied approaches to knowledge acquisition, and show how scientists disseminate knowledge through peer reviewed journals and other professional publications.

- **A new Chapter 21, Clinical Exercise Physiology for Health-Related Professionals,** developed in response to requests for more complete information linking the components of exercise physiology to clinical assessments and disease rehabilitation. This chapter focuses on the role of exercise in identifying and treating selected disease conditions. We emphasize the health-fitness professional's role in exercise testing, exercise evaluation, exercise prescription, and exercise program implementation.

- **Expanded coverage** of topics related to the preventive and rehabilitative roles of exercise in diabetes and coronary heart disease, the use and abuse of ergogenic substances, and cardiovascular adaptations to exercise training.

- **Incorporated relevant "basics"** from biology and chemistry from Chapter 1 of the first edition throughout the text where applicable.

- **Upgraded and expanded art and tables** within each chapter, with nearly 100 new figures and tables to enhance text information.

- **New material from the most current research,** and new research findings in basic and applied exercise physiology connect clinical applications for health-related areas.

- **Emphasized conceptual understanding** and interpretation of information within each chapter.

- **Focused text material on practical applications** related to exercise training and evaluation of physical fitness and performance.

- **Added new features,** such as *How to* boxes, to spark student interest and facilitate learning.

- **Added two new Appendices:** *Reliable Sources of Information* (Appendix A), and *The Internet and Exercise Physiology* (Appendix B). This appendix provides almost 500 unique sites of interest grouped into six categories that include search engines, government-related sites, general science sites, science and technology news sites, useful resource sites, and 150 sites germain to exercise physiology (including links to the emerging fields of molecular biology and molecular genetics).

Special Features that Promote Learning

We include a variety of features throughout our book to facilitate student learning:

- *How to Boxes.* Approximately 50 *How to* boxes present practical applications to related topics of interest. This material, often showcased in a step-by-step, illustrated format, provides relevance to the practice of exercise physiology. Some *How to* boxes consist of self assessment and/or laboratory-type activities.

- *Close up Boxes.* This popular feature focuses on timely and important exercise, sport, and clinical topics in exercise physiology that relate to the chapter content.

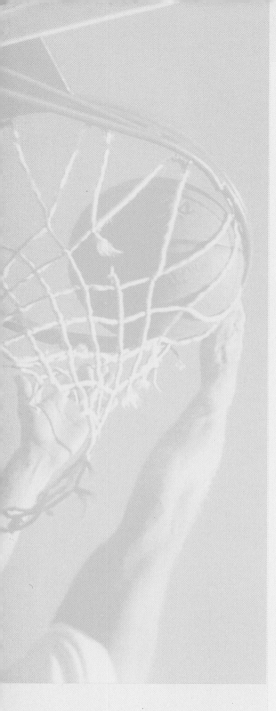

- **FYI Boxes.** FYI are incorporated throughout the text to highlight key information about different exercise physiology areas. We designed these boxes to help bring topics to life and make them relevant to student learning.

- **Thought Questions.** We include Thought Questions at the end of each chapter to encourage integrative, critical thinking and help the student apply information from the chapter. The instructor can use these questions to stimulate class discussion about chapter content and possible application of material to practical situations.

- **Appendices.** Useful current information is at the student's fingertips:

Appendix A. Reliable Sources of Information
Appendix B. The Internet and Exercise Physiology
Appendix C. The Metric System and Conversion Constants in Exercise Physiology
Appendix D. Metabolic Computations in Open-Circuit Spirometry
Appendix E. Frequently Cited Journals in Exercise Physiology
Appendix F. Evaluation of Body Composition — Girth Method
Appendix G. Evaluation of Body Composition — Skinfold Method

Teaching/Learning Package

- The integrated **Student Workbook and Study Guide** actively involves students in the learning process. The book includes four different sections:

- **Section I** facilitates student understanding of text content by focusing on key terms and concepts (student-generated glossary), and poses specific questions for each topic heading within each chapter. To answer the questions, students must read and understand key points presented within the chapter. A practice quiz is also included to test students' comprehension. Crossword puzzles provide a unique and challenging means of linking key words and concepts.

- **Section II** includes the nutritive values of 2025 common foods, including fast-food items, and the energy cost values for more than 240 physical activities. These data provide a tangible means to objectify energy intake and output and overall energy balance.

- **Section III** contains practical tests for self-assessment or group assignments, including Health-Related Physical Fitness Testing; Healthy Lifestyle Assessment; Physical Readiness; and Determining Desirable Body Weight, among others. These self-assessment tests can be used as laboratory experiences.

- **Section IV** provides solutions to the chapter practice quizzes and crossword puzzles.

For the Exercise Physiology Instructor:

- **Test generator.** A CD-ROM (MAC/PC compatible) test bank with a total of approximately 2000 multiple-choice and true-false questions, organized by chapter, makes test generation simple for the busy instructor.

- **Image Bank.** A compilation of textbook figures and tables on CD-ROM supplements lecture presentations and can be used with Macintosh- and PC-based slide-show software such as Powerpoint.

- **Student Workbook** facilitates learning objectives. For example, several instructors award extra credit when students submit the completed glossary and practice quiz portions of the workbook. This type of "directed studying" represents a valued tool that offers structure to a chapter's major content concepts. The assessment tests also serve as a laboratory-type assignments that engage students in active learning, often requiring collecting meaningful personal data.

Acknowledgments

Producing a book requires the coordinated efforts of many professionals. We are indebted to our publishing team at Lippincott Williams & Wilkins for their outstanding contributions during the text development and production processes.

We thank Eric Johnson, our acquisitions editor, who helped everyone keep their eye on the ball; Nancy Peterson, our developmental editor, who provided keen insight, suggestions, and a sense of calmness; Karen Gulliver, our managing editor, gave consistent, thoughtful, and firm direction, while helping us bend some rules as the process progressed; Susan Rockwell for heroic efforts during production; Lisa Manhart, editorial assistant, facilitated communications and meetings; Sam Collins, our graphic artist and medical illustrator, produced a beautiful art program; Bert Vander Mark created an elegant internal design; and Susan Hermansen, Lippincott Williams & Wilkins, created the final cover design. We thank everyone at Lippincott Williams & Wilkins who either directly or indirectly gave a welcome, helping hand to the book's development and production.

A special thanks also to our friends, students, colleagues, and family members for their ongoing support and encouragement throughout this project. We also thank the many reviewers and users of the first edition for their critical and helpful comments and suggestions.

WILLIAM D. MCARDLE
FRANK I. KATCH
VICTOR L. KATCH

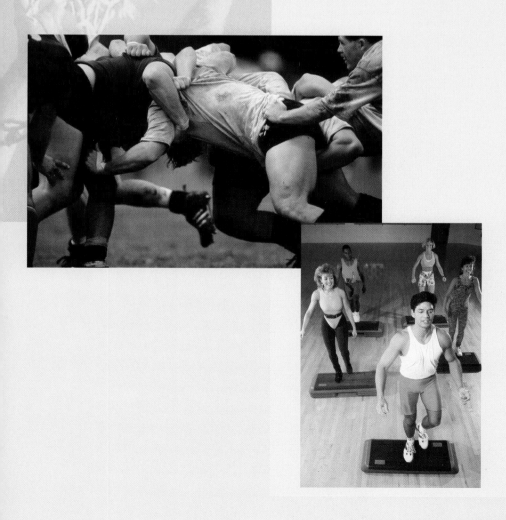

Contents

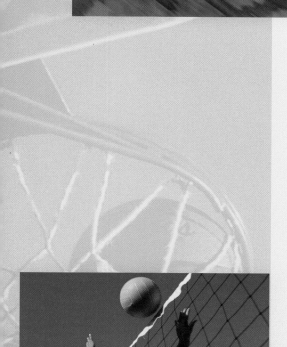

Section 1:
Introduction to Exercise Physiology 3

1. Origins of Exercise Physiology: Foundations for the Field of Study 5

Earliest Development 8

Early United States Experience 8

Contributions of the Harvard Fatigue Laboratory (1927–1946) 18

Nordic Connection (Denmark, Sweden, Norway, and Finland) 19

Other Contributors to Exercise Physiology 22

Contemporary Developments 22

A Common Link 23

General Goals of Science 25

Hierarchy in Science 25

Casual and Causal Relationships 26

Factors That Affect Relationships Among Variables 29

Establishing Laws 32

Developing Theories 32

Certainty of Science 33

Publishing Results of Experiments 34

Empirical vs. Theoretical Research; Basic vs. Applied Research 34

Thought Questions 36

Selected References 37

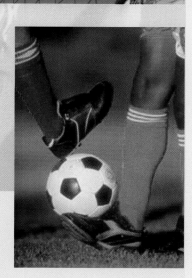

Section 2:
Nutrition and Energy Transfer 38

2. Macronutrients and Food Energy 40

Carbohydrates 41

Lipids 47

Proteins 51

Recommended Dietary Allowance 56

Calorie—A Measurement of Food Energy 61

Gross Energy Value of Foods 61

Net Energy Value of Foods 62

Calories Equal Calories 65

Thought Questions 65

Selected References 66

3. Micronutrients and Water 67

Vitamins 68

Vitamin Supplements: The Competitive Edge? 74

Minerals 75

Minerals and Exercise Performance 82

Water in the Body 84

Water Requirement in Exercise 86

Thought Questions 92

Selected References 93

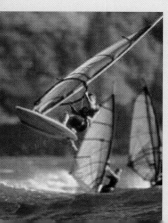

4. Fundamentals of Human Energy Transfer   95

  Adenosine Triphosphate: The Energy Currency   98
  Phosphocreatine: The Energy Reservoir   100
  Intramuscular High-Energy Phosphates   101
  Energy Source Important   101
  Cellular Oxidation   102
  Energy Release From Carbohydrate   105
  Energy Release From Fat   112
  Energy Release From Protein   114
  The Metabolic Mill   116
  Fats Burn in a Carbohydrate Flame   116
  Regulation of Energy Metabolism   117
  Acid-Base Regulation and pH   118
  Buffering and Strenuous Exercise   120
  Thought Questions   122
  Selected References   122

5. Human Energy Transfer During Exercise   124

  Immediate Energy: The ATP-PCr System   125
  Short-Term Energy: The Lactic Acid System   126
  Long-Term Energy: The Aerobic System   127
  Fast- and Slow-Twitch Muscle Fibers   132
  Energy Spectrum of Exercise   132
  Oxygen Uptake During Recovery: The So-Called
    "Oxygen Debt"   135
  Thought Questions   141
  Selected References   141

**6. Measurement of Human Energy
   Expenditure   142**

  Heat Produced by the Body   143
  Direct Versus Indirect Calorimetry   148
  Respiratory Quotient (RQ)   148
  Respiratory Exchange Ratio (R)   149
  Thought Questions   152
  Selected References   153

**7. Energy Expenditure During Rest and Physical
   Activity   154**

  Energy Expenditure at Rest: Basal Metabolic Rate   155
  Influence of Body Size on Resting Metabolism   156
  Estimating Resting Daily Energy Expenditure   157
  Factors Affecting Energy Expenditure   157
  Energy Cost of Recreational and Sport Activities   162
  Average Daily Rates of Energy Expenditure   163
  Classification of Work   163

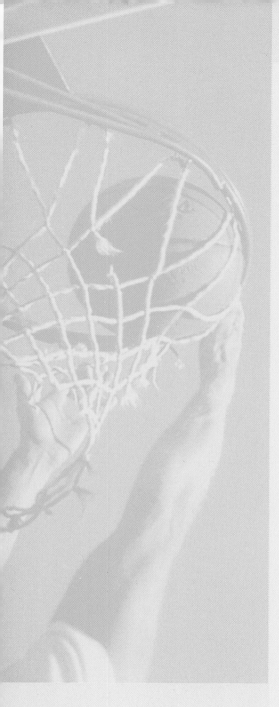

Economy of Movement 166

⋆ Mechanical Efficiency 167

Energy Expenditure During Walking 168

Energy Expenditure During Running 170

Energy Expenditure During Swimming 174

Thought Questions 177

Selected References 178

8. **Evaluating Energy-Generating Capacities During Exercise 179**

Overview of Energy Transfer Capacity During Exercise 180

Anaerobic Energy: Immediate and Short-Term Energy Systems 181

Aerobic Energy: Long-Term Energy System 188

Maximal Oxygen Uptake Measurement 189

Maximal Oxygen Uptake Predictions 198

Thought Questions 204

Selected References 205

9. **Optimal Nutrition for Exercise and Sport 206**

Nutrient Requirements 207

Exercise and Food Intake 209

The Precompetition Meal 214

Carbohydrate Intake Before, During, and After Intense Exercise 216

Glucose Intake, Electrolytes, and Water Uptake 218

Recommended Oral Rehydration Beverage 219

Post-Exercise Carbohydrate Intake 219

Carbohydrate Needs in Intense Training 221

Diet, Glycogen Stores, and Endurance 221

Carbohydrate Loading 224

Thought Questions 225

Selected References 226

Section 3:
The Physiologic Support Systems 228

10. **The Pulmonary System and Exercise 230**

Anatomy of Ventilation 231

Lung Volumes and Capacities 234

Pulmonary Ventilation 237

Disruptions in Normal Breathing Patterns 239

Respired Gases: Concentrations and Partial Pressures 241

Movement of Gas in Air and Fluids 242

Gas Exchange in the Body 243

Oxygen Transport in the Blood   245
Carbon Dioxide Transport in Blood   248
Ventilatory Control   250
Ventilatory Control in Exercise   252
Pulmonary Ventilation and Energy Demands   254
Does Ventilation Limit Aerobic Capacity?   258
Thought Questions   260
Selected References   261

11. The Cardiovascular System and Exercise   262
Components of the Cardiovascular System   264
Blood Pressure   268
Heart's Blood Supply   271
Heart Rate Regulation   275
Blood Distribution   280
Integrated Response in Exercise   282
Cardiac Output   284
Resting Cardiac Output   285
Exercise Cardiac Output   285
Exercise Stroke Volume   286
Exercise Heart Rate   288
Cardiac Output Distribution   288
Cardiac Output and Oxygen Transport   289
Extraction of Oxygen: The a-$\bar{v}O_2$ Difference   290
Cardiovascular Adjustments to Upper-Body Exercise   291
"Athlete's Heart"   292
Thought Questions   294
Selected References   294

12. The Neuromuscular System and Exercise   296
Neuromotor System Organization   297
Motor Unit Physiology   307
Proprioceptors in Muscles, Joints, and Tendons   310
Comparison of Skeletal, Cardiac, and
   Smooth Muscle   314
Gross Structure of Skeletal Muscle   315
Skeletal Muscle Ultrastructure   316
Chemical and Mechanical Events During Contraction
   and Relaxation   319
Muscle Fiber Type   322
Thought Questions   326
Selected References   327

13. Hormones, Exercise, and Training   328
Endocrine System Overview   329
Endocrine System Organization   329
Resting and Exercise-Induced Endocrine Secretions   331

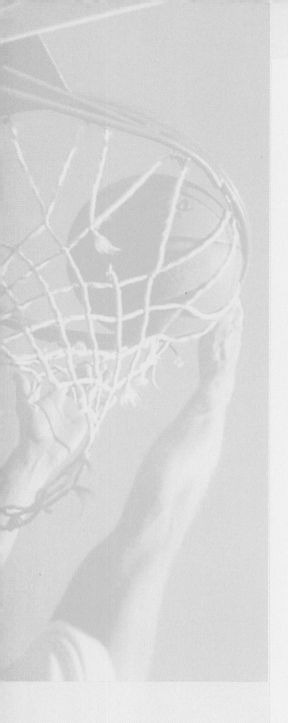

Anterior Pituitary Hormones   334
Posterior Pituitary Hormones   336
Thyroid Hormones   337
Parathyroid Hormone   337
Adrenal Hormones   338
Pancreatic Hormones   340
Diabetes Mellitus   342
Endurance Training and Endocrine Function   346
Resistance Training and Endocrine Function   351
Thought Questions   352
Selected References   352

Section 4:
Exercise Training and Adaptations in Functional Capacity   354

14. Training the Anaerobic and Aerobic Energy Systems   356

Training Must Focus on Energy Requirements   357
General Training Principles   358
Anaerobic Training   360
Aerobic Training   362
Factors That Affect Aerobic Conditioning   366
Adaptations to Exercise Training   368
Formulating an Aerobic Training Program   375
Continuous Versus Intermittent Aerobic Training   380
Maintaining Aerobic Fitness   382
Exercise Training During Pregnancy   382
Thought Questions   386
Selected References   387

15. Training Muscles to Become Stronger   388

Foundations for Studying Muscular Strength   389
Measurement of Muscular Strength   390
Strength Testing Considerations   393
Training Muscles to Become Stronger   393
Gender Differences in Muscular Strength   399
Resistance Training for Children   402
Systems of Resistance Training   402
Neural Adaptations   411
Muscle Adaptations   412
Connective Tissue and Bone Adaptations   415
Cardiovascular Adaptations   415
Metabolic Stress of Resistance Training   417

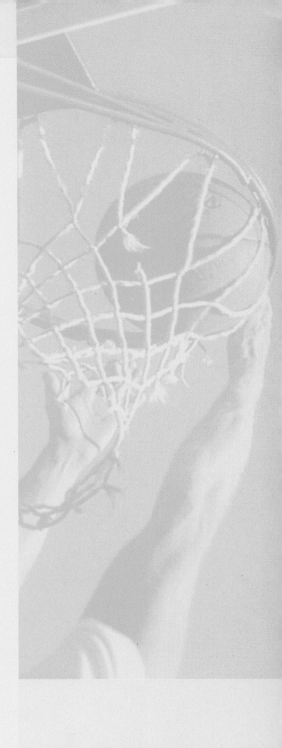

Body Composition Adaptations 419
Muscle Soreness and Stiffness 419
Thought Questions 424
Selected References 425

Section 5:
Factors Affecting Physiological Function, Energy Transfer, and Exercise Performance 426

16. Environment and Exercise 428
Thermoregulation 429
Thermal Balance 429
Hypothalamic Regulation of Body Temperature 430
Thermoregulation in Cold Stress 431
Thermoregulation in Heat Stress 431
Integration of Heat Dissipating Mechanisms 434
Effects of Clothing on Thermoregulation 434
Nutritional Aspects of Exercise in Extreme
    Environments 437
Exercise in the Heat 438
Circulatory Adjustments 438
Core Temperature During Exercise 439
Water Loss in the Heat 439
Factors That Improve Heat Tolerance 443
Evaluating Environmental Heat Stress 446
Exercise in the Cold 447
Evaluating Environmental Cold Stress 447
Stress of Altitude 449
Acclimatization 450
Altitude-Related Medical Problems 453
Exercise Capacity at Altitude 455
Altitude Training and Sea Level Performance 456
Thought Questions 458
Selected References 459

17. Ergogenic Aids 461
Anabolic Steroids 463
Androstenedione: A Legal Supplement in
    Some Sports 466
Clenbuterol: Anabolic Steroid Substitute 468
Growth Hormone: The Next Magic Pill? 469
DHEA: New Drug On the Circuit 469
Amphetamines 471
Caffeine 471

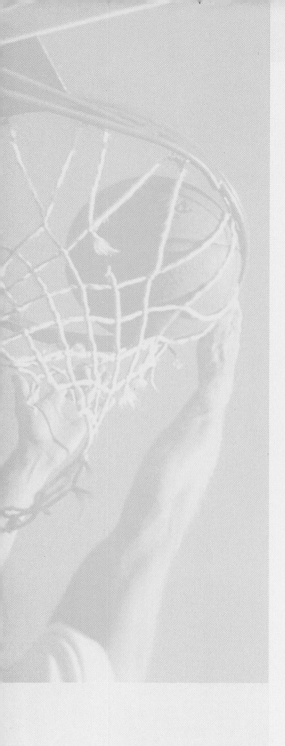

Alcohol   476
Pangamic Acid   478
Buffering Solutions   478
Phosphate Loading   480
Anti-Cortisol Producing Compounds   480
Chromium   481
Creatine   484
Red Blood Cell Reinfusion   489
Warm-Up   491
Breathing Hyperoxic Gas   492
Thought Questions   495
Selected References   495

Section 6:
Optimizing Body Composition, Aging, and Health-Related Exercise Benefits   498

18. Body Composition: Components, Assessment, and Human Variability   500
Gross Composition of the Human Body   501
Leaness, Exercise, and Menstrual Irregularities   505
Methods to Assess Body Size and Composition   506
Body Mass Index   518
Average Values for Body Composition   520
Body Composition of Champion Athletes   522
Thought Questions   526
Selected References   526

19. Obesity, Exercise, and Weight Control   528
Obesity: A Long-Term Process   529
Not Necessarily Overeating   529
Health Risks of Obesity   532
How Fat is Too Fat?   533
The Energy Balance Equation   540
Dieting to Tip the Energy Balance Equation   541
Exercising to Tip the Energy Balance Equation   545
Diet Plus Exercise: The Ideal Combination   549
Gaining Weight   550
Thought Questions   552
Selected References   552

20. Exercise, Aging, and Cardiovascular Health   554
Surgeon General's Report on Physical Activity and Health   555

Safety of Exercising   556

The New Gerontology   557

Concept of Successful Aging   558

Aging and Bodily Function   558

Regular Exercise: A Fountain of Youth?   568

Coronary Heart Disease   571

Risk Factors for Coronary Heart Disease   574

Behavioral Changes Improve Overall Health Profile   582

Thought Questions   583

Selected References   584

21. Clinical Exercise Physiology for Health-Related Professionals   587

The Exercise Physiologist/Health-Fitness Professional
In the Clinical Setting   588

Sports Medicine and Exercise Physiology: A
Vital Link   588

Training and Certification by Professional
Organizations   590

Exercise Programs for Special Populations   593

Oncology   593

Cardiovascular Diseases   595

Cardiac Disease Assessment   598

Stress Test Protocols   605

Maximal Treadmill, Cycle Ergometer, and
Swimming Tests   606

Safety of Stress Testing   607

Exercise-Induced Indicators of CHD   610

Invasive Physiologic Tests   611

Patient Classification for Cardiac Rehabilitation   611

Phases of Cardiac Rehabilitation   612

Exercise Prescription   612

The Rehabilitation Program   614

Cardiac Medications   616

Pulmonary Diseases   616

Pulmonary Assessments   624

Pulmonary Rehabilitation and Exercise Prescription   625

Pulmonary Medications   626

Thought Questions   628

Selected References   628

Appendices

**A.   Reliable Information Resources and Exercise
Physiology   632**

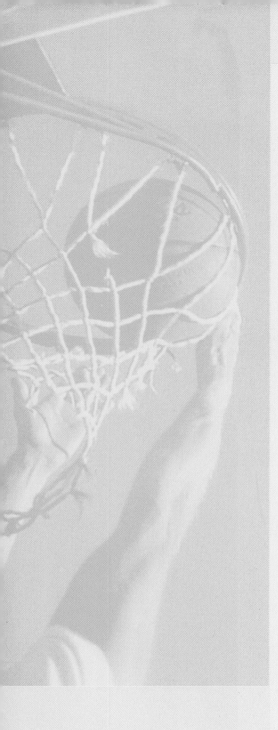

B. The Internet and Exercise
    Physiology   635

C. The Metric System and Conversion Constants in
    Exercise Physiology   645

D. Metabolic Computations in Open-Circuit
    Spirometry   648

E. Frequently Cited Journals in Exercise
    Physiology   653

F. Evaluation of Body Composition—
    Girth Method   654

G. Evaluation of Body Composition—Skinfold
    Method   661

Index   663

SECTION

1

Introduction to Exercise Physiology

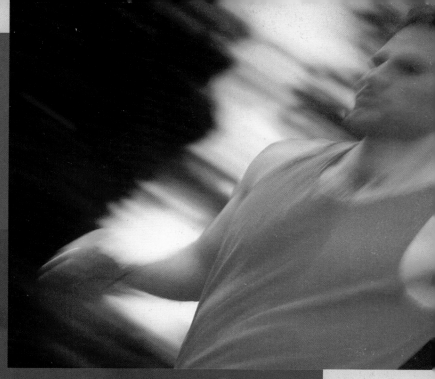

Introduction à l'étude de la medecine expérimentale (The Introduction to the Study of Experimental Medicine. 1865 (translated by H. C. Greene; Henry Schuman, Inc., New York, 1927).

Exercise physiology enjoys a rich historical past, filled with engaging stories about important discoveries in anatomy, physiology, and medicine. Fascinating people and events have shaped our field. The ancient Greek physician Galen (131-201) wrote 87 detailed essays about improving health (proper nutrition), aerobic fitness (walking), and strengthening muscles (rope climbing and weight training). From 776 B. C. to 393 A. D., the ancient Greek "sports nutritionists" planned the training regimens and diets for Olympic competitors, which included high-protein, meat diets believed to improve overall fitness. New ideas about body functioning emerged during the Renaissance as anatomists and physicians exploded every notion inherited from antiquity. Gutenberg's printing press in the 15th century disseminated both classic and newly acquired knowledge. The average could learn about local and world events, and education became more accessible as universities flourished throughout Europe.

The new anatomists went beyond simplistic notions of the early Greek scholar Empedocles' (ca. 500-c. 430 B.C.) four "bodily humors" and elucidated the complexities of the circulatory, respiratory, and digestive systems. Although the supernatural still influenced discussions of physical phenomena, many people turned from dogma to experimentation as their source of knowledge. By the middle of the 19th century, fledgling medical schools in the United States began to graduate their students, many of whom assumed positions of leadership in academia and allied medical sciences. The pioneer physicians taught in medical school, conducted research, and wrote textbooks. Some affiliated with departments of physical education and hygiene where they would oversee programs of physical training for students and athletes. These efforts helped to shape the origin of modern exercise physiology.

In our brief tour of the 2300-year history of exercise physiology in Part 1 of Chapter 1, we chronicle the achievements of several American physician-scientists. The writing and research efforts (begun in 1860) by a college president and his physician son at Amherst College gave birth to exercise physiology as we know it today. Our history in America also includes the first exercise physiology laboratory at Harvard University begun in 1891 (and the rigorous course of study for students in the Department of Anatomy, Physiology and Physical Training). We also highlight scientific contributions of current American and Nordic scientists.

The study of these pioneers in exercise physiology, and their two millennia of contributions in chemistry, nutrition, metabolism, physiology, and physical fitness, helps us to more clearly understand our historical underpinnings, and places in proper perspective the current state and direction of our field.

In Part 2 of the opening chapter, we explore the fundamentals of the scientific process, the basic notions about the scientific method and experimentation, and the way in which science enables us to more fully comprehend the nature of the diverse phenomena related to exercise physiology. Understanding a systematic approach to problem solving hopefully will provide the means for both practitioner and budding scholar to critically evaluate the scientific and popular literature related to the field.

CHAPTER 1

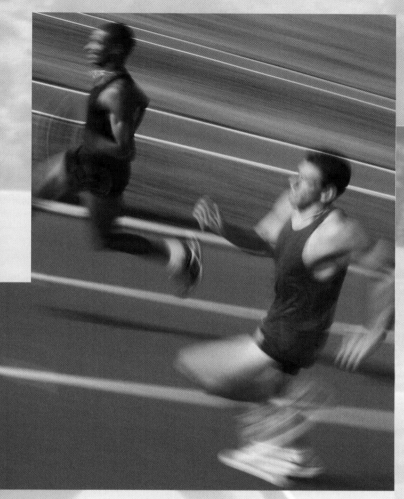

Origins of Exercise Physiology: Foundations for the Field of Study

Topics covered in this chapter

Introduction

PART 1 Origins of Exercise Physiology: From Ancient Greece to the United States

Earliest Development
Early United States Experience
Contributions of the Harvard Fatigue Laboratory (1927–1946)
Nordic Connection (Denmark, Sweden, Norway, and Finland)
Other Contributors to Exercise Physiology
Contemporary Developments
A Common Link
Summary

PART 2 Scientific Method and Exercise Physiology

General Goals of Science
Hierarchy in Science
Casual and Causal Relationships
Factors That Affect Relationships Among Variables
Establishing Laws
Developing Theories
Certainty of Science
Publishing Results of Experiments
Empirical vs. Theoretical Research; Basic vs. Applied Research
Summary
Thought Questions
Selected References

- Briefly outline Galen's contributions to health and scientific hygiene.

- Discuss the beginnings of the scientific development of exercise physiology in the United States. What roles did Austin Flint, Jr., and Edward Hitchcock, Jr., play?

- Discuss the contributions of George Wells Fitz to the academic evolution of exercise physiology.

- Outline the course of study for the first academic 4-year program in the United States from the Department of Anatomy, Physiology, and Physical Training at Harvard University.

- Identify the Harvard Fatigue Laboratory, its major scientists, and its contributions to exercise physiology.

- List the contributions of Nordic scientists to exercise physiology.

- Describe source materials and evaluative procedures in historical research.

- Outline the general goals of science.

- Discuss the role of fact finding in the scientific process.

- Describe differences between causal and casual relationships.

- Identify important factors that determine the quality of experimental research in exercise physiology.

- Identify six factors that affect relationships among variables.

- Describe differences and similarities among empirical, theoretical, basic, and applied research.

- Discuss applications of the World Wide Web for the exercise sciences.

Introduction

The ability to impact the environment depends on our capacity for physical activity. Movement represents more than just a convenience; it is fundamental to our evolutionary development—no less important than the complexities of intellect and emotion.

In this century, we have amassed so much new knowledge about physical activity that exercise physiology is now a separate academic field of study within the biological sciences. Exercise physiology, as an **academic discipline**, consists of three distinct components (Fig. 1.1):

1. Body of knowledge built on facts and theories derived from research
2. Formal course of study in institutions of higher learning
3. Professional preparation of practitioners and future investigators and leaders in the field

The current academic discipline of exercise physiology emerged from the influences of several traditional fields—primarily anatomy, physiology, and medicine. Each of these disciplines uniquely contributes to our understanding of human structure and function in health and disease. Human physiology integrates aspects of chemistry, biology, and physics to explain biological events and their sites of occurrence. Physiologists grapple with questions such as "What factors regulate body functions?", and "What sequence of events occurs between the stimulus and the response in the regulatory process?" The discipline of physiology compartmentalizes into subdisciplines, usually based on either a systems approach (renal, cardiovascular, neuromuscular, pulmonary) or a broad area of study (viral, cell, invertebrate, vertebrate, comparative, human).

Part 1 of this chapter briefly outlines the genesis of exercise physiology in the United States—from antiquity to

Exercise Physiology

Much like biochemistry represents a field distinct from biology and chemistry, exercise physiology has become a separate field of study from physiology because of its focus on functional dynamics and consequences of movement. Exercise physiologists try to determine how the body (subcell, cell, tissue, organ, system) responds in function and structure to 1) acute exercise stress, and 2) chronic physical activity. The exercise physiologist also studies exercise and training responses related to environmental factors—heat, cold, altitude, microgravity, and underwater conditions.

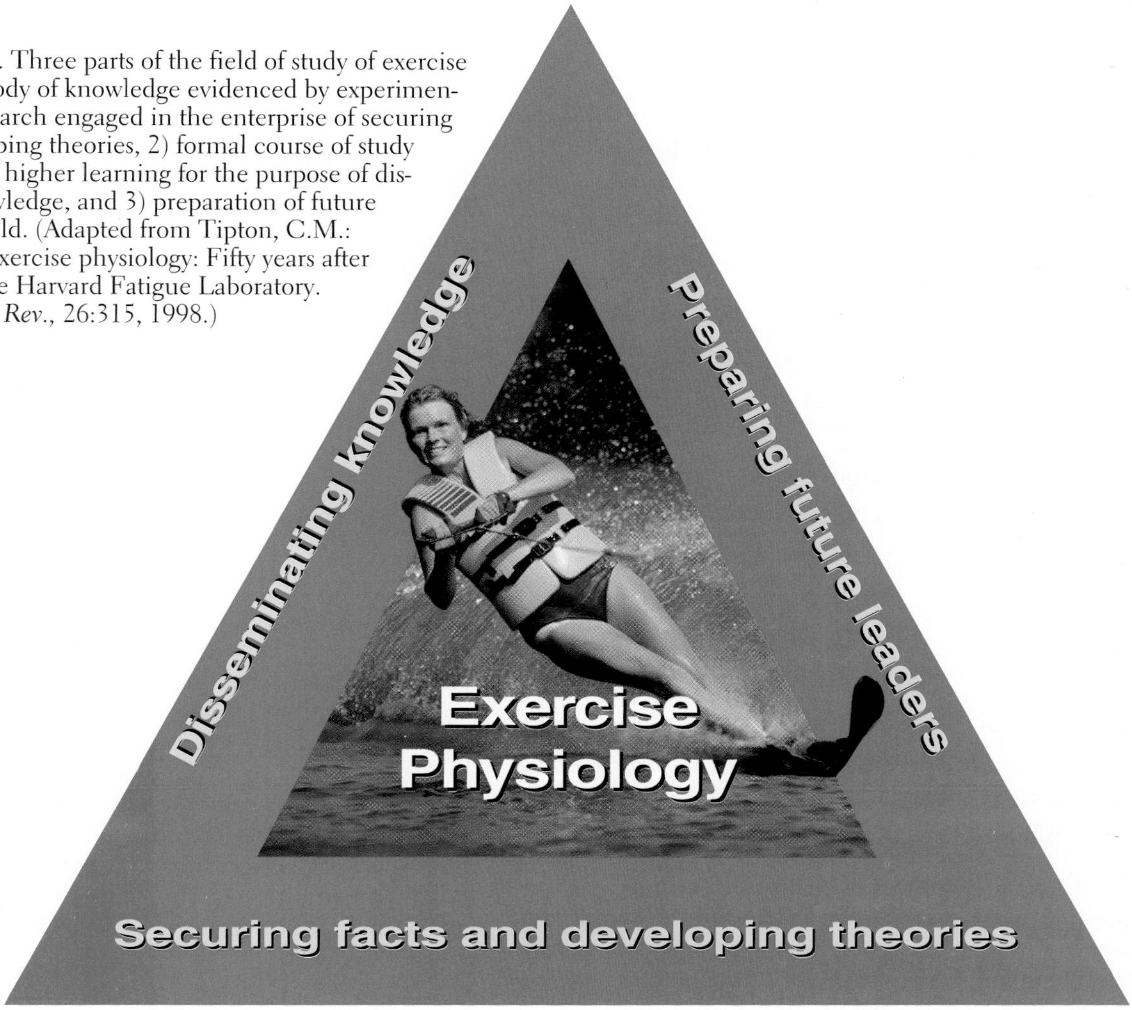

Figure 1.1
Science triangle. Three parts of the field of study of exercise physiology: 1) body of knowledge evidenced by experimental and field research engaged in the enterprise of securing facts and developing theories, 2) formal course of study in institutions of higher learning for the purpose of disseminating knowledge, and 3) preparation of future leaders in the field. (Adapted from Tipton, C.M.: Contemporary exercise physiology: Fifty years after the closure of the Harvard Fatigue Laboratory. *Exerc. Sport Sci. Rev.*, 26:315, 1998.)

the present. We emphasize the growth of formal research laboratories and the publication of textbooks in the field. Although the roots of exercise physiology link to antiquity, the knowledge explosion of the late 1950s greatly increased the number of citations in the research literature. Consider the terms *exercise* and *exertion*. In 1946, only 12 citations appeared in 5 journals. By 1962, the number increased to 128 in 51 journals, and by 1981, 655 citations occurred in 224 journals. Since then, citations have increased progressively. In 1994, more than 3558 citations and topic headings appeared in 1288 journals. By October 1999, more than 6000 citation listings appeared in over 1400 different journals. Today, exercise physiology represents a mature field of study.

The historical underpinnings of exercise physiology should be complemented by an introduction about the goals and process of science. This clarifies how scholars identify reliable information (facts) and generate hypotheses, laws, and theories related to a field, and also explains how to critically evaluate the quality of information about a specific topic area. To this end, Part 2 of this chapter introduces basic concepts of the scientific process that guide the field of exercise physiology.

PART 1

Origins of Exercise Physiology: From Ancient Greece to the United States

The origins of exercise physiology begin with the influential Greek physicians of antiquity. We also highlight contributions from scholars in the United States and Nordic countries, which fostered the scientific assessment of sport and exercise as a respectable field.

Earliest Development

The first real focus on the physiology of exercise probably began in early Greece and Asia Minor. Exercise, sports, games, and health concerned even earlier civilizations; the Minoan and Mycenaean cultures, the great biblical empires of David and Solomon, Assyria, Babylonia, Media, and Persia, and the empires of Alexander. The ancient civilizations of Syria, Egypt, Greece, Arabia, Mesopotamia , Persia, India, and China also recorded references to sports, games, and health practices (personal hygiene, exercise, training). The greatest influence on Western Civilization, however, came from the Greek physicians of antiquity—Herodicus (ca. 480 BC), Hippocrates (460–377 BC), and Claudius Galenus or **Galen** (131–201 AD). Herodicus, a physician and athlete, strongly advocated proper diet in physical training. His early writings and devoted followers influenced Hippocrates, the famous physician and "father of preventive medicine" who contributed 87 treatises on medicine, including several on health and hygiene.

Five centuries after Hippocrates, Galen emerged as the most well-known and influential physician that ever lived. Galen began studying medicine at about age 16. Over the next 50 years, he enhanced current thinking about health and scientific hygiene, an area some might consider applied exercise physiology. Throughout his life, Galen taught and practiced "laws of health" (Table 1.1).

Galen wrote at least 80 treatises and about 500 essays related to human anatomy and physiology, nutrition, growth and development, benefits of exercise and deleterious consequences of sedentary living, and diverse diseases and their treatment. One of the first laboratory-oriented physiologists, Galen conducted original experiments in physiology, comparative anatomy, and medicine; he dissected animals (e.g., goats, pigs, cows, horses, and elephants). As physician to the gladiators (probably the first in sports medicine), Galen treated torn tendons and muscles using surgical procedures that he invented, and recommended rehabilitation therapies and exercise regimens. Galen followed the Hippocratic school of medicine that believed in logical science grounded in observation and experimentation, not superstition or deity dictates. Galen wrote detailed descriptions about the forms, kinds, and varieties of "swift" vigorous exercises, including their proper quantity and duration. Galen's writings about exercise and its effects might be considered the first formal "how to" manuals about such topics, which remained influential for the next 15 centuries.

The beginnings of "modern day" exercise physiology include the periods of Renaissance, Enlightenment, and Scientific Discovery in Europe. During this time, Galen's ideas influenced the writings of the early physiologists, doctors, and teachers of hygiene and health. For example, in Venice in 1539, the Italian physician Hieronymus Mercurialis (1530–1606) published *De Arte Gymnastica Apud Ancientes* (The Art of Gymnastics Among the

TABLE 1.1
Laws of Health According to Galen, circa A.D. 140

1. Breathe fresh air
2. Eat proper foods
3. Drink the right beverages
4. Exercise
5. Get adequate sleep
6. Have a daily bowel movement
7. Control one's emotions

Ancients). This text, influenced by Galen and other Greek and Latin authors, profoundly affected subsequent writings about gymnastics (*physical training and exercise*) and health (*hygiene*) in Europe and 19th century America. The panel in Figure 1.2, redrawn from *De Arte Gymnastica*, acknowledges the early Greek influence of one of Galen's famous essays, "Exercise with the Small Ball," showing his regimen of specific strength exercises, which included discus throwing and rope climbing.

Early United States Experience

By the early 1800s in the United States, European science-oriented physicians and experimental anatomists and physiologists strongly promoted ideas about health and hygiene. Before 1800, only 39 first-edition American-authored medical books had been published; several medical schools were founded (e.g., Harvard Medical School, 1782); seven medical societies existed (the first was the New Jersey State Medical Society in 1766); and only one medical journal existed (*Medical Repository*, initially published in 1797). Outside the United States, 176 medical journals were published, but by 1850, the number in the United States had increased to 117.

Medical journal publications in the United States increased tremendously during the first half of the 19th century. Steady growth in the number of scientific contributions from France and Germany influenced the thinking and practice of American medicine. An explosion of information reached the American public through books, magazines, newspapers, and traveling "health salesmen" who sold an endless variety of tonics and elixirs, promising to optimize health and cure disease. Many health reformers

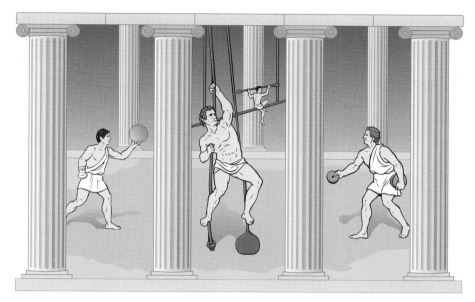

Figure 1.2

The early Greek influence of Galen's famous essay, "Exercise With the Small Ball" clearly appears in Mercurialis' *De Arte Gymnastica*, a treatise about the many uses of exercise for preventive and therapeutic medical and health benefits. Mercurialis favored discus throwing to aid patients who had arthritis and to improve muscular strength in the trunk and arm muscles. He also advocated muscle strengthening with rope climbing because it did not pose health problems. He firmly believed in walking (a mild pace stimulated conversation, but a faster pace stimulated appetite and helped with digestion). He also believed that climbing mountains helped those with leg problems, long jumping was desirable (but not for pregnant women), but he did not recommend tumbling and handsprings because they would produce adverse effects from the intestines pushing against the diaphragm. The three panels represent the exercises as they might have been performed during Galen's time.

information about exercise, how to best develop overall fitness, training (gymnastic) exercises for recreation and preparation for sport, and personal health and hygiene. Although many health faddists actually practiced "medicine" without a license, some enrolled in newly created medical schools (without entrance requirements), obtaining the M.D. degree in as little as 16 weeks. Despite this brief training, some pioneer physicians contributed to medical practice and the development of exercise physiology as we know it today.

By the middle 19th century, fledgling medical schools began to graduate their students, many of whom assumed positions of leadership in academia and allied medical sciences. Interestingly, physicians either taught in medical school and conducted research (and wrote textbooks) or affiliated with departments of physical education and hygiene. Here, they would oversee programs of physical training for students and athletes.

Austin Flint, Jr., M.D.: American Physician–Physiologist

and physicians from 1800 to 1850 used "strange" procedures to treat disease and bodily discomforts. To a large extent, scientific knowledge about health and disease was in its infancy. Lack of knowledge and factual information spawned a new generation of "healers," who fostered quackery and primitive practices on a public who wanted almost anything that seemed to work. If a salesman could offer a "cure" to combat gluttony (digestive upset) and other physical ailments, the product or procedure would become the common remedy.

The "hot topics" of the early 19th century (also true today) included nutrition and dieting (slimming), general

Austin Flint, Jr., M.D. (1836–1915), a pioneer American physician—scientist, contributed significantly to the burgeoning literature in physiology (Fig. 1.3). A respected physician, physiologist, and successful textbook author, he fostered the belief among 19th century American physical education teachers that muscular exercise should be taught from a strong foundation of science and experimentation. Flint, professor of physiology and physiological anatomy in the Bellevue Hospital Medical College of New York, chaired the Department of Physiology and Microbiology from 1861 to 1897. In 1866, he published a series of five classic textbooks,

Early Licensing Laws

Except for three states, licensing laws for physicians had been repealed in 1845, enabling vigorous promotion of homeopathic and botanical medicine (bleeding, blistering, and purgation) by health reformers, dietary faddists, water-cure specialists, animal magnetizers, electromagnetizers, revivalist ministers, and evangelists.

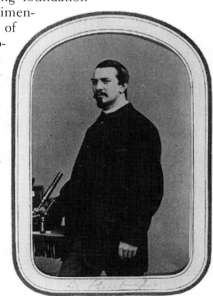

Figure 1.3
Austin Flint, Jr., M.D. American physician–physiologist.

How to Discern Reliable Historical Research

The purpose of historical research has changed through the ages. The earliest writers of history focused on literary rather than scientific objectives; they preserved beloved folktales, created epics to entertain or inspire, defended and promoted numerous causes, zealously protected the privilege of a class, and glorified the state and exalted the church. In contrast, ancient Greek scholars envisioned history as a search for the truth—the application of exacting methods to select, verify, and classify facts according to specific standards that endure the test of critical examination and preserve an accurate record of past events. Historical research enlarges our world of experience; it provides deeper insights into what has been successfully and unsuccessfully tried.

Historical scholars collect and validate source materials to formulate and verify hypotheses. Unlike experimental research, their methods feature observations and insights that cannot be repeated under conventional laboratory conditions.

Collecting Source Material

The historian's initial and most important problem-solving task seeks to obtain the best available data. The historian must distinguish between **primary source** and **secondary source** materials.

Primary Sources

Primary sources comprise the basic materials of historical research. This prized form of "data" derives from:

- Testimony from reliable eyewitnesses and earwitnesses to past events
- Direct examination of actual "objects" used in the past

A historian collects evidence from the closest witness to the past event or condition. Primary source materials include records preserved with the conscious intent of transmitting information. For example, a newspaper account of what transpired at a meeting has less intrinsic historical value than the meeting's official minutes. Records of past ideas, conditions, and events exist in written form (e.g., official records or executive documents, health records, licenses, annual reports, catalogs, and personal records—diaries, autobiographies, letters, wills, deeds, contracts, lecture notes, original drafts of speeches, articles, and books), visual (pictorial) form (photographs, movies, microfilms, drawings, paintings, etchings, coins, and sculpture), mechanical form (tape recordings, phonograph records, dictations), electronic form (digital "memory" on disc or tape), and sometimes oral form (myths, folktales, family stories, dances, games, ceremonies, reminiscences by eyewitnesses to events).

Secondary Sources

Secondary sources include information provided by a person who did not directly observe the event, object, or condition. The original publication of a research report in a scientific journal represents a primary source (often used by modern researchers to provide context to their experiments), summaries in encyclopedias, newspapers, periodicals, Internet, and other references qualify as secondary materials. The more interpretations

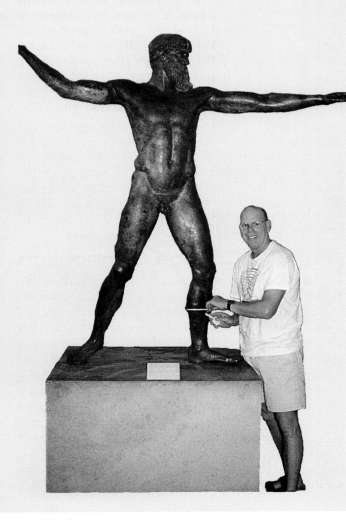

One of the authors taking anthropometric measurements on the original ancient Greek bronze statue Poseidon (460/450 B.C.; primary source—sculpted by either Kalamis or Onatas, and recovered intact in 1928 off Cape Artemision, Euboia, Greece) to determine anthropometric proportions compared with the modern reference man. For a stature of 207 cm, Poseidon's projected body mass using a prediction equation based on stature and six diameters equaled 133.7 kg. (Cooperative research project with Dr. Konstantine Pavlou, College of Sport Sciences and Hellenic Sport Science Institute, Athens, Greece and the National Archeological Museum of Athens.)

that separate a past event from the reader, the less trustworthy the evidence becomes; the transition often distorts and changes the facts. For this reason, secondary sources are less reliable. However, secondary sources acquaint a neophyte historian with major theoretical issues and suggest locations for uncovering primary source materials.

Criticizing Source Material

Historians critically examine the trustworthiness of their source material. Through **external criticism,** the historian checks the authenticity and textual integrity of the "data" to determine its admissibility as reliable evidence (time, place, and authorship). Enterprising and exacting investigation becomes part of external criticism—tracking down anonymous and undated documents, ferreting out forgeries, discovering plagiarism, uncovering incor-

rectly identified items, and restoring documents to their original forms.

After completing external criticism, the historian engages in **internal criticism** to establish the meaning and trustworthiness of a document's contents. Internal criticism determines the following:

- Conditions that produced the document
- Validity of the writer's intellectual premises
- Competency, credibility, and possible author bias
- Correctness of data interpretation

Careful historical research provides insight about how past facts influence current events. Whether an accurate record of the past predicts and influences future circumstances remains a hotly debated topic among historians.

the first entitled *The Physiology of Man; Designed to Represent the Existing State of Physiological Science as Applied to the Functions of the Human Body.* Eleven years later, Flint published *The Principles and Practice of Medicine,* a synthesis of his first five textbooks consisting of 987 pages of meticulously organized sections with supporting documentation. This tome included illustrations of equipment used to record physiological phenomena, including the Frenchman Marey's early cardiograph for registering the wave form and frequency of the pulse and a refinement of Marey's *sphygmograph,* an instrument for making pulse measurements—the forerunner of modern cardiovascular instrumentation (Fig. 1.4).

Dr. Flint, well trained in the scientific method, received the American Medical Association's prize for basic research on the heart in 1858. He published his medical school thesis, "The Phenomena of Capillary Circulation," in an 1878 issue of the *American Journal of the Medical Sciences.* His 1877 textbook included many exercise-related details about the influence of posture and exercise on pulse rate, the influence of muscular activity on respiration, and the influence of muscular exercise on nitrogen

elimination. Flint was well aware of scientific experimentation in France and England and cited the experimental works of leading European physiologists and physicians including the incomparable François Magendie (1783–1855), Claude Bernard (1813–1878), and the influential German physiologists Justis von Liebig (1803–1873), Edward Pflüger (1829–1910), and Carl von Voit (1831–1908). He also discussed the important contributions to metabolism of Antoine Lavoisier (1743–1784) and to digestive physiology from American physician–physiologist William Beaumont (1785–1853).

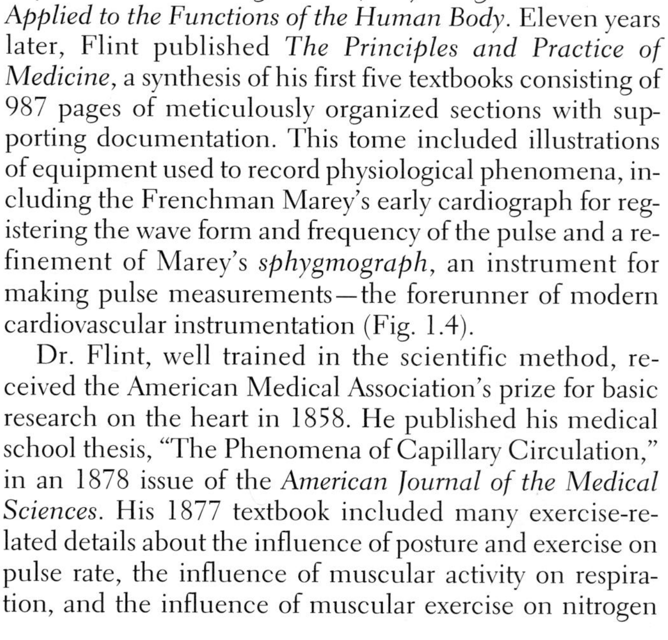

Through his textbooks, Austin Flint, Jr., influenced the first medically trained and science-oriented professor of physical education, Edward Hitchcock, Jr., M.D. (see next section). Hitchcock quoted Flint about the muscular system in his syllabus of *Health Lectures,* which became required reading for all students enrolled at Amherst College between 1861 and 1905.

Amherst College Connection

Two physicians, father and son, pioneered the American sports science movement (Fig. 1.5). **Edward Hitchcock, D.D., LL.D.** (1793–1864), served as professor of chemistry and natural history at Amherst College and as president of the College from 1845 to 1854. He convinced the college president in 1861 to allow his son Edward (1828–1911), an Amherst graduate (1849) [Harvard medical degree (1853)] to assume the duties of his anatomy course. On August 15, 1861, **Edward Hitchcock, Jr.,** became Professor of Hygiene and Physical Education with full academic rank in the *Department of Physical Culture* at an annual salary of $1000—a position he held almost continuously to 1911. Hitchcock's professorship became the second such appointment in physical education in an American col-

Figure 1.4
Marey's advanced sphygmograph.

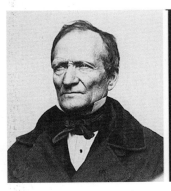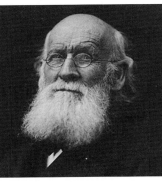

Figure 1.5
Drs. Edward Hitchcock (left), 1793–1864, and Edward Hitchcock, Jr., 1828–1911.

lege. The first, to John D. Hooker a year earlier at Amherst College in 1860, was short lived due to Hooker's poor health. Hooker resigned in 1861, and Hitchcock (Jr.) was appointed in his place.

The original idea of a Department of Physical Education with a professorship had been proposed in 1854 by William Augustus Stearns, D.D., the fourth President of Amherst College. Stearns considered physical education instruction essential for the health of students and useful to prepare them physically, spiritually, and intellectually. In 1860, the Barrett Gymnasium at Amherst College was completed and served as the training facility where all students were required to perform systematic exercises for 30 minutes daily, 4 days a week (Fig. 1.6). A unique feature of the gymnasium was Hitchcock's scientific laboratory that included strength and anthropometric equipment, and a spirometer to measure lung function, which he used to

measure the vital statistics of all Amherst students. Dr. Hitchcock was first to statistically record basic data on a large group of subjects on a yearly basis. These measurements provided solid information for his counseling duties concerning health, hygiene, and exercise training.

In 1860, the Hitchcocks coauthored an anatomy and physiology textbook geared to college physical education (Hitchcock, E., and Hitchcock, E., Jr.: *Elementary Anatomy and Physiology for Colleges, Academies, and Other Schools*. New York: Ivison, Phinney & Co., 1860); 29 years earlier, the father had published a science-oriented hygiene textbook. Interestingly, the anatomy and physiology book predated Flint's similar text by 6 years. This illustrated that an American-trained physician, with an allegiance to the implementation of health and hygiene in the curriculum, helped set the stage for the study of exercise and training well before the medical establishment focused on this aspect of the discipline. A pedagogical aspect of the Hitchcocks' text included questions at the bottom of each page about topics under consideration. In essence, the textbook also served as a "study guide" or "workbook." Figure 1.7 shows sample pages from the 1860 book on muscle structure and function.

An 1880 reprint of the book contained 373 woodcut drawings about the body's physiological systems, including detailed drawings of exercise apparatus (bars, ladders, ropes, swings) and different exercises performed with Indian clubs or "scepters," one held in each hand. Figure 1.8 shows examples of exercises with Indian clubs and those performed on a balance beam and pommel horse by Amherst College students from 1860 to the early 1890s.

Anthropometric Assessment of Body Build

From 1861 to 1888, Dr. Hitchcock, Jr., measured all students enrolled at Amherst College for 6 measures of segmental height, 23 girths, 6 breadths, 8 lengths, 8 measures of muscular strength, lung capacity, and pilosity (amount of

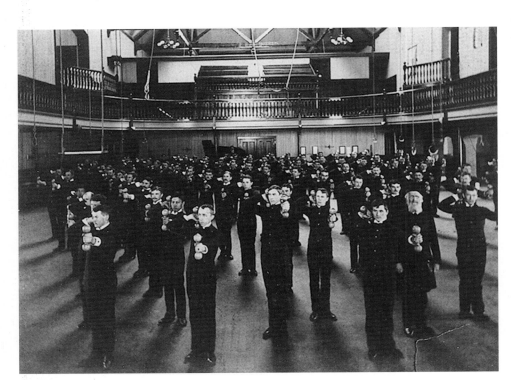

Figure 1.6
Dr. Edward Hitchcock, Jr., (second from right, with beard) with the entire class of students perform barbell exercises in the Pratt Gymnasium of Amherst College. (Photo courtesy of Amherst College Archives, and by permission of the Trustees of Amherst College, 1995 inside.)

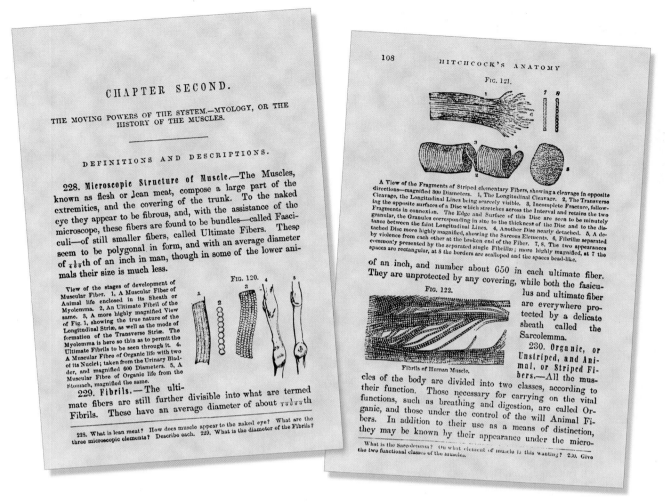

Figure 1.7
Examples from the Hitchcock text on structure and function of muscles. Note that study questions appear at the bottom of each page. (Reproduced from Hitchcock, E., and Hitchcock, E., Jr.: *Elementary Anatomy and Physiology for Colleges, Academies, and Other Schools.* New York: Ivison, Phinney & Co., 1860: pp., 132, 137. (Materials courtesy of Amherst College Archives, and permission of the Trustees of Amherst College, 1995.)

hair on the body). In 1889, Dr. Hitchcock, Jr., and Hiram H. Seelye, M.D., his colleague who also served as college physician from 1884 to 1896 in the Department of Physical Education and Hygiene, published a 37-page anthropometric manual that included five tables of anthropometric statistics based on measurements of students from 1861 to 1891.

While Hitchcock, Jr., performed pioneering anthropometric studies at the college level, the military made the first detailed anthropometric, spirometric, and muscular strength measurements on Civil War soldiers in the early 1860s. Trained military anthropometrists used a unique device, the **andrometer** (Fig. 1.9), to secure the physical dimensions of soldiers for purposes of fitting uniforms. The andrometer, originally devised in 1855 by a tailor in Edinburgh, Scotland, determined the proper clothing size for British soldiers. Special "sliders" measured total height,

breadth of the neck, shoulders, and pelvis, and length of the legs and height to the knees and crotch. Most current university exercise physiology research laboratories (and numerous medical school and military exercise research laboratories) include assessment procedures to routinely evaluate aspects of muscular strength, anthropometry, and body composition.

George Wells Fitz, M.D.: A Major Influence

George Wells Fitz, M.D. (1860–1934), early exercise physiology researcher (Fig. 1.10), helped establish the Department of Anatomy, Physiology, and Physical Training at Harvard University in 1891, shortly after he received his M.D. degree from Harvard Medical School (1891). One year later, Fitz developed the first formal ex-

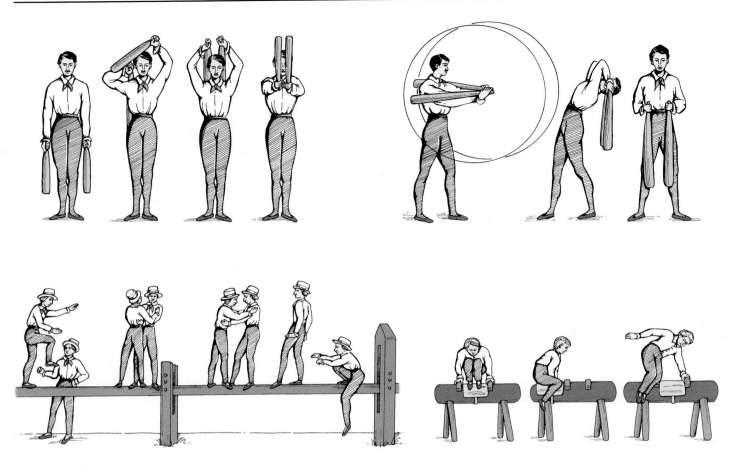

Figure 1.8
Top. Exercises with Indian clubs. **Bottom.** Exercise on a balance beam and pommel horse. These kinds of exercises were performed routinely in physical activity classes at Amherst College from 1860 to 1920.

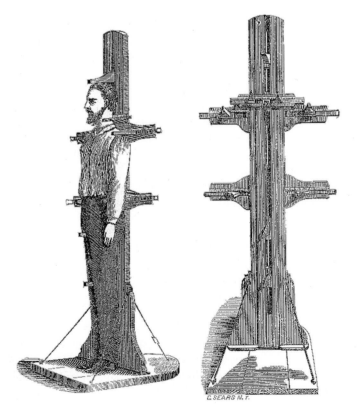

ercise physiology laboratory where students investigated the effects of exercise on cardiorespiratory function, including muscular fatigue, metabolism, and nervous system functions. Fitz, uniquely qualified to teach this course based on his sound experimental training at Harvard's Medical School, also designed new recording and measuring devices. Fitz published his research in the prestigious *Boston Medical and Surgical Journal*, including studies on muscle cramping, efficacy of protective clothing, spinal curvature, respiratory function, carbon dioxide measurement, and speed and accuracy of simple and complex movements. He also wrote two textbooks (*Principles of Physiology and Hygiene* [New York: Holt, 1908]; and revised physiologist H. N. Martin's *The Human Body. Textbook of Anatomy, Physiology and Hygiene; with Practical Exercises* [Holt, 1911]). Well-known researchers in the new program included distinguished Harvard Medical School physiologists Henry Pickering Bowditch,

Figure 1.9
The United States Sanitary Commission first used the andrometer at numerous military installations along the Atlantic seaboard during the early 1860s to size soldiers for clothing.

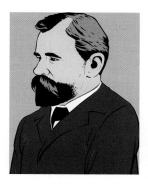

Figure 1.10
George Wells Fitz, M.D.

whose research produced the "all or none principle" of cardiac contraction and "treppe" (staircase phenomenon of muscle contraction), and William T. Porter, internationally recognized experimental physiologist. Charles S. Minot, Massachusetts Institute of Technology-educated chemist with European training in physiology, taught the histology course, and acclaimed Harvard psychologist William James offered the fourth year psychology course. The new four-year course of study, well grounded in the basic sciences even by today's standards, provided students with a rigorous, challenging curriculum in what Fitz hoped would be a new science of physical education. The third year of study was taken at the Medical School (see table in accompanying *Close up*).

Prelude to Exercise Science: Harvard's Department of Anatomy, Physiology, and Physical Training (B.S. Degree, 1891–1898)

Harvard's new physical education major and exercise physiology research laboratory focused on three objectives:

1. Prepare students, with or without subsequent training in medicine, to become directors of gymnasia or instructors in physical training.
2. Provide general knowledge about the science of exercise, including systematic training to maintain health and fitness.
3. Provide suitable academic preparation to enter medical school.

Physical education students took general anatomy and physiology courses in the medical school; after 4 years of study, graduates could enroll as second-year medical students and graduate in 3 years with an M.D. degree. Dr. Fitz taught the physiology of exercise course; thus, he deserves recognition as the first person to formally teach such a course. The new degree included experimental investigation and original work and a thesis, including 6 hours a week of laboratory study. The prerequisite for Fitzs' physiology of exercise course included general physiology or its equivalent taken at the medical school. The physiology of exercise course introduced students to the fundamentals of physical education and provided training in experimental methods related to exercise physiology. In addition to the remedial exercise course, students took a required course in applied anatomy and animal mechanics. This thrice weekly course, taught by Dr. Dudley Sargent, was the forerunner of modern biomechanics courses. Its prerequisite was general anatomy or its equivalent taken at the medical school.

Before its dismantling in 1900, nine men graduated with B.S. degrees from the Department of Anatomy, Physiology and Physical Training. The first graduate, James Francis Jones (1893), became instructor in Physiology and Hygiene, and Director of Gymnasium at Marietta College, Marietta, Ohio. One year after Fitz's untimely resignation from Harvard in 1899, the department changed its curricular emphasis to anatomy and physiology (dropping the term physical training from the department title). This terminated (at least temporarily) a unique experiment in higher education. For almost a decade before the turn of the century, the field of physical education was moving forward on a strong scientific foundation like other more developed disciplines. Unfortunately, this occasion to nurture the next generation of students in exercise physiology (and physical education) was momentarily stymied. Twenty years would pass before the visionary efforts of Dr. Fitz to "study the physiological and psychological effects of exercise," and establish exercise physiology as a bona fide field of investigation would revive, but outside of a formal physical education curriculum.

One of the legacies of the Fitz-directed "Harvard experience" between 1891 and 1899 was the mentoring it provided specialists who began their careers with a strong scientific basis in exercise and training and its relationship to health. They were taught that experimentation and discovery of new knowledge about exercise and training furthered the development of a science-based curriculum. Unfortunately, it would take another 60 years before the next generation of science-oriented physical educators (led by physiologists like A.V. Hill and D.B. Dill, not educators) would again exert strong influence on the physical education curriculum and propel exercise physiology to the forefront of scientific investigation. By 1927, 135 institutions in the United States offered bachelors degree programs in Physical Education with coursework in the basic sciences; this included four masters degree programs and two doctoral programs (Teachers College, Columbia University and New York University). Since then, programs of study with differing emphasis in exercise physiology have proliferated. Currently, approximately 172 programs in the United States and 19 in Canada offer masters or doctoral degrees with specialization in a topic related to some aspect of exercise physiology.

Exercise Studies in Research Journals

In 1898, three articles on physical activity appeared in the first volume of the *American Journal of Physiology*. Other articles and reviews subsequently appeared in prestigious journals, including the first published review in *Physiological Reviews* (2:310, 1922) on the mechanisms of muscular contraction by Nobel laureate A.V. Hill. The German applied physiology publication, *Internationale Zeitschrift für angewandte Physiologie einschliesslich*

What's in a Name?

A lack of unanimity exists for the name of the departments offering degrees (or even coursework) in exercise physiology. As of October, 1999, only one program offers an undergraduate degree titled "Exercise Physiology." Table 1.2 lists examples of 45 names of departments in the United States that offer essentially the same area of study. Each provides some undergraduate or graduate emphasis in exercise physiology (e.g., one or several courses, internships, work-study programs, laboratory rotations, or inservice programs).

Arbeitsphysiologie (1929–1940; now *European Journal of Applied Physiology and Occupational Physiology*), became a significant journal for research about exercise physiology-related topics. The *Journal of Applied Physiology*, first published in 1948, contained the classic paper by J.M. Tanner on ratio expressions of physiological data with reference to body size and function (a "must read" for exercise physiologists). The official journal of the American College of Sports Medicine, *Medicine and Science in Sports*, first appeared in 1969. It aimed to integrate both medical and physiological aspects of the emerging fields of sports medicine and exercise science. The official name of this journal changed in 1980 to *Medicine and Science in Sports and Exercise*. Publications emphasizing applied and basic exercise physiology research have increased as the

TABLE 1.2
Examples of Names for Departments Offering Courses, Degrees, and Specialization in Exercise Physiology in the United States

Allied Health	Leisure Science
Allied Health Sciences	Movement and Exercise Science
Exercise and Movement Science	Movement Studies
Exercise and Sport Science	Nutrition and Exercise Science
Exercise and Sport Studies	Nutritional and Health Sciences
Exercise Science	Performance and Sport Science
Exercise Science and Human Movement	Physical Culture
Exercise Science and Physical Therapy	Physical Education
Health and Human Performance	Physical Education and Exercise Science
Health and Physical Education	Physical Education and Human Movement
Health, Physical Education, Recreation and Dance	Physical Education and Sport Programs
Human Biodynamics	Physical Education and Sport Science
Human Kinetics	Physical Therapy
Human Kinetics and Health	Recreation
Human Movement	Recreation and Wellness Programs
Human Movement Sciences	Science of Human Movement
Human Movement Studies	Sport and Exercise Science
Human Movement Studies and Physical Education	Sport Management
Human Performance	Sport, Exercise, and Leisure Science
Human Performance and Health Promotion	Sports Science
Human Performance and Leisure Studies	Sport Science and Leisure Studies
Human Performance and Sport Science	Sport Science and Movement Education
Interdisciplinary Health Studies	Sport Studies
Integrative Biology	Wellness and Fitness
Kinesiology	Wellness Education
Kinesiology and Exercise Science	

c l o s e   u p

Course of Study: Department of Anatomy, Physiology, and Physical Training, Lawrence Scientific School, Harvard University, 1893

Few of today's undergraduate physical education major programs could match the strong science core required at Harvard in 1893. The accompanying table lists the 4-year course of study, including a detailed description of the Department's fourth year requirements listed in the 1893 course catalog. Along with core courses, Professor Fitz established an exercise physiology laboratory. The following describes the laboratory's objectives.

"A well-equipped laboratory has been organized for the experimental study of the physiology of exercise. The object of this work is to exemplify the hygiene of the muscles, the conditions under which they act, the relation of their action to the body as a whole affecting blood supply and general hygienic conditions, and the effects of various exercises on muscular growth and general health."

First Year

Experimental Physics
Elementary Zoology
Morphology of Animals
Morphology of Plants
Elementary Physiology and Hygiene (Fitz; **1**)
General Descriptive Chemistry
Rhetoric and English Composition
Elementary German
Elementary French
Gymnastics and Athletics (Sargent & Lathrop)

Second Year

Comparative Anatomy of Vertebrates
Geology
Physical Geography and Meteorology
Experimental Physics
General Descriptive Physics
Qualitative Analysis
English Composition
Gymnastics and Athletics (Sargent & Lathrop)

Third Year (at Harvard Medical School)

General Anatomy and Dissection
General Physiology (Bowditch & Porter)
Histology (Minot & Quincy)
Hygiene
Foods and Cooking [Nutrition] (at Boston Cooking School)
Medical Chemistry
Auscultation and Percussion
Gymnastics and Athletics (Sargent & Lathrop)

Fourth Year

Psychology (James)
Anthropometry (Sargent; **4**)
Applied Anatomy and Animal Mechanics [Kinesiology] (Sargent; **5**)
Physiology of Exercise (Fitz; **3**)
Remedial Exercise (Fitz; **6**)
History of Physical Education (Sargent & Fitz; **2**)
Forensics
Gymnastics and Athletics (Sargent & Lathrop; **7**)

Course	Explanation
(1) The Elementary Physiology of and Hygiene of Common Life, Personal Hygiene, Emergencies. Half-course. One lecture and one laboratory hour each week throughout the year (or three times a week, first half-year). Dr. G.W. Fitz.	This is a general introductory course intended to give the knowledge of human anatomy, physiology and hygiene which should be possessed by every student; it is suitable also for those not intending to study medicine or physical training.
(2) History of Physical Education. Half-course. Lecture once a week and a large amount of reading. Drs. Sargent and G.W. Fitz.	The student is made acquainted with the literature of physical training; the history of the various sports is traced and the artistic records (statuary, etc.) studied.
(3) Physiology of Exercise. Experimental work, original work and thesis. Laboratory work six hours a week. Dr. G.W. Fitz.	This course is intended to introduce the student to the fundamental problems of physical education and to give him the training in use of apparatus for investigation and in the methods in such work. This course is preceded by the course in General Physiology at the Medical School, or its equivalent

continued on next page

Course	Explanation
(4) Anthropometry. Measurements and Tests of the Human Body, Effects of Age, Nurture and Physical Training. Lectures and practical exercises. Half-course. Three times a week (first half-year). Dr. Sargent.	This course affords systematic training in making measurements and tests of persons for the purpose of determining individual strength and health deficiencies. Practice is also given in classifying measurements, forming typical groups, etc., and in determining the relation of the individual to such groups. This course must be preceded by the course in General Anatomy at the Medical School, or its equivalent.
(5) Applied Anatomy and Animal Mechanics. Action of Muscles in Different Exercises. Lectures and Demonstrations. Half-course. Three times a week (second half-year). Dr. Sargent.	The muscles taking part in the different exercises and the mechanical conditions under which they work are studied. The body is considered as a machine. The development of force, its utilization and the adaptation of the different parts to these ends are made prominent in the work. This course must be preceded by the course in General Anatomy at the Medical School, or its equivalent.
(6) Remedial Exercises. The Correction of Abnormal Conditions and Positions. Lectures and Demonstrations. Half-course. Twice a week (second half-year). Dr. G.W. Fitz.	Deformities such as spinal curvature are studied and the corrective effects of different exercises observed. The students are trained in the selection and application of proper exercises, and in the diagnosis of cases when exercise is unsuitable.
(7) Gymnastics and Athletics. Dr. Sargent and Mr. J.G. Lathrop.	Systematic instruction is given throughout the four years in these subjects. The students attend the regular afternoon class in gymnastics conducted by Dr. Sargent, work with the developing appliances to remedy up their own deficiencies and take part in the preliminary training for the various athletic exercises under Mr. Lathrop's direction. Much work is also done with the regular apparatus of the gymnasium.

field expands into different areas. The World Wide Web offers unique growth potential in this regard.

First Textbook in Exercise Physiology

Debate exists over the question: "What was the first textbook in exercise physiology?" Several textbook authors give the distinction of being "first" to the English translation of Fernand Lagrange's, *The Physiology of Bodily Exercise*, originally published in French in 1888. We disagree. To deserve such historical recognition, a textbook should meet the following three criteria:

1. Provide sound scientific rationale for major concepts
2. Provide summary information (based on experimentation) about important prior research in a particular topic area (e.g., contain scientific references to research in the area)
3. Provide sufficient "factual" information about a topic area to give it academic legitimacy

The Lagrange book represents a popular book about health and exercise with a "scientific" title. Based on the aforementioned criteria, the book does not exemplify a bona fide exercise physiology text; it contains fewer than 20 reference citations (based on observations of friends performing exercise). By disqualifying the Lagrange book, what text qualifies as the first exercise physiology text? Possible pre 1900 candidates for "first" include these four choices:

1. Combe's 1843 text, *The Principles of Physiology Applied to the Preservation of Health, and to the Improvement of Physical and Mental Education.* New York: Harper & Brothers, 1843
2. Hitchcock and Hitchcock's 1860 book, *Elementary Anatomy and Physiology for Colleges, Academies, and Other Schools.* New York: Ivison, Phinney & Co., 1860
3. Kolb's insightful 1893 book, *Physiology of Sport.* London: Krohne and Sesemann, 1893
4. Martin's text (1896), *The Human Body. An Account of its Structure and Activities and the Conditions of its Healthy Working.* New York: Holt & Co., 1896

Contributions of the Harvard Fatigue Laboratory (1927–1946)

The real impact of laboratory research in exercise physiology (along with many other research specialties) occurred in 1927, again at Harvard University, 27 years af-

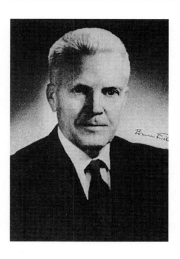

Figure 1.11
David Bruce Dill
(1891–1986).

ter Harvard closed the first exercise physiology laboratory in the United States. The 800-square foot **Harvard Fatigue Laboratory** in the basement of Morgan Hall of Harvard University's Business School legitimized exercise physiology as an important area of research and study.

Many of 20th century's great scientists with an interest in exercise affiliated with the Fatigue Laboratory. Renowned Harvard chemist and professor of biochemistry, **Lawrence J. Henderson, M.D.** (1878–1942), established the laboratory. **David Bruce Dill** (1891–1986), a Stanford Ph.D. in physical chemistry (Fig. 1.11), became the first and only scientific director of the Laboratory. While at Harvard, Dill refocused his efforts from biochemistry to experimental physiology and became the driving force behind the Laboratory's numerous scientific accomplishments. His early academic association with physician Arlie Bock (a student of famous high-altitude physiologist Sir Joseph F. Barcroft at Cambridge, England, and Dill's closest friend for 59 years), and contact with 1922 Nobel laureate **Archibald Vivian Hill** provided Dill with the confidence to successfully coordinate the research efforts of dozens of scholars from 15 different countries. Hill convinced Bock to write a third edition of Bainbridge's text, *Physiology of Muscular Activity*, and Bock invited Dill to coauthor this 1931 book.

Similar to the legacy of the first exercise physiology laboratory established in 1891 at Harvard's Lawrence Scientific School 31 years earlier, the Harvard Fatigue Laboratory demanded excellence in research and scholarship. Cooperation among scientists from around the world fostered lasting collaborations. Many of its charter scientists influenced a new generation of exercise physiologists worldwide.

Other Early Exercise Physiology Research Laboratories

Other notable research laboratories helped exercise physiology become an established field of study at colleges and universities. The Nutrition Laboratory at the Carnegie Institute in Washington, D.C. (established 1904) initiated experiments in nutrition and energy metabolism. The first research laboratories established in a department of physical education in the United States originated at George Williams College (1923), University of Illinois (1925), Springfield College (1927), and Laboratory of Physiological Hygiene at the University of California,

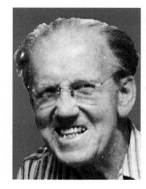

Figure 1.12
F. M. Henry (1904–1993).

Berkeley (1934). The syllabus for the Physiological Hygiene course contained 12 laboratory experiments. In 1936, **Franklin M. Henry** (Fig.1.12) assumed responsibility for the laboratory; shortly thereafter, his research appeared in various physiology-oriented journals.

Nordic Connection (Denmark, Sweden, Norway, and Finland)

Denmark and Sweden also pioneered the field of exercise physiology. In 1800, Denmark became the first European country to require physical training (military-style gymnastics) in the school curriculum. Since then, Danish and Swedish scientists continue to contribute to research in both traditional physiology and exercise physiology.

Danish Influence

In 1909, the University of Copenhagen endowed the equivalent of a Chair in Anatomy, Physiology, and Theory of Gymnastics. The first Docent, **Johannes Lindhard, M.D.** (1870–1947), later teamed with **August Krogh, Ph.D.** (1874–1949), an eminent scientist who specialized in physiological chemistry and research instrument design and construction, to conduct many of the classic experiments in exercise physiology (Fig. 1.13). For example, Lindhard and Krogh investigated gas exchange in the lungs, pioneered studies of the relative contribution of fat and carbohydrate oxidation during exercise, measured

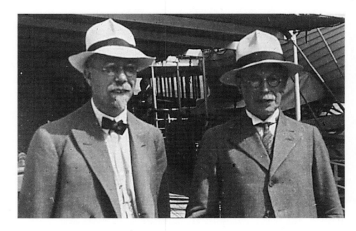

Figure 1.13
Professors August Krogh and Johannes Lindhard, early 1930s.

The Harvard Fatigue Laboratory

Over a 20-year span, Harvard Fatigue Laboratory scientists published at least 352 research papers, monographs, and a book dealing with basic and applied exercise physiology, including methodologic refinements in blood chemistry analysis, and simplified methods for analyzing fractional concentrations of expired air. Other research included acute responses and chronic adaptations to exercise under the environmental stress of altitude, heat, and cold exposure. Most of the physical activity experiments used humans exercising on either a treadmill or bicycle ergometer. These studies formed the cornerstone for future research efforts in exercise physiology; they included assessment of working capacity and physical fitness, cardiovascular and hemodynamic responses during maximal exercise, oxygen uptake and substrate utilization kinetics, exercise and recovery metabolism, and maximal oxygen uptake.

blood flow redistribution during different exercise intensities, and quantified cardiorespiratory dynamics in exercise.

By 1910, Krogh and his physician-wife Marie (Fig. 1.14) had proven through a series of ingenious, decisive experiments that diffusion governed pulmonary gas exchange during exercise and altitude exposure, not oxygen secretion from lung tissue into the blood as postulated by British physiologists Sir John Scott Haldane and James Priestley. Krogh published a series of experiments (three appearing in the 1919 *Journal of Physiology*) concerning the mechanism of oxygen diffusion and transport in skeletal muscles. He won the Nobel Prize in physiology or medicine in 1920 for discovering the mechanism for capillary control of blood flow in resting and exercising muscle. To honor the achievements of this renowned scientist, an institute for physiological research in Copenhagen bears his name (August Krogh Institute).

Three other Danish researchers—physiologists Erling Asmussen (1907–1991; ACSM Citation Award, 1976 and ACSM Honor Award, 1979), Erik Hohwü–Christensen (1904–1996; ACSM Honor Award, 1981), and Marius Nielsen (b. 1903)—conducted significant exercise physiology studies (Fig. 1.15). These "three musketeers," as Krogh called them, published voluminously during the 1930s to 1970s. Asmussen, initially an assistant in Lindhard's laboratory, became a prolific researcher, specializing in muscle fiber architecture and mechanics. He also published papers with Nielsen and/or Christensen on many applied topics, including muscular strength and performance, ventilatory and cardiovascular response to changes in posture and exercise intensity, maximum working capacity during arm and leg exercise, changes in oxidative response of muscle during exercise, comparisons of positive and negative work, hormonal and core temperature response during different intensities of exercise, and respiratory function in response to decreased ambient oxygen levels

Christensen became Lindhard's student in Copenhagen in 1925. In his 1931 doctoral thesis, Christensen reported studies of cardiac output, body temperature, and blood sugar concentration during heavy exercise on a cycle ergometer, compared arm versus leg exercise, and quantified the effects of training. Together with Krogh and Lindhard, Christensen published an important 1936 review article describing physiological dynamics during maximal exercise. With J. W. Hansen, he used oxygen uptake and the respiratory quotient to describe how diet, state of training, and exercise intensity and duration affected carbohydrate and fat utilization. Discovery of the concept of "carbohydrate loading" actually occurred in 1939. Experiments by physician Olé Bang in 1936, inspired by his mentor Ejar Lundsgaard, described the fate of blood lactate during exercise of different intensities and durations. The research of Christensen, Asmussen, Nielsen,

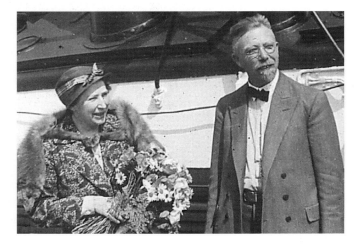

Figure 1.14
Marie and August Krogh.

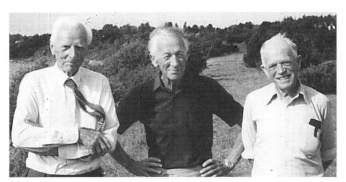

Figure 1.15
Drs. Erling Assmusen (left), Erik Hohwü-Christensen (center), and Marius Nielson (right), 1988.

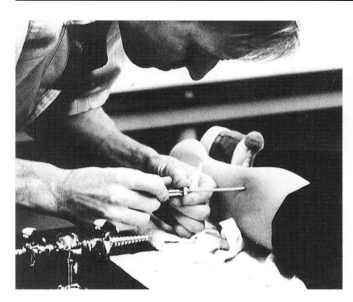

Figure 1.16
Bengt Saltin taking a muscle biopsy of gastrocnemius muscle (Photo courtesy of Dr. David Costill).

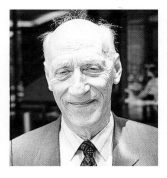

Figure 1.17
Per-Olof Åstrand, Department of Physiology, Karolinska Institute, Stockholm.

and Hansen took place at the Laboratory for the Theory of Gymnastics at the University of Copenhagen. Today, the August Krogh Institute continues the tradition of basic and applied research in exercise physiology. Since 1973, Swedish-trained scientist **Bengt Saltin** (Fig. 1.16) (the only Nordic researcher besides Erling Asmussen to receive the ACSM Citation Award [1980], and ACSM Honor Award [1990]; former student of Per-Olof Åstrand, discussed in the next section) continues his significant scientific studies at the Muscle Research Institute in Copenhagen.

Swedish Influence

Modern exercise physiology in Sweden can be traced to **Per Henrik Ling** (1776–1839), who in 1813 became the first director of Stockholm's Royal Central Institute of Gymnastics. Ling, a specialist in fencing, developed a system (incorporating his studies of anatomy and physiology) of "medical gymnastics," which became part of Sweden's school curriculum in 1820. Ling's son, Hjalmar, published a book on the kinesiology of body movements in 1866. As a result of the Lings' philosophy and influence, physical education graduates from the Stockholm Central Institute were well schooled in the basic biological sciences, in addition to proficiency in sports and games. Currently, the College of Physical Education (Gymnastik-Och Idrottshögskolan) and the Department of Physiology in the Karolinska Institute Medical School in Stockholm continue to sponsor studies in exercise physiology.

Per-Olof Åstrand, M.D., Ph.D. (b. 1922) is the most famous graduate of the College of Physical Education (1946); in 1952, he presented his doctoral thesis at the Karolinska Institute Medical School (Fig. 1.17). Åstrand taught in the Department of Physiology in the College of Physical Education from 1946–1977; it then became a department at the Karolinska Institute, where he served as

professor and department head from 1977 to 1987. Christensen, Åstrand's mentor, supervised his thesis, which evaluated physical working capacity of men and women ages 4 to 33 years. This important study, among others, established a line of research that propelled Åstrand to the forefront of experimental exercise physiology for which he achieved worldwide fame. Four of his papers, published in 1960 with Christensen as coauthor, stimulated further studies on the physiological responses to intermittent exercise. Åstrand has mentored an impressive group of exercise physiologists, including "superstar" Bengt Saltin.

Two Swedish scientists from the Karolinska Institute, **Drs. Jonas Bergström** and **Erik Hultman** (Fig. 1.18), conducted important needle biopsy experiments. With this procedure, muscle could be studied under various conditions of exercise, training, and nutritional status. Collaborative work with other Scandinavian researchers (Saltin and Hultman from Sweden and Hermanson from Norway) and researchers in the United States (e.g., Gollnick [d. 1994], Washington State University) provided new vistas from which to view the physiology of exercise.

Norwegian and Finnish Influence

The new generation of exercise physiologists trained in the late 1940s analyzed respiratory gases with a highly accurate sampling apparatus that measured minute quantities of carbon dioxide and oxygen in expired air. Norwegian sci-

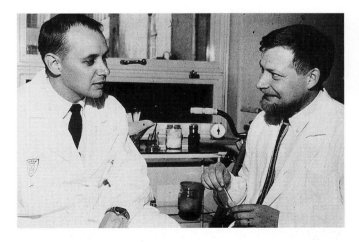

Figure 1.18
Drs. Jonas Bergström (left) and Eric Hultman, Karolinska Institute, Stockholm, mid 1960s.

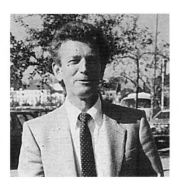

Figure 1.19
Lars A. Hermansen, Institute of Work Physiology, Oslo (1933–1984).

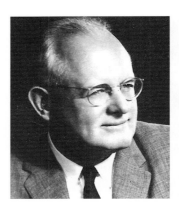

Figure 1.20
Dr. Thomas Kirk Cureton (1901–1993).

entist Per Scholander (1905–1980) developed the method of analysis (and analyzer) in 1947.

Another prominent Norwegian researcher, **Lars A. Hermansen** (1933–1984; ACSM Citation Award, 1985) from the Institute of Work Physiology, made many contributions including a classic 1969 article entitled "Anaerobic energy release," which appeared in the initial volume of *Medicine and Science in Sports* (Fig. 1.19).

In Finland, Martti Karvonen, M.D., Ph.D. (ACSM Honor Award, 1991) from the Physiology Department of the Institute of Occupational Health, Helsinki, achieved notoriety for a method to predict optimal exercise training heart rate, now called the "Karvonen formula" (see Chapter 14). Paavo Komi, Department of Biology of Physical Activity, University of Jyväskylä, has been Finland's most prolific researcher with numerous experiments published in the combined areas of exercise physiology and sport biomechanics. Table 1.3 lists the Nordic researchers who have received the prestigious ACSM Honor Award or ACSM Citation Award.

Other Contributors to Exercise Physiology

In addition to the American and Nordic scientists who achieved distinction as exercise scientists, many other "giants" in the fields of physiology and experimental sci-

TABLE 1.3
Nordic Researchers[a] Awarded the ACSM Honor Award and ACSM Citation Award

ACSM Honor Award	ACSM Citation Award
Per-Olof Åstrand, 1973	Erling Asmussen, 1976
Erling Asmussen, 1979	Bengt Saltin, 1980
Erik Hohwü-Christensen, 1981	Lars A. Hermansen, 1985
Bengt Saltin, 1990	C. Gunnar Blomqvist, 1987
Martti J. Karvonen, 1991	Paavo V. Komi, 1999

[a]Born and educated in a Nordic country.

ence made monumental contributions that indirectly contributed to the knowledge base in exercise physiology. These include physiologists Antoine Laurent Lavoisier (1743–1794; fuel combustion), Sir Joseph Barcroft (1872–1947; altitude), Christian Bohr (1855–1911; oxygen–hemoglobin dissociation curve), John Scott Haldane (1860–1936; respiration), Otto Myerhoff (1884–1951; Nobel Prize, cellular metabolic pathways), Nathan Zuntz (1847–1920; portable metabolism apparatus), Carl von Voit (1831–1908) and his student, Max Rubner (1854–1932; direct and indirect calorimetry, and specific dynamic action of food), Max von Pettenkofer (1818–1901; nutrient metabolism), Eduard F.W. Pflüger (1829–1910; tissue oxidation).

Closer to home, the field of exercise physiology owes a debt of gratitude to the pioneers of the physical fitness movement in the United States, notably **Thomas K. Cureton** (1901–1993; ACSM charter member, 1969 ACSM Honor Award) at the University of Illinois, Champaign (Fig. 1.20). Cureton, a prolific researcher, trained four generations of students beginning in 1941 who later established their research programs and influenced many of today's top exercise physiologists. These early graduates with an exercise physiology specialty soon assumed leadership positions as professors of physical education with teaching and research responsibilities in exercise physiology at numerous colleges and universities in the United States and throughout the world.

Contemporary Developments

Exercise Physiology and the World Wide Web

For exercise physiology, the World Wide Web (www) rapidly disseminates information throughout the world. Direct communication by electronic mail (e-mail) and electronic discussion groups rapidly communicates ideas heretofore impossible.

Numerous electronic discussion groups exist in exercise physiology and related areas, many with thousands of subscribers. New bulletin boards with specific areas of interest (e.g., pediatric exercise immunology, and molecular biology and exercise) enable subscribers to receive and reply to the same inquiry. Many of the field's top scientists routinely participate in discussion groups, which makes "lurking" (computer slang for following the interchanges but rarely participating) a productive pastime. Anyone with an Internet connection and e-mail address can participate in a discussion group. Appendix 1 presents examples of discussion groups of interest to exercise physiologists along with the message needed to join the group and Internet address (known as a universal resource locator or *URL*) to send the message. Joining an online group can increase one's involvement in the field. Hundreds of scientific journals appear on the Internet permitting almost instant access to the latest research information.

Professional Exercise Physiology Organizations

Just as knowledge dissemination via publications in research and professional journals signals expansion of a field of study, development of professional organizations to certify and monitor professional activities becomes critical to continued growth. The American Association for the Advancement of Physical Education (AAAPE), formed in 1885, represented the first professional organization in the United States to include topics related to exercise physiology. This association predated the current **American Alliance for Health, Physical Education, Recreation, and Dance (AAHPERD)**.

Until the early 1950s, AAHPERD represented the predominate professional organization for exercise physiologists. As the field began to expand and diversify its focus, a separate professional organization was needed to more fully respond to professional needs. In 1954, Joseph Wolffe, M.D., and 11 other physicians, physiologists, and physical educators, founded the **American College of Sports Medicine (ACSM)**. Presently, with more than 17,500 members in more than 70 countries (July, 1999), ACSM now represents the largest professional organization in the world for exercise physiology (including allied medical and health areas). ACSM's mission "promotes and integrates scientific research, education, and practical applications of sports medicine and exercise science to maintain and enhance physical performance, fitness, health, and quality of life." ACSM publishes the research journal, *Medicine and Science in Sport and Exercise* and other publications including the *ACSM's Health & Fitness Journal*, and *Guidelines for Exercise Testing and Prescription*, a recognized reference standard for professionals in the field.

Other important professional organizations related to exercise physiology include the International Council of Sport Science and Physical Education (ICSSPE), founded in 1958 in Paris, France, originally under the name International Council of Sport and Physical Education. ICSSPE serves as an international umbrella organization concerned with promoting and disseminating results and findings in the field of sport science. Its main professional publication, *Sport Science Review*, deals with thematic overviews of sport sciences research. The Federation Internationale de Medicine Sportive (FIMS), comprised of the national sports medicine associations of more than 100 countries, originated in 1928 during a meeting of Olympic medical doctors in Switzerland. FIMS promotes the study and development of sports medicine throughout the world and hosts major international conferences in sports medicine every 3 years; it also produces position statements on topics related to health, physical activity, and sports medicine. A joint 1995 position statement with the World Health Organization (WHO), entitled *Physical Activity and Health*, denotes one of their best-known documents. Other organizations representing exercise physiologists include the newly formed European College of Sport Science (ECSS) and British Association of Sport and Exercise Sciences (BASES). The most recent organization, the American Society of Exercise Physiology (ASEP), was formed in 1997 and held its first meeting in October 1998.

A Common Link

One theme unites the 2300-year history of exercise physiology: the value of mentoring by visionaries who spent an extraordinary amount of time "infecting" students with a love for science. These demanding but inspiring relationships developed researchers who nurtured the next generation of productive scholars. This nurturing process from mentor to student remains fundamental to the continued academic development of exercise physiology. The connection between mentor and student remains the hallmark of most fields of inquiry—from antiquity to the present. The mentoring process includes a love of discovery through the scientific method. In Part 2, we explore the fundamentals of the scientific process. The pioneers in our field (and contemporary researchers) incorporated these principles in their quest toward new discoveries.

summary

1. Exercise physiology as an academic field of study consists of three distinct components: 1) a body of knowledge built on facts and theories derived from research, 2) a formal course of study at institutions of higher learning, and 3) professional preparation of practitioners and future leaders in the field.

2. Exercise physiology has emerged as a field separate from physiology because of its unique focus on the study of the functional dynamics and consequences of movement.

3. Galen, one of the first "sports medicine" physicians, wrote prolifically, producing at least 80 treatises and perhaps 500 essays on topics related to human anatomy and physiology, nutrition, growth and development, the benefits of exercise and deleterious consequences of sedentary living, and diseases and their treatment.

4. Austin Flint, Jr., M.D. (1836–1915), one of the first American pioneer physician–scientists, incorporated studies about physiological responses to exercise in his influential medical physiology textbooks.

5. Edward Hitchcock, Jr., (1828–1911), Amherst College Professor of Hygiene and Physical Education, devoted his academic career to the scientific study of physical exercise and training and body size and shape. His 1860 text on anatomy and physiology, coauthored with his father, significantly influenced the sports science movement in the United States after 1860. Hitchcock's insistence on the need for science applied to physical education undoubtedly influenced Harvard's commitment to create an academic Department of Anatomy, Physiology, and Physical Training in 1891.

6. George Wells Fitz, M.D. (1860–1934) created the first departmental major in Anatomy, Physiology, and Physical Training at Harvard University in 1891; the following year, he started the first formal exercise physiology laboratory in the United States. Fitz probably was first to teach a formal exercise physiology course at the university level.

7. The real impact of laboratory research in exercise physiology (along with many other research specialties) occurred in 1927 with the creation of the Harvard Fatigue Laboratory at Harvard University's business school. Two decades of outstanding work by this laboratory legitimized exercise physiology as a key area of research and study.

8. The Nordic countries (particularly Denmark and Sweden) played an important historical role in developing the field of exercise physiology. Danish physiologist August Krogh (1874–1949) won the 1920 Nobel Prize in physiology or medicine for discovering the mechanism that controlled capillary blood flow in resting or active muscle; Krogh's basic experiments led him to conduct other experiments with exercise scientists worldwide. His pioneering work in exercise physiology continues to inspire exercise physiology studies in many areas including oxygen uptake kinetics and metabolism, muscle physiology, and nutritional biochemistry.

9. Publications of applied and basic exercise physiology research have increased as the field expands into different areas. The World Wide Web offers unique growth potential for information dissemination in this area.

10. The American College of Sports Medicine with over 17,500 members from North America and more than 70 other countries represents the largest professional organization in the world for exercise physiology (including allied medical and health areas).

11. One theme unites the 2300-year history of exercise physiology: the value of mentoring by professors who spent an extraordinary amount of time "infecting" students with a love for science.

PART 2
Scientific Method and Exercise Physiology

As the academic discipline of exercise physiology emerged, research strategies for objective measurement and problem solving and the need to report discoveries of new knowledge also developed. The beginning exercise physiology student should become familiar with the methods of science to help separate fact from "hype"—most often encountered in advertising health, fitness, and nutrition products. How does one know whether a product really works? Does warming up really "warm" the muscles to prevent injury and enhance subsequent performance? Will breathing oxygen on the sidelines during a football game help the athlete recover? Do vitamins "supercharge" energy metabolism during exercise? Will creatine, chromium, or vanadium supplements add muscle mass during resistance training? Understanding the role of science in problem solving helps to decide these and many other questions. The following section examines the goals of science, including different aspects of the scientific method of structured problem solving.

Figure 1.21
Foundations of science: facts, laws, and theories.

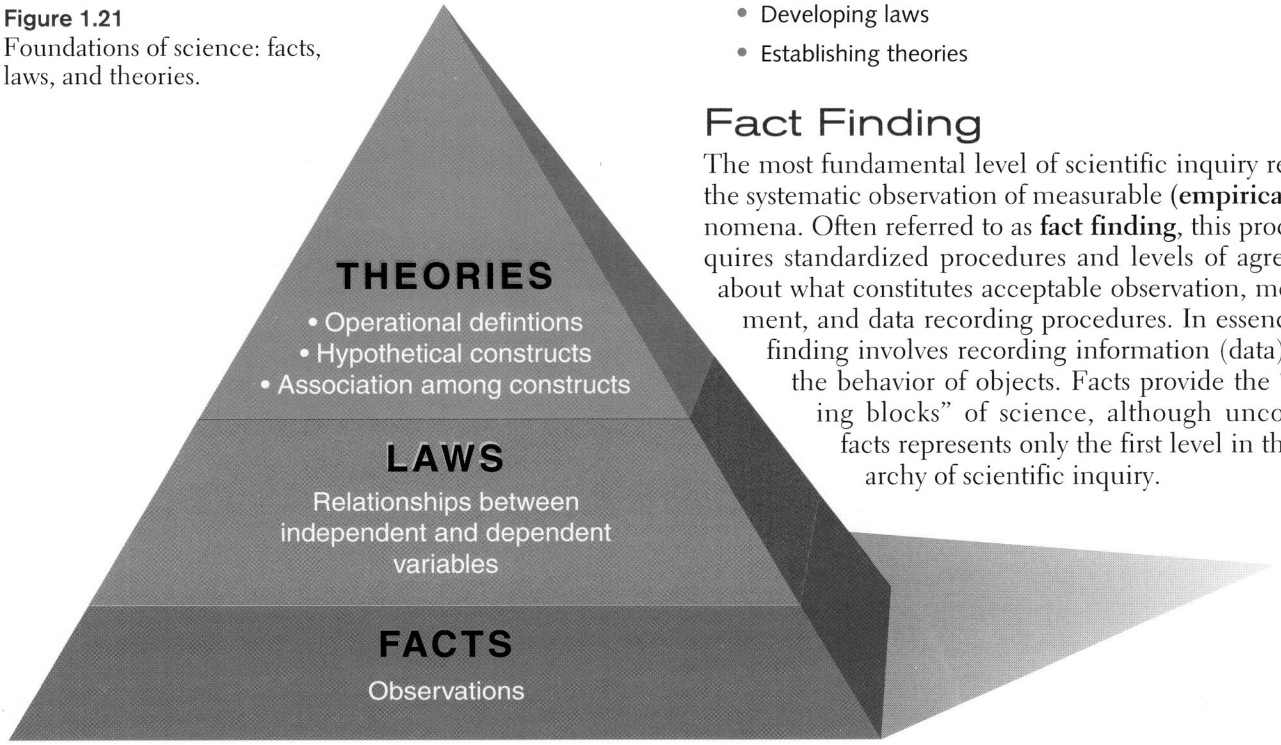

THEORIES
• Operational defintions
• Hypothetical constructs
• Association among constructs

LAWS
Relationships between independent and dependent variables

FACTS
Observations

General Goals of Science

The two distinct goals of science often seem at odds. One goal serves mankind: to provide solutions to important problems and improve life's overall quality. This view of science, most prevalent among *nonscientists*, maintains that all scientific endeavors should exhibit practicality and immediate application. The opposing goal, predominant among *scientists*, maintains that science should describe and understand all occurrences without necessity for practical application—understanding phenomena becomes a worthy goal in itself. The desire for full knowledge implies being able to 1) account for (explain) behaviors or events, and 2) predict (and ultimately control) future occurrences and outcomes. Regardless of one's position concerning the goal of science, its ultimate aims include:

• Explanation
• Understanding
• Prediction
• Control

Hierarchy in Science

Full appreciation of science requires understanding its structure and its three levels of conceptualization (Fig. 1.21):

• Finding facts
• Developing laws
• Establishing theories

Fact Finding

The most fundamental level of scientific inquiry requires the systematic observation of measurable (**empirical**) phenomena. Often referred to as **fact finding**, this process requires standardized procedures and levels of agreement about what constitutes acceptable observation, measurement, and data recording procedures. In essence, fact finding involves recording information (data) about the behavior of objects. Facts provide the "building blocks" of science, although uncovering facts represents only the first level in the hierarchy of scientific inquiry.

A Fact Is a Fact . . .

Facts exhibit no moral quality; once established, any question about facts arises only from interpretation. Although some may disagree with the meaning and implications of an established fact (e.g., the average woman possesses 50% less upper-body strength than the average man), no question exists about the "correctness" of the observation (that women have less upper-body strength than men). In essence, a fact is a fact . . . .

Fact gathering occurs in many ways. We usually observe phenomena through visual, auditory, and tactile sensory input. Regardless of the observation method, to establish something as fact demands that different researchers reproduce observations under identical conditions on different occasions. For example, the healthy human heart's four chambers and the average sea level barometric pressure of 760 mm Hg represent indisputable, easily verifiable "facts." Facts usually take the form of objective statements about the observation such as: "Jesse's body mass measured on a balance scale equals 70 kg (154 lb), or "Jesse's heart rate on rising after 8 hours of sleep averages 63 beats per minute."

Interpreting Facts

Fact finding evaluates the observed object, occurrence, or phenomenon along a continuum, either imagined or real, that represents its underlying measurable "dimension." The term **variable** identifies this measurable characteristic. Frequently, quantification of the variable results from assigning numbers to objects or events to describe their properties. For example, consider the variable percent body fat with numerical values ranging from 3 to 60% of total body mass. Other examples include the weight of an object along a "heaviness" continuum, order of team finish in the NFL's American Conference, or heart rate from rest to maximal exercise.

Some variables like 50-m swim time or blood cholesterol level distribute in a continuous nature; they can take on any numerical value, depending on the precision of the measuring instrument. **Continuous variables** are further classified into ordinal, interval, and ratio numerical data. **Ordinal variables** have rank-ordered values (e.g., small, medium, large bone frame size; first through tenth place finish in a race; standings in league competition) according to some property about each person, group, object, or event compared with others studied. In ordered ranking, no inference exists of equal differences between specific ranks (e.g., race time difference between first and second place finish equals difference between ninth and tenth place). **Interval variables** exhibit similar properties as ordinal variables, except the distance between successive values on an unbroken scale from low to high represents the same amount of change. For example, in marathon running, the temporal 20-minute difference between a finish time of 2 h:10 min and 2 h:30 min equals that of 3 h:50 min and 4 h:10 min. The ratio scale possesses properties of interval and ordinal scoring, but also contains an absolute zero point. Thus, a variable scored on a ratio basis with a value of 4 represents twice as much characteristic as a value of 2; this does not occur with interval-scored variables like temperature, in which 30°F is not twice as "hot" as 15°F.

In addition to continuous variables, some variables possess discrete properties. Scores for **discrete variables** fall only at certain points along a scale, like scores in most sporting events—"almost in" does not count in golf, soccer, basketball, or lacrosse. Discrete variables occur when the score's value simply reflects some characteristic of the object (e.g., male or female, hit or miss, win or lose, true or false, infected or not infected).

Casual and Causal Relationships

A fundamental scientific process involves observing and objectively measuring the quantity of a variable. However, it sometimes becomes important to consider how data from one variable relate to data from another variable. Understanding how variables change in relation to each other represents a higher level of science than merely describing and quantifying diverse isolated variables. For example, quantifying the degree of association between maximal oxygen uptake capacity (abbreviated $\dot{V}O_{2max}$) and chronological age reflects a higher level of understanding than describing the "facts" concerning each variable separately.

Figure 1.22, a scatter diagram between age and $\dot{V}O_{2max}$, shows that older people tend to have lower $\dot{V}O_{2max}$ values, whereas younger individuals possess higher scores. A science neophyte might interpret this inverse relationship as an indication that aging *causes* a decrease in $\dot{V}O_{2max}$, without considering an alternative possibility that decreases in $\dot{V}O_{2max}$ are caused by other variables like a sedentary lifestyle and/or chronic disease that usually accompany aging. A more extreme example to illustrate that association between variables does not necessarily **infer causality** considers the strong direct association in western culture between the length of one's trousers and stature (i.e., taller individuals wear longer-length pants than shorter counterparts). It seems highly unlikely that increasing trouser length increases stature. In reality, this association is **casual**, not causal, being driven more by cultural mores that "require" trousers to descend to ankle level—and leg length relates closely with overall body stature.

The well-established positive relationship between increasing age and increasing systolic blood pressure among adults does not mean that hypertension remains inevitable

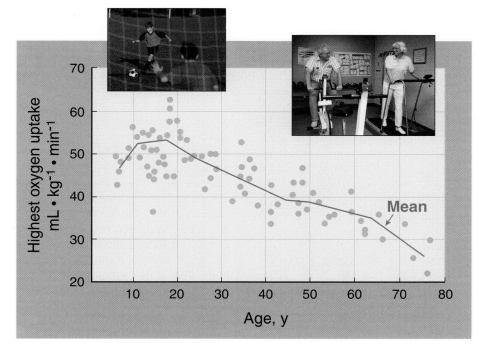

Figure 1.22
Decline in peak $\dot{V}O_{2max}$ with age. (Modified from Robinson, S.: Experimental studies of physical fitness in relation to age. *Arbeitsphysiologie*, 10:18, 1938.)

with age. Rather, the relationship between aging and blood pressure exists because other factors—sedentary lifestyle, obesity, arteriosclerosis, increased stress, and poor diet—often increase with age. Each of these variables independently can elevate blood pressure. From a scientific perspective, a change in one variable (X) does not necessarily cause changes in the other variable (Y), simply because X and Y relate in a manner that seems to "makes sense."

Independent and Dependent Variables

Two categories of variables, independent and dependent, define the nature of relationships among occurrences. This categorization relates to the manner of the variable's use, not the nature of the variable itself. For causal relationships, manipulation of the value of the **independent variable** (X-variable) changes the value of the **dependent variable** (Y-variable). For example, increases in dietary intake of saturated fatty acids (independent X-variable) increases levels of serum cholesterol (dependent Y-variable), whereas decreases in saturated fatty acid intake reduce serum cholesterol levels. In other words, the value of the dependent variable literally "depends on" the value of the independent variable.

For noncausal relationships, the distinction between dependent and independent variables becomes less clear. In such cases, the independent variable (e.g., the sum of five skinfolds or recovery heart rate on a step test) usually becomes the predictor variable, whereas the dependent variable (percent body fat or maximal oxygen uptake) represents the quality predicted. In some cases, an independent variable becomes the dependent variable, and vice versa. For example, body temperature represents the independent variable when used to predict change in regional blood flow or sweating response; body temperature assumes a dependent variable role when evaluating effectiveness of thermoregulation during heat stress.

Establishing Causality Between Variables

Scientists attempt to establish cause and effect relationships between independent and dependent variables by one of two methods:

1. Experimental studies
2. Field studies

Causality

To infer causality, science requires that a change in the X-variable (independent manipulated variable) precedes a change in the Y-variable (dependent variable expected to change), with due consideration for controlling other variables that might actually cause the relationship. Understanding causal factors in relationships among variables enhances one's understanding about observed facts.

Experimental Studies

An **experiment** represents a set of operations to determine the underlying nature of the causal relationship between independent and dependent variables. *Systematically changing the value of the independent variable and measuring the effect on the dependent variable characterizes experimentation.* In some cases, the experiment evaluates the effect of combinations of independent variables (e.g., anabolic steroid administration plus resistance training; preexercise warmup plus creatine supplementation) relative to one or more dependent variables. Regardless of the number of variables studied, an experiment's ultimate goal attempts to systematically isolate the effect of at least one independent variable related to at least one dependent variable. Only when this occurs can one decide which variable(s) really explains the phenomenon.

To illustrate the experimental method, consider two examples of seemingly straightforward studies of the effects of caffeine supplementation on endurance running performance. In one study, the researcher randomly assigns (chance selection of one subject does not affect selection of another subject) 200 subjects to one of two independent groups of 100 subjects each. One group (experimental group) receives a known dose of caffeine in pill form 30 minutes before running to exhaustion at 75% of maximum heart rate; the other group (control group) performs the identical endurance test without consuming caffeine. If time to exhaustion of the caffeine-supplemented experimental group exceeds the caffeine-free control group, caffeine may have enhanced performance. In this case, the results reflect a true effect of the independent variable and not chance occurrence.

Another way to conduct the same experiment entails having only 100 subjects perform two run trials, one with and one without caffeine. For example, in the first trial, a subject consumes caffeine before running. On another day, with sufficient time for recovery and for caffeine's effects to dissipate, the same subject runs without taking caffeine. Each of the 100 subjects would follow this procedure. To eliminate familiarization or training effects influencing test results, the order of testing alternates so that one-half of the subjects exercise first with caffeine, while the other 50 subjects perform first without caffeine.

The important feature of each of the above experiments requires the researcher's ability to manipulate the independent variable (caffeine or no caffeine), while attempting to control for other important aspects like test sequencing, environmental conditions, and perhaps even normal caffeine use before testing. *The control conditions imposed by the experimenter represents the key feature of experimental research.* Control increases the likelihood that manipulation of the independent variable causes any observed change in the dependent variable.

Often times, experimental results are not always as they appear. The two prior example experiments can be criticized on several grounds. Each of the research designs did not permit full control of potential intervening variables; a likelihood exists that variables other than the independent (treatment) variable could influence the observed change in performance. In both experiments, for example, subjects knew in which trial they received a treatment (regardless if they knew about caffeine). This creates the possibility of a **"placebo effect,"** in which a subject's performance improves largely from "expectation" or psychological factors. Many individuals perform at a higher level simply because of the suggestive power of believing the substance or procedure should produce an effect. To attribute a change in endurance to caffeine, unaffected by the subject's expectations, the researcher must use a placebo to provide appropriate control. In both preceding experiments, subjects in the no-caffeine trial should also receive an inert pill that looks, weighs, tastes, and smells the same as the caffeine-containing pill. An appropriate placebo condition controls the expectation effect, and strengthens any conclusion that caffeine enhances endurance performance should this occur.

Factors other than caffeine or a placebo effect must also be considered and controlled. For example, the experimenter needs to account for subjects' normal "background" level of caffeine consumption, particularly in the noncaffeine trials. Having subjects abstain from normal caffeine use for a predetermined duration before testing accomplishes this objective. To eliminate any possible effect of normal daily variation in performance, all testing should take place at the same time of day. To remove the potential for experimenter bias, subjects and researchers must remain unaware of the treatment condition (called a **double-blind** procedure). Some individuals might be "nonresponders" to caffeine's effects (habituation effect) because they regularly consume caffeine-containing foods and beverages. Thus, prior caffeine use becomes a potential confounding variable.

Controlling all potential factors that influence the effects of the independent variable(s) on the dependent variable(s) requires considerable effort and creativity.

Field Studies

Field studies investigate events as they occur in normal living. Under such "natural" conditions, it becomes impossible to experimentally vary the independent variable, or exert full control over potential interacting factors that might affect the relationships. In medical areas, field studies (termed **epidemiologic research**) investigate the characteristics of a group as they relate to the risks, prevalence, and severity of specific diseases. To a large extent, "risk profiles" for coronary artery disease, various cancers, and AIDS have emerged from associations generated from field studies. In exercise physiology, a field study might involve collecting data during a "real world" test of a new piece of exercise equipment (Fig. 1.23). The subject wears a wristwatch that receives signals from a chest strap transmitter that sends the heart's electrical signals to the watch. The subject then pedals the "Surfbike" at differ-

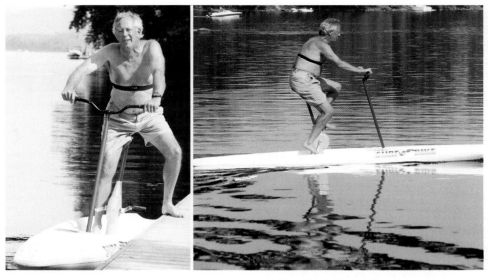

Figure 1.23
Field study in exercise physiology to estimate energy expenditure during Surfbike exercise from the heart rate-oxygen uptake relationship determined in the laboratory. Pedaling Surfbike during 400-m ride produced a heart rate of 178 beats per minute (equivalent to 10.4 kcal per minute energy expenditure). (Courtesy of F. Katch and P. Lagasse, Physical Activity Sciences, School of Medicine, Laval University, Québec City, Canada.)

ent speeds to determine heart rate during different exercise intensities. Before the aquatic experiments, the subject's heart rate and oxygen uptake were determined in the laboratory while pedaling a bicycle ergometer at different speeds. A linear relationship between laboratory determined heart rate and oxygen uptake allowed the researcher to "predict" the subject's oxygen uptake from heart rate measured during Surfbike exercise. An estimate of oxygen uptake permits calculation of caloric expenditure. In this particular experiment, Surfbike exercise at a heart rate of 178 beats per minute translated to 10.4 kcal expended per minute.

Although field studies provide objective insight about possible causes for observed phenomena, the lack of full control inherent in such research limits their ability to infer causality. Because neither active manipulation of the independent variable by the experimenter nor control over potential intervening factors occurs, no certainty exists that any observed variation in the dependent variable will result from variations in the independent variable.

Factors That Affect Relationships Among Variables

Many factors interact to causally affect relationships among variables. An understanding of the dynamics of relationships enables the educated science "consumer" to better evaluate research findings and possible limitations.

Experimental Testing Effects

Taking part in an experiment often changes subjects' behaviors, particularly if they know beforehand someone is evaluating their performance. The potential for altered behavior raises the question whether generalizability of results under structured laboratory conditions translates to behaviors in the "real world." Certainly, an appropriate control group that experiences the same laboratory environment and measurement procedures as the experimental group goes a long way in equalizing such effects across groups.

Measurement Errors

Measurement errors during data collection can be categorized into **technological error** and **recording error.** Technological errors include inherent instability of measuring devices (all mechanical and electronic instruments exhibit technological errors of different magnitudes), and the differential effects of external factors (temperature, humidity, electric current variations, air quality, proper calibration) on an instrument. Sometimes, technological errors remain constant in relation to a standard—the machine always reads high or low —or they vary and the machine randomly reads either high or low. Therefore, the researcher must identify the source of variable errors and minimize their effects; once identified, the constant error can be removed by calibrating the instrument or subtracting or adding the error component in subsequent computations. Proper and frequent instrument calibration minimizes most technological errors of measurement.

Recording errors include inaccuracies associated with improper observation and recording of phenomena. For

How to Discern Reliable Exercise Physiology Research

The following factors provide a frame of reference for evaluating the quality of research. Although the focus considers claims about chemical, pharmacologic, and nutritional ergogenic aids, the principles apply to a broad array of research in exercise physiology. ■

DISCERNING GOOD EXERCISE PHYSIOLOGY RESEARCH

Area	What to Evaluate
Scientific Rationale	Does the research represent a "fishing expedition" or does a sound rationale exist that the specific treatment should produce an effect? For example, a theoretical basis exists to believe that ingesting creatine elevates intramuscular creatine and phosphocreatine levels to augment short-term power outpt capacity. On the other hand, no theoretical basis exists to hypothesize that hyperhydration, breathing hyperoxic gas, or ingesting medium-chain triglycerides should enhance performance in the 100-m dash.
Subjects	Animals or Humans? Many diverse mammals exhibit similar physiological and metabolic processes and responses, yet significant species differences often limit direct applicability of findings to humans. For example, the models for disease processes, nutrient requirements, hormone dynamics, and growth and development can differ greatly between humans and animals.
Gender	Gender-specific responses to the interactions among exercise, training, and nutrient requirements and supplementation may limit generalizability of findings to the gender studied.
Age	Age often influences the outcome of an experimental treatment. Effective interventions for the elderly may have little or no benefit to growing children or young and middle-aged adults, and vice-versa.
Training Status	Fitness status and level of training often influence effectiveness (or ineffectiveness) of a particular diet or supplement intervention. Treatments that benefit the untrained (e.g., chemicals that enhance neurological disinhibition) often confer little effect to elite athletes. Through years of training and competition, athletes perform routinely at maximal levels of neuromuscular activation.
Baseline Level	Research must carefully establish subjects' nutritional status prior to an experimental treatment. Clearly, a nutrient supplement administered to a malnourished group would most likely cause exercise performance and training responsiveness to improve. Such nutrient intervention, however, does not demonstrate whether the same effect occurs if subjects received the supplement with baseline nutrient intake at recommended levels.
Health Status	Nutritional, hormonal, and pharmacologic interventions can profoundly affect the diseased and infirmed, yet confer little or no benefit to individuals in good health. Research findings from studies of diseased groups are often improperly generalized to the well population.
Random Assignment or Self-Selection	Research findings generalize to groups similar to the sample studied. If volunteers "self-select" into an experimental treatment (e.g., strong subjects volunteer for strength training), it becomes difficult to determine whether the experimental treatment produced the results, or the individual's motivation to take part in the study caused any observed changes. Great difficulty exists in assigning truly random samples of subjects to experimental and control groups. The researcher must randomly assign volunteer subjects to either control or experimental conditions, a process termed **randomization.** When all subjects receive the experimental supplement and the placebo treatment (see below), administrating the supplement becomes **counterbalanced**; one-half of the subjects receive the supplement first, while the other half takes the placebo first.
Double-Blind, Placebo-Controlled	The ideal experiment to evaluate the performance-enhancing influence of an exogenous supplement requires that subjects in both treatment and control groups remain unaware or "blinded" to the substance they receive. To achieve this goal, subjects should receive a similar quantity and/or form of the proposed aid, except that control group subjects receive an inert compound or placebo. The placebo treatment evaluates the possibility of subjects performing well or responding better simply because they receive a substance they believe should benefit them (the so-called psychological or "placebo effect"). To further reduce experimental bias from influencing an outcome, the researcher who administers the treatment and records responses must not know which subjects receive the treatment or placebo. The experiment becomes **double-blind** when both researcher and subject remain unaware of the treatment condition.

DISCERNING GOOD EXERCISE PHYSIOLOGY RESEARCH *continued*

Area	What to Evaluate
Control of Extraneous Factors	Under ideal experimental conditions, past experiences should be similar for both experimental and control groups, with the exception of the treatment variable. For example, if experimental subjects in a strength training experiment averaged three years more of prior resistance training experience than control subjects, any change in strength outcome could be due partly to prior experience lifting weights, not the treatment per se. Random assignment of subjects to a control or experimental group goes a long way to neutralize factors that could influence the study's outcome.
Appropriateness of Measurements	Reproducible, objective, and valid measurements must be applied to study the research question. For example, a step test to predict aerobic capacity or skinfolds to evaluate components of body composition represent imprecise tools to answer meaningful research questions about the efficacy of an ergogenic aid.
Findings Should Dictate Conclusions	The conclusions of a research study must logically follow from research findings. Frequently, investigators who study ergogenic aids extrapolate conclusions beyond the scope of their data. The implications and generalizations of research findings must be viewed within the context of the measurements made, subjects studied, and response magnitude. For example, increases in anabolic hormone levels in response to a dietary supplement reflect just that; they do not necessarily indicate an augmented training responsiveness or an improved level of muscular function. Similarly, significant improvement in brief anaerobic power output capacity with creatine supplementation does not justify the conclusion that exogenous creatine improves "physical fitness."
Statistical Versus Practical Significance	The finding of statistical significance for a particular experimental treatment only means a high probability exists that a real effect took place, not a chance occurrence. However, the magnitude of an effect must be evaluated for its real impact on physiology and/or performance. A three-beat per minute reduction in heart rate during submaximal exercise may meet some statistical test about its significance, yet have little practical effect on aerobic fitness or cardiovascular function.
Published in Peer-Reviewed Journal	Quality research withstands the rigors of critical review and evaluation by colleagues with expertise in the specific area of investigation. Peer review assures quality control over the level of scholarship and interpretation of research findings. Publications in popular health and fitness magazines with glitzy covers or quasi professional journals do not undergo the rigor of the peer-review process. In fact, self-appointed "experts" in sport nutrition and physical fitness often pay eager publishers for magazine space to promote their particular viewpoint or efficacy of a product they manufacture. The same applies to articles penned by athletes who give their reasons why a product or method works or does not work. Opinions of so-called fitness "experts" do not qualify as a peer review.
Findings Reproduced by Other Investigators	The findings from one study do not necessarily establish scientific fact. Conclusions become stronger and more generalizable when support emerges from the laboratories of other independent investigators. Consensus reduces the influence of chance, flaws in experimental design, and investigator bias in accounting for experimental effects.

example, measuring heart rate by pulse rate creates several potential sources of error: 1) location and timing of measurement, and 2) accuracy of measurement duration. Using a caliper to measure skinfolds can introduce errors due to nonstandardization of measurement sites, differences in technique for "pinching" the skinfold, accurate caliper placement, and precisely when to read the caliper dial after the pinch. The most experienced researcher attempts to eliminate all errors, but realizes this is nearly impossible.

Within-Subject (Intraindividual) Variability

Another source of measurement error relates to the inherent tendency for humans to exhibit a variable response from moment-to-moment and trial-to-trial. In a sense, **bio-logical variation** should not be considered error, but rather a "fact" of life. All biological systems exhibit inherent variability, albeit small in some cases, depending on the variable. Resting blood flow, heart rate, and blood pressure fluctuate up to ±20% within the same person from day to day, even when measured under identical conditions. One explanation for normal variation in biological function lies in the body's ability to achieve an identical physiological result through diverse mechanisms. For example, blood flow from the heart (cardiac output) occurs from the interaction of heart rate and stroke volume (blood volume pumped from the left ventrical with each beat). Consequently, increases or decreases in heart rate may have little impact on cardiac output if compensated by a proportionate alteration in the heart's stroke volume. All biological functions exhibit natural oscillations. These include easily measured variables like heart rate, breathing rate, and body temperature, to more internal measures of electrical and chemical phenomena. These do not reflect error per se, but rather fluctuations of a normal state. Repeated measurements, or a single measurement for a prolonged duration, often dampen the variation effect and provide a more representative indication of normal functioning.

Individual Differences

Individuals differ from each other in subtle and complex ways. A sampling of exercise physiology variables showing considerable between-subject variation (**individual differences**) includes muscular strength, aerobic and anaerobic capacity, body composition, muscle fiber type, heart size, running economy, and training responsiveness. Individual differences in physiological and performance responses reflect the existence of true biological differences among individuals.

Experimenter Expectation Effect

When the researcher anticipates (wishes) a particular outcome for an experiment, subtle "messages" and alterations in the testing environment may occur, which in themselves influence subject behavior to achieve a desired outcome. Perception of researcher neutrality must be maintained during the research process.

Hawthorne Effect

The **Hawthorne effect** emerged from a series of experiments in the 1930s on worker productivity at the Western Electric Company in Hawthorne, New York. The research evaluated how work hours, pay, modification of lighting, and introduction of music related to job productivity. The data revealed that introducing a change produced noticeable productivity increases. Productivity increased even when reestablishing the original working conditions. In essence, care and attention shown to workers, not the nature of the specific change in working conditions, improved job performance. In this regard, researchers must remain vigilant to guard against a "Hawthorne effect." Personal attention to subjects, or the nature of the study and measurement variables, can cause subjects to modify behaviors and change the dependent variable regardless of the influence of the independent variable. One approach to minimize a Hawthorne effect allows experimental and control groups to interact equally among themselves and the research team.

Establishing Laws

Fact gathering does not generate much controversy; after all, facts are facts. Interpretation of facts, however, raises science to a level rife for debate. Interpreting facts

leads to the second level of the scientific process—creating statements that describe, integrate, or summarize facts and observations. Such statements are known as **laws**. More precisely, a law represents a statement describing the relationships among independent and dependent variables. Laws generate from inductive reasoning (moving from specific facts to general principles). Many examples of laws exist in physiology. For example, blood flows through the vascular circuit in general accord with the physical laws of hydrodynamics applied to rigid, cylindrical vessels. Although true only in a qualitative sense when applied to the body, one law of hydrodynamics, termed Poiseuille's law, describes the interacting relationships among a pressure gradient, vessel radius, vessel length, and fluid viscosity on the force impeding blood flow (see Chapter 11 for a description of Poiseuille's law in action).

Laws are purposely not very specific; thus, they remain powerful because they generalize to many different situations. One variation of Hooke's law of springs, made in 1678 by Robert Hooke (1635–1703), a contemporary of Sir Isaac Newton, states that elongation of a spring relates in direct proportion to the force needed to produce the elongation. Engineers apply this law to design springs for different kinds of instruments via simple calculations in accordance with Hooke's law. Figure 1.24 shows a common application of Hooke's law to an everyday occurrence—measuring body weight on a spring scale.

A good (useful) law accounts for all of the facts among variables. Many laws have limits because they apply to only certain situations. A limited law proves less useful in predicting new facts. *A fundamental aspect of science tests predictions generated from a particular law.* If the prediction holds up, the law expands to additional situations; if not, the law becomes restated in more restrictive terms. Developing new technologies often permits testing laws in situations heretofore thought impossible; this allows for development of a more comprehensive law.

Laws do not provide an explanation *why* variables behave the way they do; laws only provide a general summary of the relationship among variables. Theories explain the hows and whys about laws.

Developing Theories

Theories attempt to explain the fundamental nature of laws. **Theories** offer abstract explanations of laws and facts. They try to explain the "why" of laws. Theories involve a more complex understanding (and explanation) of variables than do laws. Examples of theories include Darwin's theory of natural selection and evolution, Einstein's theory of relativity, Canon's theory of emotions, Freud's theory of personality formation and development, and Helmholtz's theories of color vision and hearing.

Theories consist of three aspects:

1. Hypothetical construct
2. Associations among constructs
3. Operational definitions

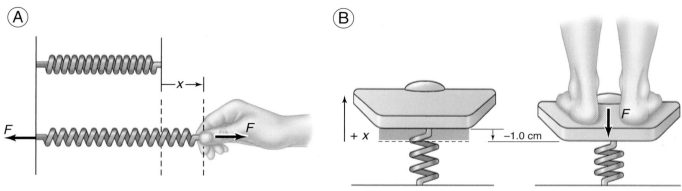

Figure 1.24
Practical application of Hooke's law. **A**. The force needed to stretch an ideal spring relates proportionally to its elongation: F = kx, where k = a proportionality constant unique to each spring. **B**. Compressing a spring in a bathroom scale. A negative force causes a negative displacement; nevertheless, it results in the production of work (W). In this example, the spring compresses 1.0 cm (0.01 m) under the weight of a person who weighs 600 Newtons (the newton, abbreviated N, represents the SI unit of force; 1 pound = 4.4482 N, or in this example, the person weighs 134.9 pounds). W = 600 × 0.01m or 6 Nm.

Hypothetical Constructs

Hypothetical constructs represent nonobservable abstract entities, consciously invented and generalized for use in theories. For example, the construct of "intelligence" emerged from observations of presumably intelligent and nonintelligent behaviors. Several constructs comprise A.V. Hill's initial theory about "oxygen debt" in recovery from exercise (see Chapter 7 for a discussion of recovery oxygen uptake). Hill proposed constructs such as "oxygen deficit," "alactacid debt" and "lactacid debt," and "steady-state" and "non–steady-state" energy transfer to explain his observations about oxygen uptake dynamics in recovery from different exercise intensities. "Physical fitness" represents another common construct in areas related to exercise physiology.

Associations Among Constructs

Scientific inquiry often requires defining relationships among constructs. For example, the construct "physical ability" becomes clarified by its association to the construct "physical fitness," which itself becomes operationally defined (see below) by numerous specific "fitness" tests. In essence, the meaning of one construct becomes understood through its relationship to other more clearly defined constructs.

Operational Definitions

The scientific process requires refinement of constructs into observable characteristics for objective quantification and recording. **Operational definitions** assign meaning to a construct by outlining the set of operations (like an instruction manual) to measure the quantity of that construct or to manipulate it. For example, the construct intelligence only becomes understood when operationally defined (i.e., score on a specific IQ test). In exercise phys-

iology, the construct anaerobic capacity becomes operationally defined as total work accomplished during 30 seconds of all-out exercise performed on an arm-crank or leg-cycle ergometer. Operational definitions permit constructs like muscular strength, aerobic capacity, flexibility, speed of movement, anaerobic power, neuromuscular reaction speed, and physical fitness to emerge from the abstract to the concrete. Operational definitions permit testing of hypotheses and theories by providing a measurement link between an abstract construct and a concrete quantity or measurement. Figure 1.25 shows the relations among theories, laws, and facts (observations).

Certainty of Science

Experimentation represents the scientific method for testing hypotheses; scientists either reject or fail to

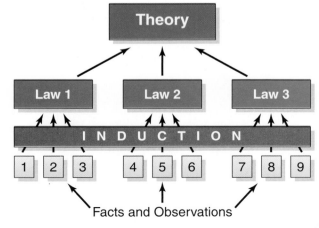

Figure 1.25
Relation among theories, laws, and facts.

reject a hypothesis. Rejecting a hypothesis represents a powerful outcome because it may nullify a theory and specific predictions generated from the theory. Failure to reject a hypothesis indicates that the observable results appear to support the theory. The terms reject and fail to reject (in contrast to prove and disprove) deserve special attention. Failure to reject does not indicate confirmation or proof, only inability to reject an hypothesis. However, if other experiments (particularly from independent laboratories) also fail to reject a given hypothesis, a strong likelihood exists (high probability) of a correct hypothesis. The structure of science makes it impossible to totally confirm a theory's absolute "correctness" because scientists may still devise a future experiment to disprove the theory. The strength of the experimental method lies in rejecting hypotheses that have direct bearing on theories or predictions from theories. *The notion of disproof represents an important distinguishing feature of the scientific method.*

Publishing Results of Experiments

Fact finding, law formulation, and theory development represent fundamental aspects of science. Allowing fellow scientists to critique one's research findings before distribution completes the process of scientific inquiry. Most journals that disseminate research rely on the researcher's peers to review and pass judgment on the suitability and quality of methods, experimental design, appropriateness of conclusions, and contribution to new knowledge. Although this aspect of science is sometimes criticized for failing to achieve true objectivity and freedom from professional bias, few would discount its importance; when executed properly, **peer review** in refereed journals

maintains a level of "quality control" in disseminating new information.

Imagine the many instances in which an experimental outcome could be influenced by self-interest and/or professional bias. Athletic shoe and nutrient supplement manufacturers sponsor sophisticated laboratories to conduct detailed "research" on the efficacy of their products. To ensure credibility, research from such laboratories must be reviewed by experts having no affiliation (direct or indirect) with the company. Without a system of "checks and balances," such studies should be viewed with skepticism and lack trustworthiness as a legitimate source of new knowledge.

Empirical vs. Theoretical Research; Basic vs. Applied Research

Different approaches lead to successful experimentation and knowledge acquisition. Figure 1.26 shows two different continuums for experimentation. The theoretical–empirical research continuum has at its foundation experimentation related to establishing laws and testing theories. Scientists doing **theoretical research** maintain that fact finding alone represents an unfocused waste of energy if the process does not emanate from and contribute to theory building. Scientists at the opposite end of the continuum collect facts and make observations with little regard for building theory. The influential psychologist B.F. Skinner exemplifies the proponent of the **empirical research** (experience related) approach. His discoveries about reinforcement—a reward for successful behavior increases the probability of success in subsequent trials—were uncovered by "accident." Skinnerian empiricists argue that theoretical scientists often do not uncover meaningful relationships because they become too "locked into" theoretical formulations and abstract models.

Basic-applied research represents another continuum. **Applied research** incorporates scientific endeavors to solve specific problems, the solution of which directly applies to medicine, business, the military, sports performance, or society's general well being. Applied research in exercise physiology might focus on methods for improving training responsiveness, facilitating fluid replenishment and temperature regulation in exercise, enhancing endurance performance, blunting the effects of fatigue byproducts, and countering the deterioration of physiological function during prolonged exposure to a weightless environment. **Basic research** lies at the other end of this continuum; no concern exists for immediate practical application of research findings. Instead,

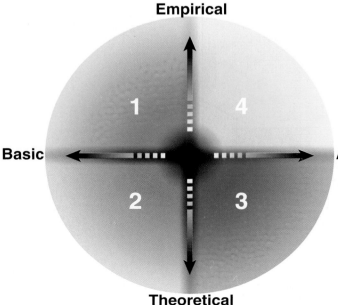

Empirical

Basic | **Applied**

1 4

2 3

Theoretical

Figure 1.26
Research continuum in science.

the researcher pursues a line of inquiry purely for the sake of discovering new knowledge. Often times, uncovering facts that initially seem of little value fill a theoretical void—and like magic, a wonderful new practical solution (or product) emerges. Nowhere has this taken place with more regularity than with research related to the space program. Facts uncovered in a weightless environment about fundamental biological and chemical processes have contributed to practical outcomes that benefit humans. Experiments on how certain chemicals react in zero gravity, for example, have resulted in the discovery of at least 25 new medicines. Manned space missions have provided fresh insights into almost every facet of medicine and physiology, from the affects of weightlessness on bone dynamics, blood pressure, and cardiac, respiratory, hormonal, neural, and muscular function, to growth of genetically engineered plants and a new generation of polymers. Each new insight and observation spawns numerous new ideas

and additional facts that help to create products with practical applications. Figure 1.27 illustrates the use of exercise as countermeasures to negate the deleterious effects of microgravity.

Research can be classified into one of four categories depicted by the quadrants in Figure 1.26. Basic-empirical research in Quadrant 1 has no immediate practical outcomes and little to do with theory. Research without immediate practical implications, but motivated by theory (establishing laws and conducting experiments that bear on theory), falls into Quadrant 2. Quadrant 3 contains theoretical-applied research primarily focused on problem solving within the framework of an existing theoretical model, whereas Quadrant 4 classifies empirical-applied research (not theory based), but aimed at solving problems. Often, lines of demarcation are not as clear-cut as in the figure, and a particular research effort spans multiple quadrants.

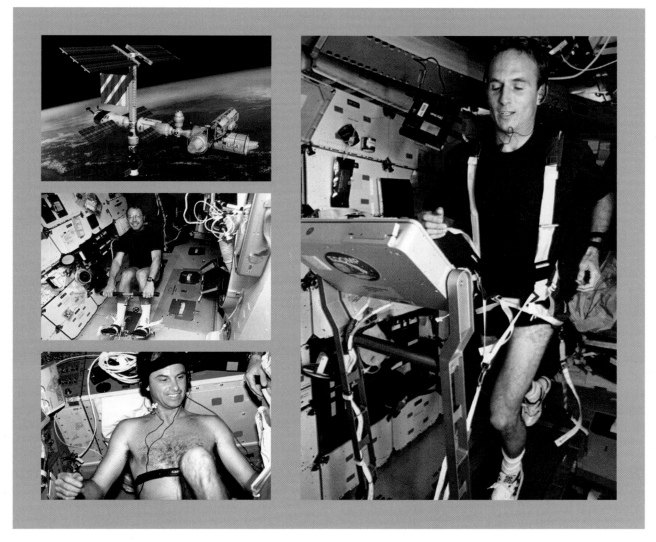

Figure 1.27
Experiments using exercise counter measures during space flight yield a wealth of new information about human physiological responses during microgravity conditions. Theoretical explorations have produced numerous serendipitous outcomes—diverse new products to help humankind. (Courtesy of the NASA Johnson Space Center.)

summary

1. The ultimate aims of science include 1) explanation, 2) understanding, 3) prediction, and 4) control.

2. Fact finding, developing laws, and establishing theories represent three levels of scientific inquiry.

3. The term variable identifies measurable characteristic of an object, occurrence, or phenomenon. The values for discrete variables fall only at certain points along a scale (e.g., scores in most sporting events); continuous variables take on any numerical value, depending on the precision of the measuring instrument.

4. Variables also categorize as either independent or dependent, depending on their use, not their inherent nature. For causal relationships, manipulation of the independent X-variable changes the value of the dependent Y-variable. Understanding how variables change in relation to each other represents a higher level of science than simply describing and quantifying individual variables. Association between variables does not necessarily infer causality.

5. An experiment represents a set of operations to determine the underlying nature of the causal relationship between independent and dependent variables. Systematically changing the value of the independent variable and measuring the effect on the dependent variable characterizes experimentation (with control of other variables that might actually cause the relationship).

6. The key feature of experimental research involves the control of conditions imposed by the experimenter. Control increases the likelihood that manipulation of an independent variable causes any observed change in a dependent variable.

7. Subject selection, appropriate use of statistics, and ability to draw meaningful inferences and conclusions from the data collected represent three important factors for evaluating the quality of research design.

8. Field or epidemiologic studies investigate events as they occur naturally. In exercise physiology, a field study might involve collecting data on the age, body mass, percent body fat, and aerobic capacity of elite triathletes and their performance time during competition. Inability of the researcher to experimentally vary the independent variable, or exert full control over potential interacting factors that might affect relationships, limits research findings.

9. Many factors interact to causally affect relationships among variables. These include experimental testing effects, measurement errors, within-subject variability, individual differences, experimenter expectation effect, and the Hawthorne effect.

10. Interpreting facts leads to the second level of the scientific process—creating statements that describe (or summarize) relationships among facts. Laws only provide a general summary of the relationship among variables; they do not provide an explanation "why" variables behave the way they do.

11. Theories attempt to clarify the fundamental nature of laws—they try to explain the "why" of laws. Theories offer abstract explanations of laws and facts.

12. A theory's absolute "correctness" remains elusive. The strength of the experimental method lies in rejecting hypotheses that have direct bearing on theories or predictions from theories. The notion of disproof represents a key distinguishing feature of the scientific method.

13. Submitting research findings for critique by fellow scientists (peer review) before their dissemination completes the process of scientific inquiry.

thought questions

1. Why should a fitness professional understand the historical roots of exercise physiology?

2. Discuss whether exercise physiology qualifies as a pure scientific area of study, or an applied subdiscipline of other specialty areas?

3. How can an understanding of the scientific method enhance professional development in areas related to exercise physiology (e.g., physical fitness program development, athletic training, personal training)?

selected references

Adams, J. A.: *Human Memory*. New York: McGraw-Hill, 1967.

American Association for Health, Physical Education, and Recreation. *Research Methods Applied to Health, Physical Education, and Recreation.* Washington, D.C., American Association for Health, Physical Education, and Recreation, 1949.

Asmussen, E.: Muscular exercise. In: *Handbook of Respiration.* Section 3. Respiration. Vol. II. Fenn, W.O. and Rahn, H. (eds.). Washington, D.C.: American Physiological Society, 1965.

Åstrand, P.O.: Influence of Scandinavian scientists in exercise physiology. *Scand. J. Med. Sci. Sports.*, 1:3, 1991.

Bang, O., et al.: Contributions to the physiology of severe muscular work. *Skand. Arch. Physiol.*, 74 (Suppl):1, 1936.

Barcroft, J.: *The Respiratory Function of the Blood. Part 1. Lesson From High Altitude.* Cambridge: Cambridge University Press, 1925.

Berryman, J.W.: The tradition of the "six things nonnatural": Exercise and medicine from Hippocrates through Ante-Bellum America. *Exerc. Sport Sci. Rev.*, 17:515, 1989.

Berryman, J.W.: *Out of Many, One. A History of the American College of Sports Medicine.* Champaign, IL: Human Kinetics, 1995.

Buskirk, E.R.: Early History of Exercise Physiology in the United States. Part 1. A contemporary historical perspective. In: *History of Exercise and Sport Science.* Messengale, J.D., and Swanson, R.A. (eds). Champaign, IL: Human Kinetics, 1997.

Buskirk, E.R.: From Harvard to Minnesota: keys to our history. *Exerc. Sport Sci. Rev.*, 20:1, 1992.

Christensen, E.H., et al.: Contributions to the physiology of heavy muscular work. *Skand. Arch. Physiol. Suppl.*, 10, 1936.

Consolazio, C.F.: *Metabolic Methods.* St. Louis: C.V. Mosby, 1951.

Consolazio, C.F.: *Physiological Measurements of Metabolic Functions in Man.* New York: McGrawHill Book Co., 1961.

Cureton, T.K., Jr.: *Physical Fitness of Champion Athletes.* Urbana, IL: University of Illinois Press, 1951.

Dill, D.B.: *Life, Heat, and Altitude: Physiological Effects of Hot Climates and Great Heights.* Cambridge, MA: Harvard University Press, 1938.

Dill, D.B.: The Harvard Fatigue Laboratory: Its development, contributions, and demise. *Circ. Res.*, 20 (Suppl I):161, 1967.

Dill, D.B.: Arlie V. Bock, pioneer in sports medicine. December 30, 1888–August 11, 1984. *Med. Sci. Sports Exerc.*, 17:401, 1985

Gerber, E.W.: *Innovators and Institutions in Physical Education.* Philadelphia: Lea & Febiger, 1971.

Green, R.M.: *A Translation of Galen's Hygiene.* IL: Charles C. Thomas, 1951.

Henry, F.M.: Aerobic oxygen consumption and alactic debt in muscular work. *J. Appl. Physiol.*, 3:427:1951.

Henry, F.M.: Lactic and alactic oxygen consumption in moderate exercise of graded intensity. *J. Appl. Physiol.*, 8:608, 1956.

Henry, F.M.: Physical education: an academic discipline. *JOHPER*, 35:32, 1964.

Hermansen, L.: Anaerobic energy release. *Med. Sci. Sports.*, 1:32, 1969.

Hermansen, L., and Andersen, K.L.: Aerobic work capacity in young Norwegian men and women. *J. Appl. Physiol.*, 20:425, 1965.

Hoberman, J.M.: The early development of sports medicine in Germany. In: *Sport and Exercise Science.* Berryman, J.W., and Park, R.J. (eds.). Urbana, IL: University of Illinois Press, 1992.

Horvath, S.M., and E.C. Horvath.: *The Harvard Fatigue Laboratory: Its History and Contributions.* Englewood Cliffs, CA: Prentice-Hall, 1973.

Johnson, R.E., et al.: *Laboratory Manual of Field Methods for the Biochemical Assessment of Metabolic and Nutrition Conditions.* Boston, MA: Harvard Fatigue Laboratory, 1946.

Katch, V.L.: The burden of disproof. *Med. Sci. Sports Exerc.*, 18:593, 1986.

Katch, V.L., et al.: *Allied Health Graduate Program Directory.* Ann Arbor, MI: Fitness Technologies Press, 1996.

Kerlinger, F.N.: *Foundations of Behavioral Research*, 2nd Ed., New York: Holt, Rinehart, and Winston, 1973.

Krogh, A.: *The Composition of the Atmosphere; An Account of Preliminary Investigations and a Programme.* Kobenhavn: A.F. Host, 1919.

Kroll, W.: *Perspectives in Physical Education.* New York: Academic Press, 1971.

Leonard, F.G.: *A Guide to the History of Physical Education.* Philadelphia: Lea & Febiger, 1923.

Lusk, G.: *The Elements of the Science of Nutrition.* 2nd Ed., Philadelphia: W.B. Saunders, 1909.

Park, R.J.: A long and productive career: Franklin M. Henry—Scientist, mentor, pioneer. *Res. Q. Exerc. Sports*, 65:295, 1994.

Park, R.J.: Concern for health and exercise as expressed in the writings of 18th century physicians and informed laymen (England, France, Switzerland). *Res. Q.*, 47:756, 1976.

Park, R.J.: The emergence of the academic discipline of physical education in the United States. In: *Perspectives on the Academic Discipline of Physical Education.* Brooks, G.A. (ed.). Champaign, IL: Human Kinetics, 1981.

Park, R.J.: Physiologists, physicians, and physical educators: nineteenth century biology and exercise, hygienic and educative. *J. Sport Hist.*, 14:28, 1987.

Park, R.J.: The rise and demise of Harvard's B.S. program in Anatomy, Physiology, and Physical Training. *Res. Q. Exerc. Sport*, 63:246, 1992.

Payne, J.F.: *Harvey and Galen. The Harveyan Oration. Oct. 19, 1896.* London: Frowde, 1897.

Ross, W.D.: Kinanthropometry: an emerging scientific technology. In: *Biomechanics of Sports and Kinanthropometry.* Book 6. Landry, F., and Orban, W.A. (eds.). Miami, FL: Symposia Specialists, Inc., 1978.

Schmidt-Nielsen, B.: August and Marie Krogh and respiratory physiology. *J. Appl. Physiol.*, 57:293, 1984.

Scholander, P.F.: Analyzer for accurate estimation of respiratory gases in one-half cubic centimeter samples. *J. Biol. Chem.*, 167:235, 1947.

Shaffel, N.: The evaluation of American medical literature. In: *History of American Medicine.* MartiIbanez, F. (ed.). New York: MD Publications, 1958.

Tipton, C.M.: Exercise physiology, part II: a contemporary historical perspective. In: *The History of Exercise and Sports Science.* Messengale, J.D., and Swanson, R.A. (eds.). Champaign, IL: Human Kinetics, 1997.

Tipton, C.M.: Contemporary exercise physiology: Fifty years after the closure of the Harvard Fatigue Laboratory. *Exerc. Sport Sci. Rev.*, 26:315, 1998.

SECTION 2

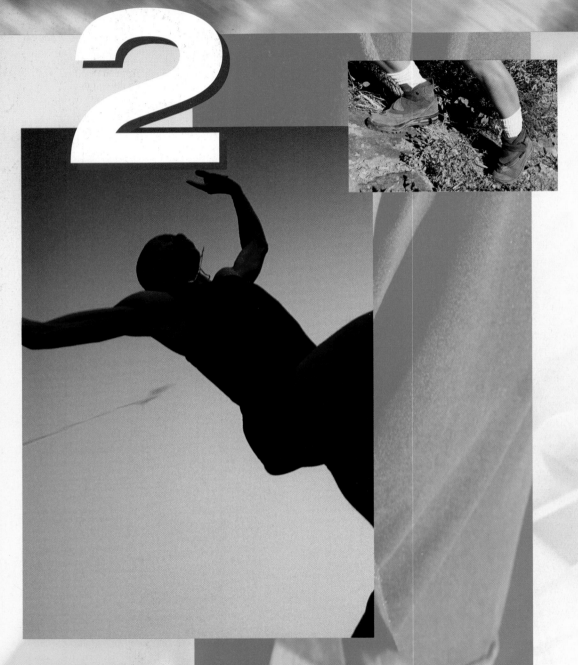

Nutrition and Energy Transfer

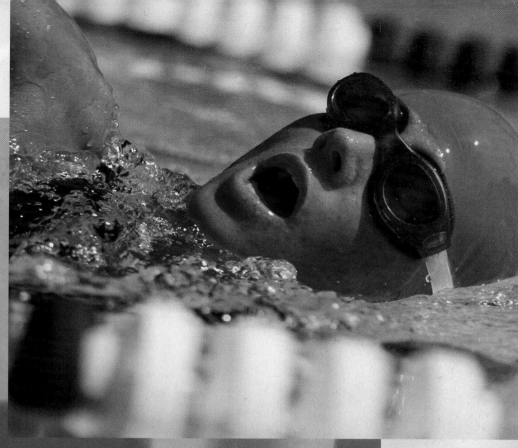

Proper nutrition forms the foundation for physical performance. The foods we consume provide fuel for biologic work and chemicals for extracting and using the potential energy within this fuel. Food also provides essential elements for synthesizing new tissue and repairing existing cells. Often, individuals exercise for optimum performance, only to fall short due to inadequate, counterproductive, and sometimes harmful nutritional practices. Sound nutritional practice and regular exercise impact a variety of disease conditions.

In the following chapters, we study how the body extracts energy from various foods we consume to become the vital fuel for exercise.

From an energy perspective, a useful analogy shows how a car and the human body obtain the energy to make them "go." In an automobile engine, igniting the proper mixture of gasoline fuel (the auto's energy "food") with oxygen provides energy to drive the pistons. Gears and linkages harness energy to turn the wheels; increasing or decreasing the energy supply either speeds up or slows down the engine. Similarly, the human machine must continuously extract energy from ingested nutrients (fuel) and harness it to perform complex functions. Besides expending considerable energy for muscular contraction during physical activity, the body generates substantial energy for these other more "quiet" forms of biologic work:

- Digest, absorb, and assimilate food nutrients
- Secrete hormones at rest and during exercise
- Maintain electrochemical gradients along cell membranes to transmit electrical signals from the brain through nerves to muscles
- Synthesize new chemical compounds like the thick and thin protein structures in skeletal muscle tissue that enlarge with resistance training

Chapters 2 and 3 in this section review the six broad categories of nutrients: carbohydrates, lipids, proteins, vitamins, minerals, and water. Understanding each nutrient's role in energy metabolism and tissue synthesis clarifies one's knowledge of the interaction between food intake and storage and exercise performance. No nutritional "magic bullets" exist per se, yet the quantity and blend of nutrients in the daily diet profoundly affect exercise capacity, training response, and overall health. Chapters 4 and 5 present an overview of areas related to energy transfer, with specific focus on 1) how cells extract chemical energy bound within the food nutrients, and 2) the dynamics of energy transfer during light, moderate, and strenuous exercise. Chapter 6 reviews the measurement of human energy expenditure at rest and during diverse physical activities, and Chapters 7 and 8 review energy expenditure and energy-generating capacities of humans. Chapter 9 deals with optimal nutrition for exercise and sport.

CHAPTER

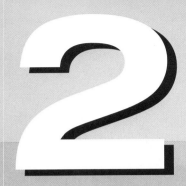

2

Topics covered in this chapter

PART 1 Macronutrients: Energy Fuel and Building Blocks for Tissue Synthesis

Carbohydrates
Lipids
Proteins
Recommended Dietary Allowance
Summary

PART 2 Energy Content of Food

Calorie—A Measurement of Food Energy
Gross Energy Value of Foods
Net Energy Value of Foods
Calories Equal Calories
Summary
Thought Questions
Selected References

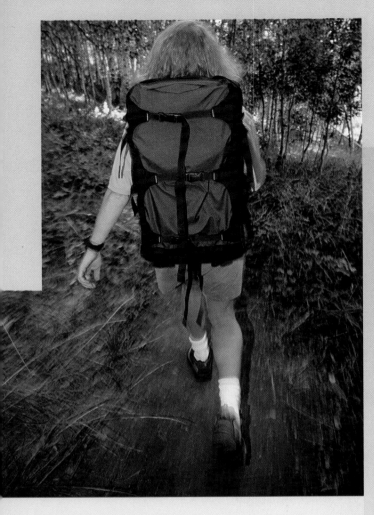

Macronutrients and Food Energy

- Distinguish among monosaccharides, disaccharides, and polysaccharides.

- Discuss carbohydrate's role as an energy source, protein sparer, metabolic primer, and central nervous system fuel.

- Define and give an example of a triglyceride, saturated fatty acid, polyunsaturated fatty acid, and monounsaturated fatty acid.

- List major characteristics of high- and low-density lipoprotein cholesterols, and discuss their roles in coronary heart disease.

- List four important functions of fat in the body.

- Define essential and non-essential amino acids, and give food sources for each.

- Describe how relative exercise intensity (low, moderate, and maximal) and duration (short and long) influence carbohydrate, fat, and protein use in energy metabolism.

- Describe the alanine-glucose cycle, and explain how the body uses protein for energy during exercise.

- Define the following: 1) heat of combustion, 2) digestive efficiency, 3) Atwater general factors.

- Compute the energy content of a meal from its macronutrient composition.

PART 1

Macronutrients: Energy Fuel and Building Blocks for Tissue Synthesis

The carbohydrate, lipid, and protein nutrients consumed daily supply the necessary energy to maintain bodily functions during rest and diverse physical activities. These nutrients (referred to as **macronutrients**) also maintain and enhance the organism's structural and functional integrity in response to exercise training. In Part 1, we discuss each macronutrient's general structure, function, and source in the diet, and emphasize their importance in sustaining physiologic function during physical activity.

Carbohydrates

All living cells contain **carbohydrates.** With the exception of lactose and a small amount of glycogen, all dietary carbohydrate originates from plant sources. Atoms of carbon, hydrogen, and oxygen combine to form a carbohydrate (sugar) molecule, always in a ratio of one atom of carbon and two atoms of hydrogen for each oxygen atom. The general formula $(CH_2O)n$ represents a simple carbohydrate, where n equals from three to seven carbon atoms. The important sugars for metabolism usually contain five and six carbons.

Monosaccharides

The **monosaccharide** molecule forms the basic unit of carbohydrates. The molecule's number of carbon atoms determines its category. The Greek name for this number, ending with "ose," indicates sugars. For example, 3-carbon monosaccharides are trioses, 4-carbon sugars are tetroses, 5-carbon pentoses, 6-carbon hexoses, and 7-carbon sugars heptoses. The hexose sugars, glucose, fructose, and galactose, represent the nutritionally important monosaccharides.

Glucose, also called dextrose or blood sugar, consists of 6 carbon, 12 hydrogen, and 6 oxygen atoms ($C_6H_{12}O_6$; Fig. 2.1). It forms as a natural sugar in food or is produced in the body through the digestion (**hydrolysis**) of more complex carbohydrates. Glyconeogenesis synthesizes glucose primarily in the liver from carbon skeletons of

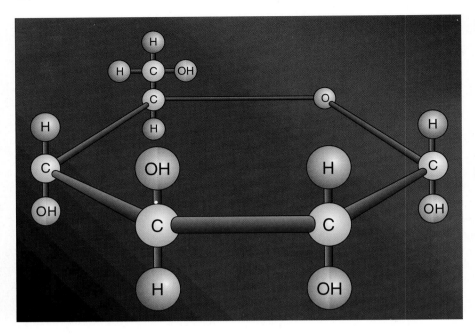

Figure 2.1
Three-dimensional ring structure of the simple sugar molecule glucose. The molecule resembles a hexagonal plate to which H and O atoms attach.

Polysaccharides

Polysaccharides include plant and animal categories.

Plant Polysaccharides

Starch and fiber represent the two common forms of plant polysaccharides.

Starch. **Starch** represents the storage form of plant polysaccharide, formed from hundreds of individual sugar molecules joined together. It appears as large granules in seed and corn cells, and in grains that make bread, cereal, spaghetti, and pastries. Large amounts also exist in peas, beans, potatoes, and roots, in which starch stores energy for the plant's future needs. The term **complex carbohydrates** commonly refers to dietary starch.

Fiber. **Fiber,** classified as a non-starch, structural polysaccharide, includes cellulose, the most abundant organic molecule on earth. Fibrous materials resist hydrolysis by human digestive enzymes. Plants *exclusively* contain fiber, which constitutes the structure of leaves, stems, roots, seeds, and fruit coverings. Fibers differ in physical and chemical characteristics and physiologic action; they occur primarily within the cell wall as cellulose, gums, hemicellulose, pectin, and noncarbohydrate lignins. Other fibers—mucilage and the gums—serve as integral components of the plant cell itself. Table 2.1 lists the fiber content of common foods.

protein. After absorption by the small intestine, glucose can be:

- Used directly by the cell for energy
- Stored as glycogen in the muscles and liver
- Converted to fats for energy storage

Fruits and honey provide the main source of **fructose** (also called levulose or fruit sugar), the sweetest of the monosaccharides. Although the small intestine absorbs some fructose directly into the blood, the liver slowly converts it to glucose. **Galactose** does not exist freely in nature; rather, it forms milk sugar (**lactose**) in the mammary glands of lactating animals. In the body, galactose converts to glucose for energy metabolism.

Disaccharides

Combining two monosaccharide molecules forms a **disaccharide** or double sugar. The monosaccharides and disaccharides collectively make up the **simple sugars**—brown sugar, corn syrup, invert sugar, honey, and "natural sweeteners."

Each of the disaccharides contains glucose as a principle component. The three disaccharides of nutritional significance include:

- **Sucrose:** glucose + fructose; the most common dietary disaccharide. It occurs naturally in most foods containing carbohydrate, particularly beet and cane sugar, brown sugar, sorghum, maple syrup, and honey
- **Lactose:** glucose + galactose; found in natural form only in milk and often called milk sugar
- **Maltose:** glucose + glucose; occurs in beer, cereals, and germinating seeds

close up

Health Implications of Dietary Fiber

Dietary fiber has received attention by researchers and the lay press because of studies that link high fiber intake with a lower occurrence of obesity, diabetes, hypertension, intestinal disorders, and heart disease. The diet of industrialized nations, high in fiber-free animal foods and low in natural plant fiber lost through processing (refining), contributes to intestinal disorders compared with a more primitive-type diet high in unrefined, complex carbohydrates. *For example, the typical American diet contains a daily fiber intake of about 12 to 15 g, far short of 20 to 35 g recommended in the dietary guidelines.*

Fibers hold considerable water and give "bulk" to the food residues in the intestines, often increasing stool weight and volume by 40 to 100%. This bulking-up action may aid gastrointestinal functioning and reduce the chances of contracting colon cancer and other gastrointestinal diseases later in life. Increased fiber intake, especially the **water-soluble fibers**, may modestly reduce serum cholesterol in humans. These include pectin and guar gum present in oats (rolled oats, oat bran, oat flour), legumes, barley, brown rice, peas, carrots, and diverse fruits.

For men with elevated blood lipids, adding 100 g of oat bran to their daily diets reduced serum cholesterol levels by 13%, and lowered the low-density lipoprotein component of the cholesterol profile. In contrast, the **water-insoluble fibers,** cellulose, hemicellulose, and lignin, and cellulose-rich products like wheat bran did not reduce cholesterol levels. The precise mechanism by which dietary fibers favorably affect serum cholesterol remains unclear. The addition of fiber may simply replace cholesterol-laden items in the diet; fiber may actually hinder cholesterol absorption, or it may reduce cholesterol metabolism in the gut. These actions would depress cholesterol synthesis and simultaneously facilitate excretion of existing cholesterol bound to the fiber in the feces. Dietary fiber slows carbohydrate digestion so it absorbs into the bloodstream more slowly by the intestine. Fiber also decreases the total number of calories consumed in subsequent meals.

Current nutritional wisdom maintains that a dietary fiber intake of about 20 to 35 g per day (ratio of 3:1 for water-insoluble to soluble fiber) plays an important part of a well-structured diet. Persons with marginal levels of nutrition should not consume excessive fiber because an increase in fiber intake can decrease the absorption of calcium, iron, magnesium, phosphorus, and trace minerals.

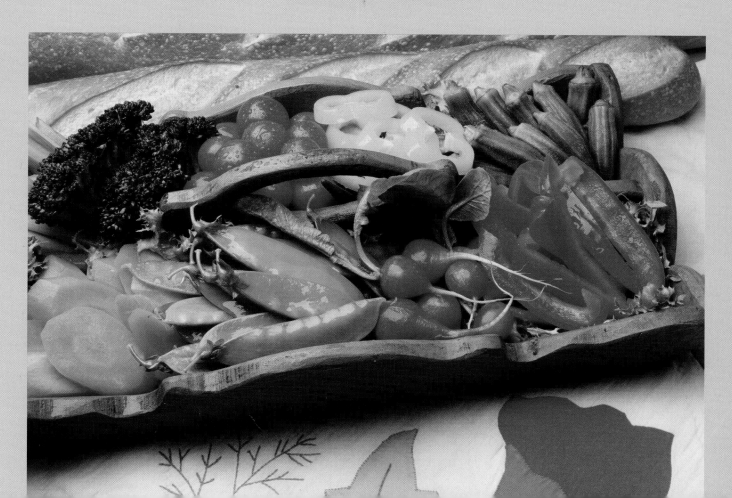

TABLE 2.1
Fiber content of some common foods listed in order of overall fiber content

	SERVING SIZE	TOTAL FIBER, g	SOLUBLE FIBER, g	INSOLUBLE FIBER, g
100% Bran cereal	1/2 cup	10.0	0.3	9.7
Peas	1/2 cup	5.2	2.0	3.2
Kidney beans	1/2 cup	4.5	0.5	4.0
Apple	1 small	3.9	2.3	1.6
Potato	1 small	3.8	2.2	1.6
Broccoli	1/2 cup	2.5	1.1	1.4
Strawberries	3/4 cup	2.4	0.9	1.5
Oats, whole	1/2 cup	1.6	0.5	1.1
Banana	1 small	1.3	0.6	0.7
Spaghetti	1/2 cup	1.0	0.2	0.8
Lettuce	1/2 cup	0.5	0.2	0.3
White rice	1/2 cup	0.5	0.0	0.5

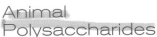

Animal Polysaccharides

During the process known as **glucogenesis,** a few hundred to thousands of glucose molecules form a large polysaccharide, **glycogen,** the storage polysaccharide in mammalian muscle and liver. Figure 2.2 illustrates that a well-nourished 80-kg person stores approximately 500 g of carbohydrate in the body. Of this, approximately 400 g exist as muscle glycogen (largest reserve), 90 to 110 g as liver glycogen (highest concentration representing between 3 to 7% of the liver's weight), but only about 2 to 3 g as blood glucose. Because each gram of carbohydrate (glycogen or glucose) contains about 4 kcal of energy, the average person stores between 1500 and 2000 kcal as carbohydrate—enough total energy to power a 20-mile run.

Muscle glycogen serves as the major source of carbohydrate energy for active muscles during exercise. In contrast to muscle glycogen, liver glycogen reconverts to glucose for transport in the blood to the working muscles. **Glycogenolysis** describes this reconversion process; it provides a rapid extramuscular supply of glucose. Unlike liver, muscle cells do not contain the enzyme to reform glucose from glycogen. Thus, glucose (or glycogen) within a muscle cell cannot supply the carbohydrate needs of surrounding cells. Depleting liver and muscle glycogen through 1) dietary restriction, or 2) heavy exercise stimulates glucose synthesis from structural components of the other macronutrients (principally protein's amino acids) through the process known as **gluconeogenesis.**

Hormones regulate liver and muscle glycogen stores by controlling the level of circulating blood sugar. Elevated blood sugar levels cause the pancreas' beta cells to secrete additional **insulin,** which facilitates the muscle cells' uptake of the glucose excess yet inhibits insulin secretion. This feedback regulation maintains blood glucose at an appropriate physiologic concentration. In contrast, if blood sugar falls below normal, the pancreas' alpha cells immediately secrete insulin's opposing hormone, **glucagon,** to normalize blood

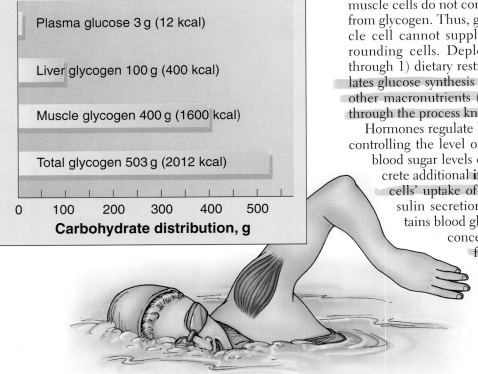

Plasma glucose 3 g (12 kcal)

Liver glycogen 100 g (400 kcal)

Muscle glycogen 400 g (1600 kcal)

Total glycogen 503 g (2012 kcal)

0   100   200   300   400   500

Carbohydrate distribution, g

Figure 2.2
Distribution of carbohydrate energy in a typical 80-kg person.

sugar level. This **"insulin antagonist"** hormone stimulates liver glycogenolysis and gluconeogenesis to increase blood glucose levels. Chapter 13 provides more detailed information about insulin and glucagon dynamics during exercise.

Diet Affects Glycogen Stores

Because the body stores comparatively little glycogen, diet can significantly affect its quantity. For example, a 24-hour fast or a low-carbohydrate, normal-calorie (isocaloric) diet dramatically reduces glycogen reserves. In contrast, maintaining a carbohydrate-rich isocaloric diet for several days doubles the body's carbohydrate stores compared with a normal, well-balanced diet. *The body's upper limit for glycogen storage equals about 15 g per kilogram (kg) of body mass, equivalent to 1050 g for the average 70-kg man, or 840 g for a typical 56-kg woman.*

Carbohydrate's Role in the Body

Carbohydrates serve important functions related to energy metabolism and exercise performance.

Energy Source

Carbohydrates act as an energy fuel mainly during high-intensity exercise. Energy from the breakdown of blood-borne glucose and muscle glycogen ultimately powers muscle action and other forms of biologic work. For physically active people, adequate daily carbohydrate intake maintains the body's relatively limited glycogen stores. In contrast, exceeding the cells' capacity to store glycogen converts excess dietary carbohydrate calories to fat, which can trigger an increase in the body's total fat content.

Protein Sparer

Spares breakdown of protein for energy

Adequate carbohydrate intake preserves tissue proteins. Normally, protein contributes to tissue maintenance, repair, and growth, and to a lesser degree serves as a nutrient energy source. With reduced glycogen reserves gluconeogenesis synthesizes glucose from protein (amino acids) and the glycerol portion of the fat (triglyceride) molecule. This metabolic process augments carbohydrate availability (and maintains plasma glucose levels) when depleted glycogen stores occur during 1) dietary restriction, 2) prolonged exercise, and 3) repeated bouts of heavy training. The price paid temporarily reduces the body's protein "stores," particularly muscle protein. In the extreme, depressed glycogen reserves significantly reduce lean tissue mass and produce an accompanying solute load on the kidneys, which must excrete the nitrogen-containing byproducts of protein breakdown.

Metabolic Primer

Carbohydrates serve as a "primer" for fat breakdown. Carbohydrate breakdown products facilitate the body's use of fat for energy. Insufficient carbohydrate metabolism (either through limitations in glucose transport into the cell as occurs in diabetes, or glycogen depletion through inad-

Important Carbohydrate Conversions

- **Glucogenesis**—glycogen synthesis from glucose
- **Gluconeogenesis**—glucose synthesis from structural components of noncarbohydrate nutrients
- **Glycogenolysis**—glucose formation from glycogen

equate diet or prolonged exercise) increases dependence on fat utilization for energy. If this happens, the body cannot generate a sustained high level of aerobic energy transfer from fat-only metabolism. This significantly reduces an individual's maximum exercise intensity.

Fuel for the Central Nervous System

The central nervous system requires carbohydrate for proper functioning. Under normal conditions, the brain uses blood glucose almost exclusively as its fuel without maintaining a backup supply of this nutrient. In poorly regulated diabetes, during starvation, or with a low carbohydrate intake, the brain adapts metabolically after about 8 days to use relatively large amounts of fat (in the form of ketones) as an alternative fuel source.

At rest and during exercise, the liver serves as the primary source to maintain normal blood glucose levels. In prolonged heavy exercise, blood glucose eventually falls below normal concentrations because of liver glycogen depletion and active muscles' continual use of available blood glucose. Symptoms of a modest blood glucose reduction (**hypoglycemia**) include feelings of weakness, hunger, and dizziness. This ultimately impacts exercise performance and may partially explain "central" or neurologic fatigue associated with prolonged exercise (or starvation). Blood sugar usually remains regulated within narrow limits because of glucose's important role in nerve tissue metabolism.

Carbohydrate Loading and Muscle Girth

Body builders who think that the extra 2.7 g of water stored with each gram of glycogen in skeletal muscle may add to muscle bulk will be disappointed by research findings. When body builders trained for 3 days on a carbohydrate loading diet (80% of total calories), no measurable difference occurred in muscle girth compared with training on a diet low in carbohydrate (10% of total calories).

Recommended Carbohydrate Intake

Figure 2.3 illustrates the carbohydrate content of selected foods. Rich carbohydrate sources include cereals, cookies, candies, breads, and cakes. Fruits and vegetables appear as less valuable sources of carbohydrates because the food's total weight (including water content) determines a food's carbohydrate percentage. The dried portions of fruits and vegetables exist as almost pure carbohydrate. For this reason, hikers and ultraendurance athletes rely on dried apricots, pears, apples, bananas, and tomatoes to provide a ready (but relatively lightweight) carbohydrate source.

Carbohydrates account for between 40 to 50% of the total calories in the typical American diet. For a sedentary 70-kg person, this translates to a daily carbohydrate intake of about 300 g. The average American consumes about one-half of carbohydrate intake as simple sugars, predominantly as sucrose and high-fructose corn syrup. Simple sugar intake represents the yearly intake equivalent to 60 pounds of table sugar (16 teaspoons of sucrose a day) and 46 pounds of corn syrup. One hundred years ago, average yearly intake of simple sugars equaled only 4 pounds per person. Consuming excessive fermentable carbohydrate (principally sucrose) contributes to tooth decay—but dietary sugar's contributing role to diabetes, obesity, and coronary heart disease remains largely unsubstantiated.

For regular exercisers, carbohydrate should supply about 60% of total daily calories (400 to 600 g), predominantly as unrefined, fiber-rich fruits, grains, and vegetables. This replenishes the carbohydrate that powered an increased physical activity level. During heavy training, carbohydrate intake should increase to 70% of total daily energy intake.

Carbohydrate Utilization in Exercise

The fuel mixture during exercise depends on intensity and duration of effort, including the exerciser's fitness and nutritional status.

Intense Exercise

Stored muscle glycogen and blood-borne glucose primarily contribute to the total energy required during high-intensity exercise, and in the early minutes of exercise when

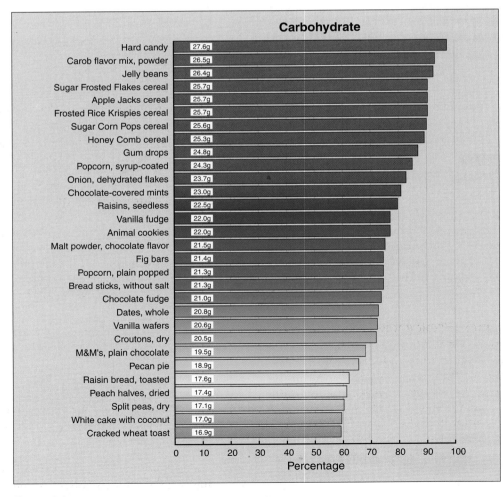

Figure 2.3
Percentage of carbohydrates in commonly served foods. The inset displays the number of grams of carbohydrate per ounce of food.

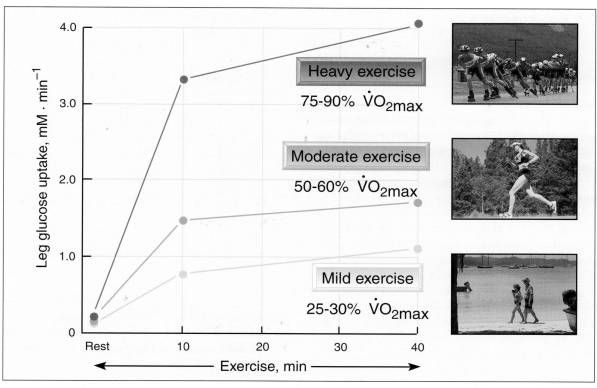

Figure 2.4
Blood glucose uptake by the leg muscles affected by exercise duration and intensity. Exercise intensity is expressed as a percent of $\dot{V}O_{2max}$. (From Felig, P., and Wahren, J.: Fuel homeostasis in exercise. *N. Engl. J. Med.*, 293:1078, 1975.)

oxygen supply fails to meet the demands for aerobic metabolism.

Figure 2.4 illustrates that early in exercise, the muscles' uptake of circulating blood glucose increases sharply and continues to increase as exercise progresses. After 40 minutes of exercise, glucose uptake increases 7 to 20 times the uptake at rest, depending on exercise intensity. Carbohydrate's large energy contribution during all-out exercise occurs because it is the only macronutrient that provides energy anaerobically. During high-intensity aerobic exercise, intramuscular glycogen becomes the preferential energy fuel. This provides an advantage because carbohydrate supplies energy for exercise *twice* as rapidly as fat and protein.

Moderate and Prolonged Exercise

During the transition from rest to submaximal exercise, almost all of the energy comes from glycogen stored in active muscles. Over the next 20 minutes, liver and muscle glycogen provide about 40 to 50% of the energy requirement, with the remaining requirement from fat breakdown plus some blood glucose utilization (Fig. 2.4). As exercise continues and glycogen stores deplete, fat catabolism increases its percentage contribution to the total energy for muscular activity. Additionally, blood glucose becomes the major source of the limited carbohydrate energy. Eventually, glucose output by the liver does not keep pace with its use, and blood glucose concentration declines.

Inability to maintain a desired level of performance (**fatigue**) may occur if exercise progresses to the point where liver and muscle glycogen decrease severely, even with sufficient oxygen available to the muscles and almost unlimited potential energy from stored fat. Endurance athletes commonly refer to fatigue under these conditions as **"bonking"** or **"hitting the wall."** Research does not explain why carbohydrate depletion coincides with the onset of fatigue in prolonged submaximal exercise. The answer may relate to 1) the key role of blood glucose in central nervous system function, 2) muscle glycogen's role as a "primer" in fat breakdown, and 3) the relatively slow rate of energy release from fat compared with carbohydrate breakdown.

Lipids

A lipid (from the Greek *lipos*, meaning fat) molecule has the same structural elements as carbohydrate except that it differs in its linkage of atoms. Specifically, the lipid's ratio of hydrogen-to-oxygen considerably exceeds that of carbohydrate. For example, the formula $C_{57}H_{110}O_6$ describes the common lipid stearin, with a H-to-0 ratio of 18.3:1; for carbohydrate the ratio equals 2:1. Lipid, a general term, refers to a heterogeneous group of compounds that includes oils, fats, and waxes and related compounds. Oils remain liquid at room temperature, whereas fats remain solid. Approximately 98% of dietary lipid exists as triglycerides (see next section). Lipids can be placed into one of three main groups: **simple lipids, compound lipids**, and **derived lipids**.

Simple Lipids

The simple lipids or "neutral fats" consist primarily of **triglycerides**. They constitute the major storage form of fat; more than 90% of the body fat exists as triglyceride predominantly in adipose (fat) cells. This molecule consists of two different clusters of atoms. A glycerol component has a 3-carbon molecule that itself does not qualify as a lipid because of its high solubility in water. The other component consists of three clusters of carbon-chained atoms, usually in an even number, termed fatty acids that attach to glycerol. Fatty acids contain straight hydrocarbon chains with as few as 4 carbon atoms or more than 20, although chain lengths of 16 and 18 carbons prevail.

Three molecules of water form when glycerol joins with the fatty acids to synthesize a triglyceride. Conversely, during hydrolysis, when the fat molecule cleaves into its constituents by lipase enzymes, three molecules of water attach at the point where the fat molecule splits. Figure 2.5 illustrates the basic structure of saturated and unsaturated fatty acid molecules. All lipid-containing foods consist of a mixture of different proportions of saturated and unsaturated fatty acids.

Saturated Fatty Acids

Saturated fatty acids contain only single bonds between carbon atoms; all of the remaining bonds attach to hydrogen. The term saturated describes the fatty acid molecule because it holds as many hydrogen atoms as chemically possible (saturated with respect to hydrogen atoms.)

Saturated fatty acids occur plentifully in animal products such as beef, lamb, pork, chicken, egg yolk, and in dairy fats of cream, milk, butter, and cheese. Saturated fatty acids from the plant kingdom include coconut and palm oil, vegetable shortening, and hydrogenated margarine; commercially prepared cakes, pies, and cookies rely heavily on saturated fatty acids in their preparation.

Unsaturated Fatty Acids

Unsaturated fatty acids contain one or more double bonds along the main carbon chain. Each double bond in the carbon chain reduces the number of potential hydrogen-binding sites; therefore, the molecule remains unsatu-

---

Sufficient Carbohydrate Intake

Athletes who do not include sufficient carbohydrate in their diet may eventually train in a state of chronic glycogen depletion. This often leads to "staleness," compromising how the athlete trains and competes at high intensity.

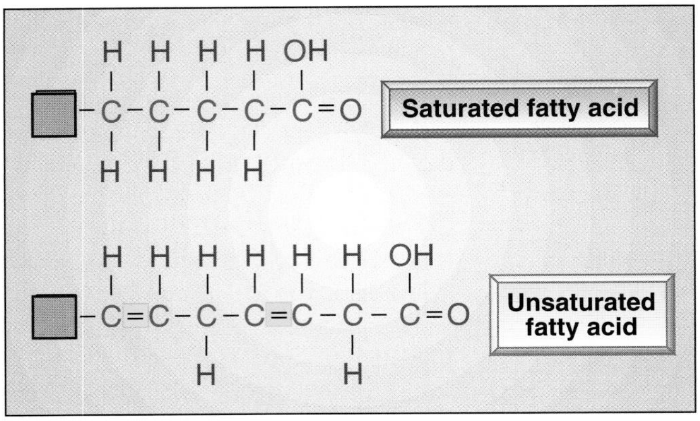

Figure 2.5
The presence or absence of double bonds between carbon atoms distinguishes the major structural difference between saturated and unsaturated fatty acids.

rated relative to hydrogen. **Monounsaturated fatty acids** contain one double bond along the main carbon chain; examples include canola oil, olive oil, peanut oil, and oil in almonds, pecans, and avocados. **Polyunsaturated fatty acids** contain two or more double bonds along the main carbon chain; this includes safflower, sunflower, soybean, and corn oil.

Fatty acids from plant sources are typically unsaturated and liquefy at room temperature. Lipids with more carbons in the fatty acid chain and containing more saturated fatty acids remain firmer at room temperature.

Fatty Acids in the Diet

The average person in the United States consumes about 15% of total calories as saturated fats (equivalent to more than 50 lb per year). This contrasts to the Tarahumara Indians of Mexico whose diet, high in complex, unrefined carbohydrate, contains only 2% of total calories as saturated fat. The relationship between saturated fatty acid intake and coronary heart disease risk has prompted health professionals to suggest replacing at least a portion of the saturated fatty acids in the diet with unsaturated fatty acids. Monounsaturated fatty acids lower coronary risk even below normal levels. Individuals should consume no more than 10% of total energy intake as saturated fatty acids. Ideally, fatty acid intake should include equal amounts of saturated, polyunsaturated, and monounsaturated fatty acids.

Compound Lipids

Compound lipids consist of a neutral fat combined with other chemicals like phosphorus (**phospholipids**) and glucose (**glucolipids**). Another group of compound fats contains the **lipoproteins**, formed primarily in the liver from the union of triglycerides, phospholipids, or cholesterol with protein. *The lipoproteins serve important functions because they constitute the main form for lipid transport in the blood.* If blood lipids did not bind to protein, they literally would float to the top like cream in nonhomogenized milk.

High- and Low-Density Lipoprotein Cholesterol

Four types of lipoproteins exist according to their gravitational densities: chylomicrons, and high-density, low-density, and very-low density lipoproteins. **Chylomicrons** form after emulsified lipid droplets leave the small intestine and enter the lymphatic vasculature. Normally, the liver takes up chylomicrons, metabolizes them, and delivers them to adipose tissue for storage.

The liver and small intestine produce **high-density lipoprotein (HDL)**. Of the lipoproteins, HDLs contain the greatest percentage of protein and the least total lipid and cholesterol. Degradation of a **very-low density lipoprotein (VLDL)** produces a **low-density lipoprotein (LDL)**. The VLDL contains the greatest percentage of lipid. VLDLs transport triglycerides (formed in the liver from fats, carbohydrates, alcohol, and cholesterol) to muscle and adipose tissue. The enzyme **lipoprotein lipase,** acts on VLDL to transform it to a denser LDL molecule, which then contains less lipid. LDL and VLDL contain the greatest lipid and least protein components.

"Bad" Cholesterol (LDL)

Among the lipoproteins, LDLs, which normally carry between 60 to 80% of the total serum cholesterol, have the greatest affinity for cells in the arterial wall. LDL delivers cholesterol to arterial tissue; here, the LDL becomes oxidized to ultimately participate in the proliferation of smooth muscle cells and other unfavorable changes that damage and narrow the artery. Regular exercise, visceral fat accumulation, and the diet's composition influence serum LDL concentration.

"Good" Cholesterol (HDL)

Unlike LDL, HDL operates as so-called "good" cholesterol to protect against heart disease. HDL acts as a scavenger in the **reverse transport of cholesterol** by removing it from the arterial wall for transport to the liver. There, it incorporates into bile where the intestinal tract excretes it.

The amounts of LDL and HDL cholesterol, and their specific ratios (e.g., HDL/total cholesterol) and subfractions, provide more meaningful indicators of coronary artery disease risk than just total cholesterol. Regular aerobic exercise and abstinence from cigarette smoking increase HDLs and favorably affect the LDL/HDL ratio. We discuss the role of exercise on the blood lipid profile more fully in Chapter 20.

Derived Lipids

Derived lipids include substances formed from simple and compound lipids. **Cholesterol,** the most widely known derived lipid, exists only in animal tissue. Cholesterol does not contain fatty acids, but shares some of the physical and chemical characteristics of lipids. Thus, from a dietary viewpoint cholesterol can be considered a lipid. Cholesterol, widespread in the plasma membrane of all cells, is obtained either through food intake (exogenous

The Leaner, the Better

Research indicates that beef fat, and not the lean portion, relates to elevated blood cholesterol. Trimming beef of all visible fat, and eating a low saturated-fat diet, enables a person to include beef in a cholesterol-lowering diet.

cholesterol) or from synthesis within the body (endogenous cholesterol). Even if an individual maintains a "cholesterol-free" diet, endogenous cholesterol synthesis usually varies between 0.5 to 2.0 g per day. *More cholesterol forms in the body with a diet high in saturated fatty acids, which facilitates cholesterol synthesis by the liver.* The rate of endogenous synthesis usually meets the body's needs; hence, severely reducing cholesterol intake, except in pregnant women and infants, would probably cause little harm.

Cholesterol participates in many complex bodily functions, including the building of plasma membranes, and as a precursor in synthesizing vitamin D, the adrenal gland hormones, and the sex hormones estrogen, androgen, and progesterone. Cholesterol serves as a component for bile (emulsifies lipids during digestion) and helps tissues, organs, and body structures form during fetal development.

Rich sources of cholesterol include egg yolk, red meats, and organ meats (liver, kidney, and brains). Shellfish, particularly shrimp, and dairy products (ice cream, cream cheese, butter, and whole milk) contain large amounts of cholesterol. *Foods of plant origin contain no cholesterol.* We discuss the relationship between cholesterol (and its lipoprotein components) and heart disease more fully in Chapter 20.

Lipids in Food

Figure 2.6 shows the approximate percentage contribution of some of the common food groups to the total lipid content of the typical American diet. Plant sources contribute about 34% to the daily lipid intake, whereas the remaining 66% comes from lipids of animal origin.

Lipid's Role in the Body

The important functions of lipids in the body include:

- Energy reserve
- Protection of vital organs and thermal insulation
- Transport medium for fat-soluble vitamins

Energy Reserve

Fat constitutes the ideal cellular fuel because each molecule 1) carries large quantities of energy per unit weight, 2) transports and stores easily, and 3) provides a ready energy source. At rest in well-nourished individuals, fat provides as much as 80 to 90% of the body's energy requirement. One gram of pure lipid contains about 9 kcal

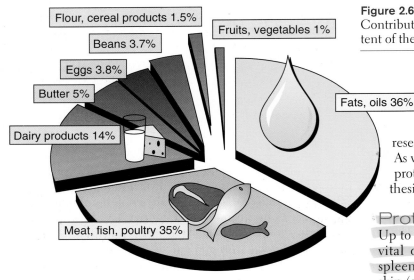

Flour, cereal products 1.5%
Beans 3.7%
Eggs 3.8%
Butter 5%
Dairy products 14%
Meat, fish, poultry 35%
Fruits, vegetables 1%
Fats, oils 36%

Figure 2.6
Contribution from the major food groups to the lipid content of the typical American diet.

would provide energy for a 20-mile run. Viewed from a different perspective, the body's energy reserves from carbohydrate could power high-intensity running for only about 1.6 hours, but the fat reserves would last 75 times longer or about 120 hours. As was the case with carbohydrates, fat as a fuel "spares" protein to carry out its important functions of tissue synthesis and repair.

Protection and Insulation

Up to 4% of the body's fat protects against trauma to the vital organs such as the heart, lungs, liver, kidneys, spleen, brain, and spinal cord. Fats stored just below the skin (subcutaneous fat) provide insulation, determining one's ability to tolerate extremes of cold exposure. Swimmers who excelled at swimming the English Channel had only slight decreases in body temperature while resting in cold water and did not have any lowering effects while swimming. In contrast, the body temperature of leaner, non-Channel swimmers decreased markedly under both conditions. The insulatory layer of fat probably affords little protection except to those in cold-related environments like deep-sea divers, ocean or channel swimmers, or Arctic inhabitants. Excess body fat hinders temperature regulation during heat stress, most notably during sustained exercise in air when the body's heat production can increase 20 times above rest-

of energy, more than twice the energy available in a gram of carbohydrate or protein due to lipid's greater quantity of hydrogen.

Approximately 15% of the body mass for men and 25% for women consists of fat. Figure 2.7 illustrates the total mass (and energy content) of fat from various sources in an 80-kg young adult man. The amount of fat in adipose tissue triglyceride translates to about 108,000 kcal. Most of this energy remains available for exercise and would fuel a run from New York City to Madison, Wisconsin, assuming an energy expenditure of about 100 kcal per mile. Contrast this to the limited 2000 kcal reserve of stored glycogen that

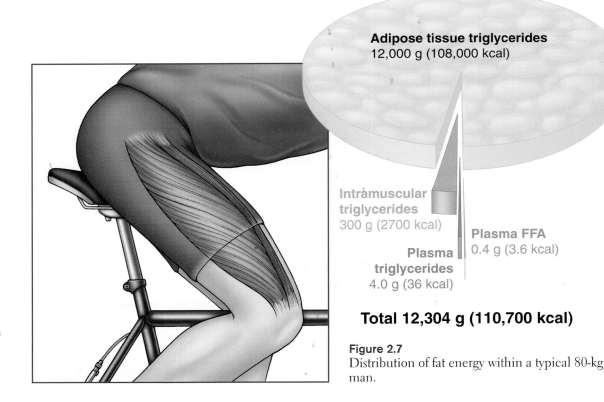

Adipose tissue triglycerides
12,000 g (108,000 kcal)

Intramuscular triglycerides
300 g (2700 kcal)

Plasma triglycerides
4.0 g (36 kcal)

Plasma FFA
0.4 g (3.6 kcal)

Total 12,304 g (110,700 kcal)

Figure 2.7
Distribution of fat energy within a typical 80-kg man.

ing. With such exercise, subcutaneous fat's shield of insulation retards heat flow from the body.

For large-sized football linemen, excess fat storage provides additional cushioning to protect the participant from the sport's normal hazards. Any possible protective benefit must be evaluated against the liability imposed by the "dead weight" of excess fat and its effect on energy expenditure, thermal regulation, and exercise performance.

Vitamin Carrier

Dietary lipid serves as a carrier and transport medium for the fat-soluble vitamins A, D, E, and K, which require an intake of about 20 g of dietary fat daily. Thus, significantly reducing lipid intake depresses the body's level of these vitamins and may ultimately lead to vitamin deficiency. In addition to a vitamin carrier, lipid in the diet can delay the onset of "hunger pangs" and contribute to satiety after the meal. This occurs because emptying of lipid from the stomach takes about 3.5 hours after its ingestion. This explains why reducing diets containing some lipid sometimes prove initially successful in blunting the urge to eat than more extreme low-fat diets.

Recommended Lipid Intake

In the United States, dietary lipid represents between 34 and 38% of total calorie intake. Most health professionals recommend that lipids should not exceed 30% of the diet's total energy content. Unsaturated fatty acids should supply at least 70% of total lipid intake.

For dietary cholesterol, the American Heart Association recommends no more than 300 mg (0.01 oz) of cholesterol be consumed each day, an intake equivalent to about 100 mg per 1000 kcal of food ingested. Three hundred mg of cholesterol almost equals the amount in the yolk of one large egg, and just about one-half the daily cholesterol consumed by the average American male. Table 2.2 presents the cholesterol and saturated fat content of common foods.

Fat Use in Exercise

The contribution of fat to the energy requirements of exercise depends on fatty acid release from triglycerides in the fat storage sites, and delivery in the circulation to muscle tissue as free fatty acids (FFA) bound to blood albumin. Triglycerides stored within the muscle cell itself also contribute to exercise energy metabolism. The data in Figure 2.8 show that active muscles' uptake of

fatty acids increases during 1 to 4 hours of moderate exercise. In the first hour of exercise, about 50% of the energy comes from fat catabolism. As exercise continues into the third hour (with accompanying glycogen depletion), fat contributes up to 70% of the total exercise energy requirement.

Proteins

The body of a normal-sized adult contains between 10 and 12 kg of protein, primarily located within the skeletal muscle mass. Structurally, proteins resemble carbohydrates and lipids because they contain atoms of carbon, oxygen, and hydrogen. They differ, however, because they also contain nitrogen (approximately 16% of the molecule) along with sulfur and occasionally phosphorous, cobalt, and iron.

Amino Acids

Just as glycogen forms from the linkage of many simple glucose subunits, the protein molecule forms from its **amino acid** "building-block" constituents. **Peptide bonds**

TABLE 2.2
Cholesterol and saturated fat content for 100 g of common foods

FOODS	SATURATED FAT (mg)	CHOLESTEROL (mg)
Butter	50.7	219
Peanut butter	8.5	0
Chocolate fudge	7.3	4
French Fries, McDonald's	6.8	13
Ice cream, vanilla	6.2	44
Taco, beef	6.2	57
Doritos, taco flavor	4.8	0
Kentucy Fried Chicken	4.2	76
Hamburger, Big Mac	3.6	36
Pizza, cheese	3.4	47
Egg, raw	3.0	410
Beef liver, fried	2.8	482
Chicken breast, fried, with skin	2.5	90
Chocolate milkshake	2.3	13
Milk, whole	2.1	14
Swordfish, broiled	1.4	50
Chicken breast, fried, without skin	1.3	91
Milk, lowfat 2%	1.2	9
Yogurt, plain low-fat	1.0	6
Shrimp, raw	0.3	152

How to Choose Between Different Fats in Your Diet

Lipids (fats) not only provide fuel for energy, they absorb fat-soluble vitamins, become a part of the cell membrane structure, provide for hormone synthesis (steroids), and insulate and protect vital organs. Most lipids store in adipose tissue for subsequent release into the blood stream as free fatty acids. Fatty acids broadly classify as monounsaturated, polyunsaturated, and saturated. Each form of fatty acid exerts different effects on lipoproteins, and on cholesterol deposition in arteries and subsequent coronary disease risk.

Choosing the Right Fats
The table shows the available food choices for different types of lipids based on how they affect total cholesterol and different lipoprotein fractions. ∎

CHOOSE THE RIGHT FAT FOR YOUR DIET

Best Choice Monounsaturated Fat	Good Choice Polyunsaturated Fat	Occasional Choice Saturated/Hydrogenated Fat
Effects on Cholesterol and Lipoproteins	**Effects on Cholesterol and Lipoproteins**	**Effects on Cholesterol and Lipoproteins**
Decreases total cholesterol	Decreases total cholesterol	Increases total cholesterol
Decreases LDL-cholesterol	Decreases LDL-cholesterol	Increases LDL-cholesterol
No effect on HDL-cholesterol	Decreases HDL-cholesterol	
Food Examples	**Food Examples**	**Food Examples**
Vegetable Oils: avocado, canola, olive, peanut	**Vegetable Oils:** corn, safflower, sesame, soybean, sunflower, *trans* fat-free margarine, mayonnaise, miracle whip	**Tropical Vegetable Oils:** coconut, palm kernel, cocoa butter **Hydrogenated Oils:** margarine, shortening
Nuts: acorns, almonds, beechnuts, cashews, chestnuts, hazelnuts, hickory, macadamia, natural peanut butter, peanuts, pecans, pistachios	**Nuts:** Brazil, butternuts, pine, walnuts	**Animal Fats:** bacon, beef fat, chicken fat, egg yolk, fatty meats, lamb fat, lard, pepperoni, pork fat, salt pork, sausage, keilbasa
Other: fish fat (Omega-3 fatty acids)	**Seeds:** sesame, pumpkin, sunflower	**Dairy Products:** butter, cheese (regular, light, lowfat), cream cheese, half & half, ice cream, sour cream, whole milk, 2% milk

link amino acids in chains representing diverse forms and chemical combinations; the joining of two amino acids produces a dipeptide, and three amino acids linked together form a tripeptide. A linear configuration of up to as many as 100 amino acids produces a polypeptide; combining more than 100 amino acids forms a protein. Single cells contain thousands of different protein molecules, while the body contains approximately 50,000 different protein-containing compounds. The biochemical functions and properties of each protein depend on the sequencing of specific amino acids.

Of the 20 different amino acids required by the body, each contains a positively charged **amine group** at one end and a negatively charged **organic acid group** at the other end. The amine group consists of two hydrogen atoms attached to nitrogen (NH_2), whereas the organic acid group (technically termed a carboxylic acid group) contains one carbon atom, two oxygen atoms, and one hydrogen atom (COOH). The remainder of the amino acid molecule, its **side chain**, may take several different forms. The specific structure of the side chain dictates the amino acid's particular characteristics. Figure 2.9 (top) shows the structure of the amino acid alanine.

The Nine Essential Amino Acids

1. Histidine (infants)
2. Leucine
3. Lysine
4. Isoleucine
5. Methionine
6. Phenylalanine
7. Threonine
8. Tryptophan
9. Valine

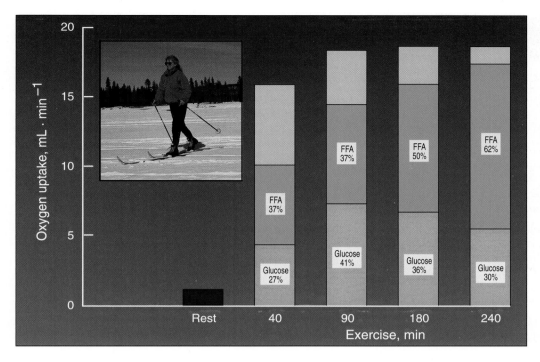

Figure 2.8
Uptake of oxygen and nutrients by the legs during prolonged exercise. (Green and orange areas represent the proportion of the total oxygen uptake caused by oxidation of free fatty acids (FFA) and blood glucose. Blue areas indicate oxidation of non–blood-borne fuels (muscle glycogen and intramuscular fats and proteins). (From Ahlborg, G., et al.: Substrate turnover during prolonged exercise in man. *J. Clin. Invest.*, 53:1080, 1974.)

Essential and Nonessential Amino Acids

The body requires 20 different amino acids, although tens of thousands of the same amino acids may combine in a single protein compound. Of the different amino acids, eight (nine in infants) cannot be synthesized in the body at a sufficient rate to prevent impairment of normal cellular function. These make up the essential or indispensable amino acids because they must be ingested preformed in foods. The body manufactures the remaining 12 **nonessential amino acids.** This does not mean they are unimportant; rather they form from compounds already existing in the body at a rate that meets demands for normal growth and tissue repair.

Animals and plants manufacture proteins that contain **essential amino acids.** *No health or physiological advantage comes from an amino acid derived from an animal compared with the same amino acid from vegetable origin.* Plants synthesize protein (and thus amino acids) by incorporating nitrogen from the soil (along with carbon, oxygen, and hydrogen from air and water). In contrast, animals do not have a broad capability for protein synthesis; they obtain much of their protein from ingested sources.

Constructing a body protein requires specific amino acid availability at the time of protein synthesis. **Complete proteins** or higher-quality proteins, come from foods with all of the essential amino acids in their correct ratio to maintain protein balance and allow for tissue growth and repair. An **incomplete protein,** or lower-quality protein, lacks one or more essential amino acids. Diets that contain mostly incomplete protein eventually produce protein malnutrition,

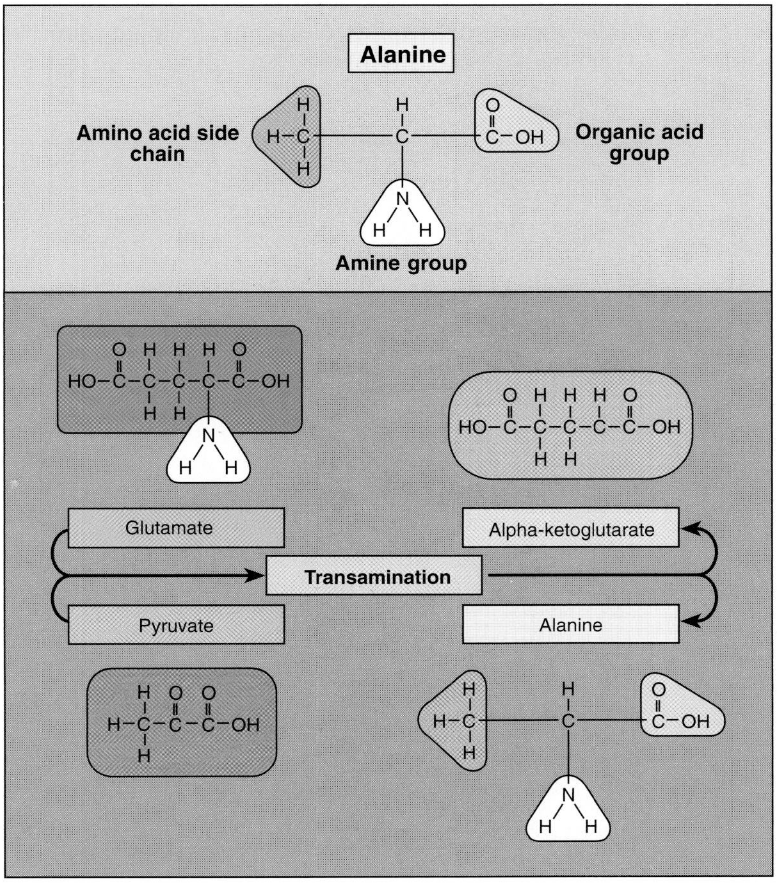

Figure 2.9
Chemical structure of alanine. In transamination, an amine group from a donor group transfers to an acceptor acid to form a new amino acid.

Mix and Match

Complete proteins can be obtained with the following complimentary combinations in a vegetarian diet:

- Beans and rice
- Peas and corn
- Bread and lentils
- Potatoes with milk or egg
- Cereals with milk or egg

despite the food source's adequacy for energy value and protein quantity.

Sources of Proteins

Dietary Sources

Sources of complete protein include eggs, milk, meat, fish, and poultry. Eggs provide the optimal mixture of essential amino acids among food sources; hence, eggs receive the highest quality rating compared with other foods. Presently, almost two-thirds of dietary protein in the U.S. comes from animal sources, whereas 80 years ago protein consumption occurred equally from plants and animals. Reliance on animal sources for dietary protein accounts for the relatively high current intake of cholesterol and saturated fatty acids.

The **"biologic value"** of food refers to its completeness for supplying essential amino acids. Animal sources contribute high-quality protein, whereas vegetables (lentils, dried beans and peas, nuts, and cereals) remain incomplete in one or more essential amino acids; thus, these have a relatively lower biologic value. Eating a variety of plant foods (grains, fruits, and vegetables), each providing a different quality and quantity of amino acids, contributes all of the required essential amino acids. Table 2.3 lists examples of excellent food sources of protein.

Synthesis in the Body

In muscle, enzymes facilitate nitrogen removal from certain amino acids and subsequently pass nitrogen to other compounds in the biochemical reactions of **transamination** (see Fig. 2.9, bottom). An amine group shifts from a donor amino acid to an acceptor acid, the acceptor thus becoming a new amino acid. *This allows amino acid formation from non–nitrogen-carrying organic compounds formed in metabolism.*

Deamination represents the process opposite to transamination. This involves removal of an amine group from the amino acid molecule and the remaining carbon skeleton converts into a carbohydrate or lipid, or used for energy. The split-off amine group forms urea in the liver, which the kidneys then excrete. Because urea must dissolve in water, excessive protein catabolism promotes fluid loss.

For deamination and transamination, the resulting carbon skeleton of the non-nitrogenous amino acid residue further degrades during energy metabolism. In well-nourished individuals at rest, protein breakdown contributes between 2 to 5% of the body's total energy requirement. During its breakdown (**catabolism**), protein first degrades into its amino acid components. The amino acid molecule then loses its nitrogen in the liver (deamination) to form urea (H_2NCONH_2) for excretion.

Protein's Role in the Body

No body "reservoirs" of protein exist; all protein contributes to tissue structures or exists as constituents of metabolic, transport, and hormonal systems. Protein constitutes between 12 to 15% of the body mass, but its content in different cells varies considerably. A brain cell, for example, contains only about 10% protein, while protein represents up to 20% of the mass of red blood cells and muscle cells. The systematic application of resistance training increases the protein content of skeletal muscle, which represents about 65% of the body's total protein.

Amino acids provide the building blocks to synthesize diverse compounds such as RNA and DNA, the heme components of the oxygen-binding hemoglobin and myoglobin compounds, the catecholamine hormones epinephrine and norepinephrine, and the neurotransmitter serotonin. Amino acids activate vitamins that play a key role in metabolic and physiologic regulation. Tissue synthesis (**anabolism**) accounts for more than one-third of the

TABLE 2.3
Rating of common sources of dietary protein

FOOD	PROTEIN RATING
Eggs	100
Fish	70
Lean beef	69
Cow's milk	60
Brown rice	57
White rice	56
Soybeans	47
Brewer's hash	45
Whole-grain wheat	44
Peanuts	43
Dry beans	34
White potato	34

protein intake during rapid growth in infancy and childhood. As growth rate declines, so does the percentage of protein retained for anabolic processes. Continual turnover of tissue protein occurs when a person attains optimal body size and growth stabilizes. Regular (and adequate) protein intake replaces the amino acids continually degraded in the turnover process.

Proteins serve as primary constituents for plasma membranes and internal cellular material. Proteins in cell nuclei (nucleoproteins) "supervise" cellular protein synthesis and transmit hereditary characteristics. Structural proteins comprise hair, skin, nails, bones, tendons, and ligaments, whereas globular proteins make up the nearly 2000 different enzymes that dramatically accelerate chemical reactions and regulate the catabolism of fats, carbohydrates, and proteins during energy release. Proteins also regulate acid-base quality of the body fluids, which contributes to neutralizing (buffering) excess acid metabolites formed during vigorous exercise.

Vegetarian Approach to Sound Nutrition

True vegetarians (**vegans**) consume nutrients from only two sources—the plant kingdom and dietary supplements. Vegans represent less than 1% of the U.S. population, although between 5 to 7% of Americans consider themselves "almost" vegetarians.

An increasing number of competitive and champion athletes consume diets consisting predominately of nutrients from varied plant sources, including some dairy and meat products. Considering the time required for training and competition, athletes often encounter difficulty planning, selecting, and preparing nutritious meals from predominantly plant sources without relying on supplementation. The fact remains that two-thirds of the world's population subsist on largely vegetarian diets with little reliance on animal protein. Well-balanced vegetarian and vegetarian-type diets can provide abundant carbohydrate, crucial in heavy training. Vegetarian-type diets have the following characteristics: usually low or devoid of choles-

> ### Diversity: Crucial for Vegetarians
>
> A vegan diet provides the essential amino acids if the RDA for protein includes 60% of protein from grain products, 35% from legumes, and the remaining 5% from green leafy vegetables. A 70-kg person who requires about 56 g of protein obtains the essential amino acids by consuming approximately 1 1/4 cups of beans, 1/4 cup of seeds or nuts, about 4 slices of whole-grain bread, 2 cups of vegetables (half being green leafy), and 2 1/2 cups from diverse grain sources like brown rice, oatmeal, and cracked wheat.

terol, high in fiber, low in saturated and high in unsaturated fatty acids, and rich in fruit and vegetable sources of antioxidant vitamins and diverse phytochemicals.

Obtaining ample high-quality protein becomes the strict vegetarian's main nutritional concern. A **lactovegetarian** diet provides milk and related products like ice cream, cheese, and yogurt. The lactovegetarian approach minimizes the problem of acquiring sufficient high-quality protein and increases the intake of calcium, phosphorus, and vitamin B_{12} (produced by bacteria in the digestive tract of animals). Good meatless sources of iron include fortified ready-to-eat cereals, soybeans, and cooked farina, whereas cereals, wheat germ, and oysters are high in zinc. Adding an egg to the diet (**ovolactovegetarian** diet) ensures an ample intake of high-quality protein.

Figure 2.10 displays the contribution of various food groups to the protein content of the American diet. By far, the greatest protein intake comes from animal sources, with only about 30% from plant sources.

Recommended Protein Intake

Despite the beliefs of many coaches, trainers, and athletes, eating excessive protein provides little benefit. Protein intakes greater than three times the recommended level do not enhance work capacity during intensive training. For athletes, muscle mass does not increase simply by eating high-protein foods. If lean tissue synthesis resulted from all of the extra protein intake consumed by the typical athlete, then muscle mass would increase tremendously. For example, eating an extra 100 g (400 kcal) of protein daily would translate into a daily 500-g (1.1 lb) in-

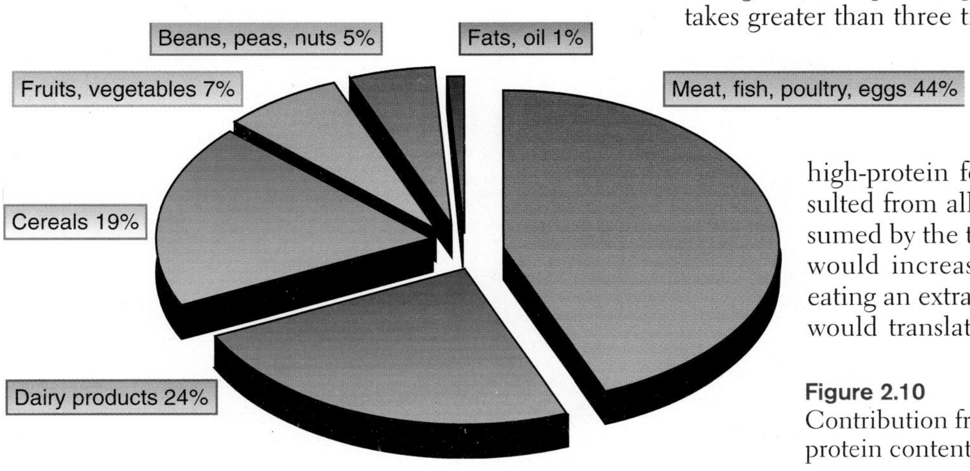

Beans, peas, nuts 5%
Fats, oil 1%
Fruits, vegetables 7%
Meat, fish, poultry, eggs 44%
Cereals 19%
Dairy products 24%

Figure 2.10
Contribution from the major food sources to the protein content of the typical American diet.

crease in muscle mass. This obviously does not happen. Additional dietary protein, after deamination (nitrogen removal), provides for energy or recycles as components of other molecules including stored fat in subcutaneous depots. Dietary protein intake significantly above recommended values can prove harmful because excessive protein breakdown strains liver and kidney function through the production and elimination of urea and other solutes.

Recommended Dietary Allowance

The **Recommended Dietary Allowance (RDA)** for protein, vitamins, and minerals represents standards for nutrient intake expressed as a daily average. *RDA levels represent a liberal yet safe excess to prevent nutritional deficiencies in practically all healthy people.*

Table 2.4 shows the protein RDAs for adolescent and adult men and women. On average, 0.83 g of protein per kg body mass represents the recommended daily intake. To determine the protein requirement for men and women ages 18 to 65, multiply body mass in kg by 0.83. Thus, for a 90-kg man, total protein requirement would equal 90 × 0.83 or 75 g. The protein RDA (and quantity of required essential amino acids) decreases with age. In contrast, the protein RDA for infants and growing children is 2.0 to 4.0 g per kg body mass. Pregnant women should increase their daily protein intake by 20 g, and nursing females should increase their intake by 10 g. Likewise, the protein requirement increases during stress, disease, and injury.

Protein Requirements For Physically Active People

Any discussion of protein requirement must include the assumption of adequate energy intake to match the added needs of exercise. *If energy intake falls below total energy expended during heavy training, even augmented protein intake may not maintain nitrogen balance.* This would occur because a disproportionate quantity of dietary protein catabolizes to balance an energy deficit rather than augment muscle development.

The common practice among weight lifters, body builders, and other power athletes of consuming liquids, powders, or pills of predigested protein represents a waste of money and may actually be counterproductive for producing the desired outcome. For example, many of these preparations contain proteins predigested to simple amino acids through chemical action in the laboratory. Available evidence does not support the belief that these simple amino acids become absorbed more easily and rapidly by the body or facilitate muscle growth brought on by training. In fact, the healthy intestine absorbes amino acids rapidly when they are part of more complex di- and tripeptide molecules. The intestinal tract handles protein best in their more complex form, whereas a concentrated amino-acid solution draws water into the small intestine, causing irritation, cramping, and diarrhea.

Current debate focuses on the necessity of a larger protein requirement for growing adolescent athletes, athletes involved in strength training (to enhance muscle growth) and endurance training programs (to counter increased protein breakdown for energy), and wrestlers and football players subjected to recurring muscle trauma. Inadequate protein intake can reduce body protein, particularly from muscle, with concomitant impairment in performance. If athletes require additional protein, then more than likely their increased food intake will compensate for training's increased energy expenditure. However, this may not occur in athletes with poor nutritional habits or who voluntarily reduce energy intake to achieve a desired aesthetic "look" to compete at a lower weight-class category to hopefully gain a competitive advantage.

TABLE 2.4
Recommended dietary allwoances of protein for adolescent and adult men and women

RECOMMENDED AMOUNT	MEN		WOMEN	
	ADOLESCENT	ADULT	ADOLESCENT	ADULT
Grams of protein per kg body weight	0.9	0.8	0.9	0.8
Grams of protein per day based on average weight[a]	59.0	56.0	50.0	44.0

[a] Average weight based on a "reference" man and woman. For adolescents (ages 14–18), average weight equals 65.8 kg (145 lb) for males and 55.7 kg (123 lb) for females. For adult men, average weight equals 70 kg (154 lb); for adult women, average weight equals 56.8 kg (125 lb).

Do Athletes Require More Protein?

Much of the current understanding of protein dynamics and exercise derives from studies that expanded the classic method of determining protein breakdown through urea excretion. For example, the output of "labeled" CO_2 from amino acids (either injected or ingested) increases during exercise in proportion to metabolic rate. As exercise progresses, the concentration of plasma urea also increases, coupled with a dramatic rise in nitrogen excretion in sweat (often occurring without changing urinary nitrogen excretion). Figure 2.11 illustrates that the sweat mechanism helps to excrete nitrogen produced from protein breakdown during exercise. Oxidation of plasma and intracellular amino acids increases significantly during moderate exercise, independent of changes in urea production.

Figure 2.11 also shows that protein use for energy reached its highest level when subjects exercised in the glycogen-depleted state. This emphasizes the important role of carbohydrate as a protein sparer, suggesting that carbohydrate availability affects the demand on protein "reserves" in exercise. Protein breakdown and accompanying gluconeogenesis undoubtedly become important factors in endurance exercise (or in frequent heavy training) when glycogen reserves diminish.

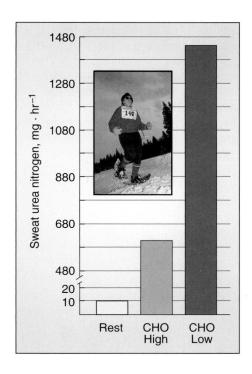

Figure 2.11
Excretion of urea in sweat at rest, and during exercise after carbohydrate loading (CHO High) and carbohydrate depletion (CHO Low). The largest utilization of protein (as reflected by sweat urea) occurs with low glycogen reserves. (From Lemon, P.W., and Nagel, F.: Effects of exercise on protein and amino acid metabolism. *Med. Sci. Sports Exerc.*, 13:141, 1981.)

Resistance Training Requires Glycogen Reserves

The potential for an increased use of protein for energy (and depressed protein synthesis) during intense aerobic exercise may explain why individuals who undertake resistance training primarily to augment muscle size refrain from glycogen-depleting, endurance-type exercise.

Increased protein catabolism during endurance exercise and heavy training often mirrors the metabolic mixture during short-term starvation. With depleted glycogen reserves, gluconeogenesis utilizing carbon skeletons from amino acids largely sustains the liver's glucose output. More than likely, greater protein breakdown reflects a homeostatic mechanism to maintain blood glucose concentration for central nervous system functioning. Eating a high-carbohydrate diet (with adequate energy intake) becomes important to preserve muscle protein in athletes who train hard and for protracted durations.

Protein degradation above the resting level occurs during endurance and resistance training exercise to a degree greater than previously acknowledged. Unfortunately, research has not pinpointed the actual protein requirements for individuals who train 2 to 6 hours daily with resistance-type exercise. Further research will determine whether the current protein RDA should be modified for specific athletic groups (e.g., body builders, weight lifters) who typically use resistance exercise to increase muscle size, strength, and power, and others involved in prolonged endurance competitions and heavy training. Until such data become available, protein should be recognized as a potential energy fuel for exercise. We do not recommend protein supplementation if an athlete's diet contains adequate calories (and protein). However, if questions remain about the nutritional adequacy of the diet, then we recommend that athletes in heavy training ($2\text{-}6\ h \cdot d^{-1}$) consume between 1.2 and 1.8 g of protein per kg of body mass daily. This level of protein intake is usually within the range of the typical protein intake of the competitive athlete, obviating the need to consume supplementary protein.

Alanine-Glucose Cycle

Although some tissue proteins do not readily contribute to energy metabolism, muscle proteins can degrade to supply energy. Figure 2.12 shows that the increased release of the amino acid alanine (and possibly glutamine) from active leg muscles relates to exercise severity; as intensity increases, alanine output correspondingly increases in proportion to exercise intensity.

Researchers have proposed that alanine indirectly serves the energy requirements of exercise. Active skeletal muscle synthesizes alanine during transamination from

c l o s e   u p

Fitness and Wellness Make Health Sense

What is Physical Fitness?

Many different definitions of physical fitness exist. Physicians sometimes define fitness as "absence of disease"; athletes may define fitness by scores on an endurance test (i.e., time to complete a marathon); and others define fitness based on appearance ("looking fit"). The President's Council on Physical Fitness and Sports states that fitness is the "measure of the body's strength, stamina, and flexibility." The American Medical Association defines fitness as "the general capacity to adapt and respond favorably to physical effort."

Defining the Wellness Construct

Wellness relates to a continual effort to remain healthy to achieve the highest potential for total well being. Within this broad framework, exercise scientists often view physical fitness from a health-related perspective involving four basic components—*cardiovascular endurance, muscular strength and endurance, joint flexibility, and body composition* (see figure below).

This approach de-emphasizes assessment of physical fitness components that stress motor performance and athletic fitness (e.g., tests of speed, power, balance, and agility) focusing instead on those fitness measures that assess functional capacity and reflect various aspects of overall good health, disease prevention, or both. A person's performance on each health-related fitness component does not remain fixed; rather, each can improve significantly through a program of regular exercise. To improve overall health-related physical fitness, a person must focus training in *each* of these categories.

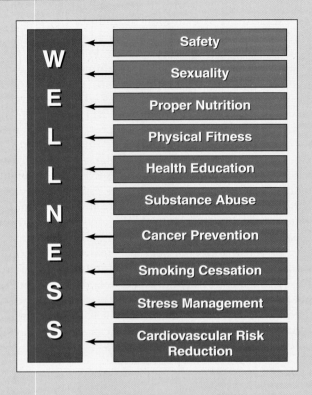

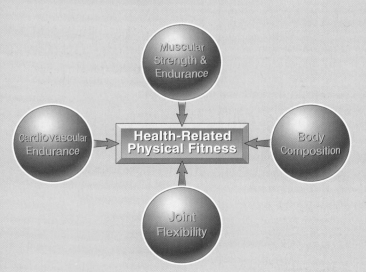

Achieving a high level of overall health-related physical fitness does not necessarily ensure attainment of good health as indicated by the wellness components illustrated in the above figure. For example, a person who runs 4 miles each day, engages in resistance exercises regularly, incorporates flexibility exercises into the warm-up and cool-down phases of the workout, and maintains a desirable level of body fat progresses toward the top of the health-related physical fitness ladder. From the perspective of wellness, if this person has high blood pressure, high cholesterol, smokes, or exhibits a high stress index, he/she would face increased risk for cardiovascular disease and clearly would not classify as being "well."

Although diverse health and fitness benefits accrue from participation in regular exercise designed to improve overall health-related physical fitness, the greatest impact relates to improved "quality of life." This person will not only have fewer health problems and functional impairments through middle and old age, but may actually live several years longer.

Fitness and Wellness Make Good Business Sense

Many businesses that offer health/fitness promotion programs have found that it costs less to keep their employees healthy then treat them when they become sick. In addition, many corporations use fitness and wellness programs as an incentive to attract, hire, and retain employees. Companies devote resources to these programs because they know they can expect less absenteeism, hospitalization, disability, job turnover rates, premature death, and health costs, and increased morale, job productivity, and satisfaction. The evidence is clear; the greater the participation, the lower the medical costs per employee.

Three Examples of Economic Benefits of Wellness

Mesa Petroleum Company, Amarillo, Texas has offered on-site fitness and wellness programs since 1979. Sixty-four percent of all employees participate. Company records indicate that after only 4 years medical costs averaged $173 per person per year for participants compared with $434 per person per year for nonparticipants. This represented more than a $200,000 yearly reduction in medical expenses. More impressively, sick leave decreased by more than 38% for participating individuals.

Tenneco Corporation in Houston, Texas significantly reduced medical care costs for men and women who participated in their on-site exercise-wellness program. Specifically, the medical care costs averaged $562 for the male and $639 for female participants compared with $1004 and $1536, re-

spectively, for nonparticipants. Sick leave decreased by about 22.5 hours per year for the participants compared with the nonparticipants. The company also reported higher job satisfaction among those participating in the wellness programs.

New York Telephone Company saved more than $5.54 million in employee absence and treatment costs, representing $69.25 per employee health care costs, with the initiation of a wellness program for its employees. This allowed the company to invest the saved money in increased employee benefits.

References
Gettman, R.L.: Cost/benefit analysis of corporate fitness program. *Fitness in Business*, 1(1):11, 1986.

Marcotte, B., and Price, J.H.: The status of health promotion programs at the worksite, a review. *Health Education*, July/Aug, 1983.

Shephard, R.J.: Worksite fitness and exercise programs: a review of methodology and health impact. *Am. J. Health Promotion*, 10:436, 1996.

Shephard R.J.: Do work-site exercise and health programs work? *Phys. Sportsmed.*, 27(2):48, 1999.

Smith, L.K.: Cost contaminant through health promotion programs. *J. Occup. Med.*, 22:36, 1980.

the glucose intermediate pyruvate. Alanine then leaves the muscle and enters the liver for deamination. The resulting carbon skeleton converts to glucose, which then enters the blood for delivery to active muscle. The residue carbon fragments from the amino acid that formed alanine oxidize for energy within the muscle cell. *The **alanine-glucose cycle** generates from 10 to 15% of the total exercise energy requirement during long-term, high-intensity exercise.*

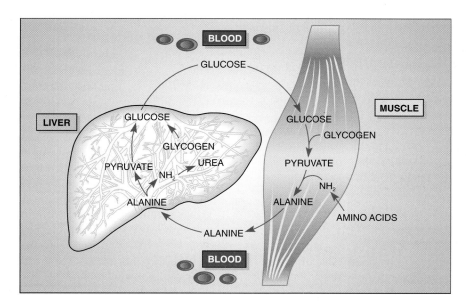

Figure 2.12
Alanine-glucose cycle. Alanine, synthesized in muscle from glucose-derived pyruvate, travels from the blood to the liver, which converts the alanine to glucose and urea. Glucose is then released back to the blood for transport to muscle as an energy substrate. During exercise, the increased production and output of alanine from muscle helps maintain blood glucose for the needs of the nervous system and active muscles.

summary

1. Carbon, hydrogen, oxygen, and nitrogen represent the primary structural units for most of the body's biologically active substances.

2. Specific combinations of carbon with oxygen and hydrogen form carbohydrates and lipids, whereas proteins consist of combinations of carbon, oxygen, and hydrogen, including nitrogen and minerals.

3. Simple sugars consist of chains from three to seven carbon atoms with hydrogen and oxygen in the ratio of 2 to 1. Glucose, the most common simple sugar, contains a six-carbon chain: $C_6H_{12}O_6$.

4. Three classifications commonly define carbohydrates: monosaccharides (sugars such as glucose and fructose); disaccharides (combinations of two monosaccharides as in sucrose, lactose, and maltose); and polysaccharides that contain three or more simple sugars to form plant starch and fiber, and the large animal polysaccharide glycogen.

5. Glycogenolysis reconverts glycogen to glucose, whereas gluconeogenesis synthesizes glucose, especially from the carbon skeletons of amino acids.

6. Fiber, a non-starch, structural plant polysaccharide, offers considerable resistance to human digestive enzymes. Although technically not a nutrient, water-soluble and water-insoluble dietary fibers confer health benefits for gastrointestinal functioning and cardiovascular disease.

7. Americans typically consume 40 to 50% of total calories as carbohydrates in fruits, grains, and vegetables.

8. Carbohydrates, stored in limited quantity in liver and muscle, serve 1) as a major source of energy, 2) to spare the breakdown of proteins, 3) as a metabolic primer for fat metabolism, and 4) as fuel for the central nervous system.

9. During intense exercise, muscle glycogen and blood glucose represent the primary fuels for exercise. The body's glycogen stores also provide energy in sustained, high levels of aerobic exercise such as marathon running, triathlon-type events, long-distance cycling, and endurance swimming.

10. A carbohydrate-deficient diet rapidly depletes muscle and liver glycogen, profoundly affecting both high-intensity anaerobic and long-duration aerobic exercise capacity. Individuals involved in heavy training should consume at least 60% of daily calories as carbohydrates (400 to 600 g), predominantly in unrefined complex form.

11. Like carbohydrates, lipids contain carbon, hydrogen, and oxygen atoms, but with a higher ratio of hydrogen to oxygen. For example, the lipid stearin has the formula $C_{57}H_{110}O_6$. Lipid molecules consist of one glycerol molecule and three fatty acid molecules.

12. Plants and animals synthesize lipids into one of three groups: 1) simple lipids (glycerol plus 3 fatty acids), 2) compound lipids (phospholipids, glycolipids, and lipoproteins) composed of simple lipids in combination with other chemicals, and 3) derived lipids like cholesterol synthesized from simple and compound lipids.

13. Saturated fatty acids contain as many hydrogen atoms as chemically possible; thus, the molecule is said to be saturated relative to hydrogen. Saturated fatty acids exist primarily in animal meat, egg yolk, dairy fats, and cheese. High intakes of saturated fatty acids elevate blood cholesterol and promote coronary heart disease.

14. Unsaturated fatty acids contain fewer hydrogen atoms attached to the carbon chain. Because double bonds connect carbon atoms.

Fatty acids exist as either monounsaturated or polyunsaturated with respect to hydrogen. Increasing the diet's proportion of unsaturated fatty acids may offer protection against heart disease.

15. Lowering blood cholesterol, especially that carried by low-density lipoprotein cholesterol, provides significant coronary heart disease protection.

16. Dietary lipid represents between 34 and 38% of the typical person's total caloric intake. Prudent recommendations suggest a 30% level or lower, of which 70 to 80% should be unsaturated fatty acids.

17. Lipids provide the largest nutrient store of potential energy for biologic work. They 1) protect vital organs, 2) provide insulation from cold, 3) transport fat-soluble vitamins, and 4) depress hunger.

18. During light and moderate exercise, fat contributes about 50% of the energy requirement. As exercise continues, stored fat becomes more important, supplying more than 80% of the body's energy needs.

19. Proteins differ chemically from lipids and carbohydrates because they contain nitrogen in addition to sulfur, phosphorus, and iron.

20. Subunits called amino acids form proteins. The body requires 20 different amino acids.

21. Eight of the 20 amino acids cannot be synthesized by the body; they must be consumed in the diet and are called essential amino acids.

22. All animal and plant cells contain protein. Complete (higher-quality) proteins contain all the essential amino acids; the other protein type represents incomplete or lower-quality proteins. Examples of higher-quality, complete proteins include animal proteins found in eggs, milk, cheese, meat, fish, and poultry.

23. Consuming a variety of plant foods provides all the essential amino acids because each food source contains a different quality and quantity of amino acids.

24. The RDA represents the recommended quantity for nutrient intake. It serves as a liberal, yet safe level of excess to meet the nutritional needs of practically all healthy people. For adults, the protein RDA equals 0.83 g per kg of body mass.

25. Protein breakdown above the resting level occurs during endurance and resistance training exercise to a degree greater than previously thought. Athletes in heavy training ($2\text{-}6 \ h \cdot d^{-1}$) should consume between 1.2 and 1.8 g of protein per kg of body mass daily.

26. Reduced carbohydrate reserves increase protein catabolism during exercise. Such findings support the wisdom of maintaining optimal levels of glycogen during strenuous training.

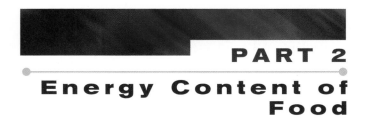

PART 2
Energy Content of Food

Calorie—A Measurement of Food Energy

One calorie expresses the quantity of heat to raise the temperature of 1 kg (1 L) of water 1° C (specifically, from 14.5 to 15.5° C). Thus, **kilogram calorie** or **kilocalorie (kcal)** more accurately defines calorie. For example, if a particular food contains 300 kcal, then releasing the potential energy trapped within this food's chemical structure increases the temperature of 300 L of water 1° C. Different foods contain different amounts of potential energy. One-half cup of peanut butter with a caloric value of 759 kcal contains the equivalent heat energy to increase the temperature of 759 L of water 1° C.

Gross Energy Value of Foods

Laboratories use **bomb calorimeters** similar to the one illustrated in Figure 2.13 to measure the total (*gross*) energy value of various food macronutrients. Bomb calorimeters operate on the principle of **direct calorimetry**, measuring the heat liberated as the food burns completely.

The bomb calorimeter works as follows:

- A small, insulated chamber filled with oxygen under pressure contains a weighed portion of food.
- The food ignites and literally explodes and burns when an electric current ignites a fuse inside the chamber.
- A surrounding water bath absorbs the heat released as the food burns (termed the heat of combustion). Insulation prevents loss of heat to the outside.

- A sensitive thermometer measures the amount of heat absorbed by the water. For example, the complete combustion of one hot dog (beef, skinless, 2 oz), bun (1.4 oz), mustard, and small french fries (2.4 oz) liberates 512 kcal of heat energy. This would raise 5.12 kg (11.3 lb) of ice water to the boiling point.

Heat of Combustion

The heat liberated by burning (oxidizing) food in a bomb calorimeter represents its **heat of combustion** or the total energy value of the food. *Burning 1 g of pure carbohydrate yields a heat of combustion of 4.20 kcal, 1 g of pure protein releases 5.65 kcal, and 1 g of pure lipid yields 9.45 kcal.* Because most foods in the diet consist of various proportions of the three macronutrients, the caloric value of a given food reflects the sum of the heats of combustion of each of the food macronutrients.

The average heats of combustion for the three nutrients (carbohydrate, $4.2 \ kcal \cdot g^{-1}$; lipid, $9.4 \ kcal \cdot g^{-1}$; protein, $5.65 \ kcal \cdot g^{-1}$) demonstrates that the complete oxidation of lipid in the bomb calorimeter liberates about 65% more energy per gram than protein oxidation, and 120% more energy than carbohydrate oxidation. Recall from Part 1 that a lipid molecule contains more hydrogen atoms than either carbohydrate or protein molecules. The common fatty acid palmitic acid, for example, has the structural formula $C_{16}H_{32}O_2$. The ratio of hydrogen atoms to oxygen atoms in

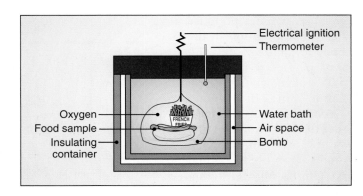

Figure 2.13
Bomb calorimeter directly measures the energy value of food.

More Lipid Equals More Calories

Lipid-rich foods contain a higher energy content than foods relatively fat-free. One glass of whole milk, for example, contains 160 kcal, whereas the same quantity of skim milk contains only 90 kcal. If a person who normally consumes one quart of whole milk each day switches to skim milk, the total calories ingested each year would be reduced by the equivalent calories in 25 pounds of body fat. Thus, following this switch for just 3 years would theoretically represent a 75-lb loss of body fat.

fatty acids always greatly exceeds the 2:1 ratio found in carbohydrates. *Simply stated, lipid molecules have more hydrogen atoms available for cleavage and subsequent oxidation for energy than carbohydrates and proteins.*

Net Energy Value of Foods

Differences exist in the energy value of foods when comparing the heat of combustion (gross energy value) determined by direct calorimetry to the *net* energy actually available to the body. This pertains particularly to proteins because the nitrogen component of this nutrient cannot be oxidized. In the body, nitrogen atoms combine with hydrogen to form urea, which urine excretes. Elimination of hydrogen in this manner represents a loss of approximately 19% of the protein molecule's potential energy. The hydrogen loss reduces protein's heat of combustion in the body to approximately 4.6 kcal per gram instead of 5.65 kcal per gram from oxidation in the bomb calorimeter. In contrast, identical physiologic fuel values exist for carbohydrates and lipids (which contain no nitrogen) compared with their heats of combustion in the bomb calorimeter.

Digestive Efficiency

The "availability" to the body of the ingested macronutrients determines their ultimate caloric yield. Availability refers to completeness of digestion and absorption. Normally about 97% of carbohydrates, 95% of lipids, and 92% of proteins become digested, absorbed, and available for energy. Large variation exists for protein ranging from a high of 97% for animal protein to a low 78% for dried peas and beans. Furthermore, less energy becomes available from a meal with high fiber content. Considering average digestive efficiencies, the net kcal value per gram for carbohydrate equals 4.0, 9.0 for lipid and 4.0 for protein. These corrected heats of combustion comprise the **Atwater general factors**, named after the scientist who first investigated the energy released from food in the calorimeter (Wilbur Olin Atwater, 1844–1907).

Energy Value of a Meal

The caloric content of any food can be determined from net Atwater kcal values, as long as one knows its composition and weight. Suppose, for example, we wanted to determine the kcal value for 1/2 cup of creamed chicken. This portion weighs 3.5 oz or about 100 g. Based on laboratory analysis of a standard recipe, the macronutrient composition of 1 g of creamed chicken contains 0.2 g of protein, 0.12 g of lipid, and 0.06 g of carbohydrate.

Using the net kcal values, 0.2 g of protein contains 0.8 kcal (0.20 × 4.0), 0.12 g of lipid equals 1.08 kcal (0.12 × 9.0), and 0.06 g of carbohydrate yields 0.24 kcal (0.06 × 4.0). The total caloric value of 1 g of creamed chicken would therefore equal 2.12 kcal (0.80 + 1.08 + 0.24). Consequently, a 100 g serving contains 100 times as much, or 212 kcal. Table 2.5 presents an example of these computations. Although this table shows the method for calcu-

TABLE 2.5
Method of calculating the caloric value of a food from its composition of macronutrients

Food: Ice cream (vanilla)
Weight: three-fourths cup = 100 grams

| | COMPOSITION | | |
	PROTEIN	LIPID	CARBOHYDRATE
Percentage	4%	13%	21%
Total grams	4	13	21
In one gram	0.04 g	0.13 g	0.21 g
Calories per gram	0.16	1.17	0.84
	(0.4 × 4.0 kcal)	(0.13 × 9.0 kcal)	(0.21 × 4.0 kcal)

Total calories per gram: 0.16 + 1.17 + 0.84 = 2.17 kcal

Total calories per 100 grams: 2.17 × 100 = 217 kcal

How to Read Food Labels

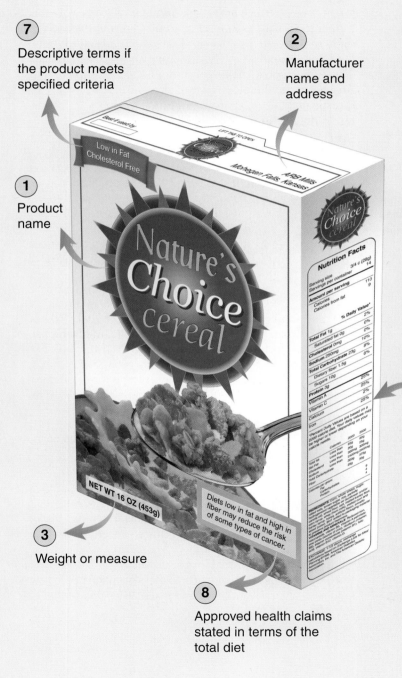

(7) Descriptive terms if the product meets specified criteria

(2) Manufacturer name and address

(1) Product name

(3) Weight or measure

(8) Approved health claims stated in terms of the total diet

Nutrition Facts

Serving size 3/4 c (28 g)
Servings per container 14

Amount per serving

Calories	110
Calories from fat	9

% Daily Value*

Total Fat 1 g	2%
Saturated fat 0 g	0%
Cholesterol 0 mg	0%
Sodium 250 mg	10%
Total Carbohydrate 23 g	8%
Dietary fiber 1.5 g	6%
Sugars 10 g	
Protein 3 g	
Vitamin A	25%
Vitamin C	25%
Calcium	2%
Iron	25%

*Percent Daily Values are based on a 2000 calorie diet. Your daily values may be higher or lower depending on your calorie needs.

		Calories	2000	2500
Total fat	Less than		65 g	80 g
Sat Fat	Less than		20 g	25 g
Cholesterol	Less than		300 mg	300 mg
Sodium	Less than		2400 mg	2400 mg
Total Carbohydrate			300 g	375 g
Fiber			25 g	30 g

Calories per gram:
Fat 9
Carbohydrates 4
Protein 4

INGREDIENTS: Corn, whole wheat, sugar, rolled oats, brown sugar, rice, partially hydrogenated vegetable oil (sunflower and/or canola oil), wheat flour, salt, malted barley flour, corn syrup, whey (from milk), malted corn and barley syrup, honey, artificial flavor, annatto etract (color), BHT added to packaging material to preserve product freshness.
VITAMINS AND MINERALS: Reduced iron, niacinamide, vitamin B6, Vitamin A palmitate zinc oxide (source of zinc), riboflavin (vitamin B2), thiamin mononitrate (vitamin B1), folic acid, vitamin B12, vitamin D.

EXCHANGE: 1-1/2 starch, exchange calculations based on *Exchange Lists for Meal Planning* ©1995, American Diabetes Association, Inc. and The American Dietetic Association.

(5) Serving size, number of servings per container, and calorie information

(6) Nutrition information panel provides quantities of nutrients per serving, in both actual amounts and as "% of Daily Values" based on a 2000-calorie energy intake

(4) Ingredients in descending order of predominance by weight

continued on next page

In 1990, the United States Congress passed the **Nutrition Labeling and Education Act** that brought sweeping changes for food labeling. All foods, except those containing only a few nutrients like plain coffee, tea, and spices, now provide consistent nutrition information. The food label must display the following information prominently, and in words an average person can understand (numbers in figure relate to numbered information below):

1. Product's common or usual name
2. Name and address of manufacturer, packer, or distributor
3. Net contents for weight, measure, or count
4. All ingredients listed in descending order of predominance by weight
5. Serving size, number of servings per container, and calorie information
6. Quantities of specified nutrients and food constituents (this includes total food energy in calories, total fat (g), saturated fat (g), cholesterol (mg), sodium (mg), total carbohydrate including starch, sugar, and fiber (g), and protein (g)
7. Descriptive terms of content
8. Approved health claims stated in terms of the total diet

Terms on Food Labels

Common terms and what they mean:

Free: Nutritionally trivial and unlikely to have physiologic consequences; synonyms include "without," "no," and "zero."

High: 20% or more of the Daily Value (DV) for a given nutrient per serving; synonyms include "rich in" or "excellent in."

Less: At least 25% less of a given nutrient or calories than the comparison food.

Low: An amount that allows frequent consumption of the food without exceeding the nutrient's DV.

Good Source: Product provides between 10% and 19% of a given nutrient's DV per serving.

Cholesterol Terms

Cholesterol-free: Less than 2 mg per serving, and 2 g or less saturated fat per serving.

Low Cholesterol: 20 mg or less cholesterol per serving, and 2 g or less saturated fat per serving.

Less Cholesterol: 25% or less cholesterol per serving and 2 g or less saturated fat per serving.

Fat Terms

Extra Lean: Less than 5 g fat, 2 g saturated fat and 95 mg cholesterol per serving, and per 100 g of meat, poultry, and seafood.

Fat Free: Less than 0.5 g fat per serving (no added fat or oil).

Lean: Less than 10 g fat, 4.5 g saturated fat, and 95 mg cholesterol per serving, and per 100 g of meat, poultry, and seafood.

Less Fat: 25% or less fat than comparison food.

Low Fat: 3 g or less fat per serving.

Light: 50% or less fat than comparison food (e.g., "50% less fat than our regular cookies").

Less Saturated Fat: 25% or less saturated fat than comparison food.

Energy Terms

Calorie Free: Fewer than 5 calories per serving.

Light: One-third fewer calories than the comparison food.

Low Calorie: 40 calories or less per serving.

Reduced Calorie: At least 25% fewer calories per serving than comparison food.

Fiber Terms

High Fiber: 5 g or more fiber per serving.

Sodium Terms

Sodium Free and *Salt Free:* Less than 5 mg sodium per serving.

Low Sodium: 140 mg or less sodium per serving.

Light: Low-calorie food with 50% sodium reduction.

Light in Sodium: No more than 50% of the sodium of comparison food.

Very Low Sodium: 35 mg or less sodium per serving.

References

The Nutrition Labeling Act of 1990. Federal Register 58(3), 1993. U.S. Government Printing Office, Superintendent of Documents, Washington, DC.

<http://www.fda.gov/opacom/backgrounders/foodlabel/new-label.html# panel> (provides complete description of the new food label and relevant terms and materials related to the label). ∎

lating the kcal value of ice cream, the same method applies for a serving of any food. Reducing the portion size by one-half would of course reduce caloric intake by 50%.

Fortunately, the need seldom exists to compute the kcal value of foods (as shown in the previous example) because the United States Department of Agriculture has already made these determinations for almost all foods. In Section IV of the Student Workbook that accompanies this text, we list the energy and nutritive values for approximately 2000 foods, expressed per ounce (28.4 g) of the food item. The specific values for each food (including specialty and fast-food items) include calories in an average portion, as well as its content of protein, lipid, carbohydrate, calcium, sodium, iron, vitamins B_1, B_2, C, and A, fiber, and cholesterol.

Calories Equal Calories

When examining the energy value of various foods, a striking observation can be made with regard to a food's energy value. Consider, for example, five common foods: raw celery, cooked cabbage, cooked asparagus spears, mayonnaise, and salad oil. To consume 100 kcal of each of these foods, one must eat 20 stalks of celery, 4 cups of cabbage, 30 asparagus spears, but only 1 tablespoon of mayonnaise or 4/5 tablespoon of salad oil. Thus, a small serving of some foods contains the equivalent energy value as a large quantity of other foods. Viewed from a different perspective, to meet daily energy needs, a sedentary young adult female would have to consume more than 420 stalks of celery, 84 cups of cabbage, or 630 asparagus spears, yet only 1.5 cups of mayonnaise or about 8 ounces of salad oil. The major difference among these foods is that high-fat foods contain more energy with little water. In contrast, foods low in fat or high in water tend to contain little energy. However, 100 kcal from mayonnaise and 100 kcal from celery are exactly the same in terms of energy.

A calorie reflects food energy regardless of the food source. *Thus, from an energy standpoint, 100 calories from mayonnaise equals the same 100 calories in 20 celery stalks.* The more one eats of any food, the more calories one consumes. However, a small quantity of fatty foods represents a considerable quantity of calories; thus, the term "fattening" often misdescribes these foods. An individual's caloric intake equals the sum of all energy consumed from either small or large quantities of foods. Celery would become a "fattening" food if consumed in excess.

summary

1. A calorie or kilocalorie (kcal) represents a measure of heat that expresses the energy value of food.

2. Burning food in a bomb calorimeter permits direct quantification of the food's energy content.

3. The heat of combustion represents the amount of heat liberated by a food's complete oxidation. Average gross energy values equal 4.2 kcal per gram for carbohydrate, 9.4 kcal per gram for lipid, and 5.65 kcal per gram for protein.

4. The coefficient of digestibility represents the proportion of food consumed actually digested and absorbed by the body.

5. Coefficients of digestibility average approximately 97% for carbohydrates, 95% for lipids, and 92% for proteins. Thus, the net energy values equal 4 kcal per gram of carbohydrate, 9 kcal per gram of lipid, and 4 kcal per gram of protein. These values, known as Atwater general factors, provide an estimate of the net energy value of foods in a diet.

6. The Atwater general factors allow one to compute the caloric content of any meal from the carbohydrate, lipid, and protein compositions of the food.

7. A calorie represents a unit of heat energy regardless of food source. From an energy standpoint, 500 kcal of chocolate ice cream topped with whipped cream and chocolate chips is no more fattening than 500 kcal of watermelon, 500 kcal of cheese and sausage pizza, or 500 kcal of a bagel with salmon, onions, and sour cream.

thought questions

1. Outline a presentation to a high school class about how to eat well for a physically active, healthy lifestyle.

2. Many college students do not eat well-balanced meals. What recommendations would you make concerning nutrient intake to ensure proper energy reserves for moderate and intense physical activities? Are nutritional supplements necessarily required?

3. Explain the importance of regular carbohydrate intake when maintaining a high level of daily physical activity. Additionally, what are some "non-exercise" benefits for a diet rich in food sources containing unrefined complex carbohydrates.

4. Discuss a rationale for recommending adequate carbohydrate intake, rather than an excess of protein, for a person who wants to increase muscle mass through heavy resistance training.

5. How would you respond to this question? "How can oxygen burning indicate the amount of calories contained in the meal I'm going to eat?"

selected references

Andrews, T.C., et al.: Effect of cholesterol reduction on myocardial ischemia in patients with coronary disease. *Circulation*, 95:324, 1997.

Brooks, G.A.: Amino acid and protein metabolism during exercise and recovery. *Med. Sci. Sports Exerc.*, 19:S150, 1987.

Brouns, F.: *Nutritional Needs of Athletes.* New York: John Wiley & Sons, 1993.

Brouns, F., and Beckers, E.: Is the gut an athletic organ? *Sports. Med.*, 15:242, 1993.

Brown, L., et al.: Cholesterol-lowering effects of dietary fiber: a meta-analysis. *Am. J. Clin. Nutr.*, 69:30, 1999.

Butterfield, G. E.: Amino acids and high protein diets. In: *Perspectives in Exercise Science and Sports Medicine, Ergonomics—The Enhancement of Exercise and Sport Performance.* Vol. 4. Williams, M., and Lamb, D. (eds.). Indianapolis: Benchmark Press, 1991.

Caggiula, A.W., and Mustak, V.A.: Effects of dietary fat and fatty acids on coronary artery disease risk and total and lipoprotein cholesterol concentrations: epidemiologic studies. *Am. J. Clin. Nutr.*, 65(Suppl):1597S, 1997.

Clarkson, P.M.: Minerals: exercise performance and supplementation in athletes. *J. Sports Sci.*, 9:91, 1991.

Clarkson, P.M., and Haymes, E.M.: Exercise and mineral status of athletes: calcium, magnesium, phosphorus, and iron. *Med. Sci. Sports Exerc.*, 27:831, 1995.

Coggan, A.R.: Plasma glucose metabolism during exercise; L effect of endurance training in humans. *Med. Sci. Sports Exerc.*, 29:620, 1997

Conroy, B.P., et al.: Bone mineral density in elite junior Olympic weight lifters. *Med. Sci. Sports Exerc.*, 25:1103, 1993.

Coyle, E. F., and Montain, S. J.: Carbohydrate and fluid ingestion during exercise: are there trade-offs? *Med. Sci. Sports Exerc.*, 24:671, 1992.

Coyle, E.F.: Substrate utilization during exercise in active people. *Am. J. Clin. Nutr.*, 61:968S, 1995.

Daly, M.E., et al.: Dietary carbohydrate and insulin sensitivity: a review of the evidence and clinical implications. *Am. J. Clin. Nutr.*, 66: 1073, 1997.

Dreon D.M., et al.: Change in dietary saturated fat intake is correlated with change in mass of large low-density-lipoprotein particles in men. *Am. J. Clin. Nutr.*, 67:828, 1998.

Economos, C.D., et al.: Nutritional practices of elite athletes: practical recommendations. *Sports Med.*, 16:381, 1993.

Fogelholm, G.M., et al.: Dietary and biochemical indices of nutritional status in male athletes and controls. *J. Am. Coll. Nutr.*, 11:181, 1992.

Food and Nutrition Board, *Recommended Dietary Allowances*, 11th Ed., National Academy of Sciences, Washington, D.C., 1999.

Hargreaves, M.: Interactions between muscle glycogen and blood glucose during exercise, *Exerc. Sport Sci. Rev.*, 25:21, 1997.

Heyward, V.H., et al.: Anthropometric, body composition and nutritional profiles of bodybuilders during training. *J. Appl. Sports Sci. Rev.*, 3:22, 1989.

Howell, W.M., et al.: Plasma lipid and lipoprotein responses to dietary fat and cholesterol: a meta-analysis. *Am. J. Clin. Nutr.*, 65:1747, 1997.

Hu, F.B., et al.: Dietary fat intake and the risk of coronary heart disease in women. *N. Engl. J. Med.*, 337:1491, 1997.

Jacobs, D.R., Jr., et al.: Is whole grain intake associated in reduced total and cause-specific death rates in older women? The Iowa Women's Health Study. *Am. J. Public Health*, 89:322, 1999.

Jeukendrup, A.E., et al.: Carbohydrate-electrolyte feedings improve 1 h time trial cycling performance. *Int. J. Sports Med.*, 18:125, 1997.

Jeukendrup, A.E., et al.: Fat metabolism during exercise: A review—Part II: Regulation of metabolism and effect of training. *Int. J. Sports Med.*, 19:293, 1998.

Katch, F.I.: U.S. government raises serious questions about reliability of U.S. Department of Agriculture's food composition database. *Int. J. Sports Nutr.*, 5:62, 1995.

Kiens, B.: Effect of endurance training on fatty acid metabolism: local adaptations. *Med. Sci. Sports Exerc.*, 29:640, 1997.

Lemon, P. W., et al.: Protein requirements and muscle mass/strength changes during intensive training in novice bodybuilders. *J. Appl. Physiol.*, 73:767, 1992.

Martin, W.H., III.: Effect of acute and chronic exercise on fat metabolism. *Exer. Sport Sci. Rev.*, 24:203, 1996.

McArdle, W.D., et al.: *Sport & Exercise Nutrition.* Baltimore: Lippincott Williams & Wilkins, 1999.

Rennie, M.J., et al.: Physical activity and protein metabolism. In: *Physical Activity, Fitness, and Health.* Bouchard, C., et al., (eds.). Champaign, IL: Human Kinetics, 1994.

Salmerón, J.E., et al.: Dietary fiber, glycemic load, and risk of non-insulin-dependent diabetes mellitus in women. *JAMA*, 277:472, 1997.

Saltin, B., and Gollnick, P.D.: Fuel for muscular exercise: role of carbohydrate. In: *Exercise, Nutrition, and Human Performance.* Horton, E.S., and Terjung, R.L., (eds.). New York: Macmillan, 1988.

Sharon, N.: Carbohydrates. *Sci. Am.*, 243:90, 1980.

Sherman, W.A., and Wimer, G.S.: Insufficient dietary carbohydrate during training: does it impair athletic performance? *Int. J. Sport Nutr.*, 1:28, 1991.

Slyper, A.H., et al.: Low-density lipoprotein and atherosclerosis. *JAMA*, 272:305, 1994.

Snyder, A.C.: Overtraining and glycogen depletion hypothesis. *Med. Sci. Sports Exerc.*, 30:1146, 1998.

Stefanick, M.I., et al.: Effects of diet and exercise in men and postmenopausal women with low levels of HDL cholesterol and high levels of LDL cholesterol. *N. Engl. J. Med.*, 339:12, 1998.

Tarnopolsky, M.A.: Protein, caffeine, and sports. *Phys. Sportsmed.*, 21:137, 1993.

Wagenmakers, A.J.M.: Muscle amino acid metabolism at rest and during exercise: Role in human physiology and metabolism. *Exerc. Sport Sci Rev.*, 26:287, 1998.

Wolk, A., et al.: Long-term intake of dietary fiber and decreased risk of coronary heart disease among women. *JAMA*, 281:1998, 1999.

CHAPTER

3

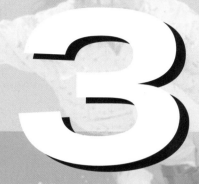

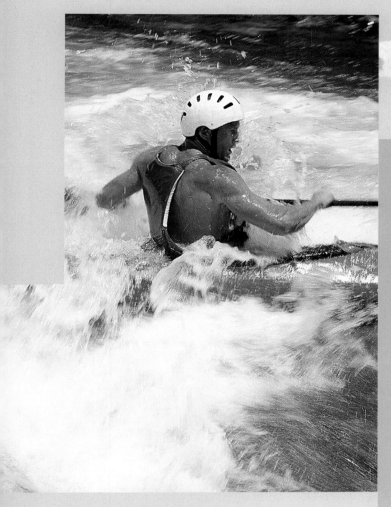

Topics covered in this chapter

PART 1 Micronutrients

Vitamins
Vitamin Supplements: The Competitive Edge?
Minerals
Minerals and Exercise Performance
Summary

PART 2 Water

Water in the Body
Water Requirements in Exercise
Summary
Thought Questions
Selected References

Micronutrients and Water

- List one function for each fat- and water-soluble vitamin, and explain the potential risks of consuming these micronutrients in excess.

- Outline three broad roles of minerals in the body.

- Define osteoporosis, exercise-induced anemia, and sodium-induced hypertension.

- Describe how regular physical activity affects bone mass and the body's iron stores.

- Outline factors related to the female athlete triad.

- List the functions of water in the body.

- Define heat cramps, heat exhaustion, and heat stroke.

- Explain factors that affect gastric emptying and fluid replacement.

Effective regulation of all metabolic processes requires a delicate blending of food nutrients in the cell's watery medium. **Micronutrients** have special significance in the metabolic mixture—they consist of the small quantities of vitamins and minerals that facilitate energy transfer and optimize normal growth and development. Consuming well-balanced meals ensures adequate nutrient intake, thus obviating the need to consume vitamin and mineral supplements. With proper food intake, vitamin and mineral supplements offer little or no physiologic benefits and could be characterized as economically wasteful. Unfortunately, consuming micronutrients in excess can also pose significant dangers to health and well-being.

Vitamins

The Nature of Vitamins

The formal discovery of vitamins showed that the body required these essential organic substances in minute amounts to perform highly specific metabolic functions. A person requires only about 350 g (12 oz) of vitamins from about 820 kg (1820 lb) of food consumed annually. Vitamins, often considered accessory nutrients, do not supply energy, are not basic building units for other compounds, and do not contribute substantially to the body's mass. Nonetheless, a prolonged inadequate intake of a particular vitamin can trigger symptoms of vitamin deficiency and lead to severe medical complications. For example, symptoms of thiamin deficiency occur after only 2 weeks on a thiamin-free diet, and after 3 or 4 weeks, symptoms of vitamin C deficiency appear. At the other extreme, consuming some fat-soluble vitamins in excess can produce a toxic overdose manifested by hair loss, irregularities in bone formation, fetal malformation, hemorrhage, bone fractures, abnormal liver function, and ultimately death.

Classification of Vitamins

Thirteen different vitamins have been isolated, analyzed, classified, and synthesized, and recommended dietary allowance (RDA) levels established. Vitamins are classified as either fat-soluble or water-soluble. Vitamins A, D, E, and K represent the **fat-soluble vitamins**; the **water-soluble vitamins** include vitamin C and the B-complex vitamins: vitamin B_6 (pyridoxine), thiamine (B_1), riboflavin (B_2), niacin (nicotinic acid), pantothenic acid, biotin, folic acid, and cobalamin (B_{12}).

No difference exists between a vitamin obtained naturally from food and a vitamin produced synthetically. Manufacturers gain huge profits in advertising vitamins as "natural" or "organically isolated," yet such vitamins are chemically identical to those synthesized in the laboratory.

Fat-Soluble Vitamins

Fat-soluble vitamins dissolve and store in the body's fatty tissues; thus, they do not require daily intake. In fact, symptoms of a fat-soluble vitamin insufficiency may not appear for years. Dietary lipid provides the source of fat-soluble vitamins, which travel to the liver for storage or dispersion to various body tissues. The liver stores vitamins A, D, and K, whereas vitamin E distributes throughout the body's fatty tissues. Prolonged intake of a "fat-free" diet accelerates a fat-soluble vitamin insufficiency. Table 3.1 lists the RDA, food sources, major bodily functions, and symptoms that result from either an excess or deficiency of fat-soluble vitamins.

Water-Soluble Vitamins

Vitamin C (ascorbic acid) and the B-complex group make up the nine water-soluble vitamins. They act largely as

Provitamin

Some vitamins in food remain in an inactive or precursor form. In the body, the **provitamins** change to the vitamin's active form. The total potential vitamin activity available from its vitamins and precursor provitamins most accurately express a specific food vitamin content.

coenzymes—small molecules that combine with a larger protein compound (apoenzyme) to form an active enzyme that accelerates the interconversion of chemical compounds. Coenzymes participate directly in chemical reactions; when the reaction runs its course, coenzymes remain intact and participate in further reactions. Water-soluble vitamins play an essential role as part of coenzymes in the cells' energy-generating reactions.

TABLE 3.1
Recommended dietary intake, food sources, major bodily functions, and symptoms of deficiency or excess of the fat-soluble vitamins for healthy adults (age 19–50)*

VITAMIN	RDA (mg) ♂	♀	DIETARY SOURCES	MAJOR BODY FUNCTIONS	DEFICIENCY	EXCESS
Vitmain A (retinol)	1.0	0.8	Provitamin A (beta-carotene) widely distributed in green vegetables. Retinol present in milk, butter, cheese, fortified margarine	Constituent of rhodopsin (visual pigment) Maintenance of epithelial tissues. Role in mucopoly-saccharide synthesis	Xerophthalmia (keratinization of ocular tissue), night blindness, permanent blindness	Headache, vomiting, peeling of skin, anorexia, swelling of long bones
Vitamin D	0.01†	0.01	Cod-liver oil, eggs, dairy products, fortified milk, and margarine	Promotes growth and mineralization of bones. Increases absorption of calcium	Rickets (bone deformities) in children. Osteomalacia in adults	Vomiting, diarrhea, weight loss, kidney damage
Vitamin E (tocopherol)	10.0	8.0	Seeds, green leafy vegetables, margarines, shortenings	Functions as an antioxidant to prevent cell damage	Possibly anemia	Relatively nontoxic
Vitamin K (phylloquinone)	0.08	0.06	Green leafy vegetables. Small amount in cereals, fruits, and meats	Important in blood clotting (helps form active prothrombin)	Conditioned deficiencies associated with severe bleeding; internal hemorrhages	Relatively nontoxic Synthetic forms at high doses may cause jaundice

*Recommended Dietary Allowances. Revised 1989. Food & Nutrition Board, National Academy of Sciences-National Research Council, Washington, D.C.

† 0.005 mg for adults 25 and older.

Because of their solubility in water, water-soluble vitamins disperse in the body fluids without appreciable storage. An excess of water-soluble vitamins is voided in the urine. If the diet regularly contains less than 50% of the recommended values for water-soluble vitamins, marginal deficiencies may develop within 4 weeks. Table 3.2 summarizes the RDA, food sources, major bodily functions, and symptoms resulting from both excess and deficiency of water-soluble vitamins.

Potential Toxicity of Vitamins

Once enzyme systems catalyzed by specific vitamins saturate, excess vitamins function as potentially harmful chemicals. A higher probability exists for overdosing with fat-soluble than water-soluble vitamins. Prolonged excessive intake of vitamins of either type can produce toxic effects, possibly leading to a fatal outcome.

Fat-soluble vitamins should not be consumed in excess without medical supervision. Adverse reactions from excessive fat-soluble vitamin intake occur at a lower multiple of the RDA than water-soluble vitamins. Women who consume excess vitamin A (as retinol but not in provitamin carotene form) early in pregnancy significantly increase risk of birth defects. Excessive vitamin A accumulation (called **hypervitaminosis A**) causes irritability, swelling of bones, weight loss, and dry itchy skin in young children. In adults, symptoms can include nausea, headache, drowsiness, loss of hair, diarrhea, and bone brittleness caused by calcium loss. Discontinuance of excessive vitamin A reverses these symptoms. Kidney damage can result from a regular excess of vitamin D. Although "overdoses" from vitamins E and K rarely occur, intakes above the recommended level provide no health or fitness benefits.

Vitamins' Role in the Body

Vitamins contain no useful energy for the body; instead, they link and regulate the sequence of metabolic reactions that release energy within food molecules. They also play an intimate role in tissue synthesis and many other biologic processes. Figure 3.1 summarizes the important biologic functions of vitamins.

Figure 3.2 illustrates the diverse routes of the macronutrients in metabolism, and the role of the water-soluble vitamins in these metabolic pathways. A vitamin participates repeatedly in metabolic reactions regardless of physical activity level; thus, the vitamin needs of athletes do not exceed those of sedentary counterparts.

Well-balanced meals provide an adequate quantity of all vitamins regardless of age and physical activity level. Individuals who expend considerable energy exercising do not need to consume special foods or supplements that increase the vitamin content above the RDA. Also, at high levels of daily physical activity, food intake usually increases to sustain the added energy requirements of exercise. Additional food consumed through a variety of nutritious meals proportionately increases vitamin and mineral intakes. This general rule has several possible exceptions. First, vitamin C and folic acid exist in foods that usually comprise only a small part of most American's total caloric intake; the availability of these foods also varies by season. Second, some athletic groups consume relatively low amounts of vitamins B_1 and B_6. If the daily diet supplies fresh fruit, grains, and uncooked or steamed vegetables, an adequate intake of these two vitamins occurs. Individuals on meatless diets should con-

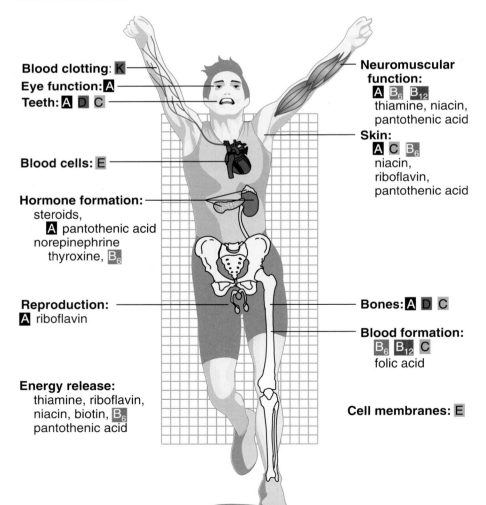

Figure 3.1
Biologic functions of vitamins.

TABLE 3.2
Recommended dietary intake, food sources, major bodily functions, and symptoms of deficiency or excess of the water-soluble vitamins for healthy adults (age 19–50)*

VITAMIN	RDA (mg) ♂	RDA (mg) ♀	DIETARY SOURCES	MAJOR BODY FUNCTIONS	DEFICIENCY	EXCESS
Vitamin B$_1$ (thiamin)	1.5	1.1	Pork, organ meats, whole grains, legumes	Coenzyme (thiamin prophosphate) in reactions involving removal of carbon dioxide	Beriberi (peripheral nerve changes, edema, heart failure)	None reported
Vitamin B$_2$	1.7	1.3	Widely distributed in foods	Constituent of two flavin nucleotide coenzymes involved in energy metabolism (FAD and FMN)	Reddened lips, cracks at mouth corner (cheilosis), eye lesions	None reported
Niacin	19	15	Liver, lean meats, grains, legumes (can be formed from tryptophan)	Constituent of two coenzymes in oxidation-reduction reactions (NAD$^+$ and NADP)	Pellagra (skin and gastrointestinal lesions, nervous, mental disorders)	Flushing, burning and tingling around neck, face, and hands
Vitamin B$_6$ (pyridoxine)	2.0	1.6	Meats, vegetables, whole-grain cereals	Coenzyme (pyridoxal phosphate) involved in amino acid and glycogen metabolism	Irritability, convulsions, muscular twitching, dermatitis, kidney stones	None reported
Pantothenic acid	4–7‡	4–7‡	Widely distributed in foods	Constituent of coenzyme A, which plays a central role in energy metabolism	Fatigue, sleep disturbances, impaired coordination, nausea	None reported
Folic acid	0.2	0.2	Legumes, green vegetables, whole-wheat products	Coenzyme (reduced form) involved in transfer of single-carbon units in nucleic acid and amino acid metabolism	Anemia, gastrointestinal disturbances, diarrhea, red tongue	None reported
Vitamin B$_{12}$	0.002	0.002	Muscle meats, eggs, dairy products, (absent in plant foods)	Coenzyme involved in transfer of single-carbon units in nucleic acid metabolism	Pernicious anemia, neurologic disorders	None reported
Biotin	0.03	0.10	Legumes, vegetables, meats	Coenzymes required for fat synthesis, amino acid metabolism, and glycogen (animal starch) formation	Fatigue, depression, nausea, dermatitis, muscular pains	None reported
Vitamin C (ascorbic acid)	60†	60	Citrus fruits, tomatoes, green peppers, salad greens	Maintains intercellular matrix of cartilage, bone, and dentine. Important in collagen synthesis	Scurvy (degeneration of skin, teeth, blood vessels, epithelial hemorrhages)	Relatively nontoxic. Possibility of kidney stones

*Recommended Dietary Allowances. Revised 1989. Food & Nutrition Board, National Academy of Sciences-National Research Council, Washington, D.C.

† 100 mg for adults who smoke.

‡ Because there is less information on which to base allowances, these figures are given in the form of ranges.

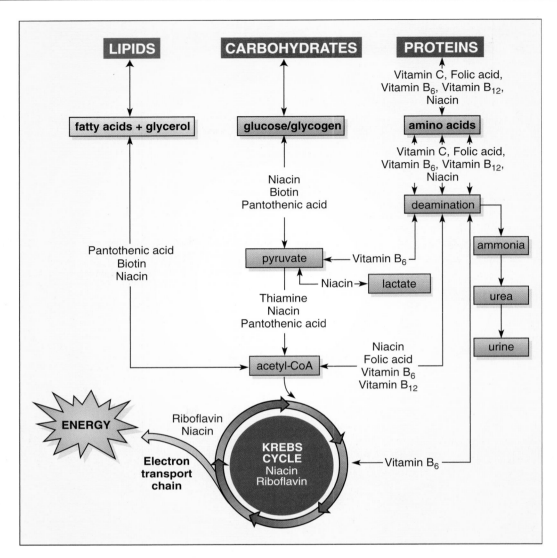

Figure 3.2
Role of water-soluble vitamins in carbohydrate, lipid, and protein metabolism.

sume a small amount of milk, milk products, or eggs because vitamin B_{12} exists only in foods of animal origin.

Antioxidant Role of Specific Vitamins

Most of the oxygen consumed in the mitochondria during energy metabolism combines with hydrogen to produce water. Normally about 2 to 5% of oxygen forms oxygen-containing free radicals like superoxide (O_2^-), hydrogen peroxide (H_2O_2), and hydroxyl (OH^-) radicals due to electron "leakage" along the electron transport chain (see Chapter 4). A **free radical** represents a highly chemically reactive molecule or molecular fragment with at least one unpaired electron in its outer orbital or valence shell. These are the same free radicals produced by heat and ionizing radiation, and carried in cigarette smoke, environmental pollutants, and even some medications.

A buildup of free radicals increases the potential for cellular damage (**oxidative stress**) to many biologically

important substances. Oxygen radicals exhibit strong affinity for the polyunsaturated fatty acids in the cell membrane's lipid bilayer. During unchecked oxidative stress, deterioration occurs in the plasma membrane's fatty acids. Membrane damage occurs through a chain-reaction series of events termed **lipid peroxidation**. These reactions, which incorporate oxygen into lipids, increase the vulnerability of the cell and its constituents. Free radicals also facilitate low density lipoprotein cholesterol oxidation, thus accelerating atherosclerosis. Oxidative stress ultimately increases the likelihood of cellular deterioration associated with advanced aging, cancer, diabetes, coronary artery disease, and a general decline in central nervous system and immune function.

Although currently nothing exists to stop oxygen reduction and free radical production, an elaborate natural defense against its damaging effects exists within the cell and extracellular space. This defense includes diverse antioxi-

c l o s e u p

Exercise, Free Radicals, and Antioxidants

The beneficial effects of physical activity are well known, but the possibility for negative effects has only recently been addressed. Potentially negative effects may occur because elevated aerobic metabolism in exercise increases the production of free radicals. Free-radical production and tissue damage cannot be directly measured in humans, but rather inferred via markers of free radical byproducts. Increased free radicals could possibly overwhelm the body's natural defenses and pose a health risk due to an increased level of oxidative stress. The opposing position maintains that while free radical production increases during exercise, the body's normal antioxidant defenses remain adequate, or concomitantly improve as natural enzymatic defenses become "upregulated" through both endurance and sprint training adaptations. This latter position is supported by research that shows the beneficial effects of regular exercise on the incidence of various forms of cancer and heart disease.

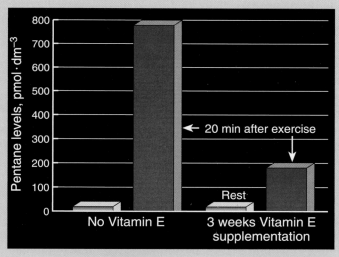

Pentane levels before and after 20-minutes of exercise at 100% VO_{2max} with and without vitamin E supplementation. Adapted from Pincemail, J., et al.: Pentane measurement in man as an index of lipoperoxidation. *Bioelectronchem. Bioenerg.*, 18:117, 1987.

Increased Metabolism and Free Radical Production. Exercise produces reactive oxygen or free radicals in at least two ways. The first occurs via an electron leak in the mitochondria, probably at the cytochrome level, which produces superoxide radicals. The second occurs during alterations in blood flow and oxygen supply—underperfusion during intense exercise followed by reperfusion in recovery, which triggers excessive free radical generation. Some argue that the potential for free radical damage may also increase during trauma, stress, muscle damage, and from environmental pollutants including smog. With exercise, the risk depends on intensity and training state because exhaustive exercise by the untrained more likely produces oxidative damage in the active muscles. The questions that arise include: 1) are physically active individuals more prone to free-radical damage, and 2) are protective agents with antioxidant properties required in increased quantities in the diets of the physically active?

In answer to the first question, research suggests that the body's natural defenses for well-nourished humans remain adequate in response to increased physical activity. Although a single bout of submaximal exercise increased oxidant production, the natural antioxidant defenses coped effectively. Even when repeating multiple bouts of exercise on consecutive days, various indices of oxidative stress did not reveal any depletion of the body's antioxidant system.

The second question provides an equivocal answer concerning the wisdom of antioxidant vitamin–mineral supplementation for active people. Some evidence with humans suggests a possible benefit from vitamin E (and possibly vitamin C) supplementation. The inset shows the effects on pentane (a primary marker of free radical production) elimination with 3 weeks of daily 200-mg vitamin E supplement on men before and after a 20-minute maximal exercise bout. Post-exercise free radical production decreased dramatically in the vitamin E-supplemented trials. For humans fed a daily antioxidant vitamin mixture of β-carotene, ascorbic acid, and vitamin E, serum and breath markers of lipid peroxidation remained lower at rest and after exercise than in subjects not receiving supplements. Five months of vitamin E supplementation in racing cyclists had a protective effect on markers of oxidative stress induced by extreme endurance exercise. *Available research suggests that if supplementation does confer benefits, then vitamin E may be the most potent antioxidant related to exercise.*

dant scavenger enzymes and metal-binding proteins. Three major antioxidant enzymes include superoxide dismutase, catalase, and glutathione peroxidase. The nutritive-reducing agents vitamins A, C, and E, and the vitamin A-precursor β–carotene also serve important protective functions. These antioxidant vitamins protect the plasma membrane by reacting with and removing free radicals, thus squelching the chain reaction. Maintaining a diet with ample antioxidant vitamins may reduce the risk of several types of cancers; a normal to above normal intake of vitamin E (in both alpha-tocopherol and gamma-tocopherol forms) and β–carotene and/or high serum levels of carotenoids may blunt the narrowing of the coronary arteries and reduce heart attack and stroke risk in men and women. The *Close up* for this chapter discusses the interaction between exercise, free radicals, and antioxidants.

We recommend consuming a well-balanced diet (recommendations of the Food Guide Pyramid, see Chapter 9) that includes fruits, grains, and vegetables. The following provide rich dietary sources of antioxidant vitamins:

- β-carotene (best known of the pigmented compounds, or carotenoids, that give color to yellow, orange, and green, leafy vegetables and fruits): carrots, dark-green leafy vegetables like spinach, broccoli, turnips, beet and collard greens; sweet potatoes; winter squash; apricots, cantaloupe, mangos, papaya
- Vitamin C: citrus fruits and juices; cabbage, broccoli, turnip greens; cantaloupe; green and red sweet peppers, berries
- Vitamin E: poultry, seafood, vegetable oils, wheat germ, fish liver oils, whole-grain breads and fortified cereals, nuts and seeds, dried beans, green leafy vegetables, and eggs

Vitamin Supplements: The Competitive Edge?

The B-complex vitamins serve as coenzymes in energy-yielding reactions during carbohydrate, fat, and protein breakdown (Fig. 3.2). They also contribute to hemoglobin synthesis and red blood cell formation. But does increasing the intake of B-complex vitamins "supercharge" energy release and improve physical performance? Over 40 years of research does *not* support using vitamin supplements to improve exercise performance or ability to train arduously in nutritionally adequate healthy people. The belief that "if a little is good, more will be better" has led many coaches, athletes, and fitness enthusiasts to advocate the use of vitamin supplements above recommended levels.

All Supplementation in Moderation

British researchers have reported that a vitamin C supplement of 500 mg daily for 6 weeks produced a pro-oxidant effect in addition to the expected antioxidant effect on DNA. The excess vitamin C promoted genetic damage by free radicals to the adenine base of DNA, not previously measured in studies of vitamin C's oxidative properties. Vitamin C in natural form in foods like orange juice does not act as a pro-oxidant.

When vitamin intake reaches recommended levels, supplements do not improve exercise performance or necessarily increase the blood levels of these micronutrients. Facts become clouded by "testimonials" from coaches and elite athletes who attribute their successes to a particular dietary modification, which usually includes specific vitamin supplements. "Buyer beware"—using testimonials to create the impression that a product "really is" effective represents pseudo-science at best and intellectual dishonesty at worst.

Megavitamins

Although physically active individuals who eat a well-balanced diet do not need to take additional vitamins, most nutritionists believe that taking a multivitamin capsule that contains the recommended allowance of each vitamin does little harm. For some people, the psychological effects may even be beneficial. However, some athletes "supercharge" with **megavitamins**, or doses of at least tenfold and up to 1000 times the RDA to improve exercise performance. This practice is potentially harmful, except in cases of a specific vitamin deficiency.

Vitamins Behave as Chemicals

Any significant excess of vitamins functions as chemicals (drugs) in the body. For example, a megadose of water-soluble vitamin C increases serum uric acid levels that precipitate gout in people predisposed to this disease. At intakes greater than 1000 mg daily, urinary excretion of oxalate (a breakdown product of vitamin C) increases, accelerating kidney stone formation in susceptible individuals. In iron-deficient individuals, megadoses of vitamin C may destroy significant amounts of vitamin B_{12}. In healthy people, vitamin C supplements frequently irritate the bowel and cause diarrhea.

Excess vitamin B_6 may induce liver and nerve damage. Excessive riboflavin (B_2) intake can impair vision, whereas a megadose of nicotinic acid (niacin) can act as a potent vasodilator and inhibit fatty acid mobilization during exercise. This could more rapidly deplete muscle glycogen. Folic acid concentrated in supplement form can trigger an allergic response producing hives, light-headedness, and breathing difficulties. Megadoses of vitamin A can induce toxicity to the nervous system, and kidney damage can result from excess vitamin D intake.

Data from the latest surveys provide troubling information; more than 30% of American adults use vitamin and/or mineral supplements, often at potentially toxic dosages. If vitamin supplementation does offer benefits to physically active individuals, the benefits may only apply to those with marginal vitamin stores. Perhaps the misuse and abuse of vitamins by individuals hoping to improve athletic performance can be put in proper perspective by the following quotation from nearly 20 years ago: "The sale of vitamins is probably the biggest rip-off in our society today. Their only effect would appear to be a highly enriched sewage around athletic training or competition sites."

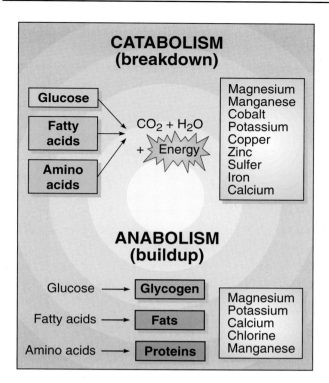

Figure 3.3
Minerals contribute to macronutrient catabolism (breakdown) and anabolism (build-up).

Minerals

The Nature of Minerals

Approximately 4% of the body's mass consists of 22 mostly metallic elements collectively called **minerals**. Minerals serve as constituents of enzymes, hormones, and vitamins; they combine with other chemicals (e.g., calcium phosphate in bone, iron in the heme of hemoglobin) or exist singularly (e.g., free calcium in body fluids). In the body, minerals are classified as **trace minerals** (those requiring less than 100 mg a day), and **major minerals** (those required in amounts greater than 100 mg a day). Excess minerals serve no useful physiologic purpose and can produce toxic effects.

Kinds, Sources, and Functions of Minerals

Most minerals, major or trace, occur freely in nature—mainly in the waters of rivers, lakes, and oceans, in topsoil, and beneath the earth's surface. Minerals exist in the root systems of plants and in the body structure of animals who consume plants and water containing minerals. Table 3.3 lists the important minerals and their functions, food sources, and daily requirements.

Whereas vitamins activate chemical processes without becoming part of the byproducts of the reactions they catalyze, minerals often become part of the body's structures and existing chemicals. Minerals serve three broad roles:

1. They provide *structure* in forming bones and teeth.
2. In terms of *function*, they help maintain normal heart rhythm, muscle contractility, neural conductivity, and acid-base balance.
3. They help *regulate* cellular metabolism by becoming part of enzymes and hormones that modulate cellular activity.

Figure 3.3 lists minerals that participate in catabolic and anabolic cellular processes. Minerals activate numerous reactions that release energy during carbohydrate, fat, and protein catabolism. In addition, minerals help to synthesize biologic nutrients—glycogen from glucose, triglycerides from fatty acids and glycerol, and proteins from amino acids. Without the essential minerals, the fine balance would be disrupted between catabolism and anabolism. Minerals also form important constituents of hormones. An inadequate thyroxine production due to iodine deficiency, for example, significantly slows the body's resting metabolism. In extreme cases, this could predispose a person to develop obesity. The synthesis of insulin, the hormone that facilitates glucose uptake by cells, requires zinc (as do approximately 100 enzymes), whereas the mineral chlorine forms the digestive acid hydrochloric acid.

Minerals and Physical Activity

The minerals required by the body can be obtained readily from food sources in a well-balanced diet. In the next sections, we describe specific functions for important minerals related to physical activity.

Calcium

Calcium, the most abundant mineral in the body, combines with phosphorus to form bones and teeth. These two minerals represent about 75% of the body's total mineral content of about 2.5% of body mass. In ionized form (about 1% of the body's 1200 mg of calcium), calcium plays an important role in muscle action, blood clotting, nerve impulse transmission, activation of several enzymes,

Major Minerals	Trace Minerals
Sodium	Iron
Potassium	Zinc
Calcium	Copper
Phosphorus	Selenium
Magnesium	Iodine
Sulfur	Fluorine
Chlorine	Chromium

Researchers are studying how boron, nickel, vanadium, arsenic, cobalt, lithium, silicon, tin, and cadmium affect body functions.

TABLE 3.3

Important major and trace minerals for healthy adults (ages 19–50) and their dietary requirements, food sources, functions, and effects of deficiencies and excesses*

MINERAL	RDA FOR ♂ AND ♀ (mg)†	DIETARY SOURCES	MAJOR BODY FUNCTIONS	DEFICIENCY	EXCESS
Major					
Calcium	1200‡ 1200	Milk, cheese, dark green vegetables, dried legumes	Bone and tooth formation Blood clotting Nerve transmission	Stunted growth Rickets, osteoporosis Convulsions	Not reported in humans
Phosphorus	1200‡ 1200	Milk, cheese, yogurt, meat, poultry, grains, fish	Bone and tooth formation Acid-base balance	Weakness, demineralization of bone Loss of calcium	Erosion of jaw (phossy jaw)
Potassium	2000	Leafy vegetables, cantelope, lima beans, potatoes, bananas, milk, meats, coffee, tea	Fluid balance Nerve transmission Acid-base balance	Muscle cramps Irregular cardiac rhythm Mental confusion Loss of appetite Can be life-threatening	None if kidneys function normally Poor kidney function causes potassium buildup and cardiac arrhythmias
Sulfur	Unknown	Obtained as part of dietary protein, and present in food preservatives	Acid-base balance Liver function	Unlikely to occur with adequate dietary intake	Unknown
Sodium	1100–3300	Common salt	Acid-based balance Body water balance Nerve function	Muscle cramps Mental apathy Reduced appetite	High blood pressure
Chlorine (chloride)	700	Part of salt-containing food. Some vegetables and fruits	Important part of extracellular fluids	Unlikely to occur with adequate dietary intake	With sodium, contributes to high blood pressure
Magnesium	350 280	Whole grains, green leafy vegetables	Activates enzymes in protein synthesis	Growth failure Behavioral disturbances Weakness, spasms	Diarrhea
Trace					
Iron	10 15	Eggs, lean meats, legumes, whole grains, green leafy vegetables	Constituent of hemoglobin and enzymes involved in energy metabolism	Iron deficiency anemia (weakness, reduced resistance to infection)	Siderosis Cirrhosis of liver
Fluorine	1.5–4.0	Drinking water, tea, seafood	May be important to maintain bone structure	Higher frequency of tooth decay	Mottling of teeth, increased bone density Neurologic disturbances
Zinc	15 12	Widely distributed in foods	Constituent of digestive enzymes	Growth failure Small sex glands	Fever, nausea, vomiting, diarrhea
Copper	1.5–3.0§ 1.5–3.0	Meats, drinking water	Constituent of enzymes associated with iron metabolism	Anemia, bone changes (rare in humans)	Rare metabolic condition (Wilson's disease)
Selenium	0.070 0.055	Seafood, meat, grains	Functions in close association with vitamin E	Anemia (rare)	Gastrointestinal disorders, lung irritation
Iodine (Iodide)	150	Marine fish and shellfish, dairy products, vegetables, iodized salt	Constituent of thyroid hormones	Goiter (enlarged thyroid)	Very high intakes depress thyroid activity
Chromium	0.075–0.25§ 0.05–0.25§	Legumes, cereals, organ meats, fats, vegetable oils, meats, whole grains	Constituent of some enzymes Involved in glucose and energy metabolism	Not reported in humans Impaired glucose metabolism	Inhibition of enzymes Occupational exposures: skin and kidney damage

*Recommended Dietary Allowances. Revised 1989. Food & Nutrition Board, National Academy of Sciences-National Research Council, Washington, D.C.

† First values are for males

‡ 800 mg for adults 25 and older

§ Beause there is less information on which to base allowances, these figures are given in the form of ranges.

synthesis of calciferol (active form of vitamin D), and fluid transport across cell membranes.

Osteoporosis: Calcium, Estrogen, and Exercise. The skeleton contains more than 99% of the body's total calcium. With calcium deficiency, the body draws on its calcium reserves in bone to replace the deficit. With prolonged imbalance, **osteoporosis** (literally meaning "porous bones") eventually develops as the bones lose their calcium mass (mineral content) and calcium concentration (mineral density) and progressively become porous and brittle. Osteoporosis afflicts 25 to 30 million Americans, of whom approximately 90% are women; shockingly, 50% of all women eventually develop osteoporosis. Men are not immune from osteoporosis; 1.5 to 2.0 million men in the United States have this disease. Among women older than age 60, this disease has reached near-epidemic proportions. Osteoporosis accounts for more than 1.5 million fractures yearly, including 700,000 spinal fractures, 250,000 wrist fractures, and more than 300,000 hip fractures and 300,000 fractures at other sites. In women, increased susceptibility relates to decreased estrogen production that accompanies menopause. Estrogen enhances calcium absorption and limits its resorption (withdrawal) from bone.

Dietary Calcium Crucial. As a general guideline, adolescents and young adults require 1200 mg of calcium daily (800 to 1000 mg for adults older than age 24) or about as much calcium in five 8-oz glasses of milk. Although growing children require more calcium per unit body mass on a daily basis than adults, many adults remain deficient in calcium intake. *Unfortunately, calcium remains one of the most frequently lacking nutrients in the diet for both non-athlete and athlete.* For an average adult, daily calcium intake ranges between 500 and 700 mg. More than 75% of adults consume less than the calcium RDA, and about 25% of females in the United States consume less than 300 mg of calcium daily. Many experts recommend a further increase to between 1200 and 1500 mg for estrogen-deprived women after menopause to ensure a positive calcium balance during this period. Among athletes, female dancers, gymnasts, and endurance competitors are most prone to calcium dietary insufficiency.

Exercise Helps. *Regular exercise slows the rate of skeletal aging.* Regardless of age or gender, young children and adults who maintain physically active lifestyles have significantly greater bone mass compared with sedentary counterparts. For men and women who remain physically active, even at ages 70 and 80 years, their bone mass exceeds that of inactive individuals of similar age. The decline in vigorous exercise with advancing age closely parallels the age-related loss of bone mass.

Exercise of moderate intensity provides a safe and potent stimulus to maintain and even increase bone mass. **Weight-bearing exercise** represents a particularly desirable form of exercise; examples include walking, running, dancing, rope

Regular Exercise and Increased Muscle Strength Slow Skeletal Aging

Moderate-to high-intensity aerobic exercise (walking, jogging, aerobic dancing, stair climbing) performed 3 days a week for 50 to 60 minutes each workout builds bone and retards its rate of loss. Muscle-strengthening exercises also benefit bone mass. Individuals with greater back strength, and those who train regularly with resistance exercise, have a greater spinal bone mineral content than weaker and untrained individuals.

skipping. Resistance-training, which generates significant muscular force against the long bones of the body, also proves beneficial. The benefits of exercise depend on adequate calcium availability for the bone-forming process.

Female Athlete Triad: An Unexpected Problem for Women Who Train Intensely

An apparent paradox exists between exercise and bone dynamics for athletic, premenopausal women. Women who train intensely and emphasize weight loss often engage in **disordered eating behaviors**—a serious ailment that in the extreme causes diverse and life-threatening complications (see *How to Recognize Warning Signs of Disordered Eating*). Disordered eating decreases energy availability, reducing body mass and body fat to a point at which the menstrual cycle becomes irregular (**oligomenorrhea**) or actually ceases, a condition termed **secondary amenorrhea**. The tightly integrated continuum that begins with disordered eating and resultant energy drain, amenorrhea, and eventual osteoporosis, reflects the clinical entity labeled the **female athlete triad** (Fig. 3.4).

Many girls and young women engaged in sports have at least one of the triad's disorders, particularly disordered eating behavior. Female athletes of the 1970 and 1980 era believed the loss of normal menstruation reflected hard training and the inevitable consequence of athletic success. The prevalence of amenorrhea among female athletes in weight-related sports (distance running, gymnastics, ballet, cheerleading, figure skating, body building) probably ranges between 25 and 65%, whereas no more than 5% of the general population experience this condition.

Sodium, Potassium, and Chlorine

The minerals sodium, potassium, and chlorine, collectively termed **electrolytes,** dissolve in the body as electrically charged particles called **ions.** Sodium and chlorine represent the chief minerals contained in blood plasma and extracellular fluid. Electrolytes modulate fluid exchange within the body's various fluid compartments, al-

Five Principles to Promote Bone Health

1. **Specificity:** exercise provides a local osteogenic effect.
2. **Overload:** progressively increasing exercise intensity promotes continued improvement.
3. **Initial Values:** individuals with the smallest total bone mass have the greatest potential for improvement.
4. **Diminishing Returns:** as one approaches the biologic ceiling for bone density, further gains require greater effort.
5. **Reversibility:** discontinuing exercise overload reverses the positive osteogenic effects of exercise.

lowing for a constant, well-regulated exchange of nutrients and waste products between the cell and its external fluid environment. Potassium represents the chief intracellular mineral.

Establishing proper electrical gradients across cell membranes represents the most important function for sodium and potassium ions. A difference in electrical balance between the cell's interior and exterior allows nerve impulse transmission, muscle stimulation and contraction, and proper gland functioning. Electrolytes also maintain plasma membrane permeability and regulate the acid and base qualities of body fluids, particularly blood.

Sodium: How Much Is Enough? The wide distribution of sodium in foods makes it easy to obtain the daily requirement without adding salt to foods. In the United States, sodium intake regularly exceeds the daily level recommended for adults of between 1100 and 3300 mg, or the amount of sodium in 0.5 to 1.5 teaspoons of table salt (sodium makes up about 40% of salt.) The typical Western diet contains about 4500 mg of sodium (8 to 12 g of salt) each day. This represents 10 times the 500 mg of sodium the body actually needs. The heavy reliance on table salt in processing, curing, cooking, seasoning, and preserving common foods accounts for the large sodium intake. Aside from table salt, common sodium-rich dietary sources include monosodium glutamate (MSG), soy sauce, condiments, canned foods, baking soda, and baking powder.

Non-Pharmacologic, Behavioral Approach to Treating Athletic Amenorrhea

- Reduce training level by 10 to 20%
- Gradually increase total energy intake
- Increase body weight by 2 to 3%
- Maintain daily calcium intake at 1500 mg

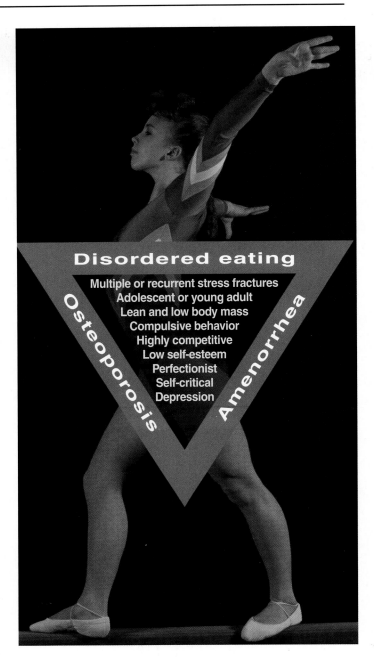

Figure 3.4
Female athlete triad: disordered eating, amenorrhea, and osteoporosis.

A normal sodium balance in the body usually occurs throughout a range of dietary intakes. For some individuals, excessive sodium intake becomes inadequately regulated. A chronic excess of dietary sodium can increase fluid volume and possibly increase peripheral vascular resistance; both factors could elevate blood pressure to levels that pose a health risk. **Sodium-induced hypertension** occurs in about one-third of hypertensive individuals in the United States.

For decades, one low-risk, first-line of defense in treating high blood pressure eliminated excess sodium from the

How to Recognize Warning Signs of Disordered Eating

Disordered eating refers to a broad spectrum of complex behaviors, core attitudes, coping strategies, and conditions that share the commonality of an emotionally based, inordinate, and often pathological focus on body shape and weight.

The athlete faces a unique set of circumstances that exacerbates the problem. Disordered eating behaviors flourish when negative aesthetic connotations associated with excess body fat blend with the athlete's belief that all body fat spells doom for success. The prevalence of disordered eating behaviors ranges between 15 and 60%, depending on the participant's sport. **Anorexia nervosa** and **bulimia nervosa** represent the two most common eating disorders. A third category, **binge-eating disorder**, does not include purging behavior.

Anorexia Nervosa

Anorexia nervosa, originally described in ancient writings, represents an unhealthy physical and mental state characterized by a crippling obsession with body size. A "nervous loss of appetite" reflects a preoccupation with dieting and thinness, and refusal to eat enough food to maintain a normal body weight (which falls below normal levels for age and stature). The relentless pursuit of thinness (present in about 1 to 2% of the general population) includes an intense fear of weight gain and fatness (despite a low body weight), and failure to menstruate regularly (amenorrhea). Anorectics have a distorted body image and actually perceive themselves as fat despite their emaciation.

Anorexia nervosa usually begins with a normal attempt to lose weight through dieting. With continued dieting, the individual continues to eat less until she practically consume no food. Eventually, food restriction becomes an obsession; the anorexic patient is not satisfied despite weight loss. As weight loss continues, the person denies the accompanying extreme emaciation. In some patients, the intense hunger that accompanies near-total food deprivation cannot be continually ignored, causing episodes of binging and subsequent purging.

Warning Signs of Anorexia Nervosa
- Preoccupation with being too fat despite maintaining a normal body weight
- Loss of menstrual cycle (amenorrhea)
- Frequent comments about body weight or shape
- Significant body weight loss
- Body weight too low for athletic performance
- Ritualistic concern and preoccupation with dieting, counting calories, cooking, and eating meals
- Excessive concern about body weight, size, and shape, even after weight loss

- Feeling of helplessness in the presence of food
- Severe mood shifts
- Guilt about eating
- Compulsive need for continuous, vigorous physical activity that exceeds training requirements for a specific sport
- Maintaining a skinny look (body weight less than 85% of expected weight)
- Preference to eat in isolation
- Refusal to eat to gain weight
- Disguise of thin-looking appearance with baggy clothes
- Episodes of binging and purging

Bulimia Nervosa

The term bulimia, literally meaning "ox hunger," refers to "gorging" or "insatiable appetite." Unlike continual semistarvation seen with anorexia nervosa, binge eating characterizes bulimia nervosa. The person consumes calorically dense food—often at night and usually between 1000 to 10,000 calories within several hours—followed by fasting, self-induced vomiting, ingesting laxatives or diuretics (water pills), or compulsive exercising solely to avoid weight gain after the binge.

Warning Signs of Bulimia Nervosa
- Excessive concern about body weight, size, and composition
- Frequent gains and losses in body weight
- Visits the bathroom after meals
- Fear of not being able to stop eating
- Eating when depressed
- Compulsive dieting after binge-eating episodes
- Severe mood shifts (depression, loneliness)
- Secretive binge eating but never overeating in front of others
- Frequent criticism of one's body size and shape
- Experiencing personal or family problems with alcohol or drugs
- Irregular menstrual cycle (oligomenorrhea)

Binge-Eating Disorder

Episodes of binging without subsequent purging behavior characterize binge-eating disorder (BED). Individuals eat more rapidly than normal until they no longer can consume additional food. The level of food intake greatly exceeds the normal level determined by physical hunger. Binge eating, in private, occurs with feelings of guilt, depression, or self-disgust. The diagnosis of BED requires that the individual experiences a lack of control over eating and a marked psychological distress when binging occurs. Binge eating differs from obesity in that the same level of

continued on next page

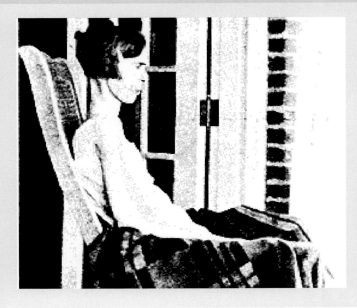

self-anger, shame, lack of control, and frustration about binge eating does not accompany obesity. Little factual information exists about the prevalence of BED.

Anorexia Athletica

The term **anorexia athletica** describes the continuum of subclinical eating behaviors of a large number of athletes who do not meet the criteria for a true eating disorder, but who exhibit at least one unhealthy method of weight control. These unhealthy methods can include fasting, vomiting (termed "instrumental vomiting" when used to make weight), and use of diet pills, laxatives, or diuretics (water pills). For many, patterns of disordered eating behaviors coincide with a specific sport season and terminate when the competitive season ends.

The first published photo of an anorexic woman in an American medical journal. *New England Journal of Medicine*, 207(5): Oct., 1932.

diet. Conventional wisdom maintains that by reducing sodium intake, perhaps the body's sodium and fluid levels become reduced, thereby lowering blood pressure. Although sodium restriction does not lower blood pressure in people with normal blood pressure (and only minimally affects those with high blood pressure), certain individuals remain "**salt sensitive**"—by reducing dietary sodium, their blood pressure decreases.

Iron

The body normally contains between 3 to 5 g (about one-sixth oz) of iron. Of this amount, approximately 80% exists in functionally active compounds, predominantly combined with hemoglobin in red blood cells. This iron-protein compound increases the oxygen-carrying capacity of blood approximately 65 times. Iron serves other important exercise-related functions besides its role in oxygen transport in blood. Iron serves as a structural component of myoglobin (about 5% of total iron), a compound similar to hemoglobin that stores oxygen for release within muscle cells. Small amounts of iron also exist in cytochromes, the specialized substances that transfer cellular energy.

Iron Stores. About 20% of the body's iron does not combine in functionally active compounds; **hemosiderin** and **ferritin** constitute the iron stores in the liver, spleen, and bone marrow. These stores replenish iron lost from the functional compounds; they also provide the iron reserve during periods of insufficient dietary iron intake. A plasma

protein, **transferrin**, transports iron from ingested food and damaged red blood cells to tissues in need. Plasma levels of transferrin often reflect the adequacy of the current iron intake.

Athletes should include normal amounts of iron-rich foods in their daily diets. People with inadequate iron intake or with limited rates of iron absorption or high rates of iron loss, often develop a reduced concentration of hemoglobin in red blood cells. This extreme condition of iron insufficiency, commonly called **iron deficiency anemia**, produces general sluggishness, loss of appetite, and reduced capacity to sustain even mild exercise. "Iron therapy" normalizes hemoglobin content of the blood and exercise capacity. Table 3.4 lists recommendations for iron intake for children and adults.

Intestinal absorption of iron varies closely with iron need, yet considerable variation in absorption (bioavailability) occurs in relation to diet composition. For example, the small intestine usually absorbs between 2 and 10% of iron from plants (**nonheme iron**), whereas iron absorption from animal sources (**heme iron**) increases to between 10 and 35%.

Of Concern to Vegetarians. *The relatively low bioavailability of nonheme iron places women on vegetarian-type diets at risk for developing iron insufficiency.* Female vegetarian runners have a poorer iron status than counterparts who consume the same quantity of iron from predominantly animal sources. Including vitamin C-rich food in the diet enhances dietary iron bioavailability. This

TABLE 3.4
Recommended dietary allowances for iron*

	AGE (y)	IRON (mg)
Children	1–10	10
Males	11–18	12
	19⁺	10
Females	11–50	15
	51⁺	10
	Pregnant	30†
	Lactating	15†

*Recommended Dietary Allowances. Revised 1989. Food & Nutrition Board, National Academy of Sciences-National Research Council, Washington, D.C.

† Generally, this increased requirement cannot be met by ordinary diets; therefore, 30 to 60 mg of supplemental iron is recommended.

occurs because ascorbic acid increases the solubility of nonheme iron making it available for absorption at the alkaline pH of the small intestine. The ascorbic acid in one glass of orange juice, for example, stimulates a threefold increase in nonheme iron absorption from a breakfast meal.

Females: A Population at Risk. Inadequate iron intake frequently occurs among young children, teenagers, and females of childbearing age, including physically active women.

Iron loss during a menstrual cycle ranges between 5 and 45 mg. This produces an additional 5-mg dietary iron requirement daily for premenopausal females, which increases the average monthly dietary iron intake need by about 150 mg. The small intestine absorbs only about 15% of ingested iron—depending on one's iron status, form of iron ingested, and composition of the meal; thus, an additional 20 to 25 mg of iron becomes available each month (from the additional 150-mg monthly dietary requirement) for synthesizing red blood cells lost during menstruation. Not surprisingly, 30 to 50% of American women experience significant dietary iron insufficiencies due to menstrual blood loss combined with a limited dietary iron intake (about 6 mg of iron per 1000 calories of food ingested).

Exercise-Induced Anemia: Fact or Fiction? Research has focused on the influence of hard training on the body's iron status, primarily due to interest in endurance sports and increased participation of women in such activities. The term "**sports anemia**" frequently describes reduced hemoglobin levels approaching **clinical anemia** (12 g per 100 mL of blood for women and 14 g per 100 mL for men) attributable to intense training. Some researchers maintain that exercise training creates an added demand for iron that often exceeds its intake. This taxes iron reserves, which eventually slows hemoglobin synthesis and/or reduces iron-containing compounds within the cell's energy transfer system. Individuals susceptible to an "iron drain" could experience reduced exercise capacity because of iron's crucial role in oxygen transport and utilization.

Heavy training could theoretically create an augmented iron demand (facilitating development of clinical anemia) from iron loss in sweat, and hemoglobin loss in urine due to red blood cell destruction with increased temperature, spleen activity and circulation rates, and from mechanical trauma (**footstrike hemolysis**) from the feet repetitively pounding the running surface. Gastrointestinal bleeding also may occur with long-distance running. Such iron loss, regardless of cause, stresses the body's iron reserves for synthesizing 260 billion new red blood cells daily in the bone marrow of the skull, upper arm, sternum, ribs, spine, pelvis, and upper legs. Iron losses pose an additional burden to women because they have the greatest iron requirement, yet lowest iron intake.

Suboptimal hemoglobin concentrations and hematocrits occur frequently among endurance athletes, thus supporting the possibility of an exercise-induced anemia. On closer scrutiny, however, transient reductions in hemoglobin concentration occur in the early phase of training and then return toward pretraining values. Figure 3.5 illustrates the response for hematologic variables for high-school female cross-country runners during a competitive season. The decrease in hemoglobin concentration with training parallels the disproportionately large expansion in plasma volume compared with total hemoglobin. For example, only 4 days of exercise training increased plasma volume by 20%, whereas the body's mass of red blood cells remained unchanged. Total hemoglobin (an important factor in endurance performance) remained the same or increased somewhat with training, yet hemoglobin concentration (expressed mg per 100 mL blood) decreased in the expanding plasma volume.

Figure 3.5
Hemoglobin, red blood cell count, and hematocrit in high-school female cross-country runners and a comparison group during the competitive season. (Adapted from Puhl, J. L., et al.: Erythrocyte changes during training in high school women cross-country runners. *Res. Q. Exerc. Sport*, 52:484, 1981.)

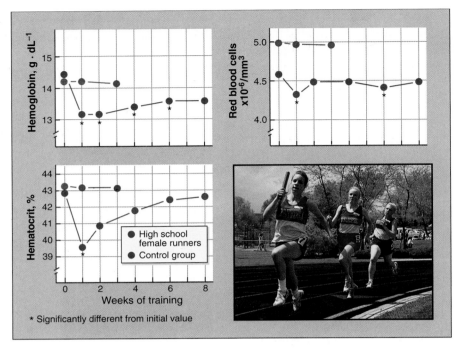

* Significantly different from initial value

Aerobic capacity and exercise performance normally improve with training despite the apparent dilution of hemoglobin. Although vigorous exercise may induce some mechanical destruction of red blood cells (including minimal iron loss in sweat), these factors do not strain an athlete's iron reserves to precipitate clinical anemia—as long as iron intake remains within the normal range. Applying stringent criteria for what constitutes anemia and insufficiency of iron reserves makes "true" sports anemia much less prevalent among highly trained athletes than believed. For male collegiate runners and swimmers, large changes in training volume and intensity during various phases of the competitive season did not reveal the early stages of anemia. Data from female athletes also confirm that the prevalence of iron deficiency anemia did *not* differ in comparisons among specific athletic groups or with nonathletic controls.

Athletes and Iron Supplements. *If an individual's diet contains the recommended iron intake, supplementing with iron does not increase hemoglobin, hematocrit, or other measures of iron status.* Any increase in iron loss with exercise training (coupled with poor dietary habits) in adolescent and premenopausal women could strain an already limited iron reserve. This does not mean that individuals involved in strenuous training should take supplementary iron, or that indicators of sports anemia result from dietary iron deficiency or exercise-induced iron loss. Iron overconsumption or overabsorption could be potentially harmful. Supplements should not be used indiscriminately; excessive iron can accumulate to toxic levels and contribute significantly to diabetes, liver disease, and heart and joint damage. Iron excess may even facilitate growth of latent cancers and infectious organisms. Athletes' iron status should be monitored by periodic evaluation of hematologic characteristics and iron reserves.

Minerals and Exercise Performance

Consuming mineral supplements above recommended levels on an acute or chronic basis does not benefit exercise performance or enhance training respon-

siveness. Loss of water and the mineral salts sodium and potassium chloride in sweat, pose an important challenge in prolonged, hot-weather exercise. Excessive water and electrolyte loss impairs heat tolerance and exercise performance and can trigger heat cramps, heat exhaustion, or heat stroke. The yearly number of heat-related deaths during spring and summer football practice provides a tragic illustration of the importance of replacing fluids and electrolytes. During practice or competition, an athlete may sweat up to 5 kg of water. This corresponds to about 8.0 g of salt depletion because each kg (1 L) of sweat contains about 1.5 g of salt (of which 40% represents sodium). Despite this potential for mineral loss during prolonged exercise in hot weather, replacement of water lost through sweating becomes the crucial and immediate need.

Defense Against Mineral Loss
Vigorous exercise triggers a rapid and coordinated release of the hormones **vasopressin**, **aldosterone**, and the enzyme **renin** to minimize sodium and water loss through the kidneys and sweat. An increase in sodium conservation by the kidneys occurs even under extreme conditions like running a marathon in warm, humid weather where sweat output often reaches $2 \text{ L} \cdot \text{h}^{-1}$. Adding a slight amount of salt to the fluid ingested or food consumed usually can replenish electrolytes lost in sweat. In one study of runners during a 20-day road race in Hawaii, plasma minerals remained normal when the athletes consumed an unrestricted diet without mineral supplements. This finding (and the findings of others) indicates that ingesting "athletic drinks" provides no special benefit in replacing the minerals lost through sweating compared with ingesting the same minerals in a well-balanced diet. Talking salt supplements may be necessary for prolonged exercise in the heat when fluid loss exceeds 4 or 5 kg. This can be achieved by drinking a 0.1 to 0.2% salt

solution (adding 0.3 tsp of table salt per L of water). Intense exercise during heat stress can produce a mild potassium deficiency. However, a diet that contains the recommended amount of this mineral corrects the deficiency.

Drinking an 8 ounce glass of orange or tomato juice replaces the calcium, potassium, and magnesium lost in 3 L (7 lb) of sweat, a sweat loss not likely to occur if an individual performs less than 60 minutes of vigorous exercise.

summary

1. Vitamins neither supply energy nor contribute to body mass. However, these organic substances serve crucial functions in almost all bodily processes, and must be obtained from food or dietary supplementation.

2. Thirteen known vitamins are classified as either water soluble or fat soluble. Vitamins A, D, E, and K comprise the fat-soluble vitamins; vitamin C and the B-complex vitamins make up the water-soluble vitamins.

3. Excess fat-soluble vitamins can accumulate in body tissues and increase to toxic concentrations. Except in relatively rare instances, excess water-soluble vitamins remain nontoxic and eventually pass in the urine.

4. Vitamins regulate metabolism, facilitate energy release, and serve important functions in bone and tissue synthesis.

5. Vitamins C and E and β-carotene serve key protective antioxidant functions. A diet with appropriate levels of these micronutrients reduces the potential for free radical damage (oxidative stress) and may protect against heart disease and cancer.

6. Vitamin supplementation (above the RDA) does not improve exercise performance or the potential for sustaining hard, physical training. In fact, serious illness occurs from regularly consuming an excess of fat-soluble and, in some instances, water-soluble vitamins.

7. Approximately 4% of body mass consists of 22 elements called minerals. They distribute in all body tissues and fluids.

8. Minerals occur freely in nature, in the waters of rivers, lakes, oceans, and in soil. The root system of plants absorbs minerals; minerals eventually incorporate into the tissues of animals that consume plants.

9. Minerals function primarily in metabolism as important parts of enzymes. Minerals provide structure to bones and teeth, and aid in the synthesis of the biologic macronutrients—glycogen, fat, and protein.

10. A balanced diet provides adequate mineral intake, except in some geographic locations that lack iodine.

11. Osteoporosis has reached epidemic proportions among older individuals, especially women. Adequate calcium intake and regular weight-bearing exercise and/or resistance training protect against bone loss at any age.

12. Women who train intensely often do not match energy intake to energy output. Reduced body weight and body fat can adversely affect menstruation, often causing advanced bone loss at an early age. Restoration of normal menses does not necessarily restore bone mass.

13. Excessive sweating during exercise produces significant losses of body water and related minerals; these should be replaced during and following exercise. Sweat loss during exercise usually does not increase mineral requirements above recommended values.

14. About 40% of American women of childbearing age have iron insufficiency. This could lead to iron-deficiency anemia, which negatively affects aerobic exercise performance and ability to perform heavy training. For women on vegetarian-type diets, the relatively low bioavailability of nonheme iron increases risk for iron insufficiency. Vitamin C (in food or supplement form) increases intestinal nonheme iron absorption.

15. Regular physical activity probably does not create a significant drain on the body's iron reserves. If it does, then females (greatest iron requirement and lowest iron intake) could show increased risk for anemia. Assessment of the body's iron status should evaluate hematologic characteristics and iron reserves.

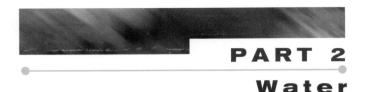

PART 2
Water

Water in the Body

Age, gender, and body composition influence an individual's body water content, which can range from 40 to 70% of total body mass. Water constitutes 72% of the weight of muscle and approximately 50% of the weight of body fat (adipose tissue). Thus, differences among individuals in the relative percentage of total body water largely result from variations in body composition (i.e., differences in lean versus fat tissue).

The body contains two fluid "compartments;" the first, **intracellular**, refers to inside the cells; the second, **extracellular** includes: 1) blood plasma (about 20% of total extracellular fluid), and 2) interstitial fluids, which primarily comprise the fluid that flows in the microscopic spaces between cells. Interstitial fluid also includes lymph, saliva, fluids in the eyes, fluids secreted by glands and the digestive tract, fluids that bathe the nerves of the spinal cord, and fluids excreted from the skin and kidneys. *Much of the fluid lost through sweating comes from extracellular fluid, predominantly blood plasma.*

Figure 3.6 illustrates the approximate partitioning of total body water between intracellular and extracellular spaces for a typical 70-kg (154-lb) man. An average of 62% (26 L) of the body's total 42 L of water represents intracellular water and 38% (16 L) comes from extracellular sources. Of the extracellular compartment, the plasma provides approximately 3 L with the remaining 13 L interstitial water.

Functions of Body Water

Water, a ubiquitous, remarkable nutrient, serves numerous functions:

- Water provides the body's transport and reactive medium.
- Diffusion of gases always takes place across surfaces moistened by water.
- Transport of nutrients and gases occurs in aqueous solution, whereas waste products leave the body through the water in urine and feces.
- Water, due to its significant heat-stabilizing qualities, absorbs considerable heat with only minimal changes in temperature.
- Watery fluids lubricate joints, keeping bony surfaces from grinding against each other.

- Being noncompressible, water provides structure and form to the body through the turgor it imparts to diverse tissues.

Water Balance: Intake Versus Output

The water content of the body remains relatively stable over time. Although considerable water loss occurs in physically active individuals, appropriate fluid intake rapidly restores any imbalance. Figure 3.7 displays the sources of water intake and water loss (output). The bottom panel illustrates that fluid balance can change dramatically during exercise, especially in a hot, humid environment.

Water Intake

In a normal environment, a fairly sedentary adult requires about 2.5 L of water each day. For an active person in a warm environment, the water requirement often increases to between 5 and 10 L daily. Three sources provide this water:

1. Liquids
2. Foods
3. Metabolic processes

The average individual normally consumes 1200 mL (41 oz) of water daily. Fluid intake can increase five or six times above normal during exercise and thermal stress. At the extreme, an individual lost 13.6 kg (30 lb) of water weight during a 2-day, 17-hour, 55-mile run across the desert in Death Valley, California. However, proper fluid ingestion with salt supplements kept body weight loss to only 1.4 kg. In this example, fluid loss and replenishment represented between 3.5 and 4 gallons of liquid!

Most foods, particularly fruits and vegetables, contain considerable water (e.g., lettuce, watermelon and cantaloupe, pickles, green beans, and broccoli); in contrast, butter, oils, dried meats, and chocolate, cookies, and cakes contain relatively little water.

Catabolizing food molecules for energy forms carbon dioxide and water. For a sedentary person, **metabolic water** provides about 25% of the daily water requirement. This includes 55 g of metabolic water from the complete breakdown of 100 g of carbohydrate, 100 g of water from 100 g of protein breakdown, and 107 g from 100 g of fat catabolism. Additionally, each gram of glycogen joins with 2.7 g of water as the glucose units link together; glycogen subsequently liberates this water during its catabolism for energy.

Water Output

The body loses water in four ways:

1. In urine
2. Through the skin
3. As water vapor in expired air
4. In feces

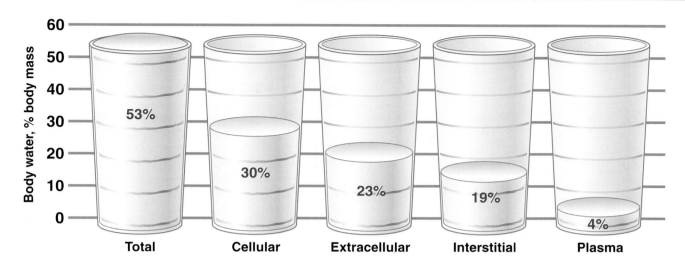

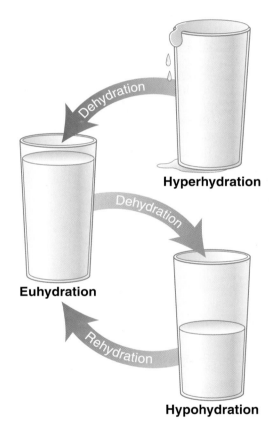

Daily euhydration variability of total body water
Temperature and climate: ±0.165 L (+0.2% body mass)
Heat exercise conditions: ±0.382 L (±0.5% body mass)

Daily plasma volume variability
All conditions: ±0.027 L (±0.6% blood volume)

Hydration Terminology

Euhydration: normal daily water hydration

Hyperhydration: new steady-state condition of increased water content

Hypohydration: new steady-state condition of decreased water content

Dehydration: process of losing water either from the hyperhydrated state to euhydration or from euhydration downward to hypohydration

Rehydration: process of gaining water from a hypohydrated state toward euhydration

Figure 3.6
Distribution of total body water between intracellular and extracellular (interstitial fluid plus plasma volume) compartments for a typical 70-kg (154-lb) man.

The kidneys normally reabsorb about 99% of the 140 to 160 L of filtrate formed each day, leaving from 1000 to 1500 mL or about 1.5 quarts of urine for excretion daily. Every 1 g of solute (e.g., the urea end-product of protein breakdown) eliminated by the kidneys requires about 15 mL of water. From a practical standpoint, using large quantities of protein for energy via a high-protein diet actually accelerates dehydration during exercise.

A small amount of water (perhaps 350 mL), termed **insensible perspiration**, continually seeps from the deeper tissues through the skin to the body's surface. Subcutan-

eous sweat glands also produce water loss through the skin. Evaporation of sweat's water component provides the refrigeration mechanism to cool the body. Daily sweat rate under most conditions amounts to between 500 and 700 mL. This by no means reflects sweating capacity; for example, a well-trained, acclimatized person can produce up to 12 L of sweat (equivalent of 12 kg) at a rate of 1 L per hour during prolonged exercise in a hot environment.

Insensible water loss of 250 to 350 mL per day occurs through small water droplets in exhaled air. This loss re-

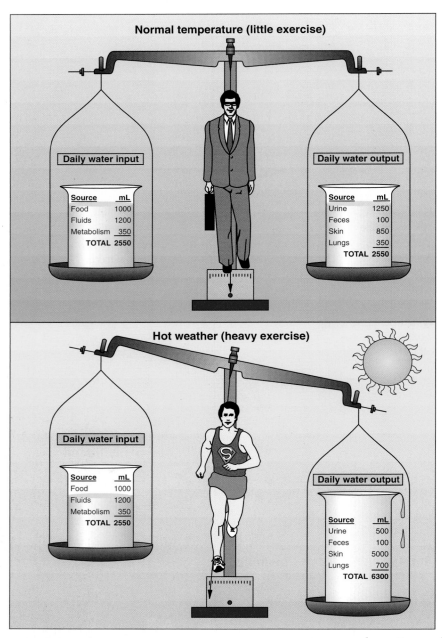

Normal temperature (little exercise)

Daily water input

Source	mL
Food	1000
Fluids	1200
Metabolism	350
TOTAL	**2550**

Daily water output

Source	mL
Urine	1250
Feces	100
Skin	850
Lungs	350
TOTAL	**2550**

Hot weather (heavy exercise)

Daily water input

Source	mL
Food	1000
Fluids	1200
Metabolism	350
TOTAL	**2550**

Daily water output

Source	mL
Urine	500
Feces	100
Skin	5000
Lungs	700
TOTAL	**6300**

Figure 3.7
Water balance in the body. **Top:** Little or no exercise in normal ambient temperature and humidity. **Bottom:** Moderate to heavy exercise in a hot, humid environment.

sults from the complete moistening of all inspired air passing down the pulmonary airways. Exercise affects this source of water loss. For physically active individuals, the respiratory passages release 2 to 5 mL of water each minute during strenuous exercise, depending on climatic conditions. Ventilatory water loss happens least in hot, humid weather and most in cold temperatures (inspired air contains little moisture), or at altitude because the less dense inspired air volumes (which require humidification) significantly increase compared with sea-level conditions.

Intestinal elimination produces between 100 and 200 mL of water loss because water constitutes approximately 70% of fecal matter. The remainder comprises nondigestible material including bacteria from the digestive process, and the residues of digestive juices from the intestine, stomach, and pancreas. With diarrhea or vomiting, water loss increases to between 1500 and 5000 mL.

Figure 3.8 shows that in addition to the 2.0 liters of water ingested daily by the average sedentary adult, saliva, gastric secretions, bile, and pancreatic and intestinal secretions contribute an additional 7 liters each day. This means that the intestinal tract takes up a total daily water quantity of about 9 liters. Of concern to athletes is the fact that ingesting concentrated solutions blunts the rate of water absorption and increases the potential for gastrointestinal distress. This can occur when ingesting salt tablets, concentrated mixtures of simple amino acids, or a "sports drink" containing a large percentage of simple sugars and minerals (see page 89).

Water Requirement In Exercise

The loss of body water represents the most serious consequence of profuse sweating. Three factors determine water loss through sweating:

1. Severity of physical activity
2. Environmental temperature
3. Humidity

Don't Rely on Oral Temperature

Oral temperature does not usually provide an accurate measure of deep body (core) temperature after strenuous exercise. Large and consistent differences occurred between oral and rectal temperatures—the average rectal temperature of 103.5°F after a 14-mile race in a tropical climate contrasted to a "normal" 98°F oral temperature. This 5.5°F discrepancy partly results from evaporative cooling of the mouth and airways during pulmonary ventilation. Considerable cooling occurs from relatively high ventilatory volumes during and immediately after heavy exercise.

The major physiologic defense against overheating comes from evaporation of sweat from the skin's surface. The evaporative loss of 1 liter of sweat releases about 600 kcal of heat energy from the body to the environment. **Relative humidity** (water content of the ambient air) impacts the efficiency of the sweating mechanism in temperature regulation. At 100% relative humidity, the ambient air becomes completely saturated with water vapor. This blocks evaporation of fluid from the skin surface to the air, thus minimizing this important avenue for body cooling. When this happens, sweat beads on the skin and eventually rolls off without providing a cooling effect. On a dry day, in contrast, the air can hold considerable moisture, and fluid evaporates rapidly from the skin. This helps the sweat mechanism to function at optimal efficiency to regulate body temperature. Interestingly, sweat loss equal to 2 to 3% of body mass causes a decrease in plasma volume. This amount of fluid loss significantly strains circulatory function, which ultimately impairs exercise capacity and thermoregulation. Chapter 16 presents a more comprehensive discussion of thermoregulatory dynamics during exercise in the heat.

Heat Disorders

From a health and safety perspective, preventing heat injury remains preferable than trying to remedy it. If one ignores the normal signs of heat stress—thirst, tiredness, grogginess, and visual disturbances—cardiovascular decompensation triggers a series of disabling complications termed **heat illness**. Heat-related disabilities become more apparent among overweight and poorly conditioned individuals, including those who exercise when dehydrated. Heat illness, in order of increasing severity, includes **heat cramps**, **heat exhaustion**, and **heat stroke**. No clear-cut demarcation exists between these maladies because symptoms often overlap. Heat illness requires immediate cor-

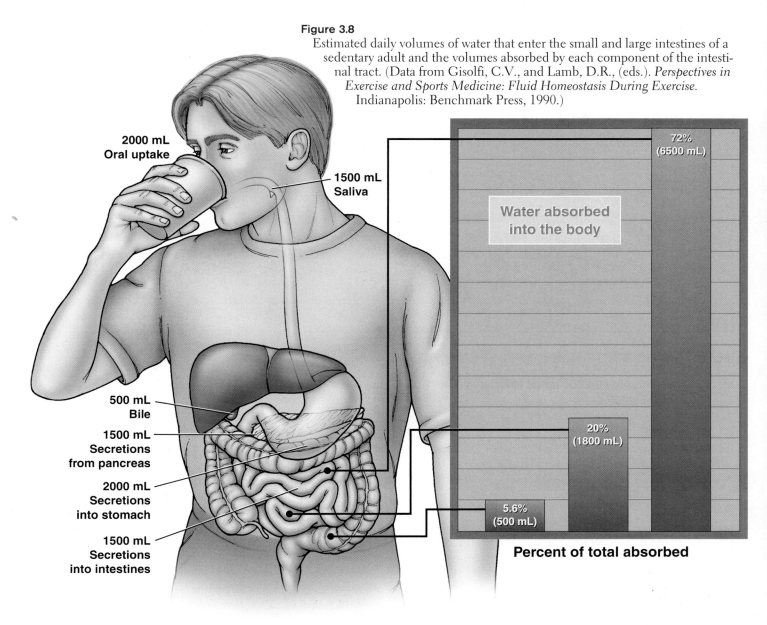

Figure 3.8

Estimated daily volumes of water that enter the small and large intestines of a sedentary adult and the volumes absorbed by each component of the intestinal tract. (Data from Gisolfi, C.V., and Lamb, D.R., (eds.). *Perspectives in Exercise and Sports Medicine: Fluid Homeostasis During Exercise.* Indianapolis: Benchmark Press, 1990.)

2000 mL
Oral uptake

1500 mL
Saliva

500 mL
Bile

1500 mL
Secretions
from pancreas

2000 mL
Secretions
into stomach

1500 mL
Secretions
into intestines

Water absorbed
into the body

72%
(6500 mL)

20%
(1800 mL)

5.6%
(500 mL)

Percent of total absorbed

How to Distinguish Between Heat Cramps, Heat Exhaustion, and Heat Stroke

Human heat dissipation occurs by 1) redistribution of blood from deeper tissues to the periphery, and 2) activation of the refrigeration mechanism provided by evaporation of sweat from the surface of the skin and respiratory passages. During heat stress, cardiac output increases, vasoconstriction and vasodilation move central blood volume towards the skin, and thousands of previously dormant capillaries threading through the upper skin layer open to accommodate blood flow. Conduction of heat away from warm blood at the skin's cooled surface provides about 75% of the body's heat dissipating functions. In contrast, heat production during physical activity often strains the body's heat-dissipating mechanisms, especially under high ambient temperature and humidity. This triggers a broad array of physical signs and symptoms collectively termed heat illness, ranging in severity from mild to life threatening.

Condition	Causes	Signs and Symptoms	Prevention
Heat Cramps	Intense, prolonged exercise in the heat; negative Na$^+$ balance	Tightening cramps, involuntary spasms of active muscles; low serum Na$^+$	Replenish salt loss; ensure acclimatization
Heat Syncope	Peripheral vasodilation and pooling of venous blood; hypotension; hypo-hydration	Giddiness; syncope, mostly in upright position during rest or exercise; pallor; high rectal temperature	Ensure acclimatization and fluid replenishment; reduce exertion on hot days; avoid standing
Heat Exhaustion	Cumulative negative water balance	Exhaustion; hypohydration, flushed skin; reduced sweating in extreme dehydration syncope, high rectal temperature	Proper hydration before exercise and adequate replenishment during exercise; ensure acclimatization
Heat Stroke	Extreme hyperthermia leading to thermoregulatory failure; aggravated by dehydration	Acute medical emergency; includes hyperpyrexia (rectal temp > 41°C), lack of sweating and neurologic deficit (disorientation, twitching, seizures, coma)	Ensure acclimatization; identify and exclude individuals at risk; adapt activities to climatic constraints

rective action to reduce heat stress and rehydrate the person until medical help arrives.

Heat Cramps

Heat cramps (involuntary muscle spasms) occur during or after intense physical activity, usually in the specific muscles exercised. Cramping probably occurs from an imbalance in hydration level and electrolyte concentrations. Sweating during heat exposure augments salt loss, increasing the chance for muscle pain and spasm (most commonly in the muscles of the abdomen and extremities) if electrolytes are not replenished. Body temperature may not necessarily increase with heat cramps. Prevention occurs in two ways: 1) providing copious amounts of water, and 2) increasing daily salt intake (adding a "pinch" of salt to foods at mealtime) several days *before* the expected heat stress.

Heat Exhaustion

Heat exhaustion, the most common heat illness among physically active individuals, usually develops in dehydrated, untrained, and unacclimatized people; it occurs mainly during the first summer heat wave or first hard training session on a hot day. Ineffective circulatory adjustments compounded by depletion of extracellular fluid (plasma volume) from excessive sweating initiates exercise-induced heat exhaustion. Blood usually pools in the dilated peripheral vessels, drastically reducing the central blood volume required to maintain adequate blood flow from the heart. Characteristics of heat exhaustion include:

weak, rapid pulse, low blood pressure in the upright position, headache, nausea, dizziness, "goose bumps" and general weakness. Sweating may become somewhat reduced, but body temperature does not increase to dangerous levels (i.e., above 104°F or 40°C). A person experiencing these symptoms should stop exercising and move to a cooler environment; fluids should be administered immediately either orally or via intravenous therapy.

Exertional Heat Stroke

Heat stroke, the most serious and complex heat-stress malady, requires immediate medical attention. Heat stroke syndrome reflects a failure of heat-regulating mechanisms triggered by excessively high body temperatures. With thermoregulatory failure, sweating usually ceases, the skin becomes dry and hot, body temperature increases to 41°C or higher, and the circulatory system becomes strained. Unfortunately, subtle symptoms often confound the complexity of exertional hyperthermia. Instead of ceasing, sweating can occur during intense exercise (e.g., 10-km running race) in young, hydrated, and highly motivated individuals. However, due to high metabolic heat production, the body's heat gain greatly exceeds avenues for heat loss. If left untreated, circulatory collapse and damage to the central nervous system and other organs can lead to death. Heat stroke represents a medical emergency. While awaiting medical treatment, only aggressive treatment to rapidly lower elevated core temperature can avert death; the magnitude and duration of hyperthermia determine organ damage and mortality. Immediate treatment includes alcohol rubs and application of ice packs. Whole-body cold- or ice-water immersion remains the most effective treatment for a collapsed hyperthermic athlete.

Practical Recommendations for Fluid Replacement in Exercise

Depending on environmental conditions, total sweat loss during a marathon run at world record pace averages about 5.3 L (12 lb). The fluid loss corresponds to an overall reduction of 6 to 8% of body mass. *Fluids must be consumed regularly during physical activity to avoid dehydration and its life-threatening consequences.*

Fluid replacement maintains plasma volume so that circulation and sweating progress at optimal levels. Ingesting "extra" water before exercising in the heat provides some thermoregulatory protection. Pre-exercise hyperhydration delays dehydration, increases sweating during exercise, and blunts the rise in body temperature compared with exercising without prior fluids. As a practical step, a person should consume 400 to 600 mL (13 to 20 oz) of cold water 10 to 20 minutes before exercising. This prudent practice should be combined with continual fluid replacement during exercise.

Gastric Emptying

The small intestine absorbs fluids after they pass from the stomach. The following important factors illustrated in Figure 3.9 influence gastric emptying:

- **Fluid temperature.** Cold fluids (5°C; 41°F) empty from the stomach at a faster rate than fluids at body temperature.

- **Fluid volume**. Keeping fluid volume in the stomach at a relatively high level speeds gastric emptying and may compensate for any inhibitory effects of the beverage's carbohydrate or electrolyte content. Optimizing the effect of stomach volume on gastric emptying occurs by consuming 400 to 600 mL of fluid immediately before exercise. Then, regularly ingesting 150 to 250 mL of fluid (at 15-minute intervals) throughout exercise continually replenishes the fluid passed into the intestine and maintains a large gastric volume during exercise.

- **Fluid osmolarity.** Gastric emptying slows when the ingested fluid contains concentrated electrolytes or simple sugars, whether in the form of glucose, fructose, or sucrose. For example, a 40% sugar solution empties from the stomach at a rate 20% slower than plain water. *As a general rule, between a 5 and 8% carbohydrate-electrolyte beverage consumed during exercise in the heat contributes to temperature regulation and fluid balance as effectively as plain water.* As an added bonus, this drink helps maintain glucose metabolism and glycogen reserves in prolonged exercise.

- **Exercise intensity.** Exercise does not negatively affect gastric emptying up to an intensity of about 75% of maximum, at which point the stomach's emptying becomes somewhat reduced.

Electrolyte Concentrations in Blood Serum and Sweat (mEq·L^{-1})

	Na$^+$	K$^+$	Cl$^-$	Mg^{++}
Blood serum	140	4.0	110	1.5–2.1
Sweat	40–45	3.9	39	3.5

Figure 3.9
Major factors that affect gastric emptying (stomach) and fluid absorption (small intestine).

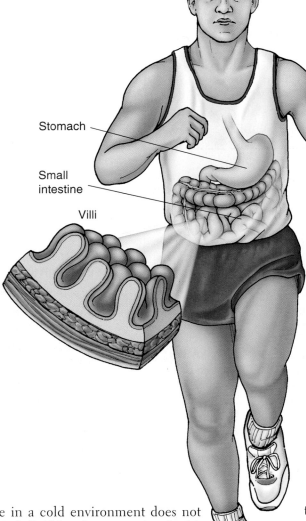

Stomach

Small intestine

Villi

Gastric emptying

- **Volume:** increased volume increases emptying rate
- **Caloric content:** increased energy content decreases emptying rate
- **Osmolality:** increased solute concentration decreases emptying rate
- **Exercise:** intensity exceeding 75% of maximum decreases emptying rate
- **pH:** marked deviations from 7.0 decrease emptying rate
- **Hydration level:** dehydration decreases gastric emptying and increases risk of gastrointestinal distress

Intestinal fluid absorption

- **Carbohydrate:** low to moderate levels of glucose + sodium increase fluid absorption
- **Sodium:** low to moderate levels of sodium increase fluid absorption
- **Osmolality:** hypotonic-to-isotonic fluids containing NaCl and glucose increase fluid absorption

Exercise in a cold environment does not produce much fluid loss from sweating. In this case, reduced gastric emptying and subsequent water absorption can be tolerated, and a more concentrated sugar solution (15 to 20 g per 100 mL of water) may be beneficial. The trade-off between ingested fluid composition and gastric emptying rate must be evaluated based on environmental stress and energy demands. *For survival, the primary concern during prolonged exercise in the heat becomes fluid replacement.* Chapter 17 addresses the desirable composition of "sports drinks" and their effects on fluid replacement.

Adequacy of Rehydration

The primary means to prevent dehydration and its consequences, especially a dangerously elevated body tempera-

ture (**hyperthermia**), requires adherence to an adequate water replacement schedule. This often becomes "easier said than done" because some individuals believe ingesting water hinders exercise performance. For wrestlers, chronic dehydration becomes a way of life during the competitive season. Competitors intentionally lose considerable fluid so they can wrestle in a lower weight class—often with fatal outcomes if dehydration becomes severe enough to precipitate cardiovascular abnormalities from electrolyte disturbances. Chronic dehydration also occurs in ballet in which dancers focus on body weight to appear thin. Many individuals on weight loss programs believe that restricting fluid intake in some way accelerates body fat loss. It does not.

Monitoring change in body weight provides a convenient method to assess: 1) fluid loss during exercise and/or heat stress, and 2) adequacy of rehydration in recovery. In addition to having athletes "weigh in" before and after

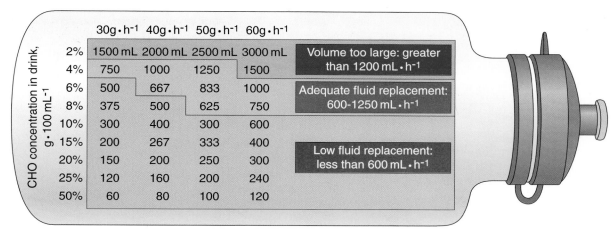

		$30g \cdot h^{-1}$	$40g \cdot h^{-1}$	$50g \cdot h^{-1}$	$60g \cdot h^{-1}$	
	2%	1500 mL	2000 mL	2500 mL	3000 mL	Volume too large: greater than $1200 mL \cdot h^{-1}$
	4%	750	1000	1250	1500	
	6%	500	667	833	1000	Adequate fluid replacement: $600-1250 mL \cdot h^{-1}$
	8%	375	500	625	750	
	10%	300	400	300	600	
	15%	200	267	333	400	Low fluid replacement: less than $600 mL \cdot h^{-1}$
	20%	150	200	250	300	
	25%	120	160	200	240	
	50%	60	80	100	120	

(Left axis label: CHO concentration in drink, $g \cdot 100 mL^{-1}$)

Figure 3.10
Volume of fluid to ingest each hour to obtain the noted amount of carbohydrate. (Modified from Coyle, E.F., and Montain, S.J.: Benefits of fluid replacement. *Med. Sci. Sports Exerc.*, 24:S324, 1992.)

practice, coaches can minimize weight loss by providing scheduled water breaks during practice/training sessions, and unrestricted access to water during competition. Each 0.45 kg (1 lb) of body weight loss corresponds to 450 mL (15 oz) of dehydration. After exercising, the thirst mechanism does not provide a precise guide to water needs. If rehydration depended entirely upon a person's thirst, it could take several days to reestablish fluid balance after severe dehydration.

Water Intoxication

Under normal conditions, a maximum of about 9.5 L (10 qt) of water can be consumed daily without unduly straining the kidneys or diluting chemical concentrations of body fluids. Consuming more than 9.5 L can produce **hyponatremia** (water intoxication), a condition related to significant dilution of the body's normal sodium concentration. Hyponatremia exists when serum sodium concentration falls below $136 mEq \cdot L^{-1}$; serum sodium below $130 mEq \cdot L^{-1}$ triggers severe symptoms. Early symptoms include headache, blurred vision, excessive sweating, and vomiting. In extreme cases, cerebral edema develops, and the individual can become delirious, convulsive, comatose, and eventually die. The most important predisposing factors to hyponatremia include:

- Prolonged high-intensity exercise in hot weather
- Poorly conditioned individuals who experience excessive sweat loss with high sodium concentration.
- Physical activity performed in a sodium-depleted state due to "salt-free" or "low-sodium" diet
- Use of diuretic medication for hypertension
- Frequent intake of large quantities of sodium-free fluid during prolonged exercise

Extreme sodium loss (through prolonged sweating) coupled with dilution of existing extracellular sodium (and accompanying reduced osmolality) from consuming fluids with low or no sodium induces hyponatremia. Hyponatremia can occur in experienced athletes. The likely scenario includes high-intensity, ultramarathon-type, continuous exercise lasting 6 to 8 hours, although it can occur in only 4 hours. Nearly 30% of athletes who competed in an Ironman Triathlon experienced symptoms of hyponatremia; these occurred most frequently late in the race or in the recovery after competition. In a large study of more than 18,000 ultraendurance athletes (including triathletes), approximately 9% of collapsed athletes during or following competition presented with symptoms of hyponatremia. An experienced ultramarathoner required hospitalization after consuming nearly 20 L of fluid during a 62-mile nonstop, 8.5 hour run.

summary

1. Water constitutes 40 to 70% of an individual's total body mass; muscle contains 72% water by weight, whereas water represents only about 50% of the weight of body fat (adipose tissue).

2. Approximately 62% of total body water exists intracellularly (inside the cells) and 38% occurs extracellularly in the plasma, lymph, and other fluids outside the cell.

3. Aqueous solutions supply food and oxygen to the cells, and waste products always leave via a watery medium. Water gives structure and form to the body and regulates body temperature.

4. The normal average daily water intake of 2.5 L comes from (a) liquid intake (1.2 L), (b) food (1.0 L), and (c) metabolic water produced during energy-yielding reactions (0.3 L).

5. Daily water loss includes: urine (1.0 to 1.5 L), through the skin as insensible perspiration (0.35L), as water vapor in expired air (0.25 to 0.35 L), and in feces (0.10 L).

6. Exercise in hot weather greatly increases the body's water requirement because of fluid loss via sweating. In extreme conditions, fluid needs increase five or six times above normal.

7. Heat cramps, heat exhaustion, and heat stroke comprise the major forms of heat illness. Heat stroke represents the most serious and complex of these maladies.

8. Several factors greatly affect the rate of gastric emptying: 1) keeping fluid volume in the stomach at a relatively high level speeds gastric emptying, 2) concentrated sugar solutions impair gastric emptying and fluid replacement, and 3) cold fluids empty from the stomach more rapidly than fluids at body temperature.

9. Maintaining plasma volume (so circulation and sweating progress optimally) represents the primary aim of fluid replacement. For the ideal replacement schedule during exercise, fluid intake should match fluid loss. Monitoring change in body weight during and following workouts indicates the effectiveness of fluid replacement.

10. Optimal gastric volume for fluid replacement occurs by consuming 400 to 600 mL of fluid immediately before exercise, followed by regular fluid ingestion during exercise (approximately 250 mL every 15 minutes).

11. Drinking concentrated sugar-containing beverages slows the rate of gastric emptying; this could disrupt the body's fluid balance in exercise, especially during heat stress.

12. The ideal oral rehydration solution contains between 5 and 8% carbohydrates. This beverage concentration replenishes carbohydrate without adversely affecting fluid balance and thermoregulation.

13. Excessive sweating and ingesting large volumes of plain water during prolonged exercise sets the stage for hyponatremia (water intoxication). A decrease in extracellular sodium concentration causes this potentially dangerous malady.

thought questions

1. Many of the foods we consume are processed and/or chemically altered, reducing their nutritional value. What dietary modifications can maintain the recommended intake of micronutrients without consuming vitamin and mineral supplements?

2. If vitamins play an important role in energy release in the body, why not 'supercharge' with supplements to enhance exercise performance?

3. A middle-age woman expresses concern about maintaining and even increasing bone mass as she ages. Advise her concerning exercise and diet to promote bone health.

4. What specific approaches might a coach establish athletes to guard against dehydration and possible heat injury? Include factors that optimize fluid replacement.

5. Many young girls and women engaged in sports have at least one of the disorders of the female athlete triad. Discuss factors related to this syndrome, and how to guard against their occurrence.

6. Give your answer to an athlete who questions: "What's wrong with taking megadoses of vitamin and mineral supplements to make sure I'm getting enough of these nutrients on a daily basis?"

selected references

Alekel, L., et al.: Contributions of exercise, body composition, and age to bone mineral density in premenopausal women. *Med. Sci. Sports Exerc.*, 27:1477, 1995.

Alessio, H.M. and Blasi, E.R.: Physical activity as a natural antioxidant booster and its effect on a healthy life span. *Res.Q. Exerc. Sport.*, 68:292, 1997.

American College of Sports Medicine. American College of Sports Medicine Position Stand on Osteoporosis and Exercise. *Med. Sci. Sports Exerc.*, 27:1, 1995.

Anderson, R.A., and Guttman, H.N.: Trace minerals and exercise. In: *Exercise, Nutrition, and Energy Metabolism.* E.S. Horton and R.L. Terjung. (eds.). New York: Macmillan, 1988.

Ashizawa, N., et al.: Tomographical description of tennis-loaded radius: reciprocal relation between bone size and volumetric BMD. *J. Appl. Physiol.*, 86:1347, 1999.

Bailey, D.A., et al.: Growth, physical activity, and bone mineral acquisition. *Exer. Sport Sci. Rev.*, 24:233, 1996.

Boot, A.M., et al.: Bone mineral density in children and adolescents: relation to puberty, calcium intake and physical activity. *J. Clin. Endocrin. Metab.*, 82:57, 1997.

Brouns, F.: *Nutritional Nedes of Athletes.* New York: John Wiley & Sons, 1993.

Brouns, F., and Beckers, E.: Is the gut an athletic organ? *Sports. Med.*, 15:242, 1993.

Buskirk, E.R., and Puhl, S.M.: *Body Fluid Balance: Exercise and Sport.* London: CRC Press, 1996.

Chung, S.-C., et al.: Effect of exercise during the follicular and luteal phases on indices of oxidative stress in healthy women. *Med. Sci. Sports Exerc.*, 31:409, 1999.

Clarkson, P.M., and Haymes, E.M.: Exercise and mineral status of athletes: calcium, magnesium, phophorus, and iron. *Med. Sci. Sports Exerc.*, 27:831, 1995.

Conroy, B.P., et al.: Bone mineral density in elite junior Olympic weight lifters. *Med. Sci. Sports Exerc.*, 25:1103, 1993.

Coyle, E. F., and Montain, S. J.: Carbohydrate and fluid ingestion during exercise: are there trade-offs? *Med. Sci. Sports Exerc.*, 24:671, 1992.

Demirel, H.A., et al.: Exercise training reduces myocardial lipid peroxidation following short-term ischemia-reperfusion. *Med. Sci. Sports Exerc.*, 30:1211, 1998.

Diaz, M.N., et al.: Antioxidants and atherosclerotic heart disease. *N. Engl. J. Med.*, 337:408, 1997.

Dook, J.E., et al.: Exercise and bone mineral density in mature female athletes. *Med. Sci. Sports Exerc.*, 29:291, 1997.

Drinkwater, B.L.: C.H. McCloy Research Lecture: Does physical activity play a role in preventing osteoporosis? *Res. Q. Exerc. Sport.* 65: 197, 1994.

Dueck, C.A., et al.: A diet and training intervention program for the treatment of athletic amenorrhea. *Int. J. Sports Nutr.*, 6:134, 1996.

Eichner, E.R.: Physical activity and free radicals. In: *Physical Activity, Fitness, and Health.* Bouchard C., et al., (eds.). Champaign, IL: Human Kinetics, 1994.

Eichner, E.R.: Sports anemia, iron supplements, and blood doping. *Med. Sci. Sports Exerc.*, 24:S315, 1992.

Ely, D.L., Overview of dietary sodium effects on and interactions with cardiovascular and neuroendocrine functions. *Am. J. Clin. Nutr.*, 65 (Suppl): 594S, 1997.

Gilsolfi, C.V., et al.: Effect of sodium concentration in a carbohydrate-electrolyte solution on intestinal absorption. *Med. Sci. Sports Exerc.*, 27:1414, 1995.

Gilsolfi, C.V., et al.: Effect of beverage osmolality on intestinal fluid absorption during exrcise. *J. Appl. Physiol.*, 85:1941, 1998.

Ginsburg, G.S., et al.: Effects of a single bout of ultraendurance exercise on lipid levels and susceptibility of lipids to peroxidation in triathletes. *JAMA*, 276:221, 1996.

Goldfarb, A.H., et al.: Antioxidants: role of supplementation to prevent exercise-induced oxidative stress. *Med. Sci. Sports Exerc.*, 25:232, 1993.

Hamdy, R.C., et al.: Regional differences in bone density of young men involved in different exercises. *Med. Sci. Sports Exerc.*, 26: 884, 1994.

Haymes, E.M.: Vitamin and mineral supplementation to athletes. *Int. J. Sport Nutr.*, 1:146, 1991.

Ji, L.L.: Exercise and oxidative stress: role of the cellular antioxidant systems. *Exerc. Sport Sci. Rev.*, 23:135, 1995.

Kanter, M.M.: Free radicals and exercise: effects of nutritional antioxidant supplementation. *Exerc. Sport Sci. Rev.*, 23:375, 1995.

Klesges, R.C., et al.: Changes in bone mineral content in male athletes: mechanisms of action and intervention effects. *JAMA*, 276:226, 1996.

Klipstein-Grobusch, K., et al.: Dietary antioxidants and risk of myocardial infarction in the elderly: the Rotterdam Study. *Am. J. Clin. Nutr.*, 69:261, 1999.

Kohrt, W.M., et al.: HRT preserves increases in bone mineral density and reductions in body fat after a supervised exercise program. *J. Appl. Physiol.*, 84:1506, 1998.

Kontulainen, S., et al.: Changes in bone mineral content with decreased training in competitive

young adult tennis players and controls: a prospective 4-yr follow-up. *Med. Sci. Sports Exerc.*, 31:646, 1999.

Layne, J.E., and Nelson, M.E.: The effects of progressive resistance training on bone density: a review. *Med. Sci. Sports Exerc.*, 31:25, 1999.

Loucks, A.B.: The reproductive system. In: *Perspectives in Exercise Science and Sports Medicine, Vol. 9: Exercise and the Female—A Life Span Approach.* Bar-Or, O., et al., (eds.). Carmel, IN: Cooper Publishing Co, 1996.

Lukaski, H.C., et al.: Iron, copper, magnesium and zinc status as predictors of swimming performance. *Int. J. Sports Med.*, 17:535, 1996.

Maughan, R.J., et al.: Restoration of fluid balance after exercise-induced dehydration: effect of food and fluid intake. *Int. J. Appl. Physiol.*, 73:317, 1996.

Nattiv, A., et al.: The female athlete triad. *Clin. Sports Med.*, 13:405, 1994.

Nieman, D.C.: Immune response to heavy exertion. *J. Appl. Physiol.*, 82:1385, 1997.

Petranick, K., and Berg, K.: The effects of weight training on bone density of premenopausal, postmenopausal, and elderly women: a review. *J. Strength and Cond. Res.*, 11:200, 1997.

Pizza, F.X., et al.: Serum haptaglobin and ferritin during a competitive running and swimming season. *Int. J. Sports Med.*, 18:233, 1997.

Rajaram, S., et al.: Effects of long-term moderate exercise on iron status in young women. *Med. Sci. Sports Exerc.*, 27:1105, 1995.

Ray, M.I., et al.: Effect of sodium in a rehydration beverage when consumed as a fluid or meal. *J. Appl. Physiol.*, 85:1329, 1998.

Rimm, E.B., et al.: Vitamin E consumption and the risk of coronary heart disease in men. *N. Engl. J. Med.*, 328: 1450, 1993.

Ryan, A.S., et al.: Aerobic exercise maintains regional bone mineral density during weight loss in postmenopausal women. *J. Appl. Physiol.*, 84:1305, 1998.

Sandor, R.P.: Heat illness: on-site diagnosis and cooling. *Phys. Sportsmed.*, 25(6):35, 1997.

Sawka, M.N., and Coyle, E.F.: Influence of body water and blood volume on thermoregulation and exercise performance in the heat. *Exerc. Sport Sci. Rev.*, 27:167, 1999.

Schmid, A., et al.: Effect of physical exercise and vitamin C on absorption of ferric sodium citrate. *Med. Sci. Sports Exerc.*, 28:1470, 1996.

Selby, G. B.: When does an athlete need iron? *Phys. Sportsmed.*, 19:97, 1991.

Singh, A., et al.: Chronic multivitamin-mineral supplementation does not enhance physical performance. *Med. Sci. Sports Exerc.*, 24:726, 1992.

Smith, A.D.: The female athlete triad: causes, diagnosis, and treatment. *Phys. Sportsmed.*, 24:67, 1996.

Speedy, D.B., et al.: Hyponatremia and weight changes in an ultradistance triathlon. *Clin. J. Sport Med.*, 7:180, 1997.

Tomten, S.E., et al.: Bone mineral density and menstrual irregularities. A comparative study of cortical and trabecular bone structures in runners with alleged normal eating behavior. *Int. J. Sports Med.*, 19:87, 1998.

Use of vitamin and mineral supplements in the United States. *Nutr. Rev.*, 70:43, 1990.

Van Loan, M.D.: What makes good bones? Factors affecting bone health. *ACSM's Health & Fitness J.*, 2:27, 1998.

Vasankari, T.J., et al.: Increased serum and low-density-lipoprotein antioxidant potential after antioxidant supplementation in endurance athletes. *Am. J. Clin. Nutr.*, 65:1052, 1997.

Vincent, H.K., et al.: Exercise training protects against contraction-induced lipid peroxidation in the diaphragm. *Eur. J. Appl. Physiol.*, 79:268, 1999.

Virk, R.S., et al.: Effects of vitamin B-6 supplementation on fuels, catecholamines, and amino acids during exercise in men. *Med. Sci. Sports Exerc.*, 31:400, 1999.

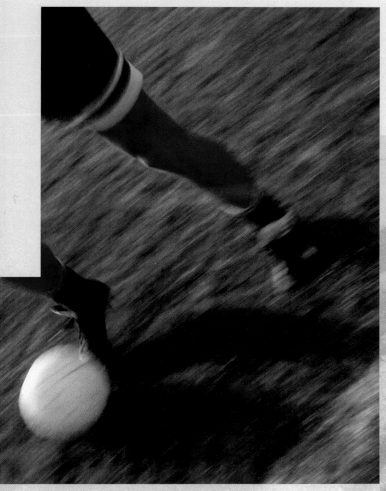

CHAPTER

4

Topics covered in this chapter

PART 1 Phosphate-Bond Energy

Adenosine Triphosphate: The Energy Currency
Phosphocreatine: The Energy Reservoir
Intramuscular High-Energy Phosphates
Energy Source Important
Cellular Oxidation
Summary

PART 2 Energy Release From Food

Energy Release From Carbohydrate
Energy Release From Fat
Energy Release From Protein
The Metabolic Mill
Fats Burn in a Carbohydrate Flame
Regulation of Energy Metabolism
Acid-Base Regulation and pH
Buffering and Strenuous Exercise
Summary
Thought Questions
Selected References

Fundamentals of Human Energy Transfer

- Identify the high-energy phosphates and discuss their roles in various forms of biological work.

- Outline the process of electron transport-oxidative phosphorylation.

- Explain oxygen's role in energy metabolism.

- Describe how anaerobic energy release occurs in cells.

- Describe lactate formation during progressively increasing exercise intensity.

- Outline the general pathways of the Krebs cycle during macronutrient catabolism.

- Contrast ATP yield from carbohydrates, fats, and proteins.

- Explain the statement, "Fats burn in a carbohydrate flame."

- Contrast the speed of energy transfer from carbohydrate versus fat combustion.

The body's capacity to extract energy from food nutrients and transfer it to the contractile elements in skeletal muscle determines the capacity to swim, run, bicycle, and ski long distances at high intensity. Energy transfer occurs through thousands of complex chemical reactions that require the proper mixture of macro- and micronutrients continually fueled by oxygen. The term **aerobic** describes such oxygen-requiring energy reactions. In contrast, **anaerobic** chemical reactions generate energy rapidly for short durations without oxygen. Rapid energy transfer allows for a high standard of performance in maximal short-term sprinting in track and swimming, or repeated stop-and-go sports like soccer, basketball, lacrosse, water polo, volleyball, field hockey, and football. The following point requires emphasis: *The anaerobic and aerobic breakdown of ingested food nutrients provides the energy source for synthesizing the chemical fuel that powers all forms of biologic work.*

In this chapter, we present an overview of how the body obtains energy to power its diverse functions. A basic understanding of carbohydrate, fat, and protein catabolism and concurrent anaerobic and aerobic energy transfer forms the basis for much of the content of exercise physiology. Knowledge about human bioenergetics provides the practical basis for formulating sport-specific exercise training regimens, recommending activities for physical fitness and weight control, and advocating prudent dietary modifications for specific sport requirements. Understanding the impact of environmental stressors on the human organism requires knowledge of energy metabolism. Furthermore, evaluating the proposed benefits of the potpourri of alleged performance-enhancing drugs, compounds, foods, and procedures necessitates an understanding of how the body generates energy. This chapter explores energy metabolism in some depth.

PART 1
Phosphate-Bond Energy

The human body receives a continual supply of chemical energy to perform its many functions. Energy derived from food oxidation does not release suddenly at some kindling temperature because the body, unlike a mechanical engine, cannot use heat energy. Rather, complex, enzymatically controlled reactions

c l o s e   u p

ATP—Nature's Powerful Ingredient

Animals and plants are as different as night and day, yet they share one important common biological trait; they each trap, store, and transfer energy through a complex series of chemical reactions that involve the compound adenosine triphosphate or ATP.

The history of the discovery of ATP reads like a mystery. It dates back to the 1860s in France, and the work of Louis Pasteur, a leading scientist of the day. During one of his experiments with yeast, Pasteur proposed that this micro–organism's ability to degrade sugar to carbon dioxide and alcohol (ethanol) was strictly a living (Pasteur termed it "vitalistic") function of the yeast cell. He hypothesized that if the yeast cell died, the fermentation process would cease.

In 1897, the German chemist, Eduard Buchner (1860–1917), made a chance observation that proved Pasteur wrong. His discovery revolutionized the study of physiologic systems and represented the beginning of the modern science of **biochemistry.** Searching for therapeutic uses for protein, he concocted a thick paste of freshly grown yeast and sand in a large mortar and pressed out the yeast cell juice. The gummy liquid proved unstable and could not be preserved by techniques available at that time. One of the laboratory assistants suggested the addition of large amounts of sugar to the mixture—his wife used this technique to preserve fruit.

To everyone's surprise, what seemed a silly solution worked; the nonliving juice from the yeast cells converted the sugar to carbon dioxide and alcohol (that directly contradicted Pasteur's prevailing theorem). The epoch finding about non-cellular fermentation earned Professor Buchner the 1907 Nobel prize in chemistry.

In 1905, British biochemists Arthur Harden and Australian biochemist William Young observed, as had their German predecessors, that the fermenting ability of yeast juice decreased gradually with time and could be restored only by adding fresh boiled yeast juice or blood serum. What revitalized the mixture? After prolonged research, inorganic phosphate, present in both liquids, was identified as the activating agent.

Other British scientists working with eventual Nobel Lauretes Harden and Young also played important roles in the final discovery of ATP. For example, crude yeast juice pressed through a gelatin film yielded a filtrate free of protein. The filtrate and protein were completely inert. But when the filtrate and protein were recombined, vigorous fermentation began. They called this combination "zymase": it consisted of the filtrate "cozymase" and the protein residue "apozymase." Many years passed before the two components were accurately analyzed and identified as containing "coenzyme" compounds. In addition, the apozymase consisted of many proteins, each a specific catalyst in the many reactions in sugar breakdown.

In 1929, the young German scientist, Karl Lohmann working in Otto Meyerhoff's laboratory, conducted a series of experiments about the "energy" source responsible for cellular reactions involving yeast and sugar. Working with yeast juice, Lohmann found that an unstable substance in the cozymase filtrate was needed to break down the sugar. This energizing substance contained the nitrogen-containing compound adenine linked to the sugar ribose and three phosphate groups. We now call this compound ATP. The potential energy stored in the "high-energy bonds," link the all-important phosphate groups in the ATP molecule. The splitting of these phosphate bonds releases the energy for *all* biologic work.

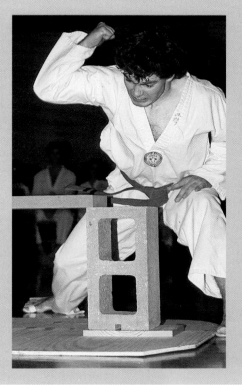

The function of ATP is amazing for the variety of processes it powers in all living cells. This ubiquitous compound is found in micro-organisms, plants, and animals ranging from nematodes to cockroaches and humans. Surprisingly, wherever ATP is found, it is always in the same structure, regardless of the organism's complexity.

within the relatively cool, watery medium of the cell extract the chemical energy trapped within the bonds of carbohydrate, fat, and protein molecules. This relatively slow extraction process reduces energy loss and enhances efficiency in energy transformations. In this way, the body makes direct use of chemical energy for biologic work. In a sense, energy becomes available to the cells as needed. The body maintains a continuous energy supply through the use of **adenosine triphosphate** or **ATP**, the special carrier for free energy.

Enzymes: Biologic Catalysts

Enzymes, highly specific protein catalysts, accelerate the forward and reverse rates of chemical reactions without being consumed or changed in the reaction. Enzymes do not induce reactions that could not otherwise occur under proper conditions. Rather, they facilitate the interaction of substances that normally would occur at a much slower rate.

Adenosine Triphosphate: The Energy Currency

The energy in food does not transfer directly to cells for biologic work. Rather, this "macronutrient energy" becomes released and funneled through the energy-rich compound ATP to power cellular needs. Figure 4.1 shows how an ATP molecule forms from a molecule of adenine and ribose (called adenosine), linked to three phosphate molecules. The bonds linking the two outermost phosphates, termed **high-energy bonds**, represent considerable stored energy within the ATP molecule.

A tight linkage or *coupling* exists between the breakdown of the macronutrient energy molecules and ATP synthesis, which "captures" a significant portion of the released energy. **Coupled reactions** occur in pairs; the breakdown of one compound provides energy for building another compound. To meet energy needs, ATP joins with water (hydrolysis) splitting the outermost phosphate bond from the ATP molecule. The enzyme **adenosine triphosphatase** accelerates this process, forming a new compound **adenosine diphosphate** or **ADP**. These reactions, in turn, couple to other reactions that use the "freed" phosphate-bond chemical energy. The body uses

ATP to transfer the energy produced during catabolic reactions to power reactions that synthesize new materials. In essence, this energy receiver-energy donor cycle represents the cells' two major energy-transforming activities:

1. Form and conserve ATP from food's potential energy
2. Use energy extracted from ATP to power biologic work

Figure 4.2 illustrates examples of the anabolic and catabolic reactions that involve the coupled transfer of chemical energy. All of the energy released from catabolizing one compound does not dissipate as heat; rather, a portion becomes harvested and conserved within the chemical structure of the newly formed compound. ATP represents the common energy transfer "vehicle" in most coupled biologic reactions.

Anabolism requires energy for synthesizing new compounds. For example, many glucose molecules join together, much like the links in a chain of sausages, to form the larger more complex glycogen molecule; similarly, glycerol and fatty acids combine to make triglycerides, and amino acids link to form proteins. Each reaction starts with simple compounds and uses them as building blocks to form larger, more complex compounds.

Catabolic reactions release energy; in many instances, this process forms ATP. During ATP catabolism, the enzyme adenosine triphosphatase catalyzes the reaction when ATP joins with water. For each mole of ATP degraded to ADP, the outermost phosphate bond splits, liberating approximately 7.3 kcal of **free energy** (i.e., energy available for work).

$$\text{ATP} + \text{H}_2\text{O} \xrightarrow{\text{ATPase}} \text{ATP} + \text{P}_i - 7.3 \text{ kcal per mol}$$

The free energy liberated in ATP **hydrolysis** reflects the energy difference between the reactant and end products. Because this reaction generates considerable energy, we refer to ATP as a **high-energy phosphate** compound. Some additional energy releases when another phosphate splits from ADP but this infrequently occurs. In some reactions of biosynthesis, ATP donates its two terminal phosphates simultaneously to construct new cellular material. Adenosine monophosphate or AMP becomes the new molecule with a single phosphate group.

The energy liberated during ATP breakdown directly transfers to other energy-requiring molecules. In muscle, this energy activates specific sites on the contractile elements causing muscle fibers to shorten. *Because energy from ATP powers all forms of biologic work, ATP constitutes the cell's "energy currency."* Figure 4.3 illustrates the general role of ATP as energy currency.

The splitting of an ATP molecule takes place immediately and without oxygen. The cell's capability for ATP breakdown generates energy for rapid use; this would not occur if energy metabolism required oxygen at all times. Think of anaerobic energy release as a back-up power

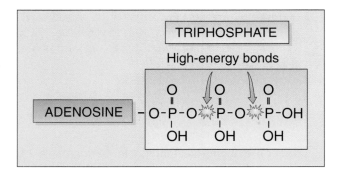

Figure 4.1
ATP, the energy currency of the cell. The starburst represents the high-energy bonds.

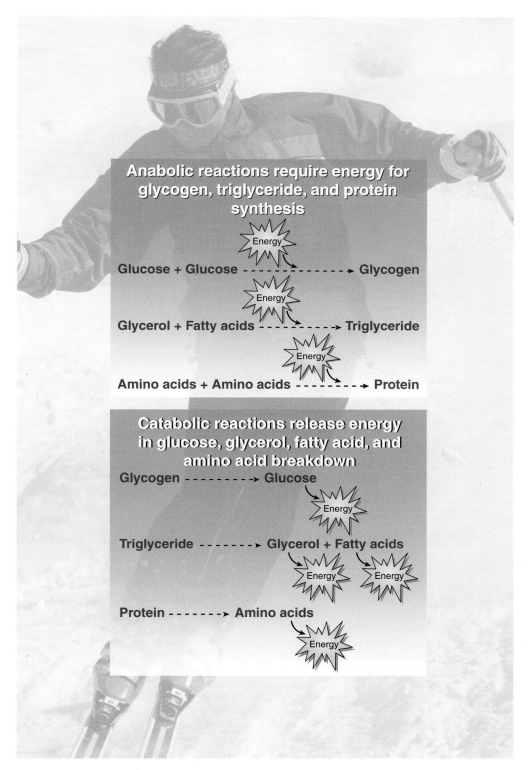

Figure 4.2
Anabolic and catabolic reactions.

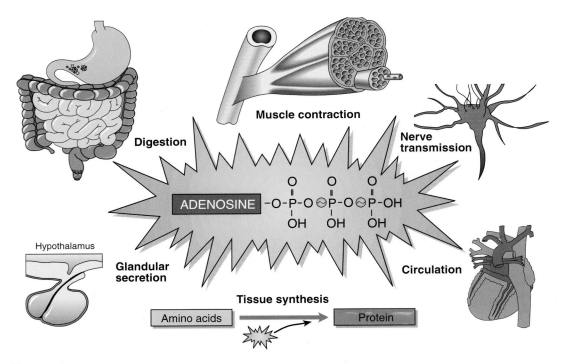

Figure 4.3
ATP represents the energy currency that powers all forms of biologic work.

source, called upon to deliver energy in excess of what can be generated aerobically. For this reason, any form of physical activity can take place immediately without instantaneously consuming oxygen; examples include sprinting for a bus, lifting a fork, driving a golf ball, spiking a volleyball, doing a pushup, or jumping up in the air. The well known practice of holding one's breath while sprint swimming provides a clear example of ATP splitting without reliance on atmospheric oxygen. Withholding air (oxygen), although not advisable, can be done during a 100-yard sprint on the track, lifting a barbell, a dash up several flights of stairs, or simply holding one's breath while rapidly flexing and extending the arms or fingers. In each case, energy metabolism proceeds uninterrupted because intramuscular anaerobic sources almost exclusively provide the energy to perform the activity.

Phosphocreatine: The Energy Reservoir

Because cells store only a small quantity of ATP, it must be resynthesized continually at its rate of use. This provides a biologically useful mechanism for regulating energy metabolism. By maintaining only a small amount of ATP, its relative concentration (and corresponding concentration of ADP) changes rapidly with any increase in a cell's energy demands. An ATP:ADP imbalance at the start of exercise immediately stimulates the breakdown of other stored energy-containing compounds to resynthesize ATP. As one might expect, increases in cellular energy transfer depend

on exercise intensity. Energy transfer increases about fourfold in the transition from sitting in a chair to walking. However, changing from a walk to an all-out sprint almost immediately accelerates energy transfer rate about 120 times within active muscle. Generating significant energy output almost instantaneously demands ATP availability and a means for its rapid resynthesis.

ATP: A Limited Currency

As we have pointed out, a limited quantity of ATP serves as the energy currency for all cells. In fact, at any one time the body stores only about 80 to 100 g (3.5 oz) of ATP. This provides enough intramuscular stored energy for several seconds of explosive, all-out exercise. A limited quantity of "stored" ATP represents an additional advantage due to the molecule's heaviness. Biochemists estimate that sedentary persons each day use an amount of ATP approximately equal to 75% of their body mass. For an endurance athlete running a marathon race and generating about 20 times the resting energy expenditure over 3 hours, total ATP usage could amount to 80 kg. Thus, with limited supplies and with high demand, ATP must be continually resynthesized to meet energy requirements.

Some energy for ATP resynthesis comes directly from the splitting (hydrolysis) of a phosphate from another intracellular high-energy phosphate compound—**phosphocreatine (PCr)**, also known as creatine phosphate or CP. PCr, similar to ATP, releases a large amount of energy when the bond splits between the creatine and phosphate molecules. The hydrolysis of PCr for energy begins at the onset of intense exercise, does not require oxygen, and

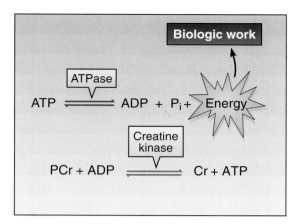

Figure 4.4
ATP and PCr are anaerobic sources of phosphate-bond energy. The energy liberated from the hydrolysis (splitting) of PCr powers the union of ADP and P to reform ATP (the creatine kinase reaction).

reaches a maximum in about 10 seconds. Thus, PCr can be considered a "reservoir" of high-energy phosphate bonds. Figure 4.4 schematically illustrates the release and use of phosphate-bond energy in ATP and PCr. The term **high-energy phosphates** describes these stored intramuscular compounds.

In both reactions, the arrows point in opposite directions to indicate reversible reactions. In other words, creatine (Cr) and inorganic phosphate (from ATP) can join again to reform PCr. This also holds true for ATP in which the union of ADP and P_i reforms ATP (see top part of figure). ATP resynthesis occurs if sufficient energy exists to rejoin an ADP molecule with one P_i molecule. Hydrolysis of PCr supplies this energy.

Cells store PCr in considerably larger quantities than ATP. Mobilization of PCr for energy takes place almost instantaneously and does not require oxygen. Interestingly, the concentration of ADP in the cell stimulates the activity level of **creatine kinase,** the enzyme that facilitates PCr breakdown. This provides a crucial feedback mechanism for rapidly forming ATP from the high-energy phosphates.

Intramuscular High-Energy Phosphates

The energy released from ATP and PCr breakdown can sustain all-out running, cycling, or swimming for 5 to 8 seconds. In the 100-m sprint, for example, the body cannot maintain maximum speed for longer than this duration. During the last few seconds of the race, runners actually slow down, with the winner often slowing the least. From an energy perspective, the winner most effectively supplies and uses the limited but rapid supply of phosphate-bond energy.

In almost all sports, the energy transfer capacity of the ATP-PCr high-energy phosphates (**immediate energy system**) plays an important role in success or failure of some phase of performance. If all-out effort continues beyond 8 seconds, or if moderate exercise continues for much longer periods, ATP resynthesis requires an additional energy source. Without this, the "fuel" supply diminishes and high-intensity movement ceases. As we discuss shortly, the foods we eat and store for ready access provide energy to continually recharge cellular supplies of ATP and PCr.

Energy Source Important

Identifying the predominant source(s) of energy required for a particular sport or physical activity provides the basis for an effective exercise training program. Football and baseball, for example, require a high energy output for brief periods. These performances rely almost exclusively on energy transfer from the intramuscular high-energy phosphates. Developing this rapid energy system becomes important when training to improve performance in movements of brief duration. Chapter 14 discusses specific training to optimize the power-output capacity of the immediate energy system.

Chemical Bonds Transfer Energy

Human energy dynamics involve transferring energy by chemical bonds. Bond splitting releases potential energy;

energy conservation occurs by new bond formation. Some energy lost by one molecule transfers to the chemical structure of other molecules without appearing as heat. In the body, biologic work takes place when compounds relatively low in potential energy "juice-up" from the transfer of energy via high-energy phosphate bonds.

Adenosine triphosphate serves as the ideal energy-transfer agent. In one respect, the phosphate bonds of ATP "trap" a large portion of the original food molecule's potential energy. ATP also readily transfers this energy to other compounds to raise them to a higher activation level. **Phosphorylation** refers to energy transfer through phosphate bonds. The energy for phosphorylation comes from **oxidation** ("biologic burning") of the carbohydrate, lipid, and protein macronutrients consumed in the diet.

Cellular Oxidation

A molecule becomes reduced when it accepts electrons from an electron donor. In turn, the molecule that gives up the electron becomes oxidized. **Oxidation reactions** (donating electrons) and **reduction reactions** (accepting electrons) remain coupled because every oxidation coincides with a reduction. *In essence, cellular oxidation-reduction constitutes the mechanism for energy metabolism.* The stored carbohydrate, fat, and protein molecules continually provide hydrogen atoms for this process. The **mitochondria,** the cell's "energy factories," contain carrier molecules that remove electrons from hydrogen (oxidation) and eventually pass them to oxygen (reduction). Synthesis of the high-energy phosphate ATP occurs during oxidation–reduction reactions.

Electron Transport

Figure 4.5 illustrates hydrogen oxidation and the accompanying electron transport to oxygen. During cellular oxidation, hydrogen atoms are not merely turned loose in the cell fluid. Rather, highly specific **dehydrogenase enzymes** catalyze hydrogen's release from the nutrient substrate. The coenzyme part of the dehydrogenase (usually the niacin-containing coenzyme, **nicotinamide adenine dinucleotide** or **NAD$^+$**) accepts pairs of electrons (energy) from hydrogen. While the substrate oxidizes and loses hydrogen (electrons), NAD$^+$ gains a hydrogen and two elec-

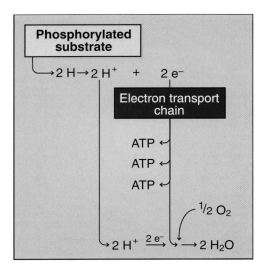

Figure 4.5
Oxidation (removal of electrons) of hydrogen and accompanying electron transport. In reduction, oxygen gains electrons and water forms.

trons and reduces to NADH; the other hydrogen appears as H$^+$ in the cell fluid.

The riboflavin-containing coenzyme, **flavin adenine dinucleotide (FAD)** is the other important electron acceptor that oxidizes food fragments. FAD also catalyzes dehydrogenations and accepts pairs of electrons. Unlike NAD$^+$, however, FAD becomes FADH$_2$ by accepting both hydrogens. This distinct difference between NAD and FAD produces a different total number of ATP in the respiratory chain (see below).

The NADH and FADH$_2$ formed in macronutrient breakdown represent energy-rich molecules because they carry electrons with a high energy transfer potential. The **cytochromes,** a series of iron-protein electron carriers, then pass, in "bucket brigade" manner, pairs of electrons carried by NADH and FADH$_2$ on the inner membranes of the mitochondria. The iron portion of each cytochrome exists in either its oxidized (ferric or Fe^{+++}) or reduced (ferrous or Fe^{++}) ionic state. By accepting an electron, the ferric portion of a specific cytochrome reduces to its ferrous form. In turn, ferrous iron donates its electron to the next cytochrome, and so on down the line. By shuttling between these two iron forms, the cytochromes transfer electrons to their ultimate destination, where they reduce oxygen to form water. The NAD$^+$ and FAD then recycle for subsequent reuse in energy metabolism.

Electron transport by specific carrier molecules constitutes the **respiratory chain,** the final common pathway where electrons extracted from hydrogen pass to oxygen. *For each pair of hydrogen atoms, two electrons flow down the chain and reduce one atom of oxygen to form water.* Of the five specific cytochromes, only the last one, cytochrome oxidase (cytochrome aa$_3$ with a strong affinity for oxygen), discharges its electron directly to oxygen. Figure 4.6A shows the route for hydrogen oxidation, electron transport, and energy transfer in the respiratory chain. The

Links in Energy Transfer

NAD$^+$ and FAD represent crucial oxidizing agents (electron acceptors) in energy metabolism. Oxidation reactions couple to reduction reactions, allowing electrons (hydrogens) picked up by NAD$^+$ and FAD to transfer to other compounds (reducing agents) during energy metabolism.

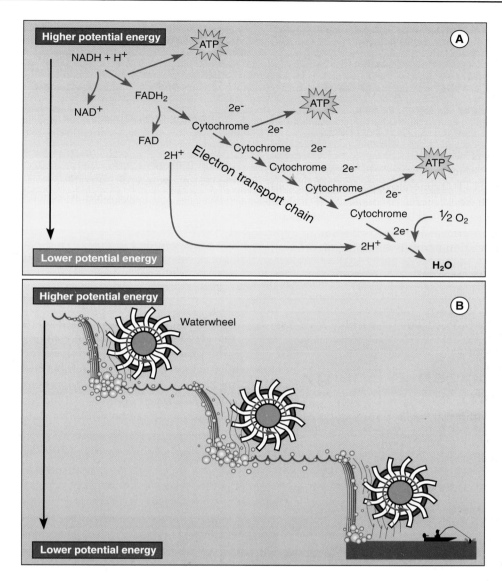

Figure 4.6
Examples of harnessing potential energy. **A,** In the body. The electron transport chain removes electrons from hydrogens and ultimately delivers them to oxygen. In this oxidation-reduction process, much of the chemical energy stored within the hydrogen atom does not dissipate to kinetic energy. Rather, it becomes conserved in forming ATP. **B,** In industry. The captured energy from falling water drives the waterwheel, which in turn performs mechanical work.

respiratory chain releases free energy in relatively small amounts. In several of the electron transfers, energy conservation occurs by forming high-energy phosphate bonds.

Oxidative Phosphorylation

Oxidative phosphorylation refers to how ATP forms during electron transfer from NADH and $FADH_2$ to molecular oxygen. This important process represents the cell's primary means for extracting and trapping chemical energy in the high-energy phosphates. *More than 90% of ATP synthesis takes place in the respiratory chain by oxidative reactions coupled with phosphorylation.*

Think of oxidative phosphorylation as a waterfall divided into several separate cascades by the intervention of

water wheels at different heights. Figure 4.6B depicts the water wheels harnessing the energy of the falling water; similarly, electrochemical energy generated via electron transport in the respiratory chain becomes harnessed and transferred (or coupled) to ADP. The energy in NADH transfers to ADP to reform ATP at three distinct coupling sites during electron transport (Fig. 4.6A). Oxidation of hydrogen and subsequent phosphorylation occurs as follows:

$$\text{NADH} + \text{H}^+ + 3\text{ADP} + 3\text{P}_i + \tfrac{1}{2}\,\text{O}_2 \rightarrow$$
$$\text{NAD}^+ + \text{H}_2\text{O} + 3\text{ATP}$$

In the above reaction, three ATP form for each NADH plus H^+. However, if $FADH_2$ originally donates hydrogen only two molecules of ATP form for each hydrogen pair oxidized. This occurs because $FADH_2$ enters the respiratory chain at a lower energy level at a point beyond the site of the first ATP synthesis.

Efficiency of Electron Transport and Oxidative Phosphorylation

Each mole of ATP stores approximately 7 kcal of energy. Because 3 moles of ATP regenerate from oxidizing 1 mole of NADH, about 21 kcal (7 kcal per mole × 3) are conserved as chemical energy. A relative efficiency of 40% occurs for harnessing chemical energy via electron transport-oxidative phosphorylation because the oxidation of a mole of NADH liberates a total of 52 kcal (21 kcal ÷ 52 kcal × 100). The remaining 60% of the energy dissipates from the body as heat. Considering that a steam engine transforms its fuel into useful energy at only about 30% efficiency, the value of 40% for the human body represents a remarkably high efficiency rate.

Role of Oxygen in Energy Metabolism

The continual resynthesis of ATP during coupled oxidative phosphorylation of the macronutrients has three prerequisites.

1. Availability of the reducing agents NADH or $FADH_2$
2. Presence of an oxidizing agent in the form of oxygen
3. Sufficient quantity of enzymes and metabolic machinery in the tissues to make the energy transfer reactions "go" at the appropriate rate

Satisfying these three conditions causes hydrogen and electrons to continually shuttle down the respiratory chain to molecular oxygen during food substrate catabolism. In strenuous exercise, inadequacy in oxygen delivery (condition #2) or its rate of utilization (condition #3) creates a relative imbalance between hydrogen release and oxygen's final acceptance of them. If either of these occur, electron-flow down the respiratory chain "backs up" and hydrogens accumulate bound to NAD^+ and FAD. In a subsequent section, we explain how lactate forms when the compound pyruvate temporarily binds these excess hydrogens (electrons); lactate formation allows electron transport-oxidative phosphorylation to continue.

For aerobic metabolism, oxygen serves as the final electron acceptor in the respiratory chain, and combines with hydrogen to form water during energy metabolism. Some might argue that the term aerobic metabolism is misleading because oxygen does not participate directly in ATP synthesis. Oxygen's presence at the "end of the line," however, largely determines one's capability for ATP production and ability to sustain high-intensity exercise. In this sense, the term aerobic seems justified.

summary

1. The energy contained within the chemical structure of carbohydrate, fat, and protein molecules does not suddenly release in the body at some kindling temperature. Rather, energy release occurs relatively slowly in small amounts during complex, enzymatically-controlled reactions, thus enabling more efficient energy transfer and conservation.

2. About 40% of the potential energy in food nutrients transfers to the high-energy compound ATP.

3. Splitting the terminal phosphate bond of ATP liberates free energy to power all forms of biologic work.

4. ATP represents the body's energy currency, although its limited quantity amounts to only about 3.5 ounces.

5. Phosphocreatine (PCr) interacts with ADP to form ATP; this non-aerobic, high-energy reservoir replenishes ATP rapidly. Collectively, ATP and PCr are referred to as "high-energy phosphates."

6. Phosphorylation represents the process by which energy is transferred in the form of phosphate bonds. In this process, ADP and Cr continually recycle into ATP and PCr

7. Cellular oxidation occurs on the inner lining of the mitochondrial membranes; it involves transferring electrons from NADH and $FADH_2$ to molecular oxygen. This releases and transfers chemical energy to form ATP from ADP plus phosphate ion.

8. During aerobic ATP resynthesis, oxygen (the final electron acceptor in the respiratory chain) combines with hydrogen to form water.

PART 2
Energy Release From Food

The energy released in macronutrient breakdown serves one crucial purpose—to phosphorylate ADP to reform the energy-rich compound ATP (Fig. 4.7). Macronutrient catabolism favors generating phosphate-bond energy, yet the specific pathways of degradation differ depending on the nutrients metabolized. In the sections that follow, we show how ATP resynthesis occurs from extracting potential energy from food macronutrients.

Energy Release from Carbohydrate

Carbohydrates' primary function supplies energy for cellular work. Our discussion of nutrient energy metabolism begins with carbohydrates for four reasons:

1. Carbohydrate represents the *only* macronutrient whose potential energy can generate ATP anaerobically. This becomes important in vigorous exercise that requires rapid energy release above levels supplied by aerobic metabolic reactions.
2. During light and moderate aerobic exercise, carbohydrate supplies about one-half of the body's energy requirements.
3. Processing fat through the metabolic mill for energy requires some carbohydrate catabolism.
4. Aerobic breakdown of carbohydrate for energy occurs at about *twice* the rate as energy generated

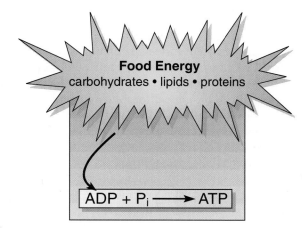

Food Energy
carbohydrates • lipids • proteins

$$ADP + P_i \longrightarrow ATP$$

Figure 4.7
Potential energy in food powers ATP resynthesis.

from fatty acid breakdown. Thus, depleting glycogen reserves significantly reduces exercise power output. In prolonged high-intensity, aerobic exercise such as marathon running, athletes often experience nutrient-related fatigue—a state associated with muscle and liver glycogen depletion.

The complete breakdown of one mole of glucose (180 g) to carbon dioxide and water yields a maximum of 686 kcal of chemical free energy available for work.

$$C_6H_{12}O_6 + 6O_2 \rightarrow 6CO_2 + 6H_2O + 689 \textbf{ kcal per mole}$$

In the body, the complete breakdown of glucose liberates the same quantity of energy, with a significant portion conserved as ATP. Synthesizing one mole of ATP from ADP and phosphate ion requires 7.3 kcal of energy. Therefore, coupling all of the energy from glucose oxidation to phosphorylation could theoretically form 94 moles of ATP per mole of glucose (686 kcal ÷ 7.3 kcal per mole = 94 moles). In the muscles, however, the phosphate bonds only conserve 38% or 263 kcal of energy, with the remainder dissipated as heat. This loss of energy represents the body's metabolic *inefficiency* for converting stored potential energy into useful energy. Consequently, glucose breakdown regenerates a net gain of 36 moles of ATP (net gain because 2 ATPs degrade to initiate glucose breakdown) per mole of glucose (263 kcal ÷ 7.3 kcal per mole = 36 ATP). An additional ATP forms if carbohydrate breakdown starts with glycogen. In the following sections, we describe ATP formation from carbohydrate, fat, and protein during energy transfer.

Anaerobic Versus Aerobic

Glucose degradation occurs in two stages. In stage one, glucose breaks down relatively rapidly into two molecules of pyruvate. Energy transfers occur without oxygen (anaerobic). In stage two of glucose catabolism, pyruvate degrades further to carbon dioxide and water. Energy transfer from these reactions require electron transport and accompanying oxidative phosphorylation (aerobic).

Anaerobic Energy from Glucose: Glycolysis (Glucose Splitting)

The first stage of glucose degradation within cells involves a series of chemical reactions collectively termed **glycolysis** (also termed the Embden-Meyerhof pathway for its discoverers); **glycogenolysis** describes these reactions when they start with stored glycogen. These series of reactions, summarized in Figure 4.8, occur in the watery medium of the cell outside of the mitochondrion. In a way, glycolytic reactions represent a more primitive form of energy transfer, well developed in amphibians, rep-

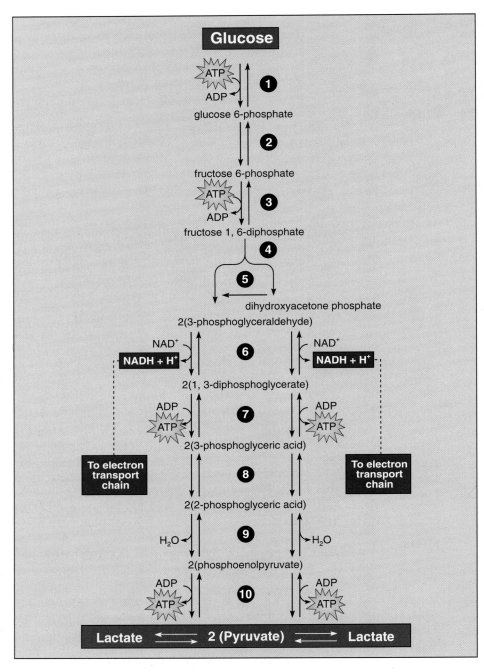

Glucose

① → glucose 6-phosphate

② → fructose 6-phosphate

③ → fructose 1, 6-diphosphate

④

⑤ dihydroxyacetone phosphate

2(3-phosphoglyceraldehyde)

⑥ NAD^+ / $NADH + H^+$

2(1, 3-diphosphoglycerate)

⑦ ADP / ATP

2(3-phosphoglyceric acid)

To electron transport chain

⑧

2(2-phosphoglyceric acid)

⑨ H_2O

2(phosphoenolpyruvate)

⑩ ADP / ATP

Lactate ⇄ 2 (Pyruvate) ⇄ Lactate

Figure 4.8

Glycolysis: Ten enzymatically controlled chemical reactions involve the anaerobic breakdown of glucose to two molecules of pyruvate. Lactate forms when NADH oxidation does not keep pace with its formation in glycolysis.

phosphorylation "primes the pump" for continued energy metabolism. The fructose 6-phosphate molecule gains an additional phosphate and changes to fructose 1, 6-diphosphate under control of the enzyme **phosphofructokinase (PFK)**. *The activity level of PFK probably places a limit on the rate of glycolysis during maximum-effort exercise.* Fructose 1, 6-diphosphate then splits into *two* phosphorylated molecules with three carbon chains; these further decompose to pyruvate in five successive reactions.

Figure 4.9 shows an overview of the glucose-to-pyruvate sequence in terms of the carbon atoms. Essentially, the 6-carbon glucose compound splits into two interchangeable 3-carbon compounds, which ultimately produce two 3-carbon pyruvate molecules and generate useful energy as ATP.

Substrate-Level Phosphorylation

Most of the energy generated in glycolysis reactions does not result in ATP resynthesis, but instead dissipates as heat. In reactions 7 and 10, however, the energy released from the glucose intermediates stimulates the direct transfer of a phosphate group to ADP, generating four molecules of ATP. Because two molecules of ATP were lost in the initial phosphorylation of the glucose molecule, glycolysis generates a *net gain* of two ATP molecules. Note that these specific phosphorylation energy transfers from substrate to ADP do not require oxygen. Rather, energy directly transfers via phosphate bonds in the anaerobic reactions called **substrate-level phosphorylation**. Energy conservation during glycolysis operates at an efficiency of about 30%.

Glycolysis accounts only for about 5% of the total ATP generated during the glucose molecule's complete break-

tiles, fish, and marine mammals. In humans, the cells' limited capacity for glycolysis assumes a crucial role during physical activities that require maximal effort for up to 90 seconds.

In the first reaction, ATP acts as a phosphate donor to phosphorylate glucose to glucose 6-phosphate. In most cells of the body, this reaction "traps" the glucose molecule. In the presence of the enzyme **glycogen synthase,** glucose can now link (become **polymerized**) with other glucose molecules to form glycogen. In energy metabolism, however, glucose 6-phosphate changes to fructose 6-phosphate. At this stage, no energy extraction occurs, yet energy incorporates into the original glucose molecule at the expense of one ATP molecule. In a sense,

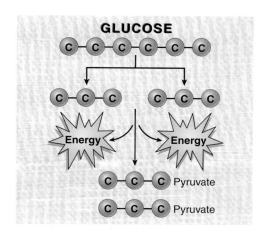

Figure 4.9
Glycolysis: Glucose-to-pyruvate pathway. A 6-carbon glucose splits into two 3-carbon compounds, which further degrade into two 3-carbon pyruvate molecules. Glucose splitting occurs under anaerobic conditions in the watery medium of the cell.

down. However, due to the high concentration of glycolytic enzymes and the speed of the glycolytic reactions, significant energy for muscle action occurs rapidly during this process. The following represent examples of activities that rely heavily on ATP generated via glycolytic anaerobic reactions: sprinting at the end of the mile run, swimming all-out from start to finish in the 50- and 100-m swim, routines on gymnastics apparatus, and sprint-running races up to 200 meters. Anaerobic energy transfer from the macronutrients occurs *only* from carbohydrate breakdown during glycolytic reactions.

Hydrogen Release in Glycolysis
During glycolysis, two pairs of hydrogen atoms become stripped from the substrate (glucose) and their electrons passed to NAD^+ to form NADH (Fig. 4.8). Normally, if the respiratory chain processed these electrons directly, three molecules of ATP would generate for each molecule of NADH oxidized. The mitochondrion in skeletal muscle, however, remains impermeable to NADH formed in

the cytoplasm during glycolysis. Consequently, the electrons from extramitochondrial NADH shuttle indirectly into the mitochondria. In skeletal muscle, this route ends with electrons passing to FAD to form $FADH_2$ at a point below the first formation of ATP (see Fig. 4.6A). Thus two, rather than three ATP molecules form when the respiratory chain oxidizes cytoplasmic NADH. Because two molecules of NADH form in glycolysis, subsequent electron transport-oxidative phosphorylation aerobically generates four ATP molecules.

Lactate Formation
Sufficient oxygen bathes the cells during light to moderate levels of energy metabolism. The hydrogens (electrons) stripped from the substrate and carried by NADH oxidize within the mitochondria to form water when they join with oxygen. In a biochemical sense, a "steady state" or more precisely "**steady rate**" exists because hydrogen oxidizes at about the same rate it becomes available. Biochemists frequently refer to this condition as **aerobic glycolysis**, with pyruvate as the end–product.

In strenuous exercise, when energy demands exceed either oxygen supply or utilization rate, the respiratory chain cannot process all of the hydrogen joined to NADH. Continued release of anaerobic energy in glycolysis depends on NAD^+ availability for oxidizing 3-phosphoglyceraldehyde (see reaction 6 in Fig. 4.8); otherwise, the rapid rate of glycolysis "grinds to a halt." In **anaerobic glycolysis**, NAD^+ "frees-up" as pairs of "excess" non-oxidized hydrogens combine temporarily with pyruvate to form lactate, catalyzed by the enzyme lactate dehydrogenase in the reversible reaction shown in Figure 4.10. Lactate does not represent the sole cause of fatigue because increased acidity by itself does not fully explain decreases in exercise performance or sensation of exhaustion.

The temporary storage of hydrogen with pyruvate represents a unique aspect of energy metabolism because it provides a ready "storage bin" to temporarily hold the end-products of anaerobic glycolysis. Once lactate forms within muscle, it diffuses rapidly into the blood for buffering and rapid removal from the site of energy metabolism. This allows glycolysis to continue supplying additional anaerobic energy for ATP resynthesis. However, this avenue for extra

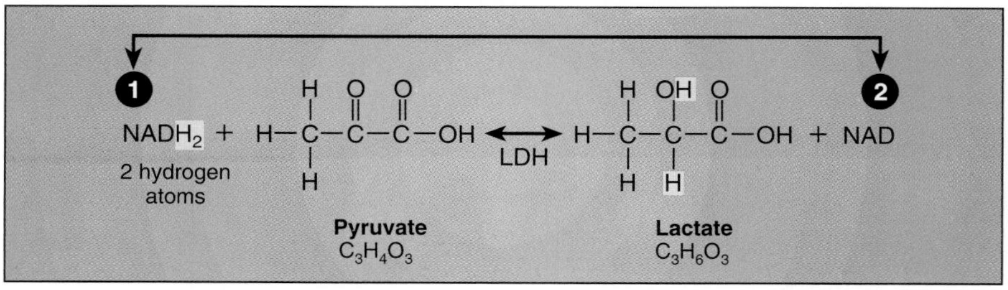

Figure 4.10
Lactate forms when excess hydrogens from NADH combine temporarily with pyruvate. This frees up $NADH_2$ to accept additional hydrogens generated in glycolysis. LDH = lactate dehydrogenase.

energy remains temporary; muscle and blood lactate levels increase and ATP regeneration cannot keep pace with its rate of utilization. Fatigue soon sets in and exercise performance diminishes. Increased acidity probably mediates the fatigue process by inactivating various enzymes involved in energy transfer and diminishing some aspect of the muscle's contractile properties.

Even at rest, energy metabolism in red blood cells forms some lactate because red blood cells contain no mitochondria and must obtain their energy from glycolysis. Lactate should not be viewed as a metabolic "waste product." To the contrary, it provides a source of chemical energy an accumulates in the body during heavy physical exercise. When sufficient oxygen once again becomes available during recovery, or when exercise pace slows, NAD$^+$ scavenges hydrogens attached to lactate; these hydrogens subsequently oxidizes to form ATP. In this regard, circulating blood lactate becomes an energy source because it readily reconverts to pyruvate for further catabolism. In addition, conserving potential energy in the lactate and pyruvate molecules occurs because the liver's **Cori cycle** synthesizes the carbon skeletons of these molecules to glucose (Fig. 4.11). The Cori cycle not only removes lactate, but uses it to resynthesize glucose and subsequently, muscle glycogen (gluconeogenesis). This pathway progresses as follows:

Muscle glycogen → Glucose → Pyruvate → Lactate (which travels to the liver) → Glucose (which returns to muscle) → Muscle glycogen

Aerobic Energy From Glucose: Krebs Cycle

Anaerobic reactions of glycolysis release only about 10% of the energy within the original glucose molecule; thus, extracting the remaining energy requires an additional metabolic pathway. This occurs when pyruvate irreversibly converts to acetyl–CoA, a form of acetic acid. Acetyl–CoA enters the second stage of carbohydrate breakdown known as the **Krebs cycle** (or more descriptively, citric acid or tricarboxylic acid cycle).

Figure 4.12 shows the pyruvate-to-acetyl–CoA reactions. Each three-carbon pyruvate molecule loses a carbon when it joins with a CoA molecule to form acetyl–CoA and carbon dioxide. The reaction from pyruvate proceeds in one direction only.

Figure 4.13 illustrates that the Krebs cycle degrades the acetyl–CoA substrate to carbon dioxide and hydrogen atoms within the mitochondria. Hydrogen atoms oxidize during electron transport-oxidative phosphorylation regenerating ATP. Figure 4.14 shows pyruvate preparing to enter the Krebs cycle by joining with the vitamin B-derivative coenzyme A (A stands for acetic acid) to form the two-carbon compound acetyl–CoA. This process releases two hydrogens and transfers their electrons to NAD$^+$, forming one molecule of carbon dioxide as follows:

$$\text{Pyruvate} + \text{NAD}^+ + \text{CoA} \rightarrow \text{Acetyl–CoA} + \text{CO}_2 + \text{NADH} + \text{H}^+$$

The acetyl portion of acetyl–CoA joins with oxaloacetate to form citrate (citric acid—the same 6-carbon com-

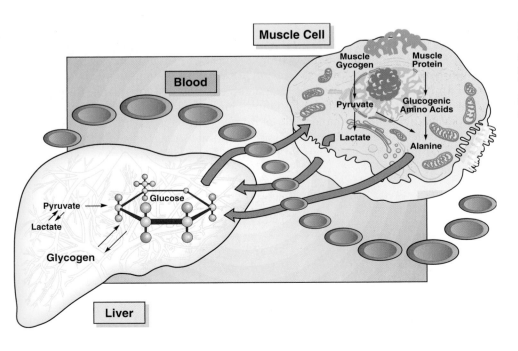

Figure 4.11
The Cori cycle in the liver synthesizes glucose from lactate released from active muscle. This gluconeogenic process maintains carbohydrate reserves.

Figure 4.12
One-way reaction of pyruvate to acetyl–CoA. Two 3-carbon pyruvate molecules join with two coenzyme A molecules to form two 2-carbon acetyl-CoA molecules with 2 carbons lost as carbon dioxide.

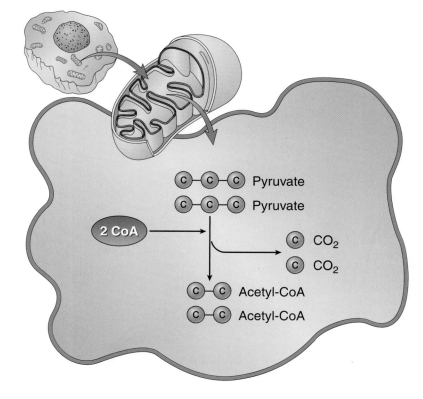

Figure 4.13
Phase 1. In the mitochondrion, Krebs cycle activity generates hydrogen atoms in acetyl–CoA breakdown. **Phase 2.** Significant ATP regenerates when hydrogens oxidize via the aerobic process of electron transport-oxidative phosphorylation (electron transport chain).

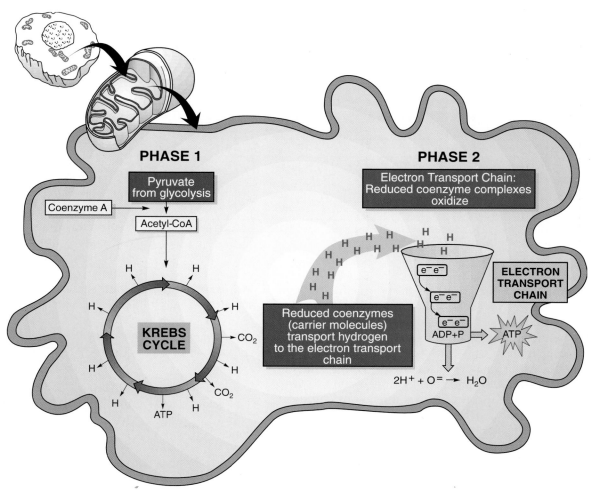

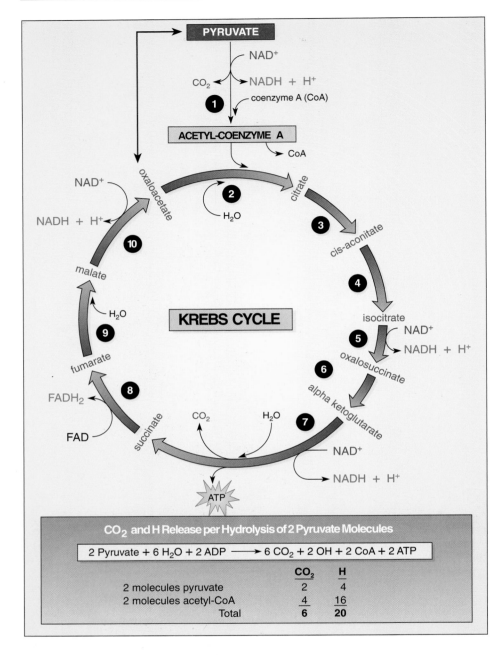

CO₂ and H Release per Hydrolysis of 2 Pyruvate Molecules

$$2 \text{ Pyruvate} + 6 \text{ } H_2O + 2 \text{ ADP} \longrightarrow 6 \text{ } CO_2 + 2 \text{ OH} + 2 \text{ CoA} + 2 \text{ ATP}$$

	CO₂	H
2 molecules pyruvate	2	4
2 molecules acetyl-CoA	4	16
Total	6	20

Figure 4.14

Release of H and CO_2 in the mitochondrion during breakdown of one pyruvate molecule. All values double when computing the net gain of H and CO2 from pyruvate breakdown because glycolysis forms two molecules of pyruvate from one glucose molecule.

cle (acetyl-CoA hydrolysis). *Generating electrons (H) for passage to the respiratory chain via NAD^+ and FAD represents the most important function of the Krebs cycle.*

Oxygen does not participate directly in Krebs cycle reactions. The aerobic process of electron transport-oxidative phosphorylation transfers a considerable portion of the chemical energy in pyruvate to ADP. With adequate oxygen, including enzymes and substrate, NAD^+ and FAD regeneration takes place allowing Krebs cycle metabolism to proceed unimpeded.

Net Energy Transfer From Glucose Catabolism

Figure 4.15 summarizes the pathways for energy transfer during glucose breakdown in skeletal muscle. Two ATP (net gain) form from substrate-level phosphorylation in glycolysis; similarly, 2 ATP come from acetyl–CoA degradation in the Krebs cycle. The 24 released hydrogen atoms (and their subsequent oxidation) can be accounted for as follows:

- Four extramitochondrial hydrogens (2 NADH) generated in glycolysis yield 4 ATP (6 ATP in heart, kidney, and liver)

- Four hydrogens (2 NADH) released as pyruvate degrade to acetyl–CoA to yield 6 ATP

- Twelve of the 16 hydrogens (6 NADH) released in the Krebs cycle yield 18 ATP

- Four hydrogens joined to FAD (2 FADH₂) in the Krebs cycle yield 4 ATP

pound found in citrus fruits) before proceeding through the Krebs cycle. The Krebs cycle continues to operate because it retains the original oxaloacetate molecule to join with a new acetyl fragment.

For each molecule of acetyl–CoA that enters the Krebs cycle, the substrate releases two carbon dioxide molecules and four pairs of hydrogen atoms. One molecule of ATP also regenerates directly by substrate-level phosphorylation from Krebs cycle reactions (see reaction 7 in Fig. 4.14). Note from the bottom of Figure 4.14 that four hydrogens release when acetyl–CoA forms from the two pyruvate molecules created in glycolysis, with an additional 16 hydrogens released in the Krebs cy-

Thirty-eight ATP represent the total ATP yield from the complete breakdown of one glucose molecule. However, because 2 ATP initially phosphorylate glucose, 36 ATP molecules represent the *net ATP yield* from complete glucose breakdown in skeletal muscle. Four ATP molecules form directly from substrate-level phosphorylation (glycolysis and Krebs cycle). In contrast, 32 ATP molecules regenerate during oxidative phosphorylation. Chapter 5 explains the specifics of carbohydrate's role in energy release under anaerobic and aerobic exercise conditions.

Carbohydrate Depletion Reduces Power Output

Carbohydrate depletion depresses work capacity (expressed as a percentage of maximum). Exercise capacity progressively decreases after 2 hours to 50% of the starting exercise intensity. Reduced power directly results from the slow rate of aerobic energy release from fat oxidation, which now becomes the energy pathway.

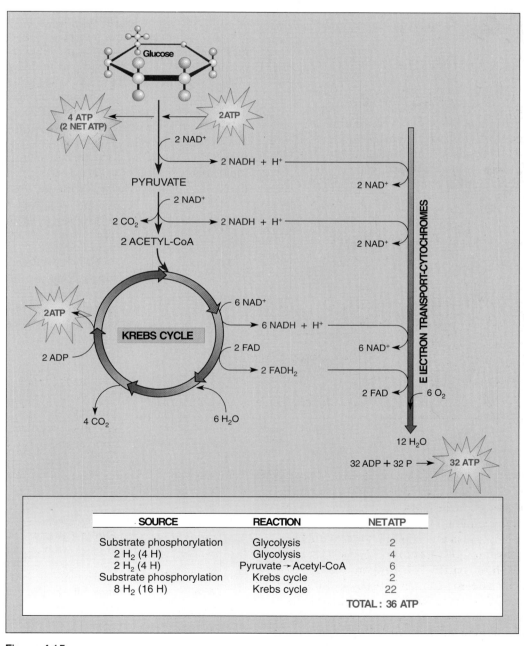

SOURCE	REACTION	NET ATP
Substrate phosphorylation	Glycolysis	2
2 H$_2$ (4 H)	Glycolysis	4
2 H$_2$ (4 H)	Pyruvate → Acetyl-CoA	6
Substrate phosphorylation	Krebs cycle	2
8 H$_2$ (16 H)	Krebs cycle	22
		TOTAL : 36 ATP

Figure 4.15
Net yield of 36 ATP from energy transfer during the complete oxidation of one glucose molecule through glycolysis, the Krebs cycle, and electron transport.

Two Different Types of Muscle Fibers

Muscle Fibers For Sprinting. Fast-twitch muscle fibers contain a rich concentration of the glycolytic enzyme phosphofructokinase. This makes them ideally suited for generating anaerobic energy via glycolysis.

Muscle Fibers For Endurance. Slow-twitch muscle fibers have an ample blood supply and large, numerous mitochondria. This makes them ideally suited for the aerobic combustion of fat and carbohydrate.

Energy Release From Fat

Stored fat represents the body's most plentiful source of potential energy. Relative to carbohydrate and protein, stored fat provides almost unlimited energy. The fuel reserves in an average young adult male represent between 60,000 and 100,000 kcal of energy from triglyceride in fat cells (**adipocytes**), and about 3000 kcal from intramuscular triglyceride stored in close proximity to the mitochondria. In contrast, the carbohydrate energy reserve only contributes about 2000 kcal.

Before energy release from fat, hydrolysis (**lipolysis**) splits the triglyceride molecule into glycerol and three water-insoluble fatty acid molecules. The enzyme lipase catalyzes triglyceride breakdown as follows:

$$\text{Triglyceride} + 3H_2O \xrightarrow{\text{Lipase}} \text{Glycerol} + 3 \text{ Fatty acids}$$

Adipocytes: Site of Fat Storage and Mobilization

All cells store some fat, but adipose tissue represents an active and major supplier of fatty acid molecules. Adipocytes synthesize and store triglycerides. Triglyceride fat droplets occupy up to 95% of the adipocyte cell's volume. Once fatty acids diffuse from the adipocyte and enter the circulation, nearly all bind to plasma albumin for transport to diverse tissues as **free fatty acids (FFA)**. Fat utilization as an energy substrate varies closely with blood flow in the active tissue. As blood flow increases with exercise, adipose tissue releases more FFA to active muscle for energy metabolism. The activity level of the enzyme **lipoprotein lipase (LPL)** facilitates the local cells' uptake of fatty acids for 1) energy use in muscle, or 2) resynthesis (reesterification) of stored triglycerides in muscle and adipose tissue.

FFA do not exist as truly "free" entities. At the muscle site, FFA releases from the albumin–FFA complex to move across the plasma membrane. Once inside the muscle cell, FFA can esterify to form intracellular triglycerides, or bind with intramuscular proteins to enter the mitochondria for energy metabolism. Medium- and short-chain fatty acids do not depend on this carrier-mediated means of transport; most diffuse freely into the mitochondrion.

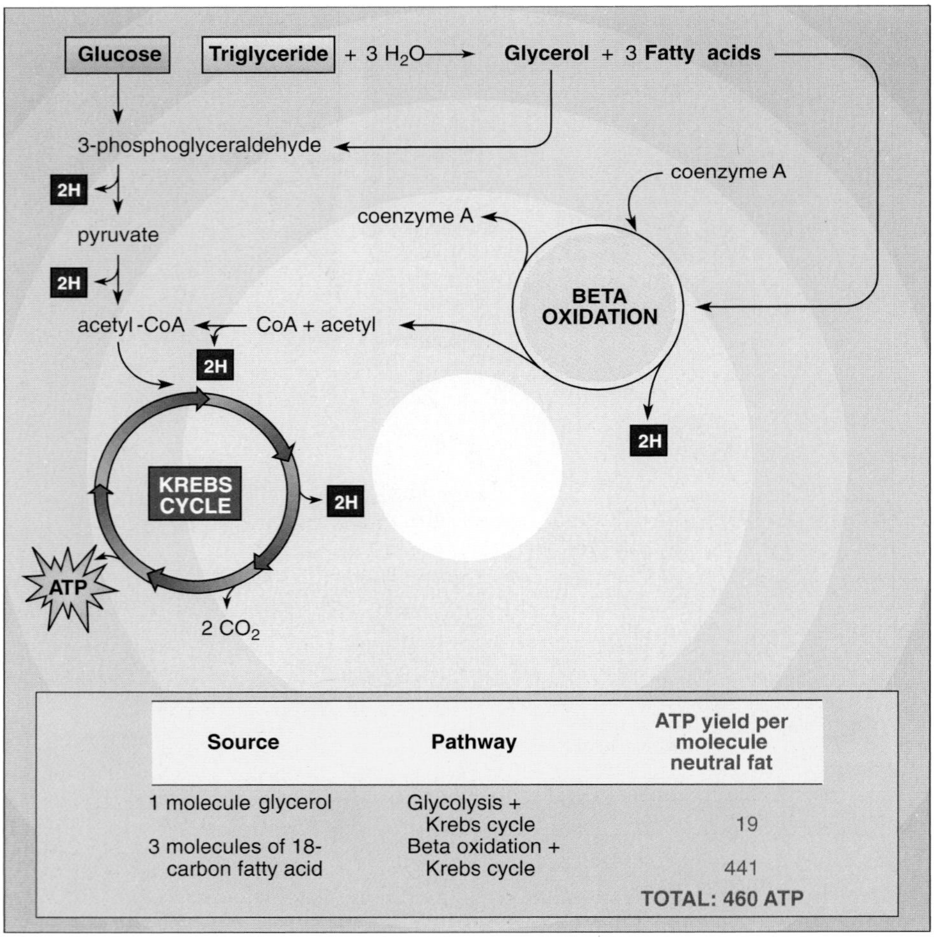

Figure 4.16
Breakdown of glycerol and fatty acid fragments of a triglyceride molecule. Glycerol enters the energy pathways of glycolysis. The fatty acid fragments enter the Krebs cycle via β-oxidation. The electron transport chain processes the released hydrogens from glycolysis, β-oxidation, and Krebs cycle metabolism to yield ATP.

Source	Pathway	ATP yield per molecule neutral fat
1 molecule glycerol	Glycolysis + Krebs cycle	19
3 molecules of 18-carbon fatty acid	Beta oxidation + Krebs cycle	441
		TOTAL: 460 ATP

Breakdown of Glycerol and Fatty Acids

Figure 4.16 summarizes the pathways for the breakdown of the triglyceride molecule's glycerol and fatty acid components.

Glycerol

The anaerobic reactions of glycolysis accept glycerol as 3–phosphoglyceraldehyde, which then degrades to pyruvate to form ATP by substrate-level phosphorylation. Hydrogen atoms pass to NAD^+, and the Krebs cycle oxidizes pyruvate. The complete breakdown of the single glycerol molecule in a triglyceride synthesizes 19 ATP molecules. Glycerol also provides carbon skeletons for glucose synthesis. *The gluconeogenic role of glycerol becomes prominent when glycogen reserves deplete due to dietary restriction of carbohydrates or extended-duration exercise or heavy training.*

Fatty Acids

The fatty acid molecule transforms to acetyl–CoA in the mitochondrion during **β–oxidation** reactions (Fig. 4.17). This involves the successive release of 2–carbon acetyl fragments split from the fatty acid's long chain. ATP phosphorylates the reactions, water is added, hydrogens pass to NAD^+ and FAD, and acetyl-CoA forms when the acetyl fragment joins with coenzyme A. *This acetyl unit is the same one generated from glucose breakdown.* β–oxidation continues until the entire fatty acid molecule degrades to acetyl-CoAs that directly enter the Krebs cycle. Hydrogens released during fatty acid catabolism oxidize through the respiratory chain. Thus, fatty acid breakdown relates directly with oxygen uptake. For β–oxidation to pro-

ceed, oxygen must be present to join with hydrogen. Without oxygen (anaerobic conditions), hydrogen remains joined with NAD^+ and FAD, causing fat catabolism to halt.

Glucose Not Retrievable from Fatty Acids. As mentioned in the previous section, cells can synthesize glucose from pyruvate and other three-carbon compounds. However, glucose cannot form from the two-carbon acetyl fragments of β–oxidation. Consequently, fatty acids cannot readily provide energy for tissues that use glucose almost exclusively for fuel (e.g., brain and nerve tissues). Just about all dietary lipid occurs in triglyceride form. Triglyceride's glycerol component can yield glucose, but the glycerol molecule contains only 3 (6%) of the 57 or so carbon atoms in the molecule (Fig. 4.18). Thus, fat from dietary sources or stored in adipocytes does not provide an adequate potential glucose source; about 95% of the fat molecule *cannot* be converted to glucose.

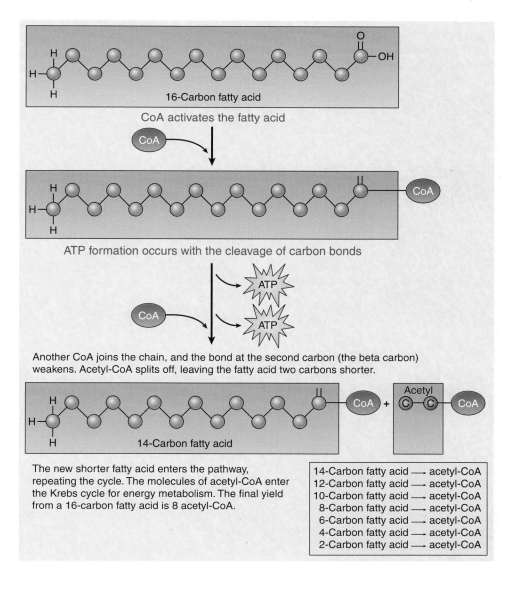

16-Carbon fatty acid

CoA activates the fatty acid

CoA

ATP formation occurs with the cleavage of carbon bonds

ATP

ATP

CoA

Another CoA joins the chain, and the bond at the second carbon (the beta carbon) weakens. Acetyl-CoA splits off, leaving the fatty acid two carbons shorter.

CoA + Acetyl C C CoA

14-Carbon fatty acid

The new shorter fatty acid enters the pathway, repeating the cycle. The molecules of acetyl-CoA enter the Krebs cycle for energy metabolism. The final yield from a 16-carbon fatty acid is 8 acetyl-CoA.

14-Carbon fatty acid ⟶ acetyl-CoA
12-Carbon fatty acid ⟶ acetyl-CoA
10-Carbon fatty acid ⟶ acetyl-CoA
8-Carbon fatty acid ⟶ acetyl-CoA
6-Carbon fatty acid ⟶ acetyl-CoA
4-Carbon fatty acid ⟶ acetyl-CoA
2-Carbon fatty acid ⟶ acetyl-CoA

Figure 4.17
Beta oxidation of a typical 16-carbon fatty acid. Fatty acids break down to 2-carbon fragments that combine with CoA to form acetyl–CoA.

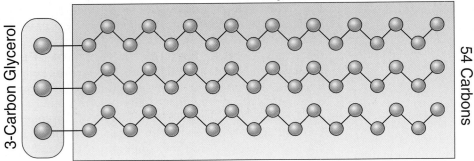

Figure 4.18
Carbon content of a typical triglyceride molecule. Note: one glycerol molecule contains 3 carbons; 3 fatty acid molecules (each with 18 carbons) contain 54 carbons. Only the glycerol portion yields glucose.

Total Energy Transfer From Fat Catabolism

For each 18-carbon fatty acid molecule, 147 molecules of ADP phosphorylate to ATP during β–oxidation and Krebs cycle metabolism. Because each triglyceride molecule contains three fatty acid molecules, 441 ATP molecules form from the triglyceride's fatty acid components (3 × 147 ATP). Also, 19 molecules of ATP form during glycerol breakdown, generating a total of 460 molecules of ATP for each triglyceride molecule catabolized. This represents a considerable energy yield because only a net of 36 ATP form during a glucose molecule's catabolism in skeletal muscle. The 40% efficiency of energy conservation for fatty acid oxidation duplicates glucose oxidation efficiency.

Fat Catabolism in Exercise

Depending on a person's state of nutrition and fitness, and intensity and duration of physical activity, intra- and extracellular fat supply between 30 to 80% of the energy for physical activity. Fat utilization for energy in light and moderate exercise varies closely with blood flow through adipose tissue (three-fold increase not uncommon) and blood flow through active muscle. Adipose tissue releases more FFA for delivery to active muscle as exercise demands increase

Exercise Intensity and Duration Affect Fat Oxidation

On a relative basis, considerable fatty acid oxidation occurs during low-intensity exercise. For example, fat combustion almost totally powers exercise at 25% of aerobic capacity. Carbohydrate and fat contribute energy equally during moderate exercise. Fat oxidation gradually increases as exercise extends to an hour or more and glycogen depletes. Toward the end of prolonged exercise (with glycogen reserves low), circulating FFAs supply nearly 80% of the total energy required.

Fat-Burning Adaptations Within Skeletal Muscle With Aerobic Training

- Facilitated rate of lipolysis and reesterification within adipocytes
- Capillary proliferation in trained muscle creates a greater total number and density of these microvessels
- Improved FFA transport through the plasma membrane of the muscle fiber
- Augmented fatty acid transport within the muscle cell by carnitine and carnitine acyl transferase
- Increased size and number of mitochondria
- Increased quantity of enzymes involved in β–oxidation, Krebs cycle metabolism, and the electron-transport chain within specifically trained muscle fibers

blood flow. Hence, somewhat greater quantities of fat from adipose tissue depots participate in energy metabolism. The energy contribution from intramuscular triglycerides probably ranges between 15 and 35%, with endurance-trained athletes using the greatest amount of intramuscular fat.

Carbohydrate availability also influences fat utilization for energy. With adequate reserves, carbohydrate becomes the preferred fuel, particularly during high-intensity aerobic exercise. Carbohydrate's utilization for energy occurs rapidly compared with fat breakdown's nearly 50% slower rate.

Energy Release From Protein

Protein acts as an energy substrate during endurance-type activities. The amino acids (primarily the **branched–chain amino acids** leucine, isoleucine, valine, glutamine, and aspartic acid) first must convert to a form

How to Estimate Individual Protein Requirement

Total body protein remains constant when nitrogen intake from food (protein) balances its excretion in feces, urine, and sweat. An imbalance in the body's nitrogen content provides 1) an accurate estimate of either protein's depletion or accumulation, and 2) a measure of the adequacy of dietary protein intake. Evaluating nitrogen balance can estimate human protein requirements under various conditions, including heavy exercise training.

> **Nitrogen Balance:** Nitrogen intake equals nitrogen output (no change in body's protein)
>
> **Positive Nitrogen Balance:** Nitrogen intake exceeds nitrogen output (body's protein increases)
>
> **Negative Nitrogen Balance:** Nitrogen intake less than nitrogen output (body's protein decreases)

The magnitude and direction of nitrogen balance in individuals engaged in exercise training depends on many factors including training status, quality and quantity of protein consumed, total energy intake, the body's glycogen levels, and intensity, duration, and type of exercise performed.

Measuring Nitrogen Balance

Nitrogen Intake. Estimate protein intake (g) by carefully measuring total food consumed over a 24-hour period. Determine nitrogen quantity (g) by assuming protein contains 16% nitrogen. Then:

Total Nitrogen Intake, g = Total Protein Intake, g × 0.16

Nitrogen Output. Researchers determine nitrogen output by collecting all of the nitrogen excreted over the same period that assessed nitrogen intake. This involves collecting nitrogen loss from urine, lungs, sweat, and feces. A simplified method estimates nitrogen output by measuring urinary urea nitrogen

(UUN; plus 4 g to account for other sources of nitrogen loss):

Total Nitrogen Output = UUN + 4 g

Example
Male: age, 22 y; total body mass, 75 kg; total energy intake (food diary), 2100 kcal; protein intake (food diary), 63 g; UUN (collection and analysis of urine output), 8 g.

Nitrogen Balance = Nitrogen Intake, g − Nitrogen Output, g
$$= (63 \text{ g} \times 0.16) - (8 \text{ g} + 4 \text{ g})$$
$$= -1.92 \text{ g}$$

This example shows that a daily negative nitrogen balance of −1.92 g occurred because protein catabolized in metabolism exceeded its replacement through dietary protein. To correct this deficiency and achieve nitrogen (protein) balance, the person would need to increase daily protein intake.

ESTIMATED DAILY PROTEIN NEEDS

Condition	Protein Needs (g protein · kg^{-1})
Normal, healthy	0.8–1.0
Fever, fracture, infection	1.5–2.0
Protein depleted	1.5–2.0
Extensive burns	1.5–3.0
Intensive training	0.8–1.5

Estimating Individual Protein Requirements
The table above estimates average protein needs under different conditions. For a healthy person who weighs 70 kg, the protein requirement equals 56 g.

$$0.8 \text{ g} \cdot \text{kg}^{-1} \times 70 \text{ kg} = 56 \text{ g}$$

The same person with a chronic infection or in a protein-depleted state would require an upper-range estimate of 140 g of protein daily.

$$2.0 \text{ g} \cdot \text{kg}^{-1} \times 70 \text{ kg} = 140 \text{ g}$$

that readily enters pathways for energy release. This conversion requires removing nitrogen from the amino acid molecule. The liver serves as the main site for **deamination**, but skeletal muscle also contains enzymes that remove nitrogen from an amino acid and pass it to other compounds during **transamination** (see Fig. 2.10). In this way, the muscle can directly use for energy the "carbon skeleton" byproducts of donor amino acids. In fact, enzyme levels for transamination adapt to exercise training; this may further facilitate protein's use as an energy substrate. Only when an amino acid loses its nitrogen containing amine group does the remaining compound (usually one of the Krebs cycle's reactive compounds) contribute to ATP formation. Some amino acids are **glucogenic**; when deaminated, they yield intermediate products for glucose synthesis via gluconeogenesis. In the liver, for example, pyruvate forms when alanine loses its amino group and gains a double-bond oxygen; this allows glucose synthesis from pyruvate. This gluconeogenic method is an important adjunct to the Cori cycle for providing glucose during prolonged exercise.

Figure 4.19 shows how protein supplies intermediates at three different levels that have energy-producing capabilities. Like fat and carbohydrate, certain amino acids are

Protein Breakdown Facilitates Water Loss

When protein provides energy, the body eliminates the nitrogen-containing amine group (and other solutes produced from protein breakdown). This requires excretion of "obligatory" water because waste products from protein catabolism leave the body dissolved in fluid (urine). For this reason, excessive protein catabolism increases the body's fluid needs.

ketogenic; they cannot synthesize to glucose, but instead when consumed in excess synthesize to fat. Amino acids that form pyruvate provide a carbon skeleton for glucose synthesis by the body, making protein a source for glucose when glycogen reserves run low.

Figure 4.19
Protein-to-energy pathways.

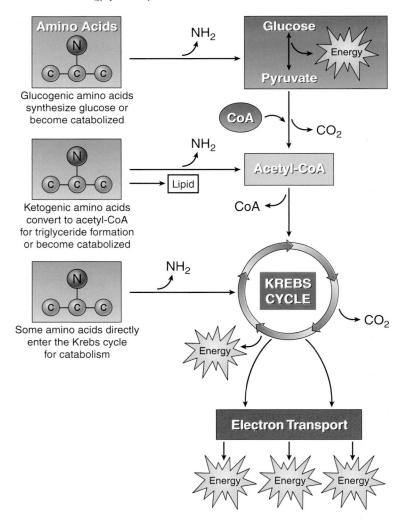

Glucogenic amino acids synthesize glucose or become catabolized

Ketogenic amino acids convert to acetyl-CoA for triglyceride formation or become catabolized

Some amino acids directly enter the Krebs cycle for catabolism

The Metabolic Mill

The Krebs cycle plays a much more important role than simply degrading the pyruvate produced during glucose catabolism. Fragments from other organic compounds formed from fat and protein breakdown provide energy during Krebs cycle metabolism. Figure 4.20 illustrates that deaminated residues of excess amino acids enter the Krebs cycle at various intermediate stages. In contrast, the glycerol fragment of triglyceride catabolism gains entrance via the glycolytic pathway. Fatty acids become oxidized via β-oxidation to acetyl–CoA, which then enters the Krebs cycle directly.

The **"metabolic mill"** depicts the Krebs cycle as the essential "connector" between energy from macronutrient energy and chemical energy of ATP. In addition the Krebs cycle (metabolic hub) provides intermediates to synthesize bionutrients for maintenance and growth. For example, excess carbohydrates provide glycerol and acetyl fragments to synthesize triglyceride. Acetyl–CoA also functions as the starting point for synthesizing cholesterol and many hormones.

In contrast, fatty acids do not contribute to glucose synthesis because pyruvate's conversion to acetyl–CoA does not reverse (notice the one-way arrow in Fig. 4.20). Many of the carbon compounds generated in Krebs cycle reactions provide the organic starting points for synthesizing nonessential amino acids. Amino acids, particularly alanine with carbon skeletons resembling Krebs cycle intermediates after deamination, synthesize to glucose (gluconeogenesis; see Chapter 2).

Fats Burn in a Carbohydrate Flame

Interestingly, fatty acid breakdown depends in part on a continual background level of carbohydrate breakdown. Recall that acetyl–CoA enters the Krebs cycle by combining with oxaloacetate to form citrate (see Fig. 4.14). Depleting carbohydrate decreases pyruvate production during glycolysis. Diminished pyruvate further reduces Krebs cycle intermediates, slowing Krebs cycle activity. Fatty acid degradation in the Krebs cycle depends on sufficient oxaloacetate availability to combine with the acetyl–CoA formed during β-oxidation (see Fig. 4.20). When carbohydrate level decreases, the oxaloacetate level may become inadequate, which reduces fat catabolism. In this sense, "*fats burn in a carbohydrate flame.*"

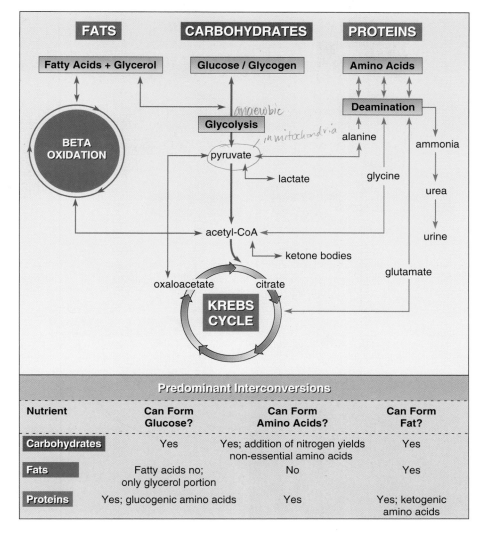

Figure 4.20
"Metabolic mill." Important interconversions between carbohydrates, fats, and proteins.

(Figure labels as shown in the diagram:)

FATS — Fatty Acids + Glycerol — BETA OXIDATION

CARBOHYDRATES — Glucose / Glycogen — Glycolysis (*anaerobic*, *in mitochondria*) — pyruvate → lactate — acetyl-CoA → ketone bodies

PROTEINS — Amino Acids — Deamination — alanine — glycine — ammonia → urea → urine — glutamate

KREBS CYCLE — oxaloacetate — citrate

Predominant Interconversions

Nutrient	Can Form Glucose?	Can Form Amino Acids?	Can Form Fat?
Carbohydrates	Yes	Yes; addition of nitrogen yields non-essential amino acids	Yes
Fats	Fatty acids no; only glycerol portion	No	Yes
Proteins	Yes; glucogenic amino acids	Yes	Yes; ketogenic amino acids

Energy Releases More Slowly From Fat

A rate limit exists for fatty acid use by active muscle. Aerobic training enhances this limit, although the rate of energy generated solely by fat breakdown represents only about one-half the value achieved with carbohydrate as the chief aerobic energy source. Thus, depleting muscle glycogen decreases a muscle's maximum aerobic power output. Just as the hypoglycemic condition coincides with a "central" or neural fatigue, exercising with depleted muscle glycogen probably causes "peripheral" or local muscle fatigue.

Excess Macronutrients Convert To Fat

Excess energy intake from any fuel source can be counterproductive. Figure 4.21 shows how too much of any macronutrient accumulates as body fat. Surplus dietary carbohydrate first fills the glycogen reserves. Once these reserves fill, excess carbohydrate converts to triglycerides for storage in adipose tissue. Excess dietary calories as fat move easily into the body's fat deposits as does any protein

excess. Once deaminated, the carbon residues of excess amino acids readily convert to fat.

Regulation of Energy Metabolism

Under normal conditions, electron transfer and subsequent energy release tightly couple to ADP phosphorylation. In general, without ADP availability for phosphorylation to ATP, electrons do not shuttle down the respiratory chain to combine with oxygen. Compounds that either inhibit or activate enzymes at key control points in the oxidative pathways modulate enzymatic regulatory control of glycolysis and the Krebs cycle. Each pathway has at least one enzyme considered "rate-limiting" because it controls the speed of that pathway's reactions. *By far, cellular ADP concentration exerts the greatest effect on the rate-limiting enzymes that control energy metabolism of the carbohydrate, fat, and protein macronutrients.* This control mechanism makes sense because any increase in ADP signals a need to supply energy to restore ATP levels. Conversely, high levels of cellular ATP signal a relatively low energy requirement, and metabolic rate slows. From a broader perspective, ADP concentrations function as a cellular feedback mechanism to maintain a relative constancy (homeostasis) in the level of energy currency available for biologic work. Other rate-limiting modulators

Excess Protein Accumulates Fat

Athletes and others who believe that taking protein supplements add to muscle beware. Extra protein consumed above what the body requires (easily achieved with a well-balanced "normal" diet) ends up as body fat! If an athlete wants to add fat, excessive protein intake achieves this end. A protein excess does not contribute to muscle tissue synthesis.

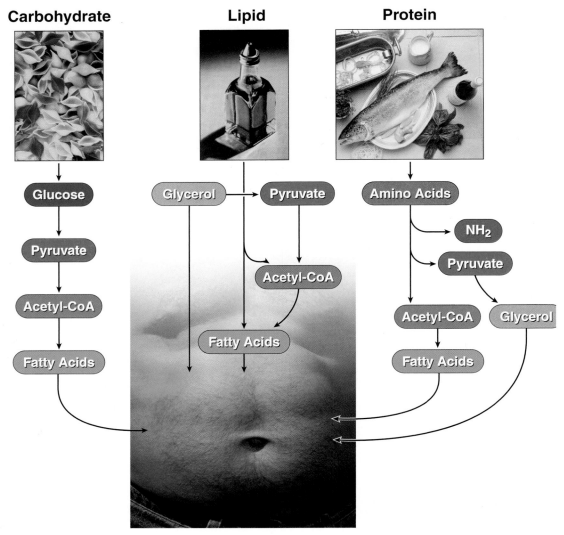

Figure 4.21
Metabolic fate of macronutrient energy surplus.

include cellular levels of phosphate, cyclic AMP, calcium, NAD^+, citrate, and pH.

Acid-Base Regulation and pH

Maintaining the acid-base balance of bodily fluids, a critical component of homeostasis, provides for optimal metabolic functioning and overall physiologic regulation.

Acid

An *acid is any substance that dissociates (ionizes) in solution and releases hydrogen ions (H^+)*. Acids have the following characteristics:

* Taste sour
* Turn litmus indicators red
* React with bases to form salts
* Cause some metals to liberate hydrogen

Examples of acids in the body include hydrochloric, lactic, phosphoric, carbonic, citric, and carboxylic acids.

Base

A *base is any substance that picks up or accepts H^+ to form hydroxide ions (OH^-) in water solutions*. Basic or alkaline solutions have the following characteristics:

* Taste bitter
* Slippery to the touch
* Turn litmus indicators blue
* React with acids to form salts

Examples of bases in the body include sodium and calcium hydroxide, and aqueous solutions of ammonia that form ammonium hydroxide.

pH

*Specifically, **pH** refers to the concentration of protons or H^+.* Solutions with relatively more OH^- than H^+ have a pH above 7.0 and are called basic or **alkaline**. Conversely, solutions with more H^+ than OH^- have a pH below 7.0 and are termed **acidic**. Chemically pure (distilled) water has a pH of 7.0 (neutral) with equal amounts of H^+ and OH^-. The pH scale shown in Figure 4.22, devised in 1909 by Danish chemist Sören Sörensen, ranges from +1.0 to +14.0.

An inverse relation exists between pH and the H^+ concentration ($[H^+]$). Because the pH scale is logarithmic, a one-unit change in pH corresponds to a tenfold change in $[H^+]$. For example, lemon juice and gastric juice (pH = 2.0) have 1000 times greater $[H^+]$ than black coffee (pH = 5.0), whereas hydrochloric acid (pH = 1.0) has approximately 1,000,000 times the $[H^+]$ of blood (pH = 7.4).

The pH of body fluids ranges from a low of 1.0 for the digestive acid hydrochloric acid to a slightly basic pH between 7.35 and 7.45 for arterial and venous blood (and most other body fluids). The term **alkalosis** refers to an increase in pH above the normal average of 7.4; this results directly from of a decrease in $[H^+]$ (increase in pH). Conversely, **acidosis** refers to an increase in $[H^+]$ (decrease in pH). The highly specific acid-base quality of various body fluids remains regulated within narrow limits because of the high sensitivity of metabolism to the $[H^+]$ of the reacting medium.

Enzymes and pH

Many chemical processes in the body occur only at a specific pH. An enzyme that works at one pH becomes inactivated when the pH of its surroundings changes. For example, the fat-digesting enzyme gastric lipase functions effectively in the stomach's highly acidic environment, but ceases to function within the slightly alkaline small intestine. The same occurs for salivary amylase, the enzyme that initiates starch breakdown in the mouth. The pH of the salivary fluids ranges between 6.4 and 7.0. When passed to the stomach (pH 1.0 to 2.0), salivary amylase ceases its digestive function and itself becomes digested by the stomach acids as does any other protein. *As a general rule, extreme changes in pH produce irreversible damage to enzymes.* For this reason, the body's pH (acid-base) balance remains within fairly narrow limits.

Buffers

*The term **buffering** designates reactions that minimize changes in $[H^+]$.* A buffer refers to chemical and physiologic mechanisms that prevent $[H^+]$ changes. If the buffer

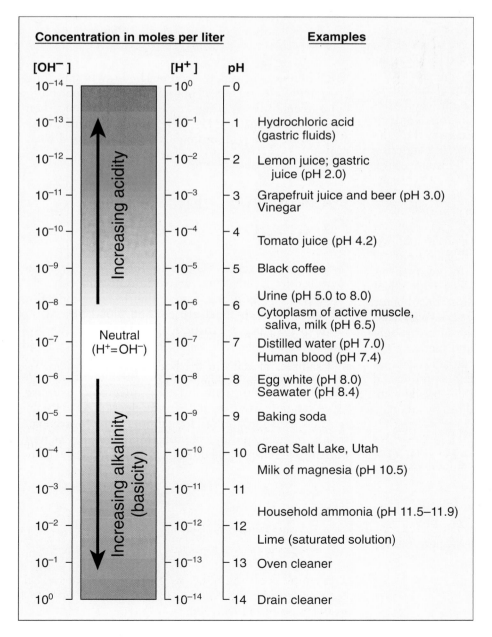

Concentration in moles per liter		Examples
$[OH^-]$	$[H^+]$	pH	
10^{-14}	10^{0}	0	
10^{-13}	10^{-1}	1	Hydrochloric acid (gastric fluids)
10^{-12}	10^{-2}	2	Lemon juice; gastric juice (pH 2.0)
10^{-11}	10^{-3}	3	Grapefruit juice and beer (pH 3.0) Vinegar
10^{-10}	10^{-4}	4	Tomato juice (pH 4.2)
10^{-9}	10^{-5}	5	Black coffee
10^{-8}	10^{-6}	6	Urine (pH 5.0 to 8.0) Cytoplasm of active muscle, saliva, milk (pH 6.5)
10^{-7}	10^{-7}	7	Distilled water (pH 7.0) Human blood (pH 7.4)
10^{-6}	10^{-8}	8	Egg white (pH 8.0) Seawater (pH 8.4)
10^{-5}	10^{-9}	9	Baking soda
10^{-4}	10^{-10}	10	Great Salt Lake, Utah Milk of magnesia (pH 10.5)
10^{-3}	10^{-11}	11	
10^{-2}	10^{-12}	12	Household ammonia (pH 11.5–11.9) Lime (saturated solution)
10^{-1}	10^{-13}	13	Oven cleaner
10^{0}	10^{-14}	14	Drain cleaner

Neutral ($H^+=OH^-$)

Increasing acidity

Increasing alkalinity (basicity)

Figure 4.22

pH scale quantitatively measures the acidity or alkalinity (basicity) of a liquid solution. Blood pH remains regulated at the slightly alkaline pH of 7.4. Values for blood pH rarely fall below a pH of 6.8, even during the most vigorous exercise.

system cannot neutralize deviations in [H$^+$], effective bodily function becomes disrupted, and coma or death ensue. Three mechanisms control the acid-base quality of the body's internal environment:

1. Chemical buffers
2. Pulmonary ventilation
3. Kidney function

Chemical Buffers

The body's chemical buffering system consists of a weak acid and a base or salt of that acid. For example, the bicarbonate buffer consists of the weak carbonic acid and its salt, sodium bicarbonate. Carbonic acid forms when the bicarbonate binds H$^+$. As long as [H$^+$] remains elevated, the reaction produces the weaker acid because the excess H$^+$ bind in the general reaction:

$$H^+ + Buffer \rightarrow H\text{-}Buffer$$

The strong stomach acid, hydrochloric acid (HCl), changes into the much weaker carbonic acid (H$_2$CO$_3$) by combining with sodium bicarbonate. This only slightly reduces the pH. When stomach acid remains elevated during digestion due to inadequacy of the body's buffer response, many individuals ingest neutralizing agents or antacids to provide buffering relief. If, however, [H$^+$] decreases and body fluids shift toward alkaline, the buffering reaction moves in the opposite direction. This process releases H$^+$ and acidity increases:

$$H^+ + Buffer \leftarrow H\text{-}Buffer$$

The body continually produces other acids in addition to digestive juices. Much of the carbon dioxide from energy metabolism reacts with water to form the relatively weak carbonic acid (CO$_2$ + H$_2$O $\rightarrow$ H$_2$CO$_3$), which then dissociates to H$^+$ and HCO$_3$ $^-$. Also, sodium bicarbonate buffers lactic acid, a stronger acid produced during anaerobic metabolism, to form sodium lactate and carbonic acid; in turn, carbonic acid dissociates and increases the [H$^+$] of extracellular fluids. Other organic acids such as fatty acids dissociate and liberate H$^+$, as do the sulfuric and phosphoric acids produced during protein breakdown. The buffering of hydrochloric acid by sodium bicarbonate occurs as follows:

$$HCl + NaHCO_3 \rightarrow NaCl + H_2CO_3 \rightarrow H^+ + HCO_3^-$$

Other chemical buffers available to the body include the phosphate buffers, phosphoric acid and sodium phosphate. These chemicals act similarly to the bicarbonate buffering system. The phosphate buffers regulate the acid-base quality of the kidney tubules and intracellular fluids, which contain a relatively high phosphate concentration. Hemoglobin and other plasma proteins also buffer carbonic acid.

Ventilatory Buffer

The respiratory center increases breathing in response to an increase in [H$^+$] in body fluids. The stimulatory adjustment causes a greater than normal exit of carbon dioxide from blood. Recall that the blood transports carbonic acid after it forms from CO$_2$ and H$_2$O. Thus, reducing the body's carbon dioxide content by hyperventilating acts directly as a ventilatory buffer by reducing carbonic acid concentration, which produces more alkaline body fluids. Conversely, reducing ventilation below normal causes carbon dioxide buildup making body fluids more acidic.

Renal Buffer

The kidneys continually excrete H$^+$ to maintain long-term acid-base quality of body fluids. The renal buffer controls acidity by altering the concentration of bicarbonate ions, ammonia, and H$^+$ secreted into the urine, while at the same time reabsorbing alkali, chloride, and bicarbonate.

Buffering and Strenuous Exercise

In strenuous exercise, large amounts of the metabolic byproduct lactate leave active muscle and enter the bloodstream. Figure 4.23 shows that lactate production dramatically alters local muscle and blood pH. At the point of physical exhaustion, the blood pH often approaches 6.8. The individual becomes disoriented and nauseated with severe headaches. The body's buffering systems continually strive to restrict fluctuations in acid-base balance throughout heavy anaerobic exercise. However, only when exercise ceases does blood pH stabilize and return to normal. In addition to the bicarbonate buffer, hemoglobin and phosphate buffers help as neutralizing agents in blood during vigorous physical activity.

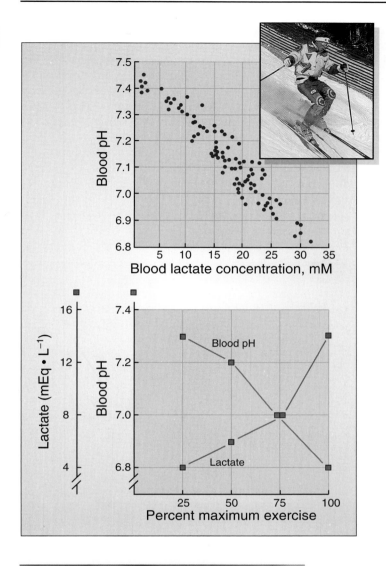

Figure 4.23
Top. Relationship between blood pH and blood lactate concentration at rest and during increasing intensities of short-duration exercise up to maximum.
Bottom. Blood pH and lactate concentration in relation to exercise intensity expressed as a percent of maximum. Decreases in blood pH accompany increases in blood lactate concentrations.

summary

1. The complete breakdown of 1 mole of glucose liberates 689 kcal of energy. Of this, ATP's bonds conserve about 263 kcal (38%), with the remainder dissipated as heat.

2. During glycolytic reactions in the cell's cytosol, a net of 2 ATP molecules form during anaerobic substrate-level phosphorylation.

3. In heavy exercise, when hydrogen oxidation does not keep pace with its production, lactate forms and pyruvate temporarily binds hydrogen. This "buys time" for anaerobic glycolysis to continue for an additional duration.

4. In the mitochondrion, the second stage of carbohydrate breakdown converts pyruvate to acetyl–CoA. Acetyl–CoA then progresses through the Krebs cycle.

5. Hydrogen atoms released during glucose breakdown oxidize via the respiratory chain; the energy generated couples to ADP phosphorylation.

6. Oxidation of one glucose molecule in skeletal muscle yields a total of 36 ATP molecules (net gain).

7. Adipose tissue serves as an active and major supplier of fatty acid molecules. Depending on a person's state of nutrition and fitness, and intensity and duration of physical activity, intra-

and extracellular fat supplies 30 to 80% of the energy for active muscles.

8. The breakdown of a triglyceride molecule yields about 457 molecules of ATP. Fatty acid catabolism requires oxygen; the term aerobic describes such reactions.

9. Protein can serve as an important energy substrate. When deamination removes nitrogen from amino acid molecules, the remaining carbon skeletons enter various metabolic pathways to produce ATP aerobically.

10. Numerous interconversions can take place among the food nutrients. Fatty acids are an exception;

they cannot be synthesized to glucose.

11. Fats require a minimum level of carbohydrate breakdown for their continual catabolism for energy in the metabolic mill. To this extent, "fats burn in a carbohydrate flame."

12. Cellular ADP concentration exerts the greatest effect on the rate-limiting enzymes that control energy metabolism.

13. The chemical and physiologic buffer systems normally regulate the acid-base quality of body fluids within narrow limits. The bicarbonate, phosphate, and protein chemical buffers provide the rapid first line of defense in acid-base regulation. These buffers consist of a weak acid and the salt of that acid. In an acidic condition, buffering action converts a strong acid to a weaker acid and a neutral salt.

14. The lungs and kidneys assist in regulating pH when the chemical buffer system becomes stressed. Changes in alveolar ventilation alter the $[H^+]$ in extracellular fluids. As acidity increases, the renal tubules act as the body's final sentinels by secreting H^+ into the urine and reabsorbing bicarbonate.

thought questions

1. How does aerobic and anaerobic energy metabolism affect optimal energy transfer capacity for a 1) 100-meter sprinter, 2) 400-meter hurdler, and 3) marathon runner.

2. How can elite marathoners run 26.2 miles at a 5-minute per mile pace, yet very few can run just one mile in 4 minutes?

3. In prolonged aerobic exercise like marathon running, explain why exercise capacity diminishes when glycogen reserves deplete, even though stored fat contains more than adequate energy reserves.

4. Is it important for weight lifters and sprinters to have a high ability to consume oxygen?

selected references

Åstrand, P.O., and Rodahl, K.: *Textbook of Work Physiology.* 3rd Ed., New York: McGraw-Hill. 1986.

Bjorntorp, P.: Importance of fat as a support nutrient for energy: Metabolism of athletes. In: *Foods, Nutrition and Sports Performance.* Williams, C., and Devlin, J.T., (eds.). London: E. & F.N. Spon, 1992.

Bodner, G.M.: Metabolism: Part I. Glycolysis, or the Embden-Myerhoff pathway. *J. Chem. Ed.,* 63:566, 1986.

Bodner, G.M.: The tricarboxyclic acid (TCA), citric acid, Krebs cycle. *J. Chem. Ed.,* 63:673, 1986.

Brooks, G.A.: Physical activity and carbohydrate metabolism. In: *Physical Activity, Fitness, and Health.* Bouchard, C., et al., (eds.). Champaign, IL: Human Kinetics, 1994.

Brooks, G.A., et al.: *Exercise Physiology: Human Bioenergetics and its Applications.* 2nd Ed., Mountain View, CA: Mayfield, 1996.

Campbell, M.K.: *Biochemistry.* Philadelphia, W.B. Saunders, 1991.

Cerretelli, P.: Energy sources for muscular exercise. *Int. J. Sports Med.,* 13(Suppl 1):S106, 1992.

Coggan, A.R., et al.: Glucose kinetics during high-intensity exercise in endurance-trained and untrained humans. *J. Appl. Physiol.,* 78:1203, 1995.

Greehnaff, P.I., and Timmons, J.A.: Interaction between aerobic and anaerobic metabolism during intense muscle contraction. *Exerc. Sport Sci. Revs.,* 26:1, 1998.

Hargreaves, M.: Interactions between muscle glycogen and blood glucose during exercise. *Exerc. Sport Sci. Revs.,* 25:21, 1997.

Horton, E.S., and Terjung, R.L.: *Exercise, Nutrition, and Energy Metabolism.* 2nd Ed., New York: Macmillan, 1994.

Jansson, E., and Kaijser, L.: Substrate utilization and enzymes in skeletal muscle of extremely endurance-trained men. *J. Appl. Physiol.,* 62:999, 1987.

Jeukendrup, A.E., et al.: Exogenous glucose oxidation during exercise in endurance-trained and untrained subjects. *J. Appl. Physiol.,* 83:835, 1997.

Lehninger, A.L., et al.: *Principles of Biochemistry.* 3rd Ed., New York: W. H. Freeman and Co., 1999.

MacRae, H.S., et al.: Effects of training on lactate production and removal during progressive exercise. *J. Appl. Physiol.,* 72:1649, 1992.

Mainwood, G.W., and Renaud, J.M.: The effect of acid-base on fatigue of skeletal muscle. *Can. J. Physiol. Pharmacol.,* 63:403, 1985.

Marieb, E.N.: *Human Anatomy and Physiology.* 4th Ed., Boston: Addison-Wesley, Co., 1997.

Martin, W.A.: Effect of acute and chronic exercise on fat metabolism. *Exerc. Sport Sci. Rev.,* 24:203, 1996.

McArdle, W.D., et al.: *Exercise Physiology: Energy, Nutrition, and Human Performance,* 4th Ed., Philadelphia: Lea & Febiger, 1995.

McCann, D.J., et al.: Phosphocreatine kinetics in humans during exercise and recovery. *Med. Sci. Sports Exerc.,* 27:378, 1995.

Mudio, D.M., et al.: Effects of dietary fat on metabolic adjustments to maximal $\dot{V}O_2$ and endurance in runners. *Med. Sci. Sports Exerc.,* 26:81, 1994.

Nicklas, B.J.: Effects of endurance exercise on adipose tissue metabolism. *Exerc. Sport Sci. Rev.,* 25:77, 1997.

Romijn, J.A., et al.: Regulations of endogenous fat and carbohydrate metabolism in relation to exercise intensity and duration. *Am. J. Physiol.,* 265:E380, 1993.

Seip, R.I., and Semenkovich, C.E.: Skeletal muscle lipoprotein lipase: Molecular regulation and physiological effects in relation to exercise. *Exerc. Sport Sci. Rev.*, 26:191, 1998.

Sherman, W.M.: Metabolism of sugars and physical performance. *Am. J. Clin. Nutr.*, 62(Suppl):228S, 1995.

Stefanick, M.L., and Wood, P.D.: Physical activity, lipid and lipoprotein metabolism, and lipid transport. In: *Physical Activity, Fitness, and Health*. Bouchard, C., et al., (eds.). Champaign, IL: Human Kinetics, 1994.

Stryer, L.: *Biochemistry*. 4th ed. San Francisco: W.H. Freeman, 1995.

Thompson, D.I., et al.: Substrate use during and following moderate- and low-intensity exercise: Implications for weight control. *Eur. J. Appl. Physiol.*, 78:43, 1998.

Trump, M.E., et al.: Importance of muscle phosphocreatine during intermittent maximal cycling. *J. Appl. Physiol.*, 80:1574, 1996.

Vander, A.J., et al.: *Human Physiology: The Mechanisms of Body Function*. 7th Ed., New York: WCB/McGraw-Hill, 1997.

Weltman, A.: *The Blood Lactate Response to Exercise*. Champaign, IL: Human Kinetics Publishers, 1995.

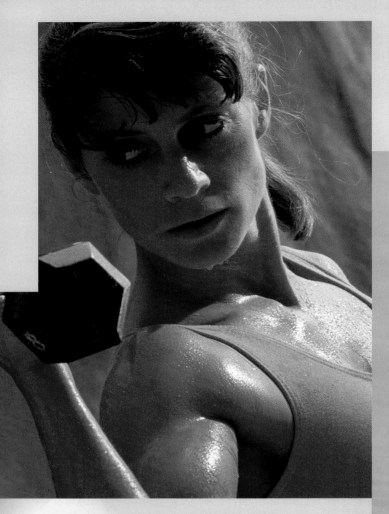

Topics covered in this chapter

Immediate Energy: The ATP-PCr System
Short-Term Energy: The Lactic Acid System
Long-Term Energy: The Aerobic System
Fast- and Slow-Twitch Muscle Fibers
Energy Spectrum of Exercise
Oxygen Uptake During Recovery: The So-Called "Oxygen Debt"
Summary
Thought Questions
Selected References

Human Energy Transfer During Exercise

- Identify the body's three energy systems, and explain their relative contributions to exercise in relation to intensity and duration.

- Describe differences in blood lactate threshold between sedentary and aerobically trained individuals.

- Outline the time course for oxygen uptake during 10 minutes of moderate exercise.

- Draw a figure for the relationship between oxygen uptake and exercise intensity during progressively increasing increments of exercise to maximum.

- Differentiate between the body's two types of muscle fibers.

- Explain differences in the pattern of recovery oxygen uptake from moderate and exhaustive exercise, including what factors account for the EPOC from each exercise mode.

- Outline optimal recovery procedures from steady-rate and non–steady-rate exercise.

- Explain the rationale for using intermittent exercise in interval training programs.

Physical activity provides the greatest stimulus to energy metabolism. In sprint running and cycling whole body energy output in world-class competitors can exceed 40 to 50 times their resting energy expenditure. In contrast, during less intense but sustained marathon running energy requirements still exceed the resting level by 20 to 25 times. This chapter explains how the body's diverse energy systems interact to transfer energy during rest and different exercise intensities.

Immediate Energy: The ATP-PCr System

Performances of short duration and high intensity such as the 100-m sprint, 25-m swim, smashing a tennis ball during the serve, or thrusting a heavy weight upwards require an immediate and rapid energy supply. The high-energy phosphates **adenosine triphosphate (ATP)** and **phosphocreatine (PCr)** stored within muscles almost exclusively provide this energy. The term **phosphagens** identifies these intramuscular energy sources.

Each kilogram of skeletal muscle stores approximately 5 millimoles (mmol) of ATP and 15 mmol of PCr. For a person with 30 kg of muscle mass, this amounts to between 570 and 690 mmol of phosphagens. If physical activity activates 20 kg of muscle, then stored phosphagen energy could power a brisk walk for 1 minute, a slow run for 20 to 30 seconds, or all-out sprint running and swimming for about 6 to 8 seconds. In the 100-meter dash, for example, the body cannot maintain maximum speed for longer than this time, and the runner may actually slow down towards the end of the race. *Thus, the quantity of intramuscular phosphagens significantly influences ability to generate "all-out" energy for brief durations.* The enzyme creatine kinase, which triggers PCr hydrolysis to resynthesize ATP, regulates the rate of phosphagen breakdown.

Although all movements utilize high-energy phosphates, many rely almost exclusively on generating energy rapidly from this "energy system." For example, success in wrestling, weight lifting, routines in gymnastics, most field events such as discus, shot put, pole vault, hammer, and javelin, and baseball and volleyball require brief but all-out, maximal effort. For longer-duration ice hockey, soccer, field hockey, lacrosse, and basketball, other energy sources continually replenish the muscles' phosphagen stores. For this purpose, the stored carbohydrate, fat, and protein macronutrients supply the necessary energy to recharge the available pool of high-energy phosphates.

Short-Term Energy: The Lactic Acid System

The intramuscular phosphagens must continually resynthesize rapidly for strenuous exercise to continue beyond a brief period. During intense exercise, intramuscular stored glycogen provides the energy source to phosphorylate ADP during anaerobic glycogenolysis, forming lactate (refer to Chapter 4, Figs. 4.8, 4.10)

Without adequate oxygen supply (or utilization) to accept all hydrogens formed in glycolysis, pyruvate converts to lactate (pyruvate + 2H → lactate). This continues rapid ATP formation by anaerobic, substrate-level phosphorylation. Anaerobic energy for ATP resynthesis from glycolysis can be viewed as "reserve fuel" that activates when the oxygen demand/oxygen utilization ratio exceeds 1.0, as occurs during the last phase "kick" of a one-mile race. Anaerobic ATP production remains crucial during a 440-m run or 100-m swim, or in **multiple-sprint sports** like ice hockey, field hockey, and soccer. These activities require rapid energy transfer that exceeds that supplied by stored phosphagens. If the intensity of "all-out" exercise decreases (thereby extending exercise duration), lactate buildup correspondingly decreases.

Blood Lactate Accumulation

Chapter 4 pointed out that some lactate continually forms even under resting conditions. However, lactate removal by heart muscle and nonactive skeletal muscle balances its production, yielding no net lactate build-up. Only when lactate removal does not match production does blood lactate begin to accumulate. *Aerobic training produces cellular adaptations that increase rates of lactate removal, so accumulation occurs only at higher exercise intensities.* Figure 5.1 illustrates the general relationship between oxygen uptake (expressed as a percentage of maximum) and blood lactate level during light, moderate, and strenuous exercise in endurance athletes and untrained individuals. During light and moderate exercise in both groups, aerobic metabolism adequately meets energy demands. Non-active tissues rapidly oxidize any lactate formed. This permits

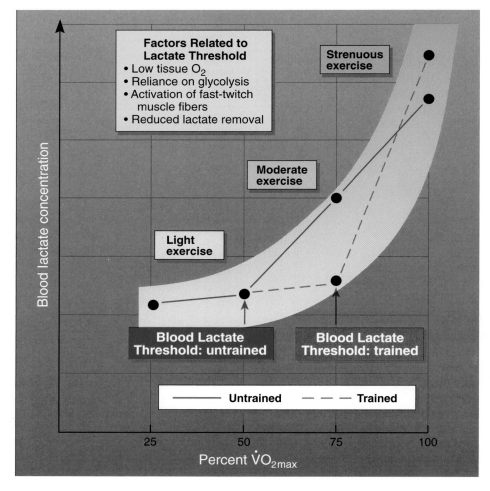

Figure 5.1
Blood lactate concentration at different levels of exercise expressed as a percentage of maximal oxygen uptake for endurance trained and untrained individuals.

blood lactate to remain fairly stable (i.e., no net blood lactate accumulates), even though oxygen uptake increases. In essence, ATP for muscular contraction comes from energy-generating reactions requiring oxidation of hydrogen.

Blood lactate begins to increase exponentially at about 55% of the healthy, untrained person's maximal capacity for aerobic metabolism. The usual explanation for increased blood lactate in heavy exercise assumes a relative tissue hypoxia (lack of oxygen). With lack of oxygen, anaerobic glycolysis partially meets the energy requirement and hydrogen release begins to exceed its oxidation down the respiratory chain. At this point, lactate forms as the excess hydrogens produced during glycolysis pass to pyruvate (see Fig. 4.10). Lactate formation increases at progressively higher levels of exercise intensity when active muscle cannot meet the additional energy demands aerobically.

As Figure 5.1 shows, trained individuals show a similar pattern of blood lactate accumulation, except for the point when blood lactate appearance sharply increases. The point of abrupt increase in blood lactate, known as the **blood lactate threshold** (also termed **onset of blood lactate accumulation**, or **OBLA**), occurs at a higher percentage of an athlete's aerobic capacity. This favorable metabolic response in the endurance athlete could result from genetic endowment (e.g., muscle fiber type distribution), specific local muscle adaptations with training that favor less lactate formation and its more rapid removal rate, or a combination of these factors.

Endurance training significantly increases capillary density and mitochondria size and number. The concentrations of the various enzymes and transfer agents involved in aerobic metabolism also increase. Such alterations enhance the cell's capacity to generate ATP aerobically, particularly via fatty acid breakdown. These training adaptations also extend exercise intensity before the onset of blood lactate accumulation. For example, world-class endurance athletes can perform at sustained high exercise intensities at 85 to 90% of their maximum capacity for aerobic metabolism.

The lactate formed in one part of an active muscle can be oxidized by other fibers in the same muscle, or by less active neighboring muscle tissue. Lactate uptake by less active muscle fibers depresses blood lactate levels during light-to-moderate exercise, and conserves blood glucose and muscle glycogen in prolonged work. The concept of the blood lactate threshold and its relation to endurance performance appears in Chapter 10.

Blood Lactate Threshold

Exercise intensity at the point of lactate buildup (blood lactate threshold) powerfully predicts aerobic exercise performance. The walking speed at which blood lactate began to build up in competitive race walkers predicted their race performance to within 0.6% of their actual race time.

Lactate-Producing Capacity

Capacity to generate high lactate levels during exercise enhances maximal power output for short durations. Because tissues continually use lactate during exercise, lactate accumulation can significantly underestimate total blood lactate production. Ability to generate a high lactate concentration in maximal exercise increases with specific sprint and power training; detraining subsequently decreases this advantage.

Well-trained "anaerobic" athletes who perform maximally for brief periods generate blood lactate levels 20 to 30% higher than untrained individuals with similar exercise. To some extent, increased intramuscular glycogen stores with training contribute a greater amount of energy via anaerobic glycolysis. Enhanced lactate-producing capacity with sprint-type training also may result from improved motivation that often accompanies the trained state (i.e., trained persons "push" themselves harder) and an approximate 20% increase in glycolytic enzyme activity (particularly phosphofructokinase). However these enzymatic changes do not match the impressive two- to three-fold increase in aerobic enzymes induced by aerobic training.

Blood Lactate as an Energy Source

Chapter 4 pointed out how blood lactate serves as substrate for glucose retrieval (gluconeogenesis), and as a direct fuel source for active muscle. Isotope tracer studies of muscle and other tissues show that lactate produced in fast-twitch muscle fibers can circulate to other fast-twitch or slow-twitch fibers for conversion to pyruvate. Pyruvate, in turn, converts to acetyl-CoA for entry to the Krebs cycle for aerobic energy metabolism. Such **lactate shuttling** between cells enables glycogenolysis in one cell to supply other cells with fuel for oxidation. *This makes muscle not only a major site of lactate production, but also a primary tissue for lactate removal via oxidation.*

A muscle oxidizes much of the lactate produced by it, without releasing lactate into the blood. Also, the liver accepts muscle-generated lactate from the blood stream and synthesizes it to glucose via the Cori cycle's gluconeogenic reactions (Chapter 4). Glucose derived from lactate takes one of two routes; it returns in the blood to skeletal muscle for energy metabolism, or it becomes synthesized to glycogen for storage. These uses of lactate make this anaerobic byproduct of intense exercise a valuable metabolic substrate.

Long-Term Energy: The Aerobic System

Although glycolysis releases anaerobic energy rapidly, only a relatively small total ATP yield results from

c l o s e   u p

Overtraining: Too Much of a Good Thing

With heavy and prolonged regular training, especially in endurance sports, certain athletes experience **overtraining**, **staleness**, or **burnout**. As a result, normal exercise performance deteriorates because the individual has difficulty recovering from a workout. The overtrained condition is more than just a short-term inability to train as hard as usual or a slight dip in competition-level performance; rather, it involves a more chronic fatigue experienced both during exercise workouts and subsequent recovery periods. It also is associated with sustained poor exercise performance, frequent infections (particular of the upper respiratory tract), and a general malaise and loss of interest in high-level training. Injuries also are more frequent in the overtrained state. Although the specific symptoms of overtraining are highly individualized, those outlined in the accompanying table generally represent the most common ones. Little is known about the etiology of this syndrome, although neuroendocrine alterations that affect the sympathetic nervous system, as well as alterations in immune function probably are involved. These symptoms persist unless the athlete rests, with complete recovery requiring weeks or even months.

Carbohydrate's Possible Role In Overtraining. A gradual depletion of the body's carbohydrate reserves with repeated strenuous training may contribute to the overtraining syndrome. The figure shows that after 3 successive days of running 16.1 km (10 miles), glycogen in the thigh muscle became nearly depleted. This occurred even though the runners' diets contained 40 to 60% of total calories as carbohydrates. In addition, glycogen use on the third day of the run averaged about 72% less than on day 1. The mechanism by which repeated occurrences of glycogen depletion may contribute to overtraining remains unclear.

Tapering Often Helps. Overtraining symptoms can range from mild to severe. They more often occur in individuals who are highly motivated, in instances where large increase in training occur abruptly, and in situations where sufficient rest and recovery have not been included in the overall training program. Overtraining symptoms are often observed before season-ending competition; therefore, to achieve peak performance, athletes should reduce their training volume and significantly increase carbohydrate intake for several days before competition—a practice called **tapering**. The goal of tapering is to provide time for muscles to resynthesize glycogen to maximal levels, and to allow them to heal from training-induced damage. The optimal length of a taper period varies. Some runners and swim-

Overtraining Signs and Symptoms

Performance-Related Symptoms
- Consistent performance decline
- Persistent fatigue and sluggishness
- Excessive recovery required after competitive events
- Inconsistent performance

Physiological-Related Symptoms
- Decrease in maximum work capacity
- Frequent headaches or stomach aches
- Insomnia
- Persistent low-grade stiffness and muscle/joint soreness
- Frequent constipation or diarrhea
- Unexplained loss of appetite and body mass
- Amenorrhea
- Elevated resting heart rate on waking

Psychological-Related Symptoms
- Depression
- General apathy
- Decreased self-esteem
- Mood changes
- Difficulty in concentrating
- Loss of competitive drive

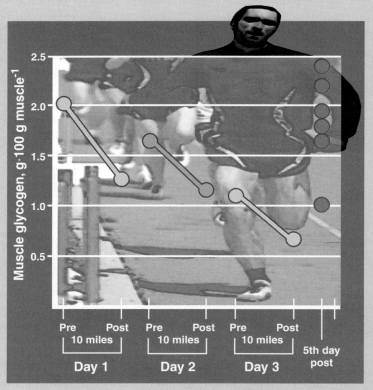

Average changes in muscle glycogen concentration for six male subjects before and after each 16.1·km run performed on three successive days. Individual values for muscle glycogen measured 5 days after the last run is referred to as "5th day post." (From Costill, D.L., et al.: Muscle glycogen utilization during prolonged exercise on successive days. *J. Appl. Physiol.*, 31:834, 1971.)

mers reduce their training load by 60% for up to 21 days without a reduction in performance. More typically, 3 to 7 days of tapering appear adequate.

References

Costill, D.L., et al.: Effects of reduced training on muscular power in swimmers. *Phys. Sportsmed.*, 13:94, 1985.
Krieder, R.B., et al.: *Overtraining in Sport*. Champaign, IL: Human Kinetics, 1998.

Kuipers, H.: Training and overtraining: an introduction. *Med. Sci. Sports Exerc.*, 30:1137, 1998.
Lehmann, M., et al.: Autonomic imbalance hypothesis and overtraining syndrome. *Med. Sci. Sports Exerc.*, 30:1140, 1998.
Raglin, J., and Bardukas, A.: Overtraining in athletes: the challenge of prevention. A consensus statement. *ACSM's Health & Fitness J.*, 3 (2)27:1999.
Raglin, J.S., and Wilson, G.S.: Overtraining in athletes. In: *Emotion in Sports*, Hanin, Y.L. (ed.). Champaign, IL: Human Kinetics, 1999.

this pathway. In contrast, aerobic metabolic reactions provide for the greatest portion of energy transfer, particularly when exercise duration extends longer than 2 to 3 minutes.

Oxygen Uptake During Exercise

The curve in Figure 5.2 illustrates oxygen uptake during each minute of a slow jog continued at a steady pace for 10 minutes. The vertical Y-axis indicates the use of oxygen by the cells (referred to as oxygen uptake or oxygen consumption); the horizontal X-axis displays exercise time. The abbreviation $\dot{V}O_2$ indicates oxygen uptake, where the $\dot{V}$ denotes the volume consumed; the dot placed above the V expresses oxygen uptake as a per minute value. Oxygen uptake during any minute can be determined easily by locating time on the X-axis and its corresponding point for oxygen uptake on the Y-axis. For example, after running 4 minutes, oxygen uptake equals approximately 17 mL·kg·min^{-1}.

From the graph, oxygen uptake increases rapidly during the first minutes of exercise and reaches a relative plateau between minutes four and six. Oxygen uptake then remains relatively stable throughout the remainder of exercise. The flat portion or plateau of the oxygen uptake curve represents the **steady rate of aerobic metabolism**—a balance between energy required by working muscles and the rate of aerobic ATP production. Oxygen-consuming reactions supply the energy for steady-rate exercise; any lactate produced either oxidizes or reconverts to glucose in the liver, kidneys, and skeletal mus-

cles. No accumulation of blood lactate occurs under these metabolic conditions.

Many Levels of Steady Rate

For some individuals, lying in bed, working around the house, and playing an occasional round of golf represent the activity spectrum for steady-rate exercise. A champion marathon runner, on the other hand, can run 26.2 miles in slightly more than 2 hours and still maintain a steady rate of aerobic metabolism. This sub–5-minute-per-mile pace represents a magnificent physiologic–metabolic accomplishment. Maintenance of the required level of aerobic metabolism necessitates well-developed functional capacities to 1) deliver adequate oxygen to active muscles, and 2) process oxygen within muscle cells for aerobic ATP production.

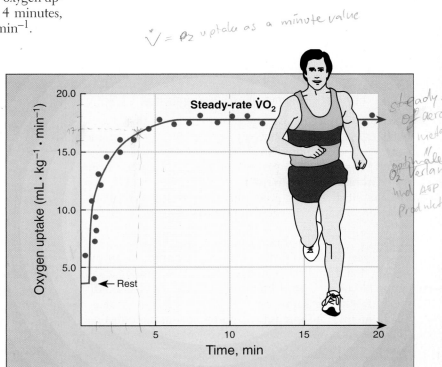

Figure 5.2
Time course of oxygen uptake during continuous jogging at a relatively slow pace. The dots along the curve represent measured values of oxygen uptake determined by open-circuit spirometry described in Chapter 4.

Limited Duration of Steady-Rate Exercise

Theoretically, exercise could continue indefinitely if performed at a steady-rate of aerobic metabolism if the person perserved. However, factors other than motivation limit the duration of steady-rate work. These include loss of important body fluids in sweat and depletion of essential nutrients, especially blood glucose and glycogen stored in liver and active muscle.

Oxygen Deficit

The upward curve of oxygen uptake shown in Figure 5.2 does not increase instantaneously to a steady-rate at the start of exercise. Instead, oxygen uptake remains considerably below the steady-rate level in the first minute of exercise, even though the exercise energy requirement stays essentially unchanged throughout the activity period. The temporary "lag" in oxygen uptake occurs because ATP provides the muscle's immediate energy requirement without the need for oxygen. Oxygen becomes important in subsequent energy transfer reactions to serve as an electron acceptor to combine with the hydrogens produced during:

* Glycolysis
* β–oxidation of fatty acids
* Krebs cycle reactions

A deficit always exists in the oxygen uptake response to a new, higher steady-rate level, regardless of activity mode or exercise intensity.

The **oxygen deficit** *quantitatively represents the difference between the total oxygen actually consumed during exercise and the amount that would have been consumed had a steady-rate, aerobic metabolism occurred immediately when exercise began.* Energy provided during the deficit phase of exercise represents a predominance of anaerobic energy transfer. Stated in metabolic terms, the oxygen deficit represents the quantity of energy produced from stored intramuscular phosphagens plus energy contributed from rapid glycolytic reactions. This yields phosphate-bond energy until oxygen uptake and energy demands reach the steady rate.

Figure 5.3 depicts the relationship between the size of the oxygen deficit and the energy contribution from the ATP-PCr and lactic acid energy systems. Exercise that generates about a 3- to 4-liter oxygen deficit substantially depletes the intramuscular high-energy phosphates. Consequently, this intensity of exercise continues only on a "pay-as-you-go" basis; ATP must be replenished continually through either glycolysis or the aerobic breakdown of car-

bohydrate, fat, and protein. Interestingly, lactate begins to increase in exercising muscle well before the phosphagens reach their lowest levels. This means that glycolysis contributes anaerobic energy early in vigorous exercise even before full utilization of the high-energy phosphates. *Energy for exercise does not merely result from a series of energy systems that "switch on" and "switch off" like a light switch. Rather, a muscle's energy supply represents a smooth transition between anaerobic and aerobic sources, with considerable overlap from one source of energy transfer to another.*

Oxygen Deficit in Trained and Untrained. Figure 5.4 shows the oxygen uptake response to submaximum cycle ergometer or treadmill exercise for a trained and untrained person. Similar values for steady-rate oxygen uptake during light and moderate exercise occur in trained and untrained individuals. The trained person, however, reaches the steady rate quicker; hence, this person has a smaller oxygen deficit for the same exercise duration compared with the untrained person. This means a greater total oxygen consumed during exercise for the trained person, with a proportionately smaller

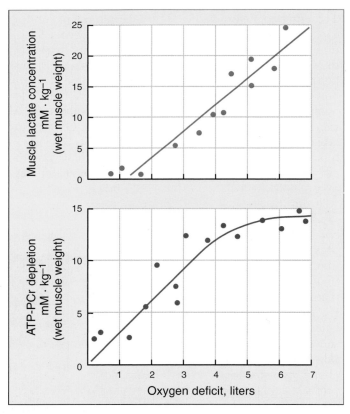

Figure 5.3

Muscle ATP and PCr depletion and muscle lactate concentration related to the oxygen deficit. (Adapted from Pernow, B., and Karlsson, J.: Muscle ATP, CP and lactate in submaximal and maximal exercise. In: *Muscle Metabolism During Exercise.* Pernow. B., and Saltin, B., (eds.). New York: Plenum Press, 1971.)

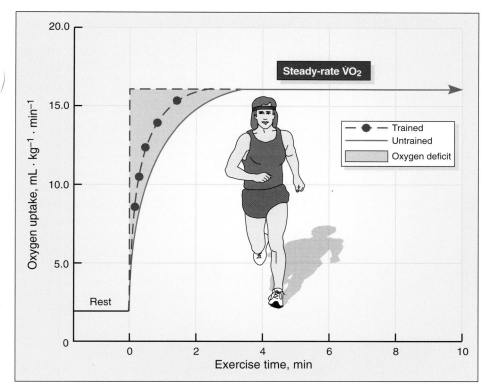

Figure 5.4
Oxygen uptake and deficit for trained and untrained individuals during submaximum cycle ergometer exercise. Both individuals reach the same steady-rate $\dot{V}O_2$ but the trained person reaches it at a faster rate, reducing the oxygen deficit.

Maximal Oxygen Uptake

Figure 5.5 depicts the curve for oxygen uptake during a series of constant-speed runs up six hills, each progressively steeper than the next. In the laboratory these "hills" are simulated by increasing treadmill elevation, raising the height of a step bench, providing greater resistance to pedaling a bicycle ergometer, or increasing the onward rush of water while a swimmer tries to maintain speed in a swim flume. Each successive hill (equivalent to an increase in exercise intensity or load) requires greater energy output, and thus an additional demand for aerobic metabolism. Increases in oxygen uptake relate linearly and in direct proportion to exercise intensity during the climb up the first several hills. The runner maintains speed up the last two hills, yet oxygen uptake does not increase by the same magnitude as in the prior hills. In fact, oxygen uptake does not increase during the run up the last hill. *The maximal oxygen uptake or simply $\dot{V}O_{2max}$ describes the region where oxygen uptake plateaus and does not increase (or increases only slightly) despite an additional increase in exercise intensity.* The $\dot{V}O_{2max}$ holds great physiologic significance because of its dependence on the functional capacity and

anaerobic energy transfer component. A likely explanation for the differences in oxygen deficit between trained and untrained individuals relates to a more highly developed aerobic bioenergetic capacity of the trained person. An augmented aerobic capacity results from either improved central cardiovascular function, or training-induced local muscular adaptations that increase a muscle's capacity to generate ATP aerobically (refer to Chapter 11). These adaptations trigger earlier aerobic ATP production in exercise with less lactate formation for the trained person.

Figure 5.5
Attainment of maximal oxygen uptake ($\dot{V}O_{2max}$) while running up hills of increasing slope. This occurs in the region where a further increase in exercise intensity does not produce an additional increase in oxygen uptake. The red dots represent measured values for oxygen uptake during the run up each hill.

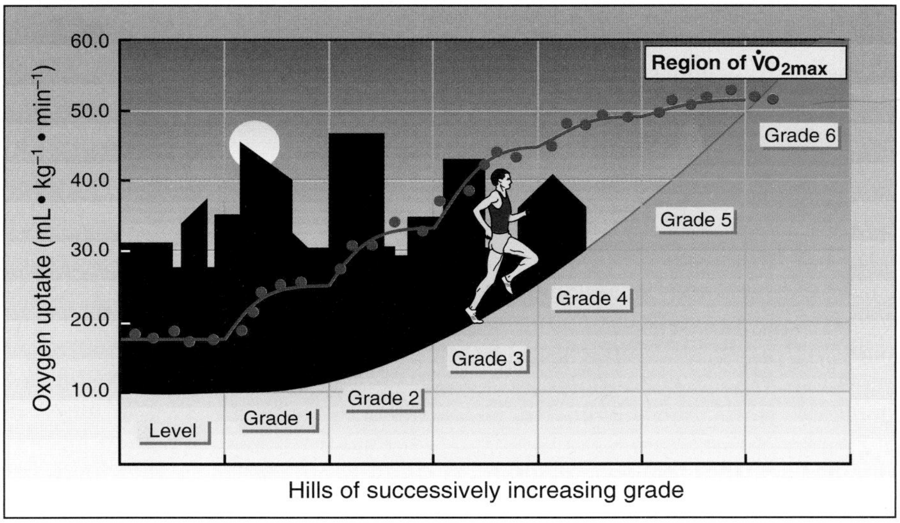

integration of the systems required for oxygen supply, transport, delivery, and utilization.

The $\dot{V}O_{2max}$ indicates an individual's capacity for aerobically resynthesizing ATP. Exercise performed above $\dot{V}O_{2max}$ can only take place by energy transfer predominantly from anaerobic glycolysis with lactate formation. Under such conditions, performance deteriorates, and the individual cannot continue at that exercise intensity. A large build up of lactate, due to the additional anaerobic muscular effort, disrupts the already high rate of energy transfer for the aerobic resynthesis of ATP. To borrow an analogy from business economics: supply (aerobic resynthesis of ATP) does not meet demand (aerobic energy required for muscular effort). An aerobic energy supply-demand imbalance affects production (lactate accumulates) and compromises exercise performance.

Because of the importance of aerobic capacity in exercise physiology, subsequent chapters cover more detailed aspects of $\dot{V}O_{2max}$, including its measurement, physiologic significance, and role in endurance performance.

Fast- and Slow-Twitch Muscle Fibers

Exercise physiologists have applied invasive biopsy techniques to study the functional and structural characteristics of human skeletal muscle (see Chapter 1, page 21). The biopsy procedure uses a special needle to puncture the muscle and obtain approximately 20 to 40 mg of tissue (the size of a grain of rice) for chemical and microscopic analysis. Two distinct fiber types have been identified in human skeletal muscle: fast-twitch and slow-twitch. The proportion of each fiber type within a particular muscle probably remains fairly constant throughout life.

Fast-Twitch Fiber

Fast-twitch muscle fibers, also known as *Type II fibers, possess a high capacity for anaerobic ATP production during glycolysis.* These fibers have a rapid contraction speed; they become activated in sprint activities that depend almost entirely on anaerobic metabolism for energy. The metabolic capabilities of fast-twitch fibers also become important in stop-and-go or change-off-pace sports like basketball, soccer, lacrosse, and field hockey. These sports often require rapid energy transfer through anaerobic metabolism.

Slow-Twitch Fiber

*The **slow-twitch muscle fibers** or Type I fibers have a contraction speed about one-half as fast as its fast-twitch counterpart.* Slow-twitch fibers possess numerous mitochondria and high enzyme concentration to sustain aerobic metabolism. They demonstrate a much greater capacity to generate ATP aerobically than fast-twitch fibers. As such, slow-twitch muscle fiber activation predominates in endurance activities that depend almost exclusively on aerobic metabolism. Middle-distance running or swimming, or basketball, field hockey, and soccer, require a blend of both

---

Oxygen Uptake and Body Size

To adjust for the effects of variations in body size on oxygen uptake (i.e., bigger people usually consume more oxygen), researchers frequently express oxygen uptake in terms of body mass (termed **relative oxygen uptake**), as milliliters of oxygen per kilogram of body mass per minute (mL $\cdot$ kg^{-1} $\cdot$ min^{-1}). At rest, this averages about 3.5 mL $\cdot$ kg^{-1} $\cdot$ min^{-1}, or 245 mL $\cdot$ min^{-1} (**absolute oxygen uptake**) for a 70-kg person. Other means of relating oxygen uptake to aspects of body size and body composition include milliliters of oxygen per kilogram of fat-free body mass per minute (mL $\cdot$ kg FFM^{-1} $\cdot$ min^{-1}), and sometimes as milliliters of oxygen per square centimeter of muscle cross-sectional area per minute (mL $\cdot$ cm MCSA^{-2} $\cdot$ min^{-1}).

---

aerobic and anaerobic capacities. Both types of muscle fibers become activated in such sports.

From the preceding discussion, do you think that the predominant fiber type in specific muscles contributes to success in a particular sport or activity? In Chapter 12, we discuss this idea and other aspects of each type of muscle fiber and their subdivisions.

Energy Spectrum of Exercise

Figure 5.6 depicts the relative contributions of anaerobic and aerobic energy sources during various durations of maximal exercise. The data represent estimates from laboratory experiments of all-out treadmill running and stationary bicycling. They also can relate to other activities by drawing the appropriate time relationships. For example, a 100-m sprint run equates to any all-out activity lasting about 10 seconds, while an 800-m run lasts approximately 2 minutes. All-out exercise for 1 minute includes the 400-m dash in track, the 100-m swim, and multiple full-court presses during a basketball game.

Intensity and Duration Determine the Blend

The body's energy transfer systems should be viewed along a continuum of exercise bioenergetics. Anaerobic sources supply most of the energy for fast movements, or during increased resistance to movement at a given speed. Also, when movement begins at either fast or slow speed (from performing a front handspring to starting a marathon run), the intramuscular phosphagens provide immediate anaerobic energy for the required muscle actions.

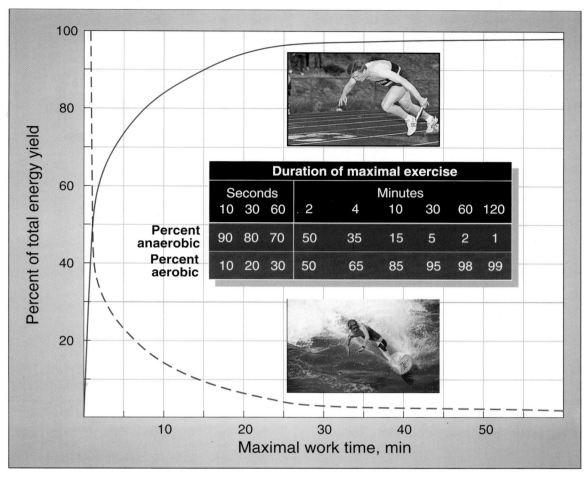

Figure 5.6
Relative contribution of aerobic and anaerobic energy metabolism during maximal physical effort of various durations; 2 minutes of maximal effort requires about 50% of the energy from both aerobic and anaerobic processes. At a world-class 4-minute mile pace, aerobic metabolism supplies approximately 65% of the energy, with the remainder generated from anaerobic processes. (Adapted from Astrand, P.O., and Rodahl, K.: *Textbook of Work Physiology.* New York: McGraw-Hill Book Company, 1977.)

At the short-duration extreme of maximum effort, the intramuscular phosphagens ATP and PCr supply the major energy for the entire exercise. The ATP-PCr and lactic acid systems provide about one-half of the energy required for "best-effort" exercise lasting 2 minutes, whereas aerobic reactions provide the remainder. For top performance in all-out, 2-minute exercise, a person must possess a well-developed capacity for both aerobic and anaerobic metabolism. Intense exercise of intermediate duration performed for 5 to 10 minutes, like middle-distance running and swimming or stop-and-go sports like basketball and soccer, demands greater aerobic energy transfer. Longer-duration marathon running, distance swimming and cycling, recreational jogging, cross-country skiing, and hiking and backpacking require a continual energy supply derived aerobically without reliance on lactate formation.

Intensity and duration determine which energy system and metabolic mixture predominate during exercise. The aerobic system predominates in low-intensity exercise with fat serving as the primary fuel source. The liver markedly increases its release of glucose to active muscle as exercise progresses from low to high intensity. Simultaneously, glycogen stored within muscle serves as the predominant carbohydrate energy source during the early stages of exercise, and when exercise intensity increases. *During high-intensity aerobic exercise, the advantage of selective dependence on carbohydrate metabolism lies in its two times more rapid energy transfer capacity compared with fat and protein fuels.* Compared with fat, carbohydrate also generates about 6% greater energy per unit oxygen consumed. As exercise continues and muscle glycogen depletes, progressively more fat (intramuscular triglycerides and circulating FFA) enters the metabolic mixture for ATP production. In maximal anaerobic effort (reactions of glycolysis), carbohydrate becomes the sole contributor to ATP production.

A sound approach to exercise training analyzes an activity for its specific energy components and then establishes a training regimen to ensure optimal physiologic and metabolic adaptations. An improved capacity for energy transfer usually improves exercise performance.

How to Measure Work On a Treadmill, Cycle Ergometer, and Step Bench

An ergometer is an exercise apparatus that quantifies and standardizes physical exercise in terms of work and/or power output. The most common ergometers include treadmill, cycle and arm-crank ergometers, stair steppers, and rowers.

Work (W) represents application of force (F) through a distance (D):

$$W = F \times D$$

For example, for a body mass of 70 kg and vertical jump score of 0.5 m, work accomplished equals 35 kilogram-meters (kg-m) (70 kg × 0.5 m). The most common units of measurement to express work include: kilogram-meters (kg-m), foot-pounds (ft-lb), joules (J), Newton-meters (Nm), and kilocalories (kcal).

Power (P) represents W performed per unit time (T):

$$P = F \times D \div T$$

Calculation of Treadmill Work

Picture the treadmill as a moving conveyor belt with variable angle of incline and speed. Work performed on a treadmill equals the product of the weight (mass) of the person (F) and the vertical distance (vert. dist) the person achieves walking or running up the incline. Vert. dist equals the sine of the treadmill angle (theta or θ) multiplied by the distance traveled along the incline (treadmill speed × time).

W = Body Mass (Force) × Vertical Distance

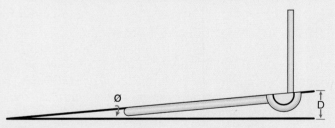

Example

For an angle θ of 8° (measured with an inclinometer or determined by knowing the percent grade of the treadmill), the sine of angle θ equals 0.1392 (see table). The vert. dist. represents treadmill speed multiplied by exercise duration multiplied by Sine θ. For example, vert. dist. on the incline while walking at 5000 m · h^{-1} for 1 hour equals 696 m (5000 × 0.1392). If a person with a body mass of 50 kg walked on a treadmill at an incline of 8° (percent grade = approximately 14%) for 60 minutes at 5000 m · h^{-1}, work accomplished computes as:

$$W = F \times \text{vert. dist. (Sine } \theta \times D)$$
$$= 50 \text{ kg} \times (0.1392 \times 5000 \text{ m})$$
$$= 34,800 \text{ kg-m}$$

The value for power equals 34,800 kg-m ÷ 60 minutes or 580 kg-m · min^{-1}.

Ø (deg)	Sine Ø	Tangent Ø	Percent grade
1	0.0175	0.0175	1.75
2	0.0349	0.0349	3.49
3	0.0523	0.0523	5.23
4	0.0698	0.0698	6.98
5	0.0872	0.0872	8.72
6	0.1045	0.1051	10.51
7	0.1219	0.1228	12.28
8	0.1392	0.1405	14.05
9	0.1564	0.1584	15.84
10	0.1736	0.1763	17.63
15	0.2588	0.2680	26.80
20	0.3420	0.3640	36.40

Calculation of Cycle Ergometer Work

The mechanically braked cycle ergometer contains a flywheel with a belt around it connected by a small spring at one end and an adjustable tension lever at the other end. A pendulum balance indicates the resistance against the flywheel as it turns. Increasing the tension on the belt increases flywheel friction, which increases resistance to pedaling. The force (flywheel friction) represents braking load in kg or kilopounds (kp = force acting on 1-kg mass at the normal acceleration of gravity). The distance traveled equals number of pedal revolutions times flywheel circumference.

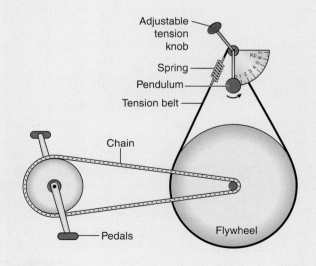

Example

A person pedaling a bicycle ergometer with a 6-m flywheel circumference at 60 rpm for 1 minute covers a distance (D) of 360 m each minute (6 m × 60). If the frictional resistance on the flywheel equals 2.5 kg, total work computes as:

$$W = F \times D$$
$$= \text{Frictional resistance} \times \text{Distance traveled}$$
$$= 2.5 \text{ kg} \times 360 \text{ m}$$
$$= 900 \text{ kg-m}$$

Power generated by the effort equals 900 kg-m in 1 min or 900 kg-m $\cdot$ min^{-1} (900 kg-m $\div$ 1 min).

Calculation of Work During Bench Stepping

Only the vertical (positive) work can be calculated in bench stepping. Distance (D) computes as bench height times the number of times the person steps; force (F) equals the person's body mass (kg).

Example

If a 70-kg person steps on a bench 0.375 meters high at a rate of 30 steps per min for 10 minutes, total work computes as:

$$W = F \times D$$
$$= \text{Body Mass, kg} \times (\text{Vertical distance (m)} \times \text{steps per min} \times 10 \text{ min})$$
$$= 70 \text{ kg} \times (0.375 \text{ m} \times 30 \times 10)$$
$$= 7875 \text{ kg-m}$$

Power generated during stepping equals 787 kg–m$\cdot$min^{-1} (7875 kg-m $\div$ 10 min). ■

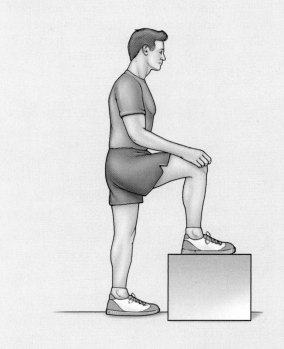

Nutrient-Related Fatigue

Severe depletion of liver and muscle glycogen during exercise induces fatigue, despite sufficient oxygen availability to muscle and an almost unlimited potential energy from stored fat. Endurance athletes commonly refer to this extreme sensation of fatigue as **"bonking"** or **hitting the wall**. (The image of hitting the wall suggests an inability to continue exercising, which in reality does not occur, although pain exists in the active muscles, and exercise intensity decreases markedly.) Skeletal muscle does not contain the **phosphatase enzyme** (present in liver) that releases glucose from cells; thus, relatively inactive muscles retain all of their glycogen. Controversy exists as to why liver and muscle glycogen depletion during prolonged exercise reduces exercise capacity. Part of the answer relates to:

- Central nervous system's use of blood glucose for energy
- Muscle glycogen's role as a "primer" in fat catabolism
- Significantly slower rate of energy release from fat compared with carbohydrate breakdown

Oxygen Uptake During Recovery: The So-Called "Oxygen Debt"

Bodily processes do not immediately return to resting levels after exercise ceases. In light exercise (e.g., golf, archery, bowling), recovery to a resting condition takes place rapidly and often progresses unnoticed. With particularly intense physical activity (running full speed for 800 m or trying to swim 200 m as fast as possible), however, it takes considerable time for the body to return to

---

It's Difficult to Excel in All Sports

An understanding of the energy requirements of various physical activities partly explains why a world-record holder in the 1-mile run does not achieve similar success as a long distance runner. Conversely, premier marathoners usually cannot run one mile in less than 4 minutes, yet they complete a 26-mile race averaging a 5-minute per mile pace.

resting levels. The difference in recovery from light and strenuous exercise relates largely to the specific metabolic and physiologic processes in each exercise mode.

A.V. Hill (1886–1977), the British Nobel physiologist (see Chapter 1), referred to oxygen uptake during recovery as the **oxygen debt**. Contemporary theory no longer uses this term. Instead, **recovery oxygen uptake** or **excess post-exercise oxygen consumption (EPOC)** defines the excess oxygen uptake above the resting level in recovery. The meaning refers to the total oxygen consumed after exercise in excess of a pre-exercise baseline level.

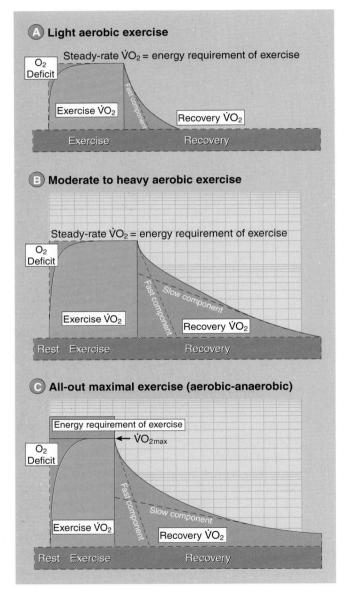

Figure 5.7
Oxygen uptake during exercise and recovery from (**A**) light steady-rate exercise, (**B**) moderate to heavy steady-rate exercise, and (**C**) exhaustive exercise with no steady-rate of aerobic metabolism. The first phase (fast component) of recovery occurs rapidly; the second phase (slow component) progresses more slowly and may take considerable time to return to resting conditions. In exhaustive exercise, the oxygen requirement of exercise exceeds the measured exercise oxygen uptake.

Panel A in Figure 5.7 shows that light exercise rapidly attains steady rate and a small oxygen deficit. Rapid recovery ensues from such exercise with an accompanying small EPOC. In moderate to heavy aerobic exercise (Panel B), it takes longer to reach steady rate, and the oxygen deficit becomes considerably larger compared with light exercise. Oxygen uptake in recovery from this relatively strenuous aerobic exercise returns more slowly to the pre-exercise resting level. Recovery oxygen uptake (similar to recovery from light exercise) initially declines rapidly followed by a more gradual decline to the baseline. In both Panels A and B, computation of the oxygen deficit and EPOC uses the steady-rate oxygen uptake to represent the exercise oxygen (energy) requirement. During exhausting exercise, illustrated in Panel C, a steady rate of aerobic metabolism cannot be attained. This produces large amounts of lactate. Blood lactate then accumulates and it takes oxygen uptake considerable time to return to the pre-exercise level. It becomes nearly impossible to determine the true oxygen deficit in such exercise because no steady rate exists, and the energy requirement exceeds the individual's maximal oxygen uptake.

No matter how intense the exercise (walking, bowling, golf, sailboarding, wrestling, cross-country skiing, or sprint running), an oxygen uptake in excess of the resting value always exists when exercise stops. The shaded area under the recovery curve in the figure indicates this quantity of oxygen; it equals the total oxygen consumed in recovery (until attaining the baseline level) minus the total oxygen that would normally be consumed at rest for an equivalent duration.

If a total of 5.5 liters equals the oxygen uptake in recovery until reaching the resting value of $0.31 \text{ L} \cdot \text{min}^{-1}$, and full recovery required 10 minutes, the EPOC would compute as 5.5 liters minus 3.1 liters ($0.31 \text{ L} \times 10 \text{ min}$), or 2.4 liters. The exercise resulted in the uptake of an additional 2.4 liters of oxygen after exercise stopped. An assumption underlying discussions of the physiologic meaning of EPOC holds that resting oxygen uptake remains essentially unchanged during exercise and recovery. This assumption may be incorrect, particularly following strenuous exercise.

The recovery curves in Figure 5.7 illustrate two fundamentals of oxygen uptake during recovery:

1. **Fast component:** In low-intensity, primarily aerobic exercise (with little increase in body temperature), about one-half the total EPOC takes place in 30 seconds; complete recovery requires several minutes.
2. **Slow component:** A second slower phase occurs in recovery from more strenuous exercise (often accompanied by considerable increases in blood lactate and body temperature). The slower phase of recovery, depending on exercise intensity and duration, may require 24 hours or more before re-establishing the pre-exercise oxygen uptake.

Metabolic Dynamics of Recovery Oxygen Uptake

Current understanding of the specific biochemical dynamics in exhaustive exercise do not permit a precise partitioning of EPOC, especially for lactate's role.

Traditional Theory: A.V. Hill's Oxygen Debt Theory

Although A.V. Hill first used the term "oxygen debt" in 1922, Danish Nobel physiologist August Krogh (1874–1949; Chapter 1) first reported the exponential decline in oxygen uptake after exercise. Hill and others discussed the dynamics of metabolism in exercise and recovery in financial-accounting terms. Based on his work with frogs, Hill likened the body's carbohydrate stores to energy "credits." Expending stored credits during exercise incurred a "debt." The larger the energy "deficit" (or use of available stored energy credits), the larger the energy debt. Recovery oxygen uptake, therefore, represented the added metabolic cost of repaying this debt—hence the term "oxygen debt."

Hill hypothesized that lactate accumulation during the anaerobic component of exercise represented the use of stored glycogen energy credits. Therefore, the subsequent oxygen debt served two purposes: 1) re-establish the original carbohydrate stores (credits) by resynthesizing approximately 80% of the lactate back to glycogen (gluconeogenesis via the Cori cycle) in the liver, and 2) catabolize the remaining lactate for energy through the pyruvate–Krebs cycle pathway. ATP generated by this latter pathway presumably powered glycogen resynthesis from the accumulated lactate. The **lactic acid theory of oxygen debt** frequently describes this early explanation of recovery oxygen uptake dynamics.

In 1933, following Hill's work, researchers at Harvard's famous Fatigue Laboratory (1927–1946; Chapter 1) attempted to explain their observations that the initial fast component of the recovery oxygen uptake occurred before blood lactate decreased. In fact, they showed that an "oxygen debt" of almost 3 liters could incur without appreciably elevating blood lactate. To resolve these discrepancies, they proposed two phases of oxygen debt:

1. Alactic or **alactacid oxygen debt** (without lactate buildup): The alactacid portion of the oxygen debt (depicted for steady-rate exercise in panels A and B of Figure 5.7, or the rapid phase of recovery from strenuous exercise in panel C), restored the intramuscular high-energy phosphates ATP and PCr depleted during exercise. The aerobic breakdown of the stored nutrients during recovery provided the energy for this restoration. A small portion of the alactacid recovery oxygen uptake reloaded the muscles' myoglobin and hemoglobin in the blood returning from previously active tissues.

2. Lactic acid or **lactacid oxygen debt** (with lactate buildup): In keeping with A.V. Hill's explanation, the major portion of the lactacid oxygen debt represented reconversion of lactate to liver glycogen.

Essentially, this model explained the energetics of oxygen debt for almost 60 years.

Testing Hill's Oxygen Debt Theory.

Acceptance of the traditional explanation for the lactacid phase of the oxygen debt requires proof that the

Early Research About "Oxygen Debt"

Hill and other researchers of the time did not have a clear understanding of human bioenergetics. They frequently applied their knowledge of energy metabolism and lactate dynamics of amphibian and reptiles to observations on humans. In frogs, for example, most of the lactate formed in active muscle reconverts to glycogen, but this may not occur in humans.

major portion of lactate produced in exercise actually resynthesizes to glycogen in recovery. This has never been proven. To the contrary, when researchers infuse radioactive-labeled lactate into rat muscle, more than 75% of this substrate appears as radioactive carbon dioxide, and only 25% becomes synthesized to glycogen. In confirming experiments with humans, no substantial replenishment of glycogen occurred 10 minutes after strenuous exercise, even though blood lactate levels decreased significantly. Contrary to the traditional theory, the heart, liver, kidneys, and skeletal muscle use a major portion of blood lactate produced during exercise as an energy substrate during exercise and recovery.

Updated Theory to Explain EPOC.

No doubt exists that the elevated aerobic metabolism in recovery helps restore the body's processes to pre-exercise conditions. Oxygen uptake after light and moderate exercise replenishes high-energy phosphates depleted in the preceding exercise and sustains the cost of a somewhat elevated overall level of physiologic function. In recovery from strenuous exercise, some oxygen resynthesizes a portion of lactate to glycogen. *However, a significant portion of recovery oxygen uptake supports physiologic functions actually taking place during recovery.* The considerably larger recovery oxygen uptake compared with oxygen deficit in high-intensity, exhaustive exercise result partly from factors such as elevated body temperature. Core temperature frequently increases by about 3°C (5.4°F) during vigorous exercise and can remain elevated for several hours into recovery. This thermogenic "boost" directly stimulates metabolism and increases EPOC.

In essence, all of the physiologic systems activated to meet the demands of muscular activity increase their need for oxygen during recovery. The recovery oxygen uptake reflects:

- Anaerobic metabolism of prior exercise
- Respiratory, circulatory, hormonal, ionic, and thermal disequilibriums caused by prior exercise

Implications of EPOC for Exercise and Recovery.

Understanding the dynamics of recovery

Causes of Excess Postexercise Oxygen Consumption (EPOC) With Heavy Exercise

- Resynthesis of ATP and PCr
- Resynthesis of blood lactate to glycogen (Cori cycle)
- Oxidation of blood lactate in energy metabolism
- Restoration of oxygen to blood, tissue fluids, and myoglobin
- Thermogenic effects of elevated core temperature
- Thermogenic effects of hormones, particularly the catecholamines epinephrine and norepinephrine
- Increased pulmonary and circulatory dynamics and other elevated levels of physiologic function

oxygen uptake provides a basis for structuring exercise intervals during training and optimizing recovery from strenuous physical activity. Blood lactate does not accumulate considerably with either steady-rate aerobic exercise or brief 5- to 10-second bouts of all-out effort powered by the intramuscular high-energy phosphates. Recovery proceeds rapidly (fast component), and exercise can begin again within a brief time. In contrast, anaerobic exercise powered mainly by glycolysis causes lactate buildup and significant disruption in physiologic processes. This requires considerably more time for complete recovery (slow component). It poses a problem in sports like basketball, hockey, soccer, tennis, and badminton because a performer pushed to a high level of anaerobic metabolism may not fully recover during brief rest periods, times out, between points, or even half-time breaks.

Procedures for speeding recovery from exercise can occur as active or passive. **Active recovery** (often called "cooling-down" or "tapering-off") involves submaximum aerobic exercise performed immediately post exercise. Many believe that continued movement prevents muscle cramps and stiffness, and facilitates the recovery process. In contrast, in **passive recovery,** a person usually lies down, assuming that complete inactivity reduces the resting energy requirements and "frees" oxygen for the recovery process. Modifications of active and passive recovery have included cold showers, massages, specific body positions, ice application, and ingesting cold fluids. Research findings have been equivocal about these recovery procedures.

Optimal Recovery From Steady-Rate Exercise

Most people can perform exercise below 55 to 60% of $\dot{V}O_{2max}$ in steady rate with little blood lactate accumulation. Recovery from such exercise resynthesizes high-energy phosphates, replenishes oxygen in the blood, body fluids, and muscle myoglobin, and supports the small energy cost

Figure 5.8
Blood lactate concentrations after maximal exercise during passive recovery and active exercise recoveries at 35% $\dot{V}O_{2max}$, 65% $\dot{V}O_{2max}$, and a combination of 35% and 65% of $\dot{V}O_{2max}$. The horizontal solid orange line indicates the level of blood lactate produced by exercise at 65% of $\dot{V}O_{2max}$ without previous exercise. (Adapted from Dodd, S., et al.: Blood lactate disappearance at various intensities of recovery exercise. *J. Appl. Physiol.: Respirat. Environ. Exercise Physiol.,* 57:1462, 1984.)

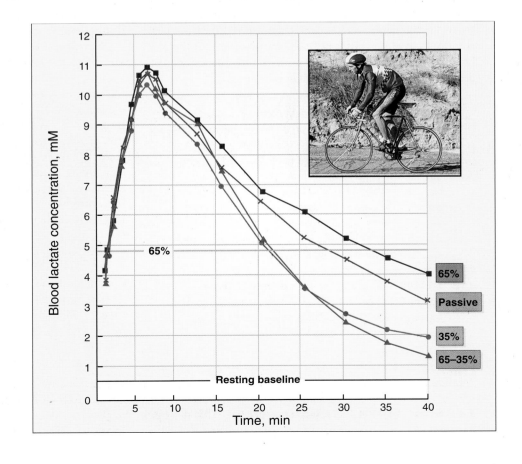

Keep Moving in Recovery From Heavy Exercise

Active recovery most likely facilitates lactate removal because of increased perfusion of blood through the "lactate-using" liver and heart. In addition, increased blood flow through the muscles in active recovery enhances lactate removal because muscle tissue oxidizes this substrate during Krebs cycle metabolism.

to sustain circulation and ventilation. Passive procedures produce the most rapid recovery in such cases because exercise elevates total metabolism and delays recovery.

Optimal Recovery from Non–Steady-Rate Exercise

Lactate formation exceeds its rate of removal and blood lactate accumulates when exercise intensity exceeds the maximum steady-rate level. As work intensity increases, the level of lactate increases sharply, and the exerciser soon becomes exhausted. The precise mechanisms of fatigue during intense anaerobic exercise are not fully understood, but the blood lactate level indicates the relative strenuousness of exercise and reflects the adequacy of the recovery.

Active aerobic exercise in recovery accelerates lactate removal. The optimal level of exercise in recovery ranges between 30 and 45% of $\dot{V}O_{2max}$ for bicycle exercise, and 55 to 60% of $\dot{V}O_{2max}$ when recovery involves treadmill running. The variation between these two forms of exercise

probably results from the more localized nature of bicycling (i.e., more intense effort per unit muscle mass), which produces a lower lactate threshold compared with running.

Figure 5.8 illustrates blood lactate recovery patterns for trained men who performed 6 minutes of supermaximum bicycle exercise. Active recovery involved 40 minutes of continuous exercise at either 35 or 65% of $\dot{V}O_{2max}$. An exercise combination of 65% $\dot{V}O_{2max}$ performed for 7 minutes followed by 33 minutes at 35% $\dot{V}O_{2max}$ evaluated whether a higher-intensity exercise interval early in recovery expedited blood lactate removal. Clearly, moderate aerobic exercise in recovery facilitated lactate removal compared with passive recovery. Combining higher-intensity exercise followed by lower-intensity exercise offered no greater benefit than a single exercise bout of moderate intensity. Recovery exercise above the lactate threshold might even prolong recovery by promoting lactate formation. In a practical sense, if left to their own choice, people voluntarily select their optimal intensity of recovery exercise for blood lactate removal.

Intermittent Exercise: The Interval Training Approach

Several approaches enable a person to perform significant amounts of normally exhaustive exercise, while simultaneously reducing the deleterious effects of anaerobic energy transfer through glycolysis. One approach requires training to improve a person's capacity to sustain exercise at a high rate of aerobic energy transfer. A high steady-rate capability exists for elite marathon runners, distance swimmers, and cross-country skiers who compete at close to 90% of $\dot{V}O_{2max}$ without significant blood lactate accumulation.

One can also exercise at an intensity that would normally prove exhausting within 3 to 5 minutes using pre-es-

TABLE 5.1
Total exercise, average oxygen uptake, and blood lactate levels during continuous and intermittent exercise

EXERCISE: REST PERIODS	TOTAL DISTANCE RUN (yd)	AVERAGE OXYGEN UPTAKE ($L \cdot min^{-1}$)	BLOOD LACTATE LEVEL ($mg \cdot 100\ mL\ blood^{-1}$)
4-min continuous	1422	5.6	150
10-s exercise 5-s rest	7294	5.1	44
10-s exercise 10-s rest	5468	4.4	20
15-s exercise 30-s rest	3642	3.6	16

*From Christenson, E.H., et al.: Intermittent and continuous running. *Acta Physiol. Scand.*, 50:269, 1960, as reported in Åstrand, P.O., and Rodahl, K.: *Textbook of Work Physiology*. New York: McGraw-Hill, 1970, p. 384.

tablished spacing of exercise and rest intervals. The utilization of exercise and rest intervals forms the basis of the **interval training** program. With this approach, the exerciser applies various work-to-rest intervals using "supermaximum" effort to overload the specific systems of energy transfer. For example, with all-out exercise of up to 8-seconds duration, intramuscular phosphagens provide the major portion of energy, with little demand on the glycolytic pathway. Rapid recovery ensues (fast component), and exercise can begin again after only a brief recovery.

Table 5.1 summarizes the results from experiments using various combinations of exercise and rest intervals during intermittent exercise. On one day, the subject ran at a speed that would normally exhaust him within 5 minutes. This continuous run covered about 0.8 mile, and the runner attained a $\dot{V}O_{2max}$ of 5.6 L · min^{-1}. The high blood lactate level shown in the last column of the table verified a relative state of exhaustion.

On another day, the runner maintained the same fast speed, but he performed the exercise intermittently with periods of 10-seconds exercise and 5-seconds recovery. With a 30-minute protocol of intermittent exercise, the actual duration of running amounted to 20 minutes and distance covered equaled 4.0 miles (5-min per mile pace) compared with 4 minutes exercise duration and 0.8 miles when running continuously. This exercise capability is more impressive considering that blood lactate remained low even though oxygen uptake averaged 5.1 L · min^{-1} (91% of $\dot{V}O_{2max}$) for the 30-minute duration. Thus, a relative balance existed between exercise energy requirements and aerobic energy transfer within the muscles during the exercise and rest intervals. These data indicate that manipulating exercise-to-rest intervals can isolate and

overload a specific energy transfer system. Extending the rest interval after a 10-second exercise bout from 5 to 10 seconds decreased the average oxygen uptake to 4.4 L · min^{-1}; with 15-second exercise and 30-second recovery intervals, only a 3.6 L · min^{-1} oxygen uptake occurred. In each case of 30 minutes of intermittent exercise, the runner achieved a longer distance and a lower blood lactate compared with the same exercise performed continuously. Coaches and athletes need to consider both exercise and rest intervals in optimizing workouts geared to train specific energy transfer systems.

One can also apply the exercise-to-rest interval (the **E-to-R method**) to improve muscular endurance. For example, two basic training approaches can improve sit-up capacity. In one method, the person performs as many sit-ups as possible for a specified time period. Suppose a person completed 40 consecutive sit-ups in 2 minutes. In each subsequent training session, the person would attempt to perform additional sit-ups. With the E-to-R method, sit-ups would be sequenced within intervals. Six sit-ups might be done within 10 seconds, followed by a 20-second rest interval. The sequence of sit-ups and rest would repeat 10 times resulting in a total of 60 sit-ups (6 sit-ups × 10 repeat bouts). Performing twenty 10-second bouts of sit-ups (total of 2-min exercise) would obviously double sit-up performance. Although the rest intervals add to the duration of training, the total number of completed sit-ups increases significantly beyond that performed in a single continuous exercise bout. The same E-to-R method can be applied to other types of performances such as push-ups, various flexibility exercises, and workouts with resistance equipment. Chapter 14 discusses the specific application of the principles of intermittent exercise to both aerobic and anaerobic training and sports performance.

summary

1. The major energy pathway for ATP production differs depending on exercise intensity and duration. Intense exercise of short duration (100-m dash, weight lifting) derives energy primarily from the intramuscular phosphagens ATP and PCr (immediate energy system). Intense exercise of longer duration (1 to 2 min) requires energy mainly from the anaerobic reactions of glycolysis (short-term energy system). The long-term aerobic system predominates as exercise progresses beyond several minutes duration.

2. The steady-rate oxygen uptake represents a balance between exercise energy requirements and aerobic ATP resynthesis. The oxygen deficit represents the difference between the exercise oxygen requirement and the actual oxygen consumed.

3. The maximum oxygen uptake or $\dot{V}O_{2max}$ represents quantitatively the maximum capacity for aerobic ATP resynthesis.

4. Humans possess different types of muscle fibers, each with unique metabolic and contractile properties. The two major fiber types are: low glycolytic-high oxidative, slow-twitch fibers, and low oxidative-high glycolytic, fast-twitch fibers.

5. Understanding the energy spectrum of exercise forms a sound basis for optimal training to improve a specific energy transfer system.

6. Bodily processes do not immediately return to resting levels after exercise ceases. The difference in recovery from light and strenuous exercise relates largely to the specific metabolic and physiologic processes in each exercise.

7. Moderate exercise performed during recovery (active recovery) from strenuous physical activity facilitates recovery compared with passive (inactive) procedures. Active recovery performed below the point of blood lactate accumulation speeds lactate removal.

8. Combining rest intervals with shorter exercise bouts (E-to-R method) allows performance of a large total amount of high-intensity exercise that normally would exhaust a person if performed continuously. Proper spacing of exercise and rest intervals can optimize workouts geared to train a specific energy transfer system.

thought questions

1. Several people attempt to run 1.5 miles as fast as possible. Part way through the run, one of them begins to slow down and walk. Explain the reasons for the fatigue and inability to maintain the original pace throughout the run.

2. If the maximal oxygen uptake represents such an important measure of a person's capacity to resynthesize ATP aerobically, why doesn't the person with the highest $\dot{V}O_{2max}$ always achieve the best marathon run performance?

3. How does an understanding of the energy spectrum of exercise help formulate optimal training to improve specific exercise performance?

4. Several members of a track team must perform repeat individual and relay events of 400-m distance during competition with only about 15 minutes rest between events. What advice provides the best way to recuperate between races?

5. Why is it so unusual to find athletes who excel at both short- and long-distance running?

selected references

Ahmaidi, S., et al.: Effects of active recovery on plasma lactate and anaerobic power following repeated intensive exercise. *Med. Sci. Sports Exerc.*, 28:450, 1996.

Bahr, R.: Effects of supramaximal exercise on excess postexercise oxygen consumption. *Med. Sci. Sports Exerc.*, 24:66, 1992.

Ball, D., et al.: The acute reversal of diet-induced metabolic acidosis does not restore endurance capacity during high-intensity exercise in man. *Eur. J. Appl. Physiol.*, 73:105, 1996.

Barstow, T.J.: Characterization of $\dot{V}O_2$ kinetics during heavy exercise. *Med. Sci. Sports Exerc.*, 26:1327, 1994.

Bogandis, G.C., et al.: Contribution of phosphocreatine and aerobic metabolism to energy supply during repeated sprint exercise. *J. Appl. Physiol.*, 80:876, 1996.

Coggan, A. R., et al.: Endurance training decreases plasma glucose turnover and oxidation during moderate-intensity exercise. *J. Appl. Physiol.*, 68:990, 1990.

Falk, B., et al.: Blood lactate concentration following exercise: effects of heat exposure and of active recovery in heat-acclimatized subjects. *Int. J. Sports Med.*, 16:7, 1995.

Gaesser, G.A., and Brooks, G.A.: Metabolic basis of excess post-exercise oxygen consumption: a review. *Med. Sci. Sports Exerc.*, 16:29, 1984.

Gladden, L.B.: Lactate uptake by skeletal muscle. In: *Exercise and Sport Sciences Reviews.* Vol. 17. Pandolf, K.B., (ed.). Baltimore: Williams & Wilkins, 1989.

Grassi, B., et al.: Faster adjustment of O_2 delivery does not affect $\dot{V}O_2$ kinetics in isolated in situ canine muscle. *J. Appl. Physiol.*, 85:1394, 1998.

Greehnaff, P.L., and Timmons, J.A.: Interaction between aerobic and anaerobic metabolism during intense muscle contraction. *Exerc. Sport Sci. Rev.*, 26:1,1998.

Hargreaves, M.: Interactions between muscle glycogen and blood glucose during exercise. *Exerc. Sport Sci. Revs.*, 25:21, 1997.

Hebestreit, H., et al.: Kinetics of oxygen uptake at the onset of exercise in boys and men. *J. Appl. Physiol.*, 85:1833, 1998.

Hochachka, P.W.: *Muscles as Molecular and Metabolic Machines.* Boca Raton, FL: CRC Press, 1994.

Holloszy, J.O., and Coyle, E.F.: Adaptations of skeletal muscle to endurance training and their metabolic consequences. *J. Appl. Physiol.*, 56:831, 1984.

Jacobs, I.: Blood lactate: Implications for training and sports performance. *Sports Med.*, 3:10, 1986.

Katz, A., and Sahlin, K.: Role of regulation of glycolysis and lactate production in human skeletal muscle. In: *Exercise and Sport Sciences Reviews.* Vol. 18. Pandolf, K.B., and Holloszy, J.O., (eds.). Baltimore: Williams & Wilkins, 1990.

Koike, A., et al.: Oxygen uptake kinetics are determined by cardiac function at onset of exercise rather than peak exercise in patients with prior myocardial infarction. *Circulation*, 90:2324, 1994.

MacRae, H.S., et al.: Effects of training on lactate production and removal during progressive exercise. *J. Appl. Physiol.*, 72:1649, 1992.

Minotti, J. R., et al.: Training-induced skeletal muscle adaptations are independent of systemic adaptations. *J. Appl. Physiol.*, 68:289, 1990.

McCann, D.J., et al.: Phosphocreatine kinetics in humans during exercise and recovery. *Med. Sci. Sports Exerc.*, 27:378, 1995.

Poole, D.C.: $\dot{V}O_2$ slow component: physiological and functional significance. *Med. Sci. Sports Exerc.*, 26:1354, 1994.

Quinn, T.J., et al.: Postexercise oxygen consumption in trained females: effect of exercise duration. *Med. Sci. Sports Exerc.*, 26:908, 1994.

Short, K.R., and Sedlock, D.A.: Excess postexercise oxygen consumption and recovery rate in trained and untrained subjects. *J. Appl. Physiol.*, 83:153, 1997.

Stainsby, W.N., and Brooks, G.A.: Control of lactic acid metabolism in contracting muscles and during exercise. In: *Exercise and Sport Sciences Reviews.* Vol 18. Pandolf, K.B., (ed.). Baltimore: Williams & Wilkins, 1990.

Starritt, E.C., et al.: Effect of short-term training on mitochrondrial ATP production rate in human skeletal muscle. *J. Appl. Physiol.*, 86:450, 1999.

Trump, M.E., et al.: Importance of muscle phosphocreatine during intermittent maximal cycling. *J. Appl. Physiol.*, 80:1574, 1996.

Tschakovsky, M.E., and Hughson, R.I.: Interaction of factors determining oxygen uptake at the onset of exercise. *J. Appl. Physiol.*, 86:1101, 1999.

Weltman, A.: *The Blood Lactate Response to Exercise. Current Issues in Exercise Science.* Monograph Number 4. Champaign, IL: Human Kinetics, 1995.

Whipp, B.J.: The slow component of O_2 uptake kinetics during heavy exercise. *Med. Sci. Sports Exerc.*, 26:1319, 1994.

Wilbur, R.L., et al.: Physiological profiles of elite off-road and road cyclists. *Med. Sci. Sports Exerc.*, 29:1090, 1997.

Wyatt, F.B.: Comparison of lactate and ventilatory threshold to maximal oxygen consumption: A meta-analysis. *J. Strength Cond. Res.*, 13:67, 1999.

CHAPTER

6

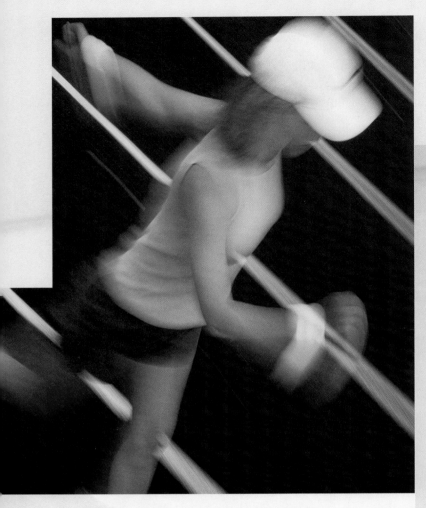

Topics covered in this chapter

Heat Produced by the Body
Direct Versus Indirect Calorimetry
Respiratory Quotient (RQ)
Respiratory Exchange Ratio (R)
Summary
Thought Questions
Selected References

Measurement of Human Energy Expenditure

- Understand the concepts of direct calorimetry, indirect calorimetry, closed-circuit spirometry, and open-circuit spirometry.

- Diagram the closed-circuit spirometry system for oxygen uptake determinations.

- Describe the portable spirometry, bag technique, and computerized instrumentation systems of open-circuit spirometry.

- Define the term respiratory quotient (RQ) including its use to quantify energy release in metabolism and the composition of the food mixture metabolized.

- Explain the difference between RQ and the respiratory exchange ratio (R), including factors that affect each.

Heat Produced by the Body

This chapter describes two techniques, direct and indirect calorimetry, to measure human energy expenditure. These procedures form the basis for accurately quantifying differences among individuals in energy metabolism at rest and during physical activity discussed in Chapter 7.

Direct Calorimetry

All of the body's metabolic processes ultimately produce heat. Consequently, we can measure human energy metabolism by measuring heat production similarly to the method for determining the energy value of foods in the bomb calorimeter (refer to Fig. 2.13).

The **human calorimeter** illustrated in Figure 6.1 consists of an airtight chamber where a person lives and works for extended periods. A known volume of water at a specified temperature circulates through a series of coils at the top of the chamber. Circulating water absorbs the heat produced and radiated by the individual. Insulation protects the entire chamber, so any change in water temperature relates directly to the individual's energy metabolism. For adequate ventilation, chemicals continually remove moisture and absorb carbon dioxide from the person's exhaled air. Oxygen added to the air recirculates through the chamber.

Professors W.O. Atwater (a chemist) and E.B. Rosa (a physicist) in the 1890s built and perfected the first human calorimeter of major scientific importance at Wesleyan University (Connecticut). Their elegant human calorimetric experiments relating energy input to energy expenditure successfully verified the *law of the conservation of energy*, and validated the relationship between direct and indirect calorimetry. The **Atwater-Rosa calorimeter** had a small chamber where the subject lived, ate, slept, and exercised on a bicycle ergometer. Experiments lasted from several hours to 13 days; during some experiments, subjects cycled continuously for up to 16 hours, expending more than 10,000 kcal. The calorimeter's operation required 16 people working in teams of 8 for 12-hour shifts.

Direct measurement of heat production (**direct calorimetry**) in humans has considerable theoretical implications, but limited practical application. Accurate measurements of heat production in the calorimeter require considerable time, expense, and formidable engineering expertise. Thus, the calorimeter cannot determine energy expenditure for most sport, occupational, and recreational activities. Also, direct calorimetry cannot be applied for large-scale studies in underdeveloped and poor countries. Total nutritional and energy balance assessments are needed for deprivation conditions, particularly undernutrition and starvation. In the 90 years since

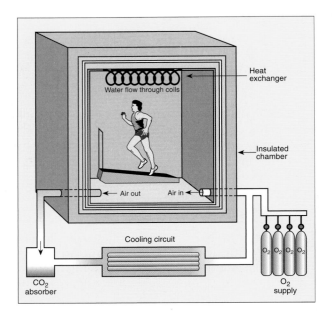

Figure 6.1
Directly measuring body's heat production in the human calorimeter.

Atwater and Rosa published their papers on human calorimetry, other methodology evolved to infer energy expenditure indirectly from metabolic gas exchange.

Indirect Calorimetry

All energy-releasing reactions in the body ultimately depend on the use of oxygen. By measuring a person's oxygen uptake during steady-rate exercise, researchers obtain an indirect yet accurate estimate of energy expenditure. **Indirect calorimetry** provides a relatively simple and a less expensive method compared with direct calorimetry. Closed-circuit and open-circuit spirometry represent two common methods of indirect calorimetry.

Closed-Circuit Spirometry

Figure 6.2 illustrates **closed-circuit spirometry** developed in the late 1800s and currently used in hospitals and research laboratories to estimate resting energy expenditure. The subject breathes 100% oxygen from a prefilled container (spirometer). The equipment consists of a "closed system" because the person rebreathes only the gas in the spirometer. A canister of soda lime (potassium hydroxide) placed in the breathing circuit absorbs the carbon dioxide in the exhaled air. A drum attached to the spirometer revolves at a known speed and records oxygen uptake from

Figure 6.2
The closed-circuit method uses a spirometer prefilled with 100% oxygen. This method works well for rest or light-intensity exercise, but not for intense exercise.

changes in the system's volume. The difference between the initial and final volumes of oxygen in the calibrated spirometer indicates oxygen uptake during the measurement interval.

During exercise, oxygen uptake measurement using closed-circuit spirometry becomes problematic. The subject must remain close to the bulky equipment, the breathing circuit resists the large gas volumes exchanged during exercise, and the slow speed of carbon dioxide removal becomes inadequate during intense exercise.

Open-Circuit Spirometry

Open-circuit spirometry represents the most widely used technique to measure oxygen uptake during exercise. A subject inhales ambient air with a constant composition of 20.93% oxygen, 0.03% carbon dioxide, and 79.04% nitrogen. The nitrogen fraction also includes a small quantity of inert gases. Changes in oxygen and carbon dioxide percentages in expired air compared with inspired ambient air indirectly reflect the ongoing process of energy metabolism. Thus, analysis of two factors—volume of air breathed during a specified time period and composition of exhaled air—measures oxygen uptake and infers energy expenditure.

Three common open-circuit, indirect calorimetric procedures measure oxygen uptake during physical activity:

1. Portable spirometry
2. Bag technique
3. Computerized instrumentation

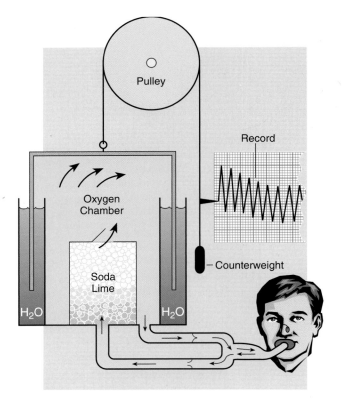

close up

A Calorie Is a Calorie Is a Calorie . . . Maybe Not!

Many obese individuals report they do not consume more food than their lean counterparts, but the food they consume results in greater fat deposition. In other words, for the same excess calories ingested, obese people store more body fat, resulting in long-term weight gain.

The possibility that obese individuals might have a defective thermogenic (heat-producing) response has been the focus of considerable research. One proposed mechanism for a blunted thermogenesis (leading to greater energy storage per quantity of excess energy consumed) is the possibility that obese individuals have increased insulin resistance and a reduced rate of non-oxidative glucose disposal, which has a greater energy cost than glucose oxidation. As a result, obese individuals who are insulin resistant may have a reduced rate of glucose storage per amount of food ingested, and a concurrent facilitated fat storage. This produces progressive weight gain over time.

To measure energy conservation groups of obese and nonobese people received the same amount of food; the energy expenditures for the groups are then measured for several hours. A blunted increase in energy expenditure in response to the meal (**thermic effect of food**) indicates greater energy storage per kcal of food ingested.

The bar graph presents the results of two experiments, one performed with obese adults and the other with obese adolescents, in addition to nonobese control groups of the same age and gender. Each group consumed the same food load, and energy expenditure was monitored for 3 hours after eating. As illustrated, both the obese adults and adolescents had a significantly smaller increase in metabolic rate than nonobese counter-

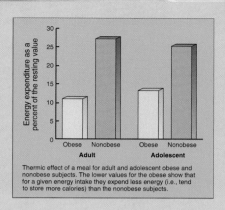

Thermic effect of a meal for adult and adolescent obese and nonobese subjects. The lower values for the obese show that for a given energy intake they expend less energy (i.e., tend to store more calories) than the nonobese subjects.

parts in response to the food challenge. This provides direct evidence for a blunted thermogenic response in obesity and explains the ease of weight gain (and difficulty for weight loss) on a given energy intake among obese people.

Consider the following example: Suppose an obese and nonobese person each consumed 2500 kcal daily, but the obese person has a blunted thermogenic response, similar to the data illustrated in the graph. Over a year, the obese person would store an extra 18,750 kcal (~50 kcal · d⁻¹) compared with the nonobese individual. This corresponds to a potential weight gain of nearly 5.5 pounds per year, or about a 27-pound difference between the obese and nonobese person over a 5-year period.

References

Katch, V.L., et al.: Reduced short-term thermic effects of a meal in obese adolescent girls. *Eur. J. Appl. Physiol.*, 65:535, 1992.

Segal, K. R., et al.: Comparison of thermic effects of constant and relative caloric loads in lean and obese men. *Am. J. Clin Nutr.*, 51:14, 1990.

Portable Spirometry. German scientists in the early 1940s perfected a lightweight, portable system to indirectly determine the energy expended during physical activity. The activities included war-related operations such as traveling over different terrain with full battle gear, operating transportation vehicles including tanks and aircraft, and simulating tasks that soldiers would encounter during actual combat. The subject carries the 3-kg box-shaped apparatus shown in Figure 6.3 on the back like a backpack. Ambient air passes through a two-way valve, and expired air exits through a gas meter. The meter measures total expired air volume and collects a small gas sample (aliquot) for later analysis of oxygen and carbon dioxide content, and subsequent determination of oxygen uptake and energy expenditure for the measurement period.

The **portable spirometer** makes it easier to estimate energy expenditure in diverse activities like mountain climbing, downhill skiing, sailing, golf, and common household activities. The equipment becomes cumbersome during vigorous activity; with rapid breathing, the meter under-records airflow measurements during heavy exercise.

Bag Technique. Figure 6.4 depicts the **bag technique**. The subject in Figure 6.4A rides a stationary bicycle ergometer wearing headgear containing a two-way, high-velocity, low-resistance breathing valve. He breathes ambient air through one side of the valve and expels it out the other side. The expired air then passes into either large canvas or plastic bags or rubber meteorologic balloons, or directly through a gas meter, which continually measures air volume. The meter collects a small sample of expired air for later analysis of oxygen and carbon dioxide composition. Figure 6.4B illustrates oxygen uptake measured by the bag technique while lifting boxes of different weights and sizes to evaluate the energy requirements of a specific occupational task.

Computerized Instrumentation. With advances in computer and microprocessor technology, the exercise scientist can accurately and rapidly measure metabolic and cardiovascular responses to exercise. A computer interfaces with at least three instruments:

1. System to continuously sample the subject's expired air

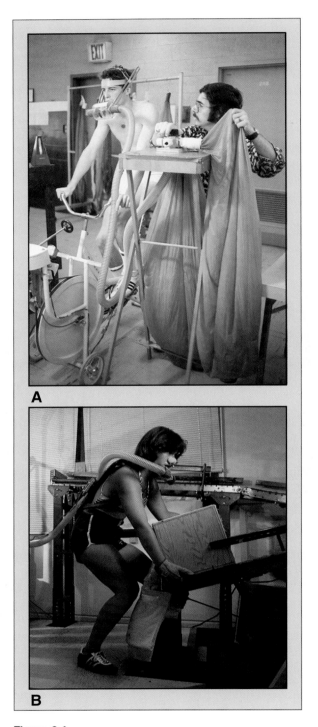

A

B

Figure 6.4
Oxygen uptake measurement by open-circuit spirometry (bag technique) during (**A**) stationary cycle ergometer exercise, and (**B**) box loading and unloading.

Figure 6.3
Portable spirometer used to measure oxygen uptake by the open-circuit method during golf and calisthenics exercise.

2. Flow-measuring device to record air volume breathed

3. Oxygen and carbon dioxide analyzers to measure the expired gas mixture's composition

The computer performs metabolic calculations based on electronic signals it receives from the instruments. A printed or graphic display of the data appears during the measurement period. More advanced systems include automated blood pressure, heart rate, and temperature monitors, and preset instructions to regulate speed, duration, and workload of a treadmill, bicycle ergometer, stepper, rower, swim flume, or other exercise apparatus. Figure 6.5 depicts **computerized instrumentation** for assessing metabolic and physiologic responses during exercise.

The system in Figure 6.6 provides wireless telemetric transmission of data for metabolic measurement—pulmonary ventilation and oxygen and carbon dioxide analysis—during a broad range of exercise, sport, and occupational activities. The lightweight (<1 lb), small device provides feedback on pacing, duration of exercise, energy expenditure, heart rate, and ventilation. The unit's

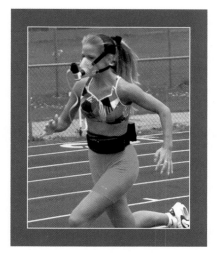

Figure 6.6
Computerized system worn by a subject during running. Easily transported during physical activity, the metabolic system weighs approximately 1 pound with a 4 × 8-inch dimension. Note the subject wears a facemask attached to the analyzer mounted on the back.

microprocessor stores all acquired data for downloading to a computer. With telemetry, data appear in "real time" on a host or network computer or the Internet. With proper calibration, commercially available miniaturized equipment can quantify the energy cost "in vivo" during diverse sport and occupational activities.

Calibration Methods.
Regardless of the apparent sophistication of a particular automated system, the output data reflect the accuracy of the measuring device. Therefore, accuracy and validity of measurement devices require careful and frequent calibration using established reference standards. Figure 6.7 illustrates two common chemical analyzers for determining the percentages of oxygen, carbon dioxide, and nitrogen

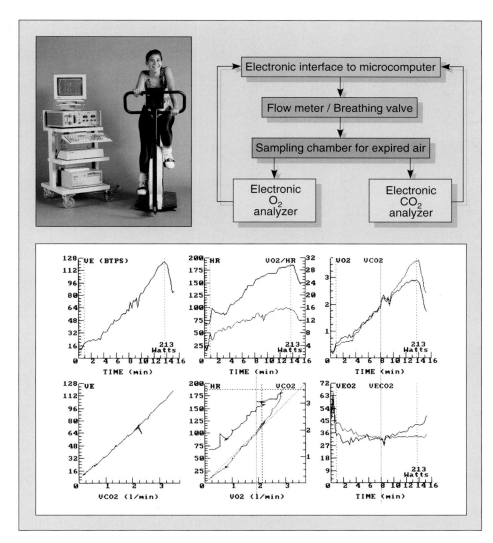

Figure 6.5
Computer systems approach to the collection, analysis, and rapid display of physiologic and metabolic data. (Photos courtesy of Fitco, a division of PhysioDyne Instrument Corporation, Farmingdale, NY.)

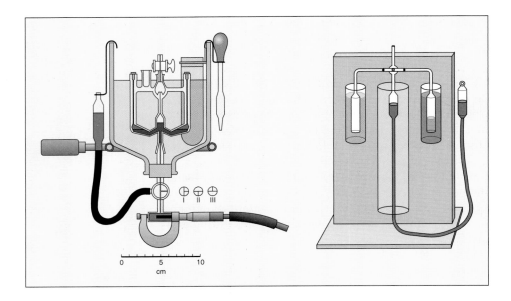

Figure 6.7
Chemical gas absorption procedures for analyzing carbon dioxide and oxygen. **Left,** Micro-Scholander gas analyzer; **Right,** Haldane gas analyzer. The Scholander uses a 0.5 mL "micro" gas sample, whereas the Haldane analyzes a 10 mL sample. Both apparatus use the force of a column of mercury to expose the gas sample to chambers containing chemicals that absorb either oxygen or carbon dioxide from the gas mixture. Subtracting the initial gas volume (before absorption) from the final volume (after absorption) determines gas individual volumes.

in an expired air sample. Many laboratories routinely use these instruments to calibrate the more sophisticated and rapid electronic analyzers. Before the widespread use of microprocessor-controlled instrumentation to analyze oxygen and carbon dioxide concentrations in expired air, all determinations of the oxygen and carbon dioxide percentages used either the **micro-Scholander** or **Haldane** methods of gas analysis. These slow methods for analyzing respiratory gases limited participation to only a few subjects in prolonged studies of exercise metabolism.

Direct Versus Indirect Calorimetry

Energy metabolism studied simultaneously using direct and indirect calorimetry provides convincing evidence for the validity of the indirect method. At the turn of the century, the two calorimetric methods were compared by Atwater and Rosa for 40 days with three men who lived in calorimeters similar to the one shown in Figure 6.1. Their daily caloric outputs averaged 2723 kcal when measured directly by heat production and 2717 kcal when computed indirectly using closed-circuit measures of oxygen uptake. Other experiments with animals and humans based on moderate exercise also demonstrated close agreement between direct and indirect methods; in most instances, the difference averaged less than ±1%. In the Atwater and Rosa calorimetry experiments, the ±0.2% method error represents a remarkable achievement, given that these experiments used hand-made instruments.

Caloric Transformation for Oxygen

Bomb calorimeter studies show that approximately 4.82 kcal release when a blend of carbohydrate, lipid, and protein burns in one liter of oxygen. Even with large variations in the metabolic mixture, this **caloric value for oxygen** varies only slightly (within ±2 to 4%).

An energy–oxygen equivalent of 5.0 kcal per liter provides a convenient yardstick to transpose any aerobic physical activity to a caloric (energy) frame of reference. Indirect calorimetry through oxygen uptake measurement provides the basis for quantifying the caloric cost of most physical activities.

Respiratory Quotient (RQ)

Complete oxidation of a molecule's carbon and hydrogen atoms to carbon dioxide and water end-products requires different amounts of oxygen due to inherent chemical differences in carbohydrate, lipid, and protein composition. Consequently, the substrate metabolized determines the quantity of carbon dioxide produced in relation to oxygen consumed. The **respiratory quotient (RQ)** refers to the following ratio of metabolic gas exchange:

$$RQ = CO_2 \text{ produced} \div O_2 \text{ consumed}$$

The RQ helps to approximate the nutrient mixture catabolized for energy during rest and aerobic exercise. Also, because the caloric equivalent for oxygen differs somewhat depending on the nutrients oxidized, precisely determining the body's heat production (kcal) requires information about oxygen uptake and RQ.

RQ for Carbohydrate

All of the oxygen consumed in carbohydrate combustion oxidizes the carbon in the carbohydrate molecule to carbon dioxide. This is because the ratio of hydrogen to oxygen atoms in carbohydrates always exists in the same ratio (2:1) as in water. The complete oxidation of one glucose molecule requires six oxygen molecules and produces six molecules of carbon dioxide and water as follows:

$$C_6H_{12}O_6 + 6\ O_2 \rightarrow 6\ CO_2 + 6\ H_2O$$

Gas exchange during glucose oxidation produces an equal number of CO_2 molecules to O_2 molecules consumed; therefore, RQ for carbohydrate equals 1.00:

$$RQ = 6CO_2 \div 6O_2 = 1.00$$

RQ for Lipid

The chemical composition of lipids differs from carbohydrates because lipids contain considerably fewer oxygen atoms in proportion to carbon and hydrogen atoms. Consequently, lipid catabolism for energy requires considerably more oxygen in relation to carbon dioxide production. Palmitic acid, a typical fatty acid, oxidizes to carbon dioxide and water, producing 16 carbon dioxide molecules for every 23 oxygen molecules consumed. The following equation summarizes this exchange to compute RQ:

$$C_{16}H_{32}O_2 + 23O_2 \rightarrow 16CO_2 + 16H_2O$$

$$RQ = 16CO_2 \div 23O_2 = 0.696$$

Generally, a value of 0.70 represents the RQ for lipid, ranging between 0.69 and 0.73, depending on the oxidized fatty acid's carbon chain length.

Kcal Equivalent for 1 L Oxygen

Assuming the combustion of a mixed diet, a rounded value of 5.0 kcal per liter of oxygen consumed designates the appropriate conversion factor for estimating energy expenditure under steady-rate conditions of aerobic metabolism.

RQ for Protein

Proteins do not simply oxidize to carbon dioxide and water during energy metabolism in the body. Rather, the liver first deaminates (removes nitrogen) the amino acid molecule; then the body excretes the nitrogen and sulfur fragments in the urine, sweat, and feces. The remaining "keto acid" fragment oxidizes to carbon dioxide and water to provide energy for biologic work. Short-chain keto acids require more oxygen in relation to carbon dioxide produced to achieve complete combustion. For example, the protein albumin oxidizes as follows:

$$C_{72}H_{112}N_2O_{22}S + 77O_2 \rightarrow 63CO_2 + 38H_2O + SO_3 + 9CO(NH_2)^2$$

$$RQ = 63CO_2 \div 77O_2 = 0.818$$

The general value 0.82 characterizes the RQ for protein.

RQ for a Mixed Diet

During activities ranging from complete bed rest to mild aerobic exercise (walking or slow jogging), the RQ seldom reflects the oxidation of pure carbohydrate or pure fat. Instead, metabolizing a mixture of nutrients occurs with an RQ intermediate between 0.70 and 1.00. *For most purposes, we assume an RQ of 0.82 from the metabolism of a mixture of 40% carbohydrate and 60% fat, applying the caloric equivalent of 4.825 kcal per liter of oxygen for the energy transformation.* Using 4.825 kcal, the maximum error possible in estimating energy metabolism from steady-rate oxygen uptake equals about 4%.

Table 6.1 presents the energy expenditure per liter of oxygen uptake for different **non-protein RQ** values, including corresponding percentages and grams of carbohydrate and fat utilized for energy. *The non-protein RQ value assumes that the metabolic mixture comprises only carbohydrate and fat.* Interpret the table as follows:

Suppose oxygen uptake during 30 minutes of aerobic exercise averages 3.22 L·min^{-1} with CO_2 production of 2.78 L · min^{-1}. The RQ, computed as $\dot{V}CO_2 \div \dot{V}O_2$ (2.78 ÷ 3.22), equals 0.86. From Table 6.1, this RQ value (left column) corresponds to an energy equivalent of 4.875 kcal per liter of oxygen uptake, or an exercise energy output of 15.7 kcal · min^{-1} (3.22 L O_2 · min^{-1} × 4.875 kcal). Based on a non-protein RQ, 54.1% of the calories come from the combustion of carbohydrate and 45.9% from fat. The total calories expended during the 30-minute exercise period equal 471 kcal (15.7 kcal · min^{-1} × 30).

Respiratory Exchange Ratio (R)

*A*pplication of the RQ requires the assumption that O_2 and CO_2 exchange measured at the lungs reflects the

How to Calculate Energy Expenditure (kcal · min^{-1}) Using the Weir Method

In 1949, J.B. Weir, a Scottish physician and physiologist from Glasgow University, presented a simple method for estimating energy expenditure from measures of pulmonary ventilation and expired oxygen percent, accurate to within ±1% of the traditional respiratory quotient (RQ) method.

Basic Equation

Weir showed that the following formula calculated caloric expenditure (kcal · min^{-1}) if energy released from protein breakdown averaged about 12.5% of total caloric expenditure (a reasonable percentage for most people):

$$\text{kcal} \cdot \text{min}^{-1} = \dot{V}_{E(STPD)} \times (1.044 - [0.0499 \times \%O_{2E}])$$

where, $\dot{V}_{E(STPD)}$ represents expired ventilation per minute corrected to standard conditions (STPD) and $\%O_{2E}$ represents expired air's oxygen percentage. The value in parenthesis (1.044 − 0.0499 × $\%O_{2E}$) represents the "**Weir factor.**" The accompanying table displays Weir factors for different $\%O_{2E}$ values.

To use the table, find the $\%O_{2E}$ and corresponding Weir factor. Compute caloric expenditure in kcal · min^{-1} by multiplying the Weir factor by $\dot{V}_{E(STPD)}$.

Example

During a steady jog on a treadmill, $\dot{V}_{E(STPD)}$ = 50 L · min^{-1} and O_{2E} = 16.0%. Energy expenditure by the Weir method computes as follows:

$$\text{kcal} \cdot \text{min}^{-1} = \dot{V}_{E(STPD)} \times (1.044 - [0.0499 \times \%O_{2E}])$$
$$= 50 \times (1.044 - [0.0499 \times 16.0])$$
$$= 50 \times 0.2456$$
$$= 12.3$$

Weir also derived the following equation to calculate kcal · min^{-1} from RQ and $\dot{V}O_2$ in L · min^{-1}:

$$\text{kcal} \cdot \text{min}^{-1} = [(1.1 \times RQ) + 3.9] \times \dot{V}O_2$$

WEIR FACTORS

%O$_{2E}$	Weir Factor	%O$_{2E}$	Weir Factor
14.50	.3205	17.00	.1957
14.60	.3155	17.10	.1907
14.70	.3105	17.20	.1857
14.80	.3055	17.30	.1807
14.90	.3005	17.40	.1757
15.00	.2955	17.50	.1707
15.10	.2905	17.60	.1658
15.20	.2855	17.70	.1608
15.30	.2805	17.80	.1558
15.40	.2755	17.90	.1508
15.50	.2705	18.00	.1468
15.60	.2556	18.10	.1308
15.70	.2606	18.20	.1368
15.80	.2556	18.30	.1308
15.90	.2506	18.40	.1268
16.00	.2456	18.50	.1208
16.10	.2406	18.60	.1168
16.20	.2366	18.70	.1109
16.30	.2306	18.80	.1068
16.40	.2256	18.90	.1009
16.50	.2206	19.00	.0969
16.60	.2157	19.10	.0909
16.70	.2107	19.20	.0868
16.80	.2057	19.30	.0809
16.90	.2007	19.40	.0769

From Weir, J.B. New Methods for calculating metabolic rate with special reference to protein metabolism. *J. Physiol.*, 109:1, 1949.

actual gas exchange from nutrient metabolism on the cellular level. This assumption is reasonably valid for rest and during steady-rate (mild-to-moderate) aerobic exercise conditions with no lactate accumulation. However, factors can alter the exchange of oxygen and carbon dioxide in the lungs so that the gas exchange ratio no longer reflects *only* the substrate mixture in cellular energy metabolism. For example, carbon dioxide elimination increases during hyperventilation because breathing increases to disproportionately high levels in relation to the actual metabolic demands. By overbreathing, the normal level of CO_2 in the blood decreases because the gas "blows off" in expired air. A corresponding increase in oxygen uptake does not accompany additional CO_2 elimination. Consequently, the exchange ratio often exceeds 1.00. *Respiratory physiologists refer to the ratio of carbon dioxide produced to oxygen con-*

sumed under such conditions as the **respiratory exchange ratio** (**R** or **RER**). This ratio computes in exactly the same manner as RQ. An increase in the respiratory exchange ratio above 1.00 cannot be attributed to foodstuff oxidation.

Exhaustive exercise presents another situation where R usually increases above 1.00. Sodium bicarbonate in the blood buffers or "neutralizes" the lactate generated during anaerobic metabolism to maintain proper acid-base balance in the reaction:

$$HLa + NaHCO_3 \rightarrow NaLa + H_2CO_3 \rightarrow H_2O + CO_2 \rightarrow Lungs$$

Lactate buffering produces the weaker carbonic acid. In the pulmonary capillaries, carbonic acid breaks down to its components, carbon dioxide and water, allowing carbon dioxide to readily exit through the lungs. The R increases above 1.00 because buffering adds "extra" CO_2 to expired air above the quantity normally released during cellular energy metabolism.

Relatively low R values can occur after exhaustive exercise when carbon dioxide remains body fluids to replenish bicarbonate that buffered the accumulating lactate. This action reduces expired carbon dioxide without affecting oxygen uptake, causing the R to go below 0.70.

TABLE 6.1
Thermal equivalents of oxygen for the non-protein respiratory quotient, including percent kcal and grams derived from carbohydrate and fat*

NON-PROTEIN RQ	Kcal PER LITER O₂ UPTAKE	PERCENTAGE Kcal DERIVED FROM		GRAMS PER LITER O₂ UPTAKE	
		CARBOHYDRATE	FAT	CARBOHYDRATE	FAT
0.707	4.686	0.0	100.0	0.000	.496
.71	4.690	1.1	98.9	.012	.491
.72	4.702	4.8	95.2	.051	.476
.73	4.714	8.4	91.6	.900	.460
.74	4.727	12.0	88.0	.130	.444
.75	4.739	15.6	84.4	.170	.428
.76	4.750	19.2	80.8	.211	.412
.77	4.764	22.8	77.2	.250	.396
.78	4.776	26.3	73.7	.290	.380
.79	4.788	29.9	70.1	.330	.363
.80	4.801	33.4	66.6	.371	.347
.81	4.813	36.9	63.1	.413	.330
.82	4.825	40.3	59.7	.454	.313
.83	4.838	43.8	56.2	.496	.297
.84	4.850	47.2	52.8	.537	.280
.85	4.862	50.7	49.3	.579	.263
.86	4.875	54.1	45.9	.621	.247
.87	4.887	57.5	42.5	.663	.230
.88	4.887	60.8	39.2	.705	.213
.89	4.911	64.2	35.8	.749	.195
.90	4.924	67.5	32.5	.791	.178
.91	4.936	70.8	29.2	.834	.160
.92	4.948	74.1	25.9	.877	.143
.93	4.961	77.4	22.6	.921	.125
.94	4.973	80.7	19.3	.964	.108
.95	4.985	84.0	16.0	1.008	.090
.96	4.998	87.2	12.8	1.052	.072
.97	5.010	90.4	9.6	1.097	.054
.98	5.022	93.6	6.4	1.142	.036
.99	5.035	96.8	3.2	1.186	.018
1.00	5.047	100.0	0	1.231	.000

* From Zuntz, N.: Ueber die Bedeutung der verschiedenen Nährstoffe als Erzeuger der Muskelkraft. *Arch. f.d. ges Physiol.*, Bonn, Ger.: LXXXIII, 557-571, 1901. *Pflügers Acrh. Physiol.*, 83:557, 1901.

summary

1. Direct and indirect calorimetry determine the body's rate of energy expenditure. Direct calorimetry measures the actual heat production in an insulated calorimeter. Indirect calorimetry infers energy expenditure from oxygen uptake and carbon dioxide production using closed-circuit or open-circuit spirometry.

2. All energy-releasing reactions in the body ultimately depend on oxygen use. By measuring a person's oxygen uptake during steady-rate exercise, researchers obtain an indirect yet accurate estimate of energy expenditure.

3. Portable spirometry, bag technique, and computerized instrumentation represent three common open-circuit, indirect calorimetric procedures to measure oxygen uptake during physical activity.

4. The complete oxidation of each nutrient requires a different quantity of oxygen uptake compared with carbon dioxide production. The ratio of carbon dioxide produced to oxygen consumed (the respiratory quotient or RQ) provides important information about the nutrient mixture catabolized for energy. The RQ averages 1.00 for carbohydrate, 0.70 for fat, and 0.82 for protein.

5. For each RQ value, a corresponding caloric value exists for one liter of oxygen consumed. The RQ-kcal relationship determines energy expenditure during exercise with a high degree of accuracy.

6. During strenuous exercise, RQ does not represent specific substrate use because of nonmetabolic production of carbon dioxide in lactate buffering (which spuriously increases the $CO_2 \div O_2$ ratio).

7. The respiratory exchange ratio (R) reflects the pulmonary exchange of carbon dioxide and oxygen under various physiologic and metabolic conditions; R does not fully mirror the macronutrient mixture catabolized for energy.

thought questions

1. Explain how an exercise physiologist determines that a marathoner derives up to 70 to 80% of total energy from fat combustion during the final 3 miles of a marathon race.

2. Explain how oxygen uptake translates to heat production during exercise.

3. A high-tech computer company wants to validate their new wrist-mounted device to measure exercise energy expenditure. The person simply exhales one breath onto the top of the instrument while exercising. The device's electronic components and microprocessor analyze expired air to compute $\dot{V}O_2$ and energy expenditure. Outline the steps necessary to perform your evaluation of the device and the criteria to determine the instrument's validity?

selected references

Atwater, W.O., and Rosa, E.B.: Description of a new respiration calorimeter and experiments on the conservation of energy in the human body. Bulletin No. 63, Washington, D.C., U.S. Department of Agriculture, Office of Experiment Stations, Government Printing Office, 1899.

Brooks, G.A., et al.: Estimation of anaerobic energy production and efficiency in rats during exercise. *J. Appl. Physiol.*, 56:520, 1984.

Brooks, G.A., et al.: *Exercise Physiology: Human Bioenergetics and its Applications.* 2nd Ed., Mountain View, CA: Mayfield, 1996.

Crandall, C.G., et al.: Evaluation of the Cosmed K2 portable telemetric oxygen uptake analyzer. *Med. Sci. Sports Exerc.*, 26:108, 1994.

Dulloo, A.G., et al.: A low-budget and easy-to-operate room respirometer for measuring daily energy expenditure in man. *Am. J. Clin. Nutr.*, 48:1367, 1988.

Ferraro, R., et al.: Energy cost of physical activity on a metabolic ward in relationship to obesity. *Am. J. Clin. Nutr.*, 53:1368, 1991.

Fogelholm, M., et al.: Assessment of energy expenditure in overweight women. *Med. Sci. Sports Exerc.*, 30:1191, 1998.

Haldane, J.S., and Priestley, J.G.: *Respiration.* New York: Oxford University Press, 1935.

Jansson, E.: On the significance of the respiratory exchange ratio after different diets during exercise in man. *Acta Physiol. Scand.*, 114:103, 1982.

Jéquier, E, and Schutz, Y.: Long-term measurements of energy expenditure in humans using a respiration chamber. *Am. J. Clin. Nutr.*, 38:989, 1983.

Kannagi, T., et al.: An evaluation of the Beckman Metabolic Cart for measuring ventilation and aerobic requirements during exercise. *J. Cardiac Rehab.*, 3:38, 1983.

Livesey, G., and Elia, M.: Estimation of energy expenditure, net carbohydrate utilization and net fat oxidization and synthesis by indirect calorimetry: evaluation of errors with special reference to detailed composition of fuels. *Am. J. Clin. Nutr.*, 47:608, 1988.

Montoye, H.J., et al.: *Measuring Physical Activity and Energy Expenditure.* Champaign, IL: Human Kinetics, 1996.

Ravussin, E., et al.: Determinants of 24-hour energy expenditure in man: methods and results using a respiratory chamber. *J. Clin. Invest.*, 78:1568, 1986.

Rumpler, W., et al.: Repeatability of 24-hour energy expenditure measurements in humans by indirect calorimetry. *Am. J. Clin. Nutr.*, 51:147, 1990.

Scholander, P.F.: Analyzer for accurate estimation of respiratory gases in one-half cubic centimeter samples. *J. Biol. Chem.*, 167:235, 1947.

Schutz, Y., and Deurenberg, P.: Energy metabolism: overview of recent methods used in human studies. *Ann. Nutr. Metab.*, 40:183, 1996.

Speakman, J.R.: The history and theory of the doubly labeled water technique. *Am. J. Clin. Nutr.*, 68(Suppl):932S, 1998.

Starling, R.D., et al.: Energy requirements and physical activity in free-living older women and men: a doubly labeled water study. *J. Appl. Physiol.*, 85:1063, 1998.

Wideman, L., et al.: Assessment of the Aerosport TEEM 100 portable metabolic measurement system. *Med. Sci. Sports Exerc.*, 28:509, 1996.

Wilmore, J.H., et al.: An automated system for assessing metabolic and respiratory function during exercise. *J. Appl. Physiol.*, 40:619, 1976.

Withers, R.T., et al.: Energy metabolism in sedentary and active 49- to 70-yr-old women. *J. Appl. Physiol.*, 84:1333, 1998.

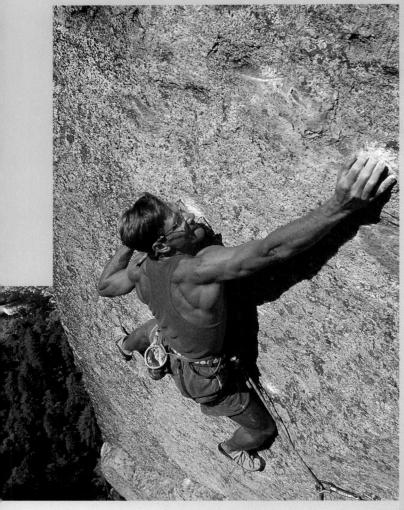

CHAPTER 7

Energy Expenditure During Rest and Physical Activity

Topics covered in this chapter

PART 1 Energy Expenditure at Rest

Energy Expenditure at Rest: Basal Metabolic Rate

Influence of Body Size on Resting Metabolism

Estimating Resting Daily Energy Expenditure

Factors Affecting Energy Expenditure

Summary

PART 2 Energy Expenditure During Physical Activity

Energy Cost of Recreational and Sport Activities

Average Daily Rates of Energy Expenditure

Classification of Work

Summary

PART 3 Energy Expenditure During Walking, Running, and Swimming

Economy of Movement

Mechanical Efficiency

Energy Expenditure During Walking

Energy Expenditure During Running

Energy Expenditure During Swimming

Summary

Thought Questions

Selected References

- Define basal metabolic rate, including factors that affect it.
- Explain the effect of body weight on the energy cost of different forms of physical activity.
- Discuss the Haldane transformation to measure oxygen uptake by open-circuit spirometry.
- Identify factors that contribute to an individual's total daily energy expenditure.
- Outline different classification systems for rating the strenuousness of physical activity.
- Describe two means to predict resting daily energy expenditure.
- Explain the concept of exercise economy, including the differences in running economy between trained and untrained children and adults.
- Graph the relationships between walking and running velocity and energy expenditure.
- List three factors that affect the energy cost of walking and running.
- Identify factors that contribute to the significantly lower exercise economy of swimming compared with running.

PART 1

Energy Expenditure at Rest

Three factors determine daily energy expenditure (Fig. 7.1):

1. Resting metabolic rate, which includes basal and sleeping conditions plus the added cost of arousal
2. Thermogenic influence of food consumed
3. Energy expended during physical activity and recovery

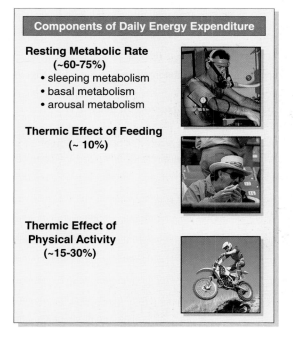

Figure 7.1
Components of daily energy expenditure.

Energy Expenditure at Rest: Basal Metabolic Rate

For each individual, a minimum energy requirement sustains the body's functions in the waking state. Measuring oxygen uptake under the following standardized conditions quantifies this requirement called the **basal metabolic rate** (BMR):

Regular Exercise Blunts a Decrease in Metabolism with Age

Differences in body composition largely explain the 2% decline in BMR per decade through adulthood. Comparisons of young and middle-aged endurance athletes, however, indicate no differences in body composition and BMR. In addition, an accompanying 8% increase in resting metabolism occurred when 50- to 65-year old men increased their fat-free body mass with heavy resistance training. These findings indicate that endurance and resistance exercise training offsets the decrease in resting metabolism usually observed with aging.

- No food consumed for at least 12 hours before measurement. The **postabsorptive state** describes this condition
- No undue muscular exertion for at least 12 hours before measurement
- Measured after the person has been lying quietly for 30 to 60 minutes in a dimly lit, temperature-controlled (thermoneutral) room

Measurement of BMR under controlled laboratory conditions provides a method to study the relationship among energy expenditure and body size, gender, and age. The BMR also establishes an important energy baseline for implementing a prudent program of weight control by food restraint, exercise, or both. In most instances, basal values measured in the laboratory remain only marginally lower than values for resting metabolic rate measured under less strict conditions, e.g., 3 to 4 hours after a light meal without physical activity. In these discussions, we use the terms basal and resting metabolism interchangeably.

Influence of Body Size on Resting Metabolism

Body surface area frequently provides a common denominator for expressing basal metabolism among individuals who differ in body size. The results of numerous experiments provide data on average values of BMR per unit surface area in men and women of different ages.

Figure 7.2 reveals that BMR averages 5 to 10% lower in females compared with males at all ages. A female's larger percentage of body fat and smaller muscle mass in relation to body size helps explain her lower metabolic rate per unit surface area. Gender differences usually disappear when expressing BMR per unit of "fat-free" mass. Whereas this observation may be of some theoretical importance, the curves in Figure 7.2 still describe the average BMR in men and women adequately. From ages 20 to 40, average values for BMR equal 38 kcal per squared meter (m^{-2}) of body surface per hour ($kcal \cdot m^{-2} \cdot hr^{-1}$) for men, and 36 $kcal \cdot m^{-2} \cdot hr^{-1}$ for women. For a more precise estimate of BMR, the actual average value for a specific age can be read directly from the curves. By using the value for heat production (BMR) in Figure 7.2 combined with the appropriate surface area value, a person's resting metabolic rate ($kcal \cdot min^{-1}$) can be estimated and converted to a total daily resting requirement.

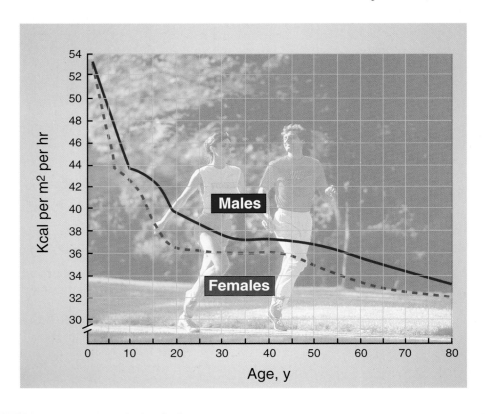

Figure 7.2
Basal metabolic rate as a function of age and gender. (Data from Altman, P. L., and Dittmer, D.: *Metabolism.* Bethesda, MD: Federation of American Societies for Experimental Biology, 1968.)

How to Calculate and Interpret Body Surface Area

Body surface area (BSA) refers to the body's external area usually expressed in square meters (m^2). Aside from using BSA to express basal metabolic rate and lung function measures, BSA sometimes serves as the frame of reference for equating different size individuals for energy expenditure during physical activity. The early measurements of BSA involved wrapping the whole body with gauze and then determining gauze area (total area, m^2 = length, m × width, m).

Calculations

Stature in m and body mass in kg predict BSA in m^2 as follows:

$$BSA = 0.20247 \times Stature^{0.725} \times Body\ mass^{0.425}$$

Example

Male: stature, 1.778 m (177.8 cm; 70 in); body mass, 75 kg (165.3 lb)

$$BSA = 0.20247 \times 1.778^{0.725} \times 75^{0.425}$$
$$= 0.20247 \times 1.51775 \times 6.02647$$
$$= 2.055\ m^2$$

The accompaning nomogram provides a simplified method to compute BSA based on stature and mass. Locate stature on Scale I and body mass on Scale II. Connect the two points with a straight edge. The intersection at Scale III gives the surface area in m^2. For example, if stature equals 185 cm and body mass equals 75 kg, BSA (Scale III) equals 1.98 m^2. ∎

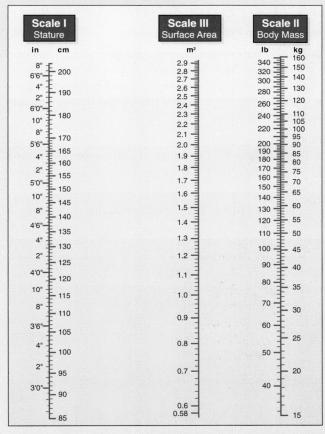

Body Surface Area Nomogram

Nomogram to estimate body surface area from stature and mass. (Reprinted from "Clinical Spirometry," as prepared by Boothby and Sandiford of the Mayo Clinic, courtesy of Warren E. Collins Inc., Braintree, MA.)

Estimating Resting Daily Energy Expenditure (RDEE)

To estimate an individual's **resting daily energy expenditure (RDEE)**, multiply the appropriate average BMR value in Figure 7.2 by surface area (see *How to Calculate and Interpret Body Surface Area*). Then multiply this hourly value by 24 to obtain a 24-hour estimate. For a 55-year-old woman, for example, the estimated BMR equals 34 kcal · m^{-2} · hr^{-1}. If her surface area were 1.40 m^2, the hourly energy expenditure equals 47.6 kcal (34 × 1.40 m^2). On a 24-hour basis, this amounts to an energy expenditure of 1142 kcal (47.6 × 24). The accompanying *"How to"* (page 158) provides a convenient means to estimate RDEE from measures of body size, body composition, and age.

Factors Affecting Energy Expenditure

The important factors that affect a person's **total daily energy expenditure** (**TDEE**) include physical activity, dietary-induced thermogenesis, and climate. Pregnancy also affects TDEE through its effect on the energy cost of many forms of physical activity.

Physical Activity

Physical activity profoundly affects human energy expenditure. World-class athletes nearly double their daily caloric outputs with 3 or 4 hours of hard training. Most people can sustain metabolic rates that average 10-times the resting value during "big muscle" exercises such as fast

How to Predict Resting Daily Energy Expenditure (RDEE) from Fat-Free Body Mass, and from Body Mass, Stature, and Age

Prediction from Fat-Free Body Mass

The fat-free body mass (FFM = body mass − fat mass) reflects total muscle mass and relates directly to the body's total energy expenditure (metabolism) during rest. Individual differences in FFM provide an estimate of resting daily energy expenditure (RDEE).

Equation

The following generalized equation, applicable to men and women, predicts RDEE (kcal · 24 h^{-1}) over a broad range of FFM to an accuracy of ±5%:

$$RDEE = 370 + 21.6 \times FFM, kg$$

Example

Calculate RDEE for a person weighing 90.9 kg (200 lb) with 21% body fat (estimated using one of the several indirect procedures described in Chapter 18), fat mass of 19.1 kg (90.9 kg×0.21), and FFM (90.9 kg − 19.1 kg) of 71.8 kg (158 lb).

$$RDEE = 370 + 21.6 \times 71.8$$
$$= 1921 \text{ kcal}$$

ESTIMATION OF RDEE (KCAL · 24h^{-1}) BASED ON FAT-FREE BODY MASS (kg)

FFM	RDEE	FFM	RDEE	FFM	RDEE
44	1320	66	1796	88	2271
45	1342	67	1817	89	2292
46	1364	68	1839	90	2314
47	1385	69	1860	91	2336
48	1407	70	1882	92	2357
49	1428	71	1904	93	2379
50	1450	72	1925	94	2400
51	1472	73	1947	95	2422
52	1493	74	1968	96	2444
53	1515	75	1990	97	2465
54	1536	76	2012	98	2487
55	1558	77	2033	99	2508
56	1580	78	2055	100	2530
57	1601	79	2076	101	2552
58	1623	80	2098	102	2573
59	1644	81	2120	103	2595
60	1666	82	2141	104	2616
61	1688	83	2163	105	2638
62	1709	84	2184	106	2660
63	1731	85	2206	107	2681
64	1752	86	2228	108	2703
65	1774	87	2249	109	2724

From Cunningham, J.J.: Body composition and resting metabolic rate: the myth of feminine metabolism. *Am. J. Clin. Nutr.*, 36:721, 1982.

Prediction from Body Mass, Stature, and Age

Body mass (BM in kg), stature (S in cm), and age (A in y) also contribute to individual differences in RDEE, making it possible to accurately estimate RDEE using these variables. The method, validated in the early 1900s by Drs. J.A. Harris and F.G. Benedict, used closed-circuit spirometry to carefully measure oxygen uptake in individuals who varied in body size and age.

Equations

Women: RDEE = 655 + (9.6 × BM) + (1.85 × S) − (4.7 × A)
Men: RDEE = 66.0 + (13.7 × BM) + (5.0 × S) − (6.8 × A)

Examples

Woman: BM= 62.7 kg; S =172.5 cm; A = 22.4 y.
RDEE = 655 + (9.6 × 62.7) + (1.85 × 172.5) − (4.7 × 22.4)
= 655 + 601.92 + 319.13 − 105.28
= 1471 kcal

Man: BM = 80 kg; S = 189.0 cm; A = 30 y.
RDEE = 66.0 + (13.7 × 80) + (5.0 × 189.0) − (6.8 × 30.0)
= 66.0 + 1096 + 945 − 204
= 1903 kcal

Harris, J.A., and Benedict, F.G.: A biometric study of basal metabolism in man. Publ. No. 279. Washington, DC: Carnegie Institute. 1919.

walking, running, cycling, and swimming. *Physical activity accounts for between 15 and 30% of a person's TDEE.*

Dietary-Induced Thermogenesis

Consuming food increases energy metabolism from the energy-requiring processes of digesting, absorbing, and assimilating nutrients. **Dietary-induced thermogenesis** (also termed **thermic effect of food**) typically reaches maximum within 1 hour after eating, depending on food quantity and type. The magnitude of dietary-induced thermogenesis ranges between 10 and 35% of ingested food energy. A meal of pure protein, for example, elicits a thermic effect often equaling 25% of the meal's total calories.

Some have touted the high thermic effect of protein consumption to promote a high-protein diet for weight loss. Advocates maintain that fewer calories ultimately become available to the body compared with a lipid- or carbohydrate-rich meal of similar caloric value. Although this point has some validity, other factors must be considered in formulating a prudent weight loss program. These include the potentially harmful strain on kidney and liver function induced by excessive dietary protein, or the cholesterol-stimulating effects of the large amount of saturated fatty acids usually contained in high-protein (meat) food from the animal kingdom. Well-balanced nutrition requires a blend of macronutrients with appropriate quantities of vitamins and minerals. When combining exercise with food restriction for weight loss, carbohydrate (not protein) intake provides energy for exercise and conserves lean tissue often lost through dieting (refer to Chapter 2).

Individuals with poor control over body weight often have a blunted thermic response to eating, most likely a genetic predisposition (see *Close up*, Chapter 6). This undoubtedly contributes to considerable body fat accumulation over a period of years. If a person's lifestyle includes regular moderate physical activity, then the thermogenic effect represents only a small portion of TDEE. Also, exercising after eating augments an individual's normal thermic response to food intake. This supports the wisdom of "going for a brisk walk" following a meal.

Climate

Environmental factors influence resting metabolic rate. The resting metabolism of people living in tropical climates averages 5 to 20% higher than counterparts in more temperate regions. Exercise performed in hot weather also imposes a small additional metabolic load, causing about a 5% elevation in oxygen uptake compared with the same work performed in a thermoneutral environment. This comes from a direct thermogenic effect of elevated core temperature, plus additional energy required for sweat-gland activity and altered circulatory dynamics.

Cold environments can also significantly affect energy metabolism, depending on a person's body fat content and the thermal quality of clothing. During extreme cold stress, resting metabolism can double or triple because shivering generates heat to maintain a stable core temperature. The effects of cold stress during exercise become most evident in cold water due to the difficulty maintaining a stable core temperature in this environment.

Pregnancy

Researchers now better understand the impact of exercise on both mother and fetus. One area of interest concerns how pregnancy affects the metabolic cost and physiologic strain imposed by exercise. *Research findings indicate that maternal cardiovascular dynamics follow normal response patterns, and that moderate exercise presents no greater physiologic stress to the mother than imposed by the additional weight gain and possible encumbrance of fetal tissue.* Pregnancy does not compromise the absolute value for aerobic capacity ($L \cdot min^{-1}$). As pregnancy progresses, increases in maternal body weight add significantly to exercise effort during weight-bearing activities like walking, jogging, and stair climbing and may reduce economy of effort. Pregnancy, particularly in the later stages, also increases pulmonary ventilation at a given submaximal exercise level. This maternal "hyperventilation" has been attributed to the direct stimulating effects of the hormone progesterone and increased sensitivity of the respiratory center to carbon dioxide.

summary

1. A person's total daily energy expenditure (TDEE) represents the sum of energy required in basal and resting metabolism, thermogenic influences (particularly thermic effect of food), and energy generated in physical activity.

2. Basal metabolic rate (BMR) reflects the minimum energy required to maintain vital functions in the waking state. BMR averages only slightly below resting metabolism, and relates proportionately to the body's surface area. BMR also relates inversely to age and gender, averaging 5 to 10% lower in women compared to men. Fat-free body (FFM) mass and percent body fat largely account for age and gender differences in BMR.

3. Body mass, stature, and age, or estimates of FFM mass provide accurate estimates resting daily energy expenditure.

4. Physical activity, dietary-induced thermogenesis, environmental factors, and pregnancy significantly affect TDEE.

5. Dietary-induced thermogenesis refers to the increase in energy metabolism attributable to digestion, absorption, and assimilation of food nutrients. A blunted thermogenic response to eating can stimulate weight gain.

6. Exposure to hot and cold environments cause a small increase in TDEE.

PART 2
Energy Expenditure During Physical Activity

An understanding of resting energy metabolism provides an important frame of reference to appreciate the potential of humans to increase daily energy output. According to numerous surveys, physical inactivity (e.g., watching television, lounging around the home, and other sedentary activities) accounts for about one-third of a person's waking hours. This means that regular physical activity can potentially provide a significant boost to the TDEE of large numbers of men and women. Actualizing this potential depends on the intensity, duration, and type of physical activity performed.

Researchers have measured the energy expended during varied activities like brushing teeth, house cleaning, mowing the lawn, walking the dog, driving a car, playing ping-pong, bowling, dancing, swimming, rock climbing, and physical activity during space flight. Consider an activity such as rowing continuously at 30 strokes a minute for 30 minutes. How can we determine the number of calories "burned" during the 30 minutes? If the amount of oxygen consumed averaged $2.0 \text{ L} \cdot \text{min}^{-1}$ during each minute of rowing, then in 30 minutes the rower would consume 60 liters of oxygen. A reasonably accurate estimate of the energy expended in rowing can be made because 1 liter of oxygen generates about 5 kcal of energy. In this example, the rower would expend 300 kcal (60 liters × 5 kcal) during the exercise period. This value represents the **gross energy expenditure** for the exercise period.

This energy cannot all be attributed solely to rowing because the 300 kcal value also includes the resting requirement during the 30-minute row. The rower's body surface area of 2.04 m^2 estimated from the nomogram in *How to Calculate and Interpret Body Surface Area* (body mass = 81.8 kg; stature = 183 cm), multiplied by the average BMR for gender ($38 \text{ kcal} \cdot \text{m}^{-2} \cdot \text{hr}^{-1} \times 2.04 \text{ m}^2$) gives the resting metabolism per hour—approximately 78 kcal per hour or 39 kcal "burned" over 30 minutes. Based on these computations, the **net energy expenditure** attributable solely to rowing equals gross energy expenditure (300 kcal) minus the requirement for rest (39 kcal), or approximately 261 kcal.

Some investigators estimate daily energy expenditure in diverse occupations by determining the time spent in each activity (usually by diary) and the activity's corresponding energy requirement. For the miner depicted in Table 7.1, who spent 12 hours during the week loading coal, the energy cost of the task ranged between 5.5 and 7.2 kcal per minute. For purposes of computation, 6.3 kcal per minute represented the energy cost during this work period. The total 26,460 kcal expended during the week aver-

TABLE 7.1
Energy expended by a coal miner during 1 week*

ACTIVITY	TIME SPENT IN 1 WEEK (hr)	(min)	RATE OF ENERGY EXPENDED (kcal·min^{-1})	ENERGY IN 1 WEEK (kcal)
Sleep in bed	58	30	1.05	3690
Nonoccupational				
Sitting	38	37	1.59	3680
Standing	2	16	1.80	250
Walking	15	0	4.90	4410
Washing and dressing	5	3	3.30	1000
Gardening	2	0	5.00	600
Cycling	2	25	6.60	960
Work				
Sitting	15	9	1.68	1530
Standing	2	6	1.80	230
Walking	6	43	6.70	2700
Cutting	1	14	6.70	500
Timbering	6	51	5.70	2340
Loading	12	6	6.30	4570
Total weekly energy expenditure				26,460
Average daily energy expenditure				3780

* Data from Garry, R. C., et al.: Expenditure of energy and the consumption of food by miners and clerks. *Medical Research Council Report No. 289.* Fife, Scotland: H.M.S.O., 1955.

c l o s e   u p

The Haldane Transformation to Calculate Oxygen Uptake

Measurement of oxygen uptake ($\dot{V}O_2$) using open-circuit spirometry provides fundamental data in the study of exercise physiology. The open-circuit method assumes that the body neither produces nor retains gaseous nitrogen during the measurement period, i.e., the quantity of nitrogen remains exactly equal in the inspired and expired air. Under this assumption, one need not collect and analyze *both* inspired and expired air volumes during measurements of oxygen consumption and carbon dioxide production. The following equation, known as the **Haldane transformation**, describes the mathematical expression about the relationship between inspired and expired air volumes based on an assumed constancy for gaseous nitrogen.

$$\dot{V}_I = \dot{V}_E \times F_E N_2 \div F_I N_2$$

where $\dot{V}_I$ equals air volume inspired, $\dot{V}_E$ equals air volume expired, and $F_E N_2$ and $F_I N_2$ equal the fractional concentrations of nitrogen in the expired and inspired air, respectively. Because the fractional concentrations for inspired oxygen ($F_I O_2$), carbon dioxide ($F_I CO_2$), and nitrogen ($F_I N_2$) are known, only $\dot{V}_E$ (or $\dot{V}_I$) and the expired air concentrations of CO_2 ($F_E CO_2$) and O_2 ($F_E O_2$) are required to calculate $\dot{V}O_2$, assuming no net production or retention of N_2.

$$\dot{V}O_2 = \dot{V}_E \times (F_E N_2 / F_I N_2) \times F_I O_2 - \dot{V}_E \times F_E O_2$$

In this formula, $F_E N_2$ equals:

$$1.00 - (F_E O_2 + F_E CO_2)$$

Comparisons of $\dot{V}O_2$ calculated from only expired ventilation (applying the Haldane transformation) versus $\dot{V}O_2$ calculated using measured inspired and expired ventilations at different exercise intensities are needed to study net nitrogen retention or production.

The data in the figure show the experimental results in which six subjects completed treadmill exercise by walking on the level at 4 mph; a 5-minute jog followed at 6 mph, followed again by a 5-minute run at 7.5 mph. Oxygen uptake was continuously monitored using open-circuit spirometry, and measures of inspired and expired pulmonary ventilations. Measurements also included barometric pressure, inspired and expired gas temperatures, relative humidity, and $F_E O_2$, $F_E CO_2$, $F_I O_2$, and $F_I CO_2$.

The figure plots $\dot{V}O_2$ estimated using only expired $\dot{V}_E$ (Y-

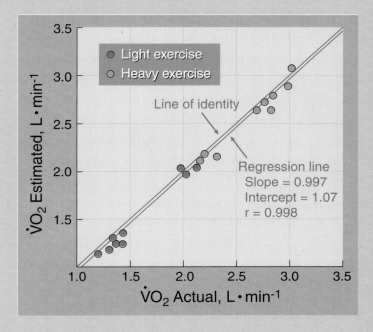

axis) versus actual $\dot{V}O_2$ calculated from both $\dot{V}_I$ and $\dot{V}_E$ (X-axis).

The solid line represents the line of identity—if all data points fall on this line, perfect association exists between the two $\dot{V}O_2$ estimates. The slope of the regression line relating the two $\dot{V}O_2$ estimates deviated only 0.003 unit from unity, and the intercept approximates zero. This indicates an impressively close relationship between the actual oxygen uptake and that predicted by the Haldane transformation. The largest difference between the actual and estimated $\dot{V}O_2$ values equaled 230 mL, an error of 7.3%. The average difference of 0.8% for all subjects occurred within the instrument's measurement error. For the nitrogen data, a difference of 1.6% occurred between the minute volume of nitrogen inspired and expired for any subject at any exercise level; 11 of 17 subject-work rates exhibited less than a ±1% difference. The largest difference, 1099 mL $N_2 \cdot min^{-1}$, occurred during heavy exercise (2.1% difference).

These findings justify the continued use of the Haldane transformation to calculate $\dot{V}O_2$ during exercise. Although production and/or retention of N_2 can occur, it has little or no effect on the $\dot{V}O_2$ computation.

Reference

Wilmore, J.H., and Costill, D.L.: Adequacy of the Haldane transformation in the computation of exercise $\dot{V}O_2$ in man. *J. Appl. Physiol.*, 35:85, 1973.

aged 3780 kcal per day. This includes the energy expended during the 8-hour work shift, the energy cost of sleeping 8 hours, and the remaining approximately 8 hours spent in nonoccupational activities.

Energy Cost of Recreational and Sport Activities

Table 7.2 lists eight examples that illustrate energy cost among diverse recreational and sport activities. Notice, for example, that volleyball requires about 3.6 kcal per minute (216 kcal per hour) for a person weighing 71 kg (157 lb). The same person expends more than twice this energy, or 546 kcal per hour, swimming the front crawl. Viewed somewhat differently, 25 minutes spent swimmig expends about the same number of calories as playing 1-hour of recreational volleyball. If the pace of the swim or volleyball game increases, energy expenditure increases proportionately.

Effect of Body Mass

Body size often plays an important role in exercise energy requirements. Figure 7.3 illustrates that heavier people expend more energy to perform the same activity than people who weigh less. This occurs because the energy expended during **weight-bearing exercise** increases directly with the body mass transported. *Such a strong relationship*

exists that one can predict energy expenditure during walking or running from body mass with almost as much accuracy as actually measuring oxygen uptake. In non–weight-bearing or **weight-supported exercise** (e.g., stationary cycling), little relationship exists between body mass and exercise energy cost.

From a practical standpoint, walking and other weight-bearing exercises expend a substantial number of calories for heavier people. Notice in Table 7.2 that playing tennis or volleyball results in considerably greater energy expenditure for a person weighing 83 kg than for someone 20-kg lighter. Expressing caloric cost of weight-bearing exercise in relation to body mass, as kcal per kilogram of body mass per minute ($kcal \cdot kg^{-1} \cdot min^{-1}$), greatly reduces the difference in energy expenditure among individuals of different body weights.

A Considerable Energy Output

The competitive efforts of elite athletes during a marathon generate a steady-rate energy expenditure of about 25 kcal per minute for the duration of the run. Among elite rowers, a 5- to 7-minute competition generates about 36 kcal per minute!

TABLE 7.2
Gross energy cost for selected recreational and sports activities in relation to body mass*

ACTIVITY	kg lb	50 110	53 117	56 123	59 130	62 137	65 143	68 150	71 157	74 163	77 170	80 176	83 183
Volleyball	12.5	2.7	2.8	3.0	3.1	3.3	3.4	3.6	3.7	3.9	4.0	4.2	
Aerobic dancing	6.7	7.1	7.5	7.9	8.3	8.7	9.2	9.6	10.0	10.4	10.8	11.2	
Cycling, leisure	5.0	5.3	5.6	5.9	6.2	6.5	6.8	7.1	7.4	7.7	8.0	8.3	
Tennis	5.5	5.8	6.1	6.4	6.8	7.1	7.4	7.7	8.1	8.4	8.7	9.0	
Swimming, slow crawl	6.4	6.8	7.2	7.6	7.9	8.3	8.7	9.1	9.5	9.9	10.2	10.6	
Touch football	6.6	7.0	7.4	7.8	8.2	8.6	9.0	9.4	9.8	10.2	10.6	11.0	
Running, 8-min mile	10.8	11.3	11.9	12.5	13.11	3.6	14.2	14.8	15.4	16.0	16.5	17.1	
Skiing, uphill racing	13.7	14.5	15.3	16.2	17.0	17.8	18.6	19.5	20.3	21.1	21.9	22.7	

* Data from *Student Study Guide and Workbook*.

Note: Energy expenditure computes as the number of minutes of participation multiplied by the kcal value in the appropriate body weight column. For example, the kcal cost of one hour of tennis for a person weighing 150 pounds equals 444 kcal (7.4 kcal × 60 min).

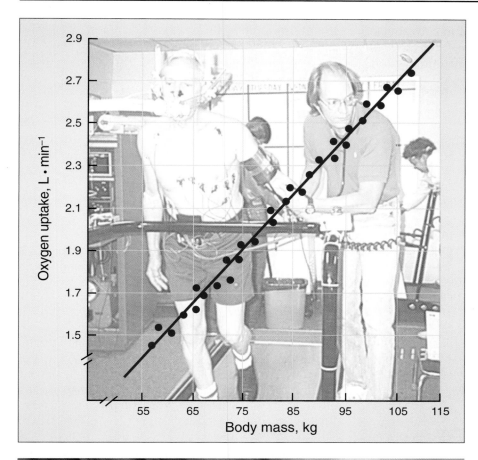

Figure 7.3
Relationship between body mass and oxygen uptake measured during submaximal, brisk treadmill walking. (From Applied Physiology Laboratory, Queens College, Flushing, NY). Photo courtesy of Dr. Jay Graves, Syracuse University.

Average Daily Rates of Energy Expenditure

committee of the United States Food and Nutrition Board proposed various norms to represent average rates of energy expenditure for men and women in the United States. These values apply to people with occupations considered between sedentary and active, and who participate in some recreational activities such as weekend swimming, golf, and tennis. Table 7.3 shows that between 2900 and 3000 kcal for males and 2200 kcal for females between the ages of 15 and 50 represent the average daily energy expenditures. As shown in the lower part of the table, the typical person spends about 75% of the day in sedentary activities. This predominance of physical *inactivity* has prompted some sociologists to refer to the modern-day American as *homo sedentarius.*

Classification of Work

ll of us at one time or another have done some type of physical work we would classify as exceedingly "difficult." This includes walking up a long flight of stairs, shoveling a snow-filled driveway, sprinting to catch a bus, loading and unloading furniture on a truck, digging trenches, skiing through a snow storm, or running in soft beach sand. Two factors affect one's rating of the difficulty of a particular task: *duration of activity* and *intensity of effort.* Both factors can vary

TABLE 7.3
Average rates of energy expenditure for men and women living in the United States[a]

	AGE (y)	BODY MASS (kg)	(lb)	STATURE (cm)	(in)	ENERGY EXPENDITURE (kcal)
Males	15–18	66	145	176	69	3000
	19–24	72	160	177	70	2900
	25–50	79	174	176	70	2900
	51+	77	170	173	68	2300
Females	15–18	55	120	163	64	2200
	19–24	58	128	164	65	2200
	25–50	63	138	163	64	2200
	50+	65	143	160	63	1900

AVERAGE TIME SPENT DURING THE DAY

ACTIVITY	TIME (hr)
Sleeping and lying down	8
Sitting	6
Standing	6
Walking	2
Recreational activity	2

Data from Food and Nutrition Board, National Research Council: *Recommended Dietary Allowances*, revised. Washington, DC, National Academy of Sciences, 1989.
[a]The information in this table was designed for the maintenance of practically all healthy people in the United States.

considerably. For example, two people of the same body size could expend an equal amount of energy to complete the same task. One might exert extreme effort over a short period, while the other exerts less effort over a longer period. Running a 26-mile marathon at various speeds illustrates this point. One runner runs at maximum pace and completes the race in a little more than 2 hours. Another runner of similar fitness selects a slower, more "leisurely" pace and completes the run in 3 hours. In these examples, the intensity of exercise distinguishes the performance. In another situation, two people run at the same speed, but one runs twice as long as the other. Here, exercise duration becomes the important consideration.

Several classification systems rate sustained physical activity for strenuousness. One system, the **physical activity ratio (PAR)**, classifies physical effort by the ratio of energy required for the task compared with the resting energy requirement. Light work for men elicits an oxygen uptake (or energy expenditure) up to three times the resting requirement; heavy work requires six to eight times the resting metabolism; maximal work consists of any task requiring metabolism to increase nine times or more above rest. *As a frame of reference, most industrial jobs and household tasks require less than three times the resting energy expenditure.*

For women, slightly lower ratios exist for the work classifications because women have lower aerobic capacities. Somewhat lower energy expenditure standards exist for categorizing the strenuousness of occupational tasks than would be applied to general exercise. Industrial work usually requires prolonged effort, often using a small muscle mass, and performed under varying and often stressful environmental conditions and physical constraints.

MET

The five-level classification system presented in Table 7.4 considers the energy required by untrained men and women performing different physical activities, including a range of occupational tasks. Because 5 kcal equals about 1 L of oxygen consumed, the five-stage classification also can be presented as liters of oxygen consumed per minute (L · min^{-1}), milliliters of oxygen per kilogram of body mass per minute (mL · kg^{-1} · min^{-1}), or **METs**, defined as a multiple of resting metabolic rate. Thus, 1 MET equals a resting oxygen uptake of about 250 mL per minute for an average-weight man and 200 mL per minute for a woman of average weight. Work performed at 2 METs requires twice the resting metabolism, or about 500 mL of oxy-

gen per minute for a man, 3 METs equals three times the resting energy expenditure, and so on. *For a more accurate classification that accounts for variations in body size, the MET should be expressed as oxygen uptake per unit of body mass, where 1 MET equals 3.5 mL · kg^{-1} · min^{-1}.*

Table 7.5 presents a system for characterizing leisure physical activity for absolute (multiples of resting metabolism) and relative (percentage of $\dot{V}O_{2max}$) intensity. The categorization for exercise intensity in terms of METs adjusts downward with age to account for a general "aging effect" on aerobic capacity.

Heart Rate to Estimate Energy Expenditure

For each person, heart rate and oxygen uptake tend to relate linearly throughout a broad range of aerobic exercise intensities. By knowing this precise relationship, exercise heart rate provides an estimate of oxygen uptake (and then energy expenditure) during physical activity. This approach serves as a substitute when oxygen uptake cannot be measured during the actual activity.

Figure 7.4 presents data for two members of a nationally ranked women's basketball team during a laboratory treadmill running test. Heart rate for each woman increased linearly with exercise intensity—a proportionate increase in heart rate accompanied each increase in oxygen uptake. However, a similar heart rate for each athlete does not correspond to the same level of oxygen uptake because the slope (rate of change) of the "HR-$\dot{V}O_2$ line" differs consid-

TABLE 7.4
Five-level classification of physical activity based on exercise intensity*

LEVEL	ENERGY EXPENDITURE			
	Men			
	kcal · min^{-1}	L · min^{-1}	mL · kg^{-1} · min^{-1}	METs
Light	2.0–4.9	0.40–0.99	6.1–15.2	1.6–3.9
Moderate	5.0–7.4	1.00–1.49	15.3–22.9	4.0–5.9
Heavy	7.5–9.9	1.50–1.99	23.0–30.6	6.0–7.9
Very heavy	10.0–12.4	2.00–2.49	30.7–38.3	8.0–9.9
Unduly heavy	12.5–	2.50–	38.4–	10.0–
	Women			
	kcal · min^{-1}	L · min^{-1}	mL · kg^{-1} · min^{-1}	METs
Light	1.5–3.4	0.30–0.69	5.4–12.5	1.2–2.7
Moderate	3.5–5.4	0.70–1.09	12.6–19.8	2.8–4.3
Heavy	5.5–7.4	1.10–1.49	19.9–27.1	4.4–5.9
Very heavy	7.5–9.4	1.50–1.89	27.2–34.4	6.0–7.5
Unduly heavy	9.5–	1.90–	34.5–	7.6–

* L·min^{-1} based on 5 kcal per liter of oxygen; ml·kg^{-1}·min^{-1} based on 65-kg man and 55-kg woman; one MET equals average resting oxygen uptake of 3.5 mL · kg^{-1} · min^{-1}.

2.2√168 × 3.5   76.36 =21.

TABLE 7.5
Characterizatiion of the intensity of leisure activity related to age

CATEGORIZATION	RELATIVE INTENSITY (% $\dot{V}O_{2MAX}$)	ABSOLUTE INTENSITY (METs)			
		YOUNG	MIDDLE-AGED	OLD	VERY-OLD
Rest	<10	1.0	1.0	1.0	1.0
Light	<35	<4.5	<3.5	<2.5	<1.5
Fairly light	<50	<6.5	<5.0	<3.5	<2.0
Moderate	<70	<9.0	<7.0	<5.0	<2.8
Heavy	>70	>9.0	>7.0	>5.0	>2.8
Maximal	100	13.0	10.0	7.0	4.0

From Bouchard, C., et al.: *Exercise, Fitness, and Health: A Consensus of Current Knowledge.* Champaign, IL: Human Kinetics, 1990.

erably between the women. For a given increase in oxygen uptake, the heart rate of subject B increases less than for subject A. However, knowing the exercise heart rate can estimate exercise oxygen uptake. For player A, an exercise heart rate of 140 b · min⁻¹ corresponds to an oxygen uptake of 1.08 L · min⁻¹, whereas the same heart rate for player B corresponds to an oxygen uptake of 1.60 L · min⁻¹. Heart rates obtained using radiotelemetry during basketball competition were applied to each player's HR-$\dot{V}O_2$ line to estimate energy expenditure under game conditions.

A major consideration when using heart rate to estimate oxygen uptake lies in the similarity between the laboratory assessment of the HR-$\dot{V}O_2$ line and the specific "in vivo" field activity applied to this relationship. For one thing, factors other than oxygen uptake influence heart rate response to exercise. These factors include environmental temperature, emotional state, previous food intake, body position, muscle groups exercised, continuous or discontinuous nature of the exercise, and whether the muscles act statically or more dynamically. During aerobic dance, for example,

significantly higher heart rates occur while dancing at a specific oxygen uptake than at the same oxygen uptake walking or running on a treadmill. Arm exercise, or when muscles act statically in a straining-type exercise, generate consistently higher heart rates compared with dynamic leg exercise at any submaximum oxygen uptake. Consequently, applying heart rates during upper-body or static exercise to a HR-$\dot{V}O_2$ line established during running or cycling *overpredicts* the criterion oxygen uptake.

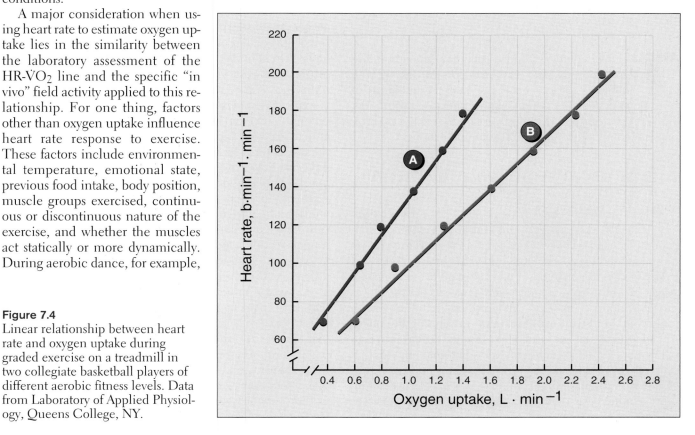

Figure 7.4
Linear relationship between heart rate and oxygen uptake during graded exercise on a treadmill in two collegiate basketball players of different aerobic fitness levels. Data from Laboratory of Applied Physiology, Queens College, NY.

summary

1. Energy expenditure can be expressed in gross or net terms. Gross (total) values include the resting energy requirement, whereas net energy expenditure reflects the energy cost of the activity per se excluding the value for resting metabolism.

2. Daily rates of energy expenditure classify different occupations and sports professions. Within any classification, variability exists due to energy expended in recreational and/or on-the-job pursuits. Heavier individuals expend more energy in most physical activities than lighter counterparts.

3. Average daily energy expenditure ranges between 2900 to 3000 kcal for males and 2200 kcal for females ages 15 to 50 years. Large individual differences in one's physical activity level affect daily energy expenditure.

4. Different classification systems rate the strenuousness of physical activities. These include ratings based on energy cost expressed in kcal · min^{-1}; oxygen requirement in L · min^{-1}; or multiples of the resting metabolic rate (METs).

5. Exercise heart rate can be used to estimate energy expenditure during physical activity from an individual's heart rate-oxygen uptake (HR-VO$_2$) line determined in the laboratory. Researchers then apply the heart rates during recreational, sport, or occupational activity to the "HR-VO$_2$ line" to estimate exercise oxygen uptake.

PART 3
Energy Expenditure During Walking, Running, and Swimming

The total energy expended each day depends on the type, intensity, and duration of physical activity. The following sections detail the energy expenditure of three popular activities,—walking, running, and swimming. These activities play an important role for weight control, physical conditioning, and cardiac rehabilitation.

Economy of Movement

The concept of economy can be viewed as the relationship between energy input and energy output. In an economic sense, economy of operation reflects the cost required to produce goods in relation to the money generated from the sale of such goods. For example, the auto industry strives to optimize a vehicle's aerodynamic design to improve economy of operation reflected by the miles-per-gallon rating. For **economy of human movement**, the quantity of energy to perform a particular task relative to performance quality represents an important concern. In a sense, many of us assess economy by visually comparing the ease of movement of highly trained athletes. It does not require a trained eye to discriminate the ease of effort in comparisons of elite swimmers, skiers, dancers, gymnasts, and divers with less proficient counterparts who seem to expend considerable "wasted energy" to perform the same tasks. Anyone who has learned a new sport recalls the difficulties encountered performing basic movements that, with practice, became automatic and seemingly "effortless."

Exercise Oxygen Uptake Reflects Economy

A common method to assess differences between individuals in economy of movement evaluates the steady-rate oxygen uptake during a specific exercise at a set power output or speed. This approach only applies to steady-rate exercise where oxygen uptake closely mirrors energy expenditure. *For example, at a given submaximum speed of running, cycling, or swimming, an individual with greater movement economy consumes less oxygen.* Economy takes on importance during longer-duration exercise, where the athlete's aerobic capability and the oxygen requirements of the task determine success. *All else being equal, a training adjustment that improves economy of effort directly translates to improved performance.* Figure 7.5 relates running economy to endurance performance in elite athletes of comparable aerobic fitness. Clearly, athletes with greater running economies (lower oxygen uptake at the same running pace) achieve better performance.

No single biomechanical factor accounts for individual differences in running economy. Significant variation in economy at a particular running speed occurs even among trained runners. In general, improved running economy results from years of arduous run training. Short-term training that emphasizes only the "proper techniques" of running (e.g., arm movements and body alignment) probably does not improve running economy. Research shows, however, that distance runners who lack an economical stride-length pattern benefit from a short-term program of audio-visual feedback that focuses on optimizing stride length.

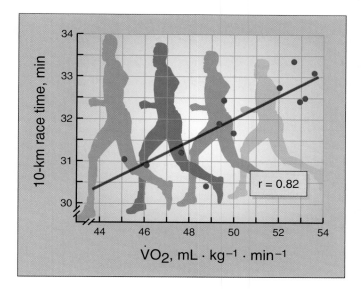

Figure 7.5
Relationship between submaximum $\dot{V}O_2$ at 16.1 km · hr^{-1} and 10-km race time in elite male runners of comparable aerobic capacity.

Mechanical Efficiency

Another way to evaluate the relationship between energy input and exercise power output estimates the **mechanical efficiency (ME)** of movement. Mechanical efficiency indicates the percentage of the total chemical energy expended that contributes to external work, the remainder being lost as heat. Within this context:

$$\text{ME (\%)} = \frac{\text{Mechanical work}}{\text{Energy input}} \times 100$$

Force, acting through a vertical distance (F × D) and usually recorded as foot-pounds or kilogram-meters (kg-m), indicates the actual external work accomplished (energy output). External work is fairly easy to determine during cycle ergometry or exercises that require lifting the body mass like stair climbing or bench stepping. In horizontal walking or running, work output cannot be computed because (technically) external work does not take place. Reciprocal leg and arm movements negate each other, and the body achieves no net gain in vertical distance. If a person walks or runs up a grade, the work component can be estimated from body mass and vertical distance (lift) achieved during the exercise period (see *How to Measure Work on a Treadmill, Cycle Ergometer, and Step Bench*, page 134). The steady-rate oxygen uptake during exercise infers the energy input portion of the efficiency equation. To obtain common units for expressing work, oxygen uptake converts to energy units (1.0 L O_2 = 5.0 kcal; see Table 6.1 for precise calorific transformations based on RQ), which can then convert to units of work.

For example, suppose a 15-minute ride on a stationary bicycle generates 13,300 kg-m of work, and net oxygen consumed to perform the work totals 25 L (RQ = 0.88). Convert the oxygen consumed to a corresponding work output to create common units of measurement. From Table 6.1, note that for an RQ of 0.88, each liter of oxygen uptake generates an energy equivalent of 4.9 kcal. Therefore, 25 L of oxygen uptake generates 122.5 kcal of energy (25 L × 4.9 kcal) during the 15-minute ride. One kcal equals the work equivalent of 426.4 kg-m in a perfectly efficient machine. Consequently, work input computes as 52,234 kg-m (122.5 kcal × 426.4 kg-m). Mechanical efficiency (%) computes as follows:

$$\text{ME(\%)} = \frac{13,300 \text{ kg-m}}{52,234 \text{ kg-m}} \times 100 = 25.5\%$$

As with all machines, the human body's efficiency for producing mechanical work falls considerably below 100%. The energy required to overcome internal and external friction becomes the biggest factor that affects mechanical efficiency. Overcoming friction represents essentially wasted energy because it accomplishes no external work; consequently, work input always exceeds work output. The efficiency of human locomotion in walking, running, and cycling ranges between 20 and 30%.

Running Economy: Children and Adults, Trained and Untrained

Boys and girls show less economy in running compared to adults; they require between 20 to 30% more oxygen per unit of body mass to run at a given speed. Differences in economy have been attributed to greater stride frequency among children, and biomechanical differences that contribute to children's inferior movement economy.

Exercise Economy and Muscle Fiber Type

Indirect evidence indicates that muscle fiber-type affects economy of cycling effort. During submaximal cycling, the exercise economies of trained cyclists varied up to 15%. Differences in muscle fiber types in the active muscles accounted for an important component of this variation. Cyclists exhibiting the most economical cycling pattern possessed the greater percentage of slow-twitch (Type I) muscle fibers in their legs. This suggests that the Type I fiber acts with greater mechanical efficiency than the faster-acting Type II fiber.

Figure 7.6
Effects of growth on (**A**) aerobic capacity and (**B**) submaximal oxygen uptake during running at 12.1 km · hr⁻¹. (Adapted from Daniels, J., et al.: Differences and changes in $\dot{V}O_2$ among runners 10 to 18 years of age. *Med. Sci. Sports*, 10:200, 1978.

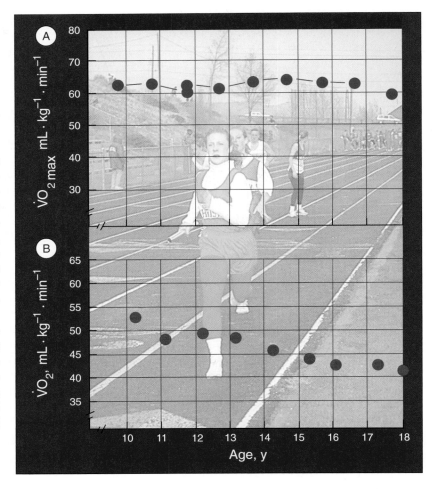

The age-related decreases in steady-rate oxygen uptake at a given speed shown in Figure 7.6B indicate that running economy improves steadily from ages 10 to 18 years. This partly explains the relatively poor performance of young children in distance running, and their progressive improvement throughout adolescence. Improved endurance occurs even though aerobic capacity relative to body mass (mL O_2 · kg⁻¹ · min⁻¹; Fig. 7.6A) remains relatively constant during this time.

At a particular speed, elite endurance runners run at a lower oxygen uptake than less trained or less successful counterparts of similar age. This holds for 8- to 11-year-old cross-country runners and adult marathoners. Elite distance athletes as a group tend to run with 5 to 10% greater economy than well-trained middle-distance runners.

Energy Expenditure During Walking

For most individuals, walking (the most common form of exercise) represents the major type of physical activity that falls outside the realm of sedentary living. Figure 7.7 displays the energy expenditure during walking at slow and fast speeds. A linear relationship exists between walking speed of 3.0 and 5.0 km · hr⁻¹ (1.9 to 3.1 mph) and oxygen uptake; at faster speeds, walking becomes less economical and the relationship curves upward to indicate a disproportionate increase in energy cost related to walking speed. This finding reveals that for a given distance travelled, greater total caloric expenditure occurs at faster but less efficient walking speeds.

Competition Walking

The energy expenditure of Olympic-caliber walkers has been studied at various speeds while walking and running on a treadmill. Their walking speeds in actual competition averaged 13.0 km · hr⁻¹ (11.5 to 14.8 km · hr⁻¹ or 7.1 to 9.2 mph) over distances ranging from 1.6 to 50 km. This represents a relatively fast speed, as the world record holder (Bernardo Segura, Mexico, 1994) averaged 14.4 km · hr⁻¹ (8.95 mph) for the 20-km (12.6-

mile) walk at the 1998 Atlanta Olympics. Figure 7.8 illustrates that the break point in economy of locomotion between walking and running for these competitive race-walkers occurred at about 8.0 km · hr⁻¹. Their data, plus biomechanical evidence, support the contention that the **crossover speed** at which running becomes more economical than walking remains about the same for both conventional walking and competitive walking styles. The oxygen uptake of racewalkers during treadmill walking at competition speeds averaged only slightly lower than the highest oxygen uptake measured for these athletes during treadmill running. Also, a linear relationship existed between oxygen uptake and walking at speeds above 8 km · hr⁻¹ (4.97 mph), but the slope of the line was *twice* as steep compared with running at the same speeds. Although the athletes could walk at velocities up to 16 km · hr⁻¹ (9.94 mph), and attain oxygen uptakes as high as those while running, the economy of walking faster than 8 km · hr⁻¹ averaged one-half of running at similar speeds.

A special gait that involves hip "rolling" allows competition walkers to achieve fast yet uneconomical rates of movement compared with conventional walking. Among elite racewalkers, the relatively large variations in walking economy relate more to performance success in this sport than competitive running.

Figure 7.7
Energy expenditures while walking on a level surface at different speeds. The line represents a compilation of values reported in the literature.

Effects of Body Mass

Body mass can predict energy expenditure with reasonable accuracy at horizontal walking speeds ranging from 3.2 to 6.4 km · hr⁻¹ (2.0 to 4.0 mph) for people of diverse body size and composition. The predicted values for energy expenditure during walking listed in Table 7.6 fall within ±15% of the energy expenditure for men and women of different sizes. On a daily basis, the estimated energy expended walking would only be in error by about 50 to 100 kcal, assuming the person walks 2 hours daily. Research supports the data in this table, which present the caloric cost of walking within the speed range indicated for a body mass up to 91 kg (200 lb). Extrapolations can be made for heavier individuals but with some loss in accuracy.

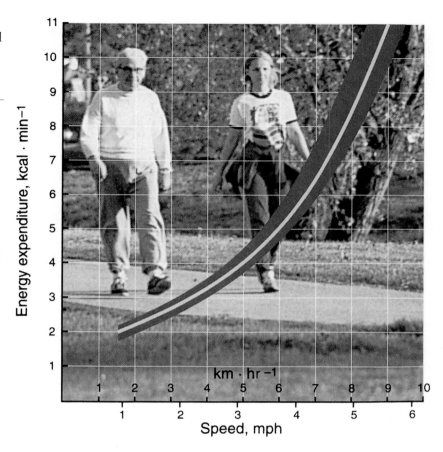

Effects of Terrain and Walking Surface

Table 7.7 summarizes the influence of terrain and surface on the energy cost of walking. Similar economies exist for level walking on a grass track or paved surface. Not surprisingly, the energy cost almost doubles walking in sand compared with walking on a hard surface; in soft snow, the metabolic cost increases 3-fold compared with treadmill walking. A brisk walk along a beach or in freshly fallen snow provides excellent exercise for programs designed to "burn up" calories or improve physiologic fitness.

Effects of Footwear

It requires considerably more energy to carry added weight on the feet or ankles than to carry similar weight

attached to the torso. For example, for a weight equal to 1.4% of body mass placed on the ankles, the energy cost of walking increases an average of 8%, or nearly 6 times more than with the same weight carried on the torso. In a practical sense, the energy cost of locomotion during walking and

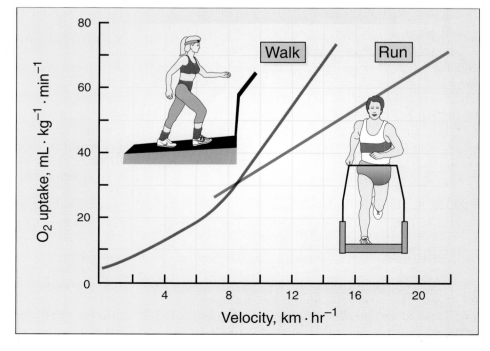

Figure 7.8
Generalized relationship between oxygen uptake and horizontal velocity for walking and running in competition walkers.

TABLE 7.6
Prediction of energy expenditure (kcal · min^{-1}) from speed of level walking and body mass

SPEED			BODY MASS						
		kg	36	45	54	64	73	82	91
mph	km · hr^{-1}	lb	80	100	120	140	160	180	200
2.0	3.22		1.9	2.2	2.6	2.9	3.2	3.5	3.8
2.5	4.02		2.3	2.7	3.1	3.5	3.8	4.2	4.5
3.0	4.83		2.7	3.1	3.6	4.0	4.4	4.8	5.3
3.5	5.63		3.1	3.6	4.2	4.6	5.0	5.4	6.1
4.0	6.44		3.5	4.1	4.7	5.2	5.8	6.4	7.0

How to use the chart: A 54-kg (120-lb) person who walks at 3.0 mph (4.83 km · hr^{-1}) expends 3.6 kcal · min^{-1}. This person would expend 216 kcal during a 60-min walk (3.6 × 60).

running significantly increases when wearing boots compared with running shoes. Simply adding an additional 100 g to each shoe causes a 1% increase in oxygen uptake during moderate running. The implication of these findings for the design of running shoes, hiking and climbing boots, and work boots traditionally required in mining, forestry, fire fighting, and the military seems clear; small changes in shoe weight produce large changes in economy of locomotion. The cushioning properties of shoes also affect movement economy. A softer-soled running shoe reduced the oxygen cost of running at moderate speed by about 2.4% compared with a similar shoe with a firmer cushioning system, even though the softer-soled shoes weighed an additional 31 g. The preceding observations about terrain, footware, and economy of locomotion indicate that at the

TABLE 7.7
Effect of different terrain on the energy expenditure of walking between 5.2 and 5.6 km · hr^{-1}

TERRAIN[a]	CORRECTION FACTOR[b]
Paved road (similar to grass track)	0.0
Plowed field	1.5
Hard snow	1.6
Sand dune	1.8

[a] First entry from Passmore, R., and Dumin, J.V.G.A.: Human energy expenditure. *Physiol. Rev.*, 35:801, 1955. Last three entries from Givoni, B., and Goldman, R.F.: Predicting metabolic energy cost. *J. Appl. Physiol.*, 30:429, 1971.

[b] The correction factor represents a multiple of the energy expenditure for walking on a paved road or grass track. For example, the energy cost of walking in a plowed field averages 1.5 times the cost of walking on the paved road.

extreme, one would dramatically elevate energy cost by walking in soft sand at rapid speed wearing heavy work boots and ankle weights. Of course, another more prudent approach would involve unweighted race-walking or running on a firm surface.

Use of Hand-Held and Ankle Weights

During running, the impact force on the legs equals about 3 times body mass, whereas the amount of leg shock with walking reaches only about 30% of this value.

Ankle weights increase the energy cost of walking to values usually observed for running. This benefits people who want to use only walking as a relatively low-impact training modality, yet require intensities of effort higher than at normal walking speeds. Hand-held weights also increase the energy cost of walking, particularly when arm movements accentuate a pumping action. However, this procedure may disproportionately elevate systolic blood pressure, due perhaps to increased intramuscular tension with gripping the weight. For individuals with hypertension or coronary heart disease, an unnecessarily "induced" elevated blood pressure would contraindicate the use of hand-held weights.

Increasing unweighted running speed or distance offers a more desirable alternative to increase energy expenditure than hand or ankle weights if running remains the preferred mode of exercise. Increasing speed certainly reduces injury potential from increased impact forces in the weighted condition and eliminates the added discomfort of carrying weights.

Energy Expenditure During Running

Terrain, weather, training goals, and the performer's fitness level influence the speed of running. Two ways quantify the energy expenditure for running:

1. During performance of the actual activity
2. On a treadmill in the laboratory, with precise control over running speed and grade

Jogging and running represent qualitative terms related to speed of locomotion. This difference relates largely to the relative aerobic energy demands required in raising and lowering the body's center of gravity and accelerating and decelerating the limbs during the run. At identical running speeds, a highly conditioned distance runner runs at a lower percentage of aerobic capacity than an untrained runner, even though the oxygen uptake during the run may be similar for both people. The demarcation between jogging and running depends on the participant's fitness; a jog for one person could be a run for another.

Independent of fitness it becomes more economical from an energy standpoint to discontinue walking and begin to jog or run at speeds greater than about 8 km · hr⁻¹ (5 mph). Figure 7.8 showed the relationship between oxygen uptake and horizontal walking and running for men and women at speeds ranging from 4 to 14 km · hr⁻¹ (2.5 to 8.7 mph). The lines relating oxygen uptake and speed of walking and running showed that the "break point" between walking and running economy occurs at about 8 km · hr⁻¹ (5.0 mph).

Economy of Running

The data in Figure 7.8 also illustrate an important principle in relation to running speed and energy expenditure. Oxygen uptake relates linearly to running speed; thus, the same total caloric cost results when running a given distance at a steady-rate oxygen uptake at a fast or slow pace. In simple terms, if one runs a mile at 10 mph, it requires about twice as much energy per minute as a 5-mph pace;

however, the runner finishes the mile in 6 minutes, whereas running at the slower speed requires twice the time or 12 minutes. Consequently, the same net energy cost for the mile exists regardless of the pace.

For horizontal running, net energy cost (i.e., excluding the resting requirement) per kilogram of body mass per kilometer traveled averages approximately 1 kcal or 1 kcal · kg⁻¹ · km⁻¹. Thus, for an individual who weighs 78 kg, the net energy requirement for running 1 km equals about 78 kcal, regardless of running speed. Expressed as oxygen uptake, this amounts to 15.6 liters of oxygen consumed per kilometer (1 L O₂ = 5 kcal).

Energy Cost Values

Table 7.8 presents values for net energy expended during running for 1 hour at various speeds. The table expresses running speed as kilometers per hour, miles per hour, and number of minutes required to complete one mile at a given running speed. The boldface values represent net calories expended to run 1 mile for a person of a given body mass; this energy requirement remains independent of running speed. For example, for a person who weighs 62 kg, running a 26.2-mile marathon requires about 2600 kcal whether the run takes just over 2 hours or 4 hours.

TABLE 7.8
Net energy expenditure per hour for horizontal running in relation to velocity and body mass[a,b]

Body Mass kg	lb	km · hr⁻¹ mph min per mile	8 4.97 12:00	9 5.60 10:43	10 6.20 9:41	11 6.84 8:46	12 7.46 8:02	13 8.08 7:26	14 8.70 6:54	15 9.32 6:26	16 9.94 6:02
		kcal per mile									
50	110	**80**	400	450	500	550	600	650	700	750	800
54	119	**86**	432	486	540	594	648	702	756	810	864
58	128	**93**	464	522	580	638	696	754	812	870	928
62	137	**99**	496	558	620	682	744	806	868	930	992
66	146	**106**	528	594	660	726	792	858	924	990	1056
70	154	**112**	560	630	700	770	840	910	980	1050	1120
74	163	**118**	592	666	740	814	888	962	1036	1110	1184
78	172	**125**	624	702	780	858	936	1014	1092	1170	1248
82	181	**131**	656	738	820	902	984	1066	1148	1230	1312
86	190	**138**	688	774	860	946	1032	1118	1204	1290	1376
90	199	**144**	720	810	900	990	1080	1170	1260	1350	1440
94	207	**150**	752	846	940	1034	1128	1222	1316	1410	1504
98	216	**157**	784	882	980	1078	1176	1274	1372	1470	1568
102	225	**163**	816	918	1020	1122	1224	1326	1428	1530	1632
106	234	**170**	848	954	1060	1166	1272	1378	1484	1590	1696

[a] Interpret the table as follows: For a 50-kg person, the *net* energy expenditure for running for 1 hour at 8 km · hr⁻¹ (4.97 mph) equals 400 kcal; this speed represents a 12-minute per mile pace. Thus, 5 miles would be run in 1 hour and 400 kcal would be expended. If the pace increased to 12 km · hr⁻¹ (7.46 mph), 600 kcal would be expended during the one-hour run.

[b] Running speeds expressed as kilometers per hour (km · hr⁻¹), miles per hour (mph), and minutes required to complete each mile (min per mile). The values in **boldface type** equal *net* calories expended to run 1 mile for a given body mass, independent of running speed.

The energy cost per mile increases proportionately with the runner's body mass. This observation certainly supports the role of weight-bearing exercise as a caloric stress for overweight individuals who want to increase energy expenditure for weight loss. For example, a 102-kg person who jogs 5 miles each day at any comfortable pace expends 163 kcal for each mile completed, or a total of 815 kcal for the 5-mile run. Increasing or decreasing the speed (within the broad range of steady-rate paces) simply alters the length of the exercise period; it has little effect on total net energy expended through exercise.

Stride Length, Stride Frequency, and Running Speed

Running speed can increase three ways:

1. Increase the number of steps each minute (stride frequency)
2. Increase the distance between steps (stride length)
3. Increase stride length and stride frequency

Although the third option may seem the obvious way to increase running speed, several experiments provide objective data concerning this question.

In 1944, researchers studied the stride pattern for the Danish champion in the 5- and 10-km running events. At a running speed of 9.3 km · hr^{-1} (5.8 mph), this athlete's stride frequency equaled 160 per minute with a corresponding stride length of 97 cm (38.2 in). When running speed increased 91% to 17.8 km · hr^{-1} (11.1 mph), stride frequency increased only 10% to 176 per minute, whereas an 83% increase to 168 cm occurred in stride length. These data illustrate that running speed increases predominantly by lengthening stride. Only at faster speeds does stride frequency become important.

Optimum Stride Length

An optimum combination of stride length and frequency exists for running at a particular constant speed. The optimum depends largely on the person's "style" of running and cannot be determined from body measurements. Running speed chosen by the person incorporates the most economical stride length. Lengthening the stride above the optimum increases oxygen uptake more than a shorter-than-optimum stride length. Thus, urging a runner who shows signs of fatigue to "lengthen your stride" to maintain speed produces counterproductive results for oxygen cost (exercise economy).

Well-trained runners run at a stride length "selected" through years of training. This produces the most economical running performance, in keeping with the concept that the body naturally attempts to achieve a level of **"minimum effort."** Consequently, no "best" style exists to characterize elite runners. Instead, individual differences in body size, inertia of limb segments, and anatomic development interact to vary one's stride.

Effects of Air Resistance

Anyone who has run into a headwind knows it requires more energy to maintain a given pace compared with running in calm weather or with the wind at one's back. Three factors influence how air resistance affects energy cost of running:

1. Air density
2. Runner's projected surface area
3. Square of headwind velocity

Depending on running speed, overcoming air resistance accounts for 3 to 9% of the total energy requirement of running in calm weather. Running into a headwind creates an additional energy expense. For example, running at 15.9 km · hr^{-1} in calm conditions produces an oxygen uptake of 2.92 L · min^{-1}. This increased by 5.5% to 3.09 L · min^{-1} against a 16-km · hr^{-1} (9.9 mph) headwind and 4.1 L · min^{-1} while running against the strongest wind (41 mph); running into the strongest wind represented a 40% additional expenditure of energy to maintain running velocity.

Some may argue that the negative effects of running into a headwind counterbalance on one's return with the tailwind. This however, does not take place because the energy cost of cutting through a headwind exceeds the reduction in exercise oxygen uptake with an equivalent wind velocity at one's back. Wind tunnel tests show that running performance significantly increases by wearing form-fitting clothing; even trimming one's hair improves aerodynamics and reduces wind resistance effects by up to 6%. In competitive cycling, manufacturers continually modify clothing and helmets (including the rider's body position on the bicycle, and frame design) to reduce the effects of air resistance on energy cost.

At altitude, wind velocity affects energy expenditure less than at sea level due to reduced air density at higher elevations. Speed skaters experience a lower oxygen require-

Calories Add Up with Regular Exercise

For distance runners who train up to 100 miles a week, or slightly less than the distance of four marathons at close to competitive speeds, the weekly caloric expenditure from exercise averages about 10,000 kcal. For the serious marathon runner who trains year-round, the total energy expended in training for 4 years before an Olympic competition exceeds two million calories—the caloric equivalent of 555 pounds of body fat. This more than likely contributes to the low levels of body fat (3 to 5% of body mass for men; 12 to 17% for women) possessed by these athletes.

How to Predict Energy Expenditure During Treadmill Walking and Running

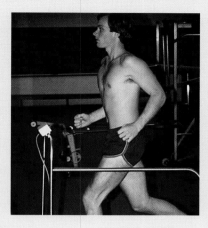

A linear relationship exists between oxygen uptake (energy expenditure) and walking speeds between 3.0 and 5.0 km · hr^{-1} (1.9 and 3.1 mph), and running at speeds faster than 8.0 km · hr^{-1} (5 to 10 mph). Adding the resting oxygen uptake to the oxygen requirements of the horizontal and vertical components of the walk or run makes it possible to estimate total (gross) exercise oxygen uptake ($\dot{V}O_2$) and energy expenditure.

Basic Equation

$\dot{V}O_2$ (mL · kg^{-1} · min^{-1}) = Resting component (1 MET; 3.5 mL O_2 · kg^{-1} · min^{-1}) + Horizontal component (speed, m · min^{-1} × oxygen cost of horizontal movement) + Vertical component (percent grade × speed, m · min^{-1} × oxygen cost of vertical movement).

[To convert mph to m · min^{-1} multiply by 26.82; to convert m · min^{-1} to mph multiply by 0.03728.]

Walking: Oxygen cost of the horizontal component of movement equals 0.1 mL · kg^{-1} · min^{-1}, and 1.8 mL · kg^{-1} · min^{-1} for the vertical component.

Running: Oxygen cost of the horizontal component of movement equals 0.2 mL · kg^{-1} · min^{-1}, and 0.9 mL · kg^{-1} · min^{-1} for the vertical component.

Predicting Energy Cost of Treadmill Walking

Problem

A 55-kg person walks on a treadmill at 2.8 mph (2.8 × 26.82 = 75 m · min^{-1}) up a 4% grade. Calculate 1) $\dot{V}O_2$ (mL · kg^{-1} · min^{-1}), 2) METs, and 3) energy expenditure (kcal · min^{-1}).
[Note: express % grade as a decimal value; i.e., 4% grade = 0.04]

Solution

1. $\dot{V}O_2$ (mL · kg^{-1} · min^{-1}) = Resting component + Horizontal component + Vertical component
   $\dot{V}O_2$ = Resting $\dot{V}O_2$ (mL · kg^{-1} · min^{-1}) + [speed (m · min^{-1}) × 0.1 mL · kg^{-1} · min^{-1}] + [% grade × speed (m · min^{-1}) × 1.8 mL · kg^{-1} · min^{-1}]
   = 3.5 + (75 × 0.1) + (0.04 × 75 × 1.8)
   = 3.5 + 7.5 + 5.4
   = 16.4 mL · kg^{-1} · min^{-1}
2. METs = $\dot{V}O_2$ (mL · kg^{-1} · min^{-1}) ÷ 3.5 mL · kg^{-1} · min^{-1}
   = 16.4 ÷ 3.5
   = 4.7
3. Kcal · min^{-1} = $\dot{V}O_2$ (mL · kg^{-1} · min^{-1}) × Body mass (kg) × 5.05 kcal · L^{-1}
   = 16.4 mL · kg^{-1} · min^{-1} × 55 kg × 5.05 kcal · L^{-1}
   = 0.902 L · m^{-1} × 5.05 kcal · L^{-1}
   = 4.6

Predicting Energy Cost of Treadmill Running

Problem

A 55-kg person runs on a treadmill at 5.4 mph (5.4 × 26.82 = 145 m · min^{-1}) up a 6% grade. Calculate 1) $\dot{V}O_2$ in mL · kg^{-1} · min^{-1}, 2) METs, and 3) energy expenditure (kcal · min^{-1}).

Solution

1. $\dot{V}O_2$ (mL · kg^{-1} · min^{-1}) = Resting component + Horizontal component + Vertical component
   $\dot{V}O_2$ = Resting $\dot{V}O_2$ (mL · kg^{-1} · min^{-1}) + [speed (m · min^{-1}) × 0.2 mL · kg^{-1} · min^{-1}] + [% grade × speed (m · min^{-1}) × 0.9 mL · kg^{-1} · min^{-1}]
   = 3.5 + (145 × 0.2) + (0.06 × 145 × 0.9)
   = 3.5 + 29.0 + 7.83
   = 40.33 mL · kg^{-1} · min^{-1}
2. METs = $\dot{V}O_2$ (mL · kg^{-1} · min^{-1}) ÷ 3.5 mL · kg^{-1} · min^{-1}
   = 40.33 ÷ 3.5
   = 11.5
3. Kcal · min^{-1} = $\dot{V}O_2$ (mL · kg^{-1} · min^{-1}) × Body mass (kg) × 5.05 kcal · L^{-1}
   = 40.33 mL · kg^{-1} · min^{-1} × 55 kg × 5.05 kcal · L^{-1}
   = 2.22 L · min^{-1} × 5.05 kcal · L^{-1}
   = 11.2

ment while skating at a particular speed at altitude compared to sea level. Overcoming air resistance at altitude only becomes important at the faster skating speeds. In all likelihood, an altitude-effect would be particularly noticeable in competitive cycling where the impeding effect of air resistance becomes considerable at the high speeds achieved by these athletes.

Drafting

To counter the negative effects of air resistance and headwind on running energy cost, athletes employ "**drafting**" by following directly behind a competitor. For example, running 1 meter behind another runner at a speed of 21.6 km · hr^{-1} decreases the total energy expenditure by about 7%. Drafting at this speed could save about 1 second for each 400 m covered during a race. The beneficial aerodynamic effect of drafting on the economy of effort also has been observed for cross-country skiing and cycling. About 90% of the power generated when cycling at 40 km · hr^{-1} on a calm day goes to overcoming air resistance. At this speed, energy expenditure decreases between 26 to 38% when a competitor follows closely behind another cyclist.

Treadmill Versus Track Running

Researchers use the treadmill almost exclusively to evaluate the physiology of running in the laboratory. A question concerns the association between treadmill running and running performance on a track or road race. For example, does it require the same energy to run a given speed or distance on a treadmill and a track in calm weather? To answer this question, researchers studied eight distance runners on both a treadmill and track at three submaximum speeds of 10.8, 12.6, and 15.6 km · hr^{-1} (6.7, 7.8, and 9.7 mph). They also studied the athletes during a graded exercise test to determine possible differences between treadmill and track running on submaximal and maximal oxygen uptake.

From a practical standpoint, no measurable differences occurred in aerobic requirements of submaximal running (up to 17.2 km · hr^{-1}) on the treadmill or track, or between the VO$_{2max}$ measured in both forms of exercise under similar environmental conditions. The possibility still exists, however, that at faster running speeds of endurance competition, air resistance could impact outdoor running, and oxygen cost may significantly exceed that of "stationary" treadmill running at the same speed.

Marathon Running

The first place finisher in the men's division of the 1998 Boston Marathon ran the course in 2h:07 min:34 s, 19 seconds under the course record set in 1994. The average speed of 4:52 minutes per mile represents an outstanding achievement in human performance. Not only does this pace require a steady-rate aerobic metabolism that greatly exceeds the aerobic capacity of the average male college

student, it also represents about 85% of the marathoners' VO$_{2max}$ maintained for just over 2 hours. Aerobic capacity of these athletes averages about 4.4 L · min^{-1} or between 70 and 84 mL · kg^{-1} · min^{-1}.

Two long-distance runners were measured during a marathon to determine energy expenditure per minute and total caloric cost. The balloon technique of open-circuit spirometry evaluated oxygen uptake every 3 miles. The two runners' achieved times of 2 h:36 min:34 s and 2 h:39 min:28 s; their VO$_{2max}$ measured during treadmill running equalled 4.43 L · min^{-1} (70.5 mL · kg^{-1} · min^{-1}) and 4.66 L · min^{-1} (73.9 mL · kg^{-1} · min^{-1}), respectively. During the race, the first runner maintained an average speed of 16.2 km · hr^{-1} (10.0 mph), which required an oxygen uptake equal to 80% of VO$_{2max}$. For the second runner, who averaged a slower speed at 16.0 km · hr^{-1} (9.92 mph), the aerobic energy requirement averaged 78.3% of maximum. Both men expended between 2300 to 2400 kcal to run the marathon.

Energy Expenditure During Swimming

Swimming exercise differs in several important respects from walking or running. For one thing, swimmers must expend energy to maintain buoyancy while at the same time generate horizontal movement using the arms and legs, either in combination or separately. Other differences include the energy requirements for overcoming drag forces that impede the movement of an object through a water medium. The amount of drag depends on the characteristics of the medium and the object's size, shape, and velocity. *These factors all contribute to a significantly lower economy in swimming compared with running. More specifically, it requires about four times more energy to swim a given distance than to run the same distance.*

Methods of Measurement

Energy expenditure has been computed from oxygen uptake measured by open-circuit spirometry during swimming. In studies conducted in the pool, the researcher walks alongside the swimmer while carrying the portable gas collection equipment. In another form of swimming exercise illustrated in Figure 7.9A, the subject remains stationary and attached ("tethered") to a cable and pulley system by a belt worn around the waist. Periodically increasing the amount of weight attached to the cable forces the swimmer to exert more effort to keep from being pulled backward.

Figure 7.9B shows a subject swimming in a flume or "swim-mill." Water circulates and its velocity can vary from a slow swimming speed to a near-record pace for a free-style sprint. Also, water temperature in the 38,000-L swim-mill can be regulated between 10 and 40°C. Win-

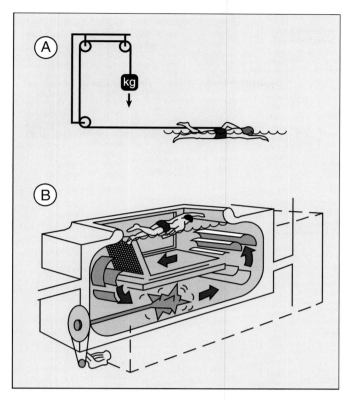

Figure 7.9
A, Tethered swimming. **B,** The swimming flume.

dows on the side of the flume beneath the water's surface enable photographic analysis of stroke mechanics. Skilled swimmers achieve essentially identical aerobic capacity values when measured by either tethered, free, or flume swimming. This means that each mode measurement evaluates the functional capacity of the aerobic system during swimming.

Energy Cost and Drag

Three components comprise the total drag force encountered by the swimmer:

1. **Wave drag**—caused by waves that build up in front of and form hollows behind the swimmer moving through the water. This component of drag does not become a significant factor until swimming at faster speeds.
2. **Skin friction drag**—produced as the water slides over the skin's surface. Research supports the common practice of swimmers "shaving down" to reduce skin friction drag. Removal of body hair reduces drag to slightly decrease the energy cost and physiologic demands during swimming.
3. **Viscous pressure drag**—contributes substantially to counter the propulsive efforts of the swimmer at slow

velocities. It results from the separation of the thin sheet of water (boundary layer) adjacent to the swimmer. The pressure differential created in front of and behind the swimmer represents viscous pressure drag. Highly skilled swimmers who "streamline" their stroke reduce this component of total drag. Streamlining with improved stroke mechanics reduces the separation region by moving the separation point closer to the trailing edge of the water. This also occurs when an oar slices through the water with the blade parallel rather than perpendicular to water flow.

Differences in total drag force between swimmers can make the difference between winning and losing, particularly in longer distance races. Wet suits worn by triathletes during the swim portion of a triathlon reduce body drag by 14%. Improved swimming economy largely explains the significantly faster swim times of athletes who wear wet suits. As in running, cross-country skiing, and cycling, drafting in ocean swimming (following closely behind the wake of a lead swimmer) reduces physiologic demands. This enables an endurance swimmer (triathlete or ocean racer) to conserve energy and possibly improve performance toward the end of the competition.

Energy Cost, Swimming Velocity, and Skill

Elite swimmers swim a particular stroke at a given velocity at a lower oxygen uptake than either less elite or recreational swimmers. Figure 7.10A illustrates oxygen uptake related to velocity for the breaststroke, front crawl, and back crawl for subjects representing three levels of ability. One subject, a recreational swimmer, did not participate in swim training; the trained subject, a top Swedish swimmer, swam on a daily basis; the elite swimmer was a European champion. Except for the breaststroke, the elite swimmer swam a given speed with a lower oxygen uptake than his trained and untrained counterparts. Figure 7.10B shows that for the two trained athletes, swimming the breaststroke "cost" the most at any speed, followed by the backstroke. The front crawl represented the least "expensive" (calorie wise) among the three strokes.

Effects of Buoyancy: Men Versus Women

Women of all ages possess on average more total body fat than men. Because fat floats and muscle and bone sink, the average woman gains a hydrodynamic lift and floats more easily than her male counterpart. This difference in buoyancy partly explains women's greater swimming economy. For example, women swim a given distance at a lower energy cost than men; expressed another way, women achieve a higher swimming velocity than men for the same level of energy expenditure.

Figure 7.10
A, Oxygen uptake as a function of speed for the breaststroke, front crawl, and back crawl in subjects who represent three different skill levels. **B,** Oxygen uptake for two trained swimmers during three competitive strokes. (From Holmér, I.: Oxygen uptake during swimming in man. *J. Appl. Physiol.*, 33: 502, 1972.) Photos courtesy of John Urbanchek, Varsity men's swim coach, University of Michigan.

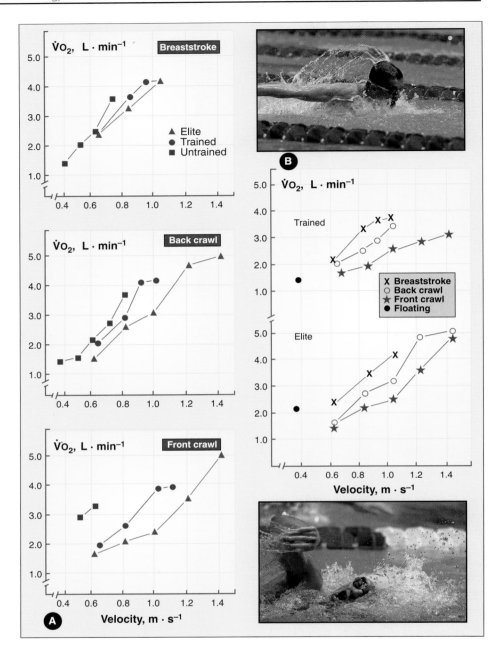

The distribution of body fat towards the periphery in women causes their legs to float higher in the water, making them more horizontal or "streamlined," whereas men's leaner legs tend to swing down in the water. Lowering the legs to a deeper position increases body drag and thus reduces swimming economy. The potential hydrodynamic benefits enjoyed by women become noteworthy in longer distances where swimming economy and body insulation take on added importance. The woman's record for swimming the 21-mile English Channel from England to France equals 7 hr: 40 min. The men's record equals 7 hr: 17 min, a difference of only 5.2%.

summary

1. The concept of economy can be viewed as the relationship between energy input and energy output. A common method to assess differences between individuals in economy of movement evaluates oxygen uptake while the subject exercises at a set power output or speed.

2. Mechanical efficiency represents the percentage of total chemical energy expended that contributes to external work, the remainder represents lost heat.

3. Children run at a given speed with less economy compared with adults because they require between 20 to 30% more oxygen per unit of body mass. This relatively lower running economy accounts for the poor endurance performance of children compared with adults with similar aerobic capacity.

4. Walking speed relates linearly to oxygen uptake between speeds of 1.9 and 3.1 mph; at faster speeds, walking becomes less economical. Walking surface also exerts an influence because walking on sand requires about twice the energy expenditure as walking on hard surfaces. The energy cost of such weight-bearing exercise becomes proportionally larger for heavier people.

5. Hand-held and ankle weights increase the energy cost of walking to values usually observed for running. This benefits those wanting to use only walking as a low-impact form of exercise training.

6. It is more economical from an energy standpoint to jog-run rather than to walk at speeds that exceed $8 \text{ km} \cdot \text{hr}^{-1}$ (5 mph). The difference between jogging and running depends on the fitness level of the participant; a jog for one person may represent a run for another.

7. An individual's total energy cost for running a given distance remains independent of running speed. For horizontal running, the net energy expenditure averages about $1 \text{ kcal} \cdot \text{kg}^{-1} \cdot \text{km}^{-1}$.

8. Shortening running stride and increasing stride frequency to maintain a constant running speed requires less energy than lengthening the stride and reducing stride frequency. An individual subconsciously "selects" the combination of stride length and frequency that favors optimal economy.

9. Overcoming air resistance accounts for 3 to 9% of running's total energy cost in calm weather. This percentage increases by the square of the wind velocity as the runner attempts to maintain pace while running into a headwind.

10. Running directly behind a competitor, a desirable aerodynamic technique called "drafting," counters the negative effect of air resistance and headwind on the energy cost of running.

11. It requires the same amount of energy to run a given distance or speed on a treadmill as on a track under identical environmental conditions.

12. It takes about four times more energy to swim than to run the same distance. In contrast to running, a swimmer must expend considerable energy to maintain buoyancy and overcome the various drag forces that impede movement.

13. Elite swimmers expend fewer calories to swim a given stroke at any velocity.

14. Significant gender differences exist for body drag, economy, and net oxygen uptake during swimming. Women swim a given distance at about 30% lower energy cost than men.

thought questions

1. A 60-kg (132-lb) elite marathoner who trains year-round expends about 4000 kcal daily over a 4-year training period before Olympic competition. Assuming body mass remains unchanged and 70% of daily caloric intake comes from carbohydrate and 1.4 g per kg body mass comes from protein, compute the runner's total 4-year calorie intake and total grams consumed from carbohydrate and protein.

2. How would you respond to this question: "Why do children who run in 10-km races never seem to perform as well as adults?"

3. A company that makes a "passive" exercise machine claims that a person using the equipment burns an average of 1.25 kcal each minute (gross cost). How well does this equipment contribute to total daily energy expenditure?

4. Most people assume they expend more total calories if they run a given distance faster. Explain why this is not true. In what way does correcting this misunderstanding contribute to a recommendation for the use of exercise for weight loss?

5. Respond to the following question: "If running 36 miles burns the calories in only 1 pound of body fat, how can anyone seriously consider regular physical activity for weight loss?"

6. You are responsible for selecting new clothing for firefighters. You can choose one of two items: an outer coat or boots. The weight of each has been reduced by 2 pounds compared with standard issue. Justify your selection based *only* from the perspective of energy expenditure during the job.

selected references

ACSM's Resource Manual for Guidelines for Exercise Testing and Prescription. 3rd Ed., Baltimore: Williams & Wilkins, 1998.

Ainsworth, B. E., et al.: Compendium of physical activities: classification of energy costs of human physical activities. *Med. Sci. Sports Exerc.*, 25: 71, 1993.

American College of Sports Medicine: *Guidelines for Exercise Testing and Prescription.* 5th Ed., Philadelphia: Lea & Febiger, 1995.

Ariens, G.A., et al.: The longitudinal development of running economy in males and females aged between 13 and 27 years: The Amsterdam Growth and Health Study. *Eur. J. Appl. Physiol.*, 76:214, 1998.

Armstrong, N., and Welsman, J.R.: Assessment and interpretation of aerobic fitness in children and adolescents. *Exerc. Sport Sci. Rev.*, 22: 435, 1994.

Belko, A., et al.: Effect of energy and protein intake and exercise intensity on the thermic effect of food. *Am. J. Clin. Nutr.*, 43: 863, 1986.

Bilodeau, B., et al.: Effect of drafting on heart rate in cross-country skiing. *Med. Sci. Sports Exerc.*, 26: 637, 1994.

Brisswalter, J., et al.: Variability in energy cost and walking gait during race walking in competitive race walkers. *Med. Sci. Sports Exerc.*, 30:1451, 1998.

Carpenter, W.H., et al.: Total energy expenditure in 4 to 6 year old children. *Am. J. Physiol.*, 27: E706, 1993.

Chatard, J-C., et al.: Performance and drag during drafting swimming in highly trained triathletes. *Med. Sci. Sports Exerc.*, 30:1276, 1998.

Clapp, J.F., III, et al.: Neonatal behavioral profile of the offspring of women who continue to exercise regularly throughout pregnancy. *Am. J. Obstet. Gynecol.*, 180:91, 1999.

Coyle, E. F., et al.: Cycling efficiency is related to the percentage of type I muscle fibers. *Med. Sci. Sports Exerc.*, 24: 782, 1992.

Cureton, K.J., et al.: Metabolic determinants of the age-related improvement in one-mile run/walk performance in youth. *Med. Sci. Sports Exerc.*, 29:259, 1997.

Dennis, S.C., and Noakes, T.D.: Advantages of a smaller body mass in humans when distance-running in warm, humid conditions. *Eur. J. Appl. Physiol.*, 79:280, 1999.

Durnin, J. V. G. A., and Passmore, R.: *Energy, Work and Leisure.* London: Heinemann, 1967.

Evans, B.W., et al.: Metabolic and hemodynamic responses to walking with hand weights in older individuals. *Med. Sci. Sports Exerc.*, 26: 1047, 1994.

Hatch, M., et al.: Maternal leisure-time exercise and timely delivery. *Am. J. Public Health*, 88:1528, 1998.

Hausswirth, C., et al.: Effects of cycling alone or in a sheltered position on subsequent running performance during a triathlon. *Med. Sci. Sports Exerc.*, 31:599, 1999.

Jansson, E.: On the significance of the respiratory exchange ratio after different diets during exercise in man. *Acta Physiol. Scand.*, 114: 103, 1982.

Keys, A., et al.: Basal metabolism and age of adult men. *Metabolism*, 22: 579, 1973.

Lake, M.J., and Cavanagh, P.R.: Six weeks of training does not change running mechanics or improve running economy. *Med. Sci. Sports Exerc.*, 28:860, 1996.

Maas, S., et al.: The validity of the use of heart rate in estimating oxygen consumption in static and in combined static/dynamic exercise. *Ergonomics*, 32:141, 1989.

Meredith, C. N., et al.: Body composition and aerobic capacity in young and middle-aged endurance-trained men. *Med. Sci. Sports Exerc.*, 19: 557, 1987.

Morgan, D.W., et al.: Variation in the aerobic demand of running among trained and untrained subjects. *Med. Sci. Sports Exerc.*, 27:404, 1995.

Nigg, B.M., and Anton, A.: Energy aspects for elastic and viscous shoe soles and playing surfaces. *Med. Sci. Sports Exerc.*, 27:92, 1995.

Piers, L.S., et al.: Is there evidence for an age-related reduction in BMR related to quantitative or qualitative change in components of lean tissue. *J. Appl. Physiol.*, 85:2196, 1998.

Poehlman, E. T., et al.: Resting metabolic rate and post prandial thermogenesis in highly trained and untrained males. *Am. J. Clin. Nutr.*, 47: 793, 1988.

Poehlman, E.T., et al.: Endurance exercise in aging humans: effects on energy metabolism. *Exerc. Sport Sci. Rev.*, 22: 75, 1994.

Porcari, J.: Pump up your walk. *ACSM's Health & Fitness J.*, 3(1):25, 1999.

Pratlaey, R., et al.: Strength training increases resting metabolic rate and norepinephrine levels in healthy 50- to 65-year-old men. *J. Appl. Physiol.*, 73:133, 1994.

Schutz, Y., et al.: Diet-induced thermogenesis measured over a whole day in obese and nonobese women. *Am. J. Clin. Nutr.*, 40: 542, 1984.

Segal, K. R., et al.: Thermic effects of food and exercise on lean and obese men of similar lean body mass. *Am. J. Physiol.*, 252: E110, 1987.

Semih, S.Y., and Feluni, T.: A comparison of the endurance training responses to road and sand running in high school and college students, *J. Strength and Cond. Res.*, 12:79, 1998.

Toussaint, H.M., and Hollander, A.P.: Energetics of competitive swimming: implications for training programs. *Sports Med.*, 18:384, 1994.

Walker, J.L., et al.: The energy cost of horizontal walking and running in adolescents. *Med. Sci. Sports Exerc.*, 31:311, 1999.

Wilmore, J. A., et al.: An automated system for assessing metabolic and respiratory function during exercise. *J. Appl. Physiol.*, 40: 619, 1976.

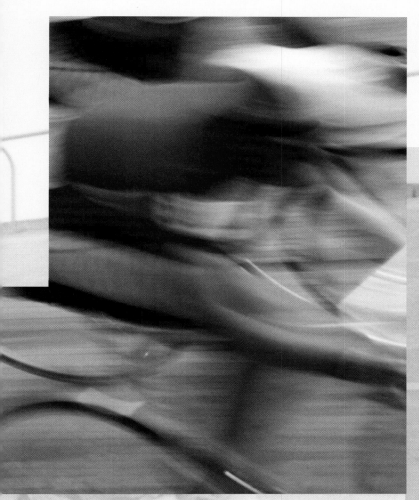

CHAPTER

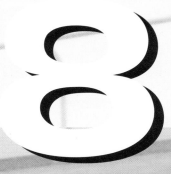

8

Topics covered in this chapter

Overview of Energy Transfer Capacity
   During Exercise
Anaerobic Energy: Immediate and Short-
   Term Energy Systems
Aerobic Energy: Long-Term Energy System
Maximal Oxygen Uptake Measurement
Maximal Oxygen Uptake Predictions
Summary
Thought Questions
Selected References

Evaluating Energy-Generating Capacities During Exercise

- Explain specificity and generality as they apply to exercise performance and physiologic function.

- Describe procedures to administer two practical "field tests" to evaluate power output capacity of the intramuscular high-energy phosphates (immediate energy system).

- Describe a commonly used test to evaluate the power output capacity of glycolysis (short-term energy system).

- Define maximal oxygen uptake ($\dot{V}O_{2max}$), including its physiological significance.

- Define graded exercise stress test.

- List criteria that indicate when a person reaches "true" $\dot{V}O_{2max}$ and $\dot{V}O_{2peak}$ during a graded exercise test.

- Outline three commonly used treadmill protocols to assess $\dot{V}O_{2max}$.

- Explain how each of the following affects $\dot{V}O_{2max}$: 1) mode of exercise, 2) heredity, 3) state of training, 4) gender, 5) body composition, and 6) age.

- Describe procedures to administer a submaximal walking "field test" to predict $\dot{V}O_{2max}$.

- Outline the procedure for administering a step test to predict $\dot{V}O_{2max}$.

- List three assumptions when predicting $\dot{V}O_{2max}$ from submaximal exercise heart rate.

- Describe one proposed nonexercise method to predict $\dot{V}O_{2max}$.

We all possess the capability for anaerobic and aerobic energy metabolism, although the capacity for each form of energy transfer varies considerably among individuals. These differences underlie the concept of **individual differences** in metabolic capacity for exercise. A person's capacity for energy transfer (and for many other physiologic functions) does not exist as some general factor for all types of exercise, but depends largely on the exercise mode used for training and evaluation. A high maximal oxygen uptake ($\dot{V}O_{2max}$) in running, for example, does not necessarily ensure a similar $\dot{V}O_{2max}$ when activating different muscle groups as in swimming and rowing. The disparity represents an example of **specificity of metabolic capacity**. In contrast, some individuals with high aerobic power in one form of exercise also possess an above average aerobic power in other diverse activities. This illustrates the **generality of metabolic capacity**. *For the most part, more specificity exists than generality in metabolic and physiologic functions.* In this chapter, we evaluate the capacity of the various energy transfer systems discussed in Chapters 4 and 5 with reference to measurement, specificity, and individual differences.

Figure 8.1 illustrates the specificity–generality concept of energy capacities. The non-overlapped areas represent specificity of physiologic function, and the overlapped areas represent generality of function. For each of the energy systems, specificity exceeds generality; rarely does one find individuals who excel in markedly different activities (e.g., sprinting and long-distance running). Yet, many world-class triathletes possess "metabolically generalized" capacities for diverse aerobic activities. What appears as a general aerobic fitness capacity results from long hours of highly specific training in *each* of the triathlon's three grueling events.

Based on the specificity principle, training for high aerobic power probably contributes little to one's capacity for anaerobic energy transfer, and vice versa. *The effects of systematic exercise training remain highly specific for neurologic, physiologic, and metabolic responses. One must therefore carefully define terms like speed, power, and endurance within the context of an activity's specific movement patterns and specific metabolic and physiologic requirements.*

Overview of Energy Transfer Capacity During Exercise

The immediate and short-term energy systems mainly power all-out exercise for up to 2 minutes in duration. Both systems operate anaerobically because their transfers of chemical energy do not require oxygen (refer to Chap-

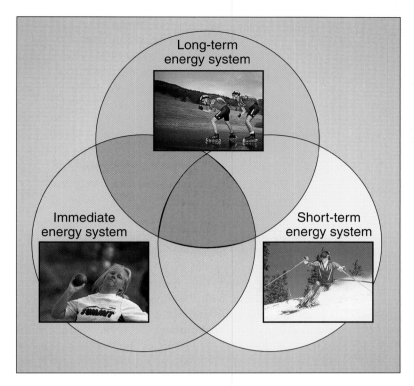

Anaerobic Energy: Immediate and Short-Term Energy Systems

Evaluation of the Immediate Energy System

Performance tests that rely on maximal activation of the intramuscular ATP-PCr energy reserves have been developed as practical "field tests" to evaluate the **immediate energy transfer system**. These maximal effort performances, referred to as **power tests**, evaluate the time-rate of doing work (i.e., work accomplished per unit time). The following formula computes power output:

$$P = \frac{F \times D}{T}$$

where, F equals force generated, D equals distance through which the force moves, and T equals exercise duration. Watts represent a common expression of power — one watt equals 0.73756 ft-lb · s⁻¹ or 6.12 kg-m · min⁻¹.

ter 4). Generally, fast movements or resistance to movement at a given speed rely primarily on anaerobic energy transfer. Figure 8.2 shows the involvement of the anaerobic and aerobic energy transfer systems for different durations of all-out exercise. At the initiation of either high- or low-speed movements, the intramuscular phosphagens, ATP and PCr, provide immediate and nonaerobic energy for muscle action. After the first few seconds of movement, the glycolytic energy system (initial phase of carbohydrate breakdown) provides an increasingly greater proportion of the total energy. Continuation of exercise, although at a lower intensity, places a progressively greater demand on aerobic metabolic pathways for ATP resynthesis.

Some activities require the capacity of more than one energy transfer system, whereas other activities rely predominately on a single system. However, all activities activate each energy system to some degree, depending on exercise intensity and duration. Of course, greater demand for anaerobic energy transfer occurs for higher-intensity and shorter-duration activities.

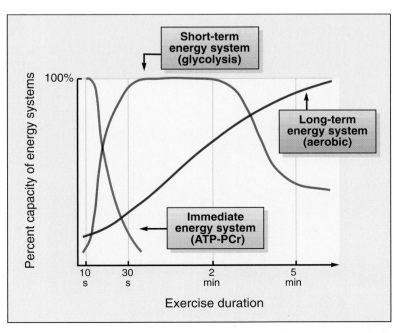

Figure 8.2
Three energy systems and their percentage contribution to total energy output during all-out exercise of different durations.

Stair-Sprinting Power Test

Researchers have measured immediate power output by a test that requires sprinting up a flight of stairs. Figure 8.3 shows a subject running up a staircase as fast as possible taking three steps at a time. The external work performed equals the total vertical distance the body rises up the stairs; for six stairs, this distance usually equals about 1.05 m.

The power output for a 65-kg woman who traverses six steps in 0.52 seconds computes as follows:

$$F = 65 \text{ kg}; D = 1.05 \text{ m}; T = 0.52 \text{ s}$$

$$P = \frac{65 \times 1.05}{0.52}$$

$$= 131.3 \text{ kg-m·s}^{-1} \text{ (1287 watts)}$$

Because body mass greatly influences the power-output score in stair-sprinting, a heavier person necessarily generates greater power at the same speed as a lighter person who covers the same vertical distance. Because of the influence of body mass, use caution in interpreting differences in stair-sprinting power scores and making inferences about individual differences in ATP-PCr energy capacity. *The test may be better suited to evaluate individuals of similar body mass, or the same people before and after a specific training regimen designed to develop immediate anaerobic leg power.*

Jumping Power Test

For years, physical fitness test batteries have included jumping tests such as the jump-and-reach test or a standing broad jump. The jump-and-reach test score equals the difference between a person's standing reach and the maximum jump-and-touch height. For the broad jump, the score represents the horizontal distance covered in a leap from a semicrouched position. Although both tests purport to measure leg power, they probably do not achieve this goal. For one thing, with the jump tests, power generated in propelling the body from the crouched position occurs only in the time the feet contact the floor's surface. This brief period does not sufficiently evaluate a person's ATP and PCr power-output capacity. Also, little relationship exists between jump-test scores and ATP-PCr levels or depletion patterns.

Other Immediate Energy Power Tests

A 6- to 8-second performance involving all-out exercise measures the person's capacity for immediate power from the intramuscular high-energy phosphates (refer to Fig. 8.2). Examples of other similar tests include sprint running or cycling, shuttle runs, and more localized movements such as arm cranking or simulated stair climbing, rowing, or skiing. In the popular **Québec 10-second test** of leg cycling power, the subject performs two all-out, 10-second rides at a frictional resistance equal

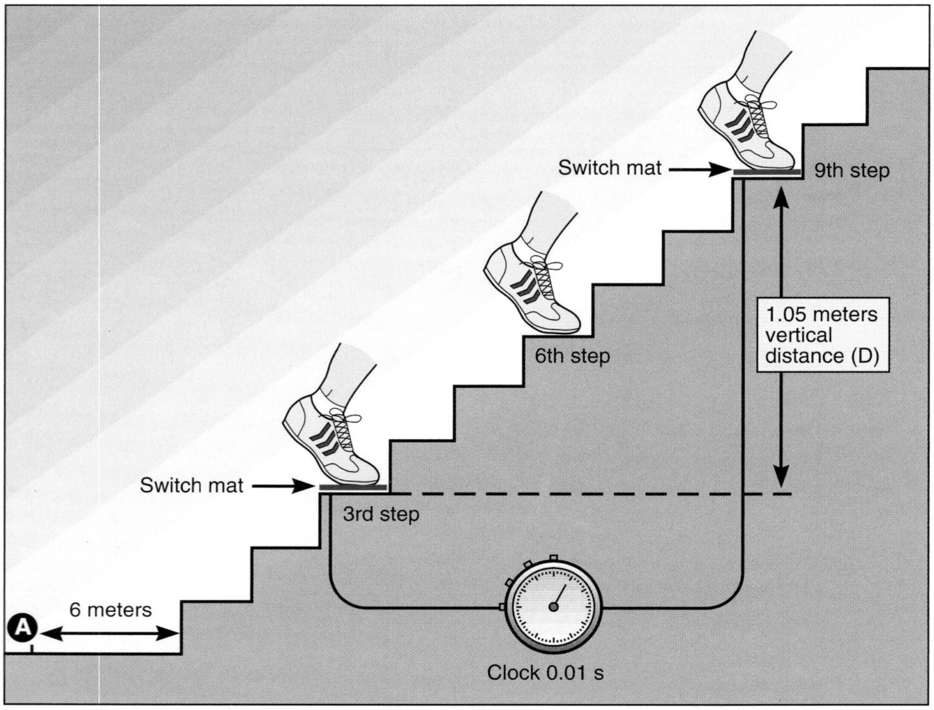

Assumptions for Interpreting All-Out Performance Estimates of the ATP-PCr Energy System

- Under conditions of maximal power output, the ATP-PCr system provides all of the ATP for exercise. Accordingly, this system generates all of the power during this time.

- Enough ATP and PCr exist to support maximal performance for approximately 6 to 8 seconds.

Figure 8.3
Stair-sprinting power test. The subject begins at point A and runs as fast as possible up a flight of stairs, taking three steps at a time. Electric switch mats placed on the steps record the time to cover the distance between stair 3 and stair 9 to the nearest 0.01 s. Power output equals the product of the subject's mass (F) and vertical distance covered (D), divided by the time (T). (Modified from Mathews, D. K., and Fox, E. L.: *The Physiological Basis of Physical Education and Athletics*. Philadelphia: W. B. Saunders, 2nd Ed., 1976.)

Interchangeable Expressions for Energy and Work

1 foot-pound (ft-lb) = 0.13825 kilogram-meters (kg-m)

1 kg-m = 7.233 ft-lb = 9.8066 joules

1 kilocalorie (kcal) = 3.0874 ft-lb = 426.85 kg-m = 4.186 kilojoules (kJ)

1 joule (J) = 1 Newton-meter (Nm)

1 kilojoule (kJ) = 1000 J = 0.23889 kcal

to 0.09 kg per kg of body mass, with 10 minutes of rest between exercise bouts. Exercise begins by pedaling as fast as possible as the friction load is applied and continues all-out for 10 seconds. Performance represents the average of the two tests reported in peak joules per kg of body mass, and total joules per kg of body mass.

Relationships Among Power Tests

If the various power tests measure the same general metabolic capacity, then one would assume individuals who rank high on one test would rank correspondingly high on a second or third test. The limited data mildly support such a hypothesis. Table 8.1 shows the interrelationships (expressed statistically as a correlation coefficient) among three tests that purport to measure immediate power output.

The relationships (ranging from poor to good) indicate some commonalty between tests and suggest that each test may be measuring a similar metabolic quality. Of practical significance, a fairly strong relationship exists between scores on the stair-sprinting power test and the 40-yard dash.

Several factors explain the low interrelationships among the other power output capacity test scores. First, a high degree of task specificity exists for human physical performance. This means that the best sprint runner may not

necessarily be the best sprint swimmer, sprint cyclist, stair sprinter, repetitive volleyball leaper, or sprint arm-cranker. Even though the same metabolic reactions generate the energy to power each performance, energy transfer takes place within the specific muscles activated by the exercise. Furthermore, each specific test requires different neurologic or skill components; the predominance of neuromuscular task specificity dictates that an individual will perform differently on each of the tests.

Power tests may be used to show changes in an athlete's performance with specific training. Such tests also serve as an excellent means for self-testing and motivation and often provide the actual movement-specific exercise for training the immediate energy system. Many football teams, for example, routinely use the 40-yard dash as a criterion to evaluate a player's speed. Although football requires many types of "speed," the 40-yard scores may provide useful information for player evaluation. Research needs to establish how 40-yard speed in a straight line relates to overall football ability for players at similar positions. A run test of shorter duration (up to 20 yd), or one with frequent changes in direction, may be equally or more important as a suitable performance measure.

Several physiologic and biochemical measures, in addition to exercise performance, can estimate the energy-generating capacity of the immediate energy system. These include:

- Size of the intramuscular ATP-PCr pool
- ATP and PCr depletion rates from all-out exercise of short duration
- Magnitude of oxygen deficit calculated from the oxygen uptake curve
- Magnitude of the alactic (fast component) portion of the recovery oxygen uptake curve

Of these measures, the most direct approach involves ATP and PCr depletion rate, which correlates highly with performance estimates of the immediate energy system. In reality, precise intramuscular biochemical data are difficult to obtain during all-out exercise of brief duration. Consequently, we must rely on the validity of specific, brief-duration exercise performance measures to reflect one's capacity for ATP-PCr energy transfer.

Evaluation of the Short-Term Energy System

Figure 8.2 showed that anaerobic reactions of glycolysis (**short-term energy system**) generate increasingly greater energy for ATP resynthesis when all-out exercise continue for longer than a few seconds. This does not mean that aerobic metabolism remains unimportant at this stage of exercise, or that the oxygen-consuming reactions have not been "switched-on." To the contrary, Figure 8.2 revealed an increase in aerobic energy contribution very early in exercise. However, the energy requirement in relatively brief

TABLE 8.1
Correlations among tests purported to measure power output from the immediate energy system[a]

VARIABLE	JUMP & REACH	STAIR-SPRINTING
40-yard dash	−0.48[b]	−0.88[b]
Jump and reach	—	−0.31[b]

[a] From the Applied Physiology Laboratory, University of Michigan (N = 31 males).

[b] Negative correlations mean faster times (lower scores) associate with higher jumps or greater power output.

How to Determine Anaerobic Power and Capacity: The Wingate Cycle Ergometer Test

Many sport and daily activities occur with rapid rest-to-exercise transitions, or at high intensities using anaerobic metabolic processes. The Wingate bicycle ergometer test represents the most popular test to assess anaerobic capacity. Developed at the Wingate Institute in Israel in the 1970s, test scores can reliably determine peak anaerobic power, anaerobic fatigue, and total anaerobic capacity.

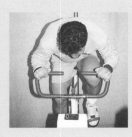

The Test

A mechanically-braked bicycle ergometer serves as the testing device. After warm-up (3-5 min), the subject begins pedaling as fast as possible without resistance. Within 3 s, a fixed resistance is applied to the flywheel; the subject continues to pedal "all out" for 30 s. An electrical or mechanical counter continuously records flywheel revolutions in 5-s intervals.

Resistance

Flywheel resistance equals 0.075 kg per kg body mass. For a 70-kg person, the flywheel resistance would equal 5.25 kg (70 kg × 0.075). Resistance often increases to 1.0 kg × body mass or higher (up to 1.3 kg) when testing power- and sprint-type athletes.

Test Scores

1. **Peak Power Output (PP)**—The highest power output, observed during the first 5-s exercise interval, indicates the energy-generating capacity of the immediate energy system (intramuscular high-energy phosphates ATP and PCr). PP, expressed in watts (1 W = 6.12 kg-m · min^{-1}), computes as: Force × Distance (number of revolutions × distance per revolution) ÷ Time in minutes (5 s = 0.0833 min).

2. **Relative Peak Power Output (RPP)**—Peak power output relative to body mass: PP ÷ Body mass, kg.

3. **Anaerobic Fatigue (AF)**—Percentage decline in power output during the test; AF represents the total capacity to produce ATP via the immediate and short-term energy systems. AF computes as: Highest 5-s PP − Lowest 5-s PP ÷ Highest 5-s PP × 100.

4. **Anaerobic Capacity (AC)**—Total work accomplished over 30 s; AC computes as the sum of each 5-s PP, or Force × Total distance in 30 s.

Example

A male weighing 73.3 kg (161.6 lb) performs the Wingate test on a Monark cycle ergometer (6.0 m traveled per pedal revolution) with an applied resistance of 5.5 kg (73.3-kg body mass x 0.075 = 5.497, rounded to 5.5 kg); pedal revolutions for each 5-s interval equal 12, 10, 8, 7, 6, and 5 (48 total revolutions in 30 s).

Calculations

1. Peak Power Output
   PP = Force × Distance ÷ Time
   = 5.5 × (12 rev × 6 m) ÷ 0.0833
   = 396 ÷ 0.0833
   = 4753.9 kg–m · min^{-1} or 776.8 W

2. Relative Peak Power Output
   RPP = PP ÷ Body mass, kg
   = 776.8 W ÷ 73.3 kg
   = 10.6 W · kg^{-1}

3. Anaerobic Fatigue
   AF = Highest PP − Lowest PP ÷ Highest PP × 100
   [Highest PP = Force × Distance ÷ Time: 5.5 kg × (12 rev × 6 m) ÷ 0.0833 min = 4753.9 kg–m · min^{-1} or 776.8 W]
   [Lowest PP = Force × Distance ÷ Time: 5.5 kg × (5 rev × 6 m) ÷ 0.0833 min = 1980.8 kg–m · min^{-1} or 323.7 W]
   = 776.8 W − 323.7 W ÷ 776.8 W × 100
   = 58. 3%

4. Anaerobic Capacity
   AC = Force × Total Distance (in 30 s)
   = 5.5 × [(12 rev + 10 rev + 8 rev + 7 rev + 6 rev + 5 rev) × 6 m]
   = 1584 kg–m · min^{-1} or 258.8 W

PERCENTILE NORMS FOR AVERAGE AND PEAK POWER FOR PHYSICALLY ACTIVE YOUNG ADULTS

	AVERAGE POWER				PEAK POWER			
	Male		**Female**		**Male**		**Female**	
% Rank	**W**	**W·kg^{-1}**	**W**	**W·kg^{-1}**	**W**	**W·kg^{-1}**	**W**	**W·kg^{-1}**
90	662	8.24	470	7.31	822	10.89	560	9.02
80	618	8.01	419	6.95	777	10.39	527	8.83
70	600	7.91	410	6.77	757	10.20	505	8.53
60	577	7.59	391	6.59	721	9.80	480	8.14
50	565	7.44	381	6.39	689	9.22	449	7.65
40	548	7.14	367	6.15	671	8.92	432	6.96
30	530	7.00	353	6.03	656	8.53	399	6.86
20	496	6.59	336	5.71	618	8.24	376	6.57
10	471	5.98	306	5.25	570	7.06	353	5.98

From Maud, P.J., and Schultz, B.B.: Norms for the Wingate anaerobic test with comparisons in another similar test. *Res. Q. Exerc. Sport*, 60:144, 1989.

all-out exercise significantly exceeds energy generated by hydrogen's oxidation in the respiratory chain. This means that the anaerobic reactions of glycolysis predominate, with large quantities of lactate accumulating within the active muscle and ultimately appearing in the blood.

Unlike tests for maximal oxygen uptake, no specific criteria exist to indicate when a person reaches a maximal anaerobic effort. In fact, one's level of self-motivation, including external factors in the test environment, likely influence test scores. *Researchers often use the blood lactate level to reveal the degree of activation of the short-term energy system.*

Performance Tests of Glycolytic Power

Activities that require substantial activation of the short-term energy system demand maximal work for up to 3 minutes. All-out runs and cycling exercise have usually tested anaerobic energy transfer capacity, although weight lifting (repetitive lifting of a certain percentage of maximum) and shuttle and agility runs have also been used. Because age, gender, skill, motivation, and body size affect maximal physical performance, selecting a suitable criterion test to develop normative standards for glycolytic energy capacity remains difficult. A test that maximally uses only leg muscles cannot adequately assess short-term anaerobic capacity for upper-body exercise such as rowing or swimming. *Considered within the framework of exercise specificity, the performance test must be similar to the activity or sport for which energy capacity is evaluated. In most cases, the actual activity serves as the test.*

In 1973, the **Katch test** used all-out leg cycling of short duration to estimate the power and capacity of the anaerobic energy systems. The frictional resistance against the bicycle's flywheel was preset at the high load of 6 kg for men and 5 kg for women. Subjects turned as many revolutions as possible in 40 seconds with pedal revolution rate recorded continuously. The peak power achieved represented **anaerobic power**, and total work accomplished reflected **anaerobic capacity**.

A subsequent modification of the Katch test, the **Wingate test**, involves 30 seconds of all-out exercise on either an arm-crank or leg-cycle ergometer. The subject's body mass determines the frictional resistance during exercise (usually 0.075 kg of resistance per kg body mass); the tester applies this resistance only after the subject overcomes the initial inertia and unloaded frictional resistance to pedaling (within about 3 s). Timing of the test then begins, with pedal revolutions counted continuously and usually reported every 5 seconds. **Peak power output** represents the highest mechanical power generated during any 3- to 5-second interval of the test; **average power output** equals the arithmetic average of total power generated during the 30-second test.

Anaerobic fatigue (percentage decline in power relative to the peak value) provides an index of anaerobic endurance; it represents the maximal capacity for ATP production via a combination of intramuscular phosphagen breakdown and the reactions of glycolysis. **Anaerobic capacity** represents the total work accomplished over the 30-second exercise period (see *How to Determine Anaerobic Power and Capacity: The Wingate Cycle Ergometer Test*).

As in the Katch test, interpretation of the Wingate test assumes that peak power output represents the energy-generating capacity of the intramuscular high-energy phosphates, while total power output reflects glycolytic capacity. Elite volleyball and ice hockey players have recorded some of the highest cycle ergometer power scores. The Wingate and Katch tests elicit reproducible performance scores with moderate validity using a variety of other "anaerobic capacity" criteria.

Figure 8.4 presents the relative contribution of each metabolic pathway during three different duration all-out cycle ergometer tests. Part A illustrates the findings as a percent of total work output, and part B presents the data in estimated kilojoules of energy (1 kJ = 4.2 kcal). Note the progressive change in the percentage contribution of each of the energy systems to the total work output as duration of effort increases.

Other Anaerobic Tests

All-out running tests ranging from 200 to 1000 m have also evaluated anaerobic power and capacity. Meaningful normative standards for these tests have been difficult to develop due to large variations among individuals in running technique and level of motivation.

Lower in Children. Children perform poorer on tests of short-term anaerobic power compared with adolescents and young adults. Perhaps children's lower muscle glycogen concentrations and rates of glycogen utilization partly account for this difference. In addition, children have less lower leg muscle strength related to body mass compared with adults, which could also diminish anaerobic exercise performance.

Gender Differences. As with most measures of physiologic capacity and exercise performance, significant gender differences exist in anaerobic power-output capacity when comparing test scores on an absolute basis. On the surface, one would assume these observations could be explained by gender differences in factors that affect power-output capacity—body mass, muscle mass, and fat-free body mass (FFM). Consequently, gender differences in anaerobic capacity should be minimized or even eliminated when expressing exercise performance relative to body mass or body composition. Such data would offer insight into whether a true gender effect exists for a muscle's capacity to generate energy anaerobically during exercise.

Available data indicate that the significant difference in anaerobic power capacity between women and men cannot be fully explained by differences in body composition, physique, muscular strength, or neuromuscular factors. For example, supermaximal cycling exercise elicited a significantly higher peak oxygen deficit (a measure of anaerobic capacity) in men than in women per unit of fat-free leg vol-

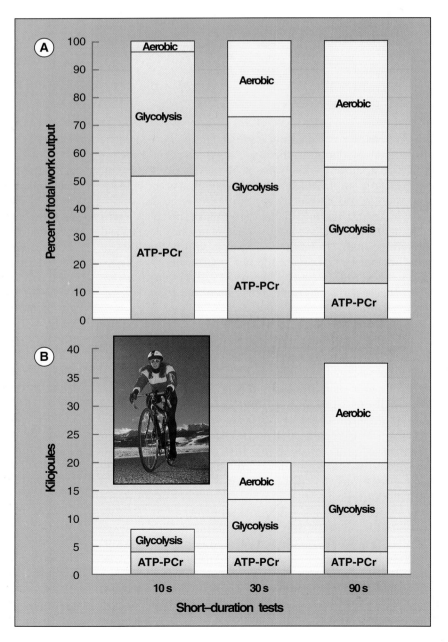

Figure 8.4
Relative contribution of each of the energy systems to the total work accomplished in three tests of short-duration. **A,** Percent of total work output. **B,** Kilojoules of energy. Test results based on the Katch test protocol. (Data from the Applied Physiology Laboratory, University of Michigan.)

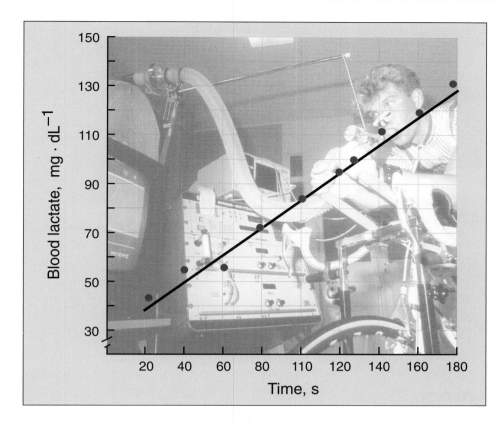

Figure 8.5
Pedaling a stationary bicycle ergometer at the highest possible power output increases blood lactate in direct proportion to the duration of exercise for up to 3 minutes. Each value represents the average of 10 subjects. (Data from the Applied Physiology Laboratory, University of Michigan.).

tate levels increased directly with duration (and total work output) of all-out exercise. The highest blood lactates occurred at the end of 3 minutes of cycling, averaging about 130 mg in each 100 mL of blood (about 16 mmol).

Glycogen Depletion

Because the short-term energy system largely depends on glycogen stored in the specific muscles activated by exercise, these muscles' pattern of glycogen depletion provides an indication of the contribution of glycolysis to exercise.

Figure 8.6 shows that the rate of glycogen depletion in the quadriceps femoris muscle during bicycle exercise closely parallels exercise intensity. With steady-rate exercise at about 30% of $\dot{V}O_{2max}$, a substantial reserve muscle glycogen remains, even after cycling for 180 minutes. Because relatively light exercise relies mainly on a low level of aerobic metabolism, large quantities of fatty acids provide energy with only moderate use of stored glycogen. The most rapid and pronounced glycogen depletion occurs at the two heaviest workloads. This makes sense from a metabolic standpoint because glycogen provides the only stored nutrient for anaerobic ATP resynthesis. Thus, glycogen has high priority in the "metabolic mill" during strenuous exercise.

Changes in total muscle glycogen illustrated in Figure 8.6 may not indicate the precise degree of glycogen breakdown in specific muscle fibers. Depending on exercise intensity, glycogen depletion occurs selectively in either fast- or slow-twitch fibers. For example, during all-out 1-minute sprints on a bicycle ergometer, activation of the fast-twitch fibers provides the predominant power for the exercise. Glycogen content in these fibers becomes almost totally depleted because of the sprint's anaerobic nature. In contrast, slow-twitch fibers become glycogen-depleted earlier than fast-twitch counterparts during moderate to heavy prolonged aerobic exercise. The specific nature of glycogen utilization (and depletion) in relation to muscle fiber type makes it difficult to evaluate the degree of glycolytic activation from changes in a muscle's total glycogen content before and after exercise.

ume. This difference persisted even though gender differences in active muscle mass had been considered. Similar observations occur for gender differences in anaerobic exercise capacity in children and adolescents.

The above findings suggest the possibility of a gender-related biologic difference in anaerobic exercise capacity. If correct, physical testing that focuses on anaerobic exercise performance would further intensify performance differences between men and women to a greater degree than typically expected. Furthermore, adjusting performance to body size or composition would not eliminate this effect. For physical testing in the occupational setting, justifiable concern exists that all-out anaerobic exercise testing exacerbates existing gender differences in performance scores; such testing adversely impacts females.

Blood Lactate Levels

Activation of the glycolytic energy pathway in maximal exercise results in a considerable accumulation of blood lactate. Blood lactate levels more than likely reflect the capacity of the short-term energy system.

Figure 8.5 presents data obtained from 10 college men who performed 10 all-out bicycle ergometer rides of different durations on the Katch test on different days. The subjects included men involved in physical conditioning programs and varsity athletics. Unaware of the duration of each test, the men were urged to turn as many revolutions as possible. The researchers measured venous blood lactate before and immediately after each test and throughout recovery. The plotted points represent the average of blood lactate values at the end of exercise for each test. Blood lac-

Figure 8.6
Glycogen depletion from the vastus lateralis portion of the quadriceps femoris muscle in bicycle exercise of different intensities and durations. Exercise at 31% of $\dot{V}O_{2max}$ (the lightest workload) caused some depletion of muscle glycogen, but the most rapid and largest depletion occurred with exercise that ranged from 83% to 150% of $\dot{V}O_{2max}$. (Adapted from Gollnick, P. D.: Selective glycogen depletion pattern in human muscle fibers after exercise of varying intensity and at varying pedaling rates. *J. Physiol.*, 241:45, 1974.)

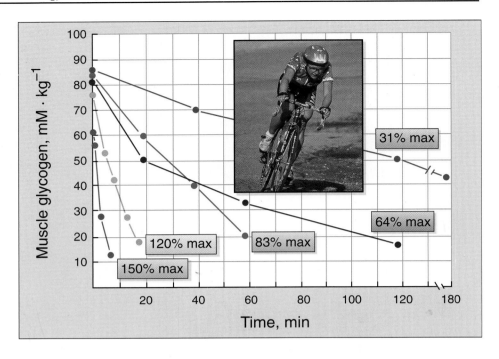

Individual Differences in Anaerobic Energy Transfer Capacity

Differences in training level, capacity to buffer acid metabolites produced in heavy exercise, and motivation contribute to individual differences in capacity to generate short-term anaerobic energy.

Effects of Training
Figure 8.7 compares the dynamics of anaerobic metabolism in trained and untrained subjects. Short-term supermaximal exercise on a bicycle ergometer in trained subjects always produced higher levels of blood and muscle lactate and greater muscle glycogen depletion compared to untrained counterparts. For all subjects, better performances usually associated with higher blood lactate levels, supporting the belief that training for brief, all-out exercise enhances the glycolytic system's capacity to generate energy. In sprint and middle-distance activities, individual differences in anaerobic capacity account for much of the variation in exercise performance.

Buffering of Acid Metabolites
Lactate accumulates when anaerobic energy transfer predominates. This increases the muscle's acidity, negatively affecting the intracellular environment. For example, decreased intracellular pH adversely affects the contractile capability of active muscles and their energy transfer enzymes. The deleterious intracellular alterations during anaerobic exercise have caused speculation that anaerobic training might enhance short-term energy transfer by increasing the body's buffering capacity (**alkaline reserve**) to enable greater lactate production (refer to discussion of performance-enhancing effects from ingestion of exogenous buffers in Chapter 17). However, only a small increase in

alkaline reserve occurs in athletes compared with sedentary individuals. Also, no appreciable change in alkaline reserve follows hard physical training. *Trained individuals have a buffering capability within the range expected for healthy untrained people.*

Motivation
Individuals with greater "pain tolerance," "toughness," or ability to "push" beyond the discomforts of fatiguing exercise definitely accomplish more anaerobic work. These people usually generate greater levels of blood lactate and glycogen depletion; they also score higher on tests of short-term energy capacity. Although difficult to categorize and quantify, motivation plays a key role in superior performance at all levels of competition.

Aerobic Energy: Long-Term Energy System

The data in Figure 8.8 illustrate that persons who engage in sports that require sustained, high-intensity exercise possess large aerobic energy transfer capacity.

Men and women who compete in distance running, swimming, bicycling, and cross-country skiing record the highest maximal oxygen uptakes. *These athletes have nearly twice the aerobic capacity as sedentary individuals.* This does not mean that only $\dot{V}O_{2max}$ determines endurance exercise capacity. Other factors, particularly those at the muscle level such as capillary density, enzymes, and muscle fiber type, strongly influence capacity to sustain exercise at a high percentage of $\dot{V}O_{2max}$ (i.e., achieve a high blood lactate threshold). However, the $\dot{V}O_{2max}$ provides useful information about long-term energy system capacity. Furthermore, attainment of $\dot{V}O_{2max}$ requires integration

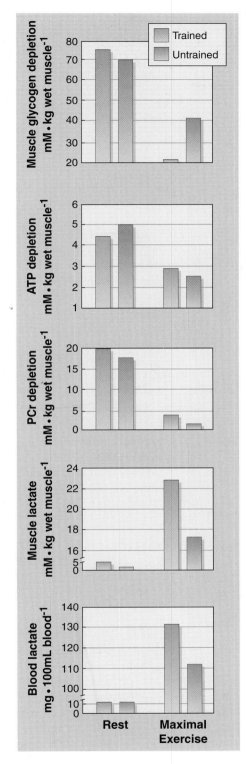

Figure 8.7
Depletion of anaerobic substrates (ATP, PCr, and glycogen) and increases in muscle and blood lactate in short-term, maximal exercise for trained and nontrained subjects. Trained subjects exhibited a greater increase in anaerobic metabolism (higher lactate levels) and a greater depletion in glycogen. Essentially the same reduction in the intramuscular high-energy phosphates ATP and PCr occurred for both groups. (From Karlsson, J., et al.: Muscle metabolites during submaximal and maximal exercise in man. *Scand. J. Clin. Invest.*, 26:382, 1971.)

Benefits of Enhanced Alkaline Reserve

Altering acid-base balance in the direction of alkalosis can temporarily but significantly enhance short-term, high-intensity exercise performance. Run times improve significantly by consuming a buffering solution of sodium bicarbonate before a high-intensity anaerobic effort. This effect is accompanied by higher blood lactate and extracellular H^+ concentrations, which indicate an increased anaerobic energy contribution.

of the ventilatory, cardiovascular, and neuromuscular systems; this gives significant physiologic "meaning" to this metabolic measure. *In essence, $\dot{V}O_{2max}$ represents a fundamental measure in exercise physiology, and serves as a standard to compare performance estimates of aerobic capacity and endurance fitness.*

Maximal Oxygen Uptake Measurement

Tests for $\dot{V}O_{2max}$ use exercise tasks that activate large muscle groups with sufficient intensity and duration to engage maximal aerobic energy transfer. Typical exercise includes treadmill walking or running, bench stepping, or cycling, tethered and flume swimming and swimbench ergometry, and simulated rowing, skiing, in-line skating, stair-climbing, ice skating, and arm-crank exercise. Considerable research effort has been directed toward 1) development and standardization of tests for $\dot{V}O_{2max}$, and 2) establishment of norms related to age, gender, state of training, and body composition.

Criteria for $\dot{V}O_{2max}$

A leveling-off or peaking-over in oxygen uptake during increasing exercise intensity (Fig. 8.9) signifies attainment of maximum capacity for aerobic metabolism (i.e., a "true" $\dot{V}O_{2max}$). When this accepted criterion is not met, or local muscle fatigue in the arms or legs rather than central circulatory dynamics limits test performance, the term "**peak oxygen uptake**" ($\dot{V}O_{2peak}$) usually describes the highest oxygen uptake value during the test.

Different Terms But the Same Fitness Component

Stamina, endurance fitness, cardiovascular fitness, and aerobic fitness all refer to the body's ability to generate ATP aerobically.

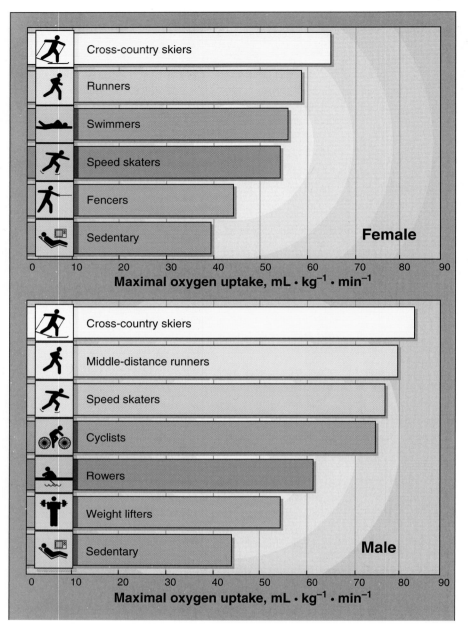

Figure 8.8
Maximal oxygen uptake of male and female Olympic-caliber athletes in different sport categories compared to healthy sedentary subjects. (Adapted from Saltin, B., and Åstrand, P. O.: Maximal oxygen uptake in athletes. *J. Appl. Physiol.*, 23:3523, 1967.)

based on metabolic and physiologic responses. These include:

- Failure for oxygen uptake versus exercise intensity to increase by some value usually expected from previous observations with the particular test ($\dot{V}O_{2max}$ criterion).

- Blood lactate levels that reach at least 70 or 80 mg per 100 mL of blood or about 8 to 10 mmol (ensures the subject has significantly exceeded the lactate threshold with a near-maximal exercise effort; $\dot{V}O_{2peak}$ criterion).

- Attainment of near age-predicted maximum heart rate, or a respiratory exchange ratio (R) in excess of 1.00 (indicates that subject exercised at close to maximum intensity; $\dot{V}O_{2peak}$ criterion).

Tests of Aerobic Power

Numerous standardized tests have measured $\dot{V}O_{2max}$. Such tests remain independent of muscle strength, speed, body size, and skill, with the exception of specialized swimming, rowing, and ice skating tests.

The data in Figure 8.9 reflect oxygen uptake with progressive increases in treadmill exercise intensity; the test terminates when the subject decides to stop even when prodded to continue. For the average oxygen uptake values of 18 subjects plotted in this figure, the highest oxygen uptake occurred before subjects attained their maximum exercise level. This peaking-over criterion substantiates attainment of a true $\dot{V}O_{2max}$.

In many instances, a peaking-over or slight decrease in oxygen uptake does not occur as exercise intensity increases. Often, the highest oxygen uptake occurs during the last minute of exercise without the plateau criterion for $\dot{V}O_{2max}$. Thus, additional criteria for establishing $\dot{V}O_{2max}$ (more precisely $\dot{V}O_{2peak}$) have been suggested

The $\dot{V}O_{2max}$ test may require a continuous 3- to 5-minute "supermaximal" effort, but it usually consists of increments in exercise intensity (referred to as a **graded exercise test** or **GXT**) until the subject stops. Some researchers have imprecisely termed the end point "exhaustion," but it should be kept in mind that the subject terminates the test (for whatever reason). A variety of psychologic or motivational factors can influence this decision, rather than true physiologic exhaustion. It can take considerable urging and encouragement to get subjects to the criterion point for $\dot{V}O_{2max}$. Children and adults encounter particular difficulty if they have had little prior experience performing strenuous exercise with its associated central (cardiorespiratory) and peripheral (local muscular)

Figure 8.9
Peaking over in oxygen uptake with increasing intensity of treadmill exercise. Each point represents the average oxygen uptake of 18 sedentary males. The point at which oxygen uptake fails to increase the expected amount or even decreases slightly with increasing exercise intensity represents the $\dot{V}O_{2max}$. (Data from the Applied Physiology Laboratory, University of Michigan).

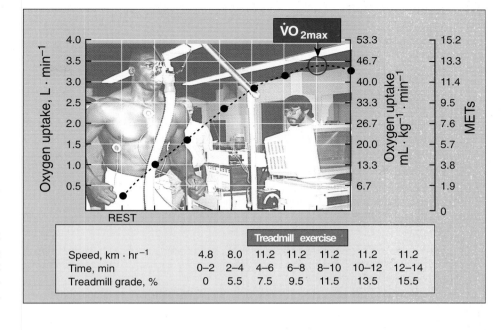

		Treadmill exercise					
Speed, km · hr^{-1}		4.8	8.0	11.2	11.2	11.2	11.2	11.2
Time, min		0–2	2–4	4–6	6–8	8–10	10–12	12–14
Treadmill grade, %		0	5.5	7.5	9.5	11.5	13.5	15.5

discomforts. *Attaining a plateau in oxygen uptake during the $\dot{V}O_{2max}$ test requires high motivation and a large anaerobic component because of the maximal exercise requirement.*

Comparison Between $\dot{V}O_{2max}$ Tests

Two types of tests determine maximal oxygen uptake:

1. **Continuous Test** — no rest between exercise increments
2. **Discontinuous Test** — several minutes rest between exercise increments

The data in Table 8.2 show a systematic comparison of $\dot{V}O_{2max}$ scores measured by six common continuous and discontinuous treadmill and bicycle procedures.

Although only a small 8 mL difference occurred in $\dot{V}O_{2max}$ between continuous and discontinuous bicycle tests, $\dot{V}O_{2max}$ averaged 6.4 to 11.2% below values on the treadmill. The largest difference among any of the three treadmill running tests equaled only 1.2%. The walking test, on the other hand, elicited $\dot{V}O_{2max}$ scores about 7% above values on the bicycle, but 5% less than the average for the three run tests.

Subjects reported intense local discomfort in the thigh muscles during heavy exercise on the continuous and discontinuous bicycle tests. In walking, subjects reported discomfort in the lower back and calf muscles, particularly at higher treadmill elevations. The running tests produced little local discomfort, yet subjects experienced a general fatigue usually categorized as feeling "winded." For ease of administration testing *healthy* subjects, we recommend a continuous treadmill run. Total time to administer the test averaged a little over 12 minutes, whereas the discontinuous running test averaged about 65 minutes. Subjects seemed to "tolerate" the continuous test well and preferred the shorter

TABLE 8.2
Average maximal oxygen uptakes for 15 college students during continuous (cont.) and discontinuous (discont.) tests on the bicycle and treadmill

VARIABLE	BIKE CONT.	BIKE, CONT.	TREADMILL, DISCONT. WALK-RUN	TREADMILL, CONT. WALK	TREADMILL, DISCONT. RUN	TREADMILL, CONT. RUN
$\dot{V}O_{2max}$, mL · min^{-1}	3691 ± 453	3683 ± 448	4145 ± 401	3944 ± 395	4157 ± 445	4109 ± 424
$\dot{V}O_{2max}$, mL · kg^{-1}·min^{-1}	50.0 ± 6.9	49.9 ± 7.0	56.6 ± 7.3	56.6 ± 7.6	55.5 ± 7.6	55.5 ± 6.8

Values are means ± standard deviations

Adapted from McArdle, W. D., et al.: Comparison of continuous and discontinuous treadmill and bicycle tests for max $\dot{V}O_2$. *Med. Sci Sports.*, 5:156, 1973.

test time. In fact, $\dot{V}O_{2max}$ can be achieved with a continuous exercise protocol where exercise intensity increases progressively in 15-second intervals. With such an approach, total test time for either bicycle or treadmill exercise averages only about 5 minutes.

Commonly Used Treadmill Protocols

Figure 8.10 summarizes six commonly used treadmill protocols to assess aerobic capacity in healthy individuals and patients with cardiovascular disease. One feature common to each test includes manipulation of exercise duration and treadmill speed and grade. The Harbor treadmill test (example F), referred to as a **ramp test**, is unique because treadmill grade increases every minute up to 10 minutes by a constant amount that ranges from 1 to 4% depending on the subject's fitness. This quick procedure linearly increases oxygen uptake to the maximum level. Healthy individuals and monitored cardiac patients tolerate the protocol without problems.

Manipulating Test Protocol to Increase $\dot{V}O_{2max}$

When a person completes a maximal oxygen uptake test, one assumes the tester has made every attempt to "push" the subject to the near-limits of performance. This effort includes verbal encouragement from laboratory staff and peers or a monetary incentive. If the test meets the usual criteria, one assumes the test score represents the subject's "true" $\dot{V}O_{2max}$.

In one study, 44 sedentary and trained men and women performed a continuous treadmill $\dot{V}O_{2max}$ test to the point where they refused to continue exercising ("exhaustion"). They recovered for 2 minutes and then performed a second $\dot{V}O_{2max}$ test. During active recovery from test 1, the researchers lowered the treadmill grade at least 2.5% below the final grade of the previous test and reduced running speed from 11.0 $km \cdot hr^{-1}$ to 9.0 $km \cdot hr^{-1}$

Figure 8.10
Six commonly used treadmill procedures. **A,** Naughton test. Three-minute exercise periods of increasing intensity alternating with 3 minutes of rest. The exercise periods vary in grade and speed. **B,** Åstrand test. Speed remains constant at 5 mph. After 3 minutes at 0% grade, grade increases 2.5% every 2 minutes. **C,** Bruce test. Grade and/or speed change every 3 minutes. Healthy subjects do not perform grades 0% and 5%. **D,** Balke test. After 1 minute at 0% grade and 1 minute at 2% grade, grade increases 1% per minute (all at a speed of 3.3 mph). **E,** Ellestad test. The initial grade is 10%, the later grade 15%, while the speed increases every 2 or 3 minutes. **F,** Harbor test. After 3 minutes of walking at a comfortable speed, grade increases at a constant preselected amount each minute (1%, 2%, 3%, or 4%), so the subject reaches $\dot{V}O_{2max}$ in approximately 10 minutes. (From Wasserman, K., et al.: *Principles of Exercise Testing and Interpretation.* 3rd Ed., Baltimore: Lippincott Williams & Wilkins, 1999.)

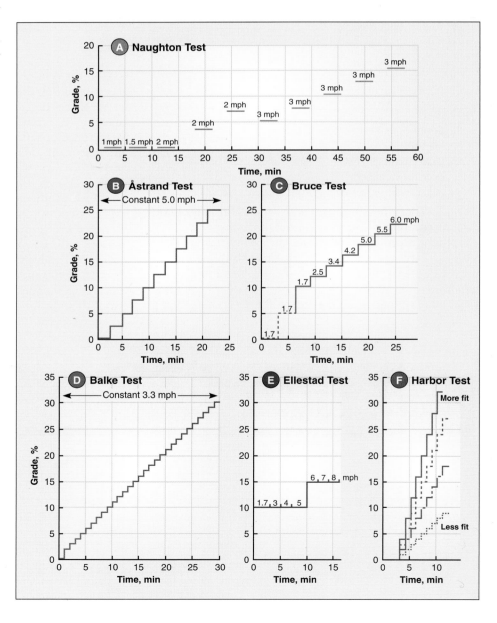

c l o s e   u p

$\dot{V}O_{2max}$ of Olympic Wheelchair-Dependent Athletes

Most able-bodied individuals have never considered the psychologic trauma, physical limitations, and societal constraints that confront the physically challenged. When an able-bodied person suffers a physical disability and loses the use of their legs, the effort to merely survive and function at a level close to "normal" becomes heroic. For many with a disability, near-normal is neither sufficient nor acceptable. Many physically-challenged individuals want to function as they did before being injured, and this includes athletic competition. A wheelchair does not pose a hindrance, but rather a support and even an exercise training device.

Athletics notwithstanding, a sedentary lifestyle represents a major cause of cardiovascular disease for wheelchair-dependent people. For these individuals, upper-body exercise training can provide an important tool for heart disease protection. The upper-body $\dot{V}O_{2max}$ of highly trained wheelchair-dependent athletes shows how well the level of physiologic function can improve in the wheelchair-dependent population.

A limited number of studies exist (utilizing diverse testing procedures) on the physical work capacity and aerobic power of wheelchair-dependent individuals. Data on 40 male French Olympic wheelchair-dependent subjects provide relevant information. The researchers tested athletes from eight different sports for $\dot{V}O_{2max}$. The athletes used their general-purpose wheelchairs for treadmill testing. Test protocol consisted of continuous exercise where intensity increased every 2 minutes. At the beginning of each 2-minute exercise bout, workload increased either by increasing speed (2.0 km $\cdot$ hr^{-1}) at a constant treadmill grade, or by increasing treadmill grade by 1% with constant velocity. The graph presents $\dot{V}O_{2max}$ (mL $\cdot$ kg$^{-1}\cdot$ min^{-1}) by sport category. Track and field athletes achieved the highest values followed by swimmers. Compare these data with the able-bodied athletes and sedentary subjects shown in Figure 8.8 of approximately the same age measured during treadmill running or stationery bicycling. When making these comparisons, remember that values for aerobic capacity during upper-body exercise among the able-bodied equal about 70% of values achieved during running and bicycling.

Legend:
- Track and field
- Swimming
- Basketball
- Table tennis
- Fencing
- Weight lifting
- Archery
- Target Shooting

Reference

Veeger, H. E. J., et al.: Peak oxygen uptake and maximal power output of Olympic wheelchair-dependent athletes. *Med. Sci. Sports Exerc.*, 23:1201, 1991.

for the trained subjects and from 9.0 km$\cdot$hr^{-1} to 6.0 km$\cdot$hr^{-1} for the sedentary subjects. After 2 minutes, treadmill speed increased to the test 1 speed for 30 seconds, at which time percent grade increased to the final grade achieved in test 1. Treadmill grade increased every 2 minutes thereafter until the subject once again terminated the test. Subjects received strong verbal encouragement particularly during the last minutes of exercise during both tests.

The $\dot{V}O_{2max}$ scores averaged 1.4% higher on the second test. The statistically significant difference of 48 mL (0.7 mL $\cdot$ kg^{-1} $\cdot$ min^{-1} for a typical subject), while small, was almost double that typically measured between the two final oxygen uptake readings on either continuous or dis-

The Importance of an Objective Standard

The consequences of not achieving a "true" $\dot{V}O_{2max}$ become apparent in training studies with $\dot{V}O_{2max}$ as a criterion. Suppose "$\dot{V}O_{2max}$" on the pretest fell 10% short of the true value (due to subject unfamiliarity or poor motivation). After aerobic training, the post-test $\dot{V}O_{2max}$ averages 25% above the pre-test score. Can one conclude that physiologic improvements per se from training induced this improvement? The answer must be "no" if solid evidence cannot establish that the initial $\dot{V}O_{2max}$ represented the true maximum. In this example, the final improvement of 25% would need adjustment to only 15% (after subtracting the 10% "failure" to achieve true $\dot{V}O_{2max}$ on the pre-test). Researchers must verify that pre-test $\dot{V}O_{2max}$ testing adequately considers *all* factors that might prevent subjects from achieving their true maximum score. Strict adherence to the criteria for $\dot{V}O_{2max}$ (or $\dot{V}O_{2peak}$) becomes crucial. Duplicate pre-tests (2-4 days apart) can provide assurance of attaining a true maximum.

continuous tests. A "booster" test after a normally administered aerobic capacity test can increase the final oxygen uptake, illustrating the need to pay careful attention to $\dot{V}O_{2max}$ administrative techniques.

Factors Affecting Maximal Oxygen Uptake

Of many factors that influence $\dot{V}O_{2max}$, the most important include exercise mode, the person's training state, heredity, gender, body composition, and age.

Exercise Mode

Variations in $\dot{V}O_{2max}$ during different modes of exercise reflect the quantity of muscle mass activated. In experiments that measured $\dot{V}O_{2max}$ on the same subjects during diverse exercise, treadmill exercise produced the highest values. Bench-stepping has generated $\dot{V}O_{2max}$ scores identical to treadmill values, and significantly higher than values on a bicycle ergometer. With arm-crank exercise, a person's aerobic capacity reaches only about 70% of treadmill $\dot{V}O_{2max}$.

For skilled but untrained swimmers, the maximal oxygen uptake during swimming falls about 20% below treadmill values. A definite test specificity exists in this form of exercise because trained collegiate swimmers achieved

$\dot{V}O_{2max}$ values swimming only 11% below treadmill values; some elite competitive swimmers equal or even exceed their treadmill $\dot{V}O_{2max}$ scores during a swimming test for aerobic capacity. Similarly, a distinct exercise and training specificity occurs among competitive racewalkers who achieve oxygen uptakes during walking that equal $\dot{V}O_{2max}$ during treadmill running. If competitive cyclists pedal at their fast rate in competition, they also achieve $\dot{V}O_{2max}$ values equivalent to treadmill scores.

The treadmill represents the laboratory apparatus of choice for determining $\dot{V}O_{2max}$ in healthy subjects. The treadmill easily quantifies and regulates exercise intensity. Compared with other forms of exercise, subjects achieve one or more of the criteria for establishing $\dot{V}O_{2max}$ or $\dot{V}O_{2peak}$ more easily on the treadmill. Bench stepping or bicycle exercise serves as suitable alternatives under non-laboratory "field" conditions.

Heredity

A question frequently raised concerns the relative contribution of natural endowment to physiologic function and exercise performance. For example, to what extent does heredity determine the extremely high aerobic capacities of the endurance athletes represented in Figure 8.8? Do these exceptionally high levels of functional capacity reflect more than the training effect? Although the answers remain incomplete, some researchers have focused on the question of how genetic variability accounts for differences among individuals in physiologic and metabolic capacity.

Early studies on this topic were conducted on 15 pairs of identical twins (same heredity since they came from the same fertilized egg) and 15 pairs of fraternal twins (did not differ from ordinary siblings because they result from separate fertilization of two eggs) raised in the same city by parents with similar socioeconomic backgrounds. The researchers concluded that heredity alone accounted for up to 93% of the observed differences in aerobic capacity assessed by $\dot{V}O_{2max}$. In addition, genetic factors accounted for 81% of the capacity of the short-term glycolytic energy system and 86% of the maximum heart rate. Subsequent investigations of larger groups of brothers, fraternal twins, and identical twins indicate a significant but much smaller effect of inherited factors on aerobic capacity and endurance performance.

Current estimates of the genetic effect ascribe about 20 to 30% for $\dot{V}O_{2max}$, 50% for maximum heart rate, and 70% for physical working capacity. Similar muscle fiber composition occurs for identical twins, whereas fiber type varies among fraternal twins and brothers. Future research will someday determine the exact upper limit of genetic determination, but present data show that inherited factors contribute *significantly* to physiologic functional capacity and exercise performance. A large genotype-dependency also exists for the potential to improve maximal aerobic and anaerobic power, and the adaptations of most muscle enzymes to training. In other words, members of the same twin-pair show the same response to exercise training. Ge-

How to Predict V̇O2max from a Walking Test

A walking test devised in the 1980s for use on large groups predicted $\dot{V}O_{2max}$ (L·min^{-1}) from the following variables (see Equation #1): body weight (W) in pounds; age (A) in years; gender (G): 0 = female, 1 = male; time (T1) for the 1-mile track walk expressed as minutes and hundredths of a minute; peak heart rate (HRpeak) in b·min^{-1} at the end of the last one-quarter mile (measured as a 15-s pulse immediately after the walk×4 to convert to b·min^{-1}). The test consisted of having individuals walk 1 mile as fast as possible without jogging or running.

For most individuals, $\dot{V}O_{2max}$ ranged within ±0.335 L·min^{-1} (±4.4 mL·kg^{-1}·min^{-1}) of actual $\dot{V}O_{2max}$. This prediction method applies to a broad segment of the general population (ages 30 to 69 y).

Equations

Equation #1

Predicts $\dot{V}O_{2max}$ in L·min^{-1}:

$$\dot{V}O_{2max} = 6.9652 + (0.0091 \times W) - (0.0257 \times A) + (0.5955 \times G) - (0.224 \times T1) - (0.0115 \times HR_{peak})$$

Equation #2

Predicts $\dot{V}O_{2max}$ in mL·kg^{-1}·min^{-1}:

$$\dot{V}O_{2max} = 132.853 - (0.0769 \times W) - (0.3877 \times A) + (6.315 \times G) - (3.2649 \times T1) - (0.1565 \times HR_{peak})$$

Example

Predict $\dot{V}O_{2max}$ (mL·kg^{-1}·min^{-1}) from the following data: gender, female; age, 30 y; body weight, 155.5 lb; T1, 13.56 min; HRpeak, 145 b·min^{-1}.

Substituting the above values in equation #2.

$$\dot{V}O_{2max} = 132.853 - (0.0769 \times 155.5) - (0.3877 \times 30.0) + (6.315 \times 0) - (3.2649 \times 13.56) - (0.1565 \times 145)$$
$$= 132.853 - (11.96) - (11.63) + (0) - (44.27) - (22.69)$$
$$= 42.3 \text{ mL} \cdot \text{kg}^{-1} \cdot \text{min}^{-1}$$

Kline, G., et al.: Estimation of $\dot{V}O_{2max}$ from a one-mile track walk, gender, age, and body weight. *Med. Sci. Sports Exerc.*, 19:253, 1987.

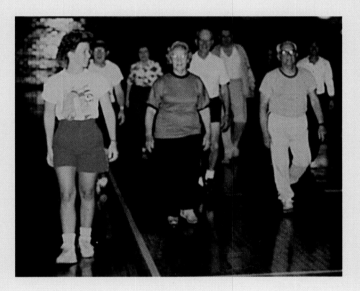

netic makeup plays such a prominent role in determining training response it is nearly impossible to predict a specific individual's response. Table 8.3 summarizes the estimated genetic contribution to important health and physical fitness components.

Training State

Maximal oxygen uptake must be evaluated relative to the person's state of training at the time of measurement. Aerobic capacity with training improves between 6 and 20%, although increases have been reported as high as 50% above pretraining levels. The largest $\dot{V}O_{2max}$ improvement occurs among the most sedentary individuals.

Gender

Maximal oxygen uptake (mL·kg^{-1}·min^{-1}) for women typically average 15 to 30% below scores for men. Even among trained athletes, this difference ranges between 10 and 20%. Such differences increase considerably when expressing $\dot{V}O_{2max}$ as an absolute value (L·min^{-1}) rather than relative to body mass (mL·kg^{-1}·min^{-1}). Among world class male and female cross-country skiers, a 43% lower $\dot{V}O_{2max}$ for women (6.54 vs. 3.75 L·min^{-1}) decreased to 15% (83.8 vs. 71.2 mL·kg^{-1}·min^{-1}) when using the athletes' body mass in the $\dot{V}O_{2max}$ ratio expression.

The apparent gender difference in $\dot{V}O_{2max}$ has been attributed to differences in body composition and hemoglobin content. Untrained young adult women possess about 25% body fat, whereas the corresponding value for men averages 15%. Although trained athletes have a lower body fat percentage, trained women still possess significantly more body fat than male counterparts. Thus, the male generates more total aerobic energy simply because he possesses a relatively large muscle mass and less fat than the female.

Probably due to higher levels of testosterone, men also

TABLE 8.3
Estimated genetic contribution to individual differences in important components of health-related physical fitness

FITNESS COMPONENT	GENETIC CONTRIBUTION
$\dot{V}O_{2max}$	20–30%
Submaximal Exercise Response	20–30%
Muscular Fitness	20–30%
Blood Lipid Profile	30–50%
Resting Blood Pressure	30%
Total Body Fat	25%
Regional Fat Distribution	30%
Habitual Activity Level	30%

Modified from Bouchard, C., and Perusse, L.: Heredity, activity level, fitness, and health. Bouchard, C., et al. (eds.). In: *Physical Activity, Fitness, and Health*. Champaign, IL: Human Kinetics, 1994.

show a 10 to 14% greater concentration of hemoglobin than women. This difference in the blood's oxygen-carrying capacity enables males to circulate more oxygen during exercise, thus giving them an edge in aerobic capacity.

Lower body fat and higher hemoglobin provide men with some advantage in aerobic power, but other factors fully explain the gender disparity. Differences in normal physical activity level between an "average" male and "average" female provide a possible explanation. Perhaps less opportunities exist for women to become as physically active as men due to social structure and constraints. Even among prepubertal children, boys exhibit more physical activity in daily life.

Despite these possible limitations, the aerobic capacity of physically active females exceeds that of sedentary males. For example, female cross-country skiers have $\dot{V}O_{2max}$ scores 40% higher than untrained males of the same age.

Body Composition

Differences in body mass explain roughly 70% of the differences in $\dot{V}O_{2max}$ scores ($L \cdot min^{-1}$) among individuals. Thus, meaningful comparisons of exercise performance or the absolute value for $\dot{V}O_{2max}$ ($L \cdot min^{-1}$) become difficult among individuals who differ in body size or body composition. This has led to the common practice of expressing oxygen uptake in terms by body surface area, body mass, FFM, or limb volume.

Table 8.4 presents typical oxygen uptake values for an untrained man and woman who differ considerably in body mass. The percent difference in $\dot{V}O_{2max}$ between these individuals, when expressing aerobic capacity in $L \cdot min^{-1}$ amounts to 43%. The woman still has about a 20% lower value when expressing $\dot{V}O_{2max}$ related to body mass ($mL \cdot kg^{-1} \cdot min^{-1}$). Expressing aerobic capacity relative to FFM reduces the difference even more.

Similar findings also occur for $\dot{V}O_{2peak}$ for men and women during arm-cranking exercise. Adjusting the arm-crank $\dot{V}O_{2peak}$ for variations in arm and shoulder size equalized values between the men and women. This suggests that gender differences in aerobic capacity largely reflect the size of the contracting muscle mass. Such observations foster the argument that essentially no gender difference exists in the capacity of active muscle mass to generate ATP aerobically. On the other hand, simply expressing aerobic capacity or endurance performance by some measure of body composition does not automatically "adjust" for observable gender differences. Researchers still must determine whether real differences exist (i.e., biological in origin), or if factors other than inherited characteristics (environmental-sociological factors) influence the difference between men and women.

Argument for Biological Differences Between Men and Women. The traditional ways of expressing oxygen uptake presented in Table 8.4 do not necessarily answer the question of whether gender differences in oxygen uptake are biologically inherent or fully attributable to differences in muscle mass and body composition. This uncertainty exists because ratio adjustments may not truly "eliminate" gender differences; they

TABLE 8.4
Different ways of expressing oxygen uptake

VARIABLE	FEMALE	MALE	% DIFFERENCE
$\dot{V}O_{2max}$, $L \cdot min^{-1}$	2.00	3.50	−43
$\dot{V}O_{2max}$, $mL \cdot min^{-1}$	40.0	50.0	−20
$\dot{V}O_{2max}$, $mL \cdot kg\ FFM^{-1} \cdot min^{-1}$	53.3	58.8	−9.0
Body mass, kg	50	70	−29
Percent body fat	25	15	+67
Fat-free body mass (FFM), kg	37.5	59.5	−37

simply express the aerobic power by using a divisor (e.g., body mass, FFM, or muscle cross-sectional area).

An experimental approach to evaluating this important topic would compare the physiologic responses and capacities of men and women of similar body size, body composition, and training history. Such a comparison eliminates the need to express oxygen uptake as a ratio score relative to body size or composition. Consequently, matching subjects on such variables should eliminate gender differences in aerobic capacity. To evaluate this hypothesis, research compared the aerobic capacity of 10 pairs of sedentary and endurance-trained men and women closely matched for age, stature, body mass, FFM, and prior training history. In addition, the observed gender difference in hemoglobin concentration provided an "adjustment" for aerobic capacity.

Figure 8.11 illustrates the effect of gender matching for either body mass or FFM on the percentage difference in $\dot{V}O_{2max}$ measured during incremental treadmill running. The higher $\dot{V}O_{2max}$ values for men versus women matched for body mass averaged 25.3% for sedentary and 22.1% for trained. After adjusting for differences in hemoglobin concentration (*adjusted* $\dot{V}O_{2max}$), gender differences persisted, decreasing to 18.4% for the sedentary group and 12.8% for the trained group. When the groups were matched for FFM, substantial gender differences still existed, averaging 18.4% for the sedentary group and 20.5% for the trained group. Adjusting for hemoglobin concentration reduced the $\dot{V}O_{2max}$ difference somewhat, but it still averaged about 11% for both groups.

These findings suggest that a portion of the gender difference in aerobic capacity may be biologically inherent and unalterable. This does not mean that aerobic capacity cannot be significantly improved by training. Rather, it may be inappropriate to expect "sex-free" differences in aerobic capacity.

Age

Changes in $\dot{V}O_{2max}$ relate to chronological age. Although limitations exist in drawing inferences from cross-sectional studies of different people at different ages, the available data provide insight into the possible effects of aging on physiologic function.

Absolute Values. Figure 8.12 shows that maximal oxygen uptake ($L \cdot min^{-1}$) increases dramatically during the growth years. Longitudinal studies (measuring the same people over a prolonged period) of children's aerobic capacity show that absolute $\dot{V}O_{2max}$ increases from about $1.0\ L \cdot min^{-1}$ at age 6 years to $3.2\ L \cdot min^{-1}$ at 16 years. $\dot{V}O_{2max}$ in girls peaks at about age 14 and declines thereafter. At age 14, the differences in $\dot{V}O_{2max}$ ($L \cdot min^{-1}$) between boys and girls approximates 25%, with the spread reaching 50% by age 16.

Relative Values. When expressed relative to body mass, the $\dot{V}O_{2max}$ remains constant at about 53 $mL \cdot kg^{-1} \cdot min^{-1}$ between the ages of 6 and 16 for boys. In contrast, relative $\dot{V}O_{2max}$ in girls gradually decreases from 52.0 $mL \cdot kg^{-1} \cdot min^{-1}$ at age 6 to 40.5 $mL \cdot kg^{-1} \cdot min^{-1}$ at age 16 years. Greater accumulation of body fat in females provides the most common explanation for this discrepancy.

Beyond age 25, $\dot{V}O_{2max}$ declines steadily at about 1% per year, so that by age 55 it averages 27% below values reported for 20-year-olds. While active adults retain a relatively high $\dot{V}O_{2max}$ at all ages (Fig. 8.12, inset graph), their aerobic capacity still declines with advancing years. However, research continues to show that one's habitual level of physical

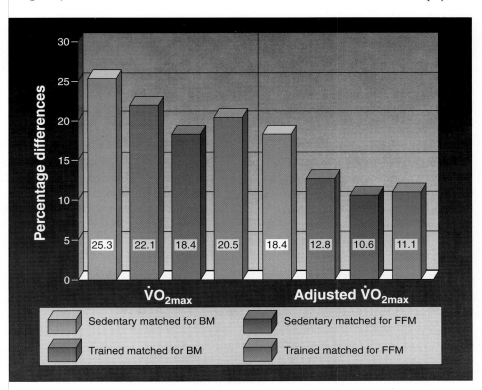

Figure 8.11
Percentage differences in $\dot{V}O_{2max}$, including the adjustment for hemoglobin (adjusted $\dot{V}O_{2max}$), in sedentary and trained men and women matched for body mass (BM) and fat-free body mass (FFM). (From Keller, B.A.: The influence of body size variables on gender differences in strength and maximum aerobic capacity. Doctoral dissertation. University of Massachusetts, Amherst, MA, 1989.)

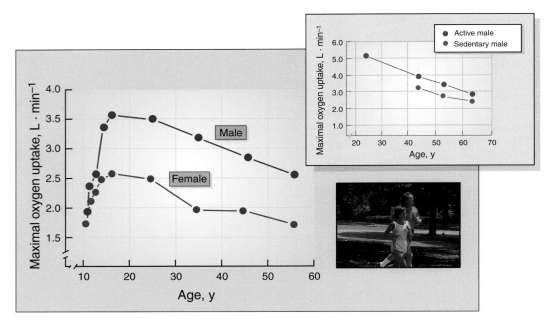

Figure 8.12
General trend for maximal oxygen uptake with age and level of activity in males and females.

activity through middle age determines changes in aerobic capacity to a greater extent than chronological age. Chapter 20 addresses this topic more fully.

Maximal Oxygen Uptake Predictions

Directly measuring $\dot{V}O_{2max}$ requires an extensive laboratory, specialized equipment, and considerable motivation on the subject's part to perform "all out." As such, $\dot{V}O_{2max}$ tests do not lend themselves to measuring large groups of untrained subjects outside of the laboratory. In addition, maximal exercise can be hazardous to adults who have not received proper medical clearance, or are tested without appropriate safeguards or supervision.

In view of these considerations, alternative tests have been devised to predict $\dot{V}O_{2max}$ from submaximal performances (*see How to Predict $\dot{V}O_{2max}$ from a Walking Test*). The most popular $\dot{V}O_{2max}$ predictions use walking and running endurance performance. Easily administered, these tests can be used with large groups of men and women without the expense and expertise required in the laboratory setting. Endurance running tests assume that maximal oxygen uptake largely determines the distance one can run in a specified time (greater than 5 or 6 min). The first of the endurance running tests required subjects to run-walk as far as possible in 15 minutes, and a 1968 revision of the test shortened the duration to 12 minutes or 1.5 miles.

Findings from many research studies suggest that the prediction of aerobic capacity should be approached with caution when using walking and running performance.

Establishing a consistent level of motivation and effective pacing becomes critical for inexperienced subjects. Some individuals may run too fast early in the run, and thus must slow down or even stop as the test progresses. Other individuals may begin too slowly and continue this way so their final run score reflects inappropriate pacing or motivation, rather than physiologic and metabolic capacity.

In addition, endurance walking-running performance results from factors other than $\dot{V}O_{2max}$. Body mass and body fatness, running economy (which continually improves during childhood), and one's percentage of aerobic capacity sustainable without blood lactate buildup (blood lactate threshold) all contribute significantly to the final score.

A Word of Caution About Predictions

All predictions involve error, referred to as the **standard error of estimate (SEE)**, derived from the original equation used to make the prediction. Errors of estimate are expressed in units of the predicted variable or as a percent. For example, say your $\dot{V}O_{2max}$ ($mL \cdot kg^{-1} \cdot min^{-1}$) prediction from a walking test equals 55 $mL \cdot kg^{-1} \cdot min^{-1}$, and the SEE of the predicted score equals ± 10 $mL \cdot kg^{-1} \cdot min^{-1}$. This means that in reality, your actual $\dot{V}O_{2max}$ probably (68% likelihood) ranges within ± 10 $mL \cdot kg^{-1} \cdot min^{-1}$ of the predicted value (in your case, between 45 and 65 $ml \cdot kg^{-1} \cdot min^{-1}$). This example represents a relatively large error.

Obviously, the larger the prediction error, the less useful the predicted score, since the true score falls within a broad range of possible values. Without know-

How to Predict V̇O₂max from Step Test Performance

Recovery heart rate from a standardized stepping exercise can classify people on cardiovascular fitness and $\dot{V}O_{2max}$ with a reasonable degree of accuracy.

The Test

Individuals step to a four-step cadence, "up-up-down-down" on a bench 16¼ inches high (height of standard gymnasium bleachers). Women perform 22 complete step-ups per minute to a metronome set at 88 beats per minute; men use 24 step-ups per minute at a metronome setting of 96 beats per minute.

Stepping begins after a brief demonstration and practice period. Following stepping, the person remains standing while another person measures pulse rate (carotid or radial artery) for a 15-s period, 5 to 20 s into recovery. Fifteen-second recovery heart rate converts to beats per minute (15-s HR × 4), which converts to a percentile ranking for predicted $\dot{V}O_{2max}$ (see table).

Equations

The following equations predict $\dot{V}O_{2max}$ ($mL\cdot kg^{-1}\cdot min^{-1}$) from step-test heart rate recovery for men and women ages 18 to 24 years:

Men: $\dot{V}O_{2max} = 111.33 - (0.42 \times$ step-test pulse rate, $b\cdot min^{-1})$

Women: $\dot{V}O_{2max} = 65.81 - (0.1847 \times$ step-test pulse rate, $b\cdot min^{-1})$

The "Predicted $\dot{V}O_{2max}$" columns of the table present the $\dot{V}O_{2max}$ values for men and women from different heart rate scores.

PERCENTILE RANKING FOR RECOVERY HEART RATE AND PREDICTED V̇O₂max (ML · KG⁻¹ · MIN⁻¹) FOR MALE AND FEMALE COLLEGE STUDENTS

Percentile	Recovery HR Females	Predicted V̇O₂max	Recovery HR Males	Predicted V̇O₂max
100	128	42.2	120	60.9
95	140	40.0	124	59.3
90	148	38.5	128	57.6
85	152	37.7	136	54.2
80	156	37.0	140	52.5
75	158	36.6	144	50.9
70	160	36.3	148	49.2
65	162	35.9	149	48.8
60	163	35.7	152	47.5
55	164	35.5	154	46.7
50	166	35.1	156	45.8
45	168	34.8	160	44.1
40	170	34.4	162	43.3
35	171	34.2	164	42.5
30	172	34.0	166	41.6
25	176	33.3	168	40.8
20	180	32.6	172	39.1
15	182	32.2	176	37.4
10	184	31.8	178	36.6
5	196	29.6	184	34.1

From McArdle, W. D., et al.: Percentile norms for a valid step test in college women. *Res. Q.*, 44:498, 1973; McArdle, W.D., et al.: Reliability and interrelationships between maximal oxygen uptake, physical work capacity, and step test scores in college women. *Med. Sci. Sports.*, 4:182, 1972.

ing the magnitude of the error, one cannot judge the usefulness of the predicted score. Whenever predictions are made, one must interpret the predicted score in light of the magnitude of the prediction error. With a small error, prediction of $\dot{V}O_{2max}$ proves useful in appropriate situations where direct measurement is not feasible.

Heart Rate Predictions of $\dot{V}O_{2max}$

Common tests to predict $\dot{V}O_{2max}$ from exercise or postexercise heart rate use a standardized regimen of submaximal exercise on a bicycle ergometer, motorized treadmill, or step test. Such tests make use of the essentially linear (straight-line) relationship between heart rate and oxygen uptake for various intensities of light to moderately heavy exercise. The slope of this line (rate of HR increase per unit $\dot{V}O_2$ increase) reflects the individual's aerobic fitness. $\dot{V}O_{2max}$ can be estimated by drawing a best-fit straight line through several submaximum points that relate heart rate and oxygen uptake (or exercise intensity), and then extending this line to an assumed maximum heart rate for the person's age.

Figure 8.13 applies this **extrapolation procedure** for a trained and untrained subject. Four submaximal measures during bicycle exercise provided the data points to draw the heart rate-oxygen uptake (HR-$\dot{V}O_2$) line. Each person's HR-$\dot{V}O_2$ line tends to be linear but the slope of the individual lines can differ considerably, largely from variations in the amount of blood the heart pumps with each beat (stroke volume). A person with relatively high aerobic fitness accomplishes more intense exercise and achieves a higher oxygen uptake before reaching a specific exercise heart rate than a less "fit" person. Also, because heart rate increases linearly with exercise intensity, the person with the lowest heart rate increase tends to have the highest exercise capacity and largest $\dot{V}O_{2max}$. The data in Figure 8.13 predict $\dot{V}O_{2max}$ by extrapolating the HR-$\dot{V}O_2$ line to a heart rate of 195 b · min^{-1} (the assumed maximum heart rate for these college-age subjects).

The following four assumptions limit the accuracy of predicting $\dot{V}O_{2max}$ from submaximal exercise heart rate:

1. **Linearity of the HR-$\dot{V}O_2$ (exercise intensity) relationship**. Various intensities of light to moderately heavy exercise meet this as-

sumption. For some subjects, the HR-$\dot{V}O_2$ line curves or asymptotes at the heavier work loads in a direction that indicates a larger than expected increase in oxygen uptake per unit increase in heart rate. Oxygen uptake increases more than predicted through linear extrapolation of the HR-$\dot{V}O_2$ line, *underestimating* the $\dot{V}O_{2max}$.

2. **Similar maximum heart rates for all subjects**. The standard deviation for the average maximum heart rate for individuals of the same age (HR$_{max}$ = 220 minus Age, y) equals ±10 b · min^{-1}. The $\dot{V}O_{2max}$ of a 25-year-old person with a maximum heart rate of 185 b · min^{-1} would be *overestimated* if the HR-$\dot{V}O_2$ line extrapolated to an assumed maximum heart rate for this age group of 195 b·min^{-1}. The opposite would occur if this subject's maximum heart rate equaled 210 b · min^{-1}. HR$_{max}$ also de-

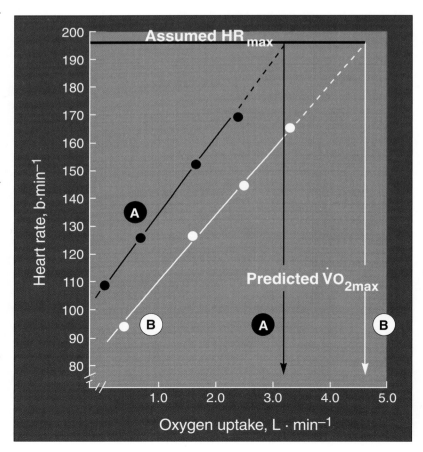

Figure 8.13
Prediction of $\dot{V}O_{2max}$ by extrapolating the linear relationship between submaximal heart rate and oxygen uptake during graded exercise in an untrained (A) and aerobically trained (B) subject.

creases with age. Without considering the age effect, older subjects would consistently be *overestimated* by assuming a maximum heart rate of 195 b · min^{-1}, which represents the appropriate estimation for 25-year-olds. Chapter 20 more fully addresses the effect of age on maximum heart rate.

3. **Assumed constant exercise economy**. The predicted $\dot{V}O_{2max}$ can vary because of variability in exercise economy when estimating submaximal oxygen uptake from exercise level. A subject with low economy (submaximal $\dot{V}O_2$ higher than assumed) is *underestimated* for $\dot{V}O_{2max}$ because heart rate increases from added oxygen cost of uneconomical exercise. The opposite occurs for a person with high exercise economy. The variation among individuals in oxygen uptake during walking, stepping, or cycling does not usually exceed ±6%. However, seemingly small modifications in test procedures profoundly affect the metabolic cost of exercise. Allowing individuals to support themselves with treadmill handrails can reduce exercise oxygen cost by 30%, and failure to maintain cadence on a bicycle ergometer or step test can dramatically alter the oxygen requirement.

4. **Day-to-day variation in exercise heart rate**. Even under highly standardized conditions, an individual's submaximal heart rate varies by about ±5 beats per minute with day-to-day testing at the same exercise intensity. This variation in exercise heart rate provides an additional source of error.

Considering these four limitations, $\dot{V}O_{2max}$ predicted from submaximal heart rate generally falls within 10 to 20% of the person's $\dot{V}O_{2max}$. Clearly, this represents too large an error for research purposes. These tests are better suited for screening and classification of aerobic fitness.

How to Predict V̇O₂max from Nonexercise Data

A V̇O$_{2max}$ prediction method uses nonexercise data from a questionnaire. This nonexercise prediction provides a useful first estimate for quick screening and possible classification of large groups of individuals.

Data to Predict V̇O$_{2max}$

1. **Sex**, (Female = 0; Male = 1)
2. **Body Mass Index (BMI), kg·m^{-2}.** Self-reported body mass (kg) and body stature (m) used to compute BMI as follows:
   BMI = Body mass, kg ÷ Stature, m^2.

3. **Physical Activity Rating (PA-R).** A point value between 0 to 10 representing overall physical activity level for previous 6 months (Table 1).
4. **Perceived Functional Ability (PFA).** Sum of the point values between 0 to 13 for questions about current level of perceived functional ability to maintain a continuous pace on an indoor track for 1 mile, and perceived pace to cover a distance of 3 miles without becoming breathless or overly fatigued (Table 2).

TABLE 1. PHYSICAL ACTIVITY RATING (PA-R)
Select the number that best describes your overall level of physical activity for the previous 6 months:

Points	Description
0	**inactive**: avoid walking or exertion; e.g., always use elevator, drive when possible instead of walking
1	**light activity**: walk for pleasure, routinely use stairs, occasionally exercise sufficiently to cause heavy breathing or perspiration
2	**moderate activity**: 10 to 60 minutes per week of moderate activity such as golf, horseback riding, calisthenics, table tennis, bowling, weight lifting, yard work, cleaning house, walking for exercise
3	**moderate activity**: over 1 hour per week of moderate activity described above
4	**vigorous activity**: run less than 1 mile per week or spend less than 30 min per week in comparable activity such as running or jogging, lap swimming, cycling, rowing, aerobics, skipping rope, running in place, or engaging in vigorous aerobic-type activity such as soccer, basketball, tennis, racquetball, or handball
5	**vigorous activity**: run 1 mile to less than 5 miles per week or spend 30 min to less than 60 min per week in comparable physical activity as described above
6	**vigorous activity**: run 5 miles to less than 10 miles per week or spend 1 hour to less than 3 hours per week in comparable physical activity as described above
7	**vigorous activity**: run 10 miles to less than 15 miles per week or spend 3 hours to less than 6 hours per week in comparable physical activity as described above
8	**vigorous activity**: run 15 miles to less than 20 miles per week or spend 6 hours to less than 7 hours per week in comparable physical activity as described above
9	**vigorous activity**: run 20 to 25 miles per week or spend 7 to 8 hours per week in comparable physical activity as described above
10	**vigorous activity**: run over 25 miles per week or spend over 8 hours per week in comparable physical activity as described above

TABLE 2. PERCEIVED FUNCTIONAL ABILITY (PFA) QUESTIONS

Suppose you exercise continuously on an indoor track for 1 mile. Which exercise pace is right for you – not too easy or not too hard? Circle the appropriate number from 1 to 13.

Points	Description
1	Walking at a slow pace (18-min mile or more)
2	
3	Walking at a medium pace (16-min mile)
4	
5	Walking at a fast pace (14-min mile)
6	
7	Jogging at a slow pace (12-min mile)
8	
9	Jogging at a medium pace (10-min mile)
10	
11	Jogging at a fast pace (8-min mile)
12	
13	Running at a fast pace (7-min mile or less)

How fast could you cover a distance of 3 miles and NOT become breathless or overly fatigued? Be realistic. Circle the appropriate number from 1 to 13.

Points	Description
1	I could walk the entire distance at a slow pace (18-min per mile or more)
2	
3	I could walk the entire distance at a medium pace (16-min per mile)
4	
5	I could walk the entire distance at a fast pace (14-min per mile)
6	
7	I could jog the entire distance at a slow pace (12-min per mile)
8	
9	I could jog the entire distance at a medium pace (10-min per mile)
10	
11	I could jog the entire distance at a fast pace (8-min per mile)
12	
13	I could run the entire distance at a fast pace (7-min per mile or less)

*The standard error of estimate (SEE) for predicting $\dot{V}O_{2max}$ = ± 3.44 mL $O_2 \cdot kg^{-1} \cdot min^{-1}$.
From George, J.D., et al.: Nonexercise $\dot{V}O_{2max}$ estimation for physically active college students. *Med. Sci. Sports Exerc.*, 29:415, 1997.

Equation

The following equation predicts $\dot{V}O_{2max}$ in $mL \cdot kg^{-1} \cdot min^{-1}$:*

$$\dot{V}O_{2max} = 44.895 + (7.042 \times sex) - (0.823 \times BMI) + (0.738 \times PFA) + (0.688 \times PA\text{-}R)$$

Example

Data:

1. Sex = female
2. BMI = 22.66 (self-reported body mass = 136 lb (61.7 kg); self-reported stature = 5 feet 5 inches (65 inches (1.65 m);
   BMI = 61.7 ÷ (1.65 × 1.65) = 22.66
3. PA-R score = 5 (see Table 1)
4. PFA score = 15 (sum of score 7 on first set of questions and score 8 on second set of questions; see Table 2)

Solution:

$$\dot{V}O_{2max} = 44.895 + (7.042 \times 0) - (0.823 \times 22.66) + (0.738 \times 15) + (0.688 \times 5)$$
$$= 44.895 + 0 - 18.65 + 11.07 + 3.77$$
$$= 41.1 \ mL \cdot kg^{-1} \cdot min^{-1}$$

summary

1. The concepts of individual differences and exercise specificity help to explain differences in capacity for anaerobic and aerobic power.

2. Individual differences refers to real differences among individuals, in contrast to variation in a physiologic response that characterizes the individual.

3. Specificity refers to a well-defined set of metabolic and physiologic responses that depend on a host of factors, including previous exercise training and method of evaluation.

4. The contribution of anaerobic and aerobic energy transfer depends largely on exercise intensity and duration. For sprint and strength-power activities, primary energy transfer involves the immediate and short-term anaerobic energy systems. The long-term aerobic energy system becomes progressively more important in activities that last longer than 2 minutes.

5. Appropriate physiologic measurements and performance tests provide estimates of each energy system's capacity. Such testing evaluates a capacity at a particular time or reveals changes consequent to specific training programs.

6. The stair-sprinting test measures power output generated by the stored intramuscular high-energy phosphates. The 30-second, all-out Wingate Test evaluates peak power and average power capacity from the glycolytic pathway. Interpretation of test results must consider the exercise specificity principle.

7. Training status, motivation, and acid–base regulation contribute to differences among individuals in the capacities of the immediate and short–term energy systems.

8. Maximal oxygen uptake ($\dot{V}O_{2max}$) provides reliable and important information on the power of the long-term aerobic energy system, including the functional capacity of various physiologic support systems.

9. Heredity, state and type of training, age, gender, and body composition all contribute uniquely to an individual's $\dot{V}O_{2max}$.

10. Tests to predict $\dot{V}O_{2max}$ from submaximal physiologic and performance data can be useful for classification purposes. The validity of prediction equations relies on the following assumptions: linearity of the HR-$\dot{V}O_2$ line, similar maximal heart rate for individuals of the same age, a constant exercise economy, and a relatively small day-to-day variation in exercise heart rate.

11. Heart rate following step-test exercise reflects the efficiency of the cardiovascular response to aerobic exercise and training. Recovery heart rate from stair-stepping can also predict $\dot{V}O_{2max}$.

12. Field methods to predict $\dot{V}O_{2max}$ provide useful information for screening purposes in the absence of the direct measurement of aerobic capacity.

13. $\dot{V}O_{2max}$ can be predicted from nonexercise data with accuracy acceptable for screening and classification purposes.

thought questions

1. How would you set-up an evaluation procedure to document aerobic fitness changes during a 6 week summer camp exercise program? How would you assess changes in fitness, and what factors must be considered?

2. Significant specificity in physiologic function and exercise performance exists. How can one reconcile the observation that certain individuals perform exceptionally well in many diverse physical activities, i.e., they appear to be "natural" athletes?

3. Why is it important for a triathlete to train in each of the sport's three events?

4. In devising training studies for aerobic fitness, why must the researcher demonstrate objectively that the true $\dot{V}O_{2max}$ was obtained in pre- and post-test measures? Describe the criteria usually applied in assessing if the subject gave appropriate effort in a graded exercise test.

5. Two individuals participate in the same aerobic training program. After 12 weeks, the $\dot{V}O_{2max}$ of one person improves 25%, while the other person only improves 7%. What factors could account for this difference in "trainability"?

selected references

Armstrong, N., and Welsman, J.R.: Assessment and interpretation of aerobic fitness in children and adolescents. *Exerc. Sport Sci. Rev.*, 22:435, 1994.

Bar-Or, O.: The Wingate anaerobic test: An update on methodology, reliability, and validity. *Sports Med.*, 4: 381, 1987.

Bouchard, C., and Perusse, L.: Heredity, activity level, fitness, and health. In: *Physical Activity, Fitness, and Health*. Bouchard, C. et al. (eds.). Champaign, IL: Human Kinetics, 1994.

Bouchard, C., et al.: Familial resemblance for $\dot{V}O_{2max}$ in the sedentary state: the HERITAGE family study. *Med. Sci. Sports Exerc.*, 30:252, 1998.

Buskirk, E.R., and Hodgson, J.L.: Age and aerobic power: the rate of change in men and women. *Fed. Proc.*, 46:1824, 1997.

Cain, S. M.: Mechanisms which control $\dot{V}O_2$ near $\dot{V}O_{2max}$: an overview. *Med. Sci. Sports Exerc.*, 27: 60, 1995.

Cooper, K.: Correlation between field and treadmill testing as a means for assessing maximal oxygen intake. *JAMA*, 203: 201, 1968.

Cureton, K.J., et al.: Metabolic determinants of the age-related improvement in one-mile run/walk performance in youth. *Med. Sci. Sports Exerc.*, 29:259, 1997.

Duncan, G.E., et al.: Applicability of $\dot{V}O_{2max}$ criteria: discontinuous versus continuous protocols. *Med. Sci. Sports Exerc.*, 29:273, 1997.

Franklin, B. A.: Exercise testing, training and arm ergometry, *Sports Med.*, 2: 109, 1985.

Gergley, T., et al.: Specificity of arm training on aerobic power during swimming and running. *Med. Sci. Sports Exerc.*, 16: 349, 1984.

Hagberg, J.M., et al.: $\dot{V}O_{2max}$ is associated with ACE genotype in postmenopausal women. *J. Appl. Physiol.*, 85:1842, 1998.

Howley, E.T., et al.: Criteria for maximal oxygen uptake: review and commentary. *Med. Sci. Sports Exerc.*, 27:1292, 1995.

Inbar, O., and Bar-Or, O.: Anaerobic characteristics in male children and adolescents. *Med. Sci. Sports Exerc.*, 18: 264, 1986.

Joyner, M. J.: Physiological limiting factors and distance running: influence of gender and age on record performances. In: *Exercise and Sport Sciences Reviews*. Vol. 21. Holloszy J.O., (ed.). Baltimore, MD: Williams & Wilkins, 1993.

Kasch, F. W., et al.: A longitudinal study of cardiovascular stability in active men aged 45 to 65 years. *Phys. Sportsmed.*, 16: 117, 1988.

Katch, V. L., et al.: Optimal test characteristics for maximal anaerobic work on the bicycle ergometer. *Res. Q.*, 48: 319, 1977.

Koziris, L.B., et al.: Relationship of aerobic power to anaerobic performance indices. *J. Strength and Cond. Res.*, 10:35, 1996.

Margaria, R., et al.: Measurement of muscular power (anaerobic) in man. *J. Appl. Physiol.*, 21: 1662, 1966.

McArdle, W. D., et al.: Specificity of run training on $\dot{V}O_{2max}$ and heart rate changes during running and swimming. *Med. Sci. Sports*, 10: 16, 1978.

Montgomery, H.E., et al.: Human gene for physical performance. *Nature*, 393:221, 1998.

Naughton, G.A., et al.: Accumulated oxygen deficit measurements during and after high-intensity exercise in trained male and female adolescents. *Eur. J. Appl. Physiol.*, 76:525, 1997.

Nindl, B.C., et al.: Lower and upper body anaerobic performance in male and female adolescent athletes. *Med. Sci. Sports Exerc.*, 27: 235, 1995.

Pelham, T. W., and Holt, L. E.: Testing for aerobic power in paddlers using sport-specific simulators. *J. Strength and Cond. Res.*, 9: 52, 1995.

Proctor, D.N., and Joyner, M.J.: Skeletal muscle mass and the reduction of $\dot{V}O_{2max}$ in trained older subjects. *J. Appl. Physiol.*, 82:1411, 1997.

Rivera, M.A., et al.: Linkage between a muscle-specific CK gene marker and $\dot{V}O_{2max}$ in the HERITAGE Family Study. *Med. Sci. Sports Exerc.*, 31:698, 1999.

Rowland, T. W.: Does peak $\dot{V}O_2$ reflect $\dot{V}O_{2max}$ in children? *Med. Sci. Sports Exerc.*, 25:689, 1993.

Rundell, K.W.: Treadmill roller ski test predicts biathlon roller ski race results of elite U.S. biathlon women. *Med. Sci. Sports Exerc.*, 27:1677, 1995.

Saavedra, C., et al.: Maximal anaerobic performance of the knee extensor muscles during growth. *Med. Sci. Sports Exerc.*, 23: 1083, 1991.

Sawka, M. N.: Physiology of upper body exercise, In: *Exercise and Sport Sciences Reviews*. Vol. 14. Pandolf K.B., (ed.). New York: Macmillan, 1986.

Sparling, P.B., et al.: The gender difference in distance running performance has plateaued: an analysis of world rankings from 1980 to 1996. *Med. Sci. Sports Exerc.*, 30:1725, 1998.

Thomas, M., et al.: Leg power in young women: relationship to body composition, strength, and function. *Med. Sci. Sports Exerc.*, 28:1321, 1996.

Vogel, J. A., et al.: Analysis of aerobic capacity in a large United States population. *J. Appl. Physiol.*, 60: 494, 1986.

Wallick, M.E., et al.: Physiological responses to in-line skating compared to treadmill running. *Med. Sci. Sports Exerc.*, 27: 242, 1995.

Wasserman, K., et al.: *Principles of Exercise Testing and Interpretation*. 3rd Ed., Baltimore: Lippincott Williams & Wilkins, 1999.

Weinstein, Y., et al.: Reliability of peak-lactate, heart rate, and plasma volume following the Wingate test. *Med. Sci. Sports Exerc.*, 30:1456, 1998.

Wells, C. L., and Plowman, S. A.: Sexual differences in athletic performance: biological or behavioral? *Phys. Sportsmed.*, 11: 52, 1983.

Weltman, A., et al.: The lactate threshold and endurance performance. *Adv. Sports Med. Fitness*, 2: 91, 1989.

Wilber, R.L., et al.: Physiological profiles of elite off-road and road cyclists. *Med. Sci. Sports Exerc.*, 29: 1090, 1997.

Zajac, A., et al.: The diagnostic value of the 10- and 30-second Wingate test for competitive athletes. *J. Strength and Cond. Res.*, 13:16, 1999.

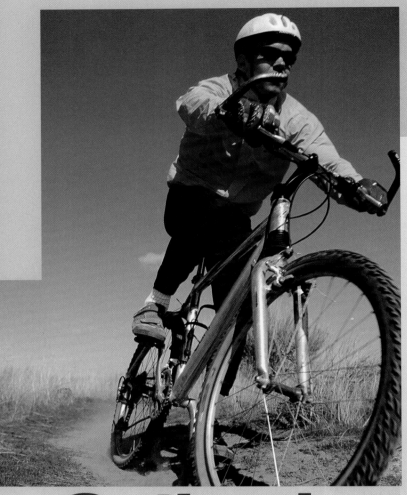

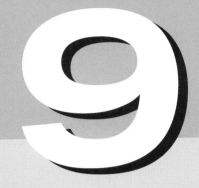

CHAPTER

9

Optimal Nutrition for Exercise and Sport

Topics covered in this chapter

Nutrient Requirements

Exercise and Food Intake

The Precompetition Meal

Carbohydrate Intake Before, During, and
  After Intense Exercise

Glucose Intake, Electrolytes, and
  Water Uptake

Recommended Oral Rehydration Beverage

Post-Exercise Carbohydrate Intake

Carbohydrate Needs in Intense Training

Diet, Glycogen Stores, and Endurance

Carbohydrate Loading

Summary

Thought Questions

Selected References

- Compare the nutrient and energy intakes of physically active men and women with sedentary counterparts.

- Outline the Food Guide Pyramid recommendations.

- Describe the timing and composition of the pre-event (pre-competition) meal, including reasons for limiting lipid and protein intake.

- Summarize the effects of low, normal, and high-carbohydrate intake on glycogen reserves and subsequent endurance performance.

- For endurance athletes, describe the: (a) potential negative effects of consuming a concentrated sugar drink 30 minutes before competition, and (b) ideal composition of a "sports drink."

- Discuss possible reasons why consuming high-glycemic carbohydrates during high-intensity aerobic exercise enhances endurance performance.

- Define "glucose polymer" and give the rationale for adding these compounds to a sports drink.

- Make a general recommendation concerning carbohydrate intake for athletes involved in heavy training.

- Describe the most effective way to replenish glycogen reserves after a hard bout of training or competition.

- Contrast classic carbohydrate loading with the modified loading procedure.

An optimal diet supplies required nutrients for tissue maintenance, repair, and growth without excessive energy intake. Only in the past decade have reasonable estimates of specific nutrient needs for individuals of different ages and body sizes been made, with considerations for individual differences in digestion, storage capacity, nutrient metabolism, and daily energy expenditure.

Establishing dietary recommendations for physically active men and women becomes complicated by the specific energy requirements of particular sports and their training demands, and individual dietary preferences. Sound nutritional guidelines form the framework for planning and evaluating food intake for individuals who exercise regularly. This chapter describes nutrient requirements of sedentary and active individuals, including optimal nutrition guidelines for physically demanding sports and heavy training.

Nutrient Requirements

Many coaches make dietary recommendations based on their "feelings" and past experiences rather than research evidence. The fact that athletes often have inadequate or incorrect information concerning dietary practices and the role of specific nutrients in exercise compounds this problem. Although research in sports and exercise nutrition continues to expand, conventional wisdom maintains that active people and athletes do *not* require additional nutrients beyond those obtained in a balanced diet. This takes on added importance because millions of adults exercise regularly to keep fit. *Active Americans, including those involved in exceptional endurance activities, consume typical diets remarkably similar in composition to those consumed by sedentary counterparts.*

Table 9.1 shows the similarity in dietary habits between athletes and nonathletes, except that athletes eat more of the same foods. This larger total quantity of food consumed (both macro- and micronutrients) supports the extra energy required by exercise. Endurance athletes and others who train heavily must maintain adequate energy and protein intakes, and necessary carbohydrate levels to match glycogen catabolism during training. Attention to proper diet does not mean an athlete must join the ranks of the more than 40% of Americans who take supplements (spending about $6 billion yearly) to micromanage their nutrient intake. *In essence, sound human nutrition represents sound nutrition for athletes.*

Recommended Nutrient Intake

Figure 9.1 shows the recommended intake for protein, lipid, and carbohydrate (expressed in g and % total kcal intake), including the general food source category for these

TABLE 9.1

Comparison of carbohydrate, lipid, protein, and energy intake of middle-aged male and female runners and sedentary controls[a]

	RUNNERS	SEDENTARY CONTROLS
Males		
Calories (kcal · d^{-1})	2959*	2361
Protein (g · d^{-1})	102.1	93.6
Protein (%)	13.8*	15.8
Lipid (g · d^{-1})	134.4*	109.0
Lipid (%)	40.8	41.5
Carbohydrate (g · d^{-1})	294.6*	225.7
Carbohydrate (%)	39.8	38.6
Cholesterol (mg · 1000 kcal^{-1})	175.0	190.0
Saturated fat (g · 1000 kcal^{-1})	16.2	16.0
Polyunsaturated fat (g · 1000 kcal^{-1})	9.0	9.3
Females		
Calories (kcal · d^{-1})	2386*	1871
Protein (g · d^{-1})	82.2	76.7
Protein (%)	14.2*	17.4
Lipid (g · d^{-1})	110.7	83.0
Lipid (%)	41.1	40.3
Carbohydrate (g · d^{-1})	234.3*	174.7
Carbohydrate (%)	39.5	39.1
Cholesterol (mg · 1000 kcal^{-1})	190.0	205.0
Saturated fat (g · 1000 kcal^{-1})	16.8	16.5
Polyunsaturated fat (g · 1000 kcal^{-1})	8.5	7.9

[a] % calories do not total 100% because alcohol calories constitute the difference.

* Values significantly different from controls.

From: Blair, S.N., et al.: Comparisons of nutrient intake in middle-aged men and women runners and controls. *Med. Sci. Sports. Exerc.*, 13:310, 1981.

Food Guide Pyramid

To more clearly reflect the current state of nutritional knowledge related to health, the U.S. Department of Agriculture (USDA) developed the **Food Guide Pyramid** as a model for good nutrition for Americans ages 2 years and older (Fig. 9.2). This approach categorizes foods that make similar nutrient contributions; it also recommends the number of servings from each food category. The guidelines emphasize diverse grains, vegetables, and fruits as major calorie sources, downplaying food sources high in animal proteins, lipids, and dairy products. Serving size and number of servings must consider needs for growth, level of physical activity, and desirable body weight maintenance.

Recommendations of the Food Guide Pyramid also apply to persons who consume a mostly vegetarian diet. Because meat, fish, and poultry represent good sources of B-vitamins and iron and zinc, vegetarians need to emphasize these nutrients in their non-meat dietary sources. Although these guidelines for healthful eating focus on the general population, they also provide a sound framework for meal planning for physically active individuals.

Diet Quality Index

The Diet Quality Index, developed by the National Research Council Committee on Diet and Health, appraises the general "healthfulness" of one's diet. The index, presented in Table 9.2, offers a simple scoring scheme based on a risk gradient associated with diet and major diet-related chronic diseases. Respondents who meet a given dietary goal receive a score of 0; a score of 1 applies to an intake within 30% of a dietary goal; the score becomes 2 when intake fails to fall within 30% of the goal.

macronutrients. The guidelines provide the necessary vitamin, mineral, and protein **recommended dietary allowances** (**RDAs**) even though total energy content amounts to only about 1200 kcal. Contrast this amount with the average energy intake for young adult Americans of 2000 kcal for women and 3000 kcal for men. By achieving the basic nutrient requirements (recommended in Fig. 9.1), a variety of food sources based on individual preference supply additional energy needs.

A prudent diet for a physically active person should provide about 60% of calories from carbohydrates, predominantly as unrefined starches (complex carbohydrates). Because glycogen synthesis in liver and muscle depends on dietary carbohydrate, some exercise physiology researchers recommend increasing daily carbohydrate intake to 70% of total calories (400 to 600 g depending on body mass) to prevent gradual depletion of glycogen stores with successive days of intense training.

Keep Them Unrefined, Complex, and Low Glycemic

Little health risk exists in subsisting chiefly on a variety of fiber-rich complex carbohydrates, as long as intake also supplies essential amino acids, fatty acids, minerals, and vitamins. The most desirable complex carbohydrates exhibit slow digestion and absorption rates. Such moderate- to low-glycemic types include whole-grain breads, cereals, pastas, legumes, most fruits, and milk and milk products.

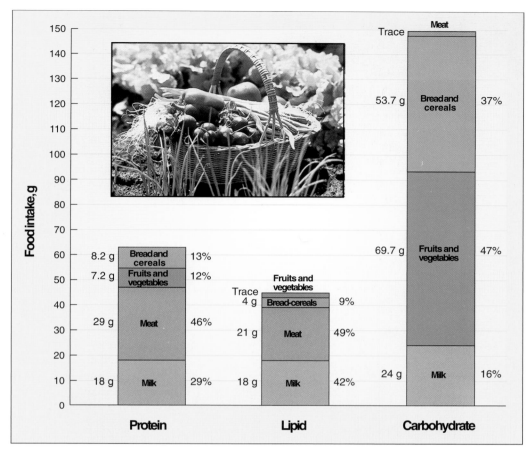

Figure 9.1
Basic recommendations for carbohydrate, lipid, and protein components, and the general categories of food sources in a balanced diet.

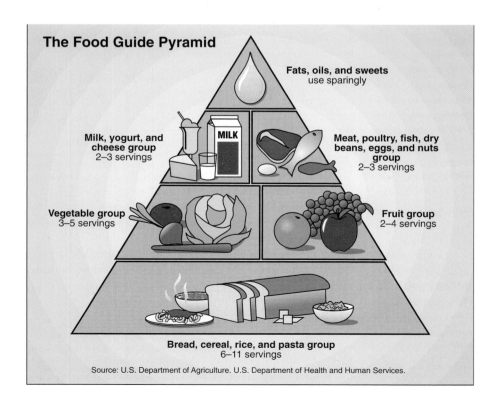

The final score equals the total for all eight categories. The index ranges from 0 to 16, with a lower score representing a higher quality diet. A score of 4 or less reflects a more healthful diet; an index of 10 or higher indicates a less healthful diet needing improvement.

Exercise and Food Intake

Figure 9.3 illustrates the average energy intakes for males and females in the U.S. population grouped by age category from 1988 to 1991. Mean energy intakes peaked between ages 16 to 29 years and declined thereafter. A similar pattern occurred for males and females, although males reported higher daily energy intakes than females at all ages. Between ages 20 to 29 years, women consumed 35% fewer kcal than men on a daily basis (3025 kcal vs. 1957 kcal). With aging, the gender difference in energy intake decreased; at age 70 years, women consumed 25% fewer kcal than men.

Physical Activity Makes a Difference

For individuals who regularly engage in moderate to intense physical activities, food intake balances easily with daily energy expenditure. Lumber workers, for example, who typically expend nearly 4500 kcal daily, unconsciously adjust energy intake to balance energy output. For them, body

Figure 9.2
The Food Guide Pyramid emphasizes grains, vegetables, and fruits as important nutrient sources.

TABLE 9.2
The Diet Quality Index

RECOMMENDATION	SCORE	INTAKE
Reduce total lipid intake to 30% or less of total energy	☐ 0 ☐ 1 ☐ 2	<30% 30–40% >40%
Reduce saturated fatty acid intake to less than 10% of total energy	☐ 0 ☐ 1 ☐ 2	<10% 10–13% >13%
Reduce cholesterol intake to less than 300 mg daily	☐ 0 ☐ 1 ☐ 2	<300 mg 300–400 mg >400 mg
Eat 5 or more servings daily of vegetables and fruits	☐ 0 ☐ 1 ☐ 2	≥5 servings 3–4 servings 0–2 servings
Increase intake of starches and other complex carbohydrates by eating 6 or more servings daily of breads, cereals, and legumes	☐ 0 ☐ 1 ☐ 2	≥6 servings 4–5 servings 0–3 servings
Maintain protein intake at moderate levels	☐ 0 ☐ 1 ☐ 2	100% RDA 100–150% RDA >150% RDA
Limit total daily sodium intake to 2400 mg or less	☐ 0 ☐ 1 ☐ 2	≤2400 mg 2400–3400 mg >3400 mg
Maintain adequate calcium intake (approximately the RDA)	☐ 0 ☐ 1 ☐ 2	≥100% RDA 67–99% RDA <67% RDA

weight remains stable despite an extremely large food intake. The balancing of food intake to meet a new level of energy output takes 1 to 2 days to attain a new energy equilibrium. The fine balance between energy expenditure and food intake does not occur in sedentary people, where caloric intake chronically exceeds daily energy expenditure. Lack of precision in regulating food intake at the low end of the physical activity spectrum contributes to "creeping obesity" in highly mechanized and technologically advanced societies.

The daily food intake of athletes in the 1936 Olympics reportedly averaged more than 7000 kcal, or roughly three times the average daily intake. These often quoted energy values justify what many believe represents the enormous food requirement of athletes in training. However, the figures represent only estimates because the original report did not present objective dietary data and probably reflect inflated estimates of energy expended (and required) by athletes. For example, distance runners who train upwards of 100 miles per week (6-min mile pace at 17 kcal · min^{-1})

probably do not expend more than 1000 to 1500 "extra" calories each day above normal energy requirements. For these endurance athletes, about 4000 kcal from daily food intake should balance increased energy expenditure.

Figure 9.4 presents data on energy intake from a large sample of elite male and female endurance, strength, and team sport athletes in the Netherlands. For males, daily energy intake ranged between 2900 and 5900 kcal, whereas female competitors consumed 1600 to 3200 kcal. Except for the high energy intake of athletes at extremes of performance and training, daily energy intake did not exceed 4000 kcal for men and 3000 kcal for women.

Extreme Energy Intake and Expenditure: The Tour de France

During competition or periods of high-intensity training, some sport activities require extreme energy output (sometimes in excess of 1000 kcal · hr^{-1} in elite marathoners and professional cyclists) and a correspondingly high energy intake. For example, the daily energy requirements of elite cross-country skiers during 1 week of training averaged 3740 to 4860 kcal for women and 6120 to 8570 kcal for men. Figure 9.5 outlines the variation in daily energy expenditure for a male competitor during the Tour de France professional cycling race. Energy expenditure averaged 6500 kcal daily for nearly 3 weeks during this event. Large daily variation occurred depending on the activity level for a particular day; the daily energy expenditure decreased to 3000 kcal on a "rest" day and increased to approximately 9000 kcal when cycling over a mountain pass. By combining liquid nutrition with normal meals, this cyclist nearly matched daily energy expenditure with energy intake.

Ultraendurance Running Competition

Energy balance (energy intake versus energy expenditure) was studied during a 1000-km (approximately 600 miles) race from Sidney to Melbourne, Australia. The Greek ultramarathon champion Kouros completed the race in 5 days, 5 hours, and 7 minutes, finishing 24 hours and 40 minutes ahead of the next competitor. Table 9.3 provides relevant features of race conditions, distance covered, average daily speed, rest and sleep patterns, and nutrient balance. Kouros did not sleep during the first 2 days of competition. He covered 463 km (288 miles) at an average speed of 11.4 km · hr^{-1} (8 min, 27 s per mile) during day 1 and 8.3 km · hr^{-1} (11 min, 37 s per mile) on day 2. During the remaining days,

Dietary Guidelines for American Adults

The USDA and the U.S. Department of Health and Human Services developed the **Dietary Guidelines for Americans** to provide practical advice for health promotion and disease prevention. They generally aim to answer the question: "What should an individual eat to stay healthy?"

- Eat a variety of foods
- Balance food intake with physical activity—maintain or improve body weight
- Choose a diet with plenty of unrefined grain products, vegetables, and fruits
- Choose a diet low in total fat, saturated fatty acids, and cholesterol
- Choose a diet moderate in sugars
- Choose a diet moderate in salt and sodium
- If you drink alcoholic beverages, do so in moderation

Some Athletes Require Supplementation

Gymnasts, ballet dancers, ice dancers, and weight-class athletes in boxing, wrestling, and judo train arduously. The nature of these sports also places an unusually high demand to maintain a lean, relatively light body mass. Energy intake often intentionally falls short of energy expenditure, and a relative state of malnutrition develops. For these athletes, nutritional supplementation proves beneficial, as suggested from the daily nutrient intake (% of RDA) data in Figure 9.6 for 97 competitive female gymnasts ages 11 to 14 years. Twenty-three percent of the girls consumed less than 1500 kcal daily, and more than 40% consumed less than two-thirds the RDA for vitamin E, folic acid, and the minerals iron, magnesium, calcium, and zinc. Clearly, the gymnasts needed either to upgrade the nutritional quality of their food intake or consider supplementation. For many athletes like these, carbohydrate intake also fails to match the glycogen requirements of intensive training. Consequently, the athlete ends up training and competing in a carbohydrate-depleted state. Some protein supplementation, to achieve a daily intake of 1.2 to 1.8 g per kg of body mass, may also be warranted to maintain normal nitrogen balance and reduce the potential for impaired training status.

he took frequent rest periods, including periodic breaks for short "naps." Weather ranged from spring to winter conditions (30°C to 8°C), and terrain varied.

The near equivalence of Kouros' estimated total energy intake (55,970 kcal) and energy expenditure (59,079 kcal) in response to physical activity represents a remarkable aspect of energy balance. Of the total energy intake, carbohydrates represented 95.3%, lipids 3%, with the remaining 1.7% as proteins. Protein intake from food averaged considerably below the RDA level (although protein in pill form provided a supplement). The unusually large daily energy intake, which ranged between 8600 and 13,770 kcal, came from Greek sweets (baklava, cookies, donuts), some chocolate, dried fruit and nuts, various fruit juices, and fresh fruits. Every 30 minutes after the first 6 hours of running, Kouros replaced sweets and fruit with a small biscuit soaked in honey or jam. He consumed a small amount of roasted chicken on day 4 and drank coffee every morning. He took a 500-mg vitamin C supplement every 12 hours and a protein pill twice daily.

Not only did Kouros perform at a pace that required a continuous energy supply averaging 49% of aerobic capacity during the first 2 days of competition (and 38% for days 3 through 5), but he finished the competition without compromising overall health (no muscle injuries or thermoregulatory problems, and body mass remained unchanged). Reported difficulties included a severe bout of constipation during the run and frequent urination that persisted for several days after the race.

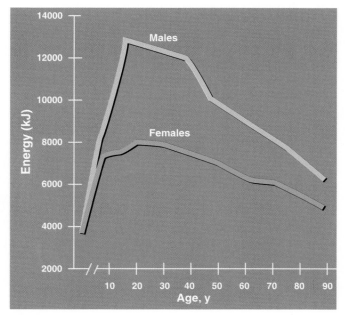

Figure 9.3

Average daily energy intake for males and females by age in the U.S. population during the years 1988 to 1991. Multiply by 0.239 to convert kJ to kcal. (From Briefel, R.R., et al.: Total energy intake of the US population: The third National Health and Nutrition Examination Survey, 1988-1991. *Am. J. Clin. Nutr.*, 62(suppl):1072S, 1995.)

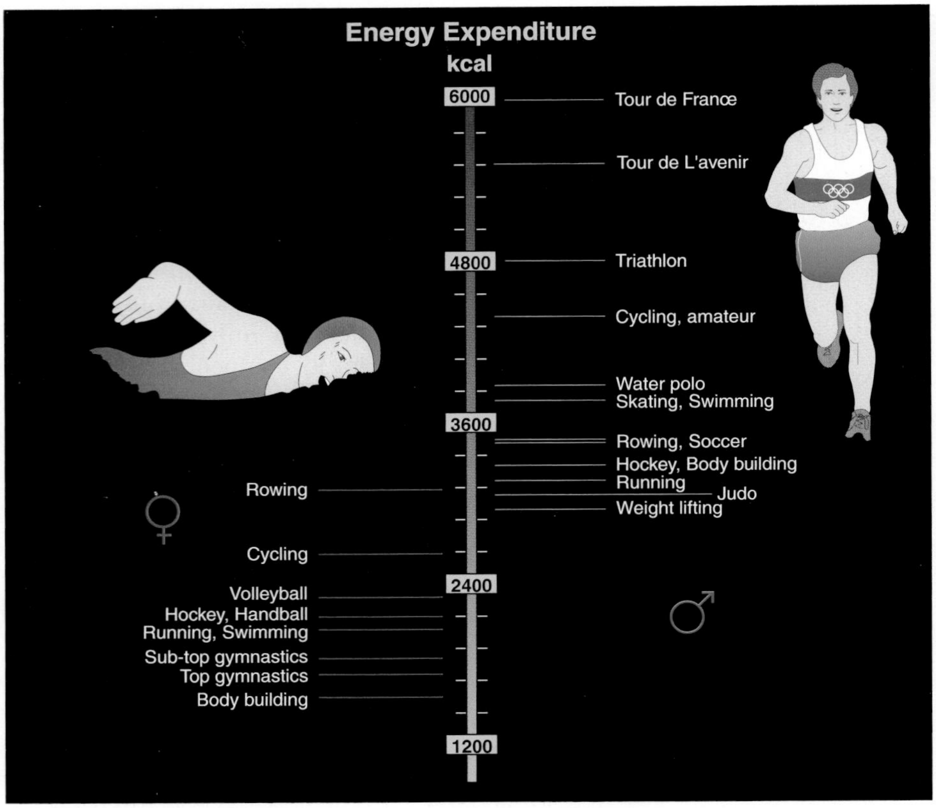

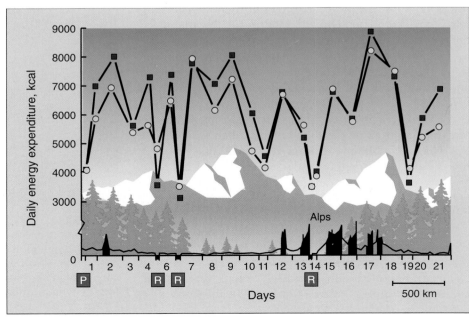

Energy Expenditure
kcal

6000 — Tour de France

— Tour de L'avenir

4800 — Triathlon

— Cycling, amateur

— Water polo
— Skating, Swimming

3600 — Rowing, Soccer
— Hockey, Body building
— Running
— Judo
— Weight lifting

Rowing —

♀

Cycling —

Volleyball — 2400
Hockey, Handball —
Running, Swimming —
Sub-top gymnastics —
Top gymnastics —
Body building —

♂

1200

Figure 9.4
Daily energy expenditure in kcal per day in elite male and female endurance, strength, and team sport athletes. (From van Erp-Baart, A. M. J., et al.: Nationwide survey on nutritional habits in elite athletes. *Int. J. Sports Med.,* 10:53, 1989.)

diture. Such data confirm other studies of physically active people, and also support the argument that regular exercise provides an effective strategy to actually "eat more yet weigh less" while maintaining a lower percentage of body fat. *Active people maintain a lighter and leaner body and a more healthful heart disease risk profile, despite an increased intake of the typical, high-fat American diet.*

Table 9.4 presents a general model for food intake for active athletes, including an example of a 2500 kcal menu containing 350 g of carbohydrates. Note the high reliance on fruits, vegetables, and grains, and the diminished emphasis on lipid. An active athlete requires about 50 kcal of food per kg of body mass (23 kcal per lb) each day to provide sufficient energy for exercise training and competition. An ideal training diet includes 60 to 70% carbohydrate, 15 to 20% protein, and less than 25% lipid. We do not encourage consuming a high-protein diet in the range of 30–35% of total calorie intake for training or the precompetition meal.

Eat More, Weigh Less

As Table 9.1 showed, the energy intake of 61 middle-age men and women who ran an average of 60 km per week averaged 40 to 60% more calories per kg of body mass than sedentary controls. The extra energy required to run between 8 and 10 km daily accounted for the runners' larger energy intake. Paradoxically, the most active men and women who ate considerably more on a daily basis weighed less than those who exercised at a lower total caloric expenditure.

Figure 9.5
Daily energy expenditure (purple squares) and energy intake (yellow circles) for a cyclist during the Tour de France competition. Note the extremely high energy expenditure values and the ability to achieve energy balance with liquid nutrition plus normal meals. P, stage; R, rest day. (Modified from Saris, W.H.M., et al.: Adequacy of vitamin supply under maximal sustained workloads: the Tour de France. In: *Elevated Dosages of Vitamins.* Walter, P. et. al., (eds.). Toronto: Huber Publishers, 1989.)

TABLE 9.3

Features of race conditions, distance covered, average daily speed, rest and sleep patterns, and nutrient balance during an elite ultraendurance performance (top).* Daily and total energy balance, nutrient distributions in food, and water intake during the race (bottom).

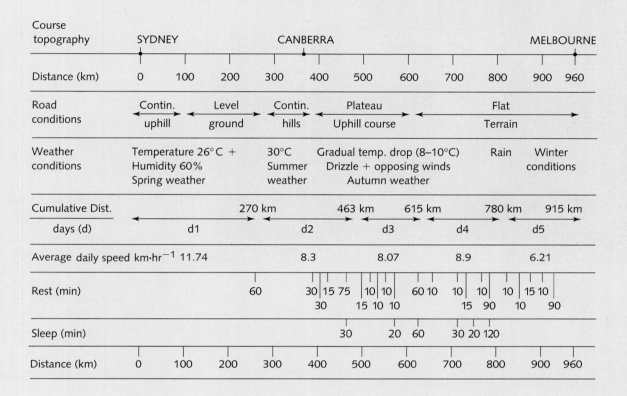

Day of the race	Distance covered	Estimated energy expenditure	Estimated energy intake	Carbohydrates			Lipids			Proteins			H_2O
	km	kcal	kcal	g	%	kcal	g	%	kcal	g	%	kcal	L
1	270	15,367	13,770	3375	98.0	15,302	20	1.3	180	22	0.7	88	22.0
2	193	10,741	8600	1981	92.2	7923	53	5.5	477	50	2.3	200	19.2
3	152	8919	12,700	3074	96.8	12,297	27	1.9	243	40	1.3	160	22.7
4	165	9780	7800	1758	90.1	7032	56	6.5	504	66	3.4	264	14.3
5	135	7736	12,500	3014	96.4	12,058	30	2.2	270	43	1.4	172	18.3
5 h	45	2536	550	138	100.0	550	—	—	—	—	—	—	3.2
Total	960	55,079	55,970	13,340		53,362	186		1674	221		734	99.7

*The runner Kouras: Body mass = 65 kg; Stature = 171 cm; % body fat = 8%; $\dot{V}O_{2max}$ = 62.5 mL · kg · min^{-1}.

Modified from Rontoyannis, G.P., et al.: Energy balance in ultramarathon running. *Am. J. Clin. Nutr.*, 49:976, 1989.

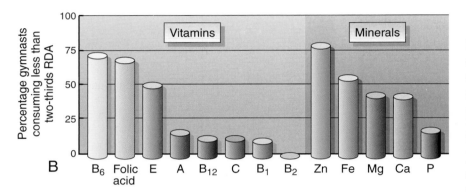

Figure 9.6
Average daily nutrient intake for 97 adolescent female gymnasts (11 to 14 y of age) in relation to recommended values. **A,** The RDA on the y-axis reflects only protein, while energy, carbohydrate (CHO), and lipid reflect "recommended" values. **B,** Percentage of gymnasts consuming less than two-thirds of the RDA. Mean age = 13.1 y, mean stature = 152.4 cm (60 in), and mean body mass = 43.1 kg (94.8 lb). (Modified from Loosli, A.R., and Benson, J.: Nutritional intake in adolescent athletes. *Sports Med.*, 37: 1143, 1990.)

The Precompetition Meal

Athletes often compete in the morning following an overnight fast. Significant depletion occurs in the body's carbohydrate reserves over a 8- to 12-hour period without eating (refer to Chapter 2), so precompetition nutrition takes on considerable importance even if the person follows appropriate dietary recommendations. *The precompetition meal provides the athlete with adequate carbohydrate energy and ensures optimal hydration.* Fasting before competition or training makes no sense physiologically because it rapidly depletes liver and muscle glycogen and ultimately impairs exercise performance. Consider the following factors when individualizing an athlete's meal plans:

- Food preference
- "Psychologic set" of competition
- Digestibility of foods

As a general rule, foods high in lipid and protein should not be consumed on competition days. These foods digest slowly and remain in the digestive tract longer than carbohydrate foods containing a similar energy content. The timing of the precompetition meal also deserves consideration. Increased emotional stress and tension depress intestinal absorption because of a significant decrease in

blood flow to the digestive tract. *Generally, 3 hours provides sufficient time to digest and absorb a carbohydrate-rich, precompetition meal.*

High Protein: Not the Best Choice

Many athletes become accustomed to and even depend on the classic "steak and eggs" precompetition meal. Although this meal may satisfy the athlete, coach, and restaurateur, its benefits to exercise performance have yet to be demonstrated. In fact, this type of low-carbohydrate meal can actually hinder optimal performance.

The high-protein precompetition meal should be modified or even abolished in favor of one high in carbohydrates for the following reasons:

- Dietary carbohydrates (not protein) replenish liver and muscle glycogen previously depleted from an overnight fast.
- Carbohydrates digest and become absorbed more rapidly than proteins or lipids. Thus, carbohydrates provide energy fuel faster and reduce the feeling of fullness following a meal.
- High-protein meals elevate resting metabolism more than high-carbohydrate meals owing to greater energy requirements for protein's digestion, absorption, and assimilation. Additional metabolic heat places demands on the body's heat-dissipating mechanisms, which impairs exercise performance in hot weather.
- Protein catabolism for energy facilitates dehydration during exercise because the byproducts of amino acid breakdown require water for urinary excretion. Approximately 50 mL of water "accompanies" the excretion of each gram of urea in urine.
- Carbohydrate provides the main energy nutrient for short-duration anaerobic exercise and prolonged, high-intensity endurance activities.

TABLE 9.4
A general model for food and energy intake for active individuals of different body weights, including a sample 2500 kcal menu containing 350 g of carbohydrate

BODY WEIGHT	110 lb (50 kg)	132 lb (60 kg)	154 lb (70 kg)	176 lb (80 kg)
Total Kcal	2500	3000	3500	4000
	Recommended Number of Daily Servings			
Milk group (90 kcal) Skim milk, 1 cup Plain, low-fat yogurt, 1 cup	4[a]	4	4	4
Meat group (55–75 kcal) Cooked, lean meat (fish, poultry), 1 oz Egg, 1 Peanut butter, 1 tbsp Low-fat cheese, 1 oz Cottage cheese, 1/4 cup	5	5	6	6
Fruits	7	9	10	12
Vegetables	3	5	6	7
Grains	16	18	20	24
Lipid	5	6	8	10

SAMPLE HIGH-CARBOHYDRATE 2500-kcal MENU (350 g)

Breakfast	Lunch	Dinner	Snack #1	Snack #2
1 cup bran cereal	3 oz lean roast beef	Chicken stir-fry:	3 cups popcorn	8 oz apple cider
8 oz low-fat milk	1 hard roll	3 oz chicken		
1 english muffin	2 tsp mayonnaise,	1 cup diced vegetables		
1 tsp margarine	mustard, lettuce	2 tsp oil		
4 oz orange juice	and tomato	2 cups rice		
	1/2 cup cole slaw	1 cup orange and		
	2 fresh plums	grapefruit sections		
	2 oatmeal cookies	1 cup vanilla yogurt		
	8 oz seltzer water	Iced tea with lemon		
	with lemon			

Modified from Carbohydrates and Athletic Performance. *Sports Science Exchange*. Vol. 7. Gatorade Sports Science Institute, Chicago, 1988.

[a]Bolded numbers below total kcal values recommended number of daily servings.

Ideal Precompetition Meal

The ideal precompetition meal maximizes muscle and liver glycogen storage, and provides glucose for intestinal absorption during exercise. The meal should: 1) contain 150 to 300 g of carbohydrate (3 to 5 g per kg of body mass) in either solid or liquid form, and 2) be consumed within 3 to 4 hours before exercising.

The benefit of a precompetition meal depends on the athlete maintaining a nutritionally sound diet throughout training. Pre-exercise intake cannot correct existing nutritional deficiencies or inadequate nutrient intake during the weeks before competition.

Liquid Meals. Commercially prepared **liquid meals** offer an alternative to the precompetition meal. Benefits include the following:

- Enhance energy and nutrient intake in training, particularly if daily energy output exceeds energy intake due to the athlete's lack of interest in food or nutrition mismanagement

- Provide a high carbohydrate content for glycogen replenishment
- Contain some lipid and protein to contribute to satiety
- Supply fluid, because these meals exist in liquid form
- Digest rapidly, leaving essentially no residue in the intestinal tract

Liquid meals prove particularly effective during daylong swimming and track meets, or tennis, ice hockey, soccer, field hockey, martial arts, wrestling, volleyball, and basketball tournaments. During tournament competition, the athlete usually has little time for or interest in food. Athletes can also use liquid meals if they experience difficulty maintaining a relatively large body mass, and as a ready source of calories to gain weight.

Carbohydrate Intake Before, During, and After Intense Exercise

High-intensity aerobic exercise continued for 1 hour *decreases liver glycogen by about 55%, whereas a 2-hour strenuous workout almost depletes the glycogen in the liver and specifically exercised muscle fibers.* Even supermaximal, repetitive, 1- to 5-minute bouts of exercise interspersed with brief rest intervals dramatically lowers liver and muscle glycogen levels (e.g., soccer, ice hockey, field hockey, European handball, and tennis). Research shows that carbohydrate supplementation improves both prolonged exercise capacity and intermittent, high-intensity exercise performance. The "vulnerability" of the body's glycogen stores during heavy exercise has focused research on the potential "high performance" benefits of carbohydrate intake just before and during exercise. Current research continues to delineate ways to optimize carbohydrate replenishment during the postexercise recovery period.

Before Exercise
The potential endurance benefits of ingesting simple sugars before exercise remain equivocal. One line of research contends that consuming rapidly absorbed, high-glycemic carbohydrates within 1 hour before exercising actually accelerates glycogen depletion and negatively affects endurance performance by: a) causing an overshoot in insulin release, thus creating low blood sugar (**rebound hypoglycemia**), which can impair central nervous system function during exercise, and b) facilitating glucose influx into muscle (through a large insulin release) to increase carbohydrate use as fuel during exercise. At the same time, high insulin levels inhibit lipolysis, which reduces free fatty acid

mobilization from adipose tissue. Both augmented carbohydrate breakdown and blunted fat mobilization contribute to premature glycogen depletion and early fatigue.

Research in the late 1970s indicated that drinking a highly concentrated sugar solution 30 minutes before exercise precipitated early fatigue in endurance activities. These findings, however, have not been replicated subsequently. More recent research indicates that consuming glucose before exercise increases muscle glucose uptake but reduces liver glucose output during exercise to a degree that actually would conserve liver glycogen reserves. The discrepancy among research findings has no clear explanation. From a practical standpoint, one way to eliminate the potential for negative effects from pre-exercise simple sugars necessitates ingesting them at least 60 minutes before exercising. This allows sufficient time to reestablish hormonal balance before beginning exercise.

Pre-Exercise Fructose
The small intestine absorbs fructose more slowly than glucose, and causes only a minimal insulin response with essentially no decline in blood glucose. These observations have stimulated debate about whether fructose might be a beneficial, immediate, pre-exercise, exogenous carbohydrate fuel source for prolonged exercise. Although the theoretical rationale for fructose use appears plausible, its exercise benefits remain inconclusive. From a practical standpoint, consuming a high-fructose beverage often produces significant gastrointestinal distress (cramping, vomiting, diarrhea), which in itself can negatively impact exercise performance. Also, once the small intestine absorbs fructose, it first must be transported to the liver for conversion to glucose. This time delay further limits fructose availability for energy.

Glycemic Index
The body does not digest and absorb all carbohydrates at the same rate. The **glycemic index** provides a qualitative indicator of how well ingested carbohydrate raises blood glucose levels. This index indicates the increase in blood glucose over a 2-hour period after consuming 50 g of a food compared with a similar amount of a carbohydrate "standard" of white bread or glucose, with a value of 100%. For example, a glycemic index of 45 indicates that ingesting 50 g of a specific food increases blood glucose concentration to 45% of the level noted for 50 g of glucose.

Figure 9.7 classifies some common foods based on their glycemic index. Interestingly, a food's glycemic rating does not directly link to its classification as a "simple" or "complex" carbohydrate. Plant starch in white rice and potatoes has a higher glycemic index than simple sugars (particularly fructose) in apples and peaches. Because a food's fiber content slows its rate of digestion, many vegetables (e.g., peas, beans, and other legumes) have a low glycemic index. Furthermore, consuming lipids and proteins slows food transport into the small intestine, reducing the glycemic index of the meal's accompanying carbohydrates.

Glycemic Index and Pre-Exercise Food Intake

The glycemic index helps formulate the composition of the immediate pre-exercise meal to provide a glucose source to maintain blood sugar and muscle metabolism with minimal increase in insulin release. Maintaining normal plasma insulin levels should theoretically stabilize blood glucose and optimize fat mobilization and catabolism, thus sparing glycogen reserves. Consuming low-glycemic index foods immediately (<30 min) before exercise allows for a relatively slow rate of glucose absorption into the blood. This eliminates an insulin surge, yet provides a steady supply of "slow-release" glucose from the digestive tract during exercise—an effect that theoretically should prove beneficial during long-term, high-intensity exercise.

During Exercise

Consuming about 60 g of liquid or solid carbohydrates each hour during exercise benefits high-intensity, long-duration exercise and repetitive, short bouts of near-maximal effort. Sustained exercise below 50% of maximum intensity relies primarily on fat oxidation, with only a relatively small demand on carbohydrate breakdown. As such, consuming carbohydrate offers little benefit during such activity. In contrast, carbohydrate intake provides supplementary glu-

Adjust Carbohydrate Intake to Body Weight

Athletes who train arduously should consume 10 g of carbohydrate per kg of body mass daily. A 100-pound (45 kg) athlete who expends 2800 kcal daily requires approximately 450 g of carbohydrate, or 1800 kcal. The athlete who weighs 150 pounds (68 kg) and expends 4200 kcal should consume about 680 g of carbohydrate (2720 kcal). In both examples, carbohydrate intake equals 64% of total energy intake.

cose during high-intensity, aerobic exercise when glycogen utilization increases greatly. Exogenous carbohydrate either 1) spares muscle glycogen because the ingested glucose powers the exercise, or 2) helps to stabilize blood glucose, which prevents headache, lightheadedness, nausea, and other symptoms of central nervous system distress. Maintaining an optimal level of blood glucose also supplies muscles with glucose when their glycogen reserves deplete in the later stages of prolonged exercise.

Consuming carbohydrates while exercising at 60 to 80% of $\dot{V}O_{2max}$ postpones fatigue by 15 to 30 minutes. This effect offers great potential for marathon runners who experience muscle fatigue within several hours after initiating exercise. Figure 9.8 shows that a single, concentrated carbohydrate intake about 2 hours into exercise (when blood glucose and glycogen reserves near depletion) restores blood glucose levels; this increases carbohydrate availability and delays fatigue because higher blood glucose levels help sustain the muscles' energy needs.

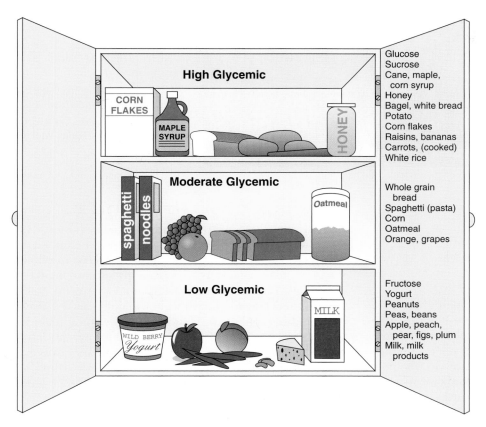

Figure 9.7
Glycemic index categories for common food sources of carbohydrates.

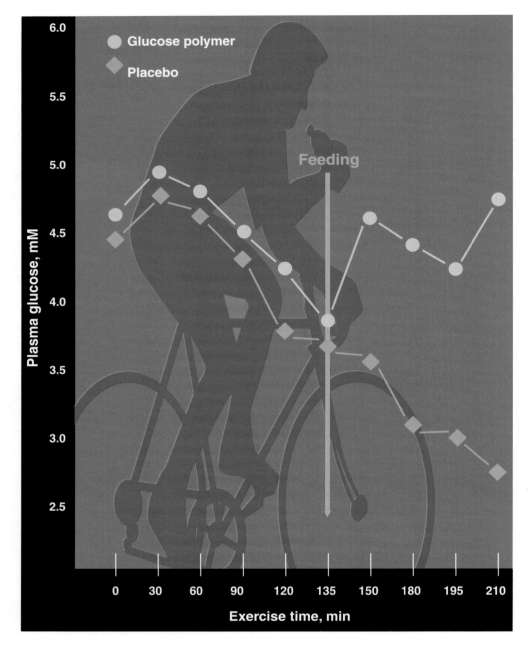

Figure 9.8
Average plasma glucose concentration during prolonged, high-intensity aerobic exercise when subjects consumed a placebo (green) or glucose polymer (gold; 3 g per kg body mass in a 50% solution). (Modified from Coggan, A.R., and Coyle, E.F.: Metabolism and performance following carbohydrate ingestion late in exercise. *Med. Sci. Sports Exerc.*, 21: 59, 1989.)

ume may lessen carbohydrate uptake, and concentrated sugar solutions diminishes fluid replacement.

The rate of stomach emptying greatly affects the absorption of fluid and nutrients by the small intestine. Exercise up to an intensity of about 75% $\dot{V}O_{2max}$ has little negative effect on gastric emptying, after which emptying rate slows considerably. *Gastric volume, however, greatly influences gastric emptying; its rate decreases as stomach volume decreases. Consequently, maintaining a relatively large fluid volume in the stomach speeds gastric emptying.*

Glucose Intake, Electrolytes, and Water Uptake

Chapter 3 explained how consuming fluids before and during exercise counters dehydration and its detrimental effects. Adding carbohydrate to the oral rehydration beverage provides additional glucose energy for exercise when the body's glycogen reserves deplete. Determining the optimal fluid/carbohydrate mixture and volume to consume during exercise takes on importance when the objectives are to reduce fatigue and prevent dehydration. Recall that consuming a large, dilute fluid vol-

Practical Recommendation

Consuming 400 to 600 mL of fluid immediately before exercise optimizes the beneficial effect of increased stomach volume on fluid and nutrient passage into the intestine. Then, regularly ingesting 250 mL of fluid throughout exercise (at 15-minute intervals) continually replenishes the fluid passed into the intestine, yet maintains a relatively large and constant gastric volume during exercise. This delivers about one liter of fluid per hour to the small intestine, a volume sufficient to meet most endurance athletes' fluid needs. Although prior research indicated that the stomach emptied colder fluid faster than fluid at room temperature, fluid temperature per se probably does not play a major role during exercise. Beverages containing alcohol or caffeine should be avoided because both com-

Glucose Polymers

If a drink contains a glucose polymer (maltodextrin) rather than simple sugars, it minimizes the negative effects of concentrated sugar molecules on gastric emptying and maintains plasma volume. Short-chain polymers (3 to 20 glucose units) derived from corn starch breakdown reduce the number of particles in solution (osmolality); this facilitates water movement from the stomach into the small intestine for absorption.

pounds induce a diuretic effect (alcohol most pronounced), facilitating water loss.

Consider Fluid Concentration

Concern exists about the possible negative effects of sugar drinks on water absorption from the digestive tract. Gastric emptying slows when ingested fluids contain an excessive concentration of particles in solution (increased osmolality), or possess high caloric content. This can negatively impact prolonged exercise in hot weather, when adequate intake and absorption play prime roles in the participant's health and safety. Ingesting up to an 8% glucose-sodium oral rehydration beverage causes little negative effect on gastric emptying. In fact, it may actually facilitate flud uptake by the intestinal lumen, because rapid, active coupled or cotransport of glucose-sodium across the intestinal mucosa stimulates water's passive uptake by osmotic action. Water not only replenishes effectively, but the additonal glucose uptake contributes to blood glucose maintenance. This glucose can then spare muscle and liver glycogen, and/or provide for blood glucose reserves during the later stage of exercise.

Rehydration solutions combining two different, transportable carbohydrate substrates (glucose, fructose, sucrose, or maltodextrins) induce greater water uptake than solutions containing only one of the substrates. Adding the second substrate into the solution stimulates more intestinal transport mechanisms, thus facilitating net water absorption by osmosis. To optimize water and carbohydrate absorption, use a 6% carbohydrate-electrolyte solution containing a combination of fructose and sucrose, each of which is absorbed by separate, noncompetitive pathways.

Sodium's Potential Benefit

Adding a moderate amount of sodium to ingested fluid maintains plasma sodium concentration. This benefits the ultraendurance athlete at risk for hyponatremia (refer to Chapter 3), which results from significant sweat-induced sodium loss coupled with an unusually large intake of plain water. *Adding sodium to the rehydration beverage maintains plasma osmolality, reduces urine output, and sustains the drive to drink.* These factors promote continued fluid intake and fluid retention during recovery from exercise.

Recommended Oral Rehydration Beverage

The ideal **oral rehydration beverage** has these five qualities:

1. Tastes good
2. Absorbs rapidly
3. Causes little or no gastrointestinal distress
4. Helps maintain extracellular fluid volume and osmolality
5. Offers potential to enhance exercise performance

Consuming a 5 to 8% carbohydrate-electrolyte beverage during exercise in the heat contributes to temperature regulation and fluid balance as effectively as plain water. The drink also maintains glucose metabolism and glycogen reserves in prolonged exercise.

To determine a drink's carbohydrate percentage, divide its carbohydrate content (in g) by the fluid volume (in mL) and multiply by 100. For example, 80 g of carbohydrate in 1000 mL (1L) of water represents an 8% solution. Of course, various environmental and exercise conditions interact to influence the optimal composition of the rehydration solution. With relatively short-duration (30 to 60 minutes), intense aerobic effort and high thermal stress, fluid replenishment takes on importance for health and safety; ingesting a more dilute carbohydrate-electrolyte solution (<5% carbohydrate) is advisable under such conditions. In cool weather, with less likelihood of significant dehydration, a more concentrated beverage of 15% carbohydrate suffices. Essentially no differences exist among liquids containing glucose, sucrose, or starch as the preferred exogenous carbohydrate fuel source during exercise.

Optimal carbohydrate replacement rate ranges between 30 to 60 g (1 to 2 oz) per hour. Table 9.5 compares the carbohydrate and mineral contents and solute concentrations (osmolality) of popular beverages used by athletes to replenish fluid during exercise.

Post-Exercise Carbohydrate Intake

Rapid replenishment of carbohydrate after prolonged exercise requires consuming foods with moderate to high glycemic indices. To speed glycogen replenishment after a hard bout of training or competition, one should immediately consume carbohydrate-rich foods. Specifically, an individual should consume 50 to 75 g (2 to 3 oz) of moderate- to high-glycemic carbohydrates every 2 hours for a total of 500 g (7 to 10 g per kg body mass), or until he or she can eat a large, high-carbohydrate meal. If consuming carbohydrate immediately after exercise is im-

TABLE 9.5
Comparison of various beverages used by athletes to replace the fluid lost in exercise

BEVERAGES	FLAVORS	CHO SOURCE	CHO (%)	SODIUM (mg)	POTAS-SIUM (mg)	OTHER MINERALS AND VITAMINS	OSMOLALITY[a] (mosmol · L⁻¹)
GATORADE* Thirst Quencher Stokely-Van Camp, Inc., a subsidiary of The Quaker Oats Company	Lemon-Lime, Lemonade, Fruit Punch, Orange, Citrus Cooler	Sucrose; Glucose (powder) Sucrose; Glucose syrup, solids (liquid)	6	110	25	Chloride, Phosphorus	280–360
Exceed* Ross Laboratories	Lemon-Lime, Orange	Glucose polymers; Fructose	7.2	50	45		
Quickick* Cramer Products, Inc.	Lemon-Lime, Fruit punch, Orange, Grape, Lemonade	Fructose; Sucrose	4.7	116	23	Chloride, Calcium Magnesium, Phosphorus Calcium, Chloride, Phosphorus	250 305
Sqwincher, The Activity Drink Universal Products, Inc.	Lemon-Lime, Fruit punch, Lemonade, Orange, Grape Strawberry, Grapefruit	Glucose; Fructose	6.8	60	36	Chloride, Phosphorus Calcium, Magnesium, Vitamin C	470
10-K Beverage Products, Inc.	Lemon-Lime, Orange, Fruit punch, Lemonade, Iced Tea	Sucrose; Glucose; Fructose	6.3	52	26	Vitamin C, Chloride Phosphorus	350
USA Wet Texas Wet, Inc.	Lemon-Lime, Orange, Fruit punch	Sucrose	6.8	62	44	Chloride, Phosphorus	450
Coca-Cola Coca-Cola, USA	Regular, Classic, Cherry	High-fructose corn syrup; Sucrose	10.7–11.3	9.2	trace		
Sprite Coca-Cola, USA	Lemon-Lime	High-fructose corn syrup; Sucrose	10.2	28	trace	Phosphorus	600–715
Cranberry Juice Cocktail		High-fructose corn syrup; Sucrose	15	10	61		695
Orange juice		Fructose; Sucrose; Glucose	11.8	2.7	510	Phosphorus, Vitamin C	890
Water		—	—	low**	low**	—	
PowerAde		High-fructose corn syrup; Maltodextrin	8	73	33	Phosphorus, Calcium, Vitamins C and A, Niacin, Riboflavin, Thiamine, Iron	690
All-Sport		High-fructose corn syrup	8–9	55	55		
10 K		Sucrose; Glucose; Fructose	6.3	54	25		
Cytomax		Fructose corn syrup; Sucrose	7–11	10	150		
Breakthrough		Maltodextrin; Fructose	8.5	60	45		
Everlast		Sucrose; Fructose	6	100	20		
Hydra Charge		Maltodextrin; Fructose	8	—	trace		
SportaLYTE		Maltodextrin; Fructose; Glucose	7.5	100	60		

[a] When reported
*Serving size = 8 fluid oz; **Depends on water source
Chart modified from Coleman, E.: Sports drink update. Gatorade Sports Science Institute, Vol. 1, No. 5, 1988.

practical, meals containing 2.5 g high-glycemic carbohydrate per kg body mass consumed at 2, 4, 6, 8, and 22 hours post exercise can rapidly restore muscle glycogen.

Legumes, fructose, and milk products should be avoided when rapidly replenishing glycogen reserves because of their slow rates of intestinal absorption. More rapid glycogen resynthesis results if the person remains inactive during the recovery period. *Under optimal carbohydrate intake conditions, glycogen replenishes at a rate of about 5% per hour. Thus, even under the best of circumstances, it requires at least 20 hours to reestablish glycogen stores after a glycogen-depleting exercise bout.*

Optimal glycogen replenishment benefits individuals involved in regular heavy training, tournament competition with qualifying rounds, and events scheduled with only 1 or 2 days for recuperation. Competitive wrestlers who lose considerable glycogen and water to "make weight" (via food and fluid restriction prior to the weigh-in) also benefit from a proper strategy of glycogen replenishment.

Carbohydrate Needs in Intense Training

Repeated days of strenuous endurance workouts for distance running, swimming, cross-country skiing, and cycling can induce a general fatigue state that makes training progressively more difficult. Often referred to as "**staleness,**" this physiologic state probably results from gradual depletion of glycogen reserves, even though the person's diet may contain the typical carbohydrate percentage. In one experiment, in which athletes ran 16.1 km (10 miles) a day for 3 successive days, glycogen in the thigh muscles became nearly depleted, even though the athletes' diets contained about 50% carbohydrate. By the third day, glycogen usage during the run was less than on the first day, and fat breakdown supplied the predominant fuel to power exercise. No further glycogen depletion occurred when daily dietary carbohydrate increased

to 600 g (70% of caloric intake). This demonstrates the importance of maintaining adequate carbohydrate intake during training.

Diet, Glycogen Stores, and Endurance

In the late 1960s, scientists observed that endurance performance significantly improved simply by consuming a carbohydrate-rich diet for 3 days prior to exercising. Conversely, endurance deteriorated if the diet consisted principally of lipids. In one series of experiments, subjects consumed one of three diets. The first maintained normal energy intake but supplied the majority of calories from lipids with only 5% from carbohydrate. The second diet provided the normal allotment for calories with the typical percentages of the three macronutrients. The third diet provided 80% of calories as carbohydrate.

The results from this classic study illustrated in Figure 9.9 show that the glycogen content of leg muscles, ex-

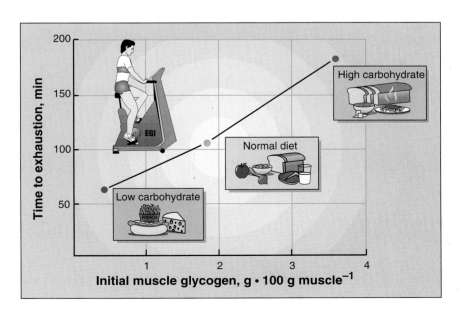

Figure 9.9
Classic experiment on the effects of a low-carbohydrate diet, mixed-diet, and high-carbohydrate diet on glycogen content of the quadriceps femoris muscle and the duration of endurance exercise on a bicycle ergometer. With a high-carbohydrate diet, endurance time tripled compared with a diet low in carbohydrate. (Adapted from Bergstrom, J., et al.: Diet, muscle glycogen and physical performance. *Acta Physiol. Scand.*, 71:140, 1967.)

close up

Optimal Replacement of Fluid and Carbohydrate During Prolonged Exercise

Intense aerobic exercise can continue uninterrupted provided 1) core temperature and plasma volume maintain relative stability, and 2) carbohydrate energy reserves remain adequate. Sweat evaporation from the skin's surface provides the main mechanism for dissipating metabolic heat generated during exercise. Dehydration, a frequent consequence of sweat-induced water loss, impairs thermoregulation and endurance performance and magnifies risk for heat injury. Consuming fluids prior to and during exercise reduces the detrimental effects of dehydration. Adding carbohydrate to a fluid replacement beverage boosts exercise energy availability in the face of progressively depleted endogenous glycogen. Determining an optimal fluid and carbohydrate mixture to reduce fatigue and prevent dehydration during an endurance activity takes on added importance because: 1) intake of large fluid volumes lessens carbohydrate uptake, and 2) concentrated sugar solutions impair fluid replacement.

The table presents a general guideline for fluid intake each hour during exercise for a given amount of carbohydrate replenishment. A trade-off exists between carbohydrate ingestion and gastric emptying. The stomach empties up to 1700 mL of water per hour, even when drinking an 8% carbohydrate solution. Consuming 1000 mL (about 1 quart) of fluid per hour probably represents an optimal volume to offset dehydration; consuming more fluid often produces gastrointestinal discomfort.

Volume of Fluid to Ingest Each Hour to Obtain the Noted Amount of Carbohydrate

CHO concentration in drink, $g \cdot 100\ mL^{-1}$	$30\ g \cdot hr^{-1}$	$40\ g \cdot hr^{-1}$	$50\ g \cdot hr^{-1}$	$60\ g \cdot hr^{-1}$	
2%	1500 mL	2000 mL	2500 mL	3000 mL	Volume too large: greater than $1200\ mL \cdot hr^{-1}$
4%	750	1000	1250	1500	
6%	500	667	833	1000	Adequate fluid replacement: $600–1250\ mL \cdot hr^{-1}$
8%	375	500	625	750	
10%	300	400	300	600	
15%	200	267	333	400	
20%	150	200	250	300	Low fluid replacement: less than $600\ mL \cdot hr^{-1}$
25%	120	160	200	240	

Practical Recommendations

- Monitor dehydration rate from changes in body weight (have athlete urinate before postexercise body weight determination to account for water lost in urine.) Each pound of weight loss corresponds to about 450 mL (15 fluid oz) of dehydration.
- Drink fluids at the same rate as their estimated rate of depletion. This means drinking at a rate close to 80% of sweating rate during prolonged exercise that produces cardiovascular stress, excessive heat, and dehydration.

- Drink between 625 to 1250 mL each hour (250 mL every 15 min) of a 4 to 8% carbohydrate beverage to meet carbohydrate (30 to 60 $g \cdot hr^{-1}$) and fluid requirements.

From Coyle, E.F., and Montain S.J.: Benefits of fluid replacement with carbohydrate during exercise. *Med. Sci Sports Exerc.*, 24:S324, 1992.

pressed as grams of glycogen per 100 g of muscle, averaged 0.6 for subjects who ate the low-carbohydrate diet, 1.75 for the typical diet, and 3.75 for the high-carbohydrate diet. Furthermore, subjects' endurance capacity varied greatly depending on the pre-exercise diet. When subjects ate the high-carbohydrate diet, endurance more than tripled compared with the low-carbohydrate diet.

These findings highlight the important role that nutrition plays in establishing appropriate energy reserves for exercise and training. A diet deficient in carbohydrate

How to Carbohydrate Load

The importance of muscle glycogen levels to enhance exercise performance remains unequivocal—time to exhaustion during intense aerobic exercise directly relates to the initial glycogen content of the liver and active musculature. In one series of experiments, muscle glycogen content increased six-fold and endurance capacity tripled for subjects fed a high-carbohydrate diet compared with feeding the same subjects a low-carbohydrate (high-fat) diet of similar energy content. Given muscle glycogen's importance in prolonged endurance performance, carbohydrate loading provides a strategy to increase initial muscle and liver glycogen levels.

Classic Carbohydrate Loading Procedure

Classic carbohydrate loading involves a two-stage procedure.

TWO-STAGE DIETARY PLAN FOR INCREASING MUSCLE GLYCOGEN

Stage 1—Depletion

  Day 1: Perform exhaustive exercise to deplete muscle glycogen in specific muscles

  Days 2, 3, 4: Maintain low-carbohydrate food intake (high percentage of protein and lipid in the daily diet)

Stage 2—Carbohydrate Loading

  Days 5, 6, 7: Maintain high-carbohydrate food intake (normal percentage of protein in the daily diet)

Competition Day

  Follow high-carbohydrate precompetition meal recommendation

Specifics of Precompetition Diet-Exercise Plan to Enhance Glycogen Storage

- Employ high-intensity, aerobic exercise for 90 minutes about 6 days before competition to reduce muscle and liver glycogen stores. Because glycogen loading occurs only in the specific muscles depleted by exercise, athletes must engage the major muscles involved in their sport.

- Maintain a low-carbohydrate diet (60 to 100 g per day) for 3 days while training at moderate intensity to further deplete glycogen stores.

- Switch to a high-carbohydrate diet (400 to 700 g per day) at least 3 days before competition, and maintain this intake up to and as part of the precompetition meal.

SAMPLE MEAL PLANS FOR CARBOHYDRATE DEPLETION (STAGE 1) AND CARBOHYDRATE LOADING (STAGE 2) PRECEDING AN ENDURANCE EVENT

Meal	Stage 1	Stage 2
Breakfast	1/2 cup fruit juice 2 eggs 1 slice whole-wheat toast 1 glass whole milk	1 cup fruit juice 1 bowl hot or cold cereal 1 to 2 muffins 1 tbsp butter coffee (cream and sugar)
Lunch	6 oz hamburger 2 slices bread 1 serving salad 1 tbsp mayonnaise and salad dressing 1 glass whole milk	2–3 oz hamburger with bun 1 cup juice 1 orange 1 tbsp mayonnaise 1 serving pie or cake
Snack	1 cup yogurt	1 cup yogurt, fruit or cookies
Dinner	2 to 3 pieces chicken, fried 1 baked potato with sour cream 1/2 cup vegetables 2 tbsp butter iced tea (no sugar)	1–1 1/2 pieces chicken, baked 1 baked potato with sour cream 1 cup vegetables 1/2 cup sweetened pineapple Iced tea (sugar) 1 tbsp butter
Snack	1 glass whole milk	1 glass chocolate milk with 4 cookies

Carbohydrate intake averages approximately 100 g or 400 kcal during Stage 1; Stage 2 carbohydrate intake increases to 400 to 700 g or about 1600 to 2800 kcal.

rapidly depletes muscle and liver glycogen. Glycogen depletion subsequently affects performance in maximal, short-term anaerobic exercise and prolonged, high-intensity aerobic effort. These observations pertain not only to athletes, but to moderately active people who eat less than the recommended quantity of carbohydrate.

Carbohydrate Loading

A particular combination of diet plus exercise produces a significant "packing" of muscle glycogen, a procedure termed "**carbohydrate loading**" or "**glycogen supercompensation**." Endurance athletes often carbohydrate load to prepare for competition. The procedure increases muscle glycogen more than the levels achieved by simply maintaining a high-carbohydrate diet. Glycogen loading packs as much as 5 g of glycogen into each 100 g of muscle (in contrast to its normal value of 1.7 g). Consuming adequate daily protein, minerals and vitamins, and abundant water must also be part of the diet. For athletes who follow the classic glycogen-loading procedure (see *How to Carbohydrate Load*), enhanced muscle glycogen levels can be maintained for at least 3 days if the diet contains about 60% of total calories as carbohydrate during the maintenance phase.

Limited Applicability

The potential benefits from carbohydrate loading apply only to intense and prolonged aerobic activities. *Unless the athlete begins competing in a state of depletion, exercise for less than 60 minutes requires only normal carbohydrate intake and glycogen reserves.* Carbohydrate loading and associated high levels of muscle and liver glycogen did not benefit athletes in a 20.9-km (13-mile) run compared with a run following a low-carbohydrate diet. A single, maximal anaerobic power output for 75-seconds also did not improve by increasing muscle glycogen availability above normal through dietary manipulation prior to exercise.

In most sport competition and exercise training, a daily diet of 60 to 70% calories as carbohydrates provides for adequate muscle and liver glycogen reserves. This diet ensures about twice the level of muscle glycogen compared with untrained counterparts who eat the typical American diet. For well-nourished athletes, any supercompensation effect from carbohydrate loading remains relatively small. During intense training, however, athletes who do not upgrade daily caloric and carbohydrate intakes to meet energy demands may experience muscle fatigue and staleness.

Athletes should experiment with carbohydrate loading before trying to manipulate their diets and exercise habits to achieve a supercompensation effect. If an athlete decides to supercompensate the plan should be attempted in stages during training, not for the first time before competition. For example, the track athlete would start with a long "depletion run" followed by a high-carbohydrate diet. A detailed log should track performance and the effects of the dietary manipulations, including subjective feelings during exercise depletion and replenishment phases. If results prove encouraging, the entire sequence of depletion, low-carbohydrate diet (maintained for only 1 day), and high-carbohydrate diet should be attempted. If no adverse effects appear, the low-carbohydrate phase should gradually extend to a maximum of 4 days.

Negative Aspects

The addition of 2.7 g of water stored with each gram of glycogen makes this a heavy fuel compared with equivalent energy as stored fat. A higher body mass due to water retention often makes the athlete feel heavy, "bloated," and uncomfortable; any extra load also directly adds to the energy cost of weight-bearing activities such as running, racewalking, or cross-country skiing. The added energy cost may actually negate the potential benefits from increased glycogen storage. On the positive side, the water liberated during glycogen breakdown aids in temperature regulation to benefit exercise in the heat.

The classic model for supercompensation would be ill-advised for individuals with specific health problems. A dietary carbohydrate overload, interspersed with periods of high lipid or protein intake, may increase blood cholesterol and urea nitrogen levels. This could pose problems for individuals predisposed to type 2 diabetes and heart disease, or with muscle enzyme deficiencies or renal disease. Failure to eat a balanced diet can produce deficiencies of some minerals and vitamins, particularly water-soluble vitamins; these deficiencies may require dietary supplementation. The glycogen-depleted state during the first phase of the glycogen-loading procedure certainly reduces one's capability to engage in intense training, possibly resulting in a detraining effect during the loading period. Dramatically reducing dietary carbohydrate for 3 or 4 days could also set the stage for lean tissue loss. This would result because muscle protein serves as gluconeogenic substrate to maintain blood-glucose levels with low glycogen reserves.

Modified Loading Procedure

The less-stringent, modified dietary protocol removes many of the negative aspects of the classic glycogen-loading sequence. This 6-day protocol does not require prior exercise to deplete glycogen. The athlete trains at about 75% of $\dot{V}O_{2max}$ (85% HR_{max}) for 1.5 hours and then gradually reduces (tapers) exercise duration on successive days. Carbohydrates represent about 50% of total caloric intake during the first three days. Three days before competition, the diet's carbohydrate content then increases to 70% of energy intake, replenishing glycogen reserves to about the same point achieved with the classic loading protocol.

summary

1. Within rather broad limits, a balanced diet from regular food intake provides the nutrient requirements of athletes and others engaged in exercise training and sports competition.

2. The Food Guide Pyramid represents a model for good nutrition for all Americans, regardless of physical activity level. The guidelines emphasize diverse grains, vegetables, and fruits as major calorie sources, downplaying foods high in animal proteins, lipids, and dairy products.

3. For physically active individuals, 60 to 70% of daily caloric intake should come from carbohydrates (400 to 600 g), particularly unrefined, low-glycemic polysaccharides.

4. Volume of daily physical activity largely determines energy intake requirements. Under most circumstances, daily energy requirements for physically active individuals probably do not exceed 4000 kcal for men and 3000 kcal for women. Under extremes of training and competition these values approach 5000 kcal for women and 9000 kcal for men.

5. The relatively high caloric intakes of physically active men and women usually increase protein, vitamin, and mineral intake above recommended values.

6. The ideal precompetition meal maximizes muscle and liver glycogen storage, and enhances glucose for intestinal absorption during exercise. High-carbohydrate and relatively low-lipid and low-protein meals generally fill this requirement. A carbohydrate-rich pre-event meal requires about 3 hours for digestion and absorption.

7. Commercially prepared liquid meals offer a practical approach to precompetition nutrition and energy supplementation. These "meals" give balance in nutritive value, contribute to fluid needs, and absorb rapidly, leaving practically no residue in the digestive tract.

8. The glycemic index provides a qualitative indication of how well ingested carbohydrate raises blood glucose levels over a 2-hour period compared with a similar amount of a carbohydrate in the form of white bread or glucose.

9. Consuming low-glycemic index foods immediately before exercise allows for a relatively slow rate of glucose absorption into the blood. This should eliminate an insulin surge, while providing a steady supply of "slow-release" glucose from the digestive tract during exercise.

10. Fluid volume within the stomach exerts the greatest effect on the rate of gastric emptying. To maintain a relatively large fluid volume in the stomach and speed gastric emptying, consume 400 to 600 mL of fluid immediately before exercise with subsequent regular ingestion of 250 mL at 15-minute intervals throughout exercise.

11. Consuming a 5 to 8% carbohydrate-electrolyte beverage during exercise in the heat contributes to temperature regulation and fluid balance as effectively as plain water. The drink also maintains blood glucose and glycogen reserves in prolonged exercise.

12. To speed glycogen replenishment after a bout of heavy training or competition, consume 50 to 75 g of moderate to high glycemic carbohydrates every 2 hours for a total of 500 g. Even under optimal conditions, it takes at least 20 hours (5% per hour) to reestablish glycogen stores.

13. Successive days of intense training gradually deplete glycogen reserves, even with the typical carbohydrate intake. This could lead to chronically reduced glycogen reserves and training "staleness."

14. A diet deficient in carbohydrate rapidly depletes muscle and liver glycogen. Glycogen depletion profoundly impairs performance in maximal, short-term anaerobic exercise and prolonged, high-intensity aerobic effort.

15. Carbohydrate loading can augment endurance performance. Athletes should become well informed about this procedure because of potential negative effects. Modifying the classic loading procedure augments glycogen storage without dramatically altering diet and exercise regimens.

thought questions

1. Among physically active men and women, how can individuals who consume the greatest number of calories weigh less than those who consume fewer calories?

2. Under what circumstances might an athlete require nutritional supplementation?

3. An athletic team has three matches scheduled on consecutive days. What should athletes consume after each day's competition, and why?

4. What advice would you give to a sprint athlete who plans to carbohydrate load for competition?

selected references

Anantaraman, R., et al.: Effects of carbohydrate supplementation on performance during 1 hour of high-intensity exercise. *Int. J. Sports Med.*, 16:461, 1995.

Bacharrach, D.W., et al.: Carbohydrate drinks and cycling performance. *J. Sports Med. Phys. Fitness*, 34:161, 1994.

Berning, J.R., and Steen, S.N.: *Nutrition for Sport and Exercise*, Gaithersburg, MD: Aspen Publishers, 1998.

Briefel, R.R., et al.: Total energy intake of the US population: The third National Health and Nutrition Examination Survey, 1988-1991. *Am. J. Clin. Nutr.*, 62(suppl):1072S, 1995.

Brouns, F., and Beckers, E.: Is the gut an athletic organ? *Sports Med*, 15:242, 1993.

Brown, R.C., and Cox, C.M.: Effects of high fat versus high carbohydrate diets on plasma lipids and lipoproteins in endurance athletes. *Med. Sci. Sports Exerc.*, 30:1677, 1998.

Bungard, L.B., et al.: Energy requirements of middle-aged men are modified by physical activity. *Am. J. Clin. Nutr.*, 68:1136, 1998.

Burelle, Y., et al.: Oxidation of an oral [^{13}C] glucose load at rest and prolonged exercise in trained and sedentary subjects. *J. Appl. Physiol.*, 86:52, 1999.

Burke, L.M., et al.: Muscle glycogen storage after prolonged exercise: effect of the frequency of carbohydrate feeding. *Am. J. Clin. Nutr.*, 64:115, 1996.

Burke, L.M., et al.: Carbohydrate intake during prolonged cycling exercise minimizes effect of glycemic index of preexercise meal. *J. Appl. Physiol.*, 85:2228, 1998.

Coggan, A.R., and Coyle, E.F.: Carbohydrate ingestion during prolonged exercise: Effects on metabolism and performance. In: *Exercise and Sport Science Reviews*. Vol. 19. Holloszy, J.O. (ed.). Baltimore, MD: Williams & Wilkins, 1991.

Coyle, E.F., and Coyle, E.: Carbohydrates that speed recovery from training. *Phys. Sportsmed.*, 21:111, 1993.

Coyle, E.F.: Substrate utilization during exercise in active people. *Am. J. Clin. Nutr.*, 61(suppl):968S, 1995.

DeMarco, H.M., et al.: Pre-exercise carbohydrate meals: application of glycemic index. *Med. Sci. Sports Exerc.*, 31:164, 1999.

Duchman, S.M., et al.: Upper limit for intestinal absorption of a dilute glucose solution in men at rest. *Med. Sci. Sports Exerc.*, 29:482, 1997.

Febbraio, M.A., and Stewart, K.L.: CHO feeding before prolonged exercise: effect of glycemic index on muscle glycogenolysis and exercise performance. *J. Appl. Physiol.*, 81:1115, 1996.

Foster-Powell, K., and Brand Miller, J. International tables of glycemic index. *Am. J. Clin. Nutr.*, 62(suppl):871S, 1995.

Gisolfi, C.V., et al.: Intestinal water absorption from select carbohydrate solutions is humans. *J. Appl. Physiol.*, 7: 2142, 1992.

Gisolfi, C.V., et al.: Effect of beverage osmolality on intestinal fluid absorption during exercise. *J. Appl. Physiol.*, 85:1941, 1998.

Glassetti, P., et al.: Enhanced muscle glucose facilitates nitrogen efflux from exercised muscle. *J. Appl. Physiol.*, 84:1952, 1998.

Goforth, Jr., H.W., et al.: Persistence of supercompensated muscle glycogen in trained subjects after carbohydrate loading. *J. Appl. Physiol.*, 82: 342, 1997.

Goodpaster, B.H., et al: The effects of pre-exercise starch ingestion on endurance performance. *Int. J. Sports Med.*, 17:366, 1996.

Grandjean, A. C.: Macronutrient intakes of US athletes compared with the general population and recommendations made for athletes. *Am. J. Clin. Nutr.*, 49:1070, 1989.

Hargreaves, M., et al.: Effect of muscle glycogen availability on maximal exercise performance. *Eur. J. Appl. Physiol.*, 75:188, 1997.

Helge, J.W., et al.: Interaction of training and diet on metabolism and endurance during exercise in man. *J. Physiol.*, 492:293, 1996.

Hickson, R.C., et al.: Muscle glycogen accumulation after endurance exercise in trained and untrained indivuduals. *J. Appl. Physiol.*, 83:897, 1997.

Hickson, J. F., Jr., and Wolinsky, I. (eds.): *Nutrition in Exercise and Sport*. 3rd Ed., Boca Raton, FL: CRC Press, 1998.

Kirwin, J.P., et al.: A moderate gycemic meal before endurance exercise can enhance performance. *J. Appl. Physiol.*, 84:53, 1998.

Horowitz, J.F., et al.: Substrate metabolism when subjects are fed carbohydrates during exercise. *Am. J. Physiol.*, 276 (5 Pt):E828, 1999.

Jeukendrup, A.E., et al.: Carbohydrate-electrolyte feedings improve 1 h time trial cycling performance. *Int. J. Sports Med.*, 18:125, 1997.

Jozsi, A.C., et al.: The influence of starch structure on glycogen resynthesis and subsequent cycling performance. *Int. J. Sports Med.*, 17:373, 1996.

Lambert, G.P., et al.: Simultaneous determination of gastric emptying and intestinal absorption during cycle exercise in humans. *Int. J. Sports Med.*, 17:48, 1996.

Leiper, J.B.: Intestinal water absorption—implications for the formulation of rehydration solutions, *Int. J. Sports Med.*, 19(Suppl. 2):s129, 1998.

Maughan, R.J., and Lieper, J.B.: Sodium intake and post-exercise rehydration in man. *Eur. J. Appl. Physiol.*, 71:311, 1995.

Maughan, R.J., et al.: Restoration of fluid balance after exercise-induced dehydration: effect of food and fluid intake. *Int. J. Appl. Physiol.*, 73:317, 1996.

McArdle, W.D., et al.: *Sport and Exercise Nutrition*. Baltimore, MD: Williams & Wilkins, 1999.

McConell, G., et al.: Effect of timing of carbohydrate ingestion on endurance exercise performance. *Med. Sci. Sports Exerc.*, 28:1300, 1996.

Nicholas, C.W., et al.: Influence of ingesting a carbohydrate-electrolyte solution on endurance capacity during intermittent, high intensity shuttle running. *J. Sports Sci.*, 13:283, 1996.

Pabkin, J.A.M., et al.: Muscle glycogen storage following prolonged exercise: effect of timing of ingestion of high glycemic index food. *Med. Sci. Sports Exerc.*, 29:220, 1997.

Pogliaghi, S., and Veicsteinas, A.: Influence of low and high dietary fat on physical performance in untrained males. *Med. Sci. Sports Exerc.*, 31:149, 1999.

Rankin, J.W., et al.: Effect of weight loss and refeeding diet composition on anaerobic performance in wrestlers. *Med. Sci. Sports Exerc.*, 28:1292, 1996.

Rauch, L.H.G., et al.: The effects of carbohydrate loading on muscle glycogen content and cycling performance. *Int. J. Sports Nutr.*, 5: 25, 1995.

Ray, M.L., et al.: Effect of sodium in a rehydration beverage when consumed as a fluid or meal. *J. Appl. Physiol.* 85:1329, 1998.

Roy, B.D., and Tarnopolsky, M.A.: Influence of differing macronutrient intakes on muscle glycogen resynthesis after resistance exercise. *J. Appl. Physiol.*, 84:890, 1998.

Ryan, A.J., et al.: Effect of hypohydration on gastric emptying and intestinal absorption during exercise. *J. Appl. Physiol.*, 84:1581, 1998.

SCAN's Guide to Nutrition and Fitness Resources: 1998. SCAN'S PULSE, suppl. *The American Dietetic Association*, Chicago, IL

Schabort, E.J., et al.: The effect of a preexercise meal on time to fatigue during prolonged cycling exercise. *Med. Sci. Sports Exerc.*, 31:464, 1999.

Schedl, H.P., et al. Intestinal absorption during rest and exercise: implications for formulating an oral rehydration solution (ORS). *Med. Sci. Sports Exerc.*, 26: 267, 1994.

Sherman, W. M., and Wimer, G. S.: Insufficient carbohydrate during training: does it impair performance? *Int. J. Sport Nutr.*, 1:28, 1991.

Shi, X., and Gisolfi, C.V.: Fluid and carbohydrate replacement during intermittent exercise. *Sports Med.*, 25:157, 1998.

Snyder, A.C.: Overtaining and glycogen depletion hypothesis. *Med. Sci. Sports Exerc.*, 30:1146, 1998.

Sparks, M.J., et al.: Pre-exercise carbohydrate ingestion: effect of the glycemic index on endurance exercise performance. *Med. Sci. Sports Exerc.*, 30:844, 1998.

Trappe, T.A., et al.: Energy expenditure of swimmers during high volume training. *Med. Sci. Sports Exerc.*, 29:950, 1997.

USDA, Center for Nutrtion policy and Promotion. USDA/HHS Dietary Guidelines for Americans. CNPP, Washington, DC, 1996.

USDA, Human Nutrition Service. The Food Guide Pyramid. Home and Garden Bulletin Number 252, HNIS, Hyattsville, MD, 1992.

Vist, G.E., and Maughn, R.J.: Gastric emptying of dilute glucose solutions in man: effect of beverage glucose concentration. *Med. Sci. Sports Exerc.*, 26: 1269, 1994.

Walberg-Rankin, J.: A review of nutritional practices and needs of bodybuilders. *J. Strength and Cond. Res.* 9:116, 1995.

Wagenmakers, A.J.M.: Carbohydrate feedings improve 1 h time trial cycling performance. *Med. Sci. Sports Exerc.*, 28:S37, 1996.

Walton, P., and Rhodes, E.C.: Glycaemic index and optimal performance. *Sports Med.*, 33:164, 1997.

Wee, S-L., et al: Influence of high and low glycemic index meals on endurance running capacity. *Med. Sci. Sports Exerc.*, 31:393, 1999.

Williams, M.H.: *Nutrition for Health, Fitness, and Sport.* Dubuque, IA. WCB/McGraw-Hill, 1998.

SECTION 3

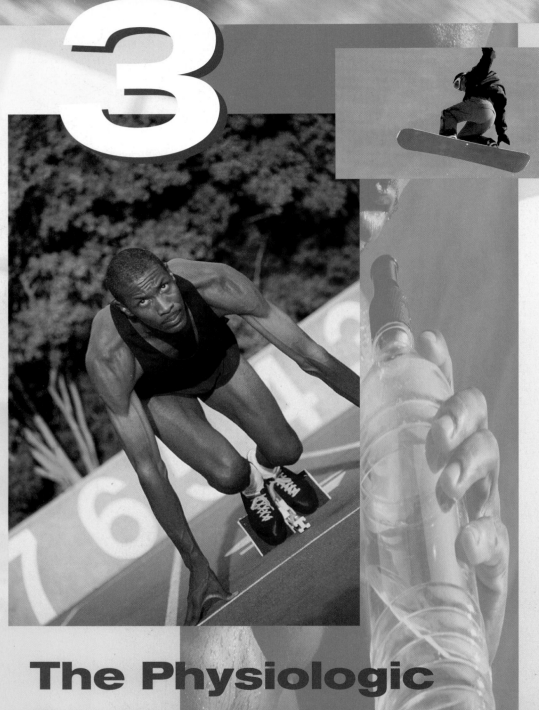

The Physiologic Support Systems

Most sport, recreational, and occupational activities require a moderately intense yet sustained energy release. The aerobic breakdown of carbohydrates, fats, and proteins generates this energy from ADP phosphorylation to ATP. Without a steady rate between oxidative phosphorylation and the energy requirements of physical activity, an anaerobic-aerobic energy imbalance develops, lactate accumulates, tissue acidity increases, and fatigue quickly ensues. Two factors limit an individual's ability to sustain a high level of exercise intensity without undue fatigue:

1. Capacity for oxygen delivery to active muscles
2. Capacity of active muscle cells to generate ATP aerobically

Understanding the role of the ventilatory, circulatory, muscular, and endocrine systems during exercise enables us to appreciate the broad range of individual differences in exercise capacity. Knowing the energy requirements of exercise, and the corresponding physiologic adjustments necessary to meet these requirements, helps formulate an effective physical fitness program and to properly evaluate physiologic and fitness status before and during such a program.

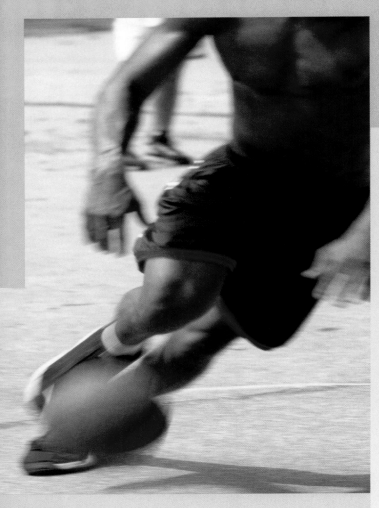

CHAPTER 10

The Pulmonary System and Exercise

Topics covered in this chapter

PART 1 Pulmonary Structure and Function

Anatomy of Ventilation
Lung Volumes and Capacities
Pulmonary Ventilation
Disruptions in Normal Breathing Patterns
Summary

PART 2 Gas Exchange

Respired Gases: Concentrations and Partial Pressures
Movement of Gas in Air and Fluids
Gas Exchange in the Body
Summary

PART 3 Oxygen and Carbon Dioxide Transport

Oxygen Transport in the Blood
Carbon Dioxide Transport in Blood
Summary

PART 4 Regulation of Pulmonary Ventilation

Ventilatory Control
Ventilatory Control in Exercise
Summary

PART 5 Pulmonary Ventilation During Exercise

Pulmonary Ventilation and Energy Demands
Does Ventilation Limit Aerobic Capacity?
Summary
Thought Questions
Selected References

- Diagram the ventilatory system, showing the glottis, larynx, trachea, bronchi, bronchioles, and alveoli.

- Describe the dynamics of inspiration and expiration during rest and exercise.

- Describe the "Valsalva maneuver" and its physiologic consequences.

- Define minute ventilation, alveolar minute ventilation, ventilation-perfusion ratio, and anatomic and physiologic dead spaces.

- Explain the "Bohr effect" and its benefit during physical activity.

- List and quantify three means for carbon dioxide transport in blood.

- Identify major factors that regulate pulmonary ventilation during rest and exercise.

- Describe how hyperventilation extends breath-holding time, but can have dangerous consequences in sport diving.

- Graph relationships among pulmonary ventilation, blood lactate, and oxygen uptake during incremental exercise, indicating the points for the lactate threshold and onset of blood lactate accumulation.

- Explain what triggers exercise-induced asthma, including factors that affect its severity.

PART 1
Pulmonary Structure and Function

If oxygen supply depended only on diffusion through the skin, it would be impossible to support the basal energy requirement, let alone the 3- to 4-liter oxygen uptake each minute to sustain a world class 5-minute per mile marathon pace. The remarkably effective **ventilatory system** meets the body's needs for gas exchange. This system, depicted in Figure 10.1, regulates the gaseous state of our "external" environment for aerating fluids of the "internal" environment during rest and exercise. The major functions of the ventilatory system include:

- Supply oxygen required in metabolism
- Eliminate carbon dioxide produced in metabolism
- Regulate hydrogen ion concentration to maintain acid-base balance

Anatomy of Ventilation

The term **pulmonary ventilation** describes how ambient air moves into and exchanges with air in the lungs. About 0.3 m (1 ft) separates the distance between ambient air just outside the nose and mouth from the blood flowing through the lungs. Air entering the nose and mouth flows into the conductive portion of the ventilatory system. Here it adjusts to body temperature and becomes filtered and almost completely humidified as it moves through the trachea. The trachea, a short 1-inch diameter tube that extends from the larynx, divides into two tubes of smaller diameter called bronchi. The bronchi serve as pri-

Ventilation's Buffering Function

The blood's hydrogen ion concentration [H^+] directly relates to plasma carbon dioxide levels because carbon dioxide combines with water to form H_2CO_3, which dissociates to produce a bicarbonate ion (HCO_3^-) and a [H^+]. The ventilatory system monitors and responds to plasma [H^+] concentration, and adjusts breathing to maintain plasma CO_2 and [H^+] at optimal levels. Regulation of [H^+] is a vital ventilatory function; the acid-base quality of the reacting medium affects all of the body's biochemical reactions.

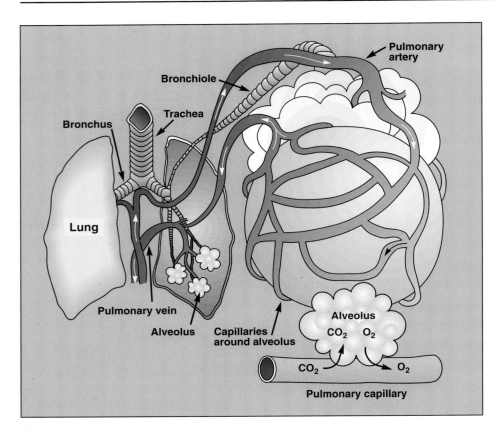

Figure 10.1
Overview of the ventilatory system showing the respiratory passages, alveoli, and gas exchange function in an alveolus.

In fact, the lungs receive the entire output of blood from the heart (cardiac output). Millions of thin-walled capillaries and alveoli lie side by side, with air moving on one side and blood on the other. The capillaries form a dense mesh that covers almost the entire outside of each alveolus (Fig. 10.3A). This web becomes so dense that blood flows as a sheet over each alveolus. Once blood reaches the pulmonary capillaries, only a single cell barrier, the **respiratory membrane**, separates blood from air in the alveolus (Fig. 10.3B). This thin tissue-blood barrier permits rapid diffusion between the alveoli gases and blood gases.

During rest, approximately 250 mL of oxygen leave the alveoli each minute and enter the blood, and about 200 mL of carbon dioxide diffuse in the reverse direction into the alveoli. When trained endurance athletes perform heavy exercise, about 20 times the resting oxygen uptake transfers across the respiratory membrane. The primary function of pulmonary ventilation during rest and exercise is to maintain fairly constant and favorable concentrations of oxygen and carbon dioxide in the alveolar chambers. This ensures effective gaseous exchange before

mary conduits within the right and left lungs. They further subdivide into numerous bronchioles that conduct inspired air through a tortuous, narrow route until it eventually mixes with the air in the **alveoli**, the terminal branches of the respiratory tract.

Lungs

The lungs provide the surface between blood and the external environment. Lung volume varies between 4 and 6 liters (amount of air in a basketball) and provides an exceptionally large moist surface. For example, the lungs of an average-sized person weigh about 1 kg, yet if spread out as in Figure 10.2, they would cover a surface of 60 to 80 m². This equals about 35 times the external surface of the person, and would cover almost one-half a tennis court or an entire badminton court. This represents a considerable interface for aeration of blood because during any 1 second of maximal exercise, no more than 1 pint of blood flows in the lung tissue's web-like, intricate network of blood vessels.

Alveoli

Lung tissue contains more than 300 million alveoli. The elastic, thin-walled, membranous sacs provide the vital surface for gas exchange between the lungs and blood. Alveolar tissue has the largest blood supply of any organ in the body.

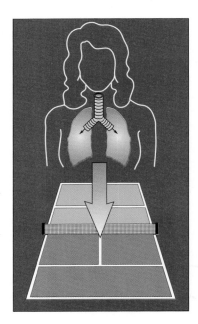

Figure 10.2
The lungs provide an exceptionally large surface for gas exchange.

Figure 10.3
A, Electron micrograph of lung capillaries (x1300). Note the extremely dense capillary bed; the dark areas represent the alveolar chambers. **B,** Electron micrograph of a pulmonary capillary (x 6000). Note the extremely thin respiratory membrane layer separating alveolar air from red blood cells. (Courtesy of Dr. R. L. Malvin, University of Michigan.)

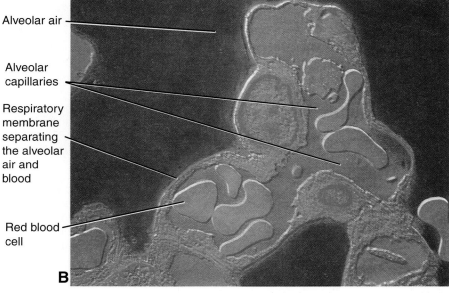

the blood exits the lungs for transit throughout the body.

Mechanics of Ventilation

Figure 10.4 illustrates the physical principle underlying the dynamics of breathing. Two balloons connect to a jar whose glass bottom has been replaced by a thin rubber membrane. When the membrane lowers, the jar's volume increases because air pressure within the jar becomes less than air pressure outside the jar. Consequently, air rushes into the balloons and they inflate. Conversely, if the elastic membrane recoils, the pressure within the jar temporarily increases, and air rushes out. Considerable air exchange occurs within the balloons as the distance and rate of descent and ascent of the rubber membrane increases. Essentially, ambient and alveolar air exchange within the lungs takes place in this manner.

The lungs do not merely suspend in the chest cavity as depicted with the balloons and jar. Rather, the difference in pressure within the lungs and the lung-chest wall interface causes the lungs to adhere to the chest wall interior and literally follow its every movement. Any change in thoracic cavity volume thus produces a corresponding change in lung volume. Lung tissue does not contain voluntary muscle, so the lungs depend on accessory means to alter their volume. Voluntary skeletal muscle action during inspiration and expiration alters thoracic dimensions to change lung volume.

Inspiration

The **diaphragm**, a large, dome-shaped sheet of muscle, serves the same purpose as the jar's rubber membrane in Figure 10.4. The diaphragm muscle makes an airtight separation between the abdominal and thoracic cavities. During inspiration, the diaphragm contracts, flattens out, and moves downward up to 10 cm toward the abdominal cavity. This enlarges and elongates the chest cavity. The air in the lungs then expands, reducing its pressure (referred to as **intrapulmonic pressure**) to about 5 mm Hg below atmospheric pressure. *The pressure differential between the lungs and ambient air literally sucks air in through the nose and mouth and inflates the lungs.* The degree of lung filling depends on two factors:

1. Magnitude of inspiratory movements
2. Pressure gradient between air inside and air outside the lung

Inspiration concludes when thoracic cavity expansion ceases and intrapulmonic pressure increases to equal atmospheric pressure.

During exercise, the scaleni and external intercostal muscles between the ribs contract, causing the ribs to rotate and lift up and away from the body—an action similar to the movement of the handle lifted up and away from the side of the bucket at the right in Figure 10.4. We breathe in air when chest cavity volume

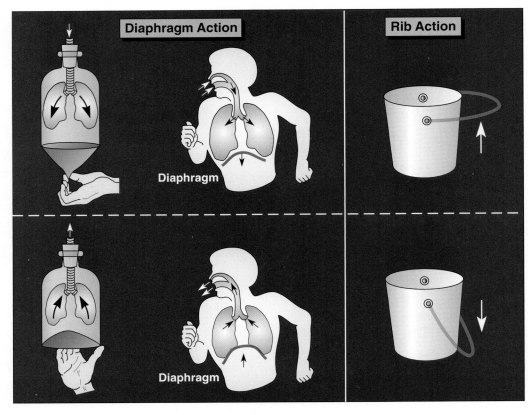

movements decrease chest cavity volume, compressing alveolar gas and moving it out through the respiratory tract to the atmosphere. During ventilation in moderate to heavy exercise, the internal intercostal muscles and abdominal muscles act powerfully on the ribs and abdominal cavity to trigger a rapid and greater depth of exhalation.

Respiratory muscle actions change thoracic dimensions to create a pressure differential between the inside and outside of the lungs to drive airflow along the respiratory tract. Greater involvement of the pulmonary musculature during progressively heavier exercise, causes larger pressure differentials and concomitant increases in air movement.

Figure 10.4
Mechanics of breathing. During inspiration, the chest cavity increases in size because the ribs rise and the muscular diaphragm lowers. During exhalation, the ribs swing down and the diaphragm returns to a relaxed position. This reduces thoracic cavity volume, and air rushes out. The movement of the jar's rubber bottom causes air to enter and leave the two balloons, simulating the diaphragm's action. The movement of the bucket handle simulates rib action.

Lung Volumes and Capacities

increases due to three factors: 1) decent of the diaphragm, 2) upward lift of the ribs, and 3) outward thrust of the sternum.

Expiration

Expiration, a predominantly passive process, occurs as air moves out of the lungs. It results from the recoil of stretched lung tissue and relaxation of the inspiratory muscles. This makes the sternum and ribs swing down, while the diaphragm moves back toward the thoracic cavity. These

Body Position Facilitates Breathing

Athletes frequently bend forward from the waist to facilitate breathing after exhausting exercise. This body position serves two purposes:

1. Facilitates blood flow to the heart
2. Minimizes antagonistic effects of gravity on inspiratory movements

Figure 10.5 depicts the various static lung volume measures. The figure also shows average values for men and women while breathing from a calibrated recording spirometer that measures oxygen uptake by the closed-circuit method (refer to Chapter 6). Two types of measurements, static and dynamic, provide information about lung volume dimensions and capacities. **Static lung volume** tests evaluate the dimensional component for air movement within the pulmonary tract, and impose no time limitation on the subject. In contrast, **dynamic lung volume** measures evaluate the power component of pulmonary performance during different phases of the ventilatory excursion.

Static Lung Volumes

During measurement of static lung function, the spirometer bell falls and rises with each inhalation and exhalation to provide a record of the ventilatory volume and breathing rate. **Tidal volume (TV)** describes air moved during either the inspiratory or expiratory phase of each breathing cycle. For healthy men and women, TV under resting conditions usually ranges between 0.4 and 1.0 L of air per breath.

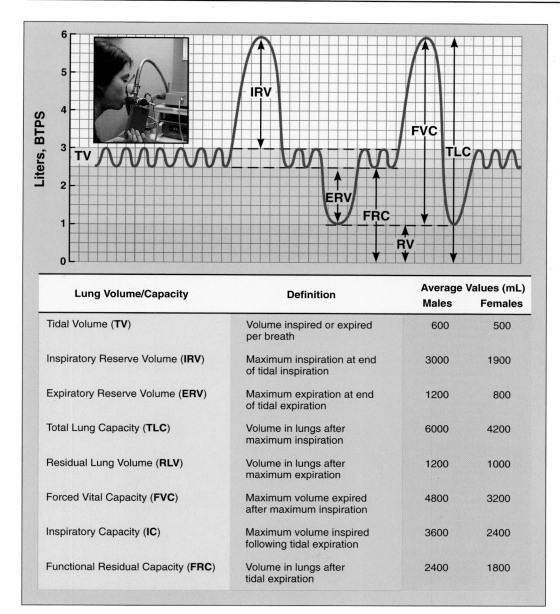

Figure 10.5
Static measures of lung volume and capacity.

Lung Volume/Capacity	Definition	Average Values (mL)	
		Males	Females
Tidal Volume (**TV**)	Volume inspired or expired per breath	600	500
Inspiratory Reserve Volume (**IRV**)	Maximum inspiration at end of tidal inspiration	3000	1900
Expiratory Reserve Volume (**ERV**)	Maximum expiration at end of tidal expiration	1200	800
Total Lung Capacity (**TLC**)	Volume in lungs after maximum inspiration	6000	4200
Residual Lung Volume (**RLV**)	Volume in lungs after maximum expiration	1200	1000
Forced Vital Capacity (**FVC**)	Maximum volume expired after maximum inspiration	4800	3200
Inspiratory Capacity (**IC**)	Maximum volume inspired following tidal expiration	3600	2400
Functional Residual Capacity (**FRC**)	Volume in lungs after tidal expiration	2400	1800

erably with body size and body position during the measurement; however, values usually average 4 to 5 L in healthy young men and 3 to 4 L in healthy young women. FVCs of 6 to 7 L are not uncommon for tall individuals, and a value of 7.6 L has been reported for a professional football player and 8.1 L for an Olympic gold medalist in cross-country skiing. Large lung volumes of some athletes probably reflect genetic influences because static lung volumes do not change appreciably with exercise training.

Residual Lung Volume

Following a forced, maximal exhalation, a volume of air that cannot be exhaled remains in the lungs. This volume, the **residual lung volume (RLV)**, averages between 1.0 and 1.2 L for college-age women and 1.2 and 1.4 L for men. RLV tends to increase with age because IRV and ERV become proportionally smaller.

After recording several representative TVs, the subject breathes in normally and then inspires maximally. An additional volume of about 2.5 to 3.5 L above TV air represents the reserve for inhalation, termed the **inspiratory reserve volume (IRV)**. The normal breathing pattern begins once again following the IRV. After a normal exhalation, the subject continues to exhale and forces as much air as possible from the lungs. This additional volume, the **expiratory reserve volume (ERV)**, ranges between 1.0 and 1.5 L for an average-size man (10 to 20% lower for a woman). During exercise, TV increases considerably because of encroachment on IRV and ERV, particularly IRV.

Forced vital capacity (FVC) represents the total air volume moved in one breath from full inspiration to maximum expiration, or vice versa. FVC varies consid-

Aging changes the various lung volumes owing to decreases in elasticity of lung tissue and a decline in pulmonary muscle power. These factors probably do not result entirely from aging per se because endurance training in older athletes slows the normal decline in lung function (see Chapter 20.) *Sedentary living, rather than true aging, most likely accounts for the greatest changes in lung volumes and pulmonary function in general.*

Dynamic Lung Volumes

Dynamic measures of pulmonary ventilation depend on two factors:

1. Volume of air moved
2. Speed of air movement

How to Predict Pulmonary Function Variables in Males and Females

Although pulmonary function variables do not directly relate to measures of physical fitness in healthy individuals, their measurement often forms part of a standard medical/health/fitness exam, particularly for individuals at risk for limited pulmonary function (e.g., chronic cigarette smokers, asthmatics). Measurement of diverse components of pulmonary dimension and lung function (with a water-filled spirometer [see figure] or electronic spirometer) also provide the framework for discussions of pulmonary dynamics during rest and exercise. Proper evaluation of measured values for pulmonary function requires comparison to norms from the clinical literature. Because pulmonary function variables associate closely with stature and age, these two variables can predict the lung function value expected average (normal) for a particular individual.

Data

Man: Age, 22 y; Stature, 182.9 cm (72 in)
Woman: Age, 22 y; Stature, 165.1 cm (65 in)

Examples

Predictions use cm for stature (ST) and years for age (A).

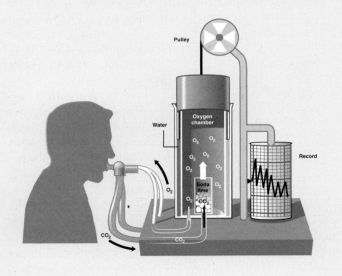

Pulley

Water

Oxygen chamber

O_2

Soda lime

CO_2

Record

CO_2

CO_2

Woman

1. Forced vital capacity (FVC)
   $$FVC, L = (0.0414 \times ST) - (0.0232 \times A) - 2.20$$
   $$= 6.835 - 0.5104 - 2.20$$
   $$= 4.12\ L$$

2. Forced expiratory volume in 1 second ($FEV_{1.0}$)
   $$FEV_{1.0}, L = (0.0268 \times ST) - (0.0251 \times A) - 0.38$$
   $$= 4.425 - 0.5522 - 0.38$$
   $$= 3.49\ L$$

3. Percentage forced vital capacity in 1 second ($FEV_{1.0}/FVC$)
   $$FEV_{1.0}/FVC, \% = (-0.2145 \times ST) - (0.1523 \times A) + 124.5$$
   $$= -35.41 - 3.35 + 124.5$$
   $$= 85.7\%$$

4. Maximum voluntary ventilation (MVV)
   $$MMV, L \cdot min^{-1} = 40 \times FEV_{1.0}$$
   $$= 40 \times 3.49\ (\text{from eq. 2})$$
   $$= 139.6\ L \cdot min^{-1}$$

Man

1. Forced vital capacity (FVC)
   $$FVC, L = (0.0774 \times ST) - (0.0212 \times A) - 7.75$$
   $$= 14.156 - 0.4664 - 7.75$$
   $$= 5.49\ L$$

2. Forced expiratory volume in 1 second ($FEV_{1.0}$)
   $$FEV_{1.0}, L = (0.0566 \times ST) - (0.0233 \times A) - 0.491$$
   $$= 10.35 - 0.5126 - 4.91$$
   $$= 4.93\ L$$

3. Percentage forced vital capacity in 1 second ($FEV_{1.0}/FVC$)
   $$FEV_{1.0}/FVC, \% = (-0.1314 \times ST) - (0.1490 \times A) + 110.2$$
   $$= -24.03 - 3.35 + 110.2$$
   $$= 82.8\%$$

4. Maximum voluntary ventilation (MVV)
   $$MMV, L \cdot min^{-1} = 40 \times FEV_{1.0}$$
   $$= 40 \times 4.93\ (\text{from eq. 2})$$
   $$= 197.2\ L \cdot min^{-1}$$

References
1. Miller, A.: *Pulmonary Function Tests in Clinical and Occupational Disease.* Philadelphia: Grune & Stratton, 1986.
2. Wasserman, K., et al.: *Principles of Exercise Testing.* Baltimore: Lippincott Williams & Wilkins, 1999.

Airflow speed depends on the pulmonary airways' resistance to the smooth flow of air and resistance offered by the chest and lung tissue to changes in shape during breathing.

Forced Expiratory Volume-to-Forced Vital Capacity Ratio

Normal values for vital capacity can occur in severe lung disease if no limit exists on the time to expel air. For this reason, a dynamic lung function measure such as the **percentage of FVC expelled in 1 second ($FEV_{1.0}$)** serves a more useful diagnostic purpose than static measures. *Forced expiratory volume-to-forced vital capacity ratio ($FEV_{1.0}/FVC$) reflects expiratory power and overall resistance to air movement in the lungs.* Normally, the $FEV_{1.0}/FVC$ averages about 85%. With severe obstructive pulmonary disease (e.g., emphysema and/or bronchial asthma), the $FEV_{1.0}/FVC$ often reaches less than 40% of vital capacity. *The clinical demarcation for airway obstruction represents the point at which a person can expel less than 70% of the FVC in 1 second.*

Maximum Voluntary Ventilation

Another dynamic assessment of ventilatory capacity requires rapid, deep breathing for 15 seconds. Extrapolation of this 15-second volume to the volume breathed had the subject continued for 1 minute represents the **maximum voluntary ventilation (MVV)**. For healthy, college-age men, the MVV usually ranges between 140 and 180 L $\cdot$min^{-1}. The average for women equals 80 to 120 L. Male members of the United States Nordic Ski Team averaged 192 L $\cdot$min^{-1}, with an individual high MVV of 239 L $\cdot$min^{-1}. Patients with obstructive lung disease achieve only about 40% of the MVV predicted normal for their age and stature. Specific pulmonary therapy benefits these patients because training the breathing musculature increases the strength and endurance of the respiratory muscles, thus enhancing MVV.

Pulmonary Ventilation

Minute Ventilation

During quiet breathing at rest, an adult's breathing rate averages 12 breaths per minute, whereas tidal volume averages about 0.5 L of air per breath. Under these conditions, the volume of air breathed each minute (**minute ventilation**) equals 6 L.

$$\text{Minute ventilation } (\dot{V}_E) = \text{Breathing rate} \times \text{Tidal volume}$$

$$6.0 \text{ L} \cdot \text{min}^{-1} = 12 \times 0.5 \text{ L}$$

An increase in depth or rate of breathing or both significantly increases minute ventilation. During maximal exercise, the breathing rate of healthy young adults usually increases to 35 to 45 breaths per minute, although elite athletes often achieve 60 to 70 breaths per minute. In addition, tidal volume commonly increases to 2.0 L and larger during heavy exercise, causing exercise minute ventilation in adults to easily reach 100 L or about 17 times the resting value. In well-trained male endurance athletes, ventilation may increase to 160 L$\cdot$min^{-1} during maximal exercise. In fact, several studies of elite endurance athletes report ventilation volumes of 200 L$\cdot$min^{-1}. *Even with these large minute ventilations, tidal volume rarely exceeds 55 to 65% of vital capacity.*

Alveolar Ventilation

Alveolar ventilation refers to the portion of minute ventilation that mixes with the air in the alveolar chambers. A portion of each breath inspired does not enter the alveoli, and thus does not engage in gaseous exchange with blood. This air that fills the nose, mouth, trachea, and other nondiffusible conducting portions of the respiratory tract constitutes the **anatomic dead space**. In healthy people, this volume averages 150 to 200 mL, or about 30% of the resting tidal volume. Almost equivalent composition exists between dead-space air and ambient air, except for dead-space air's full saturation with water vapor.

Because of dead-space volume, approximately 350 mL of the 500 mL of ambient air inspired in each tidal volume at rest mixes with existing alveolar air. This does not mean that only 350 mL of air enters and leaves the alveoli with each breath. To the contrary, if tidal volume equals 500 mL, then 500 mL of air enters the alveoli but only 350 mL represents fresh air (about one-seventh of the total air in the alveoli). The relatively small, seemingly inefficient alveolar ventilation prevents drastic changes in alveolar air composition; this ensures a consistency in arterial blood gases throughout the breathing cycle.

Table 10.1 shows that minute ventilation does not always reflect the actual alveolar ventilation. In the first example of shallow breathing, tidal volume decreases to 150 mL, yet a 6-L minute ventilation occurs when breathing rate increases to 40 breaths per minute. The same 6-L

TABLE 10.1
Relationships among tidal volume, breathing rate, and minute and alveolar minute ventilation

CONDITION	TIDAL VOLUME (mL)	× BREATHING RATE (Breaths $\cdot$min^{-1})	= MINUTE VENTILATION (mL $\cdot$ min^{-1})	− DEAD SPACE VENTILATION (mL $\cdot$ min^{-1})	= ALVEOLAR VENTILATION (mL $\cdot$ min^{-1})
Shallow breathing	150	40	6000	(150 ml × 40)	0
Normal breathing	5000	12	6000	(150 ml × 12)	4200
Deep breathing	1000	6	6000	(150 ml × 6)	5100

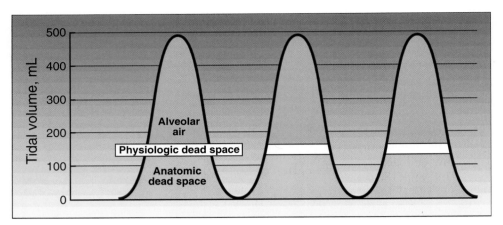

Figure 10.6
Distribution of tidal volume in the lungs of a healthy subject at rest. Tidal volume includes about 350 mL of ambient air that mixes with alveolar air, 150 mL of air in the larger air passages (anatomic dead space), and a small portion of air distributed to either poorly ventilated or poorly perfused alveoli (physiologic dead space).

minute volume results by decreasing breathing rate to 12 breaths per minute and increasing tidal volume to 500 mL. Doubling tidal volume and cutting ventilatory rate in half, as in the example of deep breathing, again produces a 6-L minute ventilation. Each ventilatory adjustment drastically affects alveolar ventilation. In the example of shallow breathing, dead-space air represents the entire air volume moved (no alveolar ventilation has taken place). The other examples involve deeper breathing; thus, a larger portion of each breath mixes with existing alveolar air. *Alveolar ventilation, not dead-space ventilation, determines gaseous concentrations at the alveolar-capillary membrane.*

Physiologic Dead Space

Some alveoli may not function adequately in gas exchange due to underperfusion of blood or inadequate ventilation relative to alveolar surface area. The term **physiologic dead space** describes that portion of the alveolar volume with poor regional perfusion (or ventilation) of tissues. Figure 10.6 illustrates that only a negligible physiologic dead space exists in the healthy lung.

Physiologic dead space can increase to 50% of resting tidal volume. This occurs with (1) inadequate perfusion during hemorrhage or blockage of the pulmonary circulation from an embolism or blood clot, or (2) inadequate alveolar ventilation in chronic pulmonary disease. *Adequate gas exchange and aeration of blood become impossible when the lung's total dead space exceeds 60% of lung volume.*

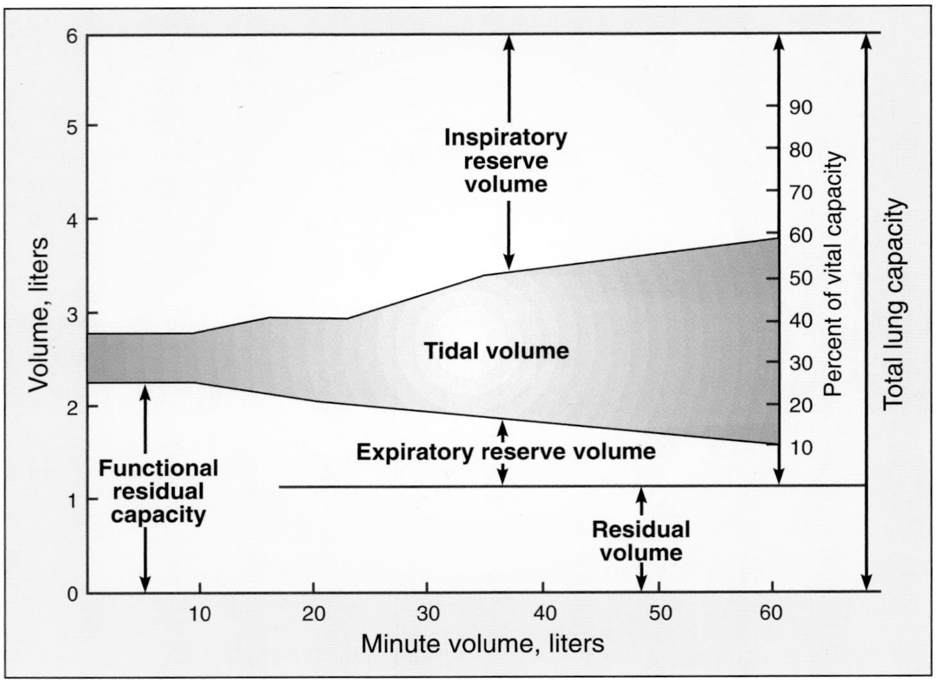

Depth Versus Rate

Increases in breathing rate and depth maintain alveolar ventilation during increasing exercise intensities. In moderate exercise, trained endurance athletes achieve adequate alveolar ventilation by increasing tidal volume and only minimally increasing breathing rate. With deeper breathing, alveolar ventilation usually increases from 70% of minute ventilation at rest to over 85% of total ventilation in exercise. *This increase occurs because deeper breathing causes a greater percentage of the incoming tidal volume to enter the alveoli.*

Figure 10.7 shows that the in-

Figure 10.7
Tidal volume and subdivisions of pulmonary air during rest and exercise.

close up

Exercise-Induced Asthma

Asthma, a chronic, obstructive respiratory disease, affects 12 million Americans, mostly children. A high fitness level does not confer immunity from this ailment. About 11% of U.S. athletes in the 1984 Olympic Games had asthma. Hyperirritability of the pulmonary airways, usually manifested by coughing, wheezing, and shortness of breath, characterizes an asthmatic condition.

With exercise, catecholamines released from the sympathetic nervous system produce a relaxation effect on smooth muscle that lines the pulmonary airways. Everyone experiences initial bronchodilation with exercise. For the asthmatic, however, bronchospasm and excessive mucus secretion follow normal bronchodilation. An acute episode of airway obstruction often appears 10 minutes after exercise; recovery usually occurs spontaneously within 30 to 90 minutes. One technique for diagnosing **exercise-induced asthma (EIA)** utilizes progressive increments of exercise on a treadmill or bicycle egometer. During a 10- to 20-minute recovery after each exercise bout, a spirometer evaluates $FEV_{1.0}/FVC$. *A 15% reduction in pre-exercise values confirms the diagnosis of EIA.*

Sensitivity to Thermal Gradients

An attractive theory to explain EIA relates to the rate and magnitude of alterations in pulmonary heat exchange as ventilation increases in exercise. As the incoming breath of air moves down the pulmonary pathways, heat and water transfer from the respiratory tract as air warms and humidifies. This form of "air-conditioning" cools and dries the respiratory mucosa; an abrupt airway rewarming occurs during recovery. The thermal gradient from cooling and subsequent rewarming (and loss of water from mucosal tissue) stimulates the release of proinflammatory chemical mediators that cause bronchospasm.

Exercise-Induced Asthma

☑ Choose appropriate type and duration of exercise

☑ Use adequate pre-exercise warm-up

☑ Reduce respiratory heat and water loss as much as possible

☑ Use medical therapy (if necessary)

Environment Makes a Difference

Exercising in a humid environment, regardless of ambient air temperature, blunts the EIA response. This is perplexing because conventional belief maintains that a dry climate best suits the asthmatic. In fact, inhaling ambient air fully saturated with water vapor in exercising patients totally abolished the bronchospastic response. This also explains why asthmatics tolerate walking or jogging on a warm, humid day or swimming in an indoor pool, whereas outdoor winter sports usually trigger an asthmatic attack. An asthmatic should perform 15 to 30 minutes of continuous warm-up because it initiates a **"refractory period"** that minimizes the severity of a bronchoconstrictive response during subsequent, more intense exercise.

In the future, researchers may better understand additional factors related to EIA. Physicians would then be able to "prescribe" an optimum environment and exercise intensity so asthmatics could benefit physically and psychologically from regular exercise. Currently, medications offer considerable relief from bronchoconstriction for individuals who want to exercise on a regular basis without affecting their performance. Exercise training cannot "cure" the asthmatic condition, but it can increase airway reserve and reduce the work of breathing during physical activity.

---

crease in tidal volume in exercise results largely from encroachment on inspiratory reserve volume, with an accompanying but smaller decrease in end-expiratory level. As exercise becomes more intense, tidal volume begins to plateau at about 60% of vital capacity; further increases in minute ventilation result from increasing breathing rate. Ventilatory adjustments occur unconsciously; each individual develops a "style" of breathing by blending breathing rate and tidal volume so alveolar ventilation matches alveolar perfusion. *Conscious attempts to modify breathing during general physical activities like running do not benefit exercise performance. In fact, conscious manipulation of breathing detracts from the exquisitely regulated ventilatory adjustments to exercise.* During rest and exercise, each individual should breathe in the manner that seems most natural.

Disruptions in Normal Breathing Patterns

Breathing patterns during exercise generally progress in an effective and highly economical manner, yet some pulmonary responses negatively impact exercise performance.

Dyspnea

Dyspnea refers to shortness of breath or subjective distress in breathing. The sense of the inability to breathe during exercise, particularly in novice exercisers, usually accompanies significantly elevated arterial carbon dioxide and [H+]. Both chemicals excite the inspiratory center to increase breathing rate and depth. Failure to adequately regulate arterial carbon dioxide and [H+] most likely relates to low aerobic fitness levels, and a poorly conditioned ventilatory musculature. The strong neural drive to breathe during exercise causes poorly conditioned respiratory muscles to fatigue, disrupting normal plasma levels of carbon dioxide and [H+]. This produces an accelerated pattern of shallow, ineffective breathing, and the individual senses an inability to breathe sufficient air.

Hyperventilation

Hyperventilation refers to an increase in pulmonary ventilation that exceeds the oxygen needs of metabolism. The "overbreathing" quickly lowers normal alveolar carbon dioxide concentration, causing excess carbon dioxide to leave body fluids via the expired air. An accompanying decrease in [H+] causes increases in plasma pH. Several seconds of hyperventilation generally produces lightheadedness; prolonged hyperventilation may lead to unconsciousness from excessive carbon dioxide unloading (see page 252).

Valsalva Maneuver

During quiet breathing, the pressure within the airways and alveoli (**intrapulmonic pressure**) decreases only 2 or 3 mm Hg below atmospheric pressure during the inspiratory cycle, while exhalation produces a similar pressure increase. However, closing the glottis following a full inspiration and then activating the expiratory muscles causes the compressive forces of exhalation to increase considerably. Maximal exhalation force against a closed glottis can increase pressure within the thoracic cavity (**intrathoracic pressure**) by more than 150 mm Hg above atmospheric pressure, with somewhat higher pressures within the abdominal cavity. A **Valsalva maneuver** describes a forced exhalation against a closed glottis. This occurs commonly in weightlifting and other activities requiring a rapid, maximum application of force for short duration. The fixation of the abdominal and thoracic cavities with this maneuver optimizes the force-generating capacity of muscles attached to the chest.

Physiologic Consequences. With the onset of a Valsalva maneuver (as often occurs in straining-type exercises; Fig. 10.8), blood pressure briefly rises abruptly as elevated intrathoracic pressure forces blood from the heart into the arterial system. At the same time, the inferior vena

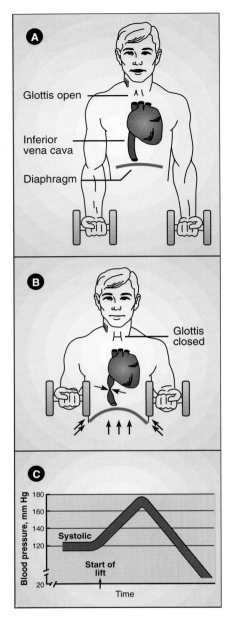

Figure 10.8
Valsalva maneuver impedes blood return to the heart because the increase in intrathoracic pressure collapses the vein (inferior vena cava) that passes through the abdominal and thoracic cavities. **A,** Normal breathing. **B,** Straining exercise with an accompanying Valsalva maneuver. **C,** Blood pressure response before and during straining-type (lifting) exercise.

cava becomes compressed because pressure within the thoracic and abdominal cavities exceed the relatively low pressures within the venous system. This significantly reduces blood flow into the heart (venous return). Reduced venous return and subsequent *fall in* arterial blood pressure can diminish the brain's blood supply, producing dizziness, "spots before the eyes," and even fainting. Normal blood flow re-establishes (with perhaps even an "overshoot") once the glottis opens and intrathoracic pressure decreases.

summary

1. The lungs provide a large interface between the body's internal fluid environment and the gaseous external environment. Probably no more than 1 pint of blood flows in the pulmonary capillaries during any 1 second.

2. Adjustments in pulmonary ventilation maintain favorable concentrations of alveolar oxygen and carbon dioxide to ensure adequate aeration of blood flowing through the lungs.

3. Pulmonary airflow depends on small pressure differences between ambient air and air within the lungs. The action of muscles that alter the dimensions of the thoracic cavity produces these pressure differences.

4. Lung volumes vary with age, gender, and body size, especially stature; they should be evaluated only in relation to norms based on these variables.

5. Tidal volume increases during exercise by encroachment on inspiratory and expiratory reserve volumes.

6. When a person breathes to vital capacity, air still remains in the lungs at maximal exhalation (residual lung volume). This allows for uninterrupted exchange of gas during all phases of the breathing cycle.

7. Forced expiratory volume in 1 second and maximum voluntary ventilation provide a dynamic picture of one's ability to sustain high airflow levels. They serve as excellent screening tests to detect lung disease.

8. Minute ventilation depends on breathing rate and tidal volume. It averages about 6 L at rest. In maximum exercise, increases in breathing rate and tidal volume produce ventilations as high as $200 \ L \cdot min^{-1}$ in large, endurance-trained individuals.

9. Alveolar ventilation represents the portion of minute ventilation entering the alveoli for gaseous exchange with the blood.

10. Healthy people have their own unique breathing styles during rest and exercise. Conscious attempts to modify breathing pattern during aerobic exercise confer no physiologic or performance benefits.

11. Disruptions in normal breathing patterns during exercise include dyspnea (shortness of breath), hyperventilation (overbreathing), and a Valsalva maneuver (forcefully trying to exhale against a closed glottis). A Valsalva maneuver generates a large pressure increase within the thoracic and abdominal cavities, which compresses the inferior vena cava and reduces venous return to the heart.

12. Exercise-induced asthma (EIA) is a relatively common obstructive lung disorder associated with the rate and magnitude of airway cooling (and drying) and subsequent rewarming. Breathing humidified air during exercise essentially eliminates EIA.

PART 2
Gas Exchange

Respired Gases: Concentrations and Partial Pressures

O ur oxygen supply depends on the oxygen concentration in ambient (atmospheric) air and its pressure. Ambient air composition remains relatively constant; 20.93% oxygen, 79.04% nitrogen (includes small quantities of inert gases that behave physiologically like nitrogen), 0.03% carbon dioxide, and usually small quantities of water vapor. The gas molecules move at great speeds and exert a pressure against any surface they contact. At sea level, the pressure of air's gas molecules raises a column of mercury to an average height of 760 mm (29.9 in). This barometric reading varies somewhat with changing weather conditions and decreases predictably at increased altitude.

G as concentration should not be confused with gas pressure:

- Gas concentration reflects the amount of gas in a given volume—determined by the product of the gas' partial pressure and solubility.

- Gas pressure represents the force exerted by the gas molecules against the surfaces they encounter.

- A mixture's total pressure equals the sum of the **partial pressures** of the individual gases.

Partial pressure computes as:

**Partial Pressure = Percent concentration ×
Total pressure of gas mixture**

TABLE 10.2
Percentages, partial pressures, and volumes of gases in 1 liter of dry ambient air at sea level

GAS	PERCENTAGE	PARTIAL PRESSURE (AT 760 mm Hg)	VOLUME OF GAS (mL · L^{-1})
Oxygen	20.93	159 mm Hg	209.3
Carbon dioxide	0.03	0.2 mm Hg	0.4
Nitrogen	79.04[a]	600 mm Hg	790.3

[a] Includes 0.93% argon and other trace rare gases.

Ambient Air

Table 10.2 presents the percentages, partial pressures, and volumes of the specific gases in 1 liter of dry, ambient air at sea level. The partial pressure of oxygen equals 20.93% of the total 760 mm Hg pressure exerted by the air mixture, or 159 mm Hg (0.2093×760 mm Hg); the random movement of the minute quantity of carbon dioxide exerts a pressure of only 0.2 mm Hg (0.0003×760 mm Hg), while nitrogen molecules exert a pressure that raises the mercury in a manometer about 600 mm (0.7904×760 mm Hg). The letter P before the gas symbol denotes partial pressure. For sea level ambient air: $P_{O_2} = 159$ mm Hg; $P_{CO_2} = 0.2$ mm Hg; $P_{N_2} = 600$ mm Hg.

Tracheal Air

Air entering the nose and mouth passes down the respiratory tract; it completely saturates with water vapor to slightly dilute the inspired air mixture. At body temperature, for example, the pressure of water molecules in humidified air equals 47 mm Hg; this leaves 713 mm Hg ($760 - 47$) as the total pressure exerted by the inspired dry air molecules at sea level. This makes the effective P_{O_2} in tracheal air decrease by about 10 mm Hg from its dry ambient value of 159 mm Hg to 149 mm Hg ($0.2093 \times [760 - 47$ mm Hg]). Humidification has little effect on inspired P_{CO_2} because of carbon dioxide's almost negligible concentration in inspired air.

Alveolar Air

Alveolar air composition differs considerably from the incoming breath of ambient air because carbon dioxide continually enters the alveoli from the blood, whereas oxygen leaves the lungs for transport throughout the body. Table 10.3 shows that moist alveolar air contains approximately 14.5% oxygen, 5.5% carbon dioxide, and 80.0% nitrogen.

After subtracting vapor pressure in moist alveolar gas, the average alveolar P_{O_2} equals 103 mm Hg ($0.145 \times [760 - 47$ mm Hg]) and 39 mm Hg ($0.055 \times [760 - 47$ mm Hg]) for P_{CO_2}. These values represent the average pressures exerted by oxygen and carbon dioxide molecules against the alveolar side of the respiratory membrane. They do not exist as physiologic constants, but vary slightly with the phase of the ventilatory cycle and adequacy of ventilation in different lung segments.

Movement of Gas in Air and Fluids

Knowledge of how gases act in air and fluids allows us to understand the mechanism for gas movement between the external environment and the body's tissues. In accord with **Henry's law**, the amount of a gas dissolved in a fluid depends on two factors:

TABLE 10.3
Percentages, partial pressures, and volumes of gases in 1 liter of moist alveolar air at sea level

GAS	PERCENTAGE	PARTIAL PRESSURE (AT 760–47 mm Hg)	VOLUME OF GAS (mL · L^{-1})
Oxygen	14.5	103 mm Hg	145
Carbon dioxide	5.5	39 mm Hg	55
Nitrogen	80.0	571 mm Hg	800
Water Vapor		47 mm Hg	

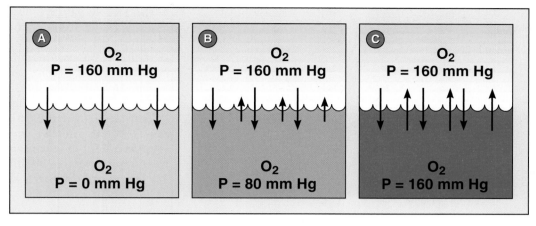

Figure 10.9
Solution of oxygen in water: **A,** When oxygen first comes in contact with pure water **B,** dissolved oxygen halfway to equilibrium with gaseous oxygen **C,** equilibrium established between the oxygen in air and oxygen dissolved in water.

1. Pressure differential between the gas above the fluid and the gas dissolved in the fluid
2. Solubility of the gas in the fluid

Pressure

Figure 10.9 shows three examples of gas movement between air and fluid. Oxygen molecules continually strike the water surface in each of the three chambers. Because the pure water in container A contains no oxygen, a large number of oxygen molecules dissolve in water. Some oxygen molecules also leave the water because the dissolved molecules move continuously in random motion. In chamber B, the pressure gradient between air and water still favors oxygen's net movement (diffusion) into the fluid from the gaseous state, but the quantity of additional oxygen dissolving in the fluid remains less than in chamber A. Eventually, the pressures for gas movement attain equilibrium, and the number of molecules entering and leaving the fluid equalize (chamber C). Conversely, if the pressure of dissolved oxygen molecules exceeds the air's oxygen pressure, oxygen leaves the fluid until it reaches a new pressure equilibrium. These examples illustrate that the net diffusion of a gas occurs only when a *difference* exists in gas pressure. A specific gas' partial pressure gradient represents the driving force for its diffusion in the body. In a similar fashion, the concentration gradient provides the driving force for diffusion of nongaseous molecules (e.g., glucose, sodium, and calcium).

Solubility

Gas solubility reflects the quantity of a gas dissolved in fluid at a particular pressure. A gas with greater solubility has a higher concentration at a particular partial pressure. For two different gases at identical pressure differentials, the solubility of each gas determines the number of molecules moving into or out of a fluid. *For each unit of pressure favoring diffusion, approximately 25 times more carbon dioxide than oxygen moves into (or from) a fluid.*

Viewed somewhat differently, equal quantities of oxygen and carbon dioxide enter or leave a fluid under significantly different pressure gradients for each gas (precisely what occurs in the body).

Gas Exchange in the Body

The exchange of gases between the lungs and blood, and their movement at the tissue level, takes place passively by diffusion. Figure 10.10 illustrates the pressure gradients favoring gas transfer in the body.

Gas Exchange in the Lungs

The first step in oxygen transport involves the transfer of oxygen from the alveoli into the blood. Three reasons account for the dilution of oxygen in inspired air as it passes into the alveolar chambers:

1. Water vapor saturates relatively dry inspired air
2. Oxygen continually leaves alveolar air
3. Carbon dioxide continually enters alveolar air

As a result, alveolar P_{O_2} averages about 100 mm Hg, a value considerably below the 159 mm Hg in ambient air. Despite this reduction in P_{O_2}, the pressure of oxygen molecules in alveolar air still averages about 60 mm Hg higher than the P_{O_2} in venous blood entering the pulmonary capillaries. Consequently, oxygen diffuses through the alveolar membrane into the blood. Carbon dioxide exists under slightly greater pressure in returning venous blood than in the alveoli, causing diffusion of carbon dioxide from the blood into the lungs. Although only a small pressure gradient of 6 mm Hg exists for carbon dioxide diffusion compared with oxygen, adequate carbon dioxide transfer occurs rapidly because of carbon dioxide's high solubility. Nitrogen, an inert gas in metabolism, remains essentially unchanged in alveolar-capillary gas.

Gas Exchange Occurs Rapidly

Diffusion in a healthy lung occurs so rapidly that blood gas and alveolar gas equilibrate in less than 1 second, equal to the midpoint of the blood's transit through the pulmonary vasculature.

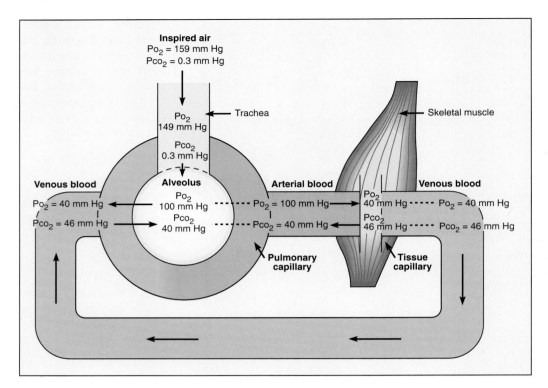

Figure 10.10

Pressure gradients for gas transfer in the body at rest, and the P_{O_2} and P_{CO_2} of ambient, tracheal, and alveolar air and these gas pressures in venous and arterial blood and muscle. Gases always diffuse at the alveolar-capillary and tissue-capillary membranes from an area of higher partial pressure to lower partial pressure.

Physiologic Adjustments Limit Blood-Flow Velocity

For most individuals who perform intense exercise, the velocity of blood flowing through the pulmonary capillaries does not exceed the speed at rest by more than 50%. This occurs despite a four- to six-fold increase in total blood flow (cardiac output) through the lungs. With increasing exercise intensity, dilation of pulmonary capillaries and opening of dormant vascular channels increase the volume of blood within the alveolar circulation by about three times

the resting value. These adjustments reduce the demand for blood flow velocity to accommodate the increased exercise cardiac output. *Thus, blood leaving the lungs for transport throughout the body in vigorous exercise contains oxygen at a pressure of approximately 100 mm Hg and carbon dioxide at 40 mm Hg.*

Gas Exchange in Tissues

In the tissues, where energy metabolism consumes oxygen at a rate almost equal to carbon dioxide production, gas pressures differ considerably from arterial blood (see Fig. 10.10). At rest, the average P_{O_2} within the muscle rarely drops below 40 mm Hg, while intracellular P_{CO_2} averages about 46 mm Hg. In contrast, vigorous exercise can reduce the pressure of

oxygen molecules in muscle tissue to 3 mm Hg, whereas the pressure of carbon dioxide approaches 90 mm Hg. The pressure differential between gases in plasma and tissues establishes the gradient for diffusion—oxygen leaves capillary blood and diffuses toward metabolizing cells, while carbon dioxide flows from the cell into the blood. Blood then enters the veins and returns to the heart for delivery to the lungs. Diffusion rapidly begins once again as venous blood enters the dense capillary network of the lungs.

summary

1. The partial pressure of a specific gas in a gas mixture varies proportionally to (a) the gas' concentration in the mixture, and (b) the total pressure exerted by the mixture.

2. Pressure and solubility determine the quantity of gas that dissolves in a fluid. Because of carbon dioxide's 25-times greater solubility than oxygen, in plasma, large numbers of carbon dioxide molecules move in body fluids down relatively small pressure (diffusion) gradients.

3. Gas molecules diffuse in the lungs and tissues down their concentration gradients from higher concentration (higher pressure) to lower concentration (lower pressure).

4. Alveolar ventilation adjusts during intense exercise so the composition of alveolar gas remains similar to resting conditions. Alveolar and arterial oxygen pressures equal about 100 mm Hg, while

carbon dioxide pressure remains at 40 mm Hg. Because venous blood contains oxygen at lower, and carbon dioxide at higher pressures than alveolar gas, oxygen diffuses into the blood and carbon dioxide diffuses into the lungs.

5. Gas exchange takes place so rapidly in a healthy lung that equilibrium occurs at about the midpoint of the blood's transit through the pulmonary circuit. Pulmonary blood flow velocity generally does not restrict complete loading of oxygen and unloading of carbon dioxide. Even with the most vigorous exercise.

6. Diffusion gradients in the tissues favor oxygen movement from the capillaries to the tissues and carbon dioxide from the cells to the blood. Exercise causes these gradients to expand, making oxygen and carbon dioxide diffuse rapidly.

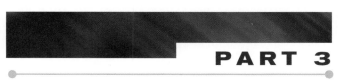

PART 3
Oxygen and Carbon Dioxide Transport

Oxygen Transport in the Blood

The blood transports oxygen in two ways:

1. **In physical solution** — dissolved in the fluid portion of the blood
2. **Combined with hemoglobin**—in loose combination with the iron-protein hemoglobin molecule in the red blood cell

Oxygen Transport in Physical Solution

Oxygen does not dissolve readily in fluids. At an alveolar PO_2 of 100 mm Hg, only about 0.3 mL of gaseous oxygen dissolves in the plasma of each 100 mL of blood (3 $mL \cdot L^{-1}$). Because the average adult's total blood volume equals about 5 liters, 15 mL of oxygen dissolves for transport in the fluid portion of the blood (3 $mL \cdot L^{-1} \times 5 = 15$ mL). This amount of oxygen could sustain life for only about 4 seconds. Viewed from a different perspective, the body would need to circulate 80 liters of blood each minute just to supply the resting oxygen requirements if oxygen were transported only in physical solution. This represents a blood flow two times higher than the maximum ever recorded for an exercising human.

Despite its limited quantity, oxygen transported in physical solution serves several important physiologic functions. The random movement of dissolved oxygen molecules establishes the PO_2 of the blood and tissue flu-

ids, which helps to regulate breathing, and determines the magnitude that hemoglobin loads with oxygen in the lungs and unloads it in the tissues.

Oxygen Combined with Hemoglobin

The blood of many animal species contains a metallic compound to augment its oxygen-carrying capacity. In humans, the iron-containing protein pigment hemoglobin constitutes the main component of the body's 25 trillion red blood cells. *Hemoglobin increases the blood's oxygen-carrying capacity 65 to 70 times above that normally dissolved in plasma.* Thus, for each liter of blood, hemoglobin temporarily "captures" about 197 mL of oxygen. Each of the four iron atoms in a hemoglobin (Hb) molecule loosely binds one molecule of oxygen to form oxyhemoglobin in the reversible **oxygenation reaction**:

$$Hb + 4\,O_2 \rightarrow Hb_4O_8$$

This reaction requires no enzymes; it progresses without a change in the valance of Fe^{++}, as occurs in the more permanent process of oxidation. *The partial pressure of oxygen in solution solely determines the oxygenation of hemoglobin to oxyhemoglobin.*

Oxygen-Carrying Capacity of Hemoglobin

In men, each 100 mL of blood contains approximately 15 to 16 g of Hb. The value averages 5 to 10% less for women, or about 14 g per 100 mL of blood. The gender difference in Hb concentration contributes to the lower aerobic capacity of women, even after adjusting statistically for gender-related differences in body mass and body fat.

Each gram of Hb can combine loosely with 1.34 mL of oxygen. Thus, we can calculate oxygen-carrying capacity of the blood from Hb concentration as follows:

Oxygen-carrying capacity = Hb (g · 100 mL blood^{-1}) × Oxygen capacity of Hb

If the blood's Hb concentration equals 15 g, then approximately 20 mL of oxygen (15 g per 100 mL × 1.34 mL

= 20.1) combine with the Hb in each 100 mL of blood if Hb achieved full oxygen saturation (i.e., if all Hb existed as Hb_4O_8).

Po_2 and Hemoglobin Saturation

Thus far, the discussion of the blood's oxygen-carrying capacity assumes that Hb achieves full saturation with oxygen when exposed to alveolar gas. Figure 10.11A shows the relationship between percent Hg saturation of Hb (left vertical axis) at various Po_2s under normal resting physiologic conditions (arterial pH 7.4, 37°C) and the effects of changes in pH (Fig. 10.11B) and temperature (Fig. 10.11C) Hb's affinity for oxygen. Percent saturation of Hb computes as follows:

Percent saturation = (Total O_2 combined with Hb ÷ Oxygen carrying capacity of Hb) × 100

This curve, termed the **oxyhemoglobin dissociation curve**, also quantifies the amount of oxygen carried in each 100 mL of normal blood in relation to plasma Po_2 (right vertical axis, Fig. 10.11A). For example, at a Po_2 of 90 mm Hg (95% Hb saturation) the normal complement of Hb in 100 mL of blood carries about 19 mL of oxygen; at 40 mm Hg (75% Hb saturation) the oxygen quantity decreases to about 15 mL, and slightly more than 2 mL at a Po_2 of 10 mm Hg. These values indicate that at relatively low partial pressures at the capillary-tissue membrane, oxygen readily dissociates (unloads) from Hb for use by the cell.

Po_2 in the Lungs

At the alveolar-capillary Po_2 of 100 mm Hg, Hb remains 98% saturated with oxygen; under these conditions the Hb in each 100 mL of blood contains about 19.7 mL of oxygen. Any additional increase in alveolar Po_2 contributes little to how much oxygen can combine with Hb. In addition to oxygen bound to Hb, each 100 mL of plasma in arterial blood contains about 0.3 mL of oxygen in solution. For healthy individuals who breathe ambient air at sea level, 100 mL of arterial blood carries 20.0 mL of oxygen (19.7 mL bound to Hb and 0.3 mL dissolved in plasma). Figure

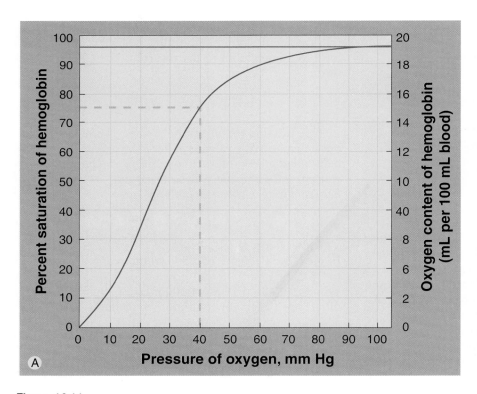
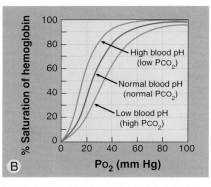
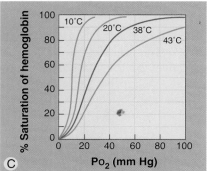

Figure 10.11
A, Oxyhemoglobin dissociation curve under physiologic conditions at rest (arterial pH 7.4, tissue temperature 37°C). The right vertical axis shows the quantity of oxygen combined with Hb in each 100 mL of blood. The bold horizontal red line indicates Hb's percent saturation at sea-level alveolar Po_2. The dashed orange line shows percent saturation at a Po_2 of 40 mm Hg (tissue and venous blood). **B,** Effects of changes in pH ([H^+]) on hemoglobin's affinity for oxygen. **C,** Effects of changes in temperature on hemoglobin's affinity for oxygen.

10.12 illustrates the percentage composition of centrifuged whole blood for red blood cells (**hematocrit**) and plasma, including representative values for oxygen carried in each component at a P_{O_2} of 100 mm Hg.

Careful examination of Figure 10.11A shows that Hb saturation changes little until oxygen pressure decreases to about 60 mm Hg. This relatively flat upper portion of the oxyhemoglobin dissociation curve provides a margin of safety to ensure near full loading of Hb despite relatively large decreases in alveolar P_{O_2}. Alveolar P_{O_2} reduction to 75 mm Hg (as occurs in certain lung diseases or when one travels to a moderate altitude) only decreases Hb saturation by about 6%. In contrast, when P_{O_2} drops below 60 mm Hg, a sharp decrease occurs in how much oxygen combines with Hb.

Tissue P_{O_2}

The P_{O_2} in the cell fluids at rest averages 40 mm Hg. Thus, dissolved oxygen in arterial plasma (P_{O_2} = 100 mm Hg) readily diffuses across the capillary membrane through tissue fluids into cells. This reduces plasma P_{O_2} below that in the red blood cell, causing Hb to release its oxygen ($HbO_2 \rightarrow Hb + O_2$). The oxygen then moves from the blood cells through the capillary membrane into the tissues.

At the tissue-capillary P_{O_2} of 40 mm Hg at rest, Hb holds about 75% of its total capacity for oxygen (see dashed orange line, Fig. 10.11A). Therefore, each 100 mL of

blood leaving the tissues carries only 15 mL of oxygen; nearly 5 mL has been released to the cells for energy metabolism. The **arteriovenous-oxygen difference (a-v O$_2$ difference)** describes the difference in oxygen content between arterial and venous blood (expressed in mL per 100 mL blood).

The a-v O_2 difference in most tissues at rest averages 5 mL. The large quantity of oxygen still remaining with Hb provides an "automatic" reserve for cells to immediately obtain oxygen should oxygen demands suddenly increase. As the cell's need for oxygen increases with any exercise above rest, tissue P_{O_2} rapidly decreases, forcing Hb to release greater quantities of oxygen to meet the exercise metabolic requirements. In vigorous exercise, tissue P_{O_2} decreases to about 15 mm Hg, and Hb retains only about 5 mL of oxygen. This expands the tissue a-v O_2 difference to 15 mL of oxygen per 100 mL of blood. When active muscles' P_{O_2} decreases to 3 mm Hg during exhaustive exercise, Hb releases virtually all of its remaining oxygen to the active tissues. Even without any increase in local blood flow, the amount of oxygen released to active muscle increases almost three times above that normally supplied at rest. It accomplishes this by a more complete unloading of Hb.

Bohr Effect

Figures 10.11B and 10.11C show that increases in acidity (H^+ concentration and CO_2) and temperature cause the oxyhemoglobin dissociation curve to shift significantly downward and to the right (enhanced unloading), particularly in the P_{O_2} range of 20 to 50 mm Hg. This phenomenon, known as the **Bohr effect** (named after its discoverer Danish physiologist Christian Bohr, 1855–1911), results from alterations in hemoglobin's molecular structure (altered state of Fe^{++} decreases its diameter).

The existence of the Bohr effect becomes important in vigorous exercise because increased metabolic heat and acidity in active tissues augments oxygen release. For example, at a P_{O_2} of 20 mm Hg and normal body temperature (37°C), percent saturation of Hb with oxygen equals 35%. At the same P_{O_2}, but with body temperature increased to 43°C (a temperature often recorded at the end of a marathon run), Hb's percent saturation decreases to about 23%. This means that more oxygen unloads from Hb for use in cellular metabolism. Similar effects take place with increased acidity during intense exercise. The lack of a negligible Bohr effect in pulmonary capillary blood at normal alveolar P_{O_2} means that Hb becomes fully loaded with oxygen as blood passes through the lungs, even during maximal exercise.

The compound **2,3-diphosphoglycerate (2,3-DPG)**, the anaerobic metabolite produced in red blood cells during glycolysis, also affects Hb's affinity for oxygen. 2,3-DPG facilitates oxygen dissociation by combining with

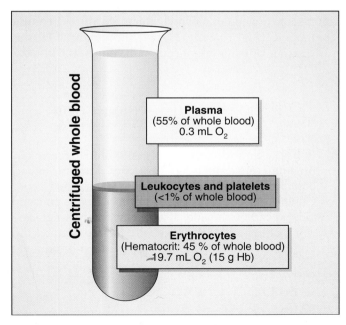

Figure 10.12
Major components of whole blood, including the quantity of oxygen carried in each 100 mL of blood (Hb = hemoglobin).

subunits of Hb to reduce its affinity for oxygen. Individuals with cardiopulmonary disease and inhabitants of high altitudes have increased levels of this metabolic intermediate. Elevated 2,3-DPG for these individuals represents a compensatory adjustment to facilitate oxygen release to the cell. In general, adaptations in 2,3-DPG occur relatively slowly compared with the immediate Bohr effect from increased temperature, acidity, and carbon dioxide. Research has yet to determine the exact effect of acute sea-level exercise (at different intensities) and chronic training on 2,3-DPG levels.

Myoglobin and Muscle Oxygen Storage

Skeletal and cardiac muscle contain the iron-protein compound **myoglobin**. Like Hb, myoglobin combines reversibly with oxygen; however, each myoglobin molecule contains only one iron atom in contrast to Hb that contains four atoms. Myoglobin adds additional oxygen to the muscle in the following reaction:

$$Mb \rightarrow MbO_2$$

Aside from its function as an "extra" source of oxygen in muscle, myoglobin facilitates oxygen transfer to the mitochondria, notably at the start of exercise and during intense exercise when cellular P_{O_2} decreases considerably. Figure 10.13 shows that the dissociation curve for myoglobin forms a rectangular hyperbola, not the s-shaped curve like that for Hb. This makes myoglobin bind and retain oxygen at low pressures much more readily than Hb. During rest and moderate exercise (when

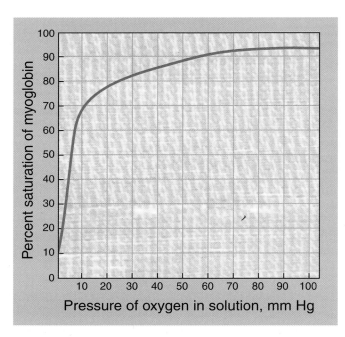

Figure 10.13
Oxymyoglobin dissociation curve.

cellular P_{O_2} remains relatively high), myoglobin remains highly saturated with oxygen. At a P_{O_2} of 40 mm Hg, for example, myoglobin retains 85% of its oxygen. MbO_2 releases its greatest quantity of oxygen when tissue P_{O_2} decreases to less than 10 mm Hg. Unlike Hb, myoglobin does not exhibit a Bohr effect.

Carbon Dioxide Transport in Blood

Once carbon dioxide forms in cells, diffusion and transport to the lungs in venous blood provides its only means for "escape." Figure 10.14 illustrates that blood transports carbon dioxide to the lungs in three ways:

1. In physical solution in plasma (7-10%)
2. In loose combination with Hb (20%)
3. Combined with water as bicarbonate (70%)

Carbon Dioxide in Solution

Plasma transports approximately 7% of carbon dioxide produced in energy metabolism as free carbon dioxide in solution (Fig. 10.14A). The random movement of this relatively small quantity of dissolved carbon dioxide molecules establishes the P_{CO_2} of the blood.

Carbon Dioxide as Carbamino Compounds

About 20% of carbon dioxide reacts directly with the amino acid molecules of blood proteins to form carbamino compounds (Fig. 10.14B). The globin portion of Hb carries a significant amount of carbon dioxide in the blood as follows:

$$CO_2 + HbNH \longrightarrow HbNHCOOH$$
$$\text{Hemoglobin} \qquad \text{Carbaminohemoglobin}$$

Formation of carbamino compounds reverses in the lungs as plasma P_{CO_2} decreases. This moves carbon dioxide into solution for diffusion into the alveoli. Concurrently, Hb's oxygenation reduces its capacity to bind carbon dioxide. The interaction between oxygen loading and carbon dioxide release, termed the **Haldane effect,** facilitates carbon dioxide removal from the lungs.

Carbon Dioxide as Bicarbonate

The major portion of carbon dioxide in solution combines with water to form carbonic acid (Fig. 10.14C).

$$CO_2 + H_2O \rightleftarrows H_2CO_3$$

A CO₂ dissolved in plasma

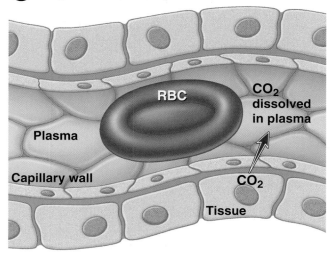

B CO₂ chemically bound to hemoglobin

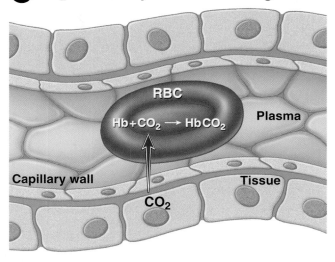

C CO₂ combined with water as bicarbonate

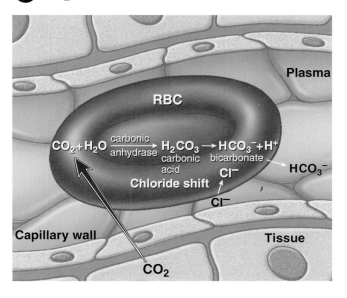

Because of the relatively slow rate of the reaction, little carbon dioxide would transport in this form without **carbonic anhydrase**, a zinc-containing enzyme within red blood cells. This catalyst accelerates the interaction of carbon dioxide and water about 5000 times.

In the Tissues. Once carbonic acid forms in the tissues, most of it ionizes to hydrogen ions (H^+) and bicarbonate ions (HCO_3^-) as follows:

$$CO_2 + H_2O \xrightarrow{\text{Carbonic anhydrase}} H_2CO_3 \rightarrow H^+ + HCO_3^-$$

The protein portion of the Hb molecule then buffers the H^+ to maintain blood pH within narrow limits. Because of bicarbonate's high solubility, it diffuses from the red blood cell into the plasma in exchange for a chloride ion (Cl^-), which then moves into the blood cell to maintain ionic equilibrium. The term **"chloride shift"** describes this exchange of Cl^- for HCO_3^-; it accounts for the higher Cl^- content of the erythrocytes in venous blood compared with arterial blood.

In the Lungs. *Plasma bicarbonate transports about 70% of the total carbon dioxide.* As tissue P_{CO_2} increases, carbonic acid forms rapidly. Conversely, in the lungs, carbon dioxide diffuses from the plasma into the alveoli; this lowers plasma P_{CO_2} and disturbs the equilibrium between carbonic acid and the formation of bicarbonate ions. As a result, H^+ and HCO_3^- recombine to form carbonic acid. In turn, carbon dioxide and water reform, and carbon dioxide exits through the lungs as follows:

$$H^+ + HCO_3^- \rightarrow H_2CO_3 \xrightarrow{\text{Carbonic anhydrase}} CO_2 + H_2O$$

Because plasma bicarbonate concentration decreases in the pulmonary capillaries, the Cl^- moves from the red blood cell back into plasma.

Figure 10.14
Carbon dioxide transport in blood. **A,** Physically dissolved in blood plasma. **B,** Chemically bound to hemoglobin (Hb). **C,** Combined with water as bicarbonate.

summary

1. Hemoglobin (Hb), the iron-protein pigment in red blood cells, increases oxygen-carrying capacity of whole blood about 65 times compared with the amount dissolved in physical solution in plasma.

2. The small quantity of oxygen dissolved in plasma exerts molecular movement and establishes the blood's P_{O_2}. Plasma P_{O_2} determines the loading of Hb at the lungs (oxygenation) and its unloading at the tissues (deoxygenation).

3. The blood's oxygen transport capacity changes only slightly with normal variations in Hb content. Gender differences in Hb concentration contribute to the lower aerobic capacity of women, even after adjusting for gender-related differences in body mass and body fat.

4. The s-shaped nature of the oxyhemoglobin dissociation curve dictates that Hb-oxygen saturation changes little until P_{O_2} decreases below 60 mm Hg. Because such low P_{O_2}s occur in the tissues, oxygen releases rapidly from capillary blood and flows into the cells to meet metabolic demands.

5. About 25% of the blood's total oxygen releases to the tissues at rest; the remaining 75% returns "unused" to the heart in the venous blood. This relatively small arteriovenous oxygen difference indicates that cells have an oxygen reserve if metabolic demands suddenly increase.

6. Increases in acidity, temperature, and carbon dioxide concentration alter hemoglobin's molecular structure, reducing its effectiveness to hold oxygen (Bohr effect). Because exercise accentuates these factors, oxygen release to tissues becomes further facilitated.

7. The iron-protein pigment myoglobin stores "extra" oxygen in skeletal and cardiac muscle. Myoglobin releases its oxygen only at a low P_{O_2}, thus facilitating oxygen transfer to the mitochondria during strenuous exercise.

8. About 7% of carbon dioxide dissolves as free carbon dioxide in plasma. This carbon dioxide in physical solution establishes the blood's P_{CO_2}.

9. About 20% of the body's carbon dioxide combines with blood proteins (including Hb), to form carbamino compounds.

10. Approximately 70% of carbon dioxide combines with water to form bicarbonate. This reaction reverses in the lungs, and carbon dioxide leaves the blood and moves into the alveoli.

PART 4

Regulation of Pulmonary Ventilation

Ventilatory Control

The body exquisitely regulates the rate and depth of breathing in response to metabolic needs. During all exercise intensities in healthy individuals, arterial pressures for oxygen and carbon dioxide, and pH remain essentially at resting values. Neural information from higher centers in the brain, from the lungs, and from mechanical and chemical sensors throughout the body regulate pulmonary ventilation. In addition, the gaseous and chemical state of the blood that bathes the brain (medulla) and the aortic and carotid chemoreceptors affect alveolar ventilation. Figure 10.15 lists the primary factors responsible for ventilatory control.

Neural Factors

The normal respiratory cycle comes from inherent, automatic activity of inspiratory neurons whose cell bodies reside in the **medial medulla**. The lungs inflate because neurons activate the diaphragm and intercostal muscles. The inspiratory neurons cease firing because of their own self-limitation, and inhibitory influence from the medulla's expiratory neurons. Stretch receptors in the bronchioles become stimulated when the lungs inflate. These receptors inhibit inspiration and stimulate expiration.

Exhalation begins by the passive recoil of the stretched lung tissue and raised ribs when the inspiratory muscles relax. Activation of expiratory neurons and associated muscles that further facilitate expiration becomes synchronized with this passive phase. As expiration proceeds, the inspiratory center is released once again from inhibition and progressively becomes active.

The respiratory center's inherent activity cannot fully account for the smooth pattern of breathing in response to the metabolic demands of exercise. Input from the hypothalamus modulates the overall ventilatory rhythm. This neural "command center" integrates input from descending neurons in the higher motor areas of the cerebral cortex, the pons, and other brain regions to affect the inspiratory cycle's duration and intensity. Concurrently, ascending neural signals from mechanical and/or chemi-

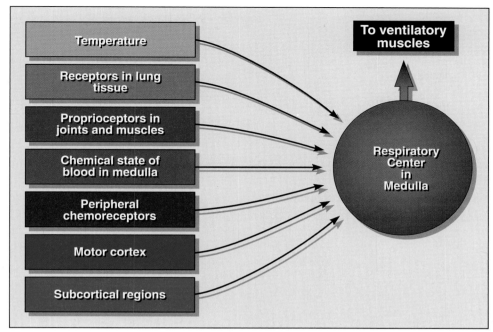

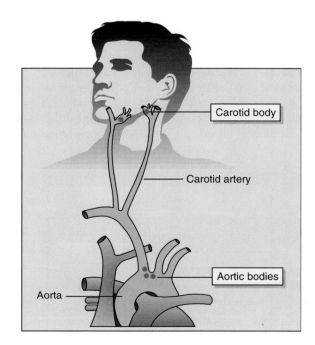

Figure 10.15
Primary factors affecting medullary control of pulmonary ventilation.

Peripheral chemoreceptors provide an "early warning system" to alert against reduced oxygen pressure, and also stimulate ventilation's response to increased carbon dioxide, temperature, acidity, a decrease in blood pressure, and perhaps a decrease in circulating potassium.

Plasma P_{CO_2} and H+ Concentration

Carbon dioxide pressure in arterial plasma provides the most important respiratory stimulus at rest. Small increases in the P_{CO_2} of inspired air stimulate the medulla and peripheral chemoreceptors to initiate large increases in minute ventilation. For example, resting ventilation almost doubles when inspired P_{CO_2} increases to just 1.7 mm Hg (0.22% CO_2 in inspired air).

cal changes in active muscles provide peripheral feedback (via the cerebellum) to the respiratory center to adjust ventilation to meet metabolic demands.

Humoral Factors

The chemical state of the blood largely regulates pulmonary ventilation at rest. Variations in arterial P_{O_2}, P_{CO_2}, acidity, and temperature activate sensitive neural units in the medulla and arterial system so ventilation adjusts to maintain arterial blood chemistry within narrow limits.

Plasma P_{O_2} and Chemoreceptors

Inhaling a gas mixture of 80% oxygen increases alveolar P_{O_2} and reduces minute ventilation by about 20%. Conversely, reducing inspired oxygen concentration increases minute ventilation, particularly if alveolar P_{O_2} falls below 60 mm Hg. Recall that at 60 mm Hg, Hb's oxygen saturation dramatically decreases. The point at which decreasing arterial P_{O_2} stimulates ventilation has been termed the **hypoxic threshold**; it usually occurs at an arterial P_{O_2} between 60 to 70 mm Hg.

Sensitivity to reduced arterial oxygen pressure (arterial hypoxia) results from stimulation of small structures located outside the central nervous system called **chemoreceptors**. Figure 10.16 shows these specialized neurons in the arch of the aorta (**arortic bodies**) and at the branching of the carotid arteries in the neck (**carotid bodies**). The carotid bodies, about 5 mm in diameter, maintain a strategic position to monitor the status of arterial blood just before it perfuses brain tissues. Nerves go from the carotid and aortic bodies to activate the brain's respiratory neurons.

Figure 10.16
Aortic and carotid cell bodies (sensitive to a reduced plasma P_{O_2}) located in the aortic arch and bifurcation of carotid arteries. These peripheral receptors defend against arterial hypoxia.

Immediate Defense at High Altitude

The decrease in arterial P_{O_2} at high altitude activates the aortic and carotid chemoreceptors to increase alveolar ventilation, thus increasing alveolar P_{O_2}. Chemoreceptors protect the organism against inspired air's reduced oxygen pressure.

Molecular carbon dioxide does not entirely account for its effect on ventilatory control. Recall that carbonic acid formed from carbon dioxide and water rapidly dissociates to bicarbonate ions and hydrogen ions. The increase in $[H^+]$ in the cerebrospinal fluid bathing the respiratory areas (which varies directly with the blood's CO_2 content) stimulates inspiratory activity. The resulting increase in ventilation eliminates carbon dioxide, which lowers arterial $[H^+]$.

Hyperventilation and Breath-Holding

If a person breath-holds after a normal exhalation, it takes about 40 seconds before breathing commences. This urge to breathe results mainly from the stimulating effects of increased arterial P_{CO_2} and $[H^+]$, and not from a decreased arterial P_{CO_2}. *The "break point" for breath-holding corresponds to an increase in arterial P_{CO_2} to about 50 mm Hg.*

If this same person consciously increased alveolar ventilation above the normal level before breath-holding, the composition of alveolar air would change and become more like ambient air. Alveolar P_{CO_2} with hyperventilation may decrease to 15 mm Hg, creating a considerable diffusion gradient for carbon dioxide run-off from venous blood entering

the pulmonary capillaries. Consequently, a larger than normal amount of carbon dioxide leaves the blood, decreasing arterial P_{CO_2} significantly below normal levels. Reduced arterial P_{CO_2} extends the breath-hold until the arterial P_{CO_2} and/or $[H^+]$ increase to a level that stimulates ventilation.

Swimmers and sport divers hyperventilate and breath-hold to improve physical performance. In sprint swimming, it is biomechanically undesirable to roll the body and turn the head during the breathing phase of the stroke. Swimmers hyperventilate on the starting blocks to prolong breath-hold time during the swim. The snorkel diver hyperventilates to extend breath-hold time, but often with tragic results. As the length and depth of the dive increase, the oxygen content of the blood can fall to critically low values before arterial P_{CO_2} increases to stimulate breathing and signal the need to ascend to the surface. Reduced arterial P_{O_2} can cause loss of consciousness before the diver reaches the surface (see Chapter 16 Close-up: *Breath-Hold Diving: Not Without its Dangers*).

Ventilatory Control in Exercise

Chemical Control

Chemical stimuli cannot fully explain the increased ventilation (**hyperpnea**) during physical activity. For example, manipulating arterial P_{O_2}, P_{CO_2}, and acidity does not increase minute ventilation nearly as much as vigorous exercise.

Arterial P_{O_2} in exercise does not decrease to the point that stimulates ventilation by chemoreceptor activation. In fact, large breathing volumes in vigorous exercise actually increase alveolar (and arterial) P_{O_2} above the average resting value of 100 mm Hg. Figure 10.17 illustrates the dynamics of venous and alveolar P_{CO_2} and alveolar P_{O_2} in relation to oxygen uptake during a graded exercise test. During light and

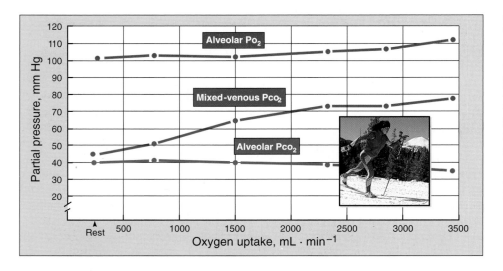

Figure 10.17
Values for P_{CO_2} in mixed-venous blood entering the lungs, and alveolar P_{O_2} and P_{CO_2} related to oxygen uptake during graded exercise. Despite increased metabolism with exercise, alveolar P_{O_2} and P_{CO_2} remain near resting levels. Increases in mixed-venous P_{CO_2} result from increased carbon dioxide production in metabolism. (Data from the Laboratory of Applied Physiology, Queens College.)

moderate exercise ($\dot{V}O_2$ = <2000 mL · min^{-1}), pulmonary ventilation closely couples to oxygen uptake and carbon dioxide production in a manner that maintains alveolar PO_2 at about 100 mm Hg and PCO_2 at 40 mm Hg. Increases in acidity (and subsequent increases in CO_2 and [H$^+$]) provide an additional ventilatory stimulus in strenuous exercise which reduces alveolar PCO_2 below 40 mm Hg and sometimes to as low as 25 mm Hg. This eliminates carbon dioxide and decreases arterial PCO_2. Concurrently, augmented ventilation slightly increases alveolar PO_2, which may facilitate oxygen loading.

Nonchemical Control

Ventilation increases so rapidly when exercise starts that it occurs almost within the first ventilatory cycle. A plateau lasting about 20 seconds follows this abrupt increase in ventilation; thereafter, minute ventilation gradually increases and approaches a steady level in relation to the demands for metabolic gas exchange. When exercise stops, ventilation decreases rapidly to a point about 40% of the final exercise value and then slowly returns to resting levels. The rapidity of the ventilatory response at the onset and cessation of exercise shows that input other than from changes in arterial PCO_2 and [H$^+$] mediate these components of exercise (and recovery) hyperpnea.

Neurogenic Factors

Cortical and peripheral factors regulate pulmonary ventilation in exercise.

- **Cortical Influence.** Neural outflow from regions of the motor cortex during exercise and cortical activation in anticipation of exercise stimulate respiratory neurons in the medulla. Cortical outflow acting in concert with the demands of exercise abruptly increases ventilation when exercise begins.

- **Peripheral Influence.** Sensory input from joints, tendons, and muscles adjust ventilation during exercise. Although the specific peripheral receptors remain unknown, experiments involving passive limb movements, electrical muscle stimulation, and voluntary exercise with the muscle's blood flow occluded support the existence of **mechanoreceptors** that produce reflex hyperpnea.

Influence of Temperature

An increase in body temperature directly excites neurons of the respiratory center and likely helps control ventilation in prolonged exercise. The rapidity of ventilatory changes at the onset and end of exercise, however, cannot be explained by the relatively slow changes in core temperature.

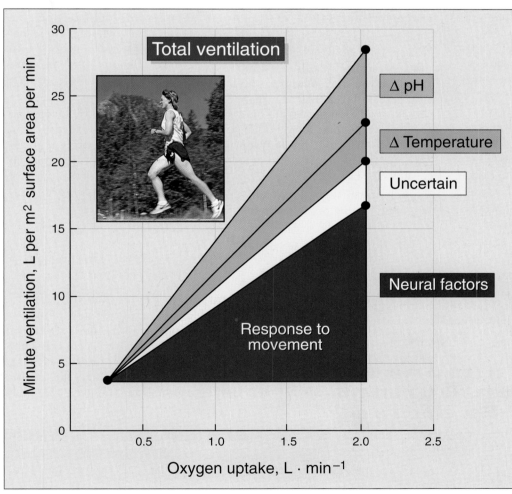

Figure 10.18
Composite of factors that influence pulmonary ventilation in exercise. The different colors estimate the contribution of changes in acidity (pH), temperature, and the effects of neurogenic stimuli from cerebral regions and/or joints and muscles. The yellow-shaded wedge represents ventilatory change not quantitatively accounted for by the other three factors. (From Lambertson, C. J.: Interactions of physical, chemical, and nervous factors in respiratory control. In *Medical Physiology*. Mountcastle V.B. (ed.). St. Louis: C.V. Mosby Co., 1974.)

Integrated Regulation

Control of breathing in exercise does not result from a single factor, but rather the combined and perhaps simultaneous effects of several chemical and neural stimuli (Fig. 10.18). The current model suggests the following scenario for ventilatory control in exercise:

1. Neurogenic stimuli from the cerebral cortex and exercising limbs cause the initial, abrupt increase in breathing when exercise begins (*Phase I*).
2. After a short plateau, minute ventilation gradually in-

creases to a steady level that adequately meets the demands for metabolic gas exchange (*Phase II*). **Central command** from the hypothalamus, plus factors intrinsic to medullary control system neurons, and peripheral stimuli from chemoreceptors and mechanoreceptors, contribute to this phase of ventilatory regulation.

3. The final phase of control (*Phase III*) involves "fine tuning" of ventilation through peripheral sensory feedback mechanism (e.g., temperature, CO_2, and $[H^+]$).

summary

1. Inherent activity of neurons in the medulla controls the normal respiratory cycle. Neural circuits that relay information from higher brain centers, the lungs themselves, and other sensors throughout the body modulate medullary activity.

2. Arterial P_{CO_2} and acidity $[H^+]$ act directly on the respiratory center or modify its activity reflexly through chemoreceptors to control alveolar ventilation at rest. Peripheral chemoreceptor activation stimulates breathing when

arterial P_{O_2} decreases during high-altitude ascent or in severe pulmonary disease.

3. Hyperventilation significantly lowers arterial P_{CO_2} and $[H^+]$. This prolongs breath-hold time until carbon dioxide and acidity increase to levels that stimulate breathing. Extended breath-hold by hyperventilation should not be practiced during underwater swimming because it could pose deadly consequences.

4. Nonchemical regulatory factors augment ventilatory adjustments

to exercise. These include: cortical activation in anticipation of exercise, and outflow from the motor cortex when exercise begins; peripheral sensory input from mechanoreceptors in joints and muscles; elevation in body temperature.

5. Neural and chemical factors that operate either singularly or in combination effectively regulate exercise alveolar ventilation. Each factor adjusts a particular phase of the ventilatory response to exercise.

PART 5
Pulmonary Ventilation During Exercise

Pulmonary Ventilation and Energy Demands

Physical activity increases oxygen uptake and carbon dioxide production more than any other physiologic stress. Large amounts of oxygen diffuse from the alveoli

into the blood returning to the lungs during exercise. Conversely, considerable carbon dioxide moves from the blood into the alveoli. Concurrently, increases in pulmonary ventilation maintain stable alveolar gas concentrations so increased oxygen and carbon dioxide exchange proceeds unimpeded. Figure 10.19 illustrates the relationship between minute ventilation and oxygen uptake

Less Breathing During Swimming

Significantly lower ventilatory equivalents occur at all levels of energy expenditure during prone swimming due to the restrictive breathing. A blunted ventilation may hinder gas exchange during maximal swimming and lower $\dot{V}O_{2max}$ when swimming compared with running.

Figure 10.19
Pulmonary ventilation, blood lactate, and oxygen uptake during graded exercise to maximum. The dashed lines extrapolate the linear relationship between $\dot{V}_E$ and $\dot{V}O_2$ during submaximal exercise. The lactate threshold indicates the oxygen uptake (or work intensity) at which blood lactate begins to increase above the resting value. It is detected at the point where the relation between $\dot{V}_E$ and $\dot{V}O_2$ deviates from linearity. (OBLA represents the point of lactate increase above a $4\ mM \cdot L^{-1}$ baseline.) Respiratory compensation indicates a further increase in pulmonary ventilation to counter the falling pH in heavy anaerobic exercise.

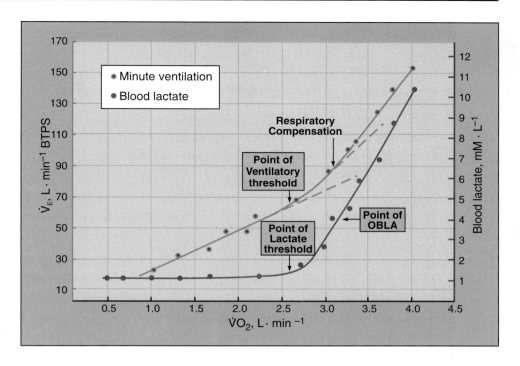

through the range of steady-rate and non–steady-rate exercise levels up to $\dot{V}O_{2max}$.

Ventilation in Steady-Rate Exercise

During light and moderate steady-rate exercise ($\dot{V}O_2 < 2.5$ $L \cdot min^{-1}$ in this example), pulmonary ventilation increases linearly with oxygen uptake; ventilation mainly increases by increases in tidal volume.

The **ventilatory equivalent for oxygen ($\dot{V}_E/\dot{V}O_2$)**, represents the ratio of minute ventilation to oxygen uptake. This index indicates breathing economy because it reflects the quantity of air breathed per amount of oxygen consumed. Healthy, young adults usually maintain $\dot{V}_E/\dot{V}O_2$ at about 25 (i.e., 25 L air breathed per L oxygen consumed) during submaximal exercise up to about 55% of $\dot{V}O_{2max}$. Higher ventilatory equivalents occur in children, averaging about 32 in 6-year-old's. Despite individual differences in the ventilatory equivalent among healthy children and among adults during steady-rate exercise, complete aeration of blood takes place because:

* Alveolar PO_2 and PCO_2 remain at near-resting values
* Transit time for blood flowing through the pulmonary capillaries proceeds slowly enough to permit complete gas exchange

During steady-rate exercise the **ventilatory equivalent for carbon dioxide ($\dot{V}_E/\dot{V}CO_2$)** also remains relatively constant because pulmonary ventilation eliminates the carbon dioxide produced during cellular respiration.

Ventilation in Non–Steady-Rate Exercise

Ventilatory Threshold

Note in Figure 10.19 (and in Fig. 2 of *How to Measure Lactate Threshold*), that as exercise $\dot{V}O_2$ increases, minute ventilation eventually takes a sharp upswing and increases disproportionately to the increase in oxygen uptake. This increases the ventilatory equivalent above the steady-rate exercise value; it may reach as high as 35 or 40 in maximal exercise. The point at which pulmonary ventilation increases disproportionately with oxygen uptake during graded exercise has been termed **ventilatory threshold (VT)**. At this exercise intensity, pulmonary ventilation no longer links tightly to oxygen demand at the cellular level. In fact, the "excess" ventilation relates directly to carbon dioxide's increased output from the buffering of lactate that begins to accumulate from anaerobic metabolism.

Recall from Chapter 6, that sodium bicarbonate in the blood buffers the lactate generated during anaerobic metabolism in the following reaction:

$$\text{Lactate} + NaHCO_3 \rightarrow \text{Na lactate} + H_2CO_3 \rightarrow H_2O + CO_2$$

Excess, nonmetabolic carbon dioxide liberated in this buffering reaction stimulates pulmonary ventilation that disproportionately increases $\dot{V}_E/\dot{V}O_2$. Additional carbon dioxide exhaled due to acid buffering causes the respiratory exchange ratio ($\dot{V}CO_2/\dot{V}O_2$) to exceed 1.00.

How to Measure Lactate Threshold

Conceptually, the **lactate threshold (LT)** represents an exercise level (power output, VO_2, or energy expenditure) where tissue hypoxia triggers an imbalance between lactate formation and its clearance, with a resulting increase in blood lactate concentration. All of the following terms refer essentially to the same LT phenomenon: expiratory compensation threshold, anaerobic threshold, onset of blood lactate accumulation, optimal ventilatory efficiency, aerobic-anaerobic threshold, onset of plasma lactate accumulation, individual anaerobic threshold, and point of metabolic acidosis.

The measurement of LT serves several important functions:

- Provides a sensitive indicator of aerobic training status
- Predicts endurance performance, often with greater accuracy than VO_{2max}
- Establishes an effective training intensity geared to the active muscles' aerobic metabolic dynamics

Different Indicators of LT

1. Fixed blood lactate concentration
2. Ventilatory threshold
3. Blood lactate–exercise VO_2 response

Fixed Blood Lactate Concentration

During low-intensity, steady-rate exercise, blood lactate concentration does not increase beyond the normal biological variation observed at rest. As exercise intensity increases, blood lactate levels exceed normal variation. The exercise intensity (or VO_2) associated with a fixed blood lactate concentration that exceeds normal resting variation denotes the LT. This often coincides with a 2.5 millimole (mM) value. A 4.0 mM lactate value indicates the **onset of blood lactate accumulation (OBLA)**. Figure 1 illustrates LT and OBLA computations from fixed blood lactate concentrations during incremental, 4.0-min exercise stages on a bicycle ergometer. Interpolation from a visual plot of power output (VO_2) versus blood lactate determines the exercise level associated with the fixed blood lactate concentrations. The decision regarding stage duration, number of stages, and interval between stages becomes important. Stages 4 minutes or longer provide better predictability than shorter ones. For the data illustrated in Figure 1, LT occurred at an exercise power output of 205 W, while 225 W predicted the fixed blood lactate concentration for OBLA.

Ventilatory Threshold

Pulmonary minute ventilation ($\dot{V}_E$) during exercise increases disproportionately in its relationship to oxygen uptake at about the same time blood lactate begins to accumulate. This **ventilatory threshold (VT)** permits prediction of LT from the $\dot{V}_E$ response during graded exercise. The mechanistic link of lactate buffering by plasma bicarbonate to produce additional CO_2 (and respiratory stimulus unrelated to VO_2) justifies the use of VT on a physiologic basis.

The test involves exercise with increments of short duration (a ramp test of 1- or 2-min increments) with continuous measurement of $\dot{V}_E$ (breath-by-breath or every 10, 20, or 30 s) to the point of fatigue (usually within 8 to 12 min). The point of non-linear increase in $\dot{V}_E$ versus VO_2 represents VT, expressed as a specific VO_2 value rather than running speed or power output common with the fixed blood lactate concentration method. Figure 2 show the relationship between $\dot{V}_E$ and VO_2 during incremental exercise; VT occurs at an exercise VO_2 of 3.04 $L \cdot min^{-1}$. It is common to express the VO_2 at LT as a percent of VO_{2max}. This represents 71% in this example.

Blood Lactate – Exercise $\dot{V}O_2$ Response

This protocol plots blood lactate concentration versus either VO_2 or exercise intensity in a manner similar to that described for determination of fixed blood lactate concentration (Fig. 1). The person exercises for 3- or 4-minute increments on a bicycle ergometer or treadmill. With treadmill exercise, blood lactate is sampled during a brief pause at the end of each stage, or without pause when using stationary cycling exercise. Figure 3 plots blood lactate versus oxygen uptake throughout the test. A best-fitting straight line depicts the linear portion of the curve; a second line describes the upward trending curve after it "breaks" from linearity. The intersection of the two lines represents LT.

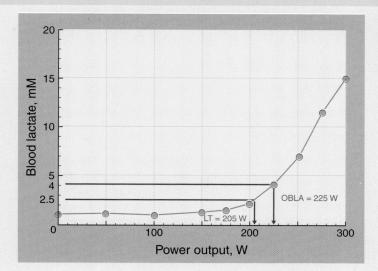

Figure 1. Fixed blood lactate concentration method for determining lactate threshold (LT) and onset of blood lactate accumulation (OBLA). This example shows LT at a fixed blood lactate of 2.5 mM and OBLA at a fixed blood lactate of 4.0 mM.

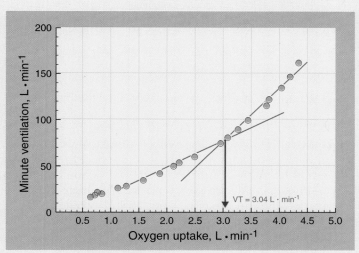

Figure 2. Determination of LT from the relationship between pulmonary minute ventilation and oxygen uptake during incremental exercise.

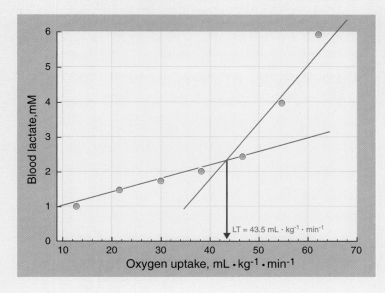

Figure 3. Determination of LT from relationship between blood lactate concentration and oxygen uptake during incremental exercise.

The term **anaerobic threshold** originally defined the abrupt increase in ventilatory equivalent caused by non-metabolic carbon dioxide production owing to lactate buffering. Some researchers believed this point signaled the body's shift to anaerobic metabolism (lactate formation) and therefore proposed the anaerobic thesbold as a non-invasive measure of the onset of anaerobiosis. Subsequent research has shown that the ratios of $\dot{V}_E/\dot{V}O_2$ or $\dot{V}CO_2/\dot{V}O_2$ do not necessarily link in a *causal* manner with lactate production (or accumulation) in exercise. Even if the association between ventilatory dynamics and cellular metabolic events is noncausal, useful information about exercise performance can be obtained by applying these indirect procedures.

Onset of Blood Lactate Accumulation

Steady-rate exercise indicates that oxygen supply and utilization satisfy the energy requirements of muscular effort. When this occurs, lactate production does not exceed its removal, and blood lactate does not accumulate. As shown in Figure 10.19, the exercise intensity or oxygen uptake at which blood lactate begins to increase above a baseline level of about $4 \text{ mM} \cdot \text{L}^{-1}$ indicates the point of **onset of blood lactate accumulation (OBLA)**. OBLA normally occurs between 55 and 65% of $\dot{V}O_{2max}$ in healthy, untrained subjects, and often equals more than 80% $\dot{V}O_{2max}$ in highly trained endurance athletes.

Causes of OBLA. The exact cause of the OBLA remains controversial. Many believe it represents the point of muscle hypoxia (inadequate oxygen) and therefore anaerobiosis. However, muscle lactate accumulation does not necessarily coincide with hypoxia because lactate forms even in the presence of adequate muscle oxygenation. The OBLA, however, does imply an imbalance between the rate of blood lactate appearance and disappearance. This imbalance may not be due to muscle hypoxia, but rather from a decreased lactate clearance in total, or increased lactate production only in specific muscle fibers. Thus, practitioners should interpret cautiously the specific metabolic significance of the OBLA and its possible relationship to tissue hypoxia.

OBLA and Endurance Performance. The point of OBLA often increases with aerobic training, without an accompanying increase in $\dot{V}O_{2max}$. This suggests that separate factors influence OBLA and $\dot{V}O_{2max}$. Traditionally, exercise physiologists have applied $\dot{V}O_{2max}$ as the main yardstick to gauge one's capacity for endurance exercise. Although this measure generally relates to long-duration exercise performance, it does not fully explain all aspects of success. Experienced distance athletes generally compete at an exercise intensity slightly above the point of OBLA. *Consequently, exercise intensity at the OBLA has emerged as a consistent and powerful predictor of aerobic exercise performance.* A study of competitive racewalkers illustrates this point. Race-walking velocity and oxygen uptake at which blood lactate began to accumulate correlated highly with 20-km race performance. In fact, the race-walking velocity at OBLA predicted race time to within 0.6% of the actual time, whereas $\dot{V}O_{2max}$ poorly predicted actual performance. *Changes in endurance performance with training often relate more closely to training-induced changes in the exercise level for OBLA than to $\dot{V}O_{2max}$ changes.*

Does Ventilation Limit Aerobic Capacity?

With inadequate breathing capacity, the line relating pulmonary ventilation and oxygen uptake in Figure 10.19 would not curve upward (increase in ventilatory equivalent) during heavy exercise; instead, it would level-off or slope downward to the right to reflect the decrease in ventilatory equivalent. Such a response would indicate a *failure* for ventilation to keep pace with increasing oxygen demands; in this case, a person truly would "run out of wind." Actually, a healthy individual tends to over-breathe in relation to oxygen uptake with increasing exercise intensity. Figure 10.17 demonstrated that the ventilatory adjustment to strenuous exercise decreases alveolar P_{CO_2} concomitant with small increases in alveolar P_{O_2}. Arterial P_{O_2} and Hb oxygen saturation remain at near-resting values during heavy exercise. This means that pulmonary function does not represent the "weak link" in the oxygen transport system of healthy individuals with average to moderately high aerobic capacity.

Work of Breathing

Two major factors determine the energy requirements of breathing:

1. Compliance of the lungs and thorax
2. Resistance of the airways to the smooth flow of air

Lung and thorax compliance refers to how "easily" these tissues stretch. The radius of the bronchi primarily establishes resistance to airflow. More specifically, airflow resistance varies inversely with a vessel's radius raised to the fourth power in accordance with Poiseuille's law. Reducing airway radius by one-half causes airway resistance to increase 16 times. Normally, bronchi and bronchiole dimensions do not impede the smooth flow of air, so breathing requires relatively little energy. In some lung diseases, however, airways constrict and/or tissues themselves lose compliance; this imposes considerable resistance to airflow. Trying to breathe through a drinking straw gives some indication of breathing difficulties encountered by the person with severe obstructive lung disease.

A healthy person rarely senses the breathing effort, even during moderate exercise. In contrast, respiratory disease often makes the work of breathing during exercise an exhausting physical task. In patients with **chronic obstructive pulmonary disease** (**COPD**; e.g., asthma, emphysema), the effort of breathing at rest can reach three times that of healthy individuals. In severe pulmonary disease, breathing's energy requirement may easily reach 40% of the total exercise oxygen uptake. This obviously encroaches on the oxygen available to the active, nonrespiratory muscles, and seriously limits the exercise capacity of these patients.

Figure 10.20 shows the relationship in healthy subjects between pulmonary ventilation and oxygen uptake during rest and submaximal exercise, and its division into respira-

Cigarette Smoke Constricts Airways

The increase in peripheral airway resistance with smoking results mainly from a vagal reflex (possibly triggered from sensory stimulation by minute particles in smoke) and partially by nicotine's stimulation of parasympathetic nerves.

tory and nonrespiratory components. At rest and in light exercise, the relatively small oxygen requirement of breathing averages between 1.9 and 3.1 mL of oxygen per liter of air breathed, or about 4% of the total energy expenditure. As the rate and depth of breathing increase during exercise, the energy cost of breathing increases to about 4 mL of oxygen per liter of ventilation. It increases to as high as 9 mL of oxygen in maximal exercise when pulmonary ventilation exceeds 100 L · min^{-1}. *At these exercise intensities, the oxygen cost of breathing represents between 10 and 20% of the total oxygen uptake.*

Effects of Cigarette Smoking

Since the initial 1964 release of the *Surgeon General's Report on Smoking and Health*, more than 20 follow-up review articles have concluded a causal link between smok-

Even the Fit Have Asthma

Champions are not immune from asthma. One of the most famous examples is 1984 Olympic marathon champion Joan Benoit Samuelson who experienced breathing problems during several races in 1991 that led to the discovery of her asthmatic condition. Despite breathing difficulties during the 1991 New York Marathon, she finished with a time of 2 hr:33 min:40 s.

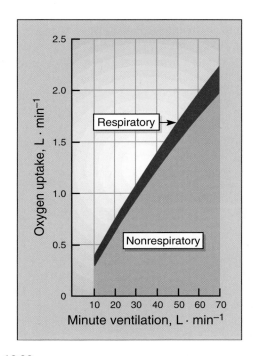

Figure 10.20
Relationship between oxygen uptake and pulmonary ventilation, and the respiratory and nonrespiratory oxygen cost components during submaximal exercise in healthy subjects. (From Levison, H., and Cherniack, R.: Ventilatory cost of exercise in chronic obstructive pulmonary disease. *J. Appl. Physiol.*, 25:21, 1968.)

ing and lung cancer, chronic bronchitis and emphysema, cardiovascular disease, and cancers of the lip, larynx, esophagus, and urinary bladder. However, little research has related cigarette smoking habits to exercise performance, although most endurance athletes avoid cigarettes for fear of hindering performance from what they consider "loss of wind." The chronic cigarette smoker shows decreases in dynamic lung function, which, in severe cases, manifests as obstructive lung disorders. Such pathologic processes usually take years to develop. Teenage and young adult smokers rarely exhibit chronic lung function deterioration of a magnitude to significantly impair exercise performance. Because of increased fitness, the young, fit smoker often believes he or she is immune from smoking's crippling effects.

Other, more acute effects of cigarette smoking adversely affect exercise capacity. For example, airway resistance at rest can increase threefold in chronic smokers and non-

smokers after 15 puffs on a cigarette during a 5-minute period. Added resistance to breathing lasts an average of 35 minutes, with only minor negative effects in light exercise in which the oxygen cost of breathing remains small. In vigorous exercise, however the residual effect of smoking on airway resistance can be detrimental because the additional cost of breathing becomes physiologically significant. In one study of habitual cigarette smokers who exercised at 80% of $\dot{V}O_2$max, breathing's energy requirement averaged 14% of the exercise oxygen uptake after smoking, but only 9% in the "nonsmoking" trials. Also, exercise heart rates averaged 5 to 7% lower after 1 day of smoking abstinence; all subjects reported they felt better exercising in the nonsmoking condition. Almost complete reversibility of the increased oxygen cost of breathing with smoking can occur in chronic smokers with only 1 day of abstinence. *Thus, athletes who cannot conquer the smoking habit should at least stop 24 hours before competition.*

summary

1. Pulmonary ventilation increases linearly with oxygen uptake during light and moderate exercise. The ventilatory equivalent at these exercise intensities averages 20 to 25 liters of air breathed per liter of oxygen consumed.

2. In non–steady-rate exercise, pulmonary ventilation increases disproportionately with increases in oxygen uptake, and the ventilatory equivalent may reach 35 or 40.

3. The eventual sharp upswing in pulmonary ventilation related to oxygen uptake during incremental exercise indicates the point of

onset of blood lactate accumulation (OBLA).

4. OBLA effectively predicts endurance performance and can be measured without significant metabolic acidosis or cardiovascular strain.

5. Breathing normally requires a relatively small oxygen cost even during exercise. In respiratory disease, the work of breathing becomes excessive, and exercise alveolar ventilation often becomes inadequate.

6. Pulmonary ventilation does not limit optimal alveolar gas ex-

change in healthy individuals who perform maximal exercise. For elite endurance athletes, pulmonary functional capacity may lag behind the exceptional training adaptations in cardiovascular and muscle function, and compromise blood's aeration during maximal exercise.

7. Airway resistance increases significantly after cigarette smoking. The added oxygen cost of breathing can impair high-intensity, aerobic exercise performance. Reversibility of these effects occurs with 1 day of cigarette abstinence.

thought questions

1. How would the relationship change between $\dot{V}_E/\dot{V}O_2$ under the following conditions: 1) aging person who remains sedentary versus aging person who performs regular aerobic exercises; 2) transition from adolescence to young adulthood; 3) person training for football?

2. As an exercise physiologist, what would you say to a person who feels the need to work on proper techniques of breathing to increase "wind" and eliminate the feelings of being "out of breath" when running continuously for 20 to 30 minutes?

3. How would you respond to the coach who asks you about the advisability of having a tank of oxygen on the

sidelines so players might breathe from it during time outs or rest breaks?

4. One of the techniques during "natural" childbirth requires the woman to breathe rapidly to effectively "work with" the normal ebb and flow of uterine contractions. How can this "hyperventilation" technique not disrupt the normal alveolar and arterial P_{CO_2} levels?

5. A person attempts to "squeeze out" a maximum lift in the standing press. After straining to complete the lift the person states: "I feel slightly dizzy and see spots before my eyes." Provide a plausible physiologic explanation. What should be done to prevent this?

selected references

Aaron, E.A., et al.: Oxygen cost of exercise hyperpnea: Implications for performance. *J. Appl. Physiol.*, 75: 1818, 1992.

Albrecht, A.E., et al: Effect of smoking cessation on exercise performance in female smokers participating in exercise training. *Am. J. Cardiol.*, 82:950, 1998.

Aliverti, A., et al.: Human respiratory muscle actions and control during exercise. *J. Appl. Physiol.*, 83:1256, 1997.

American Thoracic Society. Lung function testing: selection of reference values and interpretative strategies. *Am. Rev. Respir. Dis.*, 144:1202, 1991.

Babcock, M.A., and Dempsey, J.A.: Pulmonary system adaptations: limitations to exercise. In: *Physical Activity, Fitness, and Health.* Bouchard, C., et al., (eds.). Champaign, IL: Human Kinetics, 1994.

Bar-Or, O., and Inbar, O.: Swimming and asthma—benefits and deleterious effects. *Sports Med.*, 14: 397, 1992.

Beck, K.C.: Control of airway function during and after exercise in asthmatics. *Med. Sci. Sports Exerc.*, 31(Suppl.):S4, 1999.

Bishop, D., et al: The relationship between plasma lactate parameters, W peak and 1-h cycling performance in women. *Med. Sci. Sports Exerc.*, 30:1270, 1998.

Boutellier, U.: Respiratory muscle fitness and exercise endurance in healthy humans. *Med. Sci. Sports Exerc.*, 30:1169, 1998.

Chapman, R.F., et al.: Degree of arterial desaturation in normoxia influences $\dot{V}O_{2max}$ decline in mild hypoxia. *Med. Sci. Sports Exerc.*, 31:658, 1999.

Clark, C.J., et al.: Low intensity peripheral muscle conditioning improves exercise tolerance and breathlessness in COPD. *Eur. Respir. J.*, 9:2590, 1996.

Coast, J.R., et al.: Ventilatory work and oxygen consumption during exercise and hyperventilation. *J. Appl. Physiol.*, 74: 793, 1993.

Courteix, D., et al.: Effects of intensive swimming training on lung volumes, airway resistances and the maximal expiratory flow-volume relationship in prepubertal girls. *Eur. J. Appl. Physiol.*, 264, 1997.

Coyle, E.F., et al.: Integration of the physiological factors determining endurance performance in athletes. *Exerc. Sport Sci. Rev.* 23: 25, 1995.

Dempsey, J.A.: Is the lung built for exercise? *Med. Sci. Sports Exerc.*, 18:143, 1986.

Dempsey, J.A., et al.: Respiratory muscle perfusion and energetics during exercise. *Med. Sci. Sports Exerc.*, 28:1123, 1996.

Drazen, J.M., et al.: Drug therapy: treatment of asthma with drugs modifying the leukotriene pathway. *N. Engl. J. Med.*, 340:197, 1999.

Eldridge, F.L.: Central integration of mechanisms in exercise hyperpnea. *Med. Sci. Sports Exerc.*, 26: 319, 1994.

Gold, D.R., et al.: Effects of cigarette smoking on lung function in adolescent boys and girls. *N Engl. J. Med.*, 331:335, 1996.

Harmon. E.A., et al.: Intra-abdominal and intra-thoracic pressures during lifting and jumping. *Med. Sci. Sports Exerc.*, 20:198, 1988.

Harms, C.A., and Dempsey, J.A.: Cardiovascular consequences of exercise hyperpnea. *Exerc. Sport Sci. Revs.*, 27:37, 1999.

Harms, C.A., et al: Exercise induced arterial hypoxemia in healthy young women. *J. Physiol. (Lond.)*, 507:619, 1998.

Hébert, J-L., et al.: Pulse pressure response to the strain of the Valsalva maneuver in humans with preserved systolic function. *J. Appl. Physiol.*, 85:817, 1998.

Hopkins, S.R., et al.: Intense exercise impairs the integrity of the pulmonary blood-gas barrier in elite athletes. *Am. Rev. Respir. Crit. Care Med.*, 155:1090, 1997.

Johnson, B.D., et al.: Exercise induced diaphragmatic fatigue in healthy humans. *J. Physiol. (Lond.)* 460: 385, 1993.

Kenyon, C.M., et al.: Rib cage mechanics during quiet breathing and exercise in humans. *J. Appl. Physiol.*, 83:1242, 1997.

Kufafka, D.S., et al.: Exercise-induced bronchospasm in high school athletes via a free running test. *Chest*, 114:1613, 1998.

Loat, C.E., and Rhodes, E.C.: Relationship between the lactate and ventilatory thresholds during prolonged exercise. *Sports Med.*, 15:104, 1993.

Matsumoto, I., et al.: Effects of swimming training on aerobic capacity of exercise induced bronchoconstriction in children with bronchial asthma. *Thorax*, 54:196, 1999.

McFadden, E.R., Jr., and Gilbert, I.A.: Current concepts in exercise-induced asthma. *N. Engl. J. Med.*, 330: 1362, 1994.

McKenzie, D.C., et al.: The protective effects of continuous and interval exercise in athletes with exercise-induced asthma. *Med. Sci. Sports Exerc.*, 26: 951, 1994.

Mink, B.D.: Exercise and chronic obstructive pulmonary disease: Modest fitness gains pay big dividends. *Phys. Sportsmed.*, 25(11):43, 1997.

Neder, J.A., et al.: Short term effects of aerobic training in the clinical management of moderate to severe asthma in children. *Thorax*, 54:202, 1999.

Oleberg, D.A., et al.: Skeletal muscle chemoreflex and pH in exercise ventilatory control. *J. Appl. Physiol.*, 84:676, 1998.

Pan, L.G., et al.: Important role of carotid afferents in control of breathing. *J. Appl. Physiol.*, 85:1299, 1998.

Powers, S.K., et al.: Effects of incomplete pulmonary gas exchange on $\dot{V}O_2max$. *J. Appl. Physiol.*, 66:2491, 1989.

Richardson, R.S.: Oxygen transport: air to muscle cell. *Med. Sci. Sports Exerc.*, 30:53, 1998.

Richardson, R.S., et al.: Myoglobin O_2 desaturation during exercise: evidence of a limited oxygen transport. *J. Clin. Invest.* 96:1916, 1995.

Sandsund, M., et al.: Effects of beathing cold and warm air on lung function and physical performance in asthmatic and nonasthmatic athletes during exercise in the cold. *Ann. N.Y. Acad. Sci.*, 813:751, 1997.

Spengler, C.M., et al.: Decreased exercise blood lactate concentrations after respiratory endurance training in humans. *Eur. J. Appl. Physiol.*, 79:299, 1999.

Ward, S.: Assessment of peripheral chemoreflex contributions to exercise hyperpnea in humans. *Med. Sci. Sports Exerc.*, 26: 303, 1994.

Wasserman, K., et al.: *Principles of Exercise Testing and Interpretation.* 3rd Ed. Baltimore: Lippincott Williams & Wilkins, 1999.

Weltman, A.: *The Blood Lactate Response to Exercise.* Champaign, IL: Human Kinetics, 1995.

Weston, A., et al.: African runners exhibit greater fatigue resistance, lower lactate accumulation, and higher oxidative enzyme activity. *J. Appl. Physiol.*, 86:915, 1999.

Wyatt, F.B.: Comparison of lactate and ventilatory threshold to maximal oxygen consumption: A meta-analysis. *J. Strength and Cond. Res.*, 13:67, 1999.

CHAPTER 11

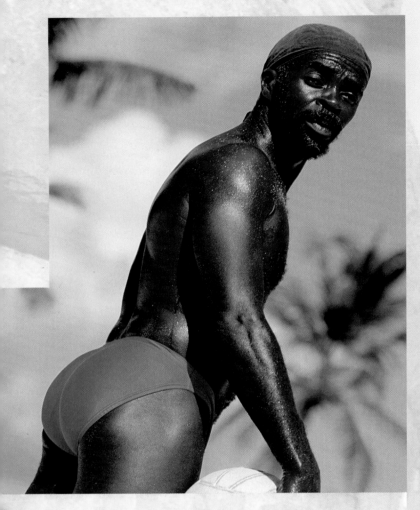

The Cardio-vascular System and Exercise

Topics covered in this chapter

PART 1 The Cardiovascular System

Components of the Cardiovascular System
Blood Pressure
Heart's Blood Supply
Summary

PART 2 Cardiovascular Regulation and Integration

Heart Rate Regulation
Blood Distribution
Integrated Response in Exercise
Summary

PART 3 Cardiovascular Dynamics During Exercise

Cardiac Output
Resting Cardiac Output
Exercise Cardiac Output
Exercise Stroke Volume
Exercise Heart Rate
Cardiac Output Distribution
Cardiac Output and Oxygen Transport
Extraction of Oxygen: The a-v̄ O_2 Difference
Cardiovascular Adjustments to Upper Body Exercise
"Athlete's Heart"
Summary
Thought Questions
Selected References

objectives

- List important functions of the cardiovascular system.

- Describe how to use the auscultatory method to measure blood pressure, and give average values for systolic and diastolic blood pressure during rest and moderate aerobic exercise.

- Describe blood pressure response during (a) resistance exercise, (b) upper-body exercise, (c) exercise in the inverted position.

- State potential benefits of aerobic exercise for a person with moderate hypertension.

- Identify intrinsic and extrinsic factors that regulate heart rate during rest and exercise.

- Identify neural and local metabolic factors that regulate blood flow during rest and exercise.

- Describe the direct Fick method to measure cardiac output. Compare average values of cardiac output during rest and maximal exercise for an endurance-trained athlete and sedentary person.

- Explain two physiologic mechanisms that affect the heart's stroke volume.

- Describe the relationship between maximal cardiac output and maximal oxygen uptake among individuals with varied aerobic fitness levels.

- Explain the meaning of "athlete's heart." Contrast structural and functional characteristics of an endurance athlete's heart with the heart of a resistance-trained athlete.

The Greek physician Galen (Chapter 1) theorized about blood flow in the body. He believed blood flowed like the tides of the sea, surging and abating into arteries, then away from the heart and back again. In Galen's view, fluid carried with it "humors," good and evil, that determined one's well-being. If a person became ill, the standard practice required blood-letting to drain off the diseased humors and restore health. This theory prevailed until the seventeenth century when physician William Harvey (Chapter 1) proposed a different scenario. Experimenting with frogs, cats, and dogs, Harvey demonstrated the existence of valves in the heart that provided for one-way movement of fluid, a finding incompatible with Galen's "ebb-and-flow" view because it suggested a circular, one-way flow of blood through the body. In a set of ingenious experiments, Harvey measured the volume of the heart's chambers and counted the number of times the heart contracted in 1 hour. He concluded that if the heart emptied only one-half its volume with each beat, the body's total blood volume would be pumped in minutes. This finding led Harvey to hypothesize that blood moved (circulated) within a closed system in a circular, unidirectional pattern throughout the body. Harvey, of course, was correct; the heart pumps the entire blood volume, approximately 5 liters, in 1 minute. Harvey's experiments changed medical science forever, although it would take nearly 200 more years for his ideas to play important roles in physiology and medicine.

From Harvey's early experiments to sophisticated research at the dawn of the twenty-first century, we know that the highly efficient ventilatory system described in Chapter 10 complements a rapid transport and delivery system comprised of blood, the heart, and more than 60,000 miles of blood vessels that integrate the body as a unit. The circulatory system serves five important functions during physical activity:

1. Delivers oxygen to active tissues
2. Aerates blood returned to the lungs
3. Transports heat, a byproduct of cellular metabolism, from the body's core to the skin
4. Delivers fuel nutrients to active tissues
5. Transports hormones, the body's chemical messengers

PART 1
The Cardiovascular System

Components of the Cardiovascular System

In essence, the cardiovascular system consists of an interconnected, continuous vascular circuit containing a pump (heart), a high-pressure distribution system (arteries), exchange vessels (capillaries), and a low-pressure collection and return system (veins). Figure 11.1 presents a schematic view of this system.

Heart

The heart provides the force to propel blood throughout the vascular circuit. This four-chambered organ, a fist-sized pump, beats at rest an average of 70 times a minute, 100,800 times a day, and 36.8 million times a year. Even for a person of average fitness, maximum output of blood from this remarkable organ exceeds fluid output from a household faucet turned wide open.

The heart muscle (**myocardium**), consists of striated muscle similar to skeletal muscle. Unlike skeletal muscle, the individual fibers interconnect in latticework fashion. As a result, stimulation (depolarization) of one myocardial cell spreads an action po-

tential throughout the myocardium causing the heart to function as a unit. Figure 11.2 shows the details of the heart as a pump. Functionally, the heart consists of two separate pumps: one pump (left heart pump) receives blood from the body and pumps it to the lungs for aeration (**pulmonary circulation**), and the other pump (right heart pump) accepts oxygenated blood from the lungs and pumps it throughout the body (**systemic circulation**).

The hollow chambers of the right heart pump perform two important functions:

1. Receives blood returning from all parts of the body
2. Pumps blood to the lungs for aeration via the pulmonary circulation

Figure 11.1
Schematic view of the cardiovascular system consisting of the heart and the pulmonary and systemic vascular circuits. The darker red shading shows oxygen-rich arterial blood, whereas deoxygenated venous blood appears somewhat paler. In the pulmonary circuit, the situation reverses, and oxygenated blood returns to the heart via the right and left pulmonary veins.

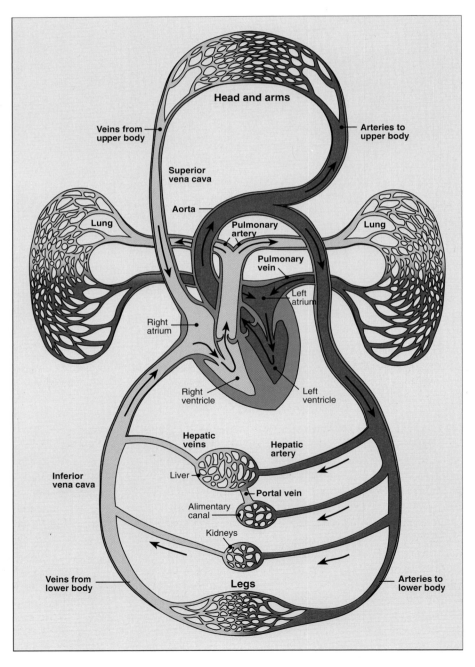

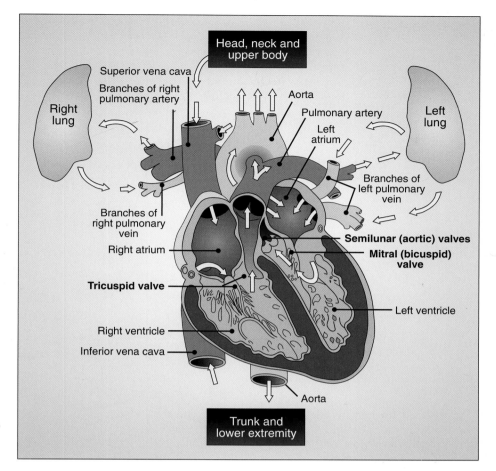

Figure 11.2
The heart's valves provide for the one-way flow of blood, indicated by the yellow arrows.

directly below. Almost immediately after atrial contraction, the ventricles contract and force blood into the arterial systems.

Arteries

The arteries provide the high-pressure tubing that conducts oxygen-rich blood to the tissues. Figure 11.3 shows the arteries composed of layers of connective tissue and smooth muscle. Because of their thickness, no gaseous exchange takes place between arterial blood and surrounding tissues. Blood pumped from the left ventricle into the highly muscular yet elastic aorta circulates throughout the body via a network of arteries and **arterioles**, or smaller arterial branches. *Arteriole walls contain circular layers of smooth muscle that either constrict or relax to regulate peripheral blood flow.* The redistribution function of arterioles becomes important during exercise because blood diverts to working muscles from areas that temporarily compromise their blood supply.

Capillaries

The arterioles continue to branch and form smaller and less muscular vessels called metarterioles. These tiny vessels end in **capillaries**, a network of microscopic blood vessels so thin they provide only enough room for blood cells to squeeze through in single file. Capillaries contain about 5% of the total blood volume at any time. Gases, nutrients, and waste products rapidly transfer across the thin, porous, capillary walls. A ring of smooth muscle (**precapillary sphincter**) encircles the capillary at its origin to control the vessel's internal diameter. This sphincter provides a local means for regulating capillary blood flow within a specific tissue to meet metabolic requirements that change rapidly and dramatically in exercise.

Capillary branching increases the total cross-sectional area of the microcirculation 800 times more than the one-inch diameter aorta. Because blood flow velocity relates inversely to the vasculature's total cross section, velocity progressively decreases as blood moves toward and into the capillaries.

The left heart pump also performs two important functions:

1. Receives oxygenated blood from the lungs
2. Pumps blood into the thick-walled, muscular aorta for distribution throughout the body via the systemic circulation

A thick, solid muscular wall (septum) separates the left and right sides of the heart. The **atrioventricular (AV) valves** situated within the heart direct the one-way flow of blood from the right atrium to the right ventricle (**tricuspid valve**) and from the left atrium to the left ventricle (**mitral valve** or **bicuspid valve**). The **semilunar valves** located in the arterial wall just outside the heart prevent blood from flowing back (regurgitation) into the heart between ventricular contractions.

The relatively thin-walled, sac-like atrial chambers receive and store blood returning from the lungs and body during ventricular contraction. About 70% of the blood returning to the atria flows directly into the ventricles before the atria contract. Simultaneous contraction of both atria forces the remaining blood into the respective ventricles

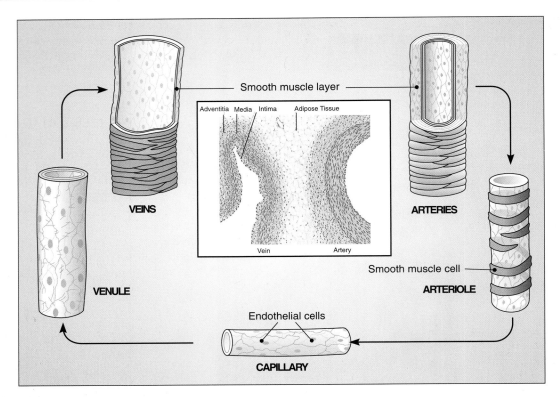

Figure 11.3
Blood vessel walls. A single layer of endothelial cells lines each vessel. Fibrous tissue wrapped in several layers of smooth muscle surrounds the arterial wall. A single layer of muscle cells envelops arterioles; capillaries consist only of one layer of endothelial cells. Fibrous tissue encases endothelial cells in venules; veins also possess a layer of smooth muscle.

Veins

The vascular system maintains continuity of blood flow as capillaries feed deoxygenated blood at almost a trickle into small veins called **venules**. Blood flow then increases slightly because the venous system's cross-sectional area becomes less than for capillaries. The lower body's smaller veins eventually empty into the largest vein, the **inferior vena cava**, that travels through the abdominal and thoracic cavities toward the heart. Venous blood draining the head, neck, and shoulder regions empties into the **superior vena cava** and moves downward to join the inferior vena cava at heart level. The mixture of blood from the upper and lower body then enters the **right atrium** and descends into the **right ventricle** for delivery through the pulmonary artery to the lungs. Gas exchange takes place in the lungs' alveolar-capillary network; here, the pulmonary veins return oxygenated blood to the left heart pump, where the journey through the body resumes.

Venous Return

A unique characteristic of veins solves a potential problem related to the low pressure of venous blood. Figure 11.4 shows that thin, membranous, flap-like valves spaced at short intervals within the vein permit one-way blood flow back to the heart. Veins compress because of low venous blood pressure, muscular contractions, or minor pressure changes within the chest cavity during breathing. Alternate venous compression and relaxation, combined with the one-way action of valves, provide a "milking" effect similar to the action of the heart. Venous compression imparts considerable energy for blood flow, whereas "diastole" (relaxation) allows vessels to refill as blood moves toward the heart. Without valves, blood would stagnate or pool (as it sometimes does) in extremity veins, and people would faint every time they stood up because of reduced blood flow to the brain.

A Significant Blood Reservoir

The veins do not merely function as passive conduits. At rest, the venous system normally contains about 65% of total blood volume; hence, veins serve as capacitance vessels or blood reservoirs. A slight increase in tension (tone) by the vein's smooth muscle layer alters the diameter of the venous tree. A generalized increase in **venous tone** rapidly redistributes blood from peripheral veins toward the central blood volume returning to the heart. *In this manner,*

Determinants of Blood Pressure

Arterial blood pressure reflects arterial blood flow per minute (cardiac output) and peripheral vascular resistance to blood flow in the following relationships:

**Blood pressure = Cardiac output ×
Total peripheral resistance**

**Total peripheral resistance = Blood
pressure ÷ Cardiac output**

*the venous system plays an important role as an **active blood reservoir** to either retard or enhance blood flow to the systemic circulation.*

Varicose Veins

Sometimes valves within a vein become defective and do not maintain one-way blood flow. This condition of **varicose veins** usually occurs in superficial veins of the lower extremities from the force of gravity that retards blood flow in an upright posture. As blood accumulates, these veins distend excessively and become painful, often impairing circulation from surrounding areas. In severe cases, the venous wall becomes inflamed and degenerates — a condition called **phlebitis**, which often requires surgical removal of the damaged vessel.

Individuals with varicose veins should avoid excessive straining exercises like heavy resistance training. During sustained, nonrhythmic muscle actions, the muscle and ventilatory "pumps" do not contribute to venous return. Increased abdominal pressure accompanying straining also impedes blood flow return. These factors cause blood to pool (temporarily stagnate) in the veins of the lower body, which could aggravate existing varicose veins. Whether regular aerobic exercise prevents the occurrence

of varicose veins remains unknown. Rhythmic physical activity could minimize complications because dynamic muscle actions continually propel peripheral blood toward the heart.

Venous Pooling

The fact that people faint when forced to maintain an upright posture without movement (e.g., standing at attention for a prolonged period) demonstrates the importance of muscle contractions to venous return. Also, changing from a lying to a standing position affects the dynamics of venous return and triggers physiologic responses. Heart rate and blood pressure stabilize during bed rest. If a person suddenly rises and remains erect, an uninterrupted column of blood exists from heart level to the toes, creating a hydrostatic force of 80 to 100 mm Hg. Swelling (edema) occurs from pooling of blood in the lower extremities and creates "back pressure" that forces fluid from the capillary bed into surrounding tissues. Concurrently, impaired venous return decreases blood pressure; at the same time, heart rate accelerates and venous tone increases to counter the hypotensive condition. Maintaining an upright position without movement leads to dizziness and eventual fainting from insufficient cerebral blood supply. Resuming a horizontal or head-down position restores circulation and consciousness.

Active Cool-Down. The potential for venous pooling justifies continued slow jogging or walking immediately following strenuous exercise. "Cooling down" with rhythmic exercise facilitates blood flow through the vascular circuit (including the heart) during recovery. An "active recovery" also speeds lactate removal from the blood. Pressurized suits worn by test pilots and special support stockings also retard hydrostatic shifts of blood to veins of the lower extremities in the upright position. A similar supportive effect occurs in upright exercise in a swimming pool because the water's external support facilitates venous return.

Figure 11.4
The valves in veins (**A**) prevent the backflow of blood, but do not hinder the normal one–way flow of blood (**B**). Contraction of nearby active muscle (**C**), or constriction of smooth muscle bands within veins (**D**) propels blood through the venous circuit.

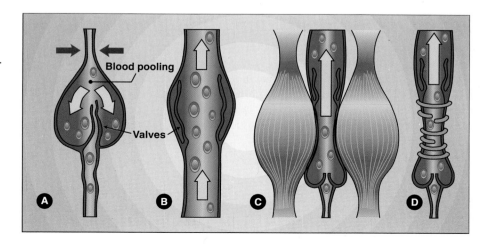

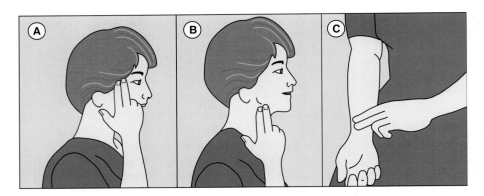

for blood flow. The alternate, rhythmic contraction and relaxation of skeletal muscles forces blood through the vessels and returns it to the heart. Increased blood flow during moderate exercise increases systolic pressure in the first few minutes; it then levels off, usually between 140 and 160 mm Hg. Diastolic pressure remains relatively unchanged.

Figure 11.6 illustrates the relationship between blood pressure during exercise of progressively increasing intensity and the quantity of blood ejected into the arterial circuit each minute (cardiac output). Various indices of arterial blood pressure increase linearly with cardiac output, with the largest increases occurring during cardiac systole. Diastolic pressure increases only about 12% during the full range of exercise intensities. Exercise-trained and sedentary subjects show similar responses. However, systolic blood pressure often increases to 200 mm Hg during max-

Blood Pressure

A surge of blood enters the aorta with each contraction of the left ventricle, distending the vessel and creating pressure within it. The stretch and subsequent recoil of the aortic wall propagates as a wave through the entire arterial system. The pressure wave readily appears as a pulse in the following areas: the superficial radial artery on the thumb side of the wrist, the temporal artery (on the side of the head at the temple), and carotid artery along the side of the trachea (Fig. 11.5). In healthy persons, pulse rate equals heart rate.

Rest

The highest pressure generated by left ventricular contraction (**systole**) to move blood through a healthy, resilient arterial system at rest usually reaches 120 mm Hg. As the heart relaxes (**diastole**) and aortic valves close, the natural elastic recoil of the aorta and other arteries provides a continuous head of pressure to move blood into the periphery until the next surge from ventricular systole. During the cardiac cycle's diastole, arterial blood pressure decreases to 70 to 80 mm Hg. Arteries "hardened" by mineral and fatty deposits within their walls, or with excessive peripheral resistance to blood flow from kidney malfunction, induce systolic pressures as high as 300 mm Hg and diastolic pressures above 120 mm Hg.

High blood pressure (**hypertension**) imposes a chronic strain on normal cardiovascular function. If left untreated, severe hypertension leads to congestive heart failure; the heart muscle weakens, unable to maintain its normal pumping ability. Degenerating, brittle vessels can obstruct blood flow, or can burst, cutting off vital blood flow to brain tissue—precipitating a stroke.

During Exercise

Rhythmic Exercise

During rhythmic muscular activities like brisk walking, hiking, jogging, swimming, and bicycling, dilation of the active muscles' blood vessels, increases the vascular area

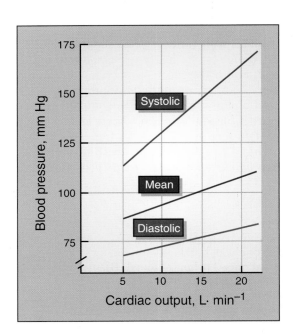

Figure 11.6
Generalized relationship between blood flow (cardiac output) and systemic arterial pressures measured at the brachial artery during exercise. Mean arterial blood pressure represents the average force exerted by the blood against the arterial walls during the entire cardiac cycle. It equals slightly less than the arithmetic average of the systolic and diastolic pressures because the heart remains in diastole longer than in systole.

How to Measure Blood Pressure

Blood pressure represents the force (pressure) exerted by blood against the arterial walls during a cardiac cycle. Systolic blood pressure, the higher of the two pressure measurements, occurs during ventricular contraction (systole) as the heart propels 70 to 100 mL of blood into the aorta. After systole, the ventricles relax (diastole), the arteries recoil, and arterial pressure continually declines as blood flows into the periphery and the heart refills with blood. The lowest pressure reached during ventricular relaxation represents diastolic blood pressure. Normal systolic blood pressure in an adult varies between 110 and 140 mm Hg, and diastolic pressure varies between 60 and 90 mm Hg. Elevated systolic or diastolic blood pressure (termed hypertension) is defined as a resting systolic blood pressure greater than 140 mm Hg and diastolic pressure exceeding 90 mm Hg. **Pulse pressure** reflects the difference between systolic and diastolic pressures.

BLOOD PRESSURE CLASSIFICATION

Systolic (mm Hg)	Diastolic (mm Hg)	Category
<130	<85	Normal
130–139	85–89	High-normal
140–159	90–99	Stage 1 hypertension
160–179	100–109	Moderate (Stage 2) hypertension
180–209	110–119	Severe (Stage 3) hypertension
>210	120	Very severe (Stage 4) hypertension

From: Fifth report of the joint committee on detection, evaluation, and treatment of high blood pressure (JNCV): *Arch. Int. Med.*, 153:154, 1993.

Measurement Procedures

Blood pressure, measured indirectly by **auscultation** (listening to sounds; described in 1902 by Russian physician N.S. Korotkoff; 1874–1920), uses a stethoscope and sphygmomanometer, consisting of a blood pressure cuff and an aneroid or mercury column pressure gauge.

1. Subject, seated in a quiet, room exposes upper arm.
2. Subject bends arm to bring the elbow to heart level.
3. Locate the brachial artery at the inner side of the upper arm, approximately 1 inch above the bend in the elbow.
4. Take the free end of the cuff and gently slide it through the metal loop (or wrap over exposed Velcro) and flap it back over so the cuff wraps around the upper arm at heart level. Align the arrows on the cuff with the brachial artery. Secure the Velcro parts of the cuff. The sphygmomanometer cuff should fit snugly (but not tight) to obtain accurate readings. Use appropriate-sized cuffs for children and the obese.
5. Place the stethoscope bell below the antecubital space over the brachial artery.
6. The cuff should now have the connecting tube (from the sphygmomanometer bulb and gauge) exiting the cuff towards the arm.
7. Before inflating the cuff, make sure the air release switch remains closed (turn the knob clockwise).
8. Inflate the cuff with quick, even pumps to about 180 mm Hg.
9. Gradually release cuff pressure (about 3 mm per s) by slowly opening the air release knob (counter-clockwise turn), noting the first sound. This sound results from turbulence from the rush of blood as the formerly closed artery briefly opens during the highest pressure in the cardiac cycle. This represents systolic blood pressure.
10. Continue to reduce pressure, noting when the sound becomes muffled (*4th phase diastolic pressure*) and when the sound disappears (*5th phase diastolic pressure*). Clinicians usually record the 5th phase as diastolic blood pressure.
11. If the measured pressure exceeds 140/90 mm Hg, allow a 10-minute rest and repeat the procedure.

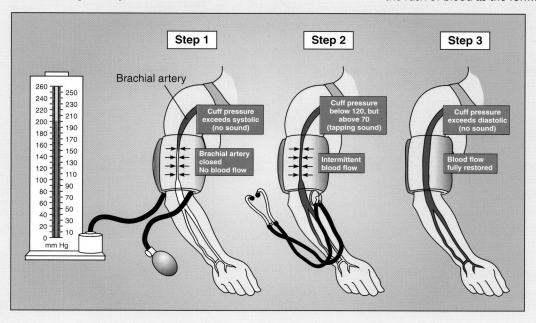

imum exercise in healthy endurance athletes owing to these athletes' large cardiac outputs.

Resistance Exercise

Straining-type exercises (e.g., heavy resistance exercise, shoveling wet snow) increase blood pressure dramatically because sustained muscular force compresses peripheral arterioles, significantly increasing resistance to blood flow. The heart's additional workload from acute elevations in blood pressure increases risk for individuals with existing hypertension or coronary heart disease. In such cases, rhythmic forms of moderate physical activity provide less risk and greater health benefits. Figure 11.7 shows blood pressure responses during rhythmic aerobic exercise and heavy resistance movements that engage small and large amounts of muscle mass.

Upper-Body Exercise

Table 11.1 shows that exercise at a given percentage of $\dot{V}O_{2max}$ increases systolic and diastolic blood pressures significantly more in rhythmic arm (upper-body) compared with leg (lower-body) exercise. The smaller arm muscle mass and vasculature offer greater resistance to blood flow than the larger and more vascularized lower-body regions. This means that blood flow to the arms during exercise requires a much larger systolic pressure head and accompanying increase in myocardial workload and vascular strain. For individuals with cardiovascular dysfunction, more prudent exercise involves larger muscle groups (walking, running, bicycling, stair climbing) rather than unregulated exercises of a limited muscle mass (shoveling, overhead hammering, or even arm-crank ergometry). If exercise training requires arm exercise, the person's response to this exercise mode (and not lower-body exercise) must formulate the exercise prescription.

Body Inversion

Inversion devices that allow a person to hang upside-down have been used for years to increase relaxation, facilitate a strength-training response, and relieve lower back pain. However, we are unaware of any research that demonstrates that body inversion provides any practical medical or physiologic benefit. On the negative side, the maneuver significantly increases blood pressure at the start and throughout the inversion period. This raises concern about possible consequences of inversion for people with hypertension, and the wisdom of performing exercises in the upside-down position, which magnifies the normal increase in exercise blood pressure. A brief period of inversion also doubles

Hypertension and Race

African Americans have twice the incidence of high blood pressure as white counterparts, and nearly seven times the rate of severe hypertension. The fact that African Americans in the United States have a much greater incidence of hypertension than blacks in Africa compounds the issue of race and hypertension. Ongoing research focuses on diet, stress, cigarette smoking, and other lifestyle and environmental factors that trigger this chronic blood pressure response in genetically susceptible blacks.

pressure within the eye (intraocular pressure) in healthy, young adults. Clearly, individuals with eye disorders should refrain from prolonged periods of inversion.

In Recovery

After a bout of sustained light- to moderate-intensity exercise, systolic blood pressure temporarily decreases below pre-exercise levels for up to 12 hours in normal and hypertensive subjects. Pooling of blood in the visceral organs and lower limbs during recovery reduces central blood volume, which contributes to lower blood pressure. The **hypotensive recovery response** further supports exercise as an important nonpharmacologic hypertension therapy. A potentially effective approach spreads several bouts of moderate physical activity throughout the day.

TABLE 11.1
Comparison of systolic and diastolic blood pressures during arm and leg exercise at similar percentages of maximal oxygen uptake

PERCENT $\dot{V}O_{2max}$	SYSTOLIC PRESSURE (mm Hg) ARMS	LEGS	DIASTOLIC PRESSURE (mm Hg) ARMS	LEGS
25	150	132	90	70
40	165	138	93	71
50	175	144	96	73
75	205	160	103	75

*From Åstrand, P. O., et al.: Intra-arterial blood pressure during exercise with different muscle groups. *J. Appl. Physiol.*, 20:253, 1965.

Heart's Blood Supply

Over 7000 gallons of blood flow from the heart each day, but none of its oxygen or nutrients pass directly to the myocardium from the heart's chambers. The myocardium maintains its own elaborate circulatory system. Figure 11.8 illustrates these vessels as a visible, crown-like network, the **coronary circulation,** that arises from the top portion of the heart.

The openings for the left and right coronary arteries emerge from the aorta just above the semilunar valves where oxygenated blood leaves the left ventricle. The arteries then curl around the heart's surface; the **right coronary artery** supplies predominantly the right atrium and ventricle, whereas the greatest blood volume flows in the **left coronary artery** to the left atrium and ventricle, and a small portion of the right ventricle. These vessels divide to eventually form a dense capillary network within the myocardium. Blood leaves the tissues of the left ventricle through the coronary sinus; blood from the right ventricle exits through the anterior cardiac veins and empties directly into the right atrium.

Myocardial Oxygen Utilization

Oxygen utilization by the heart muscle remains high in relation to its blood flow. At rest, the myocardium extracts 70 to 80% of the oxygen from the blood flowing in the coronary vessels. In contrast, most other tissues use only about 25% of the blood's available oxygen. Because near-maximal oxygen extraction occurs at rest, increases in coronary blood flow provide the only means to meet myocardial oxygen demands in exercise. In vigorous exercise, coronary blood flow increases four to six times above the resting level because of elevated myocardial metabolism and increased aortic pressure.

Profuse myocardial vascularization supplies each muscle fiber with at least one capillary. Adequate oxygenation becomes so crucial that impairment in coronary blood flow can trigger chest discomfort and pain, a condition termed **angina pectoris.** The pain increases during exercise when myocardial oxygen demand rises considerably. A blood clot (**thrombus**) lodged in one of the coronary vessels can severely impair normal heart function. This form of "heart attack" (**myocardial infarction**) often injures the myocardium; severe damage to this muscle can result in death. Chapter 21 discusses diseases of the myocardium and the role exercise testing plays in evaluating cardiac function.

Rate-Pressure Product: An Estimate of Myocardial Work

Three important mechanical factors determine myocardial oxygen uptake:

1. Tension development within the myocardium
2. Myocardial contractility
3. Heart rate

When each of the above factors increases during exercise, myocardial blood flow adjusts to balance oxygen supply with demand. The product of peak systolic blood pressure (SBP; measured at the brachial artery) and heart rate (HR) provides a convenient estimate of myocardial workload (oxygen uptake). This index of *relative* cardiac work, called the **double product** or **rate-pressure product (RPP)**, closely reflects directly measured myocardial oxygen uptake and coronary blood flow in healthy subjects over a range of exercise intensities. RPP computes as:

$$RPP = SBP \times HR$$

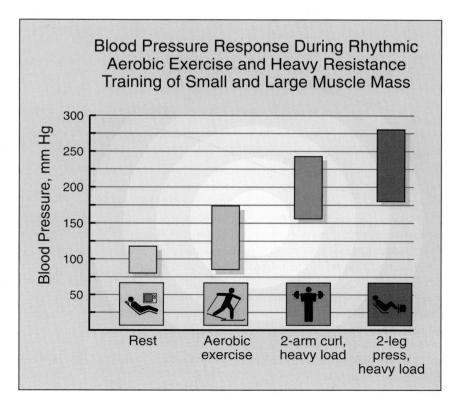

Figure 11.7
Blood pressure response during rhythmic aerobic exercise and heavy resistance training of a small and large muscle mass. The top of each bar represents systolic blood pressure; the bottom represents diastolic blood pressure.

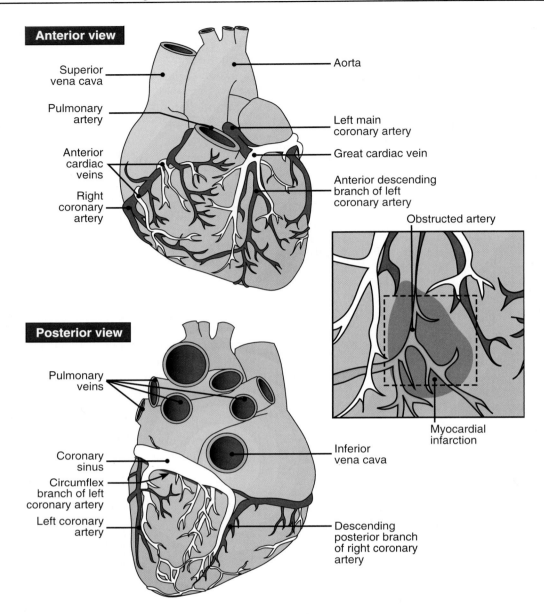

Figure 11.8
Anterior and posterior views of the coronary circulation, with arteries shaded dark and veins unshaded. Inset figure illustrates a myocardial infarction resulting from the blockage (occulsion) of a coronary vessel.

Exercise studies of people with coronary heart disease have linked the RPP to the onset of angina and/or electrocardiographic abnormalities. RPP has also assessed various clinical, surgical, and exercise interventions for their effects on cardiac performance. The reductions in exercise heart rate and systolic blood pressure with endurance training improve cardiac patients' exercise capacity because of the reduced myocardial oxygen requirement. Prolonged, intense aerobic training significantly increases the RPP of patients before they experience the onset of heart disease symptoms. In nine patients, followed over a 7-year peiod of exercise training, RPP increased 11.5% before ischemic abnormalities appeared. These important findings provide indirect evidence for a training-in- duced improvement in myocardial oxygenation, perhaps from greater coronary vascularization, reduced obstruction, or a combination of both factors. Typical values for RPP range from 6000 at rest (HR = 50 b·min^{-1}; SBP = 120 mm Hg) to 40,000 during intense exercise (HR = 200 b·min^{-1}; SBP = 200 mm Hg). Changes in heart rate and blood pressure contribute equally to a change in RPP.

Heart's Energy Supply

The heart relies almost exclusively on aerobic energy metabolism. Myocardial fibers have the greatest mitochondrial concentration of all body tissues. Glucose, fatty

close up

Exercising after Cardiac Transplantation

The prognosis for living is not good for patients with severe left ventricular dysfunction (referred to as **end-stage heart disease**). Although some minimally symptomatic or asymptomatic patients may function in a near-normal manner and survive for several years taking medication, most symptomatic patients die within 1 year of diagnosis. **Cardiac transplantation** becomes the accepted form of treatment for some of these patients. The first successful human heart transplant was performed in 1967. Although long-term survival (>1 y) was rare before the 1980s, survival rates have progressively increased due to improved immunosuppressive drug combinations, and use of transvenous endomyocardial biopsy techniques for early detection of tissue rejection.

Orthotopic transplantation involves removing the recipient's diseased heart and connecting the donor heart to the remaining great vessels and atria. For selected patients, a "piggy back" transplant uses a donor heart placed in the recipient's chest without removing the diseased heart. Regardless of the form of transplantation, patients often have complicated recoveries with recurrent hospitalization and prolonged medical care. The most common complications include infection and rejection of the donor heart, both leading causes of death.

After successful transplantations, patients report a favorable quality of life, and approximately 50% return to work. Successful pregnancy and vaginal delivery in a cardiac transplant patient has occurred, as well as completion of a full marathon run in under 6 hours. However, cardiac transplant patients have significantly impaired exercise capacity with diminished physiological and hemodynamic function. Transplant patients show an abnormal acute response to exercise. They exhibit a diminished cardiac output and oxygen uptake during exercise, and have an elevated resting heart rate and reduced left ventricular ejection fraction. Transplant patients respond positively to exercise training. The increase in peak $\dot{V}O_2$ ranges from a high of 40% to a low of 17%. This indicates that transplant patients can dramatically improve cardiorespiratory fitness, probably because of their poor initial fitness levels.

Guidelines for exercise prescription for cardiac transplant patients are essentially the same as for other post-cardiac surgery patients—with the following exception: target heart rate guidelines do not apply because of the delayed heart rate response of the denervated transplanted organ. Most often, exercise intensity is prescribed using the Borg scale for rating of perceived exertion (RPE) using ratings between "fairly light" to "somewhat hard" (RPE scale between 11 and 14). Because of the blunted heart rate response with the onset of exercise, a graded warm-up becomes particularly important for the cardiac transplant patient. Furthermore, because the transplanted heart has no connections to the nervous system, patients who have exercise-induced ischemia do not experience the painful warnings of angina pectoris.

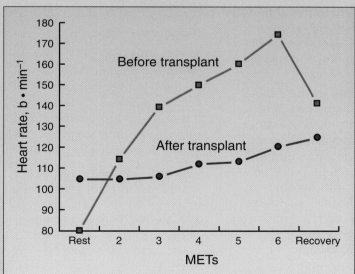

Heart rates of a patient during graded exercise before and after orthotopic cardiac transplantation. Note the elevated resting heart rate and the delayed increases in exercise heart rate and blunted recovery rate after transplantation.

Squires, R. W.: Exercise training after cardiac transplantation. *Med. Sci. Sports Exerc.*, 23:686, 1991

References

Daida, H., et al.: Sequential assessment of exercise tolerance in heart transplantation compared with coronary artery bypass surgery after Phase II cardiac rehabilitation. *Am. J. Cardiol.*, 77:696, 1996.

Hunt, S.A.: Current status of cardiac transplantation. *JAMA*, 280:1692, 1998.

Notaricus, C.F., et al.: Cardiac versus noncardiac limits to exercise after heart transplantation. *Am. Heart J.*, 135(2 Pt 1):339, 1998.

Osada, N., et al.: Long-term cardiopulmonary exercise performance after heart transplantation. *Am. J. Cardiol.*, 79:451, 1997.

Osada, N., et al.: Cardiopulmonary exercise testing identifies low risk patients with heart failure and severely impaired exercise capacity considered for heart transplantation. *J. Am. Coll. Cardiol.*, 31:577, 1998.

acids, and lactate formed in skeletal muscle during anaerobic glycolysis provide energy for proper myocardial functioning. The heart uses whatever energy substrate it "sees" on a physiologic level. When lactate efflux from skeletal muscle into blood increases during heavy exercise, the heart derives as much as 50% of its total energy by oxidizing circulating lactate. During prolonged submaximal exercise, myocardial free fatty acid catabolism increases to nearly 70% of the heart's total energy requirement.

summary

1. The striated fibers of the myocardium interconnect to make large portions of the heart contract in a unified manner. The heart functions as two separate pumps: one pump receives blood from the body and pumps it to the lungs for aeration (pulmonary circulation); the other pump accepts oxygenated blood from the lungs and pumps it throughout the body (systemic circulation).

2. Pressure changes during the cardiac cycle act on the heart's valves to provide one-way blood flow through the vascular circuit.

3. The dense capillary network provides a large, effective surface for exchange between blood and tissues. These microscopic vessels adjust blood flow in response to the tissue's metabolic activity.

4. When skeletal muscle contracts, vein compression and relaxation impart considerable energy for venous return. "Muscle-pump" action justifies use of active recovery from vigorous exercise.

5. Nerves and hormones constrict or stiffen the smooth muscle layer in venous walls. Alterations in venous tone profoundly affect redistribution of total blood volume.

6. The surge of blood with ventricular contraction (and subsequent run-off during relaxation) creates pressure changes within the arterial vessels. Systolic pressure represents the highest pressure generated during the cardiac cycle; diastolic pressure describes the lowest pressure before the next ventricular contraction.

7. Hypertension imposes a chronic stress on cardiovascular function. Regular aerobic training modestly reduces systolic and diastolic blood pressures during rest and submaximal exercise.

8. During graded exercise, systolic blood pressure increases in proportion to oxygen uptake and cardiac output, whereas diastolic pressure remains unchanged or increases slightly. The same relative exercise intensity ($\%VO_{2max}$) produces a larger pressure response with upper-body compared with lower-body exercise.

9. During recovery from light and moderate exercise, blood pressure falls below pre-exercise levels (hypotensive response) and remains lower for up to 12 hours.

10. Peak systolic and diastolic blood pressures mirror the hypertensive state during standard resistance exercises. Inordinately high blood pressure (and rate-pressure product) in such exercise poses a risk to individuals with hypertension and coronary heart disease. Regular resistance exercise training blunts the hypertensive response to straining-type exercise.

11. At rest, the myocardium extracts about 80% of the oxygen from coronary blood flow. Consequently, increased myocardial oxygen demands in exercise depend on proportionate increases in coronary blood flow.

12. The aerobic nature of myocardial tissue requires a continual oxygen supply. Impaired coronary blood flow causes chest discomfort and pain (angina pectoris); blockage of a coronary artery (myocardial infarction) can irreversibly damage heart muscle.

13. Cardiac transplantation provides a viable treatment for patients with end-stage heart disease, with approximately 50% of patients returning to work. Because of the transplanted heart's lack of direct innervation, these patients show an abnormally sluggish heart rate response to exercise.

14. The product of heart rate and systolic blood pressure (rate-pressure product) estimates relative myocardial workload. Clinicians use this index to study exercise training effects on cardiac performance in heart disease patients.

15. Glucose, fatty acids, and lactate represent the heart's main substrates for energy metabolism. As with skeletal muscle, percentage utilization of these substrates varies with exercise intensity and duration.

PART 2
Cardiovascular Regulation and Integration

Heart's Rest Period

The heart's relatively long depolarization period requires about 0.30 seconds before the myocardium can receive another impulse and contract again. This "rest" or **refractory period**, provides sufficient time for ventricular filling between beats.

At rest in a comfortable environment, the skin receives 250 mL (5%) of the 5 L of blood pumped from the heart each minute. In contrast, 20% of the total cardiac output flows to the body's surface for heat dissipation with exercise in a hot, humid environment. The rapid redistribution ("shunting") of blood to meet metabolic and physiologic requirements (with appropriate maintenance of blood pressure) requires a closed circulatory system with both central and local control of pump output and vascular dimensions.

Heart Rate Regulation

Cardiac muscle possesses intrinsic rhythmicity. Without external stimuli, the adult heart would beat steadily between 50 and 80 times each minute. Within the body, nerves that directly supply the myocardium and chemicals within the blood rapidly alter heart rate. Extrinsic control of cardiac function causes the heart to speed up in "anticipation," even before exercise begins. To a large extent, extrinsic regulation can adjust heart rate to as slow as 40 b·min^{-1} at rest in some endurance athletes, and as fast as 220 b·min^{-1} during maximum exercise.

Intrinsic Regulation

A mass of specialized muscle tissue, the **sinoatrial (S-A) node**, lies within the posterior wall of the right atrium. The S-A node spontaneously depolarizes and repolarizes to provide an "innate" stimulus to the heart. For this reason, the term "**pacemaker**" describes the S-A node. Figure 11.9 shows the normal route for transmitting the electrical impulse across the myocardium.

Heart's Electrical Impulse

Rhythms originating at the S-A node spread across the atria to another small knot of tissue, the **atrioventricular (A-V) node**. The node delays the impulse about 0.10 seconds to provide suf-ficient time for the atria to contract and force blood into the ventricles. The A-V node gives rise to the **A-V bundle (bundle of His)**, which speeds the impulse rapidly through the ventricles over specialized conducting fibers called the **Purkinje system**. The fibers form distinct branches that penetrate the right and left ventricles. Each ventricular cell becomes stimulated within 0.06 seconds from passage of the impulse into the ventricles; this causes simultaneous contraction of both ventricles. Cardiac impulse transmission progresses as follows:

$$S\text{-}A \text{ node} \rightarrow Atria \rightarrow A\text{-}V \text{ node} \rightarrow A\text{-}V \text{ bundle (Purkinje fibers)} \rightarrow Ventricles$$

Electrocardiogram

The electrical activity generated by the myocardium creates an electrical field throughout the body. Because salty body fluid conducts well, electrodes placed on the skin's surface detect the sequence of electrical events during each cardiac cycle. The **electrocardiogram (ECG)** provides a graphic

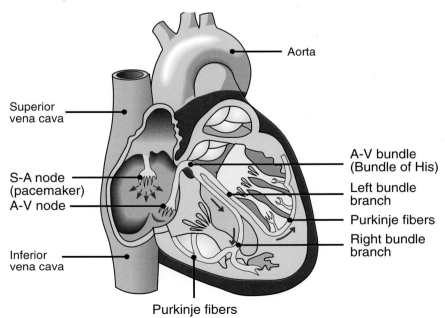

Figure 11.9
Normal route for excitation and conduction of the cardiac impulse. This impulse originates at the S-A node, travels to the A-V node, and then flows throughout the ventricular mass.

record of voltage changes during the heart's electrical activity. Figure 11.10 illustrates a normal ECG with important sequences of major myocardial electrical activity.

The ECG provides a means to monitor heart rate during exercise. Radiotelemetry allows ECG transmission while a person freely performs diverse physical activities including football, weightlifting, basketball, ice hockey, dancing, and even swimming. Electrocardiography can uncover abnormalities in heart function related to cardiac rhythm, electrical conduction, myocardial oxygen supply, and actual tissue damage (see Chapter 21, and *How to Place Electrodes for Bipolar and Twelve-Lead ECG Recordings*, p. 281).

Extrinsic Regulation

Neural impulses override the inherent myocardial rhythmicity. The signals originate in the cardiovascular center in the medulla and travel through the sympathetic and parasympathetic components of the autonomic nervous system. Figure 11.11 shows the atria supplied with large numbers of sympathetic and parasympathetic neurons, whereas the ventricles receive sympathetic fibers almost exclusively.

Sympathetic Influence

Stimulation of the sympathetic cardioaccelerator nerves releases the **catecholamines** epinephrine and norepinephrine.

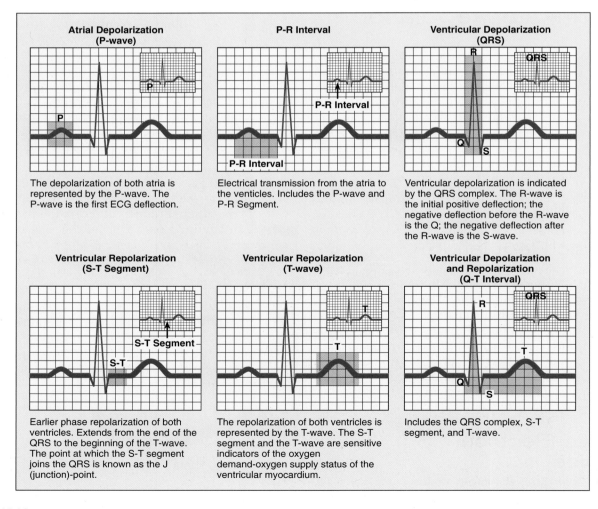

Atrial Depolarization (P-wave)
The depolarization of both atria is represented by the P-wave. The P-wave is the first ECG deflection.

P-R Interval
Electrical transmission from the atria to the venticles. Includes the P-wave and P-R Segment.

Ventricular Depolarization (QRS)
Ventricular depolarization is indicated by the QRS complex. The R-wave is the initial positive deflection; the negative deflection before the R-wave is the Q; the negative deflection after the R-wave is the S-wave.

Ventricular Repolarization (S-T Segment)
Earlier phase repolarization of both ventricles. Extends from the end of the QRS to the beginning of the T-wave. The point at which the S-T segment joins the QRS is known as the J (junction)-point.

Ventricular Repolarization (T-wave)
The repolarization of both ventricles is represented by the T-wave. The S-T segment and the T-wave are sensitive indicators of the oxygen demand-oxygen supply status of the ventricular myocardium.

Ventricular Depolarization and Repolarization (Q-T Interval)
Includes the QRS complex, S-T segment, and T-wave.

Figure 11.10
Different phases of the normal electrocardiogram (ECG) from atrial depolarization (upper left) to repolarization of the ventricles (lower right).

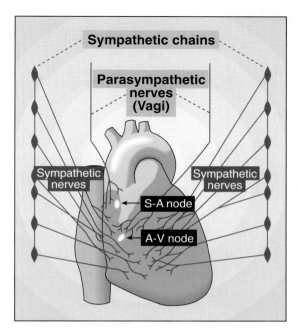

Figure 11.11
Distribution of sympathetic and parasympathetic nerve fibers to the heart.

These neural hormones increase myocardial contractility and accelerate S-A node depolarization to increase heart rate, a response termed **tachycardia**. Epinephrine, released from the medullary portion of the adrenal glands in response to general sympathetic activation, also produces a similar though slower-acting effect on cardiac function.

Parasympathetic Influence

Acetylcholine, the parasympathetic nervous system hormone, retards the sinus discharge rate, which slows heart rate. This response, termed **bradycardia**, comes from the **vagus nerve** whose cell bodies originate in the cardioin-

hibitory portion of the medulla. Vagal stimulation does not affect myocardial contractility.

Training Effects on Catecholamines

Endurance training creates an imbalance between sympathetic accelerator and parasympathetic depressor activity in favor of greater vagal (parasympathetic) dominance. The effect occurs primarily from increased parasympathetic activity, with some decrease in sympathetic discharge. Training may also decrease the S-A node's intrinsic firing rate. These adaptations account for the significant bradycardia frequently observed among highly conditioned endurance athletes or sedentary individuals who undertake aerobic training.

Cortical Influence

Impulses originating in the brain's higher somatomotor **central command system** pass via small afferent nerves to directly modulate the activity of the cardiovascular center in the **ventrolateral medulla**. This provides the coordinated and rapid response of the heart and blood vessels to optimize tissue perfusion and maintain central blood pressure in relation to motor cortex involvement. The central command exerts its effect not only during exercise but also at rest and in the pre-exercise period. Thus, variation in emotional state can significantly affect cardiovascular responses, often obscuring "true" resting values for heart rate and blood pressure. Cortical input also causes heart rate to rise rapidly in anticipation of exercise. The combined effects of an increase in sympathetic discharge and reduction of vagal tone produce the **anticipatory heart rate**.

Figure 11.12 demonstrates the extent of the anticipatory heart rate response. Radiotelemetry monitored the heart rates of trained sprint runners at rest, at the starting commands, and during a 60-, 220-, and 440-yard race. Heart rate averaged 148 b·min^{-1} at the starting commands in anticipation of the 60-yard sprint; this represented 74% of the total heart rate adjustment to the run before exercise even began. The shortest sprint event generated the greatest anticipatory response, with successively lower heart rates for longer sprint distances.

Running events of longer duration than sprints produced a similar pattern of anticipatory heart rate. For example, anticipatory heart rates of four middle-distance athletes averaged 122 b·min^{-1} during start-

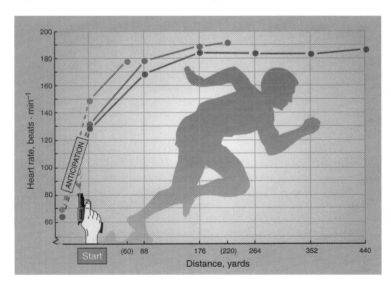

Figure 11.12
Heart rate response of sprint-trained runners. The greatest anticipatory heart rate (heart rate immediately prior to exercising) increase occurs in short sprint events and becomes successively lower just before beginning longer sprint distances.

ing commands for the 880-yard run, 118 beats for the one-mile run, and 108 beats for the two-mile run. Intense neural outflow in anticipation of all-out activity of short duration (such as sprinting) initiates rapid mobilization of bodily reserves. On the other hand, this mechanism for "revving the body's engine" might prove physiologically inefficient in longer distance events.

The heart "turns on" for exercise from four sources: 1) increased sympathetic activity, 2) decreased parasympathetic activity, combined with 3) input from the brain's central command, and 4) activation of receptors in joints and muscles as exercise begins. Even for nonsprint events, heart rate reaches 180 b·min^{-1} within 30 seconds of 1- and 2-mile runs. Further heart rate increases progress gradually, with plateaus attained several times during the runs.

Figure 11.13 depicts major factors controlling heart rate and myocardial contractility. The medulla receives continual input about blood pressure from baroreceptors within the carotid arteries and aorta. The medulla also acts as an integrating and coordinating center, receiving stimuli from the cortex and peripheral tissues, and routing an appropriate response to the heart and blood vessels.

Peripheral Input. The cardiovascular center in the medulla receives sensory input from mechanical receptors (**mechanoreceptors**) and chemical receptors in blood vessels, joints, and muscles. Stimuli from these peripheral receptors monitor the state of active muscle; they modify either vagal or sympathetic outflow to create an appropriate cardiovascular response. Reflex neural input from active muscle (termed the **exercise pressor reflex**), in conjunction with output originating in the brain's higher motor areas, assess the nature and intensity of exercise and the quantity of muscle recruited. Input from mechanoreceptors provides particularly important feedback for the central nervous system's regulation of blood flow and blood pressure during dynamic exercise. Receptors in the aortic arch and carotid sinus respond to changes in arterial blood pressure. As blood pressure increases, the stretch of arterial vessels activates these **baroreceptors**, which reflexly slows heart rate and dilates peripheral vasculature. This lowers blood pressure toward normal levels. Exercise overrides this particular feedback mechanism because heart rate and blood pressure both increase. Baroreceptors likely prevent abnormally high blood pressure levels in exercise.

A Responsive Vasculature

The capacity of the vasculature to either constrict or dilate provides rapid redistribution of blood to meet tissue's metabolic requirements while maintaining appropriate blood pressure throughout the entire system.

Carotid Artery Palpation. For healthy adults and cardiac patients, **carotid artery palpation** has little effect on heart rate during rest, exercise, and recovery. Certain vascular diseases, however, affect carotid sinus sensitivity. Under these conditions, strong external pressure against the carotid artery slows heart rate — probably from direct stimulation of carotid artery baroreceptors.

Accurate heart rate measurement provides the basis for establishing "target heart rates" during exercise training (refer to Chapter 14). If heart rate measurement consistently underestimated actual values, the person would exercise at higher levels than prescribed, certainly an undesirable effect when prescribing exercise for cardiac patients. An excellent substitute method involves determining pulse rate at the radial or temporal arteries (see Fig. 11.5) because palpation at these sites does not change heart rate.

Arrhythmias

The exquisite regulation of heart rate by intrinsic and extrinsic mechanisms generally progresses unnoticed and without adverse consequence. However, electrocardiographic and heart rate irregularities do occur and can herald significant myocardial disease. The term **arrhythmia** describes heart rhythm irregularities.

Heart Rate Irregularities

Interruption of regular heart rate pattern often occurs as extra beats (**extrasystoles**). Parts of the atria can become prematurely electrically active and depolarize spontaneously prior to S-A node excitation, a condition called **premature atrial contraction** or **PAC**. Premature excitation of ventricles (**premature ventricular contraction** or **PVC**) also occurs during the interval between two regular beats. Occasional extrasystoles appear during rest and usually progress unnoticed. Psychological stress, anxiety, and caffeine consumption can trigger extrasystoles, probably from catecholamine's effect on the rate of change of the S-A node's membrane potential. Removal of such stimuli usually reestablishes normal heart rhythm. If this fails, medication that blocks norepinephrine's action on the beta receptors of atrial cells (**beta blockers**) effectively treats this condition. Atrial arrhythmias do not compromise the heart's pumping ability (recall that atrial contraction contributes little to ventricular filling). A potentially dangerous situation arises when PACs link successively to create **atrial fibrillation**.

Ventricular fibrillation is the most serious arrhythmia. With this condition, foci of stimulation continually affect different parts of the ventricle, rather than the normal single stimulus from the A-V node. *Portions of the ventricle contract in an uncoordinated manner with repetitive PVCs, thus hindering the ventricle's ability to pump blood. Cardiac output and blood pressure decrease, and the person rapidly loses consciousness.*

Resuscitation takes two forms: 1) reestablish normal heart pumping action to restore blood pressure, and 2) halt fibrillation and reestablish normal electrical rhythm. **Car-**

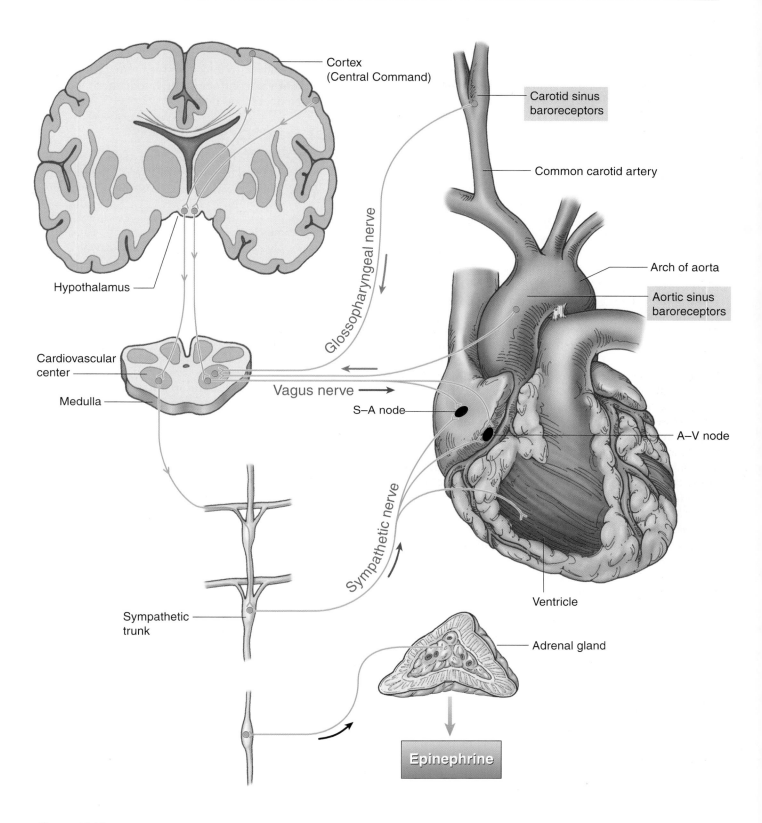

Figure 11.13
Pathways in reflex control of heart rate. The cardiovascular center in the medulla receives input from 1) baroreceptors in the carotid sinus and aortic arch, and 2) cortical stimulation (central command). Efferent pathways from the medulla activate the heart by the vagus (parasympathetic) and sympathetic nerves.

diopulmonary resuscitation (CPR) mechanically simulates the heart's pumping action and often reverses fibrillation. If this fails, a defibrillator applies a strong burst of electric current across the entire myocardium. This depolarizes the heart, which can initiate normal rhythm from the S-A node upon repolarization. All exercise specialists need to be CPR certified (and re-certified each year). The American Red Cross maintains CPR testing and certification programs for all interested persons.

Blood Distribution

Exercise Effects

Increased energy expenditure requires rapid readjustments in blood flow that affect the entire cardiovascular system. For example, nerves and local metabolic conditions act on the smooth muscle bands of arteriole walls, causing them to alter their internal diameter almost instantaneously. Concurrently, neural stimulation of venous capacitance vessels causes them to "stiffen," moving blood from peripheral veins into the central circulation.

During exercise, the vascular portion of active muscles increases through dilation of local arterioles; at the same time, vessels "shut down" blood flow to tissues that can temporarily compromise blood supply. Kidney function vividly illustrates regulatory capacity for adjusting regional blood flow. Renal circulation at rest normally averages $1100 \text{ mL} \cdot \text{min}^{-1}$ or about 20% of cardiac output. In maximal exercise, renal blood flow decreases to $250 \text{ mL} \cdot \text{min}^{-1}$, which represents only 1% of a 25-L exercise cardiac output.

Blood Flow Regulation

Pressure differentials and resistances determine fluid movement through a vessel. Resistance varies directly with the length of the vessel and inversely with its diameter; greater driving force increases flow while increased resistance impedes it. The following equation expresses the interaction between pressure, resistance, and fluid flow:

$$\text{Flow} = \text{Pressure} \div \text{Resistance}$$

Three factors determine resistance to blood flow:

1. Viscosity, or blood thickness
2. Length of conducting tube
3. Radius of blood vessel

The following equation, referred to as **Poiseuille's law**, expresses the general relationship between pressure differential (gradient), resistance, and flow in a cylindrical vessel:

$$\text{Flow} = \text{Pressure gradient} \times \text{Vessel radius}^4 \div \text{Vessel length} \times \text{Fluid viscosity}$$

Blood viscosity and transport vessel length remain relatively constant in the body. Consequently, blood vessel radius represents the most important factor affecting blood flow. *Resistance to flow changes with vessel radius raised to the fourth power.* Reducing a vessel's radius by one-half decreases flow by a factor of 16; conversely, doubling the radius increases volume 16 fold. This means that a relatively small degree of vasoconstriction or vasodilation dramatically alters regional blood flow.

Local Factors

One of every 30 to 40 capillaries actually remains open in muscle tissue at rest. Thus, opening of large numbers of "dormant" capillaries with exercise serves three important functions:

1. Increases muscle blood flow
2. Increases blood-flow volume through muscle with relatively small increases in velocity
3. Increases effective surface for gas and nutrient exchange between blood and individual muscle fibers

A decrease in tissue oxygen supply stimulates local vasodilation in skeletal and cardiac muscle. Local increases in temperature, carbon dioxide, acidity, adenosine, nitric oxide, and magnesium and potassium ions also enhance regional blood flow. These **autoregulatory mechanisms** for blood flow make sense physiologically because they reflect elevated tissue metabolism and increased oxygen need. Rapid, local vasodilation provides the most effective, immediate step for increasing a tissue's oxygen supply.

Neural Factors

Central vascular control via sympathetic, and to a minor degree parasympathetic, portions of the autonomic nervous system overrides vasoregulation afforded by local factors. For example, muscles contain small sensory nerve fibers highly sensitive to chemical substances released in active muscle during exercise. Stimulation of these fibers

A Physiologic Role for Nitric Oxide

Physiologists originally believed that acetylcholine acted singularly on arterial smooth muscle to effect dilation. We now know that nitric oxide (NO) gas functions as a potent neurotransmitter to facilitate acetylcholine's action. NO, produced by the endothelium lining of blood vessels, relaxes arterial smooth muscle in neighboring blood vessels. Vascular wall receptors for NO control important functions, particularly blood pressure regulation in response to central cardiovascular center stimulation. The degree to which the release and action of this gas affects cardiovascular dynamics in exercise remains unknown.

How to Place Electrodes for Bipolar and 12-Lead ECG Recordings

The electrocardiogram (ECG) represents a composite record of the heart's electrical events during a cardiac cycle. These events provide a means to monitor heart rate during different physical activities and exercise stress testing. The ECG can detect contraindications to exercise including previous myocardial infarction, ischemic S-T segment changes, conduction defects, and left ventricular enlargement (hypertrophy). A valid ECG tracing requires proper electrode placement. The term **ECG lead** indicates the specific placement of *a pair* of electrodes on the body that transmits the electrical signal to a recorder. The record of electrical differences across diverse ECG leads creates the composite electrical "picture" of myocardial activity.

Skin Preparation

Proper skin preparation reduces extraneous electrical "noise" (interference and skeletal muscle artifact). Abrade the skin with fine sandpaper or commercially available pads and alcohol to remove surface epidermis and oil; the skin should appear red, slightly irritated, dry, and clean.

Bipolar (3-electrode) Configuration

The left figure shows the typical electrode placement for a bipolar configuration. This positioning provides less sensitivity for diagnostic testing but proves useful for routine ECG monitoring in functional exercise testing and radiotelemetry of the ECG during physical activity. The ground (green or black) electrode attaches over the sternum, the positive (red) electrode attaches on the left side of the chest in the V_5 position (level of the 5th intercostal space adjacent to the midaxillary line), and the positive (white) electrode attaches on the right side of the chest, just below the nipple at the level of the 5th intercostal space. Placement of the positive electrode can be altered to optimize the recording (e.g.,

3rd and 4th intercostal spaces, anterior portion of the right shoulder, or near the clavicle). Correct electrode placement can be remembered as follows: *white to right, green to ground, red to left.*

Modified 12-lead (10-electrode torso-mounted) Configuration for Exercise Stress Testing

The standard 12-lead ECG consists of three limb leads, three augmented unipolar leads, and six chest leads. For improved exercise ECG recordings, electrodes mounted on the torso (abdominal level) replace the conventional ankle (leg) and wrist electrodes. This "torso-mounted limb lead system" (right figure) reduces electrical artifact introduced by limb movement during exercise.

Electrode Positioning in the Modified 10-Electrode, Torso-Mounted System

1. RL (right leg): just above right iliac crest on midaxillary line
2. LL (left leg): just above left iliac crest on midaxillary line
3. RA (right arm): just below right clavicle medial to deltoid muscle
4. LA (left arm): just below left clavicle medial to deltoid muscle
5. V_1: on right sternal border in 4th intercostal space
6. V_2: on left sternal border in 4th intercostal space
7. V_3: at midpoint of a straight line between V_2 and V_4
8. V_4: on midclavicular line in 5th intercostal space
9. V_5: on anterior axillary line and horizontal to V_4
10. V_6: on midaxillary line and horizontal to V_4 and V_5

Reference

Phibbs, B., and Buckels, L.: Comparative yields of ECG leads in multistage stress testing. *Am. Heart J.*, 90:275, 1985.

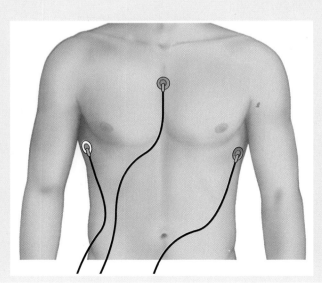

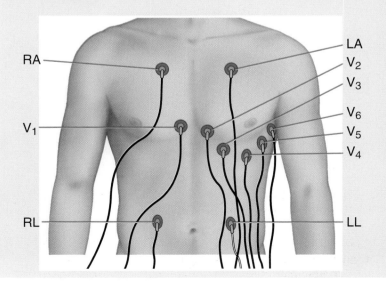

provides input to the central nervous system to bring about appropriate cardiovascular responses. With central regulation, blood flow in one area cannot dominate when a concurrent oxygen need exists in other, more "needy" tissues.

Figure 11.14 shows the distribution of sympathetic outflow. These nerve fibers end in the muscular layers of small arteries, arterioles, and precapillary sphincters. Norepinephrine acts as a general vasoconstrictor released at certain sympathetic nerve endings (**adrenergic fibers**). Other sympathetic neurons in skeletal and heart muscle release acetylcholine; these **cholinergic fibers** dilate the vessel.

Continual sympathetic constrictor neuron activity maintains a relative state of vasoconstriction termed **vasomotor tone**. Dilation of blood vessels regulated by adrenergic neurons results more from reduced vasomotor tone than increased sympathetic or parasympathetic dilator fiber activity. Powerful local vasodilation induced by metabolic byproducts also maintains blood flow in active tissue.

Hormonal Factors

Sympathetic nerves terminate in the medullary portion of the adrenal glands. With sympathetic activation, this glandular tissue releases large quantities of epinephrine and a small amount of norepinephrine into the blood. These hormones cause a constrictor response *except* in blood vessels of the heart and skeletal muscles. Adrenal hormones provide relatively minor control of regional blood flow during exercise compared with the more rapid and powerful local sympathetic neural drive.

Integrated Response in Exercise

Table 11.2 summarizes the integrated chemical, neural, and

hormonal adjustments immediately before and during exercise.

At the start of exercise (or even slightly before exercise begins), nerve centers above the medullary region initiate cardiovascular activity. The adjustments significantly increase the rate and pumping strength of the heart and alter regional blood flow in direct proportion to exercise intensity. As exercise continues and becomes more intense, sympathetic cholinergic outflow plus local metabolic factors (acting on chemosensitive nerves and directly on blood vessels) dilate resistance vessels in active musculature. Reduced peripheral resistance permits muscle tissue to accommodate greater blood flow. Constrictor adjustments in less active tissues maintain adequate perfusion pressure despite dilation of the muscle's vasculature. Vasoconstriction in non-active

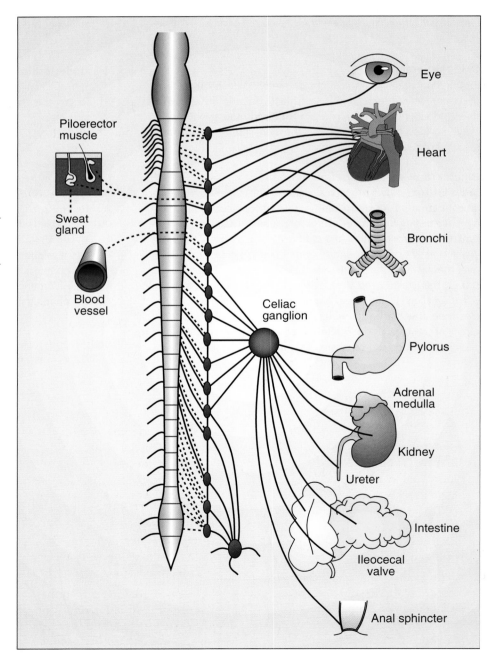

Figure 11.14
Schematic view of vascular regulation from sympathetic outflow to various organs and tissues.

TABLE 11.2
Summary of integrated chemical, neural, and hormonal adjustments prior to and during exercise

CONDITION	ACTIVATOR	RESPONSE
Pre-exercise "anticipatory" response	Activation of motor cortex and higher areas of brain causes increase in sympathetic outflow and reciprocal inhibition of parasympathetic activity	Acceleration of heart rate; increased myocardial contractility; vasodilation in skeletal and heart muscle (cholinergic fibers); vasoconstriction in other areas, especially skin, gut, spleen, liver, and kidneys (adrenergic fibers); increase in arterial blood pressure
Exercise	Continued sympathetic colinergic outflow; alterations in local metabolic conditions due to hypoxia ($\downarrow$ph, $\uparrow$PCO_2, $\uparrow$ADP, $\uparrow$Mg^{++}, $\uparrow$Ca^{++}, $\uparrow$NO, $\uparrow$temperature)	Further dilation of muscle vasculature
	Continued sympathetic adrenergic outflow in conjunction with epinephrine and norepinephrine from the adrenal medullae	Concomitant constriction of vasculature in inactive tissues to maintain adequate perfusion pressure throughout the arterial system
		Venous vessels stiffen to reduce their capacity. Venoconstriction facilitates venous return and maintains the central blood volume

areas also promotes blood redistribution to meet specific tissues' metabolic requirements during exercise.

Factors that affect venous return play an equally important role as those regulating arterial flow. Muscle and ventilatory pump action and stiffening of veins through neural stimulation propel blood into the central circulation and toward the right ventricle. This balances cardiac output and venous return.

summary

1. The cardiovascular system rapidly regulates heart rate and distributes blood while maintaining blood pressure in response to the metabolic and physiologic demands of increased physical activity.

2. The cardiac impulse begins at the S-A node. It then travels across the atria to the A-V node; after a brief delay it spreads rapidly across the large ventricular mass. With a normal conduction pattern, atria and ventricles contract effectively to provide the impetus for blood flow.

3. The electrocardiogram displays a record of the sequence of myocardial electrical events during a cardiac cycle. Electrocardiography detects abnormalities in heart function during rest and physical activity.

4. The majority of heart rhythm irregularities (arrhythmias) involve extra beats (extrasystoles). Atrial arrhythmias generally do not compromise the heart's pumping ability. Ventricular fibrillation, the most serious arrhythmia, results from repetitive, spontaneous discharge of portions of the ventricular mass. This affects the ventricle's ability to contract in a unified manner, decreasing cardiac output. Death results without immediate medical attention.

5. The sympathetic catecholamines epinephrine and norepinephrine accelerate heart rate and increase myocardial contractility. Acetylcholine, a parasympathetic neurotransmitter, slows heart rate via the vagus nerve.

6. Local increases in temperature, carbon dioxide, acidity, adenosine, nitric oxide, and magnesium and potassium ions provide potent stimuli to autoregulate blood flow in active tissues. Of these, nitric oxide occupies a role of considerable importance as a "relaxor" of arteriole smooth muscle.

7. The heart "turns on" in transition from rest to exercise from increased sympathetic and decreased parasympathetic activity. These events integrate with input from the brain's central command center.

8. Neural and hormonal extrinsic factors modify the heart's inherent rhythmicity. The heart can accelerate rapidly in anticipation of exercise and increase to 200 to 210 $b \cdot min^{-1}$ in maximum exercise.

9. Carotid artery palpation accurately measures heart rate during and immediately after exercise. In certain medical conditions, pressure against the carotid artery reflexly slows the heart, which underestimates the heart rate during exercise.

10. Cortical stimulation immediately prior to and during the initial stages of physical activity accounts for a substantial part of the heart rate adjustment to exercise.

11. Regulation of blood flow occurs when nerves, hormones, and local metabolic factors alter the internal diameter of smooth muscle bands in blood vessels. Vasoconstriction occurs when adrenergic sympathetic fibers release norepinephrine; cholinergic sympathetic neurons secrete acetylcholine that triggers vasodilation.

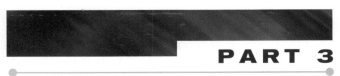

PART 3
Cardiovascular Dynamics During Exercise

Cardiac Output

Cardiac output provides the most significant indicator of the circulatory system's functional capacity to meet the demands for physical activity. As with any pump, the rate of pumping (**heart rate**) and quantity of blood ejected with each stroke (**stroke volume**) determine the heart's output of blood:

$$\text{Cardiac output} = \text{Heart rate} \times \text{Stroke volume}$$

Cardiac Output Measurement

To measure the output from a hose, pump, or faucet, one need only open a valve and collect the volume of fluid ejected during a given period. Surgical application of this direct technique by sectioning the aorta to measure blood flow in animals dramatically alters the pump's output. Measurement of human **cardiac output** requires much greater ingenuity. Three common techniques assess cardiac output in humans:

1. Direct Fick method
2. CO_2 rebreathing method
3. Indicator dilution method

Direct Fick Method
Oxygen uptake during 1 minute, and the average difference between the oxygen content of arterial and **mixed-venous blood** (**a-$\bar{v}O_2$ difference**) determine cardiac output. The question becomes: How much blood must circulate during the minute to account for the observed oxygen uptake, given the observed a-$\bar{v}O_2$ difference? The relationship between cardiac output, oxygen uptake, and a-$\bar{v}O_2$ difference embodies the principle discovered by German physiologist Adolph Fick (1829–1901) in 1870, called the **Fick equation** to honor his research.

$$\frac{\text{Cardiac output,}}{mL \cdot min^{-1}} = \frac{\text{Oxygen uptake, } mL \cdot min^{-1}}{\text{a-}\bar{v}O_2 \text{ diff, } mL \cdot dL \text{ blood}^{-1}} \times 100$$

Figure 11.15 illustrates the direct **Fick's method** to determine cardiac output. In this example, the person consumes 250 mL of oxygen during a minute at rest; the a-$\bar{v}O_2$ difference during this time averages 5 mL of oxygen per dL (100 mL) of blood. Substituting these values in the Fick equation results in a cardiac output of 5000 $mL \cdot min^{-1}$:

$$\frac{\text{Cardiac output,}}{mL \cdot min^{-1}} = \frac{250 \text{ mL } O_2}{5 \text{ mL } O_2} \times 100$$

The Fick method appears straightforward, yet the actual technique requires complex measurements usually limited to a clinical setting where the benefits exceed potential risks. Oxygen uptake measurement involves open-circuit spirometry (see Chapter 6). The more difficult aspect requires assessment of a-$\bar{v}O_2$ difference. A representative sample of arterial blood must come from a convenient systemic artery such as the femoral, radial, or brachial artery. Although these arteries are easily located, an arterial puncture can traumatize the patient. An accurate estimate of the average oxygen content of mixed-venous blood ($\bar{v}$) requires sampling from an anatomic "mixing chamber" like the pulmonary artery. This necessitates threading a flexible tube (catheter) through the antecubital vein in the arm into the right atrium, then right ventricle, and finally the pulmonary artery. Arterial and mixed-venous blood sampling occur during the same measurement period as oxygen uptake.

The Fick method has evaluated cardiovascular dynamics under a variety of experimental conditions including exercise. The method validates other techniques for cardiac output measurement. Critics of the method maintain

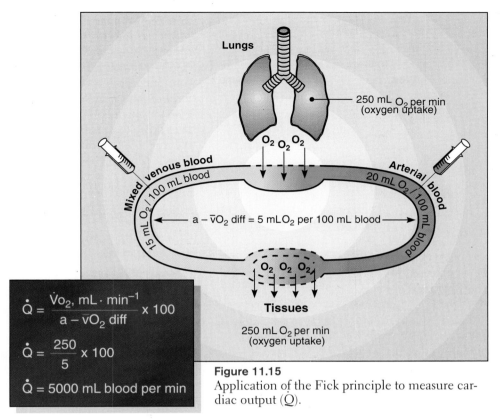

$$\dot{Q} = \frac{\dot{V}o_2, mL \cdot min^{-1}}{a - \bar{v}O_2 \ diff} \times 100$$

$$\dot{Q} = \frac{250}{5} \times 100$$

$$\dot{Q} = 5000 \ mL \ blood \ per \ min$$

Figure 11.15
Application of the Fick principle to measure cardiac output ($\dot{Q}$).

Resting Cardiac Output

Untrained Persons

Each minute, the left ventricle ejects the entire 5-L blood volume of an average-sized adult male. This value pertains to most individuals, but stroke volume and heart rate vary considerably depending on cardiovascular fitness status. A heart rate of about 70 b · min^{-1} sustains the average adult's 5-L resting cardiac output. Substituting this heart rate value in the cardiac output equation (cardiac output = stroke volume × heart rate; stroke volume = cardiac output ÷ heart rate), yields a calculated stroke volume of 71 mL per beat.

that its invasive nature alters cardiovascular dynamics—despite its accuracy, the measured cardiac output may not truly reflect a person's "normal" cardiovascular response pattern.

Less Invasive Methods

Two "noninvasive" procedures, CO_2 rebreathing and indicator dilution, do not require cardiac catheterization to estimate cardiac output. The **CO_2 rebreathing method** estimates mixed-venous and arterial carbon dioxide levels with a rapid carbon dioxide gas analyzer that measures CO_2 concentrations throughout the breathing cycle. This noninvasive, or "bloodless" technique requires only a breath-by-breath analysis of carbon dioxide.

The **indicator dilution method** determines cardiac output by injecting a known quantity of inert dye into a large vein. The indicator material remains in the vascular stream, usually bound to plasma proteins or red blood cells. It mixes as blood travels to the lungs and back to the heart before entering the systemic circuit. With continuous arterial blood sampling measures, the area under the dilution-concentration curve indicates the average concentration of indicator material in blood ejected from the heart. The cardiac output computation considers the dilution of a known quantity of dye in the unknown quantity of blood. While indicator dilution requires arterial puncture for blood sampling, it does not require sampling of blood from the right atrium, right ventricle, or pulmonary artery as required by the direct Fick method.

Endurance Athletes

Resting heart rate for an endurance athlete averages close to 50 b · min^{-1}. Because the athlete's resting cardiac output also averages 5 L · min^{-1}, blood circulates with a proportionately larger stroke volume of 100 mL per beat (5000 mL ÷ 50). Stroke volumes for women usually average 25% below values for men with equivalent training. The smaller body size of the average woman chiefly accounts for this "sex difference."

The underlying mechanisms for the heart rate and stroke volume differences between trained and untrained individuals remain unclear. Does the bradycardia that accompanies increased aerobic fitness "cause" a larger stroke volume, or vice versa, because the myocardium becomes strengthened and internal ventricular dimensions increase with training? The two factors probably interact as aerobic fitness improves:

1. Increased vagal tone slows the heart, allowing more time for ventricular filling
2. Enlarged ventricular volume and a more powerful myocardium eject a larger volume of blood with each systole

Exercise Cardiac Output

B *lood flow from the heart increases in direct proportion to exercise intensity*. From rest to steady-rate exercise,

Cardiac Output Components in Endurance-trained and Untrained Subjects During Rest and Maximal Exercise

	Cardiac output	=	Heart rate	×	Stroke volume
Untrained					
Rest	5000 mL	=	70 b · min⁻¹	×	71 mL · b⁻¹
Maximal exercise	22,000 mL	=	195 b · min⁻¹	×	113 mL · b⁻¹
Endurance trained					
Rest	5000 mL	=	50 b · min⁻¹	×	100 mL · b⁻¹
Maximal exercise	35,000 mL	=	195 b · min⁻¹	×	179 mL · b⁻¹

cardiac output increases rapidly, followed by a more gradual increase until it plateaus as blood flow matches exercise metabolic requirements.

In sedentary, college-age men, cardiac output in strenuous exercise increases about four times the resting level to an average maximum of 22 L of blood per minute. Maximum heart rate for these young adults averages 195 b · min⁻¹. Consequently, stroke volume averages 113 mL of blood per beat during maximal exercise (22,000 mL ÷ 195). In contrast, world-class endurance athletes generate maximum cardiac outputs of 35 L · min⁻¹, with a similar or slightly lower maximum heart rate than untrained counterparts. The difference between maximum cardiac output of both individuals relates *solely* to differences in stroke volume. The cardiac output of a Nordic Olympic medal winner in cross-country skiing increased eight times above rest to 40 L · min⁻¹ during a maximum exercise test. The accompanying stroke volume averaged 210 mL per beat, twice the volume of blood pumped per beat as the maximum stroke volume of a healthy, sedentary person of the same age.

Exercise Stroke Volume

Figure 11.16 plots the relationship between stroke volume and percent $\dot{V}O_{2max}$ (to better equate exercise intensity among subjects) for 8 healthy, college-age men during graded exercise on a cycle ergometer. Stroke volume increases progressively with exercise to about 50% $\dot{V}O_{2max}$ and then gradually levels off until termination of exercise. For several subjects, stroke volume decreased slightly at near maximal exercise intensities.

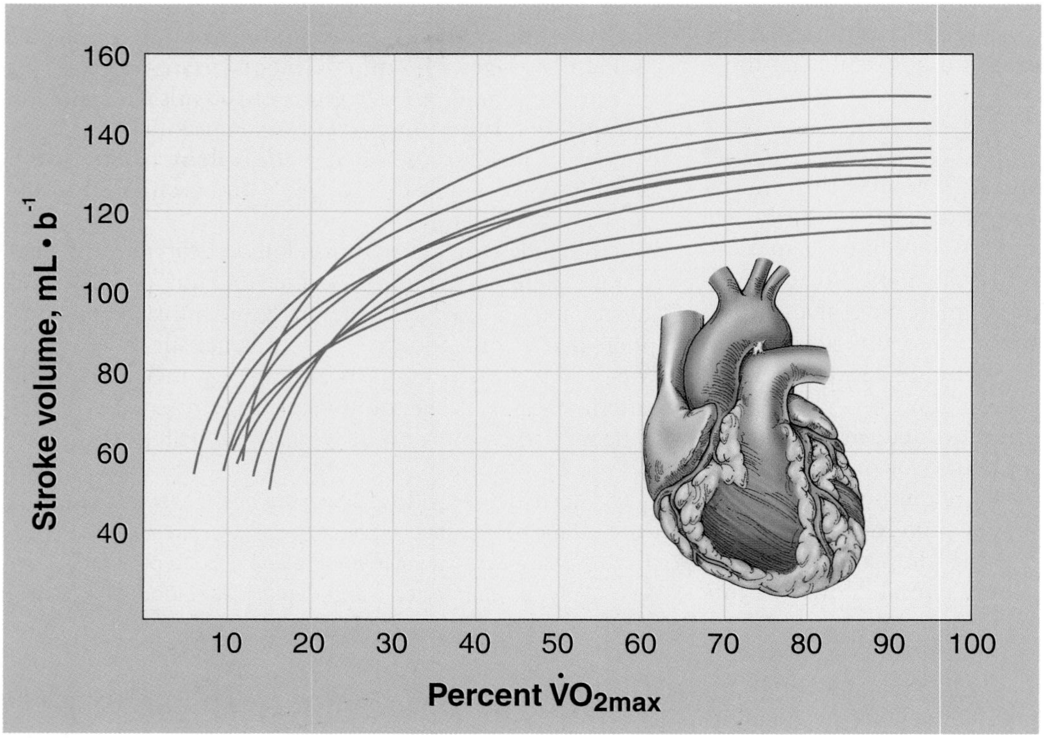

Stroke Volume and $\dot{V}O_{2max}$

Table 11.3 shows the importance of stroke volume in differentiating people with high and low $\dot{V}O_{2max}$. The subjects represented three groups: 1) patients with mitral stenosis, a valvular disease that causes inadequate emptying of the left ventricle, 2) healthy

Figure 11.16
Stroke volume related to increasing exercise intensity (percent $\dot{V}O_{2max}$) for 8 male subjects. (Data from the Applied Physiology Laboratory, University of Michigan.)

TABLE 11.3
Maximal values for oxygen uptake ($\dot{V}O_{2max}$), heart rate (HR_{max}), stroke volume (SV_{max}), and cardiac output (CO_{max}) in three groups having low, normal, and high aerobic capacities

GROUP	$\dot{V}O_{2max}$ (L · min^{-1})	HR_{max} (b · min^{-1})	SV_{max} (mL · b^{-1})	CO_{max} (L · min^{-1})
Mitral stenosis	1.6	190	50	9.5
Sedentary	3.2	200	100	20.0
Athlete	5.2	190	160	30.4

*Modified from Rowell, L. B.: Circulation. *Med. Sci. Sports*, 1:15, 1969.

but sedentary men, and 3) athletes. Differences in VO_{2max} among groups closely paralleled differences in maximal stroke volume. Aerobic capacity and maximum stroke volume of mitral stenosis patients averaged one-half the values of sedentary subjects. This close linkage also emerged in comparisons between healthy subjects; a 60% larger stroke volume in athletes compared with sedentary men paralleled their 62% larger VO_{2max}. All groups showed fairly similar maximum heart rates; thus, stroke volume differences accounted for the variations in maximum cardiac output and VO_{2max} among groups.

Stroke Volume Increases

Two physiologic mechanisms regulate stroke volume and contribute in varying degrees to stroke volume increases in exercise. The first mechanism, intrinsic to the myocardium, requires greater diastolic filling followed by a forceful systolic ejection. The second, governed by neurohormonal influence, involves normal ventricular filling followed by a forceful systolic ejection to cause greater systolic emptying.

Greater Systolic Emptying versus Enhanced Diastolic Filling

Greater ventricular filling during diastole in the cardiac cycle occurs through any factor that increases venous return (**preload**), or slows heart rate. An increase in end-diastolic volume stretches myocardial fibers, causing a powerful ejection stroke as the heart contracts. This expels the normal stroke volume plus the additional blood that entered the ventricles and stretched the myocardium.

German physiologist Otto Frank (1865–1944) and British colleague Ernest H. Starling's (1866–1927) experiments with animals in the early 1900s first described relationships between muscle force and resting fiber length. Improved contractility of a stretched muscle (within a limited range) probably relates to a more optimum arrangement of intracellular myofilaments as the muscle stretches. **Frank-Starling's law of the heart** describes this phenomenon applied to the myocardium.

For many years, physiologists taught the Frank-Starling mechanism as the "modus operandi" for all increases in stroke volume during exercise. They believed that enhanced venous return in exercise caused greater cardiac filling, which stretched the ventricles in diastole to produce a more forceful ejection. In all likelihood, this pattern describes the stroke volume response in transition from rest to exercise, or when a person moves from the upright to recumbent position. Enhanced diastolic filling probably also occurs in activities like swimming, in which the body's horizontal position optimizes venous return and myocardial preload.

The data in Table 11.4 show that body position significantly affects circulatory dynamics. Cardiac output and stroke volume reach the highest and most stable levels in the horizontal position. Near-maximal stroke volume occurs at rest in the horizontal position and increases only slightly during exercise. In contrast, gravity's effect in the upright position counters venous return and lowers stroke volume. This postural effect becomes prominent when comparing circulatory dynamics at rest in the upright and supine positions. As upright exercise intensity increases, stroke volume also increases to approach the maximum value in the supine position.

In most forms of upright exercise, the heart does not fill to an extent that significantly increases cardiac volume to values observed in the recumbent position. The increase in stroke volume during exercise likely results from the *combined effects* of enhanced diastolic filling and more complete systolic emptying. In both recumbent and upright positions, the heart's stroke volume increases in exercise despite resistance to flow from increased systolic pressure (**afterload**).

At rest in the upright position, 40 to 50% of the total end-diastolic blood volume remains in the left ventricle after systole; this **residual volume of the heart** amounts to 50 to 70 mL of blood. The sympathetic hormones epinephrine and norepinephrine enhance myocardial stroke power and systolic emptying during exercise, which reduces the heart's residual blood volume.

TABLE 11.4
Effect of body position on cardiac output, stroke volume, and heart rate during rest and exercise in well-trained endurance athletes

	REST		MODERATE EXERCISE		STRENUOUS EXERCISE	
	SUPINE	UPRIGHT	SUPINE	UPRIGHT	SUPINE	UPRIGHT
Cardiac output, L · min⁻¹	9.2	6.6	19.0	16.9	26.3	24.5
Stroke volume, mL · b⁻¹	141	103	163	149	164	155
Heart rate, b · min⁻¹	65	64	115	112	160	159
Oxygen uptake, mL · min⁻¹	345	384	1769	1864	3364	3387

Data from Bevegård, S., et al.: Circulatory studies in well-trained athletes at rest and during heavy exercise, with special reference to stroke volume and the influence of body position. *Acta physiol. Scand.*, 57:26, 1963.

Exercise Heart Rate

Graded Exercise

Figure 11.17 depicts the relationship between heart rate and oxygen uptake during increasing intensity exercise (graded exercise) to maximum for endurance athletes and sedentary college students. A straight line relates heart rate and oxygen uptake for both groups throughout the major portion of the exercise range. Heart rate for the untrained person accelerates relatively rapidly with increasing exercise demands; a much smaller heart rate increase occurs for the athlete (i.e., the slope or rate of change of the lines dif-

fers considerably between groups). Consequently, the athlete (or trained person) achieves a higher level of exercise oxygen uptake at a particular submaximal heart rate than a sedentary person. At an oxygen uptake of 2.0 L · min⁻¹, for example, the athletes' heart rate averages 70 b · min⁻¹ lower than the heart rate of sedentary students. Maximum heart rate and the heart rate-oxygen uptake relationship remain fairly consistent for a particular individual from day to day, although the slope of the relationship decreases considerably with aerobic training (see Chapter 14). Day-to-day consistency makes it possible to estimate oxygen uptake from submaximal exercise heart rate (see Chapter 8).

Submaximum Exercise

Heart rate increases rapidly and levels off within several minutes during submaximum steady-rate exercise. A subsequent increase in exercise intensity increases heart rate to a new plateau as the body attempts to match the cardiovascular response to metabolic demands. Each increment in exercise intensity requires progressively more time to achieve heart rate stabilization.

Cardiac Output Distribution

Blood flow to specific tissues increases in proportion to their metabolic activities.

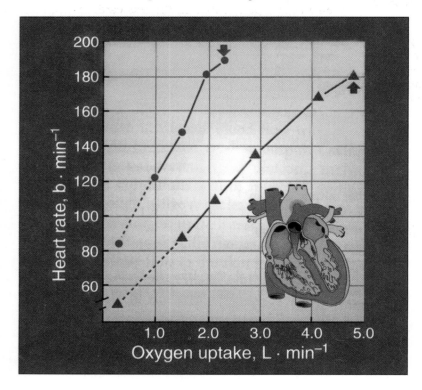

Figure 11.17
Heart rate in relation to oxygen uptake during upright exercise in endurance athletes (▲) and sedentary college students (●)(⬆= maximal values). (From Saltin, B.: Physiological effects of physical conditioning. *Med. Sci. Sports*, 1: 50, 1969.)

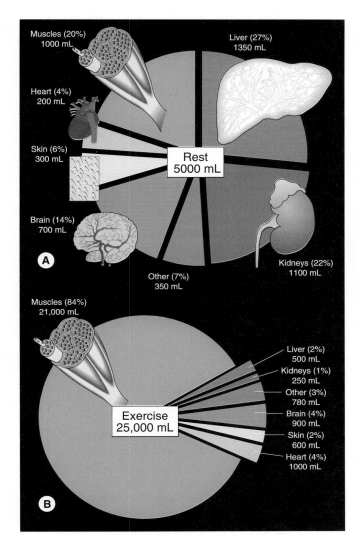

the cardiac output. Each 100 g of muscle receives 4 to 7 mL of blood per minute during rest. Muscle blood flow increases steadily during exercise to reach a maximum of between 50 to 75 mL per 100 g of tissue.

Blood Flow Redistribution

The increase in muscle blood flow with exercise comes largely from increased cardiac output. Owing to neural and hormonal vascular regulation, including local metabolic conditions within muscles, additional blood moves through active muscles from areas that temporarily tolerate a reduction in their normal blood flow. **Shunting blood** away from specific tissues occurs primarily in heavy exercise. Blood flow to the skin increases during light and moderate exercise so metabolic heat generated in muscle can dissipate at the skin's surface. During intense, short-duration exercise, cutaneous blood flow becomes compromised even when exercising in a hot environment.

In some tissues, blood flow during exercise decreases as much as four-fifths of the flow at rest. The kidneys and splanchnic tissues use only 10 to 25% of the oxygen available in their blood supply at rest. Consequently, these tissues tolerate a considerably reduced blood flow before oxygen demand exceeds supply and compromises organ function. With reduced blood flow, increased oxygen extraction from available blood maintains a tissue's oxygen needs. Visceral organs can tolerate substantially reduced blood flow for more than an hour during heavy exercise. This "frees" as much as 600 mL of oxygen each minute for use by active musculature.

Blood Flow to the Heart and Brain

The myocardium and brain tissues cannot compromise their blood supplies. At rest, the myocardium normally uses 75% of the oxygen in the blood flowing through the coronary circulation. With such a limited "margin of safety," increased coronary blood flow primarily meets the heart's oxygen demands. Cerebral blood flow increases up to 30% with exercise compared to rest; the largest portion of any "extra" blood probably moves to areas related to motor functions.

Cardiac Output and Oxygen Transport

Rest

Each 100 mL of arterial blood normally carries approximately 20 mL of oxygen or 200 mL of oxygen per liter of blood at sea level conditions (see Chapter 10). Trained and untrained adults circulate 5 L of blood each minute at rest, so potentially 1000 mL of oxygen becomes available during 1 minute (5 L blood × 200 mL O_2). Resting oxygen uptake averages only about 250 mL · min^{-1}; this means 750 mL of oxygen returns "unused" to the heart. This does not represent an unnecessary waste of cardiac

Figure 11.18
Relative distribution of cardiac output during rest (**A**) and strenuous endurance exercise (**B**). The numbers in parentheses indicate percent of total cardiac output. Despite its large mass, muscle tissue receives about the same amount of blood as the much smaller kidneys at rest. In strenuous exercise, however, nearly 85% of the total cardiac output diverts to active muscles.

Rest

Figure 11.18A shows the approximate distribution of a 5-L cardiac output at rest. More than one-fourth of the cardiac output flows to the liver, one-fifth to kidney and muscles, and the remainder diverts to the heart, skin, brain and other tissues.

During Exercise

Figure 11.18B illustrates the distribution of cardiac output to various tissues during intense aerobic exercise. *Although regional blood flow varies considerably depending on environmental conditions, level of fatigue, and exercise mode, active muscles receive a disproportionately large portion of*

The Amazing Heart

Here's a straightforward calculation with an amazing answer about the heart.

"How many cars with 20-gallon capacity gas tanks would 60 years of resting cardiac output fill-up? (Hint: Use an average resting cardiac output of 5 L · min⁻¹.)

output. To the contrary, extra oxygen in the blood above the resting needs maintains oxygen in reserve—a margin of safety for immediate release should the tissue's metabolic needs suddenly demand it.

During Exercise

A person with a maximum heart rate of 200 b · min⁻¹ and a stroke volume of 80 mL per beat generates a maximum cardiac output of 16 L (200 × 80 mL). Even during maximum exercise, hemoglobin remains fully saturated with oxygen, so each liter of arterial blood carries about 200 mL of oxygen. Consequently, 3200 mL of oxygen circulate each minute via a 16 L cardiac output (16 L × 200 mL O_2). If the body extracted all of the oxygen delivered in a 16-L cardiac output, $\dot{V}O_{2max}$ would equal 3200 mL. This represents the theoretical upper limit because the oxygen needs of tissues like the brain do not increase greatly with exercise, yet they require an uninterrupted blood supply.

An increase in maximum cardiac output directly improves a person's capacity to circulate oxygen. If the heart's stroke volume increased from 80 to 200 mL while maximum heart rate remained unchanged at 200 b · min⁻¹, maximum cardiac output would dramatically increase to 40 L · min⁻¹. This means that the amount of oxygen circulated in maximum exercise each minute would increase approximately 2.5 times from 3200 to 8000 mL (40 L × 200 mL O_2).

Maximum Cardiac Output and $\dot{V}O_{2max}$

Figure 11.19 displays the relationship between maximum cardiac output and $\dot{V}O_{2max}$ and includes values representative of sedentary individuals and elite endurance athletes. An unmistakable relationship emerges. A low aerobic capacity links closely to a low maximum cardiac output, whereas a 30- to 40-L cardiac output always accompanies ability to generate a 5- or 6-L $\dot{V}O_{2max}$.

Gender Differences in Cardiac Output

A similar response pattern for cardiac output during exercise exists between boys and girls and men and women. However, teenage and adult females require 5 to 10% larger cardiac output at any submaximal oxygen uptake than males. The gender difference in submaximal cardiac output relates to the 10% lower blood hemoglobin concentrations of women compared with men. A proportionate increase in submaximal exercise cardiac output generally compensates for the females' slightly lower oxygen transport capacity owing to reduced hemoglobin.

Extraction of Oxygen: The a-$\bar{v}O_2$ Difference

If blood flow were the only means for increasing a tissue's oxygen supply, cardiac output would need to increase from 5 L · min⁻¹ at rest to 100 L in maximum exercise to achieve a 20-fold increase in oxygen uptake (an oxygen uptake increase common among endurance athletes). Fortunately, intense exercise does not require such a large cardiac output increase be-

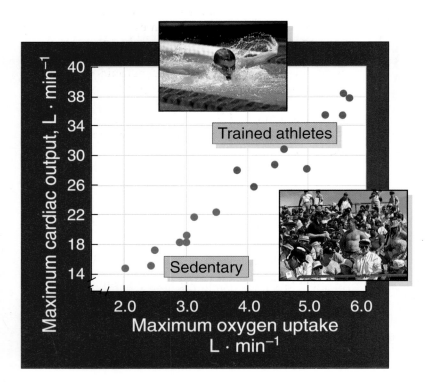

Figure 11.19
Relationship between maximal cardiac output and maximal oxygen uptake in trained and untrained individuals. Maximal cardiac output relates to $\dot{V}O_{2max}$ in a ratio of about 6:1. (Swimmer photo courtesy of Jim Richardson, University of Michigan.)

cause hemoglobin releases its considerable "extra" oxygen from blood perfusing active tissues.

Two mechanisms for oxygen supply increase a person's oxygen uptake capacity:

1. Increased tissue blood flow
2. Use of the relatively large quantity of oxygen that remains unused by tissues at rest (i.e., expand the a-$\bar{v}O_2$ difference)

The following rearrangement of the Fick equation summarizes the important relationship between maximum cardiac output, maximum a-$\bar{v}O_2$ difference, and $\dot{V}O_{2max}$:

$$\dot{V}O_{2max} = \text{Max cardiac output} \times \text{Max a-}\bar{v}O_2 \text{ difference}$$

During Rest and Exercise

Figure 11.20 shows a representative pattern for changes in a-$\bar{v}O_2$ difference from rest to maximum exercise for physically active men. A similar pattern emerges for women except that the arterial oxygen content averages 5 to 10% lower owing to lower hemoglobin concentrations in women. The figure includes values for the oxygen content of arterial and mixed-venous blood during different exercise intensities. Arterial blood oxygen con-

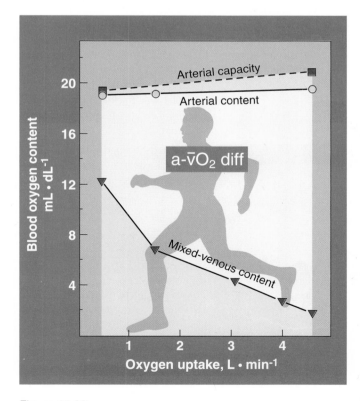

Figure 11.20
Changes in a-$\bar{v}O_2$ difference from rest to maximal exercise in physically active men.

tent varies little from its value of 20 mL · dL^{-1} at rest throughout the full exercise intensity range. In contrast, mixed-venous oxygen content varies between 12 to 15 mL · dL^{-1} at rest to a low of 2 to 4 mL · dL^{-1} during maximum exercise. The difference between arterial and mixed-venous blood oxygen content at any time (a-$\bar{v}O_2$ difference) represents oxygen extraction from blood as it circulates through the body's tissues. At rest, for example, a-$\bar{v}O_2$ difference equals 5 mL of oxygen, or only 25% of the blood's oxygen content (5 mL ÷ 20 mL × 100); 75% of the oxygen returns "unused" to the heart bound to hemoglobin.

The progressive expansion of the a-$\bar{v}O_2$ difference to at least three times the resting value occurs from a reduced venous oxygen content, which in maximal exercise approaches 20 mL in the active muscle (all oxygen extracted). The oxygen content of a true mixed-venous sample from the pulmonary artery rarely falls below 2 to 4 mL · dL^{-1} because blood returning from active tissues mixes with oxygen-rich venous blood from metabolically less active regions.

Figure 11.20 also indicates that the capacity of each 100 mL of arterial blood to carry oxygen actually increases during exercise. This results from an increased concentration of red blood cells (hemoconcentration) owing to the progressive movement of fluid from the plasma to the interstitial space with (1) increases in capillary hydrostatic pressure as blood pressure rises, and (2) metabolic byproducts of exercise metabolism that create an osmotic pressure drawing fluid from the plasma into tissue spaces.

In Heart Disease
The heart muscle of patients with advanced coronary artery disease often exhibits impaired capacity to perform work or improve with regular exercise. This negates training adaptations for maximal stroke volume and cardiac output. Patients, however, still experience improvements in exercise tolerance and aerobic capacity because aerobic training increases skeletal muscles' oxygen usage. Improved delivery and utilization of oxygen expand the a-$\bar{v}O_2$ difference (and increase the lactate threshold), enabling patients to exercise comfortably at higher intensities.

Cardiovascular Adjustments to Upper-Body Exercise

The highest oxygen uptake during upper-body exercise generally averages between 70 to 80% of the $\dot{V}O_{2max}$ in bicycle and treadmill exercise. Similarly, maximal heart rate and pulmonary ventilation remain lower in arm exercise. The relatively smaller muscle mass of the upper body largely accounts for these physiologic differences. The lower maximal heart rate in exercise that activates a smaller muscle mass most likely results from the following:

- Reduced output stimulation from the motor cortex central command to the cardiovascular center in the medulla (feedforward stimulation)
- Reduced feedback stimulation to the medulla from the smaller active musculature

In submaximal exercise, the response pattern reverses. Figure 11.21 shows that any level of submaximal power output produces a higher oxygen uptake with arm compared with leg exercise. This difference remains small during light exercise but becomes progressively larger as intensity of effort increases. Lower economy of effort in arm-crank exercise probably results from static muscle actions that do not produce external work but consume extra oxygen. In addition, extra musculature activated to stabilize the torso during most forms of arm exercise adds to the oxygen requirement. Upper-body exercise also produces greater physiologic strain (heart rate, blood pressure, pulmonary ventilation, and perception of physical effort) for any level of oxygen uptake (or percent of maximal oxygen uptake) than primarily lower-body leg exercise.

Understanding differences in physiologic response between upper- and lower-body exercise enables the physician and exercise specialist to formulate prudent exercise programs using both exercise modes. Because a standard exercise load produces greater metabolic and physiologic strain with the arms, exercise prescriptions based on running and bicycling *cannot* be applied to upper-body exer-

cise. Low correlations exists between $\dot{V}O_{2max}$ for arm exercises and $\dot{V}O_{2max}$ for leg exercise; thus, one cannot predict accurately one's aerobic capacity for arm exercise from a test using the legs, and vice versa. This further substantiates the concept of aerobic fitness specificity.

"Athlete's Heart"

A *modest increase in heart size (**cardiac hypertrophy**) represents a fundamental adjustment of the healthy heart to exercise training.* Regular aerobic exercise stimulates myocardial protein synthesis; individual muscle fibers thicken, and a fiber's contractile elements increase in number. When exercise overload ceases, heart size returns to pretraining levels.

Ultrasonic **echocardiography** applies sound waves to "map" the dimensions of the myocardium and volume of its chambers. Echocardiography has evaluated structural characteristics of the hearts of diverse athletes, and determined whether different patterns of enlargement accompany different training modes. Table 11.5 clearly shows that the heart's structural characteristics of apparently healthy athletes differ considerably from untrained individuals. Structural differences also vary with the nature of the chronic exercise training overload. For example:

- Left ventricular volume averaged 181 mL and mass averaged 308 g for swimmers, and 160 mL and 302 g for runners. Nonathletic controls averaged 101 mL for ventricular volume and 211 g for ventricular mass. Despite their large internal ventricular volume dimensions (**eccentric hypertrophy**), ventricular wall thickness for the endurance athletes remained normal.

- Athletes trained with resistance exercise (weight lifters, shot putters, and wrestlers), who regularly experience acute episodes of signifi-

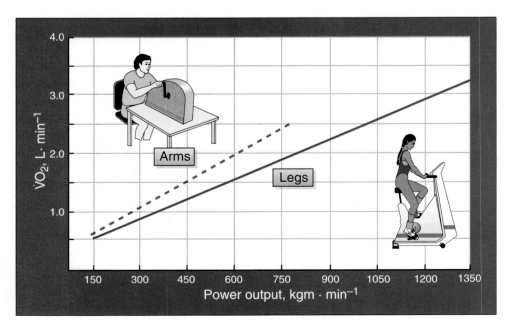

Figure 11.21
Arm (upper-body) exercise requires a greater oxygen uptake compared with leg (lower-body) exercise at any power output throughout the comparison range. The largest differences occur during intense exercise. Average data for men and women. (From Laboratory of Applied Physiology, Queens College, NY)

TABLE 11.5
Comparative average cardiac dimensions in college athletes, world-class athletes, and untrained subjects[a]

DIMENSION[b]	COLLEGE RUNNERS (N = 15)	COLLEGE SWIMMERS (N = 15)	WORLD CLASS RUNNERS (N = 10)	COLLEGE WRESTLERS (N = 12)	WORLD CLASS SHOT PUTTERS (N = 4)	NORMALS (N = 16)
LVID	54	51	48–59[c]	48	43–52[c]	46
LVV, mL	160	181	154	110	122	101
SV, mL	116	—[d]	113	75	68	—[d]
LV wall, mm	11.3	10.6	10.8	13.7	13.8	10.3
Septum, mm	10.9	10.7	10.9	13.0	13.5	10.3
LV mass, g	302	308	283	330	348	211

[a] From Morganroth, J., et al.: Comparative left ventricular dimensions in trained athletes. *Ann. Intern. Med.*, 82:521, 1975.

[b] LVID, left ventricular internal dimension at end diastole; LVV, left ventricular volume; SV, stroke volume; LV wall, posterobasal left ventricular wall thickness; Septum, ventricular septal thickness; LV mass, left ventricular mass.

[c] Range.

[d] Values not reported.

cantly elevated arterial pressure with straining-type exercises, show normal ventricular volume but a thickened ventricular wall (**concentric hypertrophy**). This undoubtedly represents compensation for the added workload resistance training imposes on the left ventricle.

The consequences of different myocardial responses to diverse training modes on long-term cardiovascular health remain unknown. *No compelling scientific evidence shows that a normal heart cannot withstand the rigors of diverse modes of arduous exercise training.*

summary

1. Cardiac output reflects the functional capacity of the circulatory system. Heart rate and stroke volume determine the heart's output capacity in the following relationship: Cardiac output = Heart rate × Stroke volume.

2. Invasive and noninvasive methods measure cardiac output. Each has specific advantages and disadvantages for use with humans, especially during exercise.

3. Cardiac output increases in proportion to exercise intensity from about 5 L · min⁻¹ at rest to a maximum in exercise of 20 to 25 L · min⁻¹ in untrained college-age men, and 35 to 40 L · min⁻¹ in elite male endurance athletes. Differences in maximum cardiac output relate to individual differences in the heart's maximum stroke volume.

4. During upright exercise, stroke volume increases during the transition from rest to moderate exercise, reaching maximum at about 50% VO_{2max}. Thereafter, increases in heart rate increase cardiac output.

5. Increases in stroke volume in upright exercise generally result from interactions between greater ventricular filling during diastole and more complete emptying during systole. Sympathetic hormones augment myocardial force generated during systole.

6. Heart rate and oxygen uptake relate linearly throughout the major portion of the exercise range in trained and untrained individuals.

Endurance training shifts the heart rate-oxygen uptake line significantly to the right because of an improved stroke volume. This reduces heart rate at any submaximal exercise level.

7. Local metabolism generally determines blood flow in specific tissues; it causes substantial diversion of cardiac output to active muscles during exercise. Kidneys and splanchnic regions also temporarily compromise their blood supplies to reroute blood to active muscles.

8. Maximum cardiac output and maximum a-v̄O_2 difference determine $\dot{V}O_{2max}$ in the following relationship: $\dot{V}O_{2max}$ = Maximum cardiac output × Maximum a-v̄O_2 difference. Large cardiac

outputs clearly differentiate endurance athletes from untrained counterparts. Training also expands the maximum a-$\bar{v}O_2$ difference.

9. Cardiac hypertrophy reflects a fundamental adaptation to increased myocardial workload imposed by exercise training. The pattern of structural and dimensional changes in the left ventricle varies with specific modes of exercise training. No scientific evidence indicates that regular exercise harms a normal heart.

thought questions

1. Provide the physiologic rationale for biofeedback and relaxation techniques to treat hypertension and stress-related disorders.

2. Discuss the following statement: "Task-specific aerobic exercise training not only trains the cardiovascular system and local musculature, but also trains the nervous system to adjust physiologically to the specific exercise mode."

3. The Romans of ancient times executed criminals by tying their arms and legs to a cross mounted in the vertical position. Discuss the physiologic responses that would cause death under these circumstances.

4. If heart transplantation surgically removes all nerves to the myocardium, why does heart rate increase for these patients during physical activity?

selected references

American College of Sports Medicine. Position stand. Physical activity, physical fitness, and hypertension. *Med. Sci. Sports Exerc.*, 25:i-x, 1993.

Balon, T.W.: Integrative biology of nitric oxide and exercise. *Exer. Sport Sci. Revs.*, 27:219, 1999.

Buckwalter, J.B., et al.: Skeletal muscle vasodilation at the onset of exercise. *J. Appl. Physiol.*, 85:1649, 1998.

Bassett, D.R., Jr., and Howley, E.T.: Maximal oxygen uptake: "classical" versus "contemporary" viewpoints. *Med. Sci. Sports Exerc.*, 29:591, 1997.

Cardillo, C., et al.: Racial differences in nitric oxide-mediated vasodilator response to mental stress in the forearm circulation. *Hypertension*, 31:1235, 1998.

Carrasco, D.I., et al.: Effect of concentric and eccentric muscle actions on muscle sympathetic nerve activity. *J. Appl. Physiol.*, 86:558, 1999.

Carter, R., et al.: Muscle pump and central command during recovery from exercise in humans. *J. Appl. Physiol.*, 87:1463, 1999.

Chen, S.Y., et al.: Cardiorespiratory response of heart transplantation recipients to exercise in the early postoperative period. *J. Formos. Med. Assoc.*, 98:165, 1999.

Delp, M.D.: Differential effects of training on the control of skeletal muscle perfusion. *Med. Sci. Sports Exerc.*, 30:361, 1998.

Dengel, D.R., et al.: Improvements in blood pressure, glucose metabolism, and lipoprotein lipids after aerobic exercise plus weight loss in obese, hypertensive middle-aged men. *Metabolism*, 47:1075, 1998.

DiBello, V., et al.: Left ventricular function during exercise in athletes and in sedentary men. *Med. Sci. Sports Exerc.*, 28:190, 1996.

Digenio, A.G., et al.: Effect of myocardial ischaemia on left ventricular function and adaptability to exercise training. *Med. Sci. Sports Exerc.*, 8:1094, 1999.

Donaldson, M. C.: Varicose veins in active people. *Phys. Sportsmed.* 18: 46, 1990.

Foster, C., et al.: Left ventricular function during interval and steady state exercise. *Med. Sci. Sports Exerc.*, 8:1157, 1999.

Franklin, B.S., et al.: Cardiac demands of heavy snow shoveling. *JAMA*, 273:880, 1995.

Gledhill, N., et al.: Endurance athletes' stroke volume does not plateau: major advantage is diastolic function. *Med. Sci. Sports Exerc.*, 26:1116, 1994.

Gordon, A., et al.: Beneficial effects of exercise training in heart failure patients with low cardiac output response to exercise—a compari-

son of two training models. *J. Intern. Med.*, 246:175, 1999.

Griffin, S.E., et al.: Blood pressure measurement during exercise: a review. *Med. Sci. Sports Exerc.*, 29:149, 1997.

Hagberg, J.M.: Physical activity, physical fitness, and blood pressure. In *Physical Activity and Cardiovascular Health*, Leon, A. (ed.). Champaign, IL: Human Kinetics, 1997.

Harms, C.A., and Dempsey, J.A.: Cardiovascular consequences of exercise hyperpnea. *Exerc. Sport Sci. Revs.*, 27:37, 1999.

Herr, M.D., et al.: Characteristics of the muscle mechanoreflex during quadriceps contractions in humans. *J. Appl. Physiol.*, 86:767, 1999.

Iellamo, F., et al.: Role of muscular factors in cardiorespiratory responses to static exercise: contribution of reflex mechanisms. *J. Appl. Physiol.*, 86:174, 1999.

Joyner, M.J., and Dietz, N.M.: Nitric oxide and vasodilation in human limbs. *J. Appl. Physiol.*, 83:1785, 1997.

Kelly, G.: Dynamic resistance exercise and resting blood pressure in adults: A meta analysis. *J. Appl. Physiol.*, 82:1559, 1997.

Leutholtz, B.C.: Exercise can reduce incidence and severity of hypertension. *ACSM's Health & Fitness J.*, 2(5):36, 1998.

MacDonald, J.R., et al.: Hypotension following mild bouts of resistance exercise and submaximal dynamic exercise. *Eur. J. Appl. Physiol.*, 79:148, 1999.

Mayo, J.J., and Kravitz, L.: A review of the acute cardiovascular responses to resistance exercise of healthy young and older adults. *J. Strength and Cond. Res.*, 13:90, 1999.

McAllister, R.M.: Adaptations in control of blood flow with training: splanchnic and renal blood flows. *Med. Sci. Sports Exerc.*, 30:375, 1998.

McCartney, N.: Acute responses to resistance training and saftey. *Med. Sci. Sports Exerc.*, 31:31, 1999.

Moore, R.L., and Palmer, B.M.: Exercise training and cellular adaptations of normal and diseased hearts. *Exerc. Sport Sci. Revs.*, 27:285, 1999.

O'Leary, D.S.: Heart rate control during exercise by baroreceptors and skeletal muscle afferents. *Med. Sci. Sports Exerc.*, 28:210, 1996.

Orbach, P., and Lowenthal, D.T.: Evaluation and treatment of hypertension in active individuals. *Med. Sci. Sports Exerc.*, 30(Suppl.):S354, 1998.

Pelliccia, A., et al.: Physiologic left ventricular cavity dilation in elite athletes. *Ann. Intern. Med.*, 130:23, 1999.

Proctor, D.N., et al.: Influence of age and gender on cardiac output-VO_2 relationship during submaximal cycle ergometry. *J. Appl. Physiol.*, 84:599, 1998.

Raven, P.B., et al.: Baroreflex regulation of blood pressure during dynamic exercise. *Exer. Sport Sci. Revs.*, 25:365, 1997.

Richardson, R.S.: Oxygen transport: air to muscle cell. *Med. Sci. Sports Exerc.*, 30:53, 1998.

Rowell, L.B., et al.: Integration of cardiovascular control systems in dynamic exercises. In: *Handbook of Physiology*, Rowell, L.B., and Shepard, J. (eds.). New York: Oxford University Press, 1996.

Rowland, T., et al.: Cardiac responses to maximal upright cycle exercise in helathy boys and men. *Med. Sci. Sports Exerc.*, 29:1146, 1997.

Saltin, B., and Strange, S.: Maximal oxygen uptake: "old" and "new" arguments for cardiovascular limitation. *Med. Sci. Sports Exerc.*, 24: 30, 1992.

Schwaiblmair, M., et al.: Cardiopulmonary exercise testing before and after lung and heart-lung transplantation. *Am. J. Respir. Crit. Care Med.*, 159:1277, 1999.

Schwaiblmair, M., et al.: Lung function and cardiopulmonary exercise performance after heart transplantation: influence of cardiac allograft vasculopathy. *Chest*, 116:332, 1999.

The Sixth report of the Joint National Committee on Prevention, Detection, Evaluation, and Treatment of High Blood Pressure. *Arch. Intern. Med.*, 157:2413, 1997.

Toner, M. M., et al.: Cardiovascular adjustment to exercise distributed between the upper and lower body. *Med. Sci. Sports Exerc.*, 22: 773, 1990.

Turley, K.R., and Wilmore, J.H.: Cardiovascular responses to treadmill and cycle ergometer exercise in children and adults. *J. Appl. Physiol.*, 83:948, 1997.

CHAPTER

12

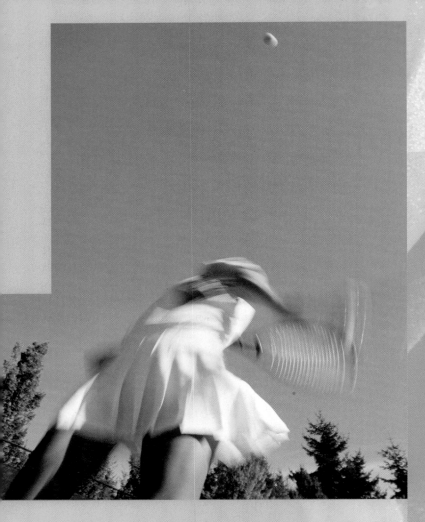

Topics covered in this chapter

PART 1 Neural Control of Human Movement

Neuromotor System Organization
Motor Unit Physiology
Proprioceptors in Muscles, Joints, and Tendons
Summary

PART 2 Muscular System: Organization and Activation

Comparison of Skeletal, Cardiac, and Smooth Muscle
Gross Structure of Skeletal Muscle
Skeletal Muscle Ultrastructure
Chemical and Mechanical Events During Contraction and Relaxation
Muscle Fiber Type
Summary
Thought Questions
Selected References

The Neuromuscular System and Exercise

- Identify the major structural components of the central nervous system that control human movement.

- Diagram the anterior motoneuron and discuss its role in human movement.

- Draw and label the basic components of a reflex arc.

- Define 1) motor unit, 2) neuromuscular junction, 3) autonomic nervous system, 4) excitatory postsynaptic potential, 5) inhibitory postsynaptic potential.

- Explain factors associated with neuromuscular fatigue.

- Describe the function of 1) muscle spindles, 2) Golgi tendon organs, 3) Pacinian corpuscles.

- Draw and label a skeletal muscle fiber's ultra-structural components.

- Describe the sequence of chemical and mechanical events during skeletal muscle contraction and relaxation.

- Contrast slow-twitch and fast-twitch (including subdivisions) muscle fiber characteristics.

- Outline muscle fiber-type distribution patterns among diverse groups of elite athletes.

- Explain modifications in muscle fibers and fiber types that result from exercise training.

PART 1
Neural Control of Human Movement

Applying appropriate force to a tennis serve, golf putt, or slap shot in hockey requires a series of coordinated neural signals that recruit specific muscle fibers. Similarities exist between a modern computer and the human body's neuromuscular circuitry, although the integrative and organizational complexity of the human nervous system far exceeds any computer. In response to changing internal and external stimuli, bits of sensory input are processed by interactive neural control mechanisms. Movements requiring little force and complex movements of great force both depend on the coordinated reception and integration of sensory neural input to transmit signals to effector organs, the muscles.

This chapter describes the neural control of human movement including:

- Structural organization of the neuromotor system, with emphasis on the central and peripheral nervous systems
- Neuromuscular transmission
- Sensory input for muscular activity
- Motor unit type, function, and activation

Neuromotor System Organization

The human nervous system consists of two major parts: 1) **central nervous system (CNS)**, which includes the brain and spinal cord, and 2) **peripheral nervous system (PNS)** comprised of cranial and spinal nerves. Figure 12.1 presents an overview of the human nervous system.

Central Nervous System – The Brain

Figure 12.2A illustrates the brain's six main areas:

1. Medulla oblongata
2. Pons
3. Midbrain
4. Cerebellum
5. Diencephalon
6. Telencephalon

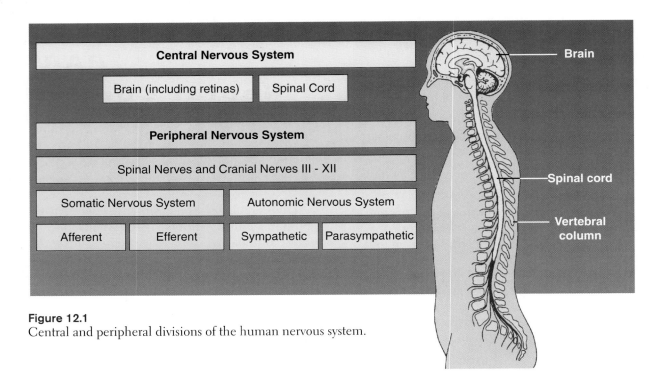

Figure 12.1
Central and peripheral divisions of the human nervous system.

Each of the 12 cranial nerves originates in one of these anatomic areas. Figure 12.2B views the brain from the top (superior view). The longitudinal fissure runs down the midline and separates the brain's right and left sides (hemispheres). Below the fissure, a large tract of nerve fibers (corpus callosum, not shown) connects the two hemispheres. The outer portion of the brain, the **cerebral cortex** or **gray matter** (nerve fibers lack a white myelin coating), consists of a series of folded convolutions. The bottom panel (Figure 12.2C) depicts the four lobes of the cerebral cortex (**occipital, parietal, temporal,** and **frontal**) and the sensory and motor areas, and cerebellum.

The bony skull and a composite of four tough membranes (meninges), which contain a jelly-like, cushioning substance, surround the brain to protect it from injury.

Organization of the Brain

The brain can be organized in a hierarchical manner with distinguishable anatomic divisions that integrate smooth functioning.

Telencephalon (Cerebrum). The telencephalon contains the two cerebral hemispheres, the **corpus striatum** and the **medulla,** which control higher levels of function like thought, intelligence, and problem solving. The cerebral cortex makes up approximately 40% of total brain weight.

Diencephalon. The **thalamus** and **hypothalamus** comprise the major structures of the diencephalon, the smallest and least distinctive of the brain divisions (i.e., containing the fewest nerve cells). The hypothalamus, situated below the thalamus, regulates functions ranging from metabolism to body temperature. The hypothalamus influences autonomic nervous system activity; input from the thalamus and limbic brain system and action of various hormones (refer to Chapter 13) affect hypothalamic activity. Changes in arterial blood pressure and gas tension, monitored by peripheral receptors in the aorta and carotid arteries, also influence the hypothalamus.

Mesencephalon (Midbrain). The **midbrain**, only 1.5 cm long and attached to the cerebellum, connects the pons (meaning bridge) and the cerebral hemispheres, relaying visual and auditory input to the cerebral cortex. The midbrain also contains parts of the extrapyramidal nuclei that integrate motor output from the cortex. The pons contains nerve tracts that connect the spinal cord with other brain areas.

Metencephalon. The metencephalon consists of the **cerebellum** and the **pons**. The cerebellum (two lateral hemispheres and a central vermis) monitors and coordinates other brain and spinal cord areas involved in motor control.

The cerebellum receives two kinds of signals: 1) motor output signals from the cortex, and 2) sensory information from receptors in muscles, tendons, joints, and skin, and visual, auditory, and vestibular end-organs. *The cerebellum's specialized brain tissue serves as the major comparing, evaluating, and integrating center for postural adjustments, locomotion, maintenance of equilibrium, perceptions of speed of body movement, and other reflex functions related to movement.*

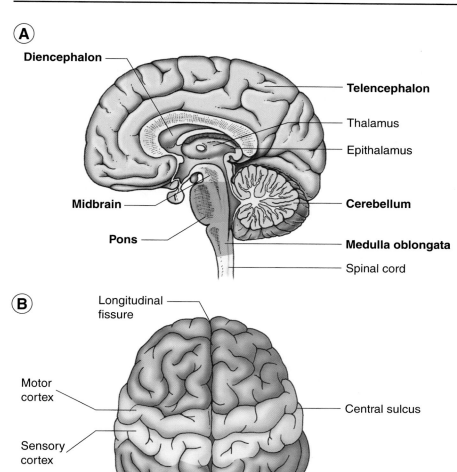

(A)
- **Diencephalon**
- **Telencephalon**
- Thalamus
- Epithalamus
- **Midbrain**
- **Cerebellum**
- **Pons**
- **Medulla oblongata**
- Spinal cord

(B)
- Longitudinal fissure
- Motor cortex
- Sensory cortex
- Central sulcus
- **Left hemisphere**
- **Right hemisphere**

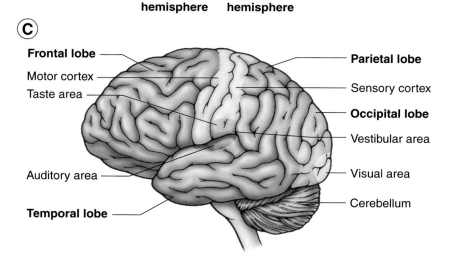

(C)
- **Frontal lobe**
- Motor cortex
- Taste area
- **Parietal lobe**
- Sensory cortex
- **Occipital lobe**
- Vestibular area
- Auditory area
- Visual area
- Cerebellum
- **Temporal lobe**

Figure 12.2

A, Principle six divisions of the brain, lateral view. **B,** Superior view of the brain. **C,** Four lobes of the cerebral cortex.

tional behavior and learning. Experiments with humans show the limbic system affects diverse automatic responses. For example, facial expressions characteristic of emotion represent "hard-wired" responses within the limbic system, not learned responses. Emotions like happiness, fear, and sadness become established within the brain's deep structures at birth.

Central Nervous System – The Spinal Cord

Figure 12.3A depicts the spinal cord (about 45 cm long and 1 cm in diameter) encased by 33 vertebrae (7 cervical, 12 thoracic, 5 lumbar, 5 sacral, and 4 coccygeal). The 12 pairs of peripheral nerves (grouped into cervical, thoracic, lumbar, and sacral sections according to their location along the spine) exit the cord through a small hole (foramen) at the juncture between each pair of vertebrae (Fig. 12.3C).

This unique anatomical design allows extreme vertebral movement without affecting spinal nerves. However, **intervertebral discs**, which separate adjacent vertebrae and provide a cushion surface, can create problems. A disc can bulge into the space occupied by that segment's spinal nerve, compressing it and causing pain in an area the nerve innervates (e.g., lower back or leg), and in some cases, loss of motor control. If this condition persists (with significant muscle weakness), surgical repair or removal of the offending disc often relieves the pressure and pain.

When viewed in cross section (Fig. 12.3B), the spinal cord shows its H-shaped core of gray matter. The limbs of this core, the ventral (anterior) and dorsal (posterior) horns, contain principally three types of nerves:

1. Interneurons
2. Sensory neurons
3. Motoneurons

Limbic System. Portions of the frontal and temporal lobes of the cerebral cortex, thalamus, and hypothalamus, and their neural connections make up the **limbic system** (a group of nerves encircling the brain stem). This configuration of neurons probably contributes to emo-

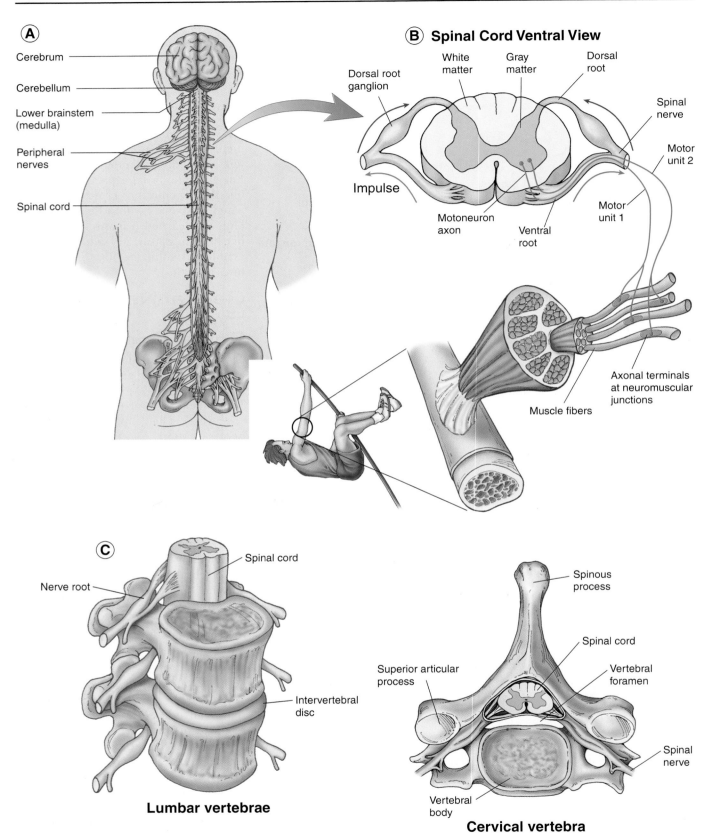

(A)
Cerebrum
Cerebellum
Lower brainstem (medulla)
Peripheral nerves
Spinal cord

(B) **Spinal Cord Ventral View**
Dorsal root ganglion
White matter
Gray matter
Dorsal root
Spinal nerve
Motor unit 2
Impulse
Motoneuron axon
Ventral root
Motor unit 1
Axonal terminals at neuromuscular junctions
Muscle fibers

(C)
Spinal cord
Nerve root
Intervertebral disc
Lumbar vertebrae

Spinous process
Spinal cord
Vertebral foramen
Superior articular process
Spinal nerve
Vertebral body
Cervical vertebra

Figure 12.3
A, Human spinal cord showing the peripheral nerves. **B,** Ventral view of spinal cord section to illustrate dorsal and ventral root neural pathways and nerve impulse direction. **C,** Junction of two lumbar vertebral bodies and a cross-section through one cervical vertebra, right.

Motor (efferent) neurons exit the cord via the ventral root to supply extrafusal and intrafusal skeletal muscle fibers. **Sensory (afferent) neurons** enter the spinal cord via the dorsal root. An area of white matter containing ascending and descending nerve tracts within the cord itself surrounds the gray core.

Ascending Nerve Tracts

Ascending nerve tracts within the spinal cord transmit sensory information from peripheral sensory receptors to the brain. Three nerves typically make up the sensory pathways:

1. The *first nerve* has its cell body in the dorsal root ganglion; its axons relay information from peripheral receptors to the spinal cord.
2. The cell body of the *second nerve* lies within the spinal cord itself; its axon passes up the spinal cord to the thalamus.
3. The thalamus contains the *third nerve* cell body; its axon transmits impulses to the cerebral cortex.

Sensory Receptors. Specialized peripheral sensory nerve endings detect conscious and subconscious sensory information. The conscious receptors detect body position, temperature, and pain, and provide for the senses of sight, sound, smell, taste, and touch. Receptors also monitor subconscious changes of the internal environment, including **chemoreceptors** that respond to changes in blood gas tension (PCO_2, PO_2) and pH, and specialized **baroreceptors** sensitive to arterial blood pressure changes.

Descending Nerve Tracts

Tracts of nerve tissue descend from the brain and terminate at neurons in the spinal cord. The **pyramidal tract** and **extrapyramidal tract** provide the two major pathways for this function.

Pyramidal Tract. Pyramidal or corticospinal tract neurons transmit impulses downward through the spinal cord. By direct routes and interconnecting spinal cord neurons, these nerves eventually excite **alpha motoneurons** that control skeletal muscles.

Extrapyramidal Tract. Extrapyramidal nerves originate in the brain stem and connect at all levels of the spinal cord. These neurons control posture; they provide a continual background level of neuromuscular tone, in contrast to discrete movements stimulated by the pyramidal tract nerves.

The **reticular formation** interconnects the spinal cord, cerebral cortex, basal ganglia, and cerebellum. Once activated, the reticular system produces either an inhibitory or facilitatory effect on other neurons.

The reticular inhibitory center transmits impulses that inhibit neurons to antigravity muscles involved in postural control. Excitation of facilitatory sensory neurons arouses the reticular nerve cells. This activates the cerebral cortex, which excites the reticular system to maintain appropriate cortical arousal. Another feedback network, superimposed on this feedback system, transmits impulses through the spinal cord to the muscles. For example, neural outflow to postural muscles increases their activity. This increased neuromuscular tone also stimulates the spindles, the muscle's own sensory modulators, to redirect excitatory impulses back to the central nervous system to arouse the reticular formation. This example of **multiple feedback control** represents one of the most complex aspects of nervous system operation.

Brain Neurotransmitters

Nerves communicate by releasing at their terminal ends chemical messengers (**neurotransmitters**) that diffuse across the junction (**synapse**) between one nerve end and the cell body of another nerve. The neurotransmitter combines with a specific receptor molecule on the postsynaptic membrane to cause depolarization, or in some instances hyperpolarization. Many of the neurons of the central nervous system, particularly in the brain, release and/or respond to these neurotransmitters. Important brain neurotransmitters include:

- Manoamines–modified amino acids including epinephrine, norepinephrine, serotonin, histamine, and dopamine.
- Neuropeptides–short chains of amino acids that include arginine, vasopressin, and angiotensin II (also act as hormones [refer to Chapter 13]). Enkephalins and endorphins (sometimes called opioid neurotransmitters) represent other neuropeptides, which produce a general sense of well-being. Release of endogenous opioid neurotransmitters with exercise contributes to the exercise "high."
- Nitric Oxide–newly discovered neurotransmitter. Neurons in the central nervous system and other cell types contain nitric oxide receptors, which modulate regulation of blood pressure and local blood flow (refer to Chapter 11).

Table 12.1 lists some currently known neurotransmitters.

Peripheral Nervous System

The **peripheral nervous system** consists of 31 pairs of spinal nerves (8 cervical, 12 thoracic, 5 lumbar, 5 sacral, and 1 coccygeal) and 12 pairs of cranial nerves. Numbers identify these nerves (e.g., C-1, first nerve from cervical re-

TABLE 12.1
Chemical neurotransmitters

PEPTIDES	NONPEPTIDES
ACTH	Acetylcholine
Angiotensin II	Dopamine
Bradykinin	Epinephrine
Endorphins	Gamma-aminobutyric
Gastrin	acid (GABA)
Glucagon	Glutamate
Growth hormone-releasing factor	Glycine
Insulin	Histamine
Oxytocin	Nitric oxide
Somatostatin	Norepinephrine
Substance P	Serotonin
Thyrotropin-releasing factor	
Vasopressin	

gion). Careful experiments have tracked their exact location and mapped the muscles they innervate. Injury to a specific spinal cord area produces predictable neurologic consequences. For example, quadriplegia almost always results from damage to the upper thoracic vertebra and corresponding descending nerve tract. Figure 12.4 shows the distribution of spinal nerves. The peripheral nervous system includes afferent nerves that relay sensory information from muscles, joints, skin, and bones *toward* the brain, and efferent nerves that transmit information *away* from the brain to glands and muscles. The somatic and autonomic nervous systems consist of efferent neurons.

Somatic Nervous System

The **somatic nervous system** innervates skeletal muscle (voluntary muscle). Somatic efferent nerve firing excites muscle activation, whereas autonomic nerve firing (see next section) can either excite or inhibit.

Autonomic Nervous System

Autonomic nervous system efferent nerves activate the viscera and other tissues on the subconscious level. Autonomic nerves innervate smooth muscle (involuntary muscle) in the intestines, sweat and salivary glands, myocardium, and some endocrine glands. Although the heart and intestines display automatic excitability, one can exert conscious control over these tissues under some circumstances. For example, individuals who practice yoga or meditation can modify their heart rate and regional blood flow on command.

Conscious modulation of aspects of the autonomic nervous system offers alternative treatment in medicine (e.g., control of hypertension and stress-related disorders through biofeedback techniques) and applies to certain sports. Competitors in archery and other target-shooting events consciously modify cardiovascular and respiratory patterns so normal breathing and pulse rate temporarily "stop" during the crucial steadying phase of performance. Some competitive power lifters go into a trance-like hypnotic state ("psyching") before an all-out lift to channel all of the muscular actions to the lift, blocking out superfluous neural input that might hinder a maximal effort.

Although the autonomic nervous system functions as a unit to maintain constancy in the internal environment, two distinct divisions exist: **sympathetic** and **parasympathetic**. Sympathetic nerve fibers mediate excitation, whereas parasympathetic activation inhibits (except for va-

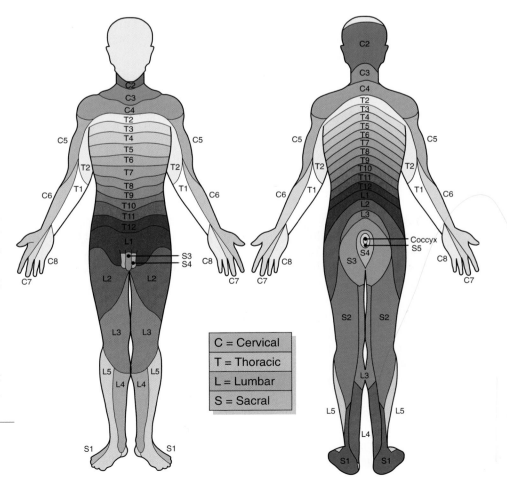

| C = Cervical |
| T = Thoracic |
| L = Lumbar |
| S = Sacral |

Figure 12.4
Location and distribution of spinal nerves.

gal parasympathetic excitation of gastrointestinal motility and tone, and secretion of insulin by the pancreas). In contrast to the somatic nervous system, some cell bodies (ganglia) of sympathetic and parasympathetic neurons exist outside the central nervous system.

Sympathetic Nervous System. Sympathetic nerve fibers supply the heart, smooth muscle, sweat glands, and viscera. These neurons exit the spinal cord and enter a series of ganglia (**sympathetic chain**) near the cord. The nerves terminate relatively far from the target organ in adrenergic endings that release norepinephrine (**adrenergic fibers**). Excitation of the sympathetic nervous system occurs during flight-or-fight situations, requiring whole body arousal for emergencies. Most of us have experienced situations marked by high anxiety or acute fear for safety. Autonomic sympathetic stimulation accelerates breathing and heart rate instantaneously; the pupils dilate; and blood flows from the skin to deeper tissues in anticipation of a perceived challenge.

Parasympathetic Nervous System. Parasympathetic nerve fibers leave the brain stem and sacral segments of the spinal cord to supply the thorax, abdomen, and pelvic regions. Parasympathetic nerve endings release acetylcholine (**cholinergic fibers**). The postganglionic parasympathetic nerve fibers, located close to the organs they innervate, produce effects *opposite* of sympathetic fibers. For example, parasympathetic neural stimulation via the vagus nerve slows heart rate, whereas sympathetic stimulation accelerates heart rate.

Most organs receive sympathetic and parasympathetic stimulation. Both systems maintain a constant degree of activation (neural tone); depending on physiologic need, one system becomes more active while the other simultaneously becomes inhibited. Dual innervation of this type permits a finer level of control at the end organs. This can be likened to hot and cold faucets being open at the same time; minor adjustment in both faucets rapidly and precisely changes tempera-

ture compared with alternately turning each of the faucets on or off. Table 12.2 compares the effects of sympathetic and parasympathetic activation on different end organs.

Autonomic Reflex Arc

Figure 12.5 illustrates a typical neural arrangement for a monosynceptic **reflex arc** in the spinal cord. Sensory input (a knee tap and the subsequent excitation of muscle spindles within the quadriceps) initiates transmission of afferent impulses to the spinal cord via the sensory (dorsal) root. This, in turn, stimulates the anterior motoneuron to the quadricep femoris causing this muscle to contract and extend the lower leg (counteracting the initial stretch). In a polysynaptic reflex arc, the nerves synapse in the cord through interneurons that distribute information to various cord levels. The impulse then passes over the motor root pathway through anterior motoneurons to the effector organ.

Another example of a simple reflex arc occurs when a person accidentally touches a hot object. Stimulation of pain receptors in the fingers sends sensory information rapidly over afferent fibers to the spinal cord to activate efferent motor fibers causing removal of the hand from the hot object. Concurrently, the signal transmits via interneurons up the cord to the sensory area in the brain that actually "feels" the pain. The various operational levels for sensory input, processing, and motor output, including the reflex action just described, explain how the hand withdraws from the hot object *before* the person perceives pain. Reflex actions in the spinal cord and other subconscious areas of the central nervous system control many muscle functions. These reflex actions even operate for people who have had their spinal cords severed above the level required for the reflex.

Complex Reflexes

Complex spinal reflexes that involve multiple synapses and muscle groups also exist. Consider the situation of stepping on a tack with the left foot. Almost simultaneously as

TABLE 12.2
Comparison of effects of sympathetic and parasympathetic activation on end organs

END ORGAN	PARASYMPATHETIC EFFECTS	SYMPATHETIC EFFECTS
Skeletal Muscle	Decrease blood flow	Increase blood flow
Ventilation	Decrease	Increase
Sweat Glands	No effect	Increase perspiration
Heart	Decrease force and contraction rate	Increase force and contraction rate
GI Tract Motility	Increase	Decrease
Eyes	Constrict pupils	Dilate pupils
Secretion of Digestive Juices	Increase	Decrease
Blood Pressure	Decrease mean pressure	Increase mean pressure
Airways	Decrease diameter	Increase diameter

Patella Tendon Reflex

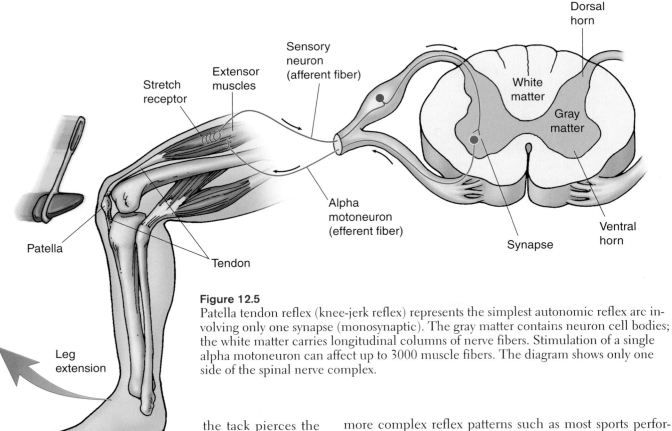

Figure 12.5
Patella tendon reflex (knee-jerk reflex) represents the simplest autonomic reflex arc involving only one synapse (monosynaptic). The gray matter contains neuron cell bodies; the white matter carries longitudinal columns of nerve fibers. Stimulation of a single alpha motoneuron can affect up to 3000 muscle fibers. The diagram shows only one side of the spinal nerve complex.

the tack pierces the skin, the right leg straightens to remove weight from the injured foot, which lifts off the ground. Figure 12.6A illustrates the neural and motor pathways activated in this complex action, termed the **crossed-extensor reflex**, in the following sequence:

1. The tack stimulates pain receptors in the skin, which transmit the message to the spinal cord via the sensory nerve.
2. Sensory neurons branch to each side of the cord to activate interneurons in the gray matter.
3. Interneurons synapse with motoneurons, innervating both flexor and extensor muscles in each leg.
4. Inhibition and stimulation of appropriate leg flexor and extensor muscles cause concurrent rapid extension of the uninjured limb and flexion (removal) of the injured limb.
5. Simultaneously, interneuron connections activate neural pathways to transmit information to appropriate sensory areas of the brain where the pain is "felt."

Learned Reflexes

The knee-jerk and crossed-extensor reflexes occur automatically and require no learning. Practice facilitates other more complex reflex patterns such as most sports performances or occupational tasks. Consider a trained office worker who types 90 words per minute. At an average of five letters per word, this requires six to eight keystrokes per second. For this person, the sight of a word to type initiates a series of rapid hand and finger movements requiring little conscious effort. A beginning typist, in contrast, proceeds slowly; thought must be given to the position of each key and the proper execution of wrist and finger movement. As neuromuscular pathways become "ingrained" through hours of practice, the typing movements progressively become reflex actions as the beginner approaches expert status.

Nerve Supply to Muscle

The terminal branches of one neuron innervate at least one of the body's approximately 250 million muscle fibers. Because only about 420,000 motor nerves exist, a single nerve usually supplies numerous individual muscle fibers. *The ratio of muscle fibers to nerve generally relates to a muscle's particular movement function.* The delicate, precise work of the eye muscles, for example, requires one neuron to control fewer than ten muscle fibers. For less complex movements of the large leg muscles, a motoneuron may innervate as many as 3000 muscle fibers. The next sections review how information processed in the central nervous system activates specific muscles to cause an appropriate motor response.

Crossed-Extensor Reflex

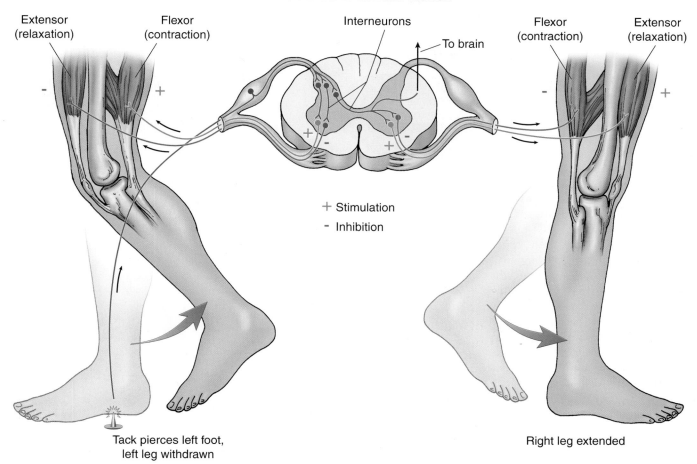

Figure 12.6
Crossed-extensor reflex involving both legs is a more complex reflex involving multiple synapses and muscle groups.

Motor Unit Anatomy

*The **motor unit**, comprised of an anterior motoneuron and the specific muscle fibers it innervates, represents the functional unit of movement.* A motor nerve can innervate many muscle fibers, because the terminal end of an axon forms numerous branches. A muscle fiber, in contrast, receives stimulation from only one nerve fiber.

Anterior Motoneuron

Figure 12.7 shows an **anterior motoneuron** consisting of a cell body, axon, and dendrites. The cell's unique design enables it to transmit electrochemical impulses from the spinal cord to muscle. The **cell body**, located within the spinal cord's gray matter, houses the **control center**—the structures involved in replicating and transmitting the genetic code. The **axon** extends from the cord and delivers an impulse to the muscle fibers it innervates. Short neural branches called **dendrites** receive impulses through numerous spinal cord connections and conduct them toward the cell body.

Nerve cells conduct impulses *in one direction only* down the axon away from the stimulation point. As the axon ap-

proaches the muscle, it branches with each terminal branch innervating a single muscle fiber. A whole muscle contains numerous motor units, each with a single motoneuron and its complement of muscle fibers. All of a motor unit's muscle fibers do not cluster within the muscle, but rather disperse over subregions of the muscle with fibers of other motor units. Consequently, the force generated by a motor unit distributes over a larger tissue area, which reduces localized mechanical stress.

Enervation Ratio

The finger contains 120 motor units controlling 41,000 muscle fibers; in contrast, the medial gastrocnemius muscle (calf) has 580 motor units innervating 1,030,000 fibers. The ratio of muscle fibers per motor unit averages 340 for muscles of the finger and 1800 for the gastrocnemius.

Figure 12.7
The anterior motoneuron consists of a cell body, dendrites, and axon. The inset illustrates a node of Ranvier that permits impulses to jump from one node to the next as the electrical current travels toward the terminal branches at the motor end-plate.

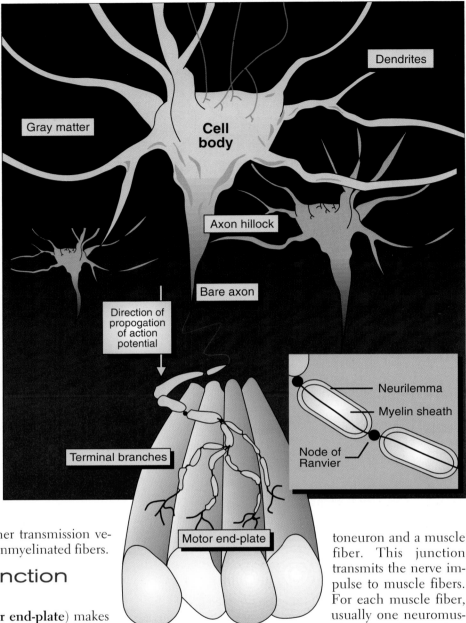

A lipid-protein membrane, the **myelin sheath**, encircles the axon of nerve fibers that are either long in length or large in diameter. In the peripheral nervous system, specialized cells (**Schwann cells**) encase the bare axon and then spiral around it. Myelin forms a large part of this sheath and insulates the axon. A thinner membrane, the **neurilemma**, covers the myelin sheath. **Nodes of Ranvier** interrupt the Schwann cells and myelin every 1 or 2 mm along the axon's length. Although the myelin sheath insulates the axon to ion flow, the nodes of Ranvier permit axon depolarization along axon segments. The alternating sequence of myelin sheath and node of Ranvier allows impulses to "jump" from node to node as electrical current travels toward the terminal branches at the motor end-plate. Nerve conduction in this manner accounts for the higher transmission velocity in myelinated compared with unmyelinated fibers.

Neuromuscular Junction (Motor End-Plate)

The **neuromuscular junction** (**motor end-plate**) makes up the interface between the end of a myelinated mo-

toneuron and a muscle fiber. This junction transmits the nerve impulse to muscle fibers. For each muscle fiber, usually one neuromuscular junction exists.

Figure 12.8 details the neuromuscular junction based on electron microscopic studies.

The terminal portion of the axon forms several smaller axon branches whose endings, the presynaptic terminals, lie close but do not contact the muscle fiber's plasma membrane (**sarcolemma**). The region of the postsynaptic membrane (**synaptic gutter**) contains infoldings that increase its surface area. Between the synaptic gutter and the presynaptic terminal of the axon lies the **synaptic cleft**, the region where actual neural impulse transmission occurs.

Excitation

Excitation normally occurs only at the neuromuscular junction. The neurotransmitter **acetylcholine** provides the chemical stimulus to change an electrical neural impulse into a chemical stimulus at the motor end-plate. Acetyl-

Types of Motoneurons

The large diameters of anterior motoneurons, termed **type A alpha fibers,** range between 8 to 20 microns (μ; 1μ = one-millionth of a m). Diameters of other smaller type A fibers (**gamma efferent motoneurons**) do not exceed 10 μ. Their conduction velocities equal about one-half that of the alpha fibers. Gamma efferent fibers connect with special stretch sensors (proprioceptors) in skeletal muscle to detect minute changes in muscle fiber length.

Figure 12.8
Microanatomy of the neuromuscular junction. Inset displays details of presynaptic and postsynaptic contact areas between the motoneuron and the muscle fiber it innervates.

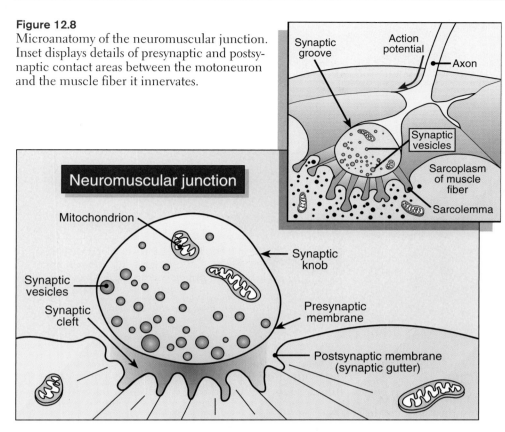

choline, released from small, sac-like vesicles within the terminal axon, increases the postsynaptic membrane's permeability to sodium and potassium ions. This spreads the impulse over the entire muscle fiber as a wave of depolarization. As depolarization progresses, the muscle fiber's contractile machinery primes for its major function—contraction.

The enzyme **cholinesterase**, concentrated at the borders of the synaptic cleft, breaks down acetylcholine within five milliseconds after its release from synaptic vesicles. This repolarizes the postsynaptic membrane. The axon resynthesizes acetylcholine from acetic acid and choline (byproducts of cholinesterase action) so the entire process can begin again when another nerve impulse arrives.

Facilitation

When a motoneuron's microvoltage decreases sufficiently to reach its threshold for excitation, it generates an action potential. **Excitatory postsynaptic potential** (**EPSP**) describes the change in membrane potential (increase in positive charges inside the cell) at the junction between two neurons. *The EPSP hypopolarizes the neuron, making it easier to fire.* With a subthreshold EPSP, the neuron does not discharge, but its resting membrane potential still lowers, temporarily increasing its tendency to fire. A neuron fires when many subthreshold excitatory impulses arrive in rapid succession, a condition termed **temporal summation**. **Spatial summation** describes the simultaneous stimulation of different presynaptic terminals on the same neuron. The "summing" of each excitatory effect often initiates an action potential.

Removing inhibitory neural influences becomes important under certain exercise conditions. In all-out strength and power activities, disinhibition and maximal activation of all motoneurons required for a movement can enhance performance. *Effective disinhibition fully activates muscle groups during maximal lifting; this accounts for the rapid, highly specific strength increases noted in the early stages of a resistance training program.* Enhanced neuromuscular activation also explains significant improvements in muscular strength without concomitant increases in muscle size. Central nervous system excitation (neuronal facilitation) also explains why intense concentration (psyching) can improve maximal strength and power performances. The amino acids glutamate and acetylcholine typically exert an excitatory neurotransmitter influence.

Inhibition

Certain presynaptic terminals generate inhibitory impulses by releasing chemicals that increase the postsynaptic membrane's permeability to potassium and chloride ions. The efflux of positively charged potassium ions (or influx of negatively charged chloride ions) increases the membrane's resting electrical potential, creating an **inhibitory postsynaptic potential** (**IPSP**). *The IPSP hyperpolarizes the neuron, making it more difficult to fire.* No action potential generates if a motoneuron encounters excitatory and inhibitory influences, or encounters a large IPSP. For example, a person can usually override (inhibit) the reflex to pull the hand away when removing a splinter. The neurotransmitter amino acids gamma aminobutyric acid (GABA) and glycine provoke an inhibitory response. Neural inhibition serves protective functions; it also reduces the input of unwanted stimuli so smooth, purposeful responses can take place.

Motor Unit Physiology

Three physiologic and mechanical properties categorize motor units and the muscle fibers they innervate (Table 12.3):

1. Twitch (speed of contraction) characteristics
2. Tension-generating (force) characteristics
3. Fatigability characteristics

TABLE 12.3
Characteristics and correspondence between motor units and muscle fiber types

MOTOR UNIT DESIGNATION	FORCE PRODUCTION	CONTRACTION SPEED	FATIGUE RESISTANCE	SAG†	MOTOR UNIT MUSCLE FIBER TYPE
Fast Fatigable (FF)	High	Fast	Low	Yes	Fast Glycolytic (FG)
Fast Fatigue-Resistant (FR)	Moderate	Fast	High	Yes	Fast Oxidative-Glycolytic (FOG)
Slow (S)	Low	Slow	High	No	Slow Oxidative (SO)

† Under repetitive stimuli, some motor units respond smoothly with a systematic increase in tension, while others first increase tension and then decrease or "sag" slightly in response to the same tetanic stimulus. These sag characteristics can classify the different motor units. Only the S motor units do not exhibit sag, which probably relates more to their lower force-generating capabilities than their fatigue characteristics.

Modified from Lieber, R.L.: *Skeletal Muscle Structure and Function: Implications for Rehabilitation and Sports Medicine*. Baltimore: Williams & Wilkins, 1992.

Twitch Characteristics

Early experiments revealed that motor units developed high, low, or intermediate tension in response to a single electrical impulse. Motor units with the capacity for low force production show slow contraction velocities, yet resist fatigue; those generating higher tension contract rapidly but fatigue early. Figure 12.9 illustrates these characteristics for the following three motor unit categories:

1. Fast-twitch, high-force, fast-fatigue (*type IIb*)
2. Fast-twitch, moderate-force, fatigue-resistant (*type IIa*)
3. Slow-twitch, low-tension, fatigue-resistant (*type I*)

Relatively large motoneurons with fast conduction velocities innervate between 300 to 500 fast-twitch muscle fibers. These fast-fatigable (FF) and fast-fatigue–resistant (FR) units reach greater peak tension and develop it nearly twice as fast as slow-twitch (S) motor units innervated by small motoneurons with slow conduction velocities. However, slow-twitch motor units exhibit less fatigue than fast-twitch units. Specific exercise training modifies the fatigue (metabolic) characteristics of motor units. With prolonged aerobic training, some fast-twitch units become almost as fatigue resistant as slow-twitch counterparts.

Tension-Generating Characteristics

All-or-None Principle

If a stimulus triggers an action potential in the motoneuron, all of the accompanying muscle fibers contract. A single motor unit cannot generate strong and weak contractions—either the impulse elicits a contraction or it does not. Once the neuron fires, and the impulse reaches the neuromuscular junction, the muscle cells always contract (to the fullest extent) in accord with the **all-or-none principle**.

Gradation of Force

The force of a muscle's action varies from slight to maximal in one of two ways:

1. Increasing the *number* of motor units recruited
2. Increasing the *frequency* of motor unit discharge

Activation of all motor units in a muscle generates considerable force compared with activating only a few units. Total tension also increases if repetitive stimuli reach a muscle before it relaxes. Blending recruitment of motor units and their firing rate permits a wide variety of graded muscle actions. The golf swing provides a good example of force gradation. Tension in hands, arms, and legs continually adjusts during the backswing, swing initiation and acceleration, club-ball contact, and follow-through. The seemingly simple task of writing with a pen involves a myriad of complex, coordinated, and diverse neuromuscular forces and actions.

Motor Unit Recruitment

Low force muscle actions activate few motor units, whereas higher force actions enlist more units. **Motor unit recruitment** describes the process of adding more motor units to increase muscular force. Motoneurons with progressively larger axons become recruited as muscle force increases. This response (termed the **size principle**) provides an anatomic basis for the orderly recruitment of specific motor units to produce a smooth action.

Figure 12.10 illustrates that not all of a muscle's motor units fire at the same time. For example, when lifting a barbell, specific muscles contract to move the limb and weight at

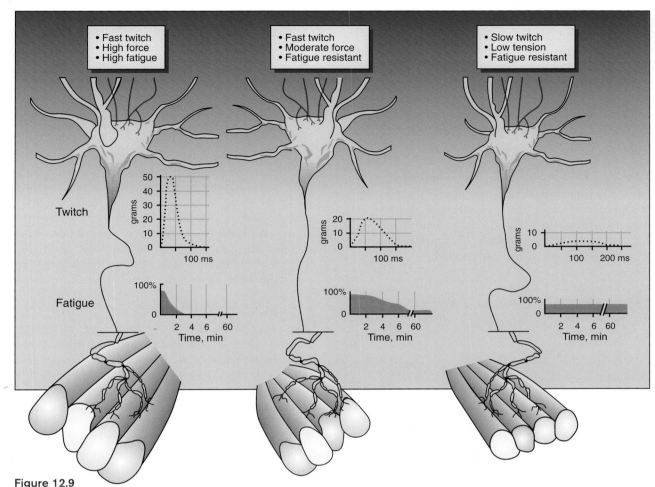

Figure 12.9
Speed, force, and fatigue characteristics of motor units. Fast-twitch motoneurons fire rapidly with short bursts; slow-twitch motoneurons fire slowly but continuously. (Modified from Edington, D.W., and Edgerton, V.R.: *The Biology of Physical Activity.* Boston: Houghton-Mifflin, 1976.)

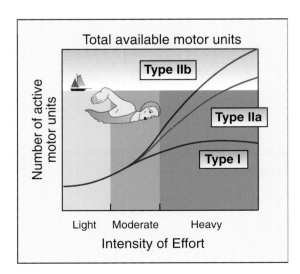

Figure 12.10
Recruitment of slow-twitch and fast-twitch muscle fibers (motor units) related to exercise intensity. Increasingly intense physical effort progressively recruits more fast-twitch fibers.

a particular speed under a given magnitude of tension development. One can lift a relatively light weight at varied speeds. With heavier weight, the speed options decrease considerably. *From the standpoint of neural control, slow-twitch and fast-twitch motor units become selectively recruited and modulated in their firing pattern to produce the desired response.*

In activities requiring varying force outputs, slow-twitch motor units with low activation thresholds become selectively recruited during lighter effort. Activation of more powerful, higher threshold, fast-twitch units progresses in accordance with the size principle as force requirements increase. Sustained, submaximal jogging, cycling, cross-country skiing on a level grade, and lifting a light weight at slow speed involve selective recruitment of slow-twitch motor units. With rapid, powerful movements like sprint running 100 m or swimming 50 m the fast-twitch fibers become activated, particularly type IIb fibers. Fast-twitch units activate when a runner or bicyclist ascends a hill or maintains a constant pace over varied terrain.

The differential control of the motor unit firing pattern distinguishes specific athletic groups and skilled from unskilled performers. Weightlifters, for example, demonstrate a synchronous pattern of motor-unit firing (many motor units recruited simultaneously during lifting), whereas endurance athletes generally exhibit an asynchronous firing pattern (some motor units fire while others recover). The synchronous firing of fast-twitch fibers certainly aids the weight lifter in generating rapid force. Conversely, asynchronous firing of slow-twitch, fatigue-resistant motor units provides a built-in recuperative period to enable the endurance performer to continue with reduced fatigue.

Neuromuscular Fatigue

Resistance to fatigue (the decline in muscle tension with repeated stimulation) represents the third quality distinguishing differences in motor units. Fatigue can result from disruption in the chain of events among any of the four components of the neuromotor system (in order of hierarchy):

1. Central nervous system
2. Peripheral nervous system
3. Neuromuscular junction
4. Muscle fiber

Factors associated with a decrease in the muscle's force-generating capacity include:

- Significant reduction in muscle glycogen and blood glucose produces fatigue during prolonged, submaximal exercise. This "nutrient-related fatigue" occurs despite availability of sufficient oxygen and fatty acid substrate for ATP regeneration through aerobic metabolic pathways.

- Muscle fatigue in short-term maximal exercise reflects insufficient oxygen availability and/or utilization, increased lactate accumulation, and an increase in [H⁺] within active muscle fibers. Extreme reliance on anaerobic metabolism ultimately: (a) inhibits the contractile mechanism; (b) depletes intramuscular high-energy phosphates; (c) impairs energy transfer via glycolysis from reduced activity of key enzymes; (d) disturbs the tubular system for transmitting the impulse throughout the cell; and (e) creates ionic imbalances. For example, disruption of intracellular Ca^{++} alters the activity of the myofilaments and impairs muscular performance.

- Impaired function (fatigue) at the neuromuscular junction causes failure of the action potential to cross from the motoneuron to the muscle fiber. The mechanism for this aspect of neural fatigue remains unknown.

With impaired muscle function during prolonged submaximal exercise, additional motor-unit recruitment maintains the required force output for the particular activity. In all-out exercise, when all motor units presumably become maximally activated, a decrease in neural activity measured by the electromyogram (EMG) accompanies fatigue. Depressed EMG activity supports the argument that failure in neural or myoneural transmission contributes to fatigue in some maximal effort muscle actions.

Proprioceptors in Muscles, Joints, and Tendons

Muscles, joints, and tendons contain specialized sensory receptors sensitive to stretch, tension, and pressure. These end-organs (**proprioceptors**) rapidly relay information about muscular dynamics, limb position, and movement (i.e., kinesthesia and proprioception) to conscious and unconscious parts of the central nervous system for processing. Continual monitoring of the progress of any movement or sequence of movements provides the basis for modifying subsequent motor patterns.

Muscle Spindles

Muscle spindles provide sensory information about changes in length and tension of muscle fibers. They primarily respond to muscle stretch and through reflex action initiate a stronger contraction to reduce the stretch.

Figure 12.11 illustrates the fusiform-shaped spindle attached in parallel to regular muscle fibers (**extrafusal fibers**). With this arrangement, any elongation of the muscle stretches the spindle. The number of spindles per gram of muscle varies depending on the muscle group. More spindles exist in muscles that routinely perform complex movements. The spindle contains two types of specialized fibers with contractile capabilities (**intrafusal fibers**).

Two afferent (sensory) and one efferent (motor) nerve fibers service the spindles. The motor spindles consist of thin gamma efferent fibers that innervate the contractile, striated ends of intrafusal fibers. These fibers, activated by higher brain centers, maintain the spindle at peak operation at all muscle lengths.

Stretch Reflex

The muscle spindle detects, responds to, and controls changes in extrafusal muscle fiber length to regulate move-

Camillo Golgi

Camillo Golgi (1843–1926), Italian neuro-histochemist, discovered the Golgi tendon organs in 1878 using a silver nitrate stain described in his masterful text, *On the Fine Anatomy of the Nervous System.* He was awarded the nobel Prize in Physiology or Medicine in 1906 with Santiago Ramón y Cajal (1852–1934) for their work on the structure of the nervous system.

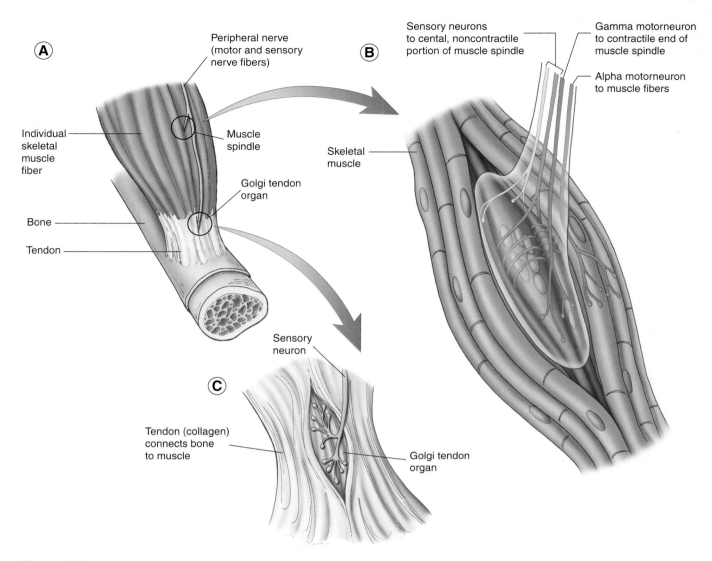

Figure 12.11
A, General location of muscle spindles and Golgi tendon end organs. **B,** Muscle spindle surrounded by skeletal muscle fibers. Two types of sensory neurons innervate the spindle's central portion: 1) fast-adapting neurons with spiral endings, and 2) slow-adapting neurons with branched endings. Gamma motoneurons innervate the contractile ends of muscle spindle cells, and alpha motoneurons activate skeletal muscle cells. **C,** Slow-adapting sensory neurons innervate Golgi tendon organs. Excessive tension or stretch on a muscle activates Golgi receptors to initiate reflex inhibition of the muscles they supply. These sensory organs provide a protective mechanism within the muscle-tendon structure to detect and inhibit undue strain.

ment and posture. Neural input continuously bombards postural muscles to maintain their readiness to respond to voluntary movements and provide continual force to counter gravity's pull and maintain upright posture. To this end, the stretch reflex represents a fundamental controlling mechanisms for neuromuscular regulation. Three main components comprise the stretch reflex:

1. Muscle spindle: responds to stretch.
2. Afferent nerve fiber: carries sensory impulses from the muscle spindle to the spinal cord.
3. Efferent motoneuron: stimulates muscle to contract.

Figure 12.12 illustrates the neural pathways involved in the stretch reflex. In part A, the biceps muscle shortens to maintain the bony lever at a 90 degree angle while holding a 1-kg book. Suddenly increasing the book's weight three-fold (part B) stretches the muscle, causing the spindles' sensory endings to direct impulses through the dorsal root to the spinal cord to activate the motoneuron. The returning motor impulses (part C) contract the muscle more forcefully, returning the limb to its original non-stretched position.

The reflex concurrently activates interneurons in the spinal cord to facilitate an appropriate "whole body" move-

How to Provide Prudent, Immediate Treatment for Soft Tissue Injuries

The most common injuries during general fitness programs include sprains (overstretching or tearing of ligamentous tissue) and strains (overstretching or tearing of muscle or tendinous tissues). The extent of tissue damage depends on the magnitude of the unusual force and duration of its application. Strains and sprains are classified as first, second, or third degree. The prudent, immediate treatment of soft tissue injury reduces further damage prior to medical treatment.

Injury Classification

1. *First degree, mild injury*. Does not compromise the ligament or tendon. Physical activity can usually begin again within 1 week. Some localized tenderness and swelling within the muscle or connective tissue may occur, accompanied by reduced normal range of motion.
2. *Second degree, moderate injury*. Involves a tear of a ligamentous or muscle section, impairing function. Joint laxity

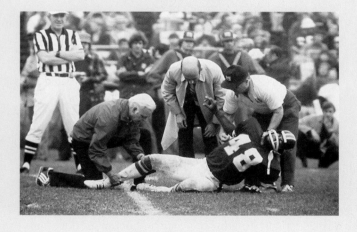

becomes noticeable under stress; significant swelling and discoloration may occur, with increased pain through the range of motion of the affected joint area.
3. *Third degree, severe injury*. Complete tear or rupture of the ligament/tendon at either end of its attachment, accompanied by joint instability. Extreme swelling, spasms, with persistent pain.

Injury Treatment

The five-letter acronym **PRICE** (Protection, Rest, Ice, Compression, Elevation) describes the preferred immediate treatment sequence for soft tissue injury.

1. *Protection*: Isolate the injured area to protect it from further damage.
2. *Rest*: Restrict further activity/use of the injured area.
3. *Ice*: Apply ice immediately to the injured area and continue application for 24 to 72 hours depending on injury severity. Surround the area with an ice pack secured with elastic wrap. Ice causes vasoconstriction, reducing internal bleeding and swelling (fluid seepage into surrounding tissues). Ice also reduces pain. The standard ice application interval lasts 15 to 20 minutes, with reapplication hourly or when pain persists. Ice or compression at bedtime is unnecessary unless the pain interferes with sleep. If the injury involves a contusion (bruise) to a muscle belly, mildly stretch the muscle before applying ice; if possible, maintain the stretched position for the duration of ice application.
4. *Compression*: Compression should be firm but not tight; the wrap should begin distal to the injury and proceed toward the injured area.
5. *Elevation*: Raise the injured area above heart level to minimize gravity's hydrostatic effect on venous pooling and fluid efflux into injured tissues. Elevate the limb when practical. During sleep, elevate the injured limb with blankets or pillows.

---

ment response. Excitatory impulses activate synergistic muscles that support the desired movement, while inhibitory impulses flow to neurons of muscles antagonistic to the movement. The stretch reflex acts as a self-regulating, compensating mechanism; it enables the muscle to adjust automatically to differences in load (and length) without immediately processing information through higher neural centers.

Golgi Tendon Organs

In contrast to muscle spindles that lay parallel to extrafusal muscle fibers, **Golgi tendon organs** connect in series to as

many as 25 extrafusal fibers. The tiny sensory receptors, also located in ligaments of joints, primarily detect differences in muscle tension rather than length. Figure 12.13 shows that Golgi tendon organs respond as a feedback monitor to discharge impulses when the muscle shortens or stretches.

When activated by excessive muscle tension or stretch, Golgi receptors rapidly conduct signals to cause reflex inhibition of the muscles they supply. This occurs because of an overriding influence of inhibitory spinal interneurons on the motoneurons supplying muscle. With extreme tension or stretch, the sensor's discharge increases to further de-

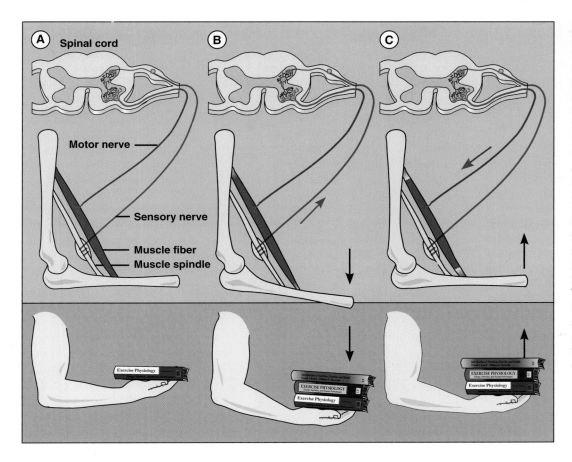

Figure 12.12
Schematic representation of the stretch reflex. Because spindle fibers (intrafusal fibers) run parallel to skeletal muscle (extrafusal) fibers, spindle fibers stretch (and fire) when extrafusal fibers stretch. Activation of the spindle's sensory receptors reflexly stimulates alpha motoneurons. Contraction of extrafusal fibers removes stretch from the intrafusal fibers and silences the spindle afferents. The diagram illustrates how the stretch reflex acts as a self-regulating mechanism to maintain relative constancy of limb position.

press motoneuron activity and reduce tension in muscle fibers. The ultimate function of the Golgi tendon organs is to protect muscle and its connective tissue from injury caused by excessive load.

Pacinian Corpuscles

Pacinian corpuscles, small, ellipsoidal bodies located near Golgi tendon organs, respond to quick movement and deep pressure. Compression of the corpuscle's onion-like capsule by mechanical stimulus transmits pressure to sensory nerve endings within its core. This changes the nerve ending's electrical potential. If this generator potential reaches sufficient magnitude, a sensory signal flows down the myelinated axon toward the spinal cord after leaving the corpuscle.

Pacinian corpuscles adapt rapidly; they discharge a few impulses at the onset of a steady stimulus and then remain electrically silent, or discharge a second volley of impulses when the stimulus ceases. These mechanical sensors detect changes in movement or pressure, rather than the magnitude of movement or pressure.

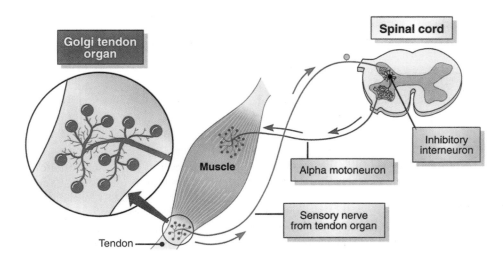

Figure 12.13
The Golgi tendon organ. Excessive tension or stretch on a muscle activates the tendon's Golgi receptors, which brings about a reflex inhibition of the muscles they supply. In this way, the Golgi tendon organ functions as a protective sensory mechanism to detect and subsequently inhibit undue strain within the muscle-tendon structure.

summary

1. Central nervous system neural control mechanisms finely regulate human movement. In response to internal and external stimuli, bits of sensory input are automatically and rapidly routed, organized, and retransmited to the effector organs, the muscles.

2. Tracts of nerve tissue descend from the brain to influence neural activity in the spinal cord. Neurons in the extrapyramidal tract control posture and furnish a continual background level of neuromuscular tone; the pyramidal tract neurons initiate discrete movements.

3. The cerebellum, the major comparing, evaluating, and integrating center, fine tunes muscular activity.

4. The spinal cord and other subconscious areas of the central nervous system control numerous muscular functions. The reflex arc processes automatic (subconscious) muscular movements and responses.

5. The number of muscle fibers in a motor unit depends on the muscle's movement function. Intricate movement patterns require a relatively small fiber-to-neuron ratio, whereas for gross movements, a single neuron may innervate several thousand muscle fibers.

6. The anterior motoneuron (cell body, axon, and dendrites) transmits the electrochemical nerve impulse from the spinal cord to muscle. Dendrites receive impulses and conduct them toward the cell body; the axon transmits the impulse in one direction only (down the axon to the muscle).

7. The neuromuscular junction interfaces between the motoneuron and its muscle fibers. Acetylcholine release at this junction activates the muscle.

8. Excitatory and inhibitory impulses continually bombard synaptic junctions between neurons. These alter a neuron's threshold for excitation by increasing or decreasing its tendency to fire. In all-out, high-power exercise, a large degree of disinhibition benefits performance because it maximally activates a muscle's motor units.

9. Motor units classify into three types, depending on speed of contraction, force generated, and fatigability: 1) fast-twitch, high-force, and high-fatigue; 2) fast-twitch, moderate-force, and fatigue-resistant; and 3) slow-twitch, low-tension, and fatigue-resistant.

10. Gradation of muscle force results from an interaction of factors that regulate the number and type of motor units recruited and their frequency of discharge. Light exercise predominantly recruits slow-twitch motor units followed by activation of fast-twitch units when force output requirements increase (size principle).

11. Alterations in motor unit recruitment and firing pattern explain a large portion of strength improvement with resistance training, particularly the first few training sessions when muscles "learn" the intricacies of highly specific neuromuscular interactions.

12. Sensory receptors in muscles, tendons, and joints relay information about muscular dynamics and limb movement to specific portions of the central nervous system. This provides crucial sensory feedback information to the central nervous system to optimize movement economy and prevent injury.

PART 2

Muscular System: Organization and Activation

Skeletal muscles transform the chemical energy in ATP into the mechanical energy of motion. Part 2 presents the architectural organization of skeletal muscle and focuses on its gross and microscopic structure. The discussion includes the sequence of chemical and mechanical events in muscular contraction and relaxation, and differences in muscle fiber characteristics among elite performers in diverse sports.

Comparison of Skeletal, Cardiac, and Smooth Muscle

Humans possess three types of muscle (cardiac, smooth, and skeletal), each of which has functional and anatomical differences. Cardiac muscle, as the name implies, occurs only in the heart. It shares several common features with skeletal muscle; both appear striated under microscopic examination and contract in a similar manner. Smooth muscle lacks a striated appearance, but shares cardiac muscle's characteristic of subconscious regulation. Table 12.4 compares the structural and functional characteristics of the three types of muscle.

Gross Structure of Skeletal Muscle

Each of the more than 430 voluntary muscles in the body contains various wrappings of fibrous connective tissue. Figure 12.14 shows the cross section of a muscle consisting of thousands of cylindrical cells called fibers. These long, slender multinucleated fibers (whose number probably becomes fixed by the second trimester of fetal development) lie parallel to one another, with the force of contraction occurring along the fiber's long axis.

A fine layer of connective tissue, the **endomysium**, wraps each fiber and separates it from neighboring fibers. Another layer of connective tissue, the **perimysium**, surrounds a bundle of up to 150 fibers to form a **fasciculus**. The **epimysium** surrounds the entire muscle with a fascia of fibrous connective tissue. This protective sheath tapers at its distal end as it blends into and joins the intramuscular tissue sheaths to form the dense, strong connective tissue of **tendons**. The tendons connect both ends of the muscle to the **periosteum**, the outermost covering of the skeleton. The force of muscle action transmits directly from the muscle's connective tissue harness to the tendons at their bony points of attachment.

Beneath the endomysium and surrounding each muscle fiber lays the **sarcolemma**, a thin, elastic membrane that encloses the fiber's cellular contents. The cell's aqueous protoplasm (**sarcoplasm**) contains contractile proteins, enzymes, energy compounds, nuclei, and specialized cellular organelles. The sarcoplasm contains an extensive interconnecting network of tubular channels and vesicles called the **sarcoplasmic reticulum**. This highly specialized, intricate support system provides the cell with structural integrity; it also helps activate and contract muscle.

Chemical Composition

Skeletal muscle contains approximately 75% water and 20% protein, with the remaining 5% inorganic salts and high-energy phosphates, urea, lactate, calcium, magnesium, and phosphorus; enzymes and pigments; sodium, potassium, and chloride ions; and amino acids, fats, and carbohydrates.

TABLE 12.4
Characteristics of the three types of human muscle

	TYPE OF MUSCLE		
CHARACTERISTICS	**SKELETAL**	**CARDIAC**	**SMOOTH**
Location	Attached to bones	Heart only	Part of blood vessel stucture: surrounds many internal hollow organs
Function	Movement	Pumps blood	Constricts blood vessels; moves contents of internal organs
Anatomical description	Large cylindrical, multinucliated cells arranged in parallel	Quadrangular cells	Small, spindle-shaped cells with long axis oriented in the same direction
Striated	Yes	Yes	No
Initiation of action potential	By neuron only	Spontaneous (pacemaker cells)	Spontaneous
Duration of electrical activity	Short (1–2 ms)	Long (~200 ms)	Very long, slow (~300 ms)
Energy source	Anaerobic, Aerobic	Aerobic	Aerobic
Energy efficiency	Low	Moderate	High
Fatigue resistance	Low to high	Low	Very low
Rate of shortening	Fast	Moderate	Very slow
Duration of action	As brief as 100 ms; prolonged tetanus	Short (~300 ms); summation and tetanus not possible	Very long; may be sustained indefinitely

Blood Supply

Because dynamic exercise often requires an oxygen uptake of 4000 mL · min^{-1} and higher, the oxygen uptake of muscle increases at least 70 times above its resting level to about 3400 mL · min^{-1}. To accommodate the increased oxygen requirement, the local vascular bed redirects blood flow through active tissues. In continuous, rhythmic exercise, such as running, swimming, and cycling, muscle blood flow fluctuates; it decreases during the shortening action and increases during muscle relaxation. Alternating contraction and relaxation provides a "milking action" to facilitate blood flow through the muscles and back to the heart. Concurrently, the rapid dilation of previously dormant capillaries within muscle increases the effective surface for nutrient and gaseous exchange.

Straining-type activities present a somewhat different picture. When a muscle contracts to about 60% of its force-generating capacity, blood flow within the muscle diminishes because of elevated intramuscular pressure. The muscle's compressive force with a maximal isometric action actually stops blood flow. As a result, stored intramuscular phosphagens and anaerobic glycolytic reactions provide the energy to sustain muscular effort.

Muscle Capillarization

Aside from delivering oxygen, nutrients, and hormones, the capillary microcirculation removes heat and metabolic byproducts from active tissues. The significant increase (as much as 40%) in skeletal muscle capillary density with aerobic training enhances these functions.

Skeletal Muscle Ultrastructure

Electron microscopy, x-ray diffraction, and histochemical staining techniques have revealed the ultrastructure of skeletal muscle. Figure 12.15 shows the different levels of subcellular organization within a muscle fiber.

Each muscle fiber contains smaller functional units that lie parallel to the fiber's long axis. The **myofibrils**, approximately 1 μ in diameter, contain even smaller subunits (**myofilaments**) that also run parallel to the myofibril's long axis. The myofilaments consist mainly of two proteins, **actin** and **myosin**, which make up about 84% of the myofibrillar complex.

The Sarcomere

At low magnification under a light microscope, the alternating light and dark bands along the length of the skeletal muscle fiber appear **striated**. Figure 12.16 illustrates the structural details of this cross-striation pattern within a myofibril.

The **I band** shows up as the lighter area, the darker zone is the **A band**. The **Z line** bisects the I band and adheres to the sarcolemma to stabilize the entire structure. *The sarcomere, the repeating unit between two Z lines, makes up the functional unit of the muscle cell.* The actin and myosin filaments within a sarcomere provide the mechanical mechanism for muscle action.

The position of the sarcomere's thin actin and thicker myosin proteins overlaps the two filaments. The center of the A band contains the **H zone**, a region of lower optical density because of the absence of actin filaments in this region. The **M line** bisects the central portion of the H zone and delineates the sarcomere's center. The M line contains the protein structures that support the arrangement of myosin filaments.

Actin-Myosin Orientation

Figure 12.17A illustrates actin-myosin orientation within a sarcomere at resting length. Part B shows the

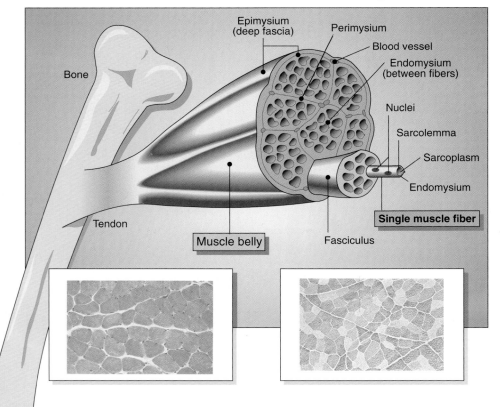

Epimysium (deep fascia)
Perimysium
Blood vessel
Endomysium (between fibers)
Bone
Nuclei
Sarcolemma
Sarcoplasm
Endomysium
Single muscle fiber
Tendon
Muscle belly
Fasciculus

Figure 12.14

Cross section of an intact muscle and its connective tissue wrappings. The inset displays transverse sections of striated muscle where different staining procedures identify different muscle fiber types. (Inset photos from Sobotta, J., and Hammersen, F.: *Histology. Color Atlas of Microscopic Anatomy.* 3rd Ed. Baltimore: Urban & Schwarzenberg, 1992.)

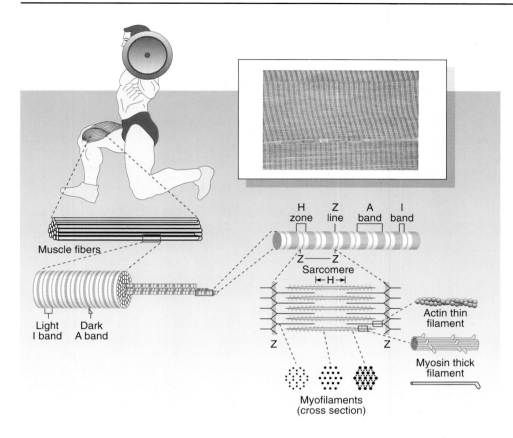

Muscle fibers

Light I band   Dark A band

H zone   Z line   A band   I band

Z — Z
Sarcomere
H

Z   Z

Actin thin filament

Myosin thick filament

Myofilaments (cross section)

Figure 12.15
Microscopic organization of skeletal muscle (microscope magnification, approximately x205,000). Muscle fibers comprise the contractile component of whole muscle; these fibers contain myofibrils (composed of actin and myosin protein filaments). The inset displays skeletal muscle fibers with prominent cross-striations.

ple, a 1 μ -diameter myofibril contains about 450 thick filaments in the center of the sarcomere and 900 thin filaments at each end. Consequently, a single muscle fiber 100 μ in diameter and 1 cm long contains about 8000 myofibrils, each with 4500 sarcomeres. This results in a total of 16 billion thick and 64 billion thin filaments in a single muscle fiber.

Figure 12.18 details the spatial orientation of various proteins that form the contractile

hexagonal arrangement of actin and myosin filaments. Six thin actin filaments, each about 50 angstroms (Å; 1Å = 100-millionths of a cm) in diameter and 1 μ long, surround a thicker myosin filament (150 Å in diameter and 1.5 μ long). This forms an impressive muscular substructure. For exam-

filaments. Projections, or **crossbridges,** spiral around the myosin filament at the region where the actin and myosin filaments overlap. Crossbridges repeat at intervals of 450 Å along the filament. Their globular, lollipop-like heads extend perpendicularly to interact with the thinner actin

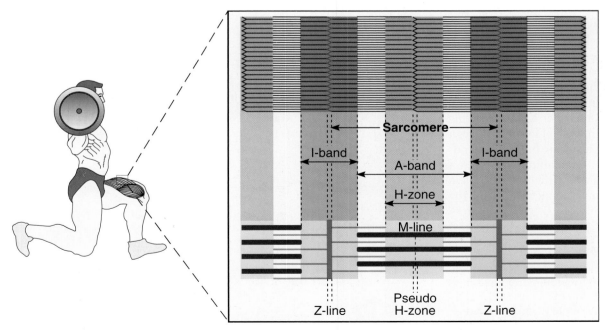

Sarcomere

I-band   A-band   H-zone   M-line   I-band

Z-line   Pseudo H-zone   Z-line

Figure 12.16
Structural orientation of myofilaments in a sarcomere. The Z line borders the sarcomere at both ends.

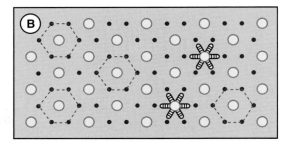

Figure 12.17
A, Ultrastructure of actin-myosin orientation within a resting sarcomere. **B,** Electron micrograph through a cross section of myofibrils in a single muscle fiber. Note the hexagonal orientation of the smaller actin and larger myosin filaments, and crossbridges that extend from a thick to thin filament.

strands; this creates the structural and functional link between myofilaments.

Tropomyosin and **troponin**, the two most important constituents of the actin helix structure, regulate the make-and-break contacts between myofilaments during muscle action. Tropomyosin distributes along the length of the actin filament in a groove formed by the double helix. It inhibits actin and myosin interaction (coupling) and prevents their permanent bonding. Troponin, embedded at fairly regular intervals along the actin strands, exhibits a high affinity for calcium ions (Ca^{++}), which play a crucial role in muscle function and fatigue. The action of Ca^{++} and troponin

Figure 12.18
Details of the thick and thin protein filaments, including tropomyosin, troponin, and the M line. The globular heads of the myosin contain the enzyme myosin ATPase; these active heads free energy from ATP to power contraction.

triggers myofibrils to interact and slide past each other. Once fiber activation occurs, troponin molecules change to tug on the tropomyosin protein strand, moving the tropomyosin deeper into the groove between the two actin strands. This uncovers actin's active molecular sites and allows muscle action to proceed.

The M line consists of transversely and longitudinally oriented proteins that maintain proper orientation of the thick filament within a sarcomere. Figure 12.18 shows that the perpendicularly oriented M-bridges connect with six adjacent thick (myosin) filaments in a hexagonal pattern.

Intracellular Tubule Systems

Figure 12.19 illustrates the tubule system within a muscle fiber. An extensive network of interconnecting tubular channels, the sarcoplasmic reticulum, runs parallel to the myofibrils. The lateral end of each tubule terminates in a sac-like vesicle that stores Ca^{++}. Another network of tubules, the transverse-tubule system (**T-tubule system**), runs perpendicular to the myofibril. The T tubules lie between the lateral-most portion of two sarcoplasmic channels; the vesicles of these structures abut the T tubule. The repeating pattern of two vesicles and T tubules in the region of each Z line forms a **triad**. Each sarcomere contains two triads; this pattern repeats regularly throughout the myofibril's length.

The T tubules pass through the fiber and open externally from the inside of the muscle cell. *The triad and T-tubule system function as a microtransportation or plumbing network for spreading the action potential (wave of depolarization) from the fiber's outer membrane inward to the deeper regions of the cell.* The triad sacs release Ca^{++} during depolarization, which diffuses a short distance to activate the actin filaments. Contraction begins when the myosin filaments' crossbridges interact with the active sites

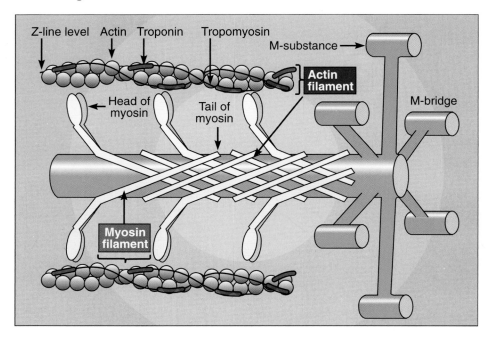

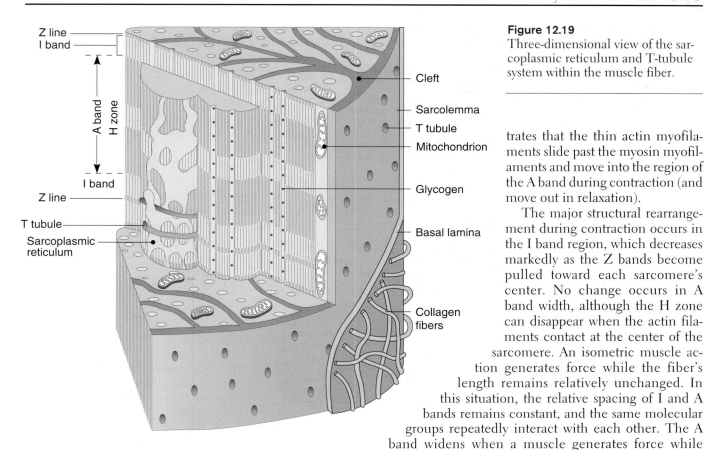

Z line
I band
A band
H zone
I band
Z line
T tubule
Sarcoplasmic reticulum

Cleft
Sarcolemma
T tubule
Mitochondrion
Glycogen
Basal lamina
Collagen fibers

Figure 12.19
Three-dimensional view of the sarcoplasmic reticulum and T-tubule system within the muscle fiber.

trates that the thin actin myofilaments slide past the myosin myofilaments and move into the region of the A band during contraction (and move out in relaxation).

The major structural rearrangement during contraction occurs in the I band region, which decreases markedly as the Z bands become pulled toward each sarcomere's center. No change occurs in A band width, although the H zone can disappear when the actin filaments contact at the center of the sarcomere. An isometric muscle action generates force while the fiber's length remains relatively unchanged. In this situation, the relative spacing of I and A bands remains constant, and the same molecular groups repeatedly interact with each other. The A band widens when a muscle generates force while lengthening in an eccentric action.

Mechanical Action of Crossbridges

The globular head of the myosin crossbridge provides the mechanical power stroke for actin and myosin filaments to slide past each other. Figure 12.21 shows the oscillating to-and-fro nature of the crossbridges, which move similar to the action of oars in water. But unlike oars the crossbridges do not all move synchronously. During muscle activation, each crossbridge undergoes repeated but independent cycles of attachment and detachment to actin. Because a single crossbridge moves only a short distance, crossbridges must attach, produce movement, and detach thousands of times to shorten the sarcomere. Only about 50% of the crossbridges contact the actin filaments at any instant to form the contractile protein complex **actomyosin**; the remaining crossbridges maintain some other position in their vibrating cycle.

on actin filaments. When electrical excitation ceases, cytoplasmic free Ca^{++} concentration decreases and the muscle relaxes.

Chemical and Mechanical Events During Contraction and Relaxation

The electron microscope has unraveled many secrets of cellular structure that have led to explanations of the chemical and mechanical events in muscular contraction and relaxation. Considerable evidence supporting a **sliding-filament theory** of muscle contraction coincides with existing knowledge about muscle ultrastructure and function.

Sliding-Filament Theory

The sliding-filament theory proposes that muscle fibers shorten or lengthen because thick and thin myofilaments slide past each other without the filaments themselves changing length. The action of myosin crossbridges, which cyclically attach, rotate, and detach from the actin filaments (energy provided by ATP hydrolysis), drives the shortening process. Muscle contraction changes the relative size of the sarcomere's various zones and bands. Figure 12.20 illus-

Like a Cocked Spring

Before the muscle action, the elongated, flexible myosin head literally bends around the ATP molecule and becomes cocked, almost like a spring. The myosin then interacts with the adjacent action filament, producing a sliding motion that initiates muscle shortening.

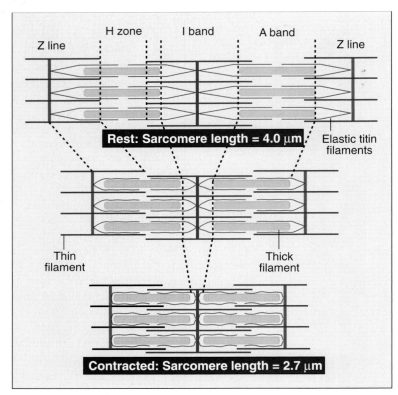

Figure 12.20
Structural rearrangement of actin and myosin filaments at resting muscle length and during contraction (1 μm = 0.000001 m).

The right side of Figure 12.21 shows that each crossbridge action contributes only a small longitudinal displacement to the filaments' total sliding action. This process has been likened to climbing a rope, with the arms and legs representing the crossbridges. Climbing occurs by first reaching with the arms, then grabbing, pulling, contacting with the legs, and breaking arm contact, and then repeating this process throughout the climb.

Link Between Actin, Myosin, and ATP

Interaction and movement of the protein filaments during a muscle action require that the myosin crossbridges continually oscillate by combining, detaching, and recombining to new sites along the actin strands (or the same sites in a static

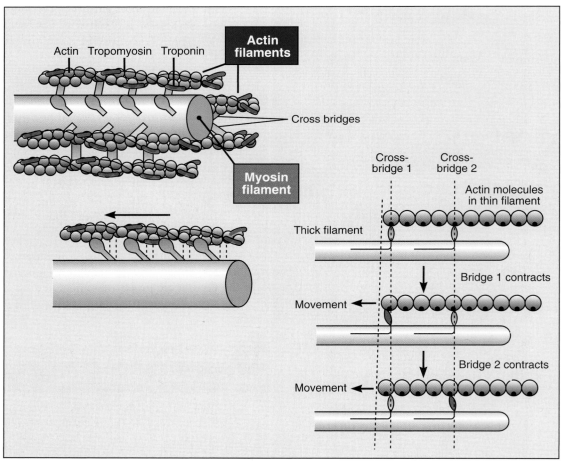

Figure 12.21
Relative positioning of actin and myosin filaments during crossbridge oscillation. The action of each bridge produces a small movement. For clarity we omitted one of the actin strands from the left-hand portion of the figure.

action.) When an ATP molecule joins the actomyosin complex, it detaches the myosin crossbridges from the actin filament. This reaction permits the myosin crossbridge to resume its original state so it can again bind to a new active actin site. The dissociation of actomyosin occurs as follows:

$$\text{Actomyosin} + \text{ATP} \rightarrow \text{Actin} + \text{Myosin-ATP}$$

ATP serves an important function in muscle action. *Splitting the terminal phosphate from ATP provides energy for crossbridge movement.* One of the reacting sites on the globular head of the myosin crossbridge binds to a reactive site on actin. The other myosin active site acts as the enzyme myofibrillar adenosine triphosphatase (**myosin-ATPase**), which splits ATP to release its energy for muscle action. ATP splits relatively slowly if myosin and actin remain apart; when joined, however, the ATP hydrolysis rate increases tremendously. Energy released from ATP changes the shape of the globular head of the myosin crossbridge so it interacts and oscillates with the appropriate actin molecule. Specific speed and power training modify enzymatic activity to facilitate the sequence of events in muscle action (see Chapter 14).

Excitation-Contraction Coupling

Excitation-contraction coupling provides the physiologic mechanism whereby an electrical discharge at the muscle initiates the chemical events that cause contraction.

An inactive muscle's Ca^{++} concentration remains relatively low. When stimulated to contract, the action potential's arrival at the transverse tubules releases Ca^{++} from the lateral sacs of the sarcoplasmic reticulum, and intracellular Ca^{++} levels increase dramatically. The rapid binding of Ca^{++} to troponin in the actin filaments releases troponin's inhibition of actin-myosin interaction. In a sense, the muscle becomes "turned on" for action.

Myosin-ATPase splits ATP when the active sites of actin and myosin join together. Energy transfer from ATP breakdown moves the myosin crossbridges, and the muscle generates tension.

$$\text{Actin} + \text{Myosin ATPase} \rightarrow \text{Actomyosin ATPase}$$

The crossbridges uncouple from actin when ATP binds to the myosin bridge. Coupling and uncoupling continue as long as Ca^{++} concentration remains at a level sufficient to inhibit the troponin-tropomyosin system. Discontinuing the nerve stimulus to the muscle moves Ca^{++} back into the lateral sacs of the sarcoplasmic reticulum. This restores the inhibitory effect of troponin-tropomyosin; the presence of ATP keeps actin and myosin separated.

$$\text{Actomyosin-ATPase} \rightarrow \text{Actomyosin} + \text{ADP} + \text{Pi} + \text{Energy}$$

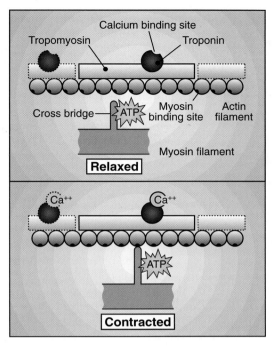

Figure 12.22
Interaction among actin-myosin filaments, Ca^{++}, and ATP in relaxed and contracted muscle. In the relaxed state, troponin and tropomyosin interact; actin prevents coupling of a myosin crossbridge to actin. During contraction, the crossbridge couples with actin because Ca^{++} binds with troponin-tropomyosin.

Figure 12.22 illustrates the interaction among actin and myosin filaments, Ca^{++}, and ATP in relaxed and contracted muscle fibers. In essence, the magnitude and duration of contraction relates directly to the presence of calcium. Contraction ceases (and relaxation begins) when calcium moves back into the sarcoplasmic reticulum, and the troponin-tropomyosin complex again inhibits the interaction of myosin and actin.

Relaxation

After muscle action, active transport mechanisms pump Ca^{++} into the sarcoplasmic reticulum, where it concentrates in the lateral vesicles. Calcium retrieval from

Rigor Mortis

Soon after death, the muscles become stiff and rigid, a condition termed *rigor mortis.* This occurs because the muscle cells no longer contain ATP. Without ATP, the myosin crossbridges and actin remain attached, and the muscle cannot return to a relaxed state.

the myofilament proteins "turns off" the active sites on the actin filament. Deactivation of troponin-tropomyosin prevents mechanical linkage between myosin crossbridges and actin filaments. This reduces myosin ATPase activity so ATP hydrolysis ceases. Return of actin and myosin filaments to their original state completes relaxation.

Sequence of Events in Muscle Excitation-Contraction

Nine important steps describe muscle activation and relaxation:

1. Initiation of an action potential by the anterior motoneuron. The impulse spreads over the muscle fiber's surface as the sarcolemma depolarizes.
2. The muscle's action potential depolarizes the transverse tubules at the sarcomere's A-I junction.
3. Depolarization of the transverse tubules releases Ca^{++} from the lateral sacs of the sarcoplasmic reticulum.
4. Ca^{++} binds to troponin-tropomyosin in the actin filaments. This releases the inhibition that prevents actin from combining with myosin.
5. Actin combines with myosin ATP. Actin also activates myosin ATPase, which then splits ATP. Energy from ATP hydrolysis powers the movement of the myosin crossbridges.
6. Binding of ATP to the myosin crossbridge breaks the actin-myosin bond and allows the crossbridge to separate from actin. This creates relative movement (sliding) of the thick and thin filaments, and the muscle shortens.
7. Crossbridge activation continues as long as Ca^{++} concentration remains high enough (owing to membrane depolarization) to inhibit the troponin-tropomyosin system.
8. Ca^{++} concentration rapidly decreases when muscle stimulation ceases and active transport pumps Ca^{++} back into the lateral sacs of the sarcoplasmic reticulum.
9. Ca^{++} removal restores the inhibitory action of troponin-tropomyosin. In the presence of ATP, actin and myosin remain in a dissociated, relaxed state.

Muscle Fiber Type

Human skeletal muscle does not consist simply of a homogeneous group of fibers with similar metabolic and functional properties. Despite considerable debate concerning the method and terminology for classifying skeletal muscle, *two* distinct fiber types have emerged for classification by their *contractile* and *metabolic* characteristics: fast twitch and slow twitch. Table 12.5 lists characteristics of these fiber types and subdivisions.

Measurement of Fiber Types

One of the first methods for classifying muscle fiber types applied histochemical staining to divide fibers into three categories based on stain shading (from dark to light, with an intermediate shade), depending on the fiber's concentrations of different types or isoforms of myosin ATPase. Slow-contracting (**type I**) fibers stained dark, and fast-contracting **type IIa** fibers remained light in color. The shade of fast-contracting **type IIb** fibers fell between type I and type IIa.

Other classification schemes for **muscle fiber typing** utilize fiber structure, biochemistry, function, and contractility. Complications inherent with muscle fiber typing include inability to generalize from a single, small sample from one muscle to the entire body musculature. Fiber types tend to layer within a muscle. Thus, a small sample of muscle secured from a single area may not represent the biopsied muscle's total fiber population. The multiple criteria for classifying and characterizing human muscle depicted in Table 12.5 may be a more appropriate classification strategy than applying only one criterion.

Fast-Twitch Fibers

Fast-twitch muscle fibers exhibit the following characteristics:

1. Rapidly transmit action potentials
2. Possess high activity level of myosin ATPase
3. Show rapid rate of calcium release and uptake by the sarcoplasmic reticulum
4. Generate rapid crossbridge turnover

These qualities relate to a fast-twitch fiber's ability to rapidly transfer energy for quick, forceful muscle actions. Recall that myosin-ATPase splits ATP to provide energy for muscle action. The fast-twitch fiber's intrinsic speed of contraction and tension development averages two to three times the speed of fibers classified as slow-twitch (see next section).

Fast-twitch fibers rely on a well-developed, short-term glycolytic system for energy transfer. They have been labeled FG fibers to signify fast glycogenolytic capabilities. Short-term, high-power output activities and other forceful muscular actions that depend almost entirely on anaerobic metabolism for energy activate fast-twitch fibers. Stop-and-go or change-of-pace sports (e.g. basketball, soccer, rugby, lacrosse, and field hockey) require rapid energy from anaerobic pathways in fast-twitch fibers.

Fast-Twitch Subdivisions

Fast-twitch fiber subdivisions exist in humans. The type IIa fiber combines a fast contraction speed with a moderately well-developed capacity for aerobic (high level of the aerobic enzyme succinic dehydrogenase [SDH]) and anaerobic (high level of the anaerobic enzyme phosphofructokinase [PFK]) energy transfer. The term **fast-oxidative-glycolytic (FOG)** also describes these fibers. Another subdivision, the type IIb fiber (considered the true **fast-glycolytic [FG] fiber**, possesses the greatest potential for anaerobic energy transfer.

TABLE 12.5
Classification of skeletal muscle fiber types

| | FIBER TYPES | | |
| | FAST-TWITCH | | SLOW-TWITCH |
CHARACTERISTIC	TYPE IIB	TYPE IIA	TYPE I
Electrical activity patterns	Phasic; High frequency		Tonic; Low frequency
Morphology	FTb	FTa	ST
Color	White	White/red	Red
Fiber diameter	Large	Intermediate	Small
Capillaries/mm^2	Low	Intermediate	High
Mitochondrial volume	Low	Intermediate	High
Histochemistry and	IIB	IIA	I
biochemistry	FG	FOG	SO
Myosin ATPase	High	High	Low
Calcium capacity	High	Medium/high	Low
Glycolytic capacity	High	High	Low
Oxidative capacity	Low	Medium/high	High
Function and	FF	FR	S
contractility	FT	FT	ST
Speed of action	Fast	Fast	Slow
Speed of relaxation	Fast	Fast	Slow
Fatigue resistance	High	Moderate/high	Low
Force capacity	High	Intermediate	Low

FT = fast-twitch; FG = fast, glycolytic; FOG = fast, oxidative, glycolytic; SO = slow, oxidative; FF = fast-contracting, fast-fatigue; FR = fast-contracting, fatigue-resistant; S = slow-contracting

From Kraus, W.: Skeletal muscle adaptation to chronic low-frequency motor nerve stimulation. *Exerc. Sport Sci. Rev.*, 22:313:1994.

Slow-Twitch Fibers

Slow-twitch muscle fibers generate energy for ATP resynthesis predominantly by aerobic energy transfer. They possess a low activity level of myosin ATPase, a slow speed of contraction, and a glycolytic capacity less well developed than fast-twitch counterparts (see Table 12.5). However, slow-twitch fibers contain relatively large and numerous mitochondria and iron-containing cytochromes of the electron transport chain (which contribute to their red appearance). A high concentration of mitochondrial enzymes also supports the enhanced aerobic metabolic machinery. Consequently, slow-twitch fibers resist fatigue and aid in prolonged aerobic exercise. These fibers have been labeled **slow-oxidative (SO) fibers** to describe their slow contraction speed and predominant reliance on oxidative metabolism.

Studies of muscle glycogen depletion patterns indicate that slow twitch muscle fibers almost exclusively power prolonged, moderate exercise. Even after exercising 12 hours, the limited but still available glycogen ex-

ists in the unused fast-twitch fibers. Differences in oxidative capacity of the two fiber types determine blood flow capacity through muscle tissues during exercise; slow-twitch fibers receive considerably more blood than fast-twitch counterparts. Exercise at near-maximum aerobic and anaerobic levels, as in middle-distance running, swimming, or multiple-sprint sports, (field hockey, lacrosse, basketball, ice hockey, soccer), activates both muscle fiber types.

Differences Between Athletic Groups

Several interesting observations emerge concerning muscle fiber type variation among individuals and sport categories, and the possible influence of specific exercise training on a muscle's fiber composition and metabolic capacity. On average, sedentary children and adults possess about 50% slow-twitch fibers. The percentage of fast-twitch fibers probably distributes equally between subdivi-

close up

Excess Muscle

Weightlifters exhibit remarkable muscular hypertrophy. These relatively large individuals often possess a fat-free body mass (FFM) in excess of 90% of total body mass compared with the average FFM of 80 to 85% for typical, non–resistance-trained men. Many athletes use resistance training to increase muscular strength and enhance specific sport performance. Bodybuilders, on the other hand, lift weights solely to improve body configuration and form.

Limited information exists about the massive muscular hyper-

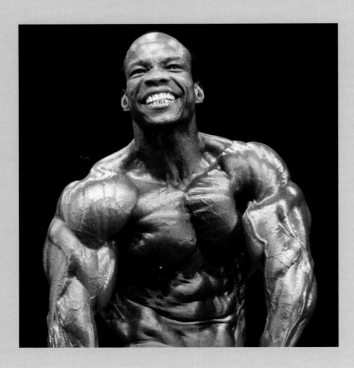

trophy of body builders and other athletic groups. One approach attempts to quantify **excess muscle** (the amount of muscle in excess of that expected based on body structure) by measuring the body's total potassium (a mineral found mainly in muscle that closely predicts muscle mass). An anthropometric technique devised by noted scientist Dr. Albert R. Behnke provides the means for computing excess muscle. Behnke maintained that because the lower trunk region (hips) does not hypertrophy with weight training to the same extent as other body areas, one could estimate a body builder's body mass before initiating weight training by calculating the weight-equivalent of the hips (designated W[hips]). Scale weight minus W[hips] provides an estimate of excess muscle resulting from resistance training.

Two of us have estimated excess muscle in bodybuilders, weightlifters, and professional football players (interior linemen). Excess muscle of 15.7 kg (34.6 lb) for body builders accounts for approximately 21% of their total FFM; for the weightlifters, 13.9 kg (30.6 lb) of excess muscle accounts for 19% of FFM. Although football players often weigh up to 32 kg (70 lb) more than the weightlifters and bodybuilders, their excess muscle (relative to expectations based on body mass) equaled only 7.6 kg (16.8 lb), accounting for only 8% of FFM. These comparisons point to the remarkable muscular development of resistance-trained athletes, particularly bodybuilders. This magnitude of muscularity demands incredible dedication to training and proper nutrition. The average elite body builder has trained for a minimum of 10 years, 2 hours a day, 5 days a week.

Reference

Katch, V. L,.and Katch, F. I., et al.: Extreme muscular development in man: Body composition of competitive Olympic lifters, power lifters, and body builders. *Med. Sci. Sports,* 12 : 340, 1980.

Muscle Fiber Training Specificity

Why do some highly trained athletes who switch to a sport requiring different muscle groups feel essentially untrained for the new activity? The answer lies in the fact that only the specific fibers used in training adapt metabolically and physiologically to exercise. Thus, swimmers or canoeists do not necessarily transfer their upper-body "fitness" to a running sport unless they specifically train the muscles required for that sport.

sions. Fiber type distribution varies considerably among individuals. Generally, one's muscle fiber type distribution remains consistent for the body's major muscle groups.

Elite athletes possess distinct patterns of fiber distribution. Successful endurance athletes, for example, have a predominance of slow-twitch fibers in the muscles activated in their sport; the fast-twitch muscle fiber predominates for sprint athletes. Figure 12.23 illustrates sport-specific tendencies for muscle fiber type among top Nordic competitors from different sports. Athletic groups with the highest aerobic and endurance capacities (e.g., distance runners and cross-country skiers) also possess the greatest percentages of slow-twitch fibers, often as high as 90%. In contrast, weightlifters, ice-hockey players, and sprinters

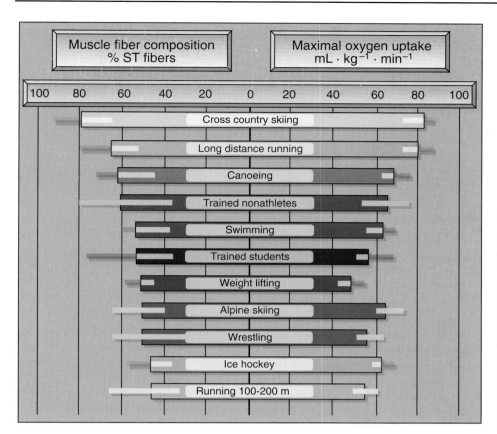

Figure 12.23
Muscle fiber composition (percent slow-twitch fibers, left side) and maximal oxygen uptake (right side) in athletes representing different sports. The outer, lightly shaded bars denote the range. (From Bergh, U., et al.: Maximal oxygen uptake and muscle fiber types in trained and untrained humans. *Med. Sci. Sports*, 10:151, 1978.)

tend to have more fast-twitch fibers and a relatively lower $\dot{V}O_{2max}$. As might be expected, middle-distance specialists (men and women) show approximately equal percentages of the two muscle fibers types. Equal fiber type distribution also exists for power athletes like throwers, jumpers, and high jumpers. Figure 12.24 presents additional data for muscle fiber composition for three muscle groups among elite U.S. male and female athletes.

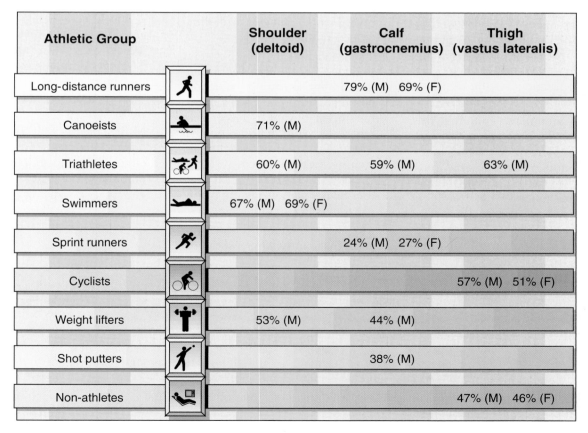

Athletic Group		Shoulder (deltoid)	Calf (gastrocnemius)	Thigh (vastus lateralis)
Long-distance runners			79% (M) 69% (F)	
Canoeists		71% (M)		
Triathletes		60% (M)	59% (M)	63% (M)
Swimmers		67% (M) 69% (F)		
Sprint runners			24% (M) 27% (F)	
Cyclists				57% (M) 51% (F)
Weight lifters		53% (M)	44% (M)	
Shot putters			38% (M)	
Non-athletes				47% (M) 46% (F)

Figure 12.24
Percentage of slow-twitch fibers in three muscle groups of male (M) and female (F) athletes. The percentage of fast-twitch fibers equals the difference between 100% and the percentage of slow-twitch fibers. Data from the research literature.

Relatively clear-cut distinctions between performance and muscle fiber composition emerge only for elite athletes who have achieved prominence in a specific sport category. Regardless of performance status, muscle fiber composition does not exclusively determine success. Within groups of trained or untrained individuals, knowledge of a person's predominant fiber type provides limited value in predicting performance outcome. Performance capacity depends on a blending of many physiologic, biochemical, neurologic, and biomechanical support systems, and not simply a single factor like muscle fiber type.

summary

1. Various wrappings of connective tissue that encase skeletal muscle eventually blend into and join the tendinous attachment to bone. This harness enables muscles to act on the bony levers to transform chemical energy of ATP into mechanical energy and motion.

2. Skeletal muscle contains approximately 75% water, 20% protein, with the remaining 5% inorganic salts, enzymes, minerals, pigments, fats, proteins, and carbohydrates.

3. Vigorous aerobic exercise increases muscle's oxygen uptake nearly 70 times above its resting level. An increase in capillary density up to 40% with aerobic training augments a muscle's oxygen supply.

4. The sarcomere contains the contractile proteins actin and myosin—the muscle fiber's functional unit. An average-sized muscle fiber contains about 4500 sarcomeres and a total of 16 billion thick (myosin) and 64 billion thin (actin) filaments. The actin and myosin filaments within the sarcomere provide the mechanical mechanism for muscle action.

5. Crossbridge projections link thin and thick contractile filaments. The globular head of the myosin crossbridge provides the mechanical power stroke for actin and myosin filaments to slide past each other.

6. Tropomyosin and troponin, two myofibrillar proteins, regulate the make-and-break contacts between filaments during muscle action. Tropomyosin inhibits actin and myosin interaction; troponin with calcium triggers the myofibrils to interact and slide past each other.

7. The triad and T-tubule system provide a microtransportation network for spreading the action potential from the fiber's outer membrane inward to deeper cell regions. Contraction occurs when calcium activates actin, attaching the myosin crossbridges to active sites on the actin filaments. Relaxation occurs when calcium concentration decreases.

8. The sliding-filament theory proposes that a muscle fiber shortens or lengthens because its protein filaments slide past each other without changing length. Excitation-contraction coupling provides the physiologic mechanism that initiates an electrical discharge, triggering the chemical events that cause contraction.

9. Two types of muscle fibers classify according to their contractile and metabolic characteristics: 1) fast-twitch fibers (type II), which predominantly generate energy anaerobically for quick, powerful contractions, and 2) slow-twitch fibers (type I), which contract at relatively slow speeds and generate energy for ATP resynthesis largely by aerobic metabolism. The predominance of specific metabolic characteristics defines the two fast-twitch fiber subdivisions.

10. Muscle fiber type distribution differs in individuals. Genetic code largely determines a person's predominant fiber type.

11. Specific exercise training improves the metabolic capacity of both fiber types.

thought questions

1. Show how knowledge about neuromuscular exercise physiology can enhance an athlete's (a) muscular strength and power, (b) sports skill performance.

2. Present the pros and cons for muscle fiber typing of children to "guide" them into sports to hopefully achieve success.

3. How might drugs that mimic neurotransmitters affect physiologic response and performance in maximal exercise?

4. In terms of neuromuscular physiology, discuss the validity of the adage, "Practice makes perfect."

selected references

Antonio, J., and Gonyea, W.J.: Skeletal muscle fiber hyperplasia. *Med. Sci. Sports Exerc.*, 25: 1333, 1993.

Armstrong, R.B.: Muscle fiber recruitment patterns and their metabolic correlates. In: *Exercise, Nutrition, and Energy Metabolism*. Horton E.S. and Terjung R.L., (eds.). New York: Macmillan, 1988.

Asmussen, E.: Muscle fatigue. *Med. Sci. Sports Exerc.*, 25:412, 1993.

Asp, S., et al.: Muscle glycogen accumulation after a marathon: roles of fiber type and pro- and macroglycogen. *J. Appl. Physiol.*, 86:474, 1999.

Baldwin J., et al.: Muscle IMP accumulation during fatiguing submaximal exercise in endurance trained and untrained men. *Am. J. Physiol.*, 277(1 Pt 2): R295, 1999.

Basmajian, J.V., and Deluca, C.J.: *Muscles Alive. Their Functions Revealed by Electromyography*. 5th Ed., Baltimore: Williams & Wilkins, 1985.

Billeter, R., and Hoppler, H.: Muscular basis of strength. In: *Strength and Power in Sport*. Komi, P. (ed.). London: Blackwell Scientific Publications, 1992.

Carins, S.P., et al.: Role of extracellular $[Ca^{2+}]$ in fatigue of isolated mammalian skeletal muscle. *J. Appl. Physiol.*, 84:1395, 1998.

Carlson, C.J., et al.: Skeletal muscle myostatin mRNA expression is fiber-type specific and increases during hindlimb unloading. *Am. J. Physiol.*, 277: (2 Pt 2): R601, 1999.

Carrasco, D.I., et al.: Effect of concentric and eccentric muscle actions on muscle sympathetic nerve activity. *J. Appl. Physiol.*, 86:558, 1999.

Davis, J.M., and Bailey, S.P.: Possible mechanisms of central nervous system fatigue during exercise. *Med. Sci. Sports Exerc.*, 29:45, 1997.

Dawson, B., et al.: Changes in performance, muscle metabolites, enzymes and fibre types after short sprint training. *Eur. J. Appl. Physiol.*, 78:163, 1998.

Demirel, H.A., et al.: Exercise induced alterations in skeletal muscle myosin heavy chain phenotype: dose-response relationship. *J. Appl. Physiol.*, 86:1002, 1999.

Green, H., et al.: Regulation of fiber size, oxidative potential, and capillarization in human muscle by resistance exercise. *Am. J. Physiol.*, 276:R591, 1999.

Hochachka, P.W.: *Muscles as Molecular and Metabolic Machines*. Boca Raton, FL: CRC Press, 1994.

Hogan, M.D., et al.: Increased [lactate] in working dog muscle reduces tension development independent of pH. *Med. Sci. Sports Exerc.*, 27:371, 1995.

Holloszy, J.O., and Coyle, E.F.: Adaptations of skeletal muscle to endurance training and their metabolic consequences. *J. Appl. Physiol.*, 56:831, 1984.

Kadi, F., et al.: Cellular adaptation of the trapezius muscle in strength-trained athletes. *Histochem. Cell Biol.*, 111:189, 1999.

Kraus, W.E., et al.: Skeletal muscle adaptation to chronic low-frequency motor nerve stimulation. *Exerc. Sport Sci. Rev.*, 22: 313, 1994.

Lewis, S.F., and Fulco, C.S.: A new approach to studying muscle fatigue and factors affecting performance during dynamic exercise in humans. *Exerc. Sport Sci. Revs.*, 26:91, 1998.

Lieber, R.L.: *Skeletal Muscle Structure and Function: Implications for Rehabilitation and Sports Medicine*. Baltimore: Williams & Wilkins, 1992.

Lutz, G.J., and Lieber, R.L.: Skeletal muscle myosin II structure and function. *Exerc. Sport Sci. Revs.*, 27:63, 1999.

MacLaren, C.P., et al: A review of metabolic and physiological factors in fatigue. In: *Exercise and Sport Sciences Reviews*. Vol. 17. Pandolf, K.B. (ed.). Baltimore: Williams & Wilkins, 1989.

Masuda, K., et al.: Changes in surface EMG parameters during static and dynamic fatiguing contractions. *J. Electromyogr. Kinesiol.*, 9:39, 1999.

Nichols, T.R., et al.: Rapid spinal mechanisms of motor coordination. *Exerc. Sport Sci. Revs.*, 27:255, 1999.

Otten, E.: Concepts and models of functional architecture in skeletal muscle. In: *Exercise and Sport Sciences Reviews*. Vol. 16. Pandolf, K.B. (ed.). New York: Macmillan, 1988.

Patel, T.J., and Lieber, R.L.: Force transmission in skeletal muscle: from actomyosin to external tendons. *Exer. Sport Sci. Revs.*, 25:321, 1997.

Putman, C.T., et al.: Satellite cell content and myosin isoforms in low-frequency-stimulated fast muscle of hypothyroid rat. *J. Appl. Physiol.*, 86:40, 1999.

Roy, R.R., et al.: Modulation of myonuclear number in functionally overloaded and exercised rat plantaris fibers. *J. Appl. Physiol.*, 87: 634, 1999.

Schunk, K., et al.: Contributions of dynamic phosphorus-31 magnetic resonance spectroscopy to the analysis of muscle fiber distribution. *Invest. Radiol.*, 34:348, 1999.

Seals, D.R., and Victor, R.G.: Regulation of muscle sympathetic nerve activity during exercise in humans. In: *Exercise and Sport Sciences Reviews*. Vol. 19. Holloszy, J.O. (ed.). Baltimore: Williams & Wilkins, 1991.

Tikkanen, H.O., et al.: Significance of skeletal muscle properties on fitness, long-term physical training and serum lipids. *Atherosclerosis*, 142:367, 1999.

Weston, A.R., et al.: African runners exhibit greater fatigue resistance, lower lactate accumulation, and higher oxidative enzyme activity. *J. Appl. Physiol.*, 86:915, 1999.

Wickham, J.B., and Brown, J.M.: Muscles within muscles: the neuromotor control of intra-muscular segments. *Eur. J. Appl. Physiol.*, 78:219, 1998.

Williams, J.H.: Contractile apparatus and sarcoplasmic reticulum function: effects of fatigue, recovery, and elevated Ca^{2+}. *J. Appl. Physiol.*, 83:444, 1997.

CHAPTER

13

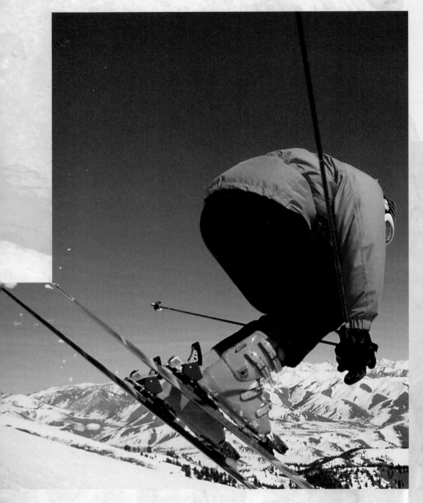

Topics covered in this chapter

Endocrine System Overview
Endocrine System Organization
Resting and Exercise-Induced Endocrine
   Secretions
Anterior Pituitary Hormones
Posterior Pituitary Hormones
Thyroid Hormones
Parathyroid Hormone
Adrenal Hormones
Pancreatic Hormones
Diabetes Mellitus
Endurance Training and Endocrine Function
Resistance Training and Endocrine Function
Summary
Thought Questions
Selected References

Hormones, Exercise, and Training

- Draw the location of the body's major endocrine glands within an outline of the human body.

- Describe how hormones alter cellular reaction rates of specific target cells.

- Describe how hormonal, humoral, and neural factors stimulate endorcrine glands.

- List the hormones secreted by the anterior and posterior pituitary glands, and describe how exercise affects these secretions.

- List the thyroid gland hormones, their functions, and response to exercise.

- List the hormones of the adrenal medulla and adrenal cortex, their functions, and response to exercise.

- List the hormones of the pancreas' alpha and beta cells, their functions, and response to exercise.

- Define type 1 and type 2 diabetes mellitus, and give 3 differences between these two diabetes subdivisions.

- List five risk factors for type 2 diabetes.

- Outline the benefits of regular exercise for a type 2 diabetic.

- Explain the general effects of exercise training on endocrine function.

- Discuss the interactions among exercise, stress, illness, and immune system function.

- Describe the functions of opioid peptides and their response to acute exercise.

Hormones, the body's chemical messengers, affect almost every aspect of human function. They regulate growth, metabolism, and reproduction, and augment the ability to respond acutely and chronically to physical and psychologic stress. Hormones maintain internal homeostasis by modulating electrolyte and acid-base balance, and adjusting energy metabolism to power biologic work.

This chapter reviews various aspects of the endocrine system (from Greek *endon*, meaning within and *krino*, meaning to separate), including its functions during rest and physical activity and response to exercise training.

Endocrine System Overview

Figure 13.1 shows the location of the major endocrine organs: the pituitary, thyroid, parathyroid, adrenal, pineal, and thymus glands. Several organs contain discrete areas of endocrine tissue that also produce hormones. These include the pancreas, gonads (ovaries and testes), and hypothalamus (also a major organ of the nervous system).

Endocrine System Organization

Three components characterize the endocrine system:

1. Host gland
2. Hormones
3. Target (receptor) cells or organs

Glands are classified as either endocrine, exocrine, or both. **Endocrine glands** secrete hormones; they lack ducts (ductless), but secrete their substances directly into the extracellular space around the gland. Hormones then diffuse into the blood for transport throughout the body. Similar to neuromuscular responses, hormone secretion must adjust rapidly to changing bodily functions. For this reason, many hormone secretions occur in a pulsatile manner rather than at a constant output.

Exocrine glands (sweat glands and glands of the upper digestive tract) have secretory ducts that lead directly to the specific compartment or surface that requires the hormone. The nervous system controls almost all exocrine glands.

Small But Crucial

Endocrine glands are small compared with other organs of the body; combined, they weigh only about 0.5 kg. Endocrine hormone secretions occur in minute amounts, measured in micrograms (μg; 10^{-6} g), nanograms (ng; 10^{-9} g), and even picograms (pg; 10^{-12} g).

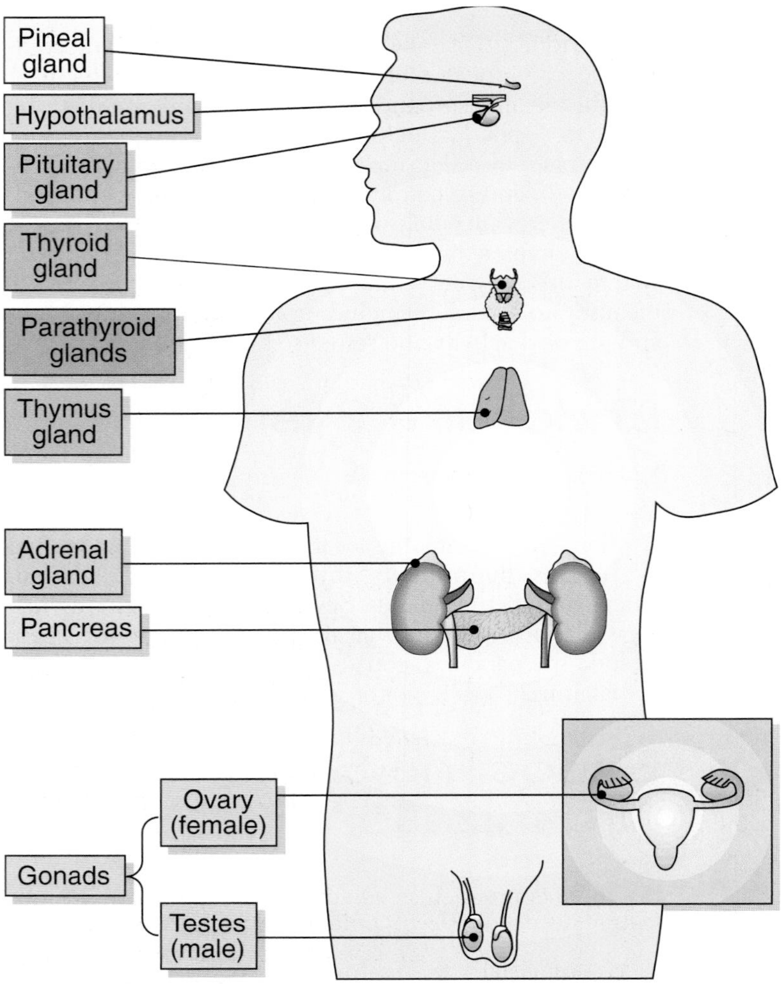

Pineal gland

Hypothalamus

Pituitary gland

Thyroid gland

Parathyroid glands

Thymus gland

Adrenal gland

Pancreas

Ovary (female)

Gonads

Testes (male)

Figure 13.1
Location of the major hormone-producing endocrine organs.

Nature of Hormones

Three distinct "chemical" classifications apply to hormones:

1. Hormones derived from steroid compounds
2. Hormones derived from amino acids or polypeptides
3. Lipid-based hormones

The adrenal cortex and gonads synthesize steroid hormones from circulating cholesterol, whereas other tissues (e.g., stomach, intestine) produce polypeptide hormones that range from small to large proteins. A third class of hormones consists of biologically active lipids found in nearly all plasma membranes. Examples of lipid-based hormones include prostaglandins that regulate blood vessel diameter, stomach secretions, and blood clotting. Another kind of hormone, the glycoprotein erythropoietin, stimulates bone marrow to produce red blood cells.

How Hormones Function

Most hormones do not directly affect cellular activity. Instead, they combine with a specific receptor molecule on the cell surface. The cell then discharges a second chemical that initiates a cascade of cellular events. The binding hormone acts as the "**first messenger**" to react with the enzyme **adenyl cyclase** in the plasma membrane to form **cyclic 3,5-adenosine monophosphate (cyclic-AMP)**. This compound acts as "**second messenger**" or mediator, to influence cellular function by initiating a predictable series of actions within the target cell.

Some hormones cross plasma membranes and act as their own second messenger. These hormones exert their effect *only* on cells that contain a receptor for that hormone. Hormone action at specific target cells occurs by:

- Changing the synthesis rate of intracellular proteins
- Altering enzyme activity
- Modifying cell membrane transport
- Inducing secretory activity

A target cell's ability to respond to a hormone depends largely on the presence of specific protein receptors on its membrane or in its interior. For example, receptors for the adrenal gland-stimulating adrenocorticotropic hormone appear only on certain adrenal cortex cells. On the other hand, all cells contain receptors for thyroxine, the principal hormone that stimulates cellular metabolism. Consequently, thyroxine produces a more general effect on bodily functions. **Up-regulation** describes a dynamic state where target cells form more receptors in response to increasing hormone levels. In contrast, prolonged exposure to high hormone concentrations desensitizes target cells, and they respond less vigorously to hormonal stimulation. The resulting **down-regulation** decreases receptor number to prevent target cells from over-reacting to persistently high hormone levels.

Caffeine Stimulates Lipolysis

Caffeine augments cyclic-AMP activity in fat cells; cyclic-AMP, in turn, activates hormone-sensitive lipases to promote lipolysis, releasing free fatty acids into the plasma. Increased plasma free-fatty acid levels stimulate fat oxidation, thus conserving liver and muscle glycogen.

The plasma concentration of a hormone depends upon:

- Sum of synthesis and release by the host gland
- Rate of receptor tissue uptake
- Rate of hormone removal from blood by the liver and kidneys

In most cases, removal rate (usually measured in the urine) equals rate of release.

Hormone Effects on Enzymes

Alteration of enzymatic activity and enzyme-mediated membrane transport constitute the major mechanisms of hormone action. Hormones affect enzyme activity in one of three ways:

1. Stimulate enzyme synthesis
2. Combine with the enzyme to change its shape through **allosteric modulation**, which increases or decreases the enzyme's ability to interact with a substrate
3. Activate many inactive enzyme forms to increase the total amount of active enzyme

In addition to altering enzyme activity, hormones facilitate or inhibit transport of substances into cells. Insulin, for example, promotes glucose uptake through the plasma membrane. In contrast, the hormone epinephrine inhibits a cell's glucose uptake.

The secondary effects of hormone action, although often indirect, remain powerful. The release of insulin increases a muscle fiber's glucose uptake for subsequent synthesis to muscle glycogen. Increased intramuscular glycogen levels contribute substantial energy to power high-intensity exercise. In contrast, an insulin deficiency causes inadequate cellular glucose uptake, which negatively impacts exercise capacity. Chronic insulin insufficiency also increases blood glucose and other metabolites so they "spill-over" into the urine.

Control of Hormone Secretion

Endocrine glands are stimulated in one of three ways:

1. Hormonal stimulation
2. Humoral stimulation
3. Neural stimulation

Target Cell Activation

The activation of a target cell by hormone-receptor interaction depends on:

1. Blood hormone levels
2. Relative number of target cell receptors for that hormone
3. Affinity or strength of the union between hormone and receptor

Other Glands and Hormones

The liver secretes the hormone somatomedin that affects growth of muscle, cartilage, and other tissues. The small intestine's mucosal lining secretes secretin, gastrin, and cholecystokinin to promote, regulate, and coordinate digestion. Parathormone, a parathyroid gland secretion, promotes calcium uptake by intestine and kidneys and calcium release from bones. The hypothalamus directly secretes several stimulating or releasing hormones. Somatoliberin stimulates somatotropin release from the anterior pituitary.

Hormonal Stimulation

Hormones influence the secretion of other hormones. For example, hormones from the hypothalamus induce the discharge of most anterior pituitary hormones. Many anterior pituitary hormones, in turn, stimulate other "target gland" endocrine organs to release their hormones into the circulation. Increased blood levels of these hormones provide feedback to inhibit release of anterior pituitary hormones, which ultimately inhibits target gland secretion.

Humoral Stimulation

Fluctuating blood levels of ions, nutrients, bile, and other body compounds stimulate hormone release. The term **humoral** denotes these stimuli to distinguish them from the fluid-borne hormonal stimuli. An increase in blood glucose (the humoral agent) stimulates insulin release from the pancreas. Because insulin promotes glucose entry into cells, blood sugar levels decline, ending the humoral initiative for insulin release.

Neural Stimulation

Nerve fibers affect hormone release. During stress, activation of the adrenal medulla by the sympathetic nervous system initiates release of the catecholamines epinephrine and norepinephrine. In this case, the nervous system augments normal endocrine control to maintain homeostasis. Activation of the hypothalamus and sympathetic nervous system during exercise blunts pancreatic insulin release. Blood sugar levels increase to ensure sufficient carbohydrate fuel for muscle and nerve tissue.

Resting and Exercise-Induced Endocrine Secretions

Table 13.1 lists the endocrine organs, secreted hormones and their action, control variables, effects of

TABLE 13.1
Endocrine glands, secreted hormones, functions, secretory control factors, effects of hypo- and hypersecretion, and effects of exercise on hormone secretion

HOST GLAND	HORMONE	HORMONE EFFECTS	CONTROL OF HORMONE SECRETION	EFFECTS OF HYPOSECRETION AND HYPERSECRETION	EXERCISE EFFECTS ON HORMONE SECRETION
Anterior pituitary	Growth hormone (hGH; somatotropin)	Stimulates tissue growth; mobilizes fatty acids for energy; inhibits CHO metabolism	Hypothalamic releasing factor (GHRF)	*Hypo-* dwarfism in children; *Hyper-*gigantism in children; acromegly in adults	↑ with increasing exercise
	Thyrotropin (TSH)	Stimulates production and release of thyroxine from thyroid gland	Hypothalamic TSH-releasing factor; thyroxine	*Hypo-*cretinism in children (stunted growth, mental retardation); myxedema in adults (low BMR, constipation, dry skin, puffy eyes, edema, lethargy); *Hyper-*Graves' disease (autoimmune disease—elevated BMR, weight loss, irregular heartbeat), heart disease	↑ with increasing exercise
	Corticotropin (ACTH)	Stimulates production and release of cortisol, aldosterone, and adrenal hormones	Hypothalamic ACTH-releasing factor; cortisol	*Hypo-* rarely seen; *Hyper-*Cushing's disease	Unknown
	Gonadotropic (FSH and LH)	LH works with FSH to stimulate production of estrogen and progesterone by ovaries and testosterone by male testes	Hypothalamic FSH- and LH-releasing factor; female-estrogen and progesterone; male-testosterone	*Hypo-* failure of sexual maturation; *Hyper-* none	No change
	Prolactin (PRL)	Inhibits testosterone; mobilizes fatty acids	Hypothalamic PRL-inhibiting factor	*Hypo-* poor milk production in nursing women, *Hyper-*galactorrhea, cessation of menses in females, impotence in males	↑ with increasing exercise
	Endorphins	Blocks pain; promotes euphoria; affects feeding and female menstrual cycle	Stress – physical/emotional (may be intensity related)	Unknown	↑ with long-duration exercise
Posterior pituitary	Vasopressin (ADH)	Controls water excretion by kidneys	Hypothalamic secretory neurons	*Hypo-* diabetes; *Hyper-*unknown	↑ with increasing exercise
	Oxytocin	Stimulates uterus and breasts muscles; important in birthing and lactation	Hypothalamic secretory neurons	Unknown	Unknown

TABLE 13.1 *(continued)*

HOST GLAND	HORMONE	HORMONE EFFECTS	CONTROL OF HORMONE SECRETION	EFFECTS OF HYPOSECRETION AND HYPERSECRETION	EXERCISE EFFECTS ON HORMONE SECRETION
Adrenal cortex	Cortisol Corticosterone	Promotes fatty acid and protein catabolism; conserves blood sugar/insulin antagonist; anti-inflammatory effects with epinephrine	ACTH; stress	*Hypo-* Addison's disease (weight loss; glucose and sodium levels drop and potassium levels rise resulting in hypotension and dehydration); *Hyper-* Cushing's disease (persistent hyperglycemia, dramatic losses in muscle and bone protein, and water and salt retention leading to hypertension)	↑ in heavy exercise only
	Aldosterone	Promotes sodium, potassium, and water retention by the kidneys	Angiotensin and plasma potassium concentration; renin	*Hypo-* Addison's disease; *Hyper-* aldosteronism (excessive sodium and water retention and accelerated excretion of potassium)	↑ with increasing exercise
Adrenal medulla	Epinephrine Norepinephrine	Facilitates sympathetic activity, increases cardiac output, regulates blood vessels, increases glycogen catabolism and fatty acid release	Stress stimulated hypothalamic sympathetic nerves	*Hypo-* unimportant; *Hyper-* hypertension, increased metabolism	Epinephrine, ↑ in heavy exercise Norepinephrine, ↑ with increasing exercise
Thyroid	Thyroxine (T_4) Triiodothyronine (T_3)	Stimulates metabolic rate; regulates cell growth and activity	TSH; whole body metabolism	*Hypo-* decreased BMR and body temperature, cold intolerance, decreased appetite, weight gain, decreased glucose metabolism, elevated cholesterol, decreased protein synthesis, hypotension, muscle cramps, growth retardation, depressed ovarian function; *Hyper-* increased BMR, temperature, heat intolerance, increased appetite, weight loss, hypertension, enhanced catabolism of glucose, fat, and protein, loss of muscle, muscle atrophy, depressed ovarian function	↑ with increasing exercise
Pancreas	Insulin	Promotes CHO transport into cells; increases CHO catabolism and decreases blood glucose; promotes fatty acid and amino acid transport into cells	Plasma glucose levels	*Hypo-* diabetes; *Hyper-* hypoglycemia, anxiety, nervousness, weakness	↓ with increasing exercise

TABLE 13.1 *(continued)*

HOST GLAND	HORMONE	HORMONE EFFECTS	CONTROL OF HORMONE SECRETION	EFFECTS OF HYPOSECRETION AND HYPERSECRETION	EXERCISE EFFECTS ON HORMONE SECRETION
	Glucagon	Promotes release of glucose from liver to blood; increases fat metabolism, reduces amino acid levels	Plasma glucose levels	*Hypo-* chronic hypo-glycemia, low circulating amino acids; *Hyper-* hyperglycemia	↑ with increasing exercise
Parathyroid	Parathormone (PTH)	Raises blood calcium; lowers blood phosphate	Plasma calcium concentration	*Hypo-* hypocalcemia, respiraory paralysis, uncontrolled spasms and convulsions; *Hyper-* hypercalcemia, extreme leaching of calcium from bones, depression of nervous system activity, muscle weakness, formation of kidney stones	↑ with long-term exercise
Ovaries	Estrogen Progesterone	Controls menstrual cycle; increases fat deposition; pro-motes female sex characteristics	FSH, LH	*Hypo* (estrogen)-; *Hyper* (progesterone)- masculinization or virilization	↑ with exercise; depends on menstrual phase
Testes	Testosterone	Controls muscle size; increases RBC; decreases body fat; promotes male sex characteristics		*Hypo-* feminization; *Hyper-* masculinization or virilization	↑ with exercise

hypo- and hypersecretion, and the effects of exercise on hormone output. The following sections review some important hormones, their functions during rest and exercise, and the specific host-gland-hormone response to exercise training.

Anterior Pituitary Hormones

Figure 13.2 shows the **pituitary gland** (**hypophysis**), its secretions and various target glands, and their hormone secretions. The pituitary gland consists of distinct anterior and posterior lobes (each with different hormone secretions). The gland attaches to the hypothalamus by neural elements that innervate the posterior pituitary. This nerve bundle (**hypophyseal stalk**) serves as a conduit for hormone movement from its site of synthesis in the hypothalamus to storage in the pituitary. Located beneath the base of the brain, the **anterior pituitary** secretes at least six different polypeptide hormones and influences the secretion of several others.

Growth Hormone

Human growth hormone (**hGH** or **somatotropin**) promotes cell division and proliferation throughout the body. This hormone facilitates protein synthesis by:

The True Master Gland

Because of its widespread influence, many consider the anterior pituitary the body's master gland. However, the hypothalamus actually controls anterior pituitary activity, making the hypothalamus the true master gland.

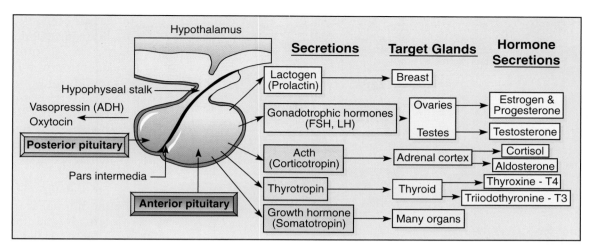

Figure 13.2
Pituitary gland and its secretions.

1. Increasing amino acid transport through plasma membranes
2. Stimulating RNA formation
3. Activating cellular ribosomes that increase protein synthesis

Release of hGH also depresses carbohydrate utilization, while increasing fat use for energy. Insufficient hGH secretion early in life blunts skeletal growth (dwarfism), whereas excess production produces extreme growth (giantism). Excessive hGH secretion in post-puberty causes continued soft tissue growth and bone thickening, a condition termed **acromegly**.

Hypothalamic secretion of hGH-releasing hormone stimulates the anterior pituitary gland's production of hGH. Another hormone, hypothalamic **somatostatin**, inhibits hGH release. *Each primary pituitary hormone has its own hypothalamic releasing factor (hormone).* Anxiety, stress, and physical activity provide neural input to the hypothalamus to discharge its releasing hormones.

Exercise, hGH, and Tissue Synthesis

Studies of exercise-induced hGH production show increased hormone secretion a few minutes after exercise begins. Increasing exercise intensity increases hGH production and total secretion. Moreover, hGH secretion relates more closely to peak exercise intensity than exercise duration or total exercise volume. The exact stimulus for hGH release with exercise remains unknown; neural factors most likely provide the primary control.

Several hypotheses suggest the mechanism of how hGH and exercise interact to increase protein synthesis and subsequent muscle hypertrophy, cartilage formation, skeletal growth, and cell proliferation. One hypothesis maintains that exercise directly activates hGH production, which in turn stimulates anabolic processes. For example,

a doubling of hGH pulse frequency and amplitude occurs in exercise. Exercise also stimulates endogenous opiate release; these hormones facilitate hGH discharge by inhibiting the liver's production of somatostatin, a hormone that blunts hGH release.

Figure 13.3 illustrates a model for describing the overall actions and regulation of hGH. An elevation in plasma hGH stimulates triglyceride release from adipose tissue while inhibiting cellular glucose uptake (anti-insulin effect). Inhibiting carbohydrate catabolism while maintaining blood glucose levels sustains prolonged exercise. Concurrently, hGH promotes its anabolic, tissue-building effects (mediated via somatomedins) on diverse tissue including bone and skeletal muscle. Elevated levels of hGH and somatomedins promote hypothalamic release of growth hormone-inhibiting hormone, which depress the release of growth hormone-releasing hormone; this inhibits anterior pituitary release of hGH.

With advances in molecular biology and genetic engineering, exogenous hGH availability has increased significantly. Consequently, its potential for abuse as a performance-enhancing drug, particularly among strength and power athletes, raises concern within the sports medicine community (see Chapter 17).

Thyrotropin

Thyrotropin (thyroid-stimulating hormone or TSH) maintains growth and thyroid gland development, including regulation of hormone output from thyroid cells. Because of the thyroid gland's important role in controlling cellular metabolism, physical activity usually increases anterior pituitary TSH output.

Corticotropin

Corticotropin (adrenocorticotropic hormone or ACTH) regulates adrenal cortex hormonal output similar to the way TSH controls thyroid secretions. ACTH directly en-

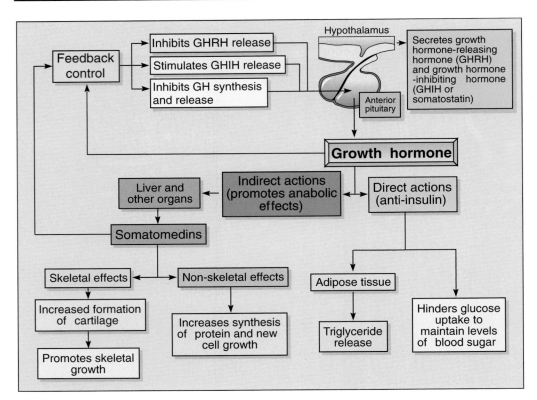

Figure 13.3
Overview for classifying the actions and regulation of human growth hormone (GH).

hances triglyceride mobilization from adipose tissue, increases the rate of gluconeogenesis, and stimulates protein catabolism. ACTH concentrations increase with exercise duration if intensity exceeds 25% of aerobic capacity.

Hypersecretion of ACTH (due to pituitary tumor) causes Cushing's disease (see Table 13.1) and associated hypertension (due to excess salt and water retention by the kidneys), reduces glucose metabolism, increases body fat (particularly in the face and trunk), and enhances masculinization (due to increased androgen production). ACTH deficiency leads to Addison's syndrome, characterized by sodium depletion, reduced extracellular and plasma fluid volume, susceptibility to infection, loss of appetite, weight loss, nausea, vomiting, and diarrhea.

Gonadotropic Hormones

Follicle-stimulating hormone (FSH) and **luteinizing hormone (LH)** comprise the gonadotropic hormones. In females, FSH initiates follicle growth in the ovaries and stimulates the ovaries to secrete estrogens, one type of female sex hormone. The combination of LH and FSH causes estrogen secretion and initiates rupture of the follicle to allow the ovum to pass through the fallopian tube for fertilization. In the male, FSH stimulates germinal epithelial growth in the testes to promote sperm development. LH also stimu-lates the testes to secrete the hormone testosterone.

The nature of gonadotropin release confounds interpretation of any exercise-associated alterations in FSH and LH. Because LH normally releases in a pulsatile manner, it becomes difficult to separate any specific exercise-related change from the normal secretion pattern. In addition, anxiety affects LH levels via action of the "stress" hormone norepinephrine. LH increases in anticipation of exercise and reaches its peak when exercise ceases.

Prolactin

Prolactin (PRL) governs milk secretion from mammary glands. PRL levels increase with higher exercise intensities and return toward baseline within 45 minutes of recovery. Owing to its important role in female sexual function, repeated exercise-induced PRL release may inhibit the ovaries and alter the menstrual cycle, a response often observed among athletic women. The significance of an increased PRL in men following acute maximal exercise remains unknown.

Endorphins

The endorphins, considered hypothalamic neurotransmitters, are split from the large prohormone precursor molecule **pro-opiomelancortin (POMC)** isolated from the anterior pituitary. The anterior pituitary then secretes these chemicals into the general circulation. Endorphins (and related compounds) act as natural opiate-like chemicals that produce an analgesic effect in response to pain. We discuss the role of these endogenous opioids in exercise later in this chapter.

Posterior Pituitary Hormones

Figure 13.2 also depicts the **posterior pituitary gland (neurohypophysis)** formed as an outgrowth of the hypothalamus. This gland stores two hormones, **antidiuretic hormone (ADH or vasopressin)** and **oxytocin**. The posterior pituitary does not synthesize its hormones, but receives them from the hypothalamus for release to the general circulation via neural stimulation.

ADH primarily limits how much urine the kidneys produce. Oxytocin stimulates uterine muscle activity and milk ejection from the breasts during lactation; thus, oxytocin contributes significantly to birthing and nursing.

Exercise stimulates ADH secretion, which increases water reabsorption by the kidney tubules during and after exercise. ADH release (stimulated by sweating) preserves body fluids, particularly in hot-weather exercise when dehydration poses a real risk. Excessive fluid intake inhibits ADH release and urine volume increases proportionately.

Thyroid Hormones

Release of TSH by the anterior pituitary gland stimulates hormone release by the thyroid gland, located in the neck just below the larynx (Fig. 13.4). The thyroid secretes two protein-iodine bound hormones, **thyroxine (T_4)** and **triiodothyronine (T_3)**. T_3 secretion occurs more rapidly then T_3; however, T_3 acts several times faster than T_4.

T_4 secretion increases metabolism of all cells through its stimulating effect on enzyme activity. For example, hypersecretion of T_4 increases basal metabolic rate (BMR) up to four times. Because of this thermogenic effect, clinicians have used significant deviations in BMR to detect thyroid gland abnormalities (refer to Chapter 4).

A person with abnormally high T_4 production (and accompanying elevated BMR) can lose weight rapidly.

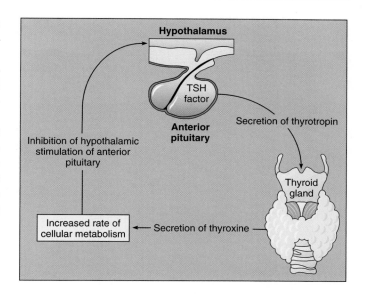

Figure 13.5
Feedback system for regulating thyroid hormone release.

Conversely, low T_4 output blunts metabolism, facilitating body fat accumulation. *However, thyroid malfunction probably accounts for no more than 3% of obesity in the population.*

Figure 13.5 illustrates the exquisite feedback system for thyroid output regulation and BMR. A decrease in whole body metabolism to some critical value stimulates hypothalamic release of TSH; this increases thyroid output, which stimulates resting metabolism. Conversely, an inordinate increase in metabolic rate blunts TSH release and decreases metabolism.

Blood levels of free T_4 (not bound to plasma protein) increase during exercise. This could result from core temperature increases with exercise that alter protein binding of several hormones including T_4. The importance of these transient alterations in hormone levels remains unknown.

Parathyroid Hormone

Four small sections of tissue comprise the **parathyroid gland** within thyroid tissue (refer to Fig. 13.4). This gland secretes the calcium-regulating parathyroid hormone (**PTH** or **parathormone**) in response to decreases in plasma calcium concentration. PTH activates intestinal uptake and renal reabsorption of calcium; it stimulates bone to increase calcium and phosphorous release into the extracellular fluid and plasma. PTH also activates a kidney enzyme that converts inactive vitamin D to its active form; active vitamin D increases calcium absorption from the small intestine.

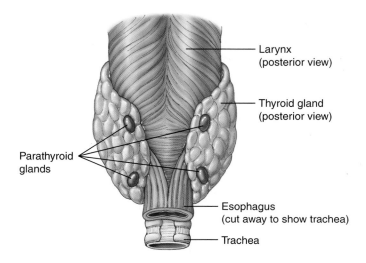

Figure 13.4
Thyroid gland located on both sides of the neck in the larynx region. Not visible externally under normal conditions.

Adrenal Hormones

Figure 13.6 shows the flattened, cap-like **adrenal glands** located just above each kidney. The glands form two distinct parts; the **adrenal medulla** (inner portion) and **adrenal cortex** (outer portion). Each secretes a different type of hormone.

Adrenal Medulla Hormones

The adrenal medulla forms part of the sympathetic nervous system. It prolongs and augments sympathetic neural effects by secreting two hormones, **epinephrine** and **norepinephrine** (collectively termed **catecholamines**). Neural outflow from the hypothalamus directly influences adrenal medulla secretions (80% as epinephrine), which affect the heart, blood vessels, and glands in the same (albeit slower) way as direct sympathetic nervous system stimulation.

Exercise intensity directly governs the quantity of adrenal medulla secretion. For example, norepinephrine levels increase two to six times throughout exercise gradations from light to maximum. Exercise duration also influences catecholamine response, as revealed by the direct relationship between plasma epinephrine and norepinephrine levels and mileage run. Other factors that determine catecholamine response to exercise include age (greater catecholamine secretion in older subjects at the same exercise intensity) and gender (greater epinephrine secretion in males than females at the same relative exercise intensity).

Adrenal Cortex Hormones

The adrenal cortex secretes **adrenocortical hormones** in response to ACTH stimulation from the pituitary gland. These steroid hormones categorize by function into one of three groups: **mineralocorticoids**, **glucocorticoids**, and **androgens**, each produced in a different zone or layer of the adrenal cortex.

Mineralocorticoids

Mineralocorticoids regulate mineral salts (sodium and potassium) in the body's extracellular fluid space. Of the three mineralocorticoids, **aldosterone**, the most physiologically important hormone, comprises almost 95% of all mineralocorticoids.

Figure 13.7 shows the major mechanisms for controlling aldosterone release from the adrenal cortex. Aldosterone regulates sodium reabsorption in the kidneys' distal tubules. Increased aldosterone secretion moves sodium ions (which also draws fluid) from renal filtrate back into the blood, with little sodium passing into the urine. Conservation of fluid via sodium reabsorption increases plasma volume, often with a concomitant increase in cardiac output and arterial blood pressure. In contrast, sodium and fluid literally pours into the urine when aldosterone secretion ceases.

Because the kidneys exchange either a potassium or hydrogen ion for each reabsorbed sodium ion, aldosterone indirectly stabilizes serum potassium and pH. Mineral balance preserves nerve transmission and muscle function; in fact, neuromuscular activity would cease without sodium and potassium regulation.

Outflow from the sympathetic nervous system during exercise constricts blood vessels to the kidneys. Reduced renal blood flow stimulates the kidneys to release the enzyme renin into the blood. Renin in turn stimulates the production of **angiotensin**, a potent vasoconstrictor that also activates aldosterone secretion from the adrenal cortex. Aldosterone secretion increases progressively during exercise, with peak plasma levels as high as six times the resting value. The **renin-angiotensin mechanism** during

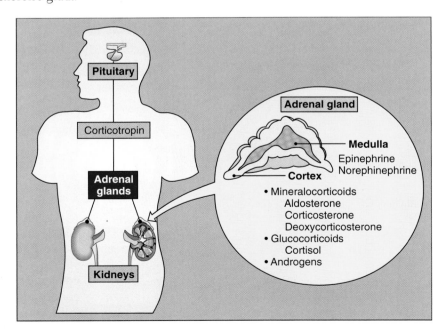

Figure 13.6
Adrenal glands and their secretions.

rest controls aldosterone secretion in response to changes in blood pressure in the kidneys' afferent arterioles.

Glucocorticoids

Cortisol (**hydrocortisone**), the major glucocorticoid of the adrenal cortex, affects energy metabolism in three ways:

1. Stimulates protein breakdown to amino acids in all cells except the liver. Once liberated, amino acids circulate to the liver to become synthesized to glucose via gluconeogenesis
2. Supports gluconeogenic action of other hormones, primarily glucagon and hGH
3. Serves as an insulin antagonist by inhibiting glucose uptake and oxidation

Obesity, Aldosterone, and Teenage Hypertension

Obese teenagers commonly have high blood pressure associated with increased aldosterone production. This form of hypertension relates to 1) decreased salt sensitivity (and hence increases in total body water), 2) increased sodium intake, and 3) decreased sensitivity to insulin's effects (hyperinsulinemia). These interrelationships suggest a direct link between obesity and hypertension.

Cortisol secretion also accelerates fat mobilization, particularly during periods of low energy intake and prolonged, moderate physical activity. The liver then splits the mobilized fat into simpler ketoacid components. Above-normal ketoacid levels in extracellular fluid can precipitate the potentially dangerous medical condition of **ketosis** (a form of acidosis). Individuals who consume very low-carbohydrate diets often experience ketosis because of the reliance on high levels of fat breakdown.

Emotional stress and physical exertion induce hypothalamic secretion of corticotropin-releasing factor that stimulates the anterior pituitary to release ACTH. ACTH, in turn, causes the adrenal cortex to release cortisol to initiate its stress-reducing responses.

Physical activity varies cortisol response, depending on exercise intensity and duration, fitness level, nutritional status, and even circadian rhythm. Cortisol output increases with exercise intensity. High cortisol levels also occur in prolonged exercise like marathon running, long-duration cycling, and hiking. Plasma

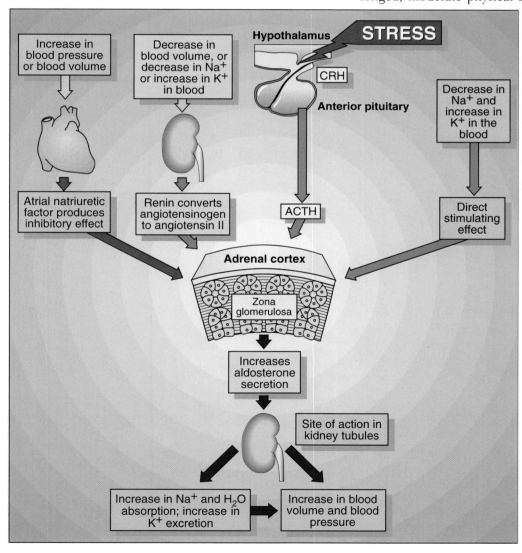

Figure 13.7
Major mechanisms that control aldosterone release from the adrenal cortex.

cortisol increases at relatively low levels of sustained exercise and remains elevated for up to 2 hours in recovery.

Androgens

The adrenal glands and ovaries (in females) and testes (in males) produce sex steroid hormones collectively term **androgens**. Specifically, the ovaries provide the primary source of **estradiol** (**estrogen**) and luteal phase **progesterone**; the adrenal glands in males and females synthesize **dehydroepiandrosterone** (**DHEA**) and its sulfate, DHEAS. The testes produce **testosterone**, also secreted in small amounts by ovaries; conversely, testosterone converts to estrogen in peripheral tissues.

Plasma testosterone concentration in females, although about one-tenth the level in males, increases with exercise (as do estradiol and progesterone). Both resistance training and moderate aerobic exercise increase serum and free testosterone levels of untrained males after about 15 to 20 minutes. Testosterone decreases below resting values during longer duration, higher intensity aerobic exercise.

Pancreatic Hormones

The pancreas, about 14 cm long and weighing 60 g, lies just below the stomach. Figure 13.8 illustrates the two different tissue types, **acini** and **islets of Langerhans**, that form this gland. The islets of Langerhans function as endocrine tissues composed of alpha cells that secrete **glucagon** and beta cells that secrete **insulin**. The acini tissue provides exocrine function and secretes digestive enzymes.

Insulin

Insulin's major function centers on regulation of glucose metabolism by facilitating cellular glucose uptake in all tissues except the brain. The pancreas releases insulin when blood glucose levels increase. This stimulates cellular glucose uptake (and glycogen formation), which lowers blood glucose levels. In essence, insulin exerts a hypoglycemic effect. Conversely, with insufficient insulin secretion, only trace amounts of glucose diffuse into cells. Blood glucose concentration increases from a normal 80 to 95 mg·dL^{-1} of blood to as high as 1000 mg·dL^{-1}; this excess glucose spills into the urine. Figure 13.9 shows insulin's role in glucose metabolism.

Insulin also influences fat metabolism. As blood glucose levels increase after a meal, insulin release transports some glucose into fat cells for triglyceride synthesis. A well-regulated insulin response maintains carbohydrate as the perferred energy source, with excess glucose synthesized to glyco-

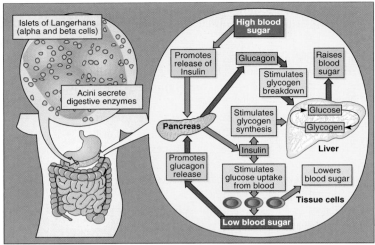

Figure 13.8
The pancreas and its secretions.

gen or triglyceride. In insulin's absence, fatty acids provide the primary energy source. Insulin also stimulates amino acid uptake and protein synthesis in muscle tissue.

Glucose-Insulin Interaction

The glucose level in blood that passes through the pancreas provides the feedback mechanism to regulate insulin secretion. Blood glucose increase stimulates insulin

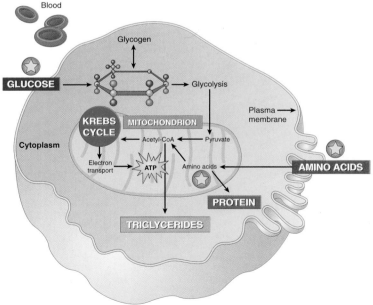

Figure 13.9
Insulin's primary functions. The circled stars show the locations where insulin influences metabolism.

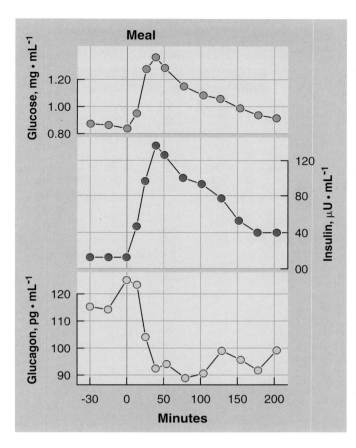

Figure 13.10
Effects of a high-carbohydrate meal on blood glucose levels and insulin and glucagon secretions.

secretion, whereas blood glucose reduction depresses insulin release.

Figure 13.10 shows the effects of a high-carbohydrate meal on the pancreas' secretion of insulin and glucagon. Shortly after a meal, insulin output increases (with a corresponding decrease in glucagon) in response to increasing blood glucose concentrations. These hormonal adjustments minimize alterations in circulating glucose. With inadequate insulin, because of an unresponsive pancreas or depressed sensitivity of peripheral tissues to insulin's action, initial glucose levels exceed the values depicted in the figure. If this occurs, plasma glucose increases considerably after a meal, signifying the condition known as **diabetes mellitus**.

Figure 13.11 illustrates that insulin levels progressively decrease during exercise

of increasing intensity and duration because of the inhibitory effects of increased catecholamine release on the pancreas. Reduced insulin enhances hepatic glucose output and sensitizes the liver to the glucose-releasing effects of glucagon and epinephrine. *Catecholamine suppression of insulin, which increases in proportion to exercise intensity, explains why the hypoglycemia sometimes observed with pre-exercise concentrated glucose intake (and accompanying oversecretion of insulin) does not occur when consuming simple sugars during exercise.* Free fatty acids provide progressively more energy as insulin output decreases during longer-duration exercise (>1 hr).

Glucagon

The alpha cells of the islets of Langerhans secrete glucagon, the **"insulin antagonist" hormone**. In contrast to insulin, glucagon increases blood glucose levels and stimulates both liver glycogenolysis and gluconeogenesis.

Similar to insulin, blood glucose level regulates glucagon release from the pancreas (see Fig. 13.10). A decline in plasma glucose concentration stimulates the alpha cells' release of glucagon, resulting in an instantaneous release of glucose from the liver. Glucagon contributes to blood glucose regulation during long-duration exercise and starvation; both conditions markedly decrease blood glucose and glycogen reserves.

Blood Glucose Homeostasis and Hormone Action

Figure 13.12 summarizes the regulatory control of blood glucose through insulin and glucagon action. Blood glucose regulation exemplifies a negative feedback system; any deviation in blood glucose from normal levels sets in motion responses that act to restore normalcy.

The right side of Figure 13.12 depicts the hypoglycemic response – those events that decrease circulating blood

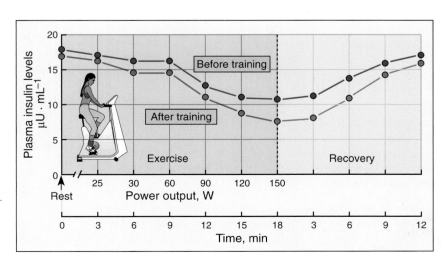

Figure 13.11
Plasma insulin levels during exercise and recovery before and after training.

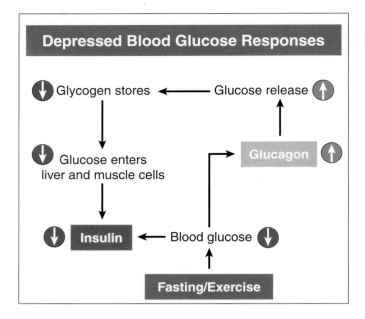

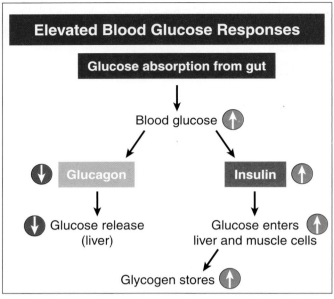

Figure 13.12

Blood glucose control via insulin and glucagon modulation. The arrows designate either an increase (↑) or decrease (↓). The left side of the figure indicates factors that increase blood glucose (hyperglycemic responses); the right side of the figure outlines responses that lower blood glucose (hypoglycemic responses).

glucose. After a meal, for example, glucose absorption from the small intestine elevates blood glucose concentration. This initiates insulin secretion by the pancreas and inhibits glucagon release. Depressed glucagon release reduces the liver's glucose output; increased insulin release stimulates glucose entry into the liver for glycogen synthesis and increases muscle uptake of glucose for energy metabolism and glycogen synthesis. These effects on glucagon and insulin decrease blood glucose concentration to normal levels and facilitate restoration of glucogen reserves.

The left side of the figure shows that a decrease in blood glucose (e.g., fasting or prolonged exercise) blunts insulin release and simultaneously increases glucagon output. Both responses elevate blood glucose concentration and reduce glycogen reserve.

Diabetes Mellitus

As early as the first century AD, the Greek physician Aretaeos of Kappadokia described the symptoms of what he termed diabetes mellitus (*mellitus* is Latin for sweetened with honey):

Diabetes is a wonderful affliction, not very frequent among men, being a melting down of the flesh and limbs into urine. The patients never stop making water. The flow is incessant, as in the opening of aqueducts. Life is short, disgusting and painful; thirst unquenchable; ex-cessive drinking, which, however, is disproportionate to the large quantity of urine, for more urine is passed; and one cannot stop them from drinking or making water; and at no distant term they expire.

The Chinese physician Chen Chuan, in the seventh century AD, recorded that the urine of those afflicted with diabetes tasted sweet. Eleven more centuries passed until the pancreas became linked to diabetes. In 1869, a German medical student, Paul Langerhans, described different looking cells in the pancreas from surrounding exocrine pancreatic cells. He referred to them as "islands in the pancreas" (named islets of Langerhans by Gustave Leguesse in 1903) that seemed different from the remaining pancreas tissue.

Twenty-one years after Langerhans discovery, researchers surgically removed the pancreas from a dog and discovered that the animal then exhibited all the symptoms of diabetes: increased thirst, increased urine flow, elevated blood glucose, glucose in the urine, and generalized wasting of body mass. In 1921, the Canadian physician Frederick Grant Banting (1891–1941) was the first to describe (in dogs) the pancreatic substance insulin and its effect on metabolism. Banting with co-recipiant John Richard Macleod (1876–1935) won the 1923 Nobel Prize in physiology or medicine for their research.

The disease of diabetes mellitus consists of subgroups of disorders that exhibit different pathophysiologies, with **type 1** and **type 2** subgroups most prevalent. Use of the for-

How to Detect Warning Signs of Diabetes Mellitus

Type 1 or Type 2 diabetes mellitus ranks among the leading causes of death in the United States. It causes blindness, kidney failure, need for amputation, and birth defects. It also contributes to atherosclerosis and hypertension. About one-half of the 725,000 people each year who learn they have diabetes go untreated. Indications of the diabetic condition include:

- Elevated blood glucose (**hyperglycemia**)
- Presence of glucose in urine (**glycosuria**)
- Increased urinary fluid loss (**polyuria**) resulting from the osmotic effect of glucose particles in renal filtrate
- Excessive levels of ketone bodies in the blood from reliance on excessive fat catabolism (**ketosis**) resulting in acetone aroma from the breath

Type 1 Diabetes

In type 1 diabetes, the pancreas loses its ability to synthesize insulin. Without insulin facilitating glucose entry into cells, any sugar absorbed in digestion accumulates in blood (spilling into the urine) and cannot enter the cells for metabolism. When this occurs, the person must take exogeneous insulin on a regular basis to maintain blood glucose concentration within the relatively narrow normal range.

Type 2 Diabetes

In type 2 diabetes, the cells resist insulin's effects. In the initial stages of the disease, the pancreas can produce excessive insulin (hyperinsulinemia) in response to increased blood glucose. Eventually, however, cells resist insulin's action, and blood glucose increases to an abnormally high level, which induces more insulin release. Finally, pancreas cells burn out and reduce their ability to produce insulin. This syndrome represents a self-aggravating condition.

DIFFERENCES BETWEEN THE TWO MAJOR FORMS OF DIABETES MELLITUS

Condition	Type 1	Type 2
Other names	Type I-IDDM	Type II-NIDDM
	Juvenile-onset	Adult-onset
	Ketosis-prone	Ketosis-resistant
	Brittle	Stable
Age of onset	<20 y (mean = 12 y)	>40 y
	<40 y in some cases	
Other condition	Viral infection	Obesity
Insulin required	Yes	Sometimes
Insulin receptors	Normal	Low or normal
Symptoms	Relatively severe	Relatively moderate
Prevalence in diabetic population	5 to 10%	90 to 95%

KEY BLOOD TESTS FOR DETECTING DIABETES MELLITUS

Substance	Normal Values	Decision Level
Fasting plasma glucose (FPG); following 8-h fast	<110 mg $\cdot$ dL^{-1}	≤ 45 mg $\cdot$ dL^{-1}–indicates **hypoglycemia** and a prediabetic condition 110–125 mg $\cdot$ dL^{-1}–indicates **impaired range** >126 mg $\cdot$ dL^{-1}–indicates **suspected diabetes**
Total cholesterol	<200 mg $\cdot$ dL^{-1}	>240 mg $\cdot$ dL^{-1}–patients with diabetes often have elevated plasma cholesterol
Triglyceride	40–160 mg $\cdot$ dL^{-1}, males 35–135 mg $\cdot$ dL^{-1}, females	>250 mg $\cdot$ dL^{-1}–patients with diabetes often have elevated plasma triglycerides

Oral Glucose-Tolerance Test*	Upper Limit of Normal	Diabetic Values
Time = 0	115 mg $\cdot$ dL^{-1}	>140 mg $\cdot$ dL^{-1}
Time = 60 min	200 mg $\cdot$ dL^{-1}	>200 mg $\cdot$ dL^{-1}
Time = 120 min	140 mg $\cdot$ dL^{-1}	>200 mg $\cdot$ dL^{-1}

*Previously perferred but an expensive, time consuming, and unpleasant test. Blood drawn following ingestion of a standard glucose load. Ordinarily, blood glucose rises initially and then returns to normal. In diabetes mellitus, however, blood glucose remains elevated during the recovery period. Many variations exist in the timing of blood sampling and quantity of glucose ingested. Fasting plasma glucose test currently recommended.

mer terms **insulin-dependent** and **noninsulin-dependent diabetes mellitus** (in addition to use of Roman numerals for subgroup identification) has been discontinued because they indicate treatments that can overlap and vary, rather than reflect the underlying pathogenesis.

Tests for Diabetes

Several tests diagnose diabetes. The American Diabetic Association recommends the **fasting plasma glucose test** (**FPG**) rather than the popular oral glucose tolerance test, which evaluates blood sugar levels over 2 hours after drinking a glucose-containing solution (see *How to Detect Warning Signs of Diabetes Mellitus*). The FPG test simply measures plasma glucose after an 8-hour fast.

The current value for suspected diabetes (FPG of >126 mg·dL^{-1}) is lower than the previous standard of 140 mg·dL^{-1} and acknowledges that patients can be asymptomatic with microvascular complications (small blood vessel damage) with FPG values in the low- to mid-120 mg·dL^{-1} range. The impaired range represents a transition between normal and diabetes where the body no longer responds properly to insulin or secretes adequate amounts. These individuals require close monitoring as they are often at high risk for developing full-blown diabetes.

Type 1 Diabetes

Type 1 diabetes includes all forms of diabetes caused by destruction of the pancreas' insulin-producing beta cells, caus-

Insulin Commercialization

Danish Nobel Laurete August Krogh (1920) (see Chapter 1) received permission in 1922 from the original patent holders (Board of Governors of the University of Toronto in the names of the those who first discovered insulin, researchers Banting, Collip, and Best) to govern the quality of insulin production in Denmark, Norway, and Sweden. In 1923, Krogh and colleagues founded the Nordisk Insulin Laboratory, which in 1989 became Novo Nordisk Pharmaceutical, Inc., the world's largest producer of insulin and diabetes care systems. (Bodil Schmidt-Nielson — daughter of August and Marie Krogh, provides intimate details about the initial discovery of insulin, including many conflicts and controversies, in her insightful book, *August & Marie Krogh. Lives in Science.* New York: American Physiological Society, 1995.)

An Array of Exercises

If no contraindications exist, personal choice dictates activity mode for the diabetic. Rhythmic aerobic exercises (swimming, bicycling, and walking) provide excellent cardiovascular conditioning and calorie-burning effects. Circuit-resistance exercise also improves cardiovascular function, glucose metabolism, and blood lipid profiles. Diabetic patients with peripheral neuropathy and microvascular degeneration should *NOT* perform exercises that traumatize the feet (e.g., jogging and high-impact aerobics).

ing insulin deficiency. The disease most frequently emerges in childhood but can present itself at any age. Tendency toward type 1 diabetes shows a strong genetic component. More than likely, the disease is triggered by an autoimmune response to something in the environment (e.g., viral infection) that destroys the beta cells' ability to synthesize insulin. Compared with the type 2 subgroup, patients have an abnormality in glucose homeostasis. Exercise produces more profound effects on the metabolic state of type 1 diabetics, and management of exercise-related problems requires greater attention.

Type 2 Diabetes

Type 2 diabetes affects an estimated 16 million people in the United States (1 of every 17 Americans). It typically arises because of **insulin resistance** (body tissues require greater than normal insulin for glucose regulation). Type 2 diabetes generally occurs among overweight, sedentary, middle-aged individuals with a family history of the disease.

Despite sufficient insulin production, adequate glucose does not enter the cells of type 2 diabetics; this increases blood glucose levels to abnormally high levels, and glucose passes into the urine (glycosuria). Excessive glucose particles in the renal filtrate create an osmotic effect that diminishes water reabsorption increasing fluid loss (polyuria). With decreased cellular glucose uptake, the type 2 diabetic relies heavily on fat catabolism for energy. This produces an excess of ketoacids and a tendency toward acidosis (ketosis). The following individuals are considered at risk for type 2 diabetes:

- Body mass in excess of 20% of ideal
- First-degree relative with diabetes
- Member of a high-risk ethnic population (black, Latino, American Indian, Asian)

Oral medications in Type 2 diabetes

Agent	Action	Brand Name	Exercise Effects
Sulfonylurea	Increases insulin secretion	Glucotrol, Micronase, Orinase, Tolinase, Diabinese, Glynase	Yes
Metformin	Decreases glucose production by liver	Glucophage	Yes
Troglitazone	Increases glucose uptake by muscle	Rezulin	Yes
Acarbose	Decreases absorption of glucose from gut	Precose	No

Young, J. C.: Exercise for clients with type 2 diabetes. *ACSM's Health & Fitness J.*, 2(2): 24, 1998.

- Delivered a baby weighing more than 9 pounds, or developed gestational diabetes
- Blood pressure at or above 140/90 mm Hg
- HDL cholesterol level of 35 mg·dL^{-1} or lower, and/or a triglyceride level of 250 mg·dL^{-1} or higher
- Impaired fasting plasma glucose or impaired glucose tolerance on previous testing

Diabetes and Exercise

Hypoglycemia during exercise represents the most common disturbance of glucose homeostasis in type 1 diabetes. During prolonged moderate exercise, hepatic glucose release does not keep pace with increased glucose utilization by active muscles. Plasma glucose reductions become severe in patients who need intensive insulin therapy to normalize glucose levels throughout the day. Sedentary lifestyle and excessive body fat reduce exercise tolerance of type 1 and type 2 diabetics, independent of blood glucose regulation.

Exercise Guidelines for Type 1 Diabetes

- Ingest 15 to 30 g of carbohydrate for each 30 minutes of intense exercise
- Consume a carbohydrate snack after exercise
- Decrease insulin dose:
   a. Intermediate-acting insulin — decrease the dose by 30 to 35% on the day of exercise.
   b. Intermediate-acting and short-acting insulin — omit the dose if it precedes exercise.
   c. Multiple doses of short-acting insulin — reduce the dose before exercise by 30% and supplement carbohydrate intake.
   d. Continuous subcutaneous insulin infusion — eliminate mealtime bolus or insulin increment that precedes or follows exercise.
- Avoid exercising for 1 hour those muscles receiving a short-acting insulin injection
- Avoid exercising in the late evening

Exercise Benefits For Diabetics

Regular physical activity for the type 2 diabetic improves glycemic control, cardiovascular function, body composition, psychological profile, and reduces a broad array of heart disease risks. Although some patients with type 1 diabetes improve their control of blood glucose (with lower daily insulin requirements) with regular exercise, the results are less consistent than for type 2 patients. Despite this limitation, type 1 and type 2 diabetic patients probably benefit equally from the exercise-related benefits to improve physical fitness, blood pressure, weight control, and blood lipid profile.

Glycemic Control. An acute exercise bout abruptly decreases plasma glucose levels in type 2 diabetics. Improved glucose regulation with exercise may persist for hours to days, and most likely results from the muscles' increased insulin sensitivity with physical activity. Improved longer-term glycemic control in the physically active diabetic probably results from the cumulative effects of each acute exercise session, rather than from changes in physical fitness per se. The hyperinsulinemic patient shows the greatest benefit from regular exercise, a response consistent with the notion that exercise reverses insulin resistance (i.e., increases insulin sensitivity).

Cardiovascular Effects. Increased morbidity (disease) and mortality in type 2 diabetes occur from coronary heart disease, stroke, and peripheral vascular and nerve disease, resulting from accelerated atherosclerosis and elevated blood glucose. Regular physical activity favorably modifies plasma lipoproteins, hyperinsulinemia, hyperglycemia, some blood coagulation parameters, local vascularization, and blood pressure.

Weight Loss. Exercise without diet therapy only moderately reduces body weight among type 2 diabetics. These effects, however, should not be underestimated because small changes in body weight with exercise may not reflect the more favorable changes in overall body composition. Exercise produces similar effects on body composition and weight loss for the diabetic and nondiabetic. For both

Figure 13.13
Potential physical and physiologic problems encountered by individuals with type 2 diabetes who begin an exercise program.

Potential problems with exercise in type 2 diabetes	
System	**Potential Problem**
Systemic	• Retinal hemorrhage • Increased proteinuria • Acceleration of microvascular lesions
Cardiovascular	• Cardiac arrhythmias • Ischemic heart disease (often silent) • Excessive rise in blood pressure • Post-exercise orthostatic hypotension
Metabolic	• Increased hyperglycemia • Increased ketosis
Musculoskeletal	• Foot ulcers (in presence of neuropathy) • Orthopedic injury related to neuropathy • Accelerated degenerative joint disease • Eye injuries and retinal hemorrhage

groups, body fat loss occurs most effectively through the prudent combination of diet *and* exercise.

Psychological Benefits. Regular exercise for diabetics and non-diabetics decreases anxiety, improves mood and self-esteem, increases sense of well-being, and enhances overall quality of life.

Exercise Risks for Diabetics

The potential complications of exercise for diabetics must be considered and minimized through proper screening of patients before they begin an exercise program and careful monitoring during exercise. Figure 13.13 lists some potential adverse effects of exercise for the diabetic.

Endurance Training and Endocrine Function

able 13.2 lists endocrine hormones and their general responses to exercise training. Because of complex interactions between endocrine secretions and central nervous system function, limited research exists concerning multiple hormone secretions and chronic exercise adaptations.

Endurance training generally decreases the magnitude of hormonal response to a standard level of exercise. Exercise at the same absolute intensity produces a lower hormonal response of trained subjects compared with untrained counterparts. However, adjusting exercise intensity to a percentage of each person's maximum capacity (i.e., same relative intensity) eliminates the training-related difference in hormonal response. With maximal exercise, trained subjects have an identical or slightly higher catecholamine and pituitary hormonal response than untrained subjects.

When the Diabetic Should Avoid Exercising

• Retinal (eye) hemorrhages or recent eye surgery
• Fever or infection
• Blood glucose <80 mg·dL^{-1}. (Eat extra carbohydrate until blood glucose increases to >120 mg·dL^{-1} before exercising).
• Blood glucose >250 mg·dL^{-1} and urine ketones present. (Decrease blood glucose to about 120 mg·dL^{-1}).

Anterior Pituitary Hormones

hGH and Long-Term Exercise Training

Most research on hGH involves responses to a single exercise session. Less information exists on hGH levels during prolonged exercise training. Research on the dynamics of hGH secretions with chronic exercise takes on significance because of the causal relationship between hGH availability and maintenance of fat-free body mass (FFM) with aging and weight loss.

Figure 13.14 shows the effects of a run training program on 24-hour integrated serum hGH concentrations in 21 healthy, eumenorrheic women. The study involved two training groups: one group ran at speeds corresponding to the lactate threshold (@LT), while the other group ran at speeds above lactate threshold (>LT). Nontraining subjects served as controls (C).

Both training groups completed similar weekly mileage. The distance covered during the first week equaled 5 miles; weekly mileage gradually increased to 24 miles by week 20 and continued at this distance until week 40. Thereafter, weekly mileage increased by 1.25 miles each additional 3 weeks. Subjects ran between 35 and 40 miles per week by the end of the study.

The year-long training program increased $\dot{V}O_{2max}$ by 9.9% for the @LT group and 11.8% for the >LT group. In addition, the @LT group increased exercise $\dot{V}O_2$ at lactate threshold ($\dot{V}O_2$ −LT) by 21.5%, while the >LT group's $\dot{V}O_2$ −LT increased by 28%. The control group did not change. No differences in body mass, percent body fat, or body fat mass emerged among groups. However, FFM increased for both training groups.

For hGH, the >LT group showed a marked 50% increase in integrated 24-hour resting hGH concentration after training. Growth hormone concentrations remained unaffected by exercise training for the @LT and control

TABLE 13.2
Hormonal response to exercise training

HORMONE	TRAINING RESPONSE
Hypothalamus-Pituitary Hormones	
hGH	Resting values increased: trained tend to have less dramatic rise during exercise
TSH	No known training effect
ACTH	Trained have increased exercise values
PRL	Some evidence that training lowers resting values
FSH, LH, and Testosterone	Trained females have depressed values; testosterone levels may increase in males with long-term strength training
Posterior Pituitary Hormones	
Vasopressin (ADH)	Some evidence that training slightly reduces ADH at a given workload
Oxytocin	No research available
Thyroid Hormones	
Thyroxine (T_4)	Reduced concentration of total T_3 and increased free thyroxine at rest
Triiodothyronine (T_3)	Increased turnover of T_3 and T_4 during exercise
Adrenal Hormones	
Aldosterone	No significant training adaptation
Cortisol	Trained exhibit slight elevations during exercise
Epinephrine	Decrease in secretion at rest and same absolute exercise intensity after training
Norepinephrine	
Pancreatic Hormones	
Insulin	Training increases sensitivity to insulin; normal decrease in insulin during exercise is greatly reduced in response to training
Glucagon	Smaller increase in glucose levels during exercise at both absolute and relative workloads
Kidney Hormones	
Renin (enzyme)	No apparent training effect
Angiotensin	

groups. The researchers hypothesized that relatively strenuous exercise above the lactate threshold increased hGH pulsatile secretion through the stimulating effect of endogenous opiates and catecholamines, while at the same time exercise inhibited somatostatin release. Further research needs to determine if training at intensities above LT counters hGH decrease in aging, and how this affects body weight loss and the associated deleterious effects on body composition.

Corticotropin (ACTH)
Corticotropin stimulates the adrenal cortex and thus increases fat mobilization for energy. Training raises ACTH levels during physical activity. Enhanced fatty acid oxidation spares glycogen, which benefits prolonged exercise performance.

PRL
It remains unclear whether long-term training alters PRL, other than training-induced changes mediated by sympathetic activity or other multiple hormone interactions. One study of male runners showed significantly lower PRL levels compared with sedentary subjects.

FSH, LH, and Testosterone
Women with a history of exercise participation have altered FSH and LH levels at different phases of the menstrual cycle. Alterations in these hormones usually cause menstrual dysfunction. FSH levels decrease in trained women throughout an abbreviated anovulatory menstrual cycle, whereas LH and progesterone concentrations rise in the cycle's follicular phase. Factors other than acute and long-term exercise can alter reproductive function in women athletes; these include weight loss, dietary changes, changes in lean-to-fat ratio, emotional stress of training and competition, and altered clearance rates of gonadal steroid hormones.

Endurance training affects pituitary-gonadal function in men, including testosterone and PRL concentrations. Figure 13.15 compares testosterone, LH, and FSH levels

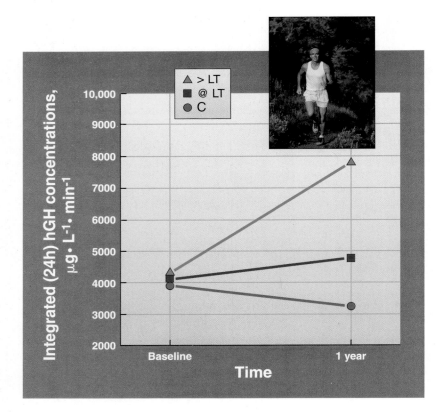

Figure 13.14
Integrated 24-hour hGH concentrations for subjects 1) training at the lactate threshold (@LT), 2) training above the lactate threshold (>LT), and 3) non-training controls (C). Note the large (50%) increase in hGH concentrations for the >LT group compared with the @LT and C groups. (Data from Weltman, A., et al.: Endurance training amplifies the pulsatile release of growth hormone: effects of training intensity. *J. Appl. Physiol.*, 72:2188, 1992.)

Resistance training presents a different picture because elite male athletes have elevated serum testosterone, LH, and FSH.

Posterior Pituitary Hormones

Vasopressin (ADH)

Maximal exhaustive exercise or prolonged submaximal exercise at the same relative intensity produces no difference in ADH response between trained and untrained individuals. However, some evidence suggests that ADH concentration decreases with training in response to submaximal exercise at the same absolute intensity.

Oxytocin

As of December, 1999, we are unaware of research on training-induced changes in this hormone.

among 46 male runners (64 km average weekly distance) and 18 nonrunners matched for age, stature, and body mass. The runners had depressed testosterone levels without significant difference in LH and FSH compared with nonrunners.

Reduced testosterone concentration (both increased clearance and decreased production) in endurance-trained men parallel the sex-steroid reductions in women who undergo endurance training and its associated lower body fat levels. Because LH and FSH do not differ between trained and untrained persons, an impaired gonadotropin release from the anterior pituitary does not account for reduced testosterone levels in the trained state.

Thyroid Hormones

Exercise training coordinates a pituitary-thyroid response that increases turnover of thyroid hormones, a response usually associated with excessive hormonal action that leads to hyperthyroidism. However, no evidence indicates this condition develops in highly trained individuals. BMR

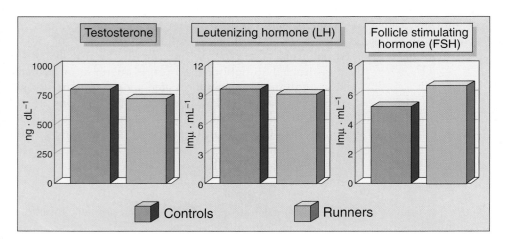

Figure 13.15
Comparison of testosterone, LH, and FSH levels among runners and untrained controls. Runners demonstrate significantly lower testosterone levels with no difference in LH and FSH compared with controls. (Data from Wheeler, G.D, et al.: Reduced serum testosterone and prolactin levels in male distance runners. *J.A.M.A.*, 252:514, 1984.)

Close up

Exercise, Infectious Illness, and Immune Response

Many people believe that excessive, strenuous exercise increases susceptibility to certain illnesses. Some also believe that more moderate regular exercise makes a person "healthy" and less susceptible to infectious illness like the common cold.

By 1918, reports indicated that most pneumonia cases among boys in boarding school occurred in athletes, and that respiratory infections seemed to progress toward pneumonia after intense sports training. Anecdotes have also related the severity of poliomyelitis to participation in heavy physical activity at a critical time of infection.

Subsequent epidemiologic and clinical data indicated that acute, unusually heavy physical activity profoundly affected immune function dynamics in a manner that *increased* susceptibility to illness, particularly upper-respiratory tract infection (URTI).

The immune system consists of a complex, well-regulated grouping of cells, hormones, and interactive modulators that defend the body against outside microbe invaders (bacterial, viral, and fungal), foreign macromolecules, and abnormal cancerous cell growth. If infection occurs, the immune system attempts to blunt the severity of illness and speed recovery.

The figure depicts the interactions among exercise, stress, illness, and immune system function. Exercise, stress, and illness represent interactive factors, each affecting the body's immune system. For example, exercise can modulate the stress response (either positively or negatively) to affect susceptibility to illness, while certain illnesses clearly influence exercise capability. More than likely, other stressors like lack of sleep, mental stress, poor nutrition, or weight loss can magnify the impact on the immune system of a single bout or repeated bouts of exhaustive exercise. Each factor (stress, illness, and acute and chronic exercise) independently affects immune status, immune function, and resistance to disease.

Researchers speculate that substances called cytokines indirectly affect tissues under attack by pathogens. When released, cytokines travel in the blood as messenger chemicals of the immune system to initiate an inflamatory alarm response to cellular abnormalities. This process marshalls macrophages (e.g., natural killer cells) and other defenders to thwart invading bacteria or virus.

Light to moderate physical activity provides some protection against URTI (and possibly diverse cancers) compared to a sedentary lifestyle, and does not appear to exacerbate the severity and duration of the illness if infection does occur. In contrast, a bout of intense physical activity (e.g., a marathon run or heavy training session) provides an "open window" (3 to 72 h) that decreases antiviral and antibacterial resistance and increases risk of respiratory infection that manifests itself within 1 or 2 weeks. Limited data indicate that aerobic exercise training positively affects natural immune functions in young and old individuals and the obese during weight loss.

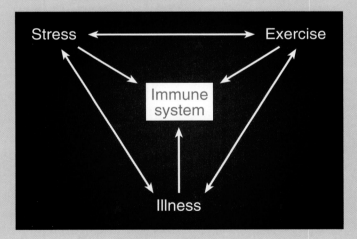

Theoretical model of the interrelationships among stress, exercise, illness, and the immune system. (Adapted from MacKinnon, L.T.: Current challenges and future expectations in exercise immunology: back to the future. *Med. Sci. Sports Exerc.*, 26: 191, 1994.)

References

1. Chandra, R.K.: Nutrition and the immune system: an introduction. *Am. J. Clin. Nutr. (Suppl.)*, 60:460S, 1997.
2. Flynn, M.G., et al.: Effects of resistance training on selected indexes of immune function in elderly women. *J. Appl. Physiol.*, 86:1905, 1999.
3. Nieman, D.C., et al.: Exercise and immune function. Recent developments. *Sports Med.*, 27:73, 1999.
4. Peters-Futre, E.M.: Vitamin C, neutrophil function, and URTI risk in distance runners: the missing link. *Exerc. Immunol. Rev.*, 3:32, 1997.
5. Shephard, R.J., and Shek, P.N.: Acute and chronic over-exertion: Do depressed immune responses provide useful markers? *Int. J. Sports Med.*, 19:159, 1998.
6. Weldner, T.G., et al.: The effect of exercise training on the severity and duration of a viral upper respiratory illness. *Med. Sci. Sports Exerc.*, 30:1578, 1998.

and resting core temperature remain normal with training, indicating that increased T4 turnover that accompanies chronic exercise occurs through a mechanism that differs from this hormone's normal dynamics.

Research on women who train to run a marathon reveals interesting responses for thyroid turnover. Moving from a baseline of relatively sedentary living to training 48 km a week mildly depressed thyroid function (reflected by *decreased* T3 and T4 levels). Extending training distance to 80 km a week significantly *increased* these hormones. Changes in body composition that accompany a high training volume may contribute to discrepancies in an exercise-induced change in thyroid function in females.

Adrenal Hormones

Aldosterone
The response of the renin-angiotensin-aldosterone system during exercise contributes to homeostatic control of fluid and electrolytes. This represents a transient response because exercise training does not affect resting levels of these compounds or their normal response to exercise.

Cortisol
Plasma cortisol levels increase less in trained compared with sedentary subjects during the same moderate exercise levels. Greater cortisol output among untrained individuals may partly result from heightened psychological stress experienced during exercise testing.

Epinephrine and Norepinephrine
A more relevant discussion about catecholamine response to exercise and training involves the **sympathoadrenal response**, rather than simply an adrenal gland response. Fig-ure 13.16 shows a large decrease in epinephrine and norepinephrine concentrations to a standard bout of intense exercise during the first 2 weeks of training. Bradycardia and a smaller increase in blood pressure during submaximal exercise after training are the most familiar responses to sympathoadrenal adaptation to training. Both responses favorably lower myocardial oxygen demands to exercise and other stressors. Some have argued that reduced catecholamine output reflects the benefits of regular physical activity in blunting the response to stress.

Pancreatic Hormones

Insulin and Glucagon
Endurance training maintains plasma insulin and glucagon levels in exercise closer to resting values. This seemingly depressed hormonal response with training occurs through several mechanisms:

- Increased muscle and fat tissue sensitivity to insulin. After training, it requires less insulin to regulate blood glucose. Improved insulin sensitivity probably relates to improved binding capacity of insulin to receptor sites on individual muscle fibers and adipocytes. Liver cells also increase their insulin sensitivity.

- Increased percentage contribution of fat catabolism for fuel during submaximal exercise; decreased carbohydrate metabolism lowers the insulin requirement.

Exercise Training in Diabetes
The clinical use of exercise training to control glucose in type 1 diabetics remains unclear, despite the clear association between regular exercise and improved insulin sensitivity by peripheral tissues. These individuals must exercise with caution because 1) increased insulin sensitivity, and 2) fast delivery of injected insulin via the

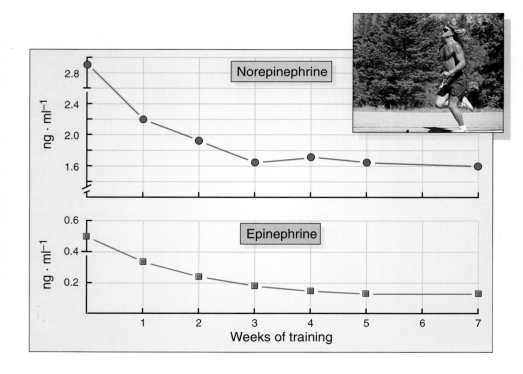

Figure 13.16
Week-by-week changes in plasma catecholamines during a five-minute exercise bout at 243 watts for six male subjects. Training consisted of running and stationary cycling 6 days a week. Catecholamine levels decreased progressively during training with the most rapid decline in the early training phase. (Data from Winder, W.W., et al.: Time course of sympathoadrenal adaptations to endurance exercise training in man. *J. Appl. Physiol.*, 45:370, 1968.)

rapid circulation with exercise accelerate glucose removal from plasma, possibly inducing serious hypoglycemia (see Exercise Guidelines for Type 1 Diabetes, page 345).

As a consequence of obesity (and possibly diet), many overweight men and women experience reduced glucose tolerance from generalized insulin resistance, which causes excessive insulin output (hyperinsulinemia). For these individuals, many of whom eventually develop type 2 diabetes, exercise training often reduces resting plasma insulin levels and lowers insulin output during fasting plasma glucose (FPG) test (thus indicating improved insulin sensitivity). *Without doubt, exercise training provides important non-pharmacologic therapy for type 2 diabetes.*

Resistance Training and Endocrine Function

The large variation among individuals in muscular strength and hypertrophy responses to resistance training implicates the possibility of significant individual differences in endocrine dynamics with regular muscle overload. Muscle remodeling with resistance training reflects a complex process involving cell receptor interaction with different hormones, which stimulates DNA synthesis of contractile proteins. The magnitude of the response links to the configuration of the exercise stimulus (e.g., frequency, intensity, volume, and mode of training) and more than likely hormonal response.

Testosterone and growth hormone are the two primary hormones involved in resistance training adaptations. Testosterone's primary role is to augment hGH release and to interact with the nervous system. The importance of these functions may exceed any direct anabolic effect of testosterone on muscle. Not all research has demonstrated a direct hGH increase with resistance training. Perhaps a hGH stimulatory response requires a threshold of exercise training intensity or training duration. *Current belief maintains that resistance training increases the frequency and amplitude of testosterone and hGH secretion, thereby contributing to hypertrophic effects on muscle.*

Available but limited data indicate that the exercise-induced increases in testosterone and hGH in men does not occur in women. Debate concerns whether this blunted hormonal response limits a woman's relative muscular hypertrophy with overload training.

Special Endocrine Considerations

Opioid Peptides and Exercise

In the 1970s, scientists studying the pain-relieving effects of opioid peptides (e.g., morphine) discovered they exhibited neurotransmitter properties that acted on specific brain opioid receptor sites. With this finding came the realization that perhaps the brain itself produced endogenous, opioid-like, mood-altering substances.

Isolation and purification of two opioid pentapeptides, methionine and leucine enkephalin (*enkephalin*, Greek meaning in the brain), provided the first evidence that endogenous substances behaved like opiates. Several other opioid substances have been identified; these include beta-lipotrophin, beta-endorphin, and dynorphin, the most potent opioid peptide. Endorphins also have been implicated in regulating menstruation and modulating the response of hGH, ACTH, PRL, catecholamines, and cortisol.

Beta-endorphin and **beta-lipotrophin** opioids generally increase with acute exercise. Plasma beta-endorphin in exercising men and women has increased five times the resting level, with higher values probably occurring in the brain itself. The most notable postulated exercise-related endorphin effect has been its role in triggering a state of euphoria and exhilaration ("**exercise high**") as duration of moderate to intense exercise increases. The endorphin effect may also increase pain tolerance, improve appetite control, and reduce anxiety, tension, anger, and confusion — all of which are proposed benefits of regular exercise.

The effect of chronic exercise on endorphin response remains controversial because of conflicting data. One could hypothesize that physical training increases an individual's sensitivity to opioid effects so it takes less of the hormone to induce a specific effect. In this sense, regular exercise could be viewed as a positive addiction. Opiates produced in the body during exercise may degrade more slowly in the blood of trained compared with untrained individuals. Certainly, a slower disposal rate would facilitate a given opiate response. It might even augment one's tolerance for extended exercise.

summary

1. The endocrine system consists of a host organ, a hormone, and a target or receptor organ. Hormones exist as either steroids or amino acid (polypeptide) derivatives.

2. Hormones alter rates of cellular reactions by acting at specific receptor sites to enhance or inhibit enzyme function.

3. Blood hormone concentration depends on the amount of hormone synthesized, the amount released, the amount taken up by the target organ, and its rate of removal from the blood.

4. The anterior pituitary secretes at least six hormones: PRL, the gonadotropic hormones FSH and LH, corticotropin, thyrotropin, and hGH. Endorphins also

are released from the anterior pituitary.

5. hGH promotes cell division and cellular proliferation; TSH controls the amount of hormone secreted by the thyroid gland; ACTH regulates the output of the hormones of the adrenal cortex; PRL affects reproduction and development of female secondary sex characteristics; FSH and LH stimulate the ovaries to secrete estrogen and progesterone in women and testosterone in men.

6. The posterior pituitary secretes antidiuretic hormone that controls the kidneys' excretion of water. It also secretes oxytocin, important in birthing and milk secretion.

7. Thyroxine elevates metabolic rate in all cells, and increases carbohydrate and fat breakdown in energy metabolism.

8. The inner (medulla) and outer (cortex) portions of the adrenal gland secrete two different types of hormones. The medulla secretes the catecholamines epinephrine and norepinephrine. The adrenal cortex secretes mineralocorticoids (regulate extracellular sodium and potassium), glucocorticoids (stimulate gluconeogenesis and serve as an insulin antagonist), and androgens (control secondary sex characteristics).

9. Insulin, secreted by the pancreas' beta cells, increases glucose transport into cells thereby controling the bodys' rate of carbohydrate metabolism. Diminished insulin production or decreased insulin sensitivity causes diabetes mellitus. The pancreas also secretes glucagon, an insulin antagonist that raises blood sugar.

10. Type 1 and type 2 diabetes represent the most prevalent diabetes subgroups. Type 1 diabetes causes insulin deficiency by destroying the pancreas' insulin-producing beta cells. Type 2 diabetes generally occurs in overweight, sedentary, middle-aged individuals with a family history of the disease. It typically arises because of insulin resistance (body tissues require greater than normal insulin for glucose regulation). Eventually, even a large insulin output does not regulate blood sugar.

11. Exercise training has differential effects on resting and exercise-induced hormone production and release. Training elevates hormone response during exercise for ACTH and cortisol, and depresses hGH, PRL, FSH, LH, testosterone, ADH, T_4, and insulin; no known training response occurs for aldosterone, renin, and angiotensin.

12. Exercise, stress, and illness represent interactive factors, each affecting the body's immune system and resistance to disease.

13. Exercise-induced elevation of beta-endorphins has been associated with euphoria, increased pain tolerance, the "exercise high," and menstrual dysfunction.

thought questions

1. Visit the local health food store and compose a list of supplements that claim to enhance exercise performance. Identify the ingredients and their alleged effects. Which supplements purport to simulate hormonal release? Based on your knowledge of hormonal regulation and function, can any of these products deliver on their claims?

2. Discuss the meaning of the following: Hormones act as silent messengers to integrate the body as a unit.

3. Hormones play crucial roles in normal growth and development and physiologic function. Give specific examples of why more is not necessarily better regarding these chemicals.

selected references

ADA/ACSM Diabetes Mellitus and Exercise. Joint Position Paper.: *Med. Sci. Sports Exerc.*, 29:1, 1997.

American College of Sports Medicine. Position Stand. The recommended quantity and quality of exercise for developing and maintaining cardiorespiratory and muscular fitness, and flexibility in healthy adults. *Med. Sci. Sports Exerc.*, 30:975, 1998.

Arciero, P.J., et al.: Comparison of short-term diet and exercise on insulin action in individuals with abnormal glucose tolerance. *J. Appl. Physiol.*, 86:1930, 1999.

Arciero, P.J., et al.: Effects of short-term inactivity on glucose tolerance, energy expenditure, and blood flow in trained subject. *J. Appl. Physiol.*, 84:1365, 1998.

Bergman, B.C., et al.: Muscle net glucose uptake and glucose kinetics after endurance training in men. *Am. J. Physiol.*, 277(1 Pt 1):E81, 1999.

Bjørnholt, J.V., et al.: Fasting blood glucose: An underestimated risk factor for cardiovascular death. *Diabetes Care*, 22:45, 1999.

Braun, B., et al.: Effects of exercise intensity on insulin sensitivity in women with non-insulin-dependent diabetes mellitus. *J. Appl. Physiol.*, 78: 300, 1995.

Bush, J.A., et al.: Exercise and recovery responses of adrenal medullary neurohormones to heavy resistance exercise. *Med. Sci. Sports Exerc.*, 31:554, 1999.

Campaigne, B.N.: Exercise and type 1 diabetes. *ACSM's Health & Fitness J.*, 2:35, 1998.

Carrol, J.F., et al.: Effect of training on blood volume and plasma hormone concentrations in the elderly. *Med. Sci. Sports Exerc.*, 27: 79, 1995.

Castell, L.M., et al.: Some aspects of the acute phase response after a marathon race, and the effects of glutamine supplementation. *Eur. J. Appl. Physiol.*, 75:47, 1997.

Cox, J.H., et al.: Effect of aging on response to exercise training in humans: skeletal muscle GLUT-4 and insulin sensitivity. *J. Appl. Physiol.*, 86:2019, 1999.

Davis, J.M., et al.: Exercise, alveolar macrophage function, and susceptibility to respiratory infection. *J. Appl. Physiol.*, 83:1461, 1997.

Del Corral, P., et al.: Metabolic effects of low cortisol during exercise in humans. *J. Appl. Physiol.*, 84:939, 1998.

Dengel, D.R., et al.: Improvements in blood pressure, glucose metabolism, and lipoprotein lipids after aerobic exercise plus weight loss in obese, hypertensive middle-aged men. *Metabolism*, 47:1075, 1998.

Després, J-P.: Visceral obesity, insulin resistance, and dyslipidemia: contribution of endurance exercise training to the treatment of the plurimetabolic syndrome. *Exer. Sport Sci. Revs.*, 25:271, 1997.

Deyssig, R., et al.: Effect of growth hormone treatment on hormonal parameters, body composition and strength in athletes. *Acta Endocrinol.*, 128: 313, 1993.

Dorion, B.A., et al.: Beta-endorphin response to high intensity exercise and music in college-age women. *J. Strength and Cond. Res.*, 13:24, 1999.

Fabbri, A., et al.: Body-fat distribution and responsiveness of the pituitary-adrenal axis to corticotropin-releasing-hormone stimulation in sedentary and exercising women. *J. Endocrinol. Invest.*, 22:377, 1999.

Flynn, M.G., et al.: Effects of resistance training on selected indexes of immune function in elderly women. *J. Appl. Physiol.* 86:1905, 1999.

Ferrara, C.M., et al.: Short-term exercise enhances insulin-stimulated GLUT-4 translocation and glucose transport into adipose cells. *J. Appl. Physiol.*, 85:2106, 1998.

Galliven, E.A., et al.: Hormonal and metabolic responses to exercise across time of day and menstrual cycle phase. *J. Appl. Physiol.*, 83:1822, 1997.

Goldfarb, A.H., et al.: Gender effect on beta-endorphin response to exercise. *Med. Sci. Sports Exerc.*, 30:1672, 1998.

Greiwe, J.S., et al.: Norepinephrine response to exercise at the same relative intensity before and after endurance training. *J. Appl. Physiol.*, 86:531, 1999.

Gu, K., et al.: Diabetes and decline in heart disease mortality in US adults. *JAMA*, 281:1291, 1999.

Hansen, P.A., et al.: Increased GLUT-4 translocation mediates enhanced insulin sensitivity of muscle glucose transport after exercise. *J. Appl. Physiol.*, 85:1218, 1998.

Houmard, J.A., et al.: Testosterone, cortisol, and creatine kinase levels in male distance runners during reduced training. *Int. J. Sports Med.*, 11: 41, 1990.

Howlett, T.A.: Hormonal responses to exercise and training: a short review. *Clin. Endocrinol.*, 26:723, 1987.

Inder, W.J., et al.: Prolonged exercise increases peripheral plasma ACTH, CRH, and AVP in male athletes. *J. Appl. Physiol.*, 85:835, 1998.

Ivy, J.L., et al.: Prevention and treatment of non-insulin-dependent diabetes mellitus. *Exerc. Sport Sci. Revs.*, 27:1, 1999.

Kanaley, J.A., et al.: Human growth hormone response to repeated bouts of aerobic exercise. *J. Appl. Physiol.*, 83:1756, 1997.

Kang, J., et al.: Substrate utilization and glucose turnover during exercise of varying intensities in individuals with NIDDM. *Med. Sci. Sports Exerc.*, 31:82, 1999.

King, D.S., et al.: Effect of oral androstenedione on serum testosterone and adaptations to resistance training in young men: a randomized controlled trial. *Jama*, 281:2020, 1999.

King, D.S., et al.: Time course for exercise-induced alterations in insulin action and glucose tolerance in middle aged people. *J. Appl. Physiol.*, 78:17, 1995.

Kraemer, W.J., et al.: Effects of different heavy-resistance exercise protocols on plasma β-endorphin concentrations. *J. Appl. Physiol.*, 74: 450, 1993.

Kraemer, W.J., et al.: The effects of short-term resistance training on endocrine function in men and women. *Eur. J. Appl. Physiol.*, 78:69, 1998.

Lindahl, B., et al.: Improved fibrinolysis by intense lifestyle intervention. A randomized trial in subjects with impaired glucose tolerance. *J. Intern. Med.*, 246:105, 1999.

Loucks, A.B., and Callister, R.: Induction and prevention of low-T3 syndrome in exercising women. *Am. J. Physiol.*, 264: R924, 1993.

MacKinnon, L.T.: Current challenges and future expectations in exercise immunology: back to the future. *Med. Sci. Sports Exerc.*, 26: 191, 1994.

Mayer-Davis, E.J., et al.: Intensity and amount of physical activity in relation to insulin sensitivity. *JAMA*, 279:669, 1998.

Nakai, N., et al.: Insulin activation of pyruvate dehydrogenase complex is enhanced by exercise training. *Metabolism.*, 48:865, 1999.

Ohannesian, J.P., et al.: Small weight gain is not associated with development of insulin resistance in healthy, physically active individuals. *Horm. Metab. Res.*, 31:323, 1999.

Pratley, R., et al.: Strength training increases resting metabolic rate and norepinephrine levels in healthy 50- to 65-yr-old men. *J. Appl. Physiol.*, 73:133, 1994.

Richter, E.A., and Sutton, J.R.: Hormonal adaptation to physical activity. In: *Physical Activity, Fitness, and Health*. Bouchard, C., et al., (eds.). Champaign, IL: Human Kinetics, 1994.

Strobel, G., et al.: Effect of severe exercise on plasma catecholamines in differently trained athletes. *Med. Sci. Sports Exerc.*, 31:560, 1999.

Struder, H.K., et al.: Neuroendocrine system and mental function in sedentary and endurance-trained elderly males. *Int. J. Sports Med.*, 20:159, 1999.

Wallace, M.B., et al.: Effects of cross-training on markers of insulin resistance/hyperinsulinemia. *Med. Sci. Sports Exerc.*, 29:1170, 1997.

Weltman, A., et al.: Exercise training decreases the growth hormone (GH) response to acute constant-load exercise. *Med. Sci. Sports Exerc.*, 29:669, 1997.

Whaley, M.H., et al.: Physical fitness and clustering of risk factors associated with the metabolic syndrome, *Med. Sci. Sports Exerc.*, 31:287, 1999.

White, R.D., and Sherman, C.; Exercise in diabetes management: maximizing benefits, controlling risks. *Phys. Sportsmed.*, 27(4):63, 1999.

Xiao-ren, P., et al.: Effects of diet and exercise in preventing NIDDM in people with impaired glucose tolerance. *Diabetes Care*, 20:537, 1997.

Young, J.C.: Exercise for clinents with type 2 diabetes. *ACSM's Health & Fitness J.*, 2:24, 1998.

Zaccaria, M., et al.: Blunted growth hormone response to maximal exercise in middle-aged versus young subjects and no effect of endurance training. *J. Clin. Endocrinol. Metab.*, 84:2303, 1999.

Zerath, E., et al.: Effect of endurance training on postexercise parathyroid hormone levels in elderly men. *Med. Sci. Sports Exerc.*, 29:1139, 1997.

SECTION

4

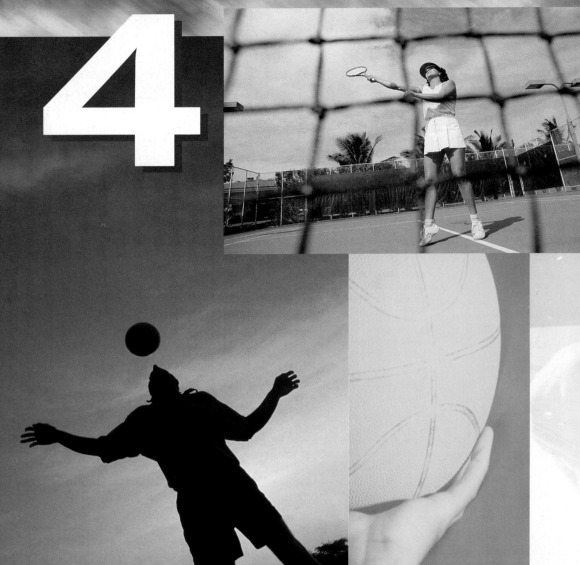

Exercise Training and Adaptations in Functional Capacity

Exercise training for sports often entails more art than science. Individual achievements or win-loss records rather than scientific inquiry and discovery frequently gauge the success of different conditioning programs. For example, basketball and soccer coaches frequently place considerable importance on developing aerobic capacity, yet may not devote enough time to vigorous anaerobic training. Although these sports require a relatively steady release of aerobic energy, crucial game situations frequently demand all-out effort.

A poorly trained anaerobic energy transfer system can prevent a player from performing at full potential. Training the anaerobic capacity of endurance athletes, on the other hand, proves wasteful because of the minimal contribution of anaerobic energy transfer to successful performance. Rather, endurance activities demand a highly conditioned heart and vascular system capable of delivering large quantities of blood (oxygen) to muscles with high capacity to generate ATP aerobically. At the other extreme, one's aerobic metabolic capacity contributes little to overall success in sprint activities and sports like football. Here, performance largely depends on muscular strength and power, which require energy generated in reactions that do not use oxygen.

Developing a training program to achieve optimum exercise and sports performance requires a clear understanding of energy transfer and how specific training affects energy delivery and utilization systems.

Chapters 14 and 15 focus on training for aerobic and anaerobic power and muscular strength, the physiologic consequences of such training, and important factors that affect training success.

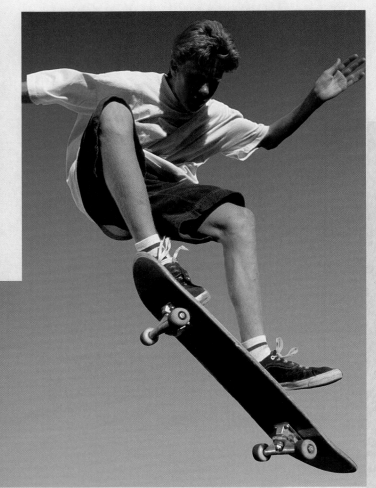

CHAPTER

14

Topics covered in this chapter

Training Must Focus on Energy
  Requirements
General Training Principles
Anaerobic Training
Aerobic Training
Factors That Affect Aerobic Conditioning
Adaptations to Exercise Training
Formulating an Aerobic Training Program
Continuous Versus Intermittent Aerobic
  Training
Maintaining Aerobic Fitness
Exercise Training During Pregnancy
Summary
Thought Questions
Selected References

Training the Anaerobic and Aerobic Energy Systems

objectives

- Define the following principles of exercise training: 1) overload, 2) specificity, 3) individual differences, and 4) reversibility.

- Discuss the overload principle for training the 1) intramuscular high-energy phosphates, and 2) glycolytic systems. Outline the specific adaptations in each system with training.

- Graph heart rate response during exercise and recovery from a 3-minute step test for an aerobically trained individual and a sedentary person. Explain the different responses.

- Describe how the following factors affect an aerobic training program: 1) initial fitness level, 2) genetics, 3) training frequency, 4) training duration, and 5) training intensity.

- List cardiovascular and pulmonary adaptations to aerobic training.

- Explain how exercise heart rate can establish an appropriate exercise intensity for aerobic training.

- Define the training-sensitive zone.

- Explain the need to adjust the training-sensitive zone for swimming and other forms of upper-body exercise.

- Explain the influence of age on 1) maximum heart rate, and 2) training-sensitive zone.

- Contrast continuous versus intermittent aerobic exercise training, including advantages and disadvantages of each.

- Outline potential benefits and risks of exercising during pregnancy.

Training Must Focus on Energy Requirements

Many forms of physical activity require rapid bursts of power during which energy requirements far exceed the oxygen delivery capacity. Even with available oxygen, cellular energy transfer from aerobic reactions progresses too slowly to match energy demands. This means that rapid anaerobic (not aerobic) energy transfer capacity determines how fast a running back plows through the line in football, a volleyball player spikes the ball over the net, and a softball player beats out an infield hit. Even longer-duration sports like basketball, tennis, field hockey, lacrosse, and soccer involve sprinting, dashing, darting, and stop-and-go where capacity to generate short bursts of anaerobic power play an important role.

At the other extreme, success in endurance activities necessitates a highly trained aerobic energy system. This requires a cardiovascular system capable of delivering large quantities of blood to active tissues for an extended time, and a musculature with high capacity to process oxygen for the aerobic resynthesis of ATP.

Energy for Exercise: Knowing What to Train For

Training for a particular sport or performance goal requires careful evaluation of the activity's energy components. This often overlooked factor forms the basis for effectively partitioning one's time for specific training of the appropriate energy transfer systems.

Figure 14.1 summarizes the involvement of anaerobic and aerobic energy transfer systems during all-out exercise of different durations. Keep in mind that the three energy systems (ATP-PCr system, lactic acid [glycolytic] system, and aerobic system) often operate concurrently during physical activity. However, their contributions to the total energy requirement can differ markedly depending on exercise duration and intensity.

A maximum burst of effort for a tennis serve, golf swing, front flip in gymnastics, and even a 60- or 100-m sprint requires immediate energy transfer. This occurs anaerobically, almost exclusively from the intramuscular high-energy phosphates ATP and PCr. In performances lasting up to 90 seconds (100-m swim or 440-m run), anaerobic energy transfer reactions still predominate. In this case, the initial glycolytic phase of carbohydrate breakdown with subsequent lactate formation provides the primary energy source. The person's capacity and tolerance for lactate accumulation determine the magnitude of energy generated from anaerobic sources.

Training for these activities must reach sufficient intensity and duration to overload the glycolytic energy transfer system. Although wrestling, boxing, ice hockey, a 200-m swim, 1500-m run, or a full-court press in basketball require rapid anaerobic energy transfer, aerobic energy

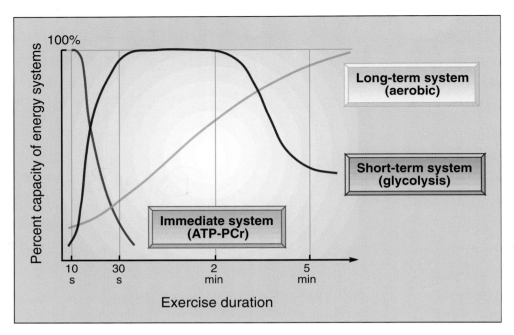

Figure 14.1
Three systems of energy transfer and their relative degree of activation during all-out exercise of different durations.

metabolism also plays an important role. As exercise intensity diminishes somewhat, and duration extends between 2 to 4 minutes, reliance on energy from anaerobic metabolism decreases, whereas energy release from oxygen-consuming reactions predominates. Beyond 4 minutes, exercise becomes progressively more dependent on aerobic metabolism; energy from aerobic reactions almost exclusively powers a marathon run, long-distance swim, or 25-mile continuous bicycle ride.

General Training Principles

*P*roper exercise training induces biologic adaptations that improve performance in specific tasks. Effective physiologic conditioning requires adherence to carefully planned and executed activities. Attention focuses on frequency and length of workouts, type of training, speed, intensity, duration, and repetition of the activity, and appropriate competition. These factors vary depending on the performance goal. However, several general principles of physiologic conditioning underlie the performance classifications shown in Figure 14.2.

Overload Principle

Enhanced physiologic improvement through training requires application of specific exercise **overload**. By exercising at a level above normal, many biological adaptations occur that improve functional efficiency. Appropriate combinations of training frequency, intensity, and duration provide individualized and progressive overload for

exercise training of the athlete, sedentary person, disabled individual, and even cardiac patient.

Specificity Principle

A common question about exercise training concerns the relative effectiveness of swimming, cycling, and running for developing aerobic/cardiovascular fitness (usually measured by $\dot{V}O_{2max}$). These "big muscle" activities prove equally effective for providing cardiovascular overload and improving aerobic power for the specific mode of exercise. Elite endurance athletes in discrete sports have high values for $\dot{V}O_{2max}$ in their particular activity (refer to Close Up: *Profile of the Real "Super" Aerobic Athletes*, page 371). However, aerobic fitness developed through one form of exercise training does not necessarily transfer to other aerobic activities that use a different musculature. In fact, training produces minimal changes in aerobic capacity unless testing and training modes are nearly identical.

Exercise training specificity refers to adaptations in metabolic and physiologic systems that depend on the type of overload imposed. In a broad sense, exercise stress, like strength-power training, induces specific strength-power adaptations; likewise, regular aerobic (cardiovascular) exercise elicits specific endurance-training adaptations with essentially no transfer effects between strength training and aerobic training. The specificity principle also encompasses activities with *identical* metabolic components. For example, aerobic fitness for swimming, bicycling, running, or rowing improves most effectively when the exerciser trains the specific muscles required for the specific activity. *In essence, specific exercise elicits specific adaptations, creating specific training effects (referred to as the* **SAID** *principle—Specific Adaptations to Imposed Demands).*

Figure 14.2
Performance classifications based on the duration of all-out exercise and corresponding predominant intracellular energy pathways.

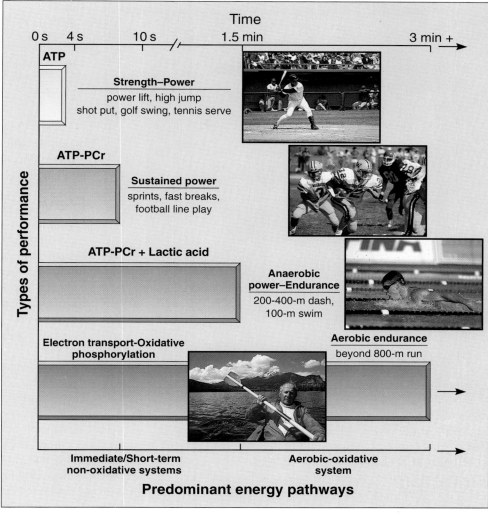

Specificity of Aerobic Power: An Example

In an experiment in one of our laboratories to study aerobic training specificity, 15 men swam 1 hour a day, 3 days a week, for 10 weeks at heart rates between 85 and 95% of maximum (HR_{max}). Measurements of VO_{2max} were made during treadmill running and tethered swimming before and after training. Because vigorous swim training elicits a *general overload* to the central circulation (as reflected by high exercise heart rates), we anticipated at least some transfer in aerobic power improvements from swim training to running. This did not occur; an almost total specificity accompanied the VO_{2max} improvement with swim training.

Figure 14.3 illustrates that swim training improved VO_{2max} 11% when measured during swimming, but only 1.5% when measured during running. If only treadmill running had been used to evaluate swim training effects, we would mistakenly have concluded that there was no training effect. For maximum performance during testing, subjects improved 34% in swim time to exhaustion but only 4.6% in run time on the treadmill test.

These findings and the research of others strongly indicate that training for specific aerobic activities must provide an appropriate general level of cardiovascular stress, and overload the specific muscles required by the activity. Little improvement results when a dissimilar exercise measures aerobic capacity or exercise performance; on the other hand, significant improvements emerge when the exercise training mode evaluates aerobic adaptations. One can appreciate the difficulty in maintaining "good shape" for diverse forms of aerobic exercise like the triathlon. The relatively large change in maximum exercise time (compared with VO_{2max}) in the above study suggests that aerobic capacity probably peaks early in training; thereafter, exercise performance improvements continue to increase through mechanisms other than improved VO_{2max}.

Adaptations within the active musculature (e.g., enhanced lactate threshold) rather than central circulatory factors provide part of the explanation.

Local Adaptations

Endurance training overload of specific muscle groups improves exercise performance and aerobic power by enhancing both oxygen transport and oxygen utilization in the trained muscles. For example, the oxidative capacity of well-trained cyclists' vastus lateralis muscle (predominant muscle in cycling) exceeds that of endurance runners and improves significantly with bicycle ergometer training. This type of local adaptation certainly increases the potential of trained muscle to generate ATP aerobically. Aerobic improvement also results from greater regional blood flow in trained tissue, owing to more effective distribution of cardiac output and increased capillary microcirculation. Such training adaptations only come into play when a specific exercise modality activates these muscles.

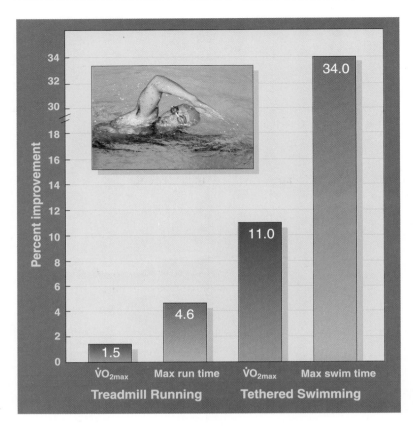

Figure 14.3
Effects of 10 weeks of interval swim training on changes in VO_{2max} during running and swimming. (From Magel, J.R., et al.: Specificity of swim training on maximum oxygen uptake. *J. Appl. Physiol.*, 38: 151: 1975.)

nize how athletes and trainees respond to a given exercise stimulus and adjust the exercise prescription based on that response.

Reversibility Principle

Detraining occurs rapidly when a person stops exercising. After only a week or two of detraining, measurable reductions occur in physiologic function and exercise capacity, with a total loss of training improvements within several months. Figure 14.4 shows average changes reported from several studies of the physiologic and metabolic variables with detraining (including bed rest).

In one experiment, VO_{2max} decreased 25% in five subjects confined to bed for 20 consecutive days; a similar decrease in maximal stroke volume and cardiac output accompanied the loss of aerobic capacity (roughly 1% per day). Capillary number within trained muscle also decreased 14 to 25% over the detraining period.

These data clearly highlight the transient and reversible nature of exercise training improvements, even among elite athletes. For this reason, athletes begin a reconditioning program several months before the start of the competitive season, or maintain some moderate level of off-season, sport-specific exercise to slow down the rate of deconditioning. Ex-athletes usually show poorer physiologic condition several years after they cease active participation than the business executive who exercises on a regular basis.

Individual Differences Principle

Many factors contribute to variations in training responses among individuals. One important factor is the person's relative fitness level at the start of training. People vary in their initial fitness and state of training at the start of a conditioning program and thus may respond to the same training stimulus differently. Insisting that all performers on a team (or even the same event) train the same way and at the same relative or absolute exercise intensity does not optimize training by recognizing individual differences in training responsiveness. Training programs must meet individual needs and capacities. Coaches and trainers should recog-

Anaerobic Training

The capacity to perform all-out exercise for up to 90-seconds duration depends mainly on anaerobic energy metabolism. Proper implementation of the overload principle improves this energy-generating capacity. Recall that anaerobic energy transfer generates from the breakdown of the intramuscular high-energy phosphates ATP and PCr, and glycolytic reactions that transform glucose into lactate.

ATP-PCr System

During the first 6 seconds of all-out exercise, the anaerobic breakdown of the energy currency ATP and the energy

Generality for Cardiac Training

A high degree of specificity in training exists for aerobic fitness, yet more general effects occur in cardiac function (e.g., ventricular contractility). This indicates that the heart muscle per se becomes conditioned through a variety of big-muscle exercise modes that increase demand for blood flow.

reservoir PCr provide energy almost immediately to power muscular effort. All-out bursts of effort for 5 to 10 seconds provide appropriate overload of the immediate energy system in specific muscles. A sprint swimmer, for example, might swim intervals of 20 m at maximal velocity to overload the arms and upper body, whereas a sprint runner obtains similar overload of the intramuscular phosphate pool of the legs by running repeat 60- to 100-m sprints. A football lineman may sprint for only 2 or 3 seconds on a given play. To increase intensity of overload during this short but intense period of exercise training, the player could run for 6 to 10 seconds with a weighted belt or vest, or sprint up hills or stairs. Because the high-energy phosphates supply almost all of the energy for this brief exercise, only a small amount of lactate forms, and recovery progresses rapidly (alactacid recovery oxygen uptake). Thus, a subsequent exercise bout can begin after only a 30- to 60-second recovery.

As a general rule, training to enhance intramuscular ATP-PCr energy transfer capacity requires repetitive bouts of intense, short-duration exercise. *The training activities selected must engage the muscles in the movement patterns for which the person desires improved anaerobic power.* This achieves two important goals: 1) enhances the metabolic capacity of specifically trained muscle fibers, and 2) facilitates neuromuscular adaptations to the sport-specific rate and pattern of movement. In Chapter 17, we discuss the efficacy of creatine supplementation to enhance the power output capacity of the intramuscular high-energy phosphates.

Glycolytic (Lactic Acid) System

To improve capacity of the short-term, lactic acid energy system, training must overload this specific form of energy

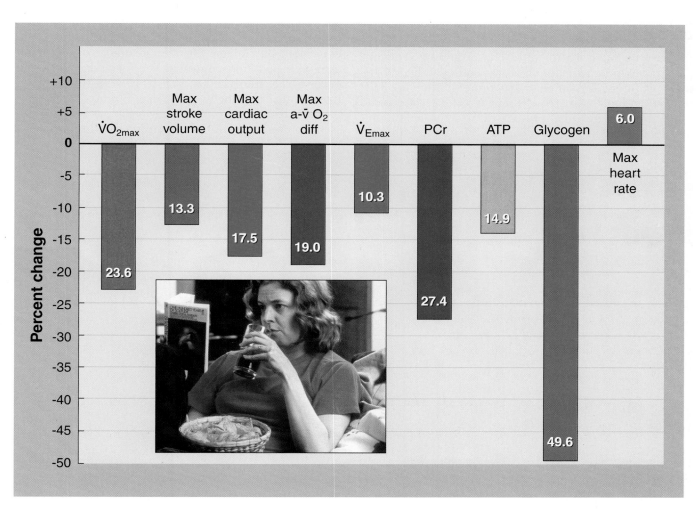

Figure 14.4
Average changes in physiologic and metabolic variables with different durations of detraining. Based on data from six studies. Values as follows: $\dot{V}O_{2max}$ in $L \cdot min^{-1}$; stroke volume in $mL \cdot b^{-1}$; cardiac output in $L \cdot min^{-1}$; a-$\bar{v}$ O_{2diff} = arteriovenous oxygen differences in $mL \cdot dL^{-1}$; $\dot{V}_{Emax}$ = maximum minute ventilation in $L \cdot min^{-1}$; PCr in $mmol \cdot g$ wet muscle wt^{-1}; ATP in $mmol \cdot g$ wet muscle wt^{-1}; glycogen in $mmol \cdot g$ wet muscle wt^{-1}; max heart rate in $b \cdot min^{-1}$.

transfer. Such training provides considerable physiologic stress and requires extreme motivation. Bouts of up to 1 minute of intense running, swimming, or cycling, stopped 30 to 40 seconds before exhaustion, activate the glycolytic energy pathways, causing a large lactate accumulation. To ensure maximum lactate production during each training session (indicative of the appropriate metabolic overload), the individual repeats the exercise bout several times, interspersed with 3 to 5 minutes of recovery. Each successive exercise interval causes "**lactate stacking**," which ultimately increases blood lactate levels above that of just one bout of all-out effort to voluntary exhaustion. As with all exercise training, the training mode must engage the specific muscle groups that require enhanced anaerobic energy capacity.

Aerobic Training

Evaluating Initial Status and Training Success

Reasons for initiating an exercise training program range from general to highly specific. Athletes train for specific performance enhancement: the baseball pitcher attempts to increase throwing velocity, the body builder focuses on enhanced muscle size and definition, and a sprint runner trains to decrease 100-m sprint time by

Prolonged Recovery

Recovery time can be considerable with intense exercise that elevates core temperature, disrupts internal equilibrium, and significantly elevates blood lactate. For this reason, apply intervals of anaerobic training at the end of workout. Otherwise, fatigue from training carries over and perhaps hinders ability to perform subsequent aerobic training.

focusing on "exploding" from the starting blocks. In contrast, the sedentary person initiates a fitness program for more general goals—to reduce body fat, lower cholesterol or blood pressure, change appearance, or improve cardiorespiratory function and overall health.

Evaluating the success of a sport-specific training program involves measuring changes in actual performance before, during, and after training. Often, one assumes that equivalent physiologic changes accompany measurable changes in performance and vice versa. This does not always occur as was illustrated in Figure 14.3. In this example, maximum swimming performance improved to a much greater extent than the accompanying increase in $\dot{V}O_{2max}$.

In contrast to training for sports-specific improvement,

TABLE 14.1
Aerobic capacity ($\dot{V}O_{2max}$) classification based on gender and age. Values in mL · kg^{-1} · min^{-1}

CATEGORY			AGE, y			
MEN	**13–19**	**20–29**	**30–39**	**40–49**	**50–59**	**60+**
1. Very Poor	<35.0	<33.0	<31.5	<30.2	<26.1	<20.5
2. Poor	35.0–38.3	33.0–36.4	31.5–35.4	30.2–33.5	26.1–30.9	20.5–26.0
3. Fair	38.4–45.1	36.5–42.4	35.5–40.9	33.6–38.9	31.0–35.7	26.1–32.2
4. Good	45.2–50.9	42.5–46.4	41.0–44.9	39.0–43.7	35.8–40.9	32.3–36.4
5. Excellent	51.0–55.9	46.5–52.4	45.0–49.4	43.8–48.0	41.0–45.3	36.5–44.2
6. Superior	>56.0	>52.5	>49.5	>48.1	>45.4	>44.3
			AGE, y			
WOMEN	**13–19**	**20–29**	**30–39**	**40–49**	**50–59**	**60+**
1. Very Poor	<25	<23.6	<22.8	<21.0	<20.2	<17.5
2. Poor	25.0–30.9	23.6–28.9	22.8–26.9	21.0–24.4	20.2–22.7	17.5–20.1
3. Fair	31.0–34.9	29.0–32.9	27.0–31.4	24.5–28.9	22.8–26.9	20.2–24.4
4. Good	35.0–38.9	33.0–36.9	31.5–35.6	29.0–32.8	27.0–31.4	24.5–30.2
5. Excellent	39.0–41.9	37.0–40.0	35.7–40.0	32.9–36.9	31.5–35.7	30.3–31.4
6. Superior	>42.0	>41.0	>40.1	>37.0	>35.8	>31.5

Data from Cooper, K. *The Aerobics Way*, New York: Bantam Books, Inc. 1982

current interest in physical activity participation arises largely from a desire to improve health-related fitness components, primarily **cardiorespiratory fitness (CR-F)**. Although most scientists believe that $\dot{V}O_{2max}$ provides the best measure of CR-F, other variables like blood pressure, heart rate, various blood chemistries (e.g., cholesterol, lactate threshold), body composition, feelings of well-being and self-esteem, and ratings of perceived exertion during exercise also provide useful information.

The Gold Standard: $\dot{V}O2max$

The $\dot{V}O_{2max}$ test represents the most often cited criterion to evaluate CR-F changes with training. Chapter 7 presented the different protocols for laboratory and field assessment and prediction of aerobic capacity. Current practice evaluates the $\dot{V}O_{2max}$ score against **criterion-referenced standards** rather than **norm-referenced standards**. Criterion-referenced standards establish a minimum $\dot{V}O_{2max}$ consistent with good health (similar to blood pressure and cholesterol standards), independent of the score's percentile ranking within a particular normative data set. Table 14.1 presents criterion-referenced $\dot{V}O_{2max}$ standards for men and women of different ages. The "very poor" category for each age group represents the lower limit of CR-F below which an individual's low cardiorespiratory fitness probably places them at an increased risk for cardiovascular disease.

Cardiorespiratory Fitness Standards for Children

Because of the relatively strong association between aerobic capacity and performance time (higher $\dot{V}O_{2max}$ relates to better performance), a valid method to evaluate CR-F in children uses time to complete a 1-mile walk-run. Table 14.2 presents criterion standards for $\dot{V}O_{2max}$ and 1-mile times for children of different ages.

The setting of CR-F standards for children requires careful attention. Although $\dot{V}O_{2max}$ ($mL \cdot kg^{-1} \cdot min^{-1}$) remains relatively stable or decreases slightly between ages 5 and 19 years, walk-run performance almost doubles due to growth and development and improved exercise economy during this period (a 12-year old runs a mile twice as fast as a 5-year old). Also, $\dot{V}O_{2max}$ improves only slightly for children who undergo aerobic training, whereas exercise performance increases significantly. This raises the question of whether aerobic capacity or exercise performance represents the "best" expression of CR-F in children and its improvement with training.

Finally, using a single equation generated from a walk-run field test to predict $\dot{V}O_{2max}$ in children poses problems because of continually increasing levels of running economy as a child ages. Variations in exercise economy alter the relationship between aerobic fitness and running performance through all stages of growth and development.

Heart Rate Response

A low heart rate during submaximal exercise generally reflects a large stroke volume and correspondingly high level of CR-F (see Chapter 11). If the heart pumps a large quantity of blood with each beat, then adequate blood (oxygen) delivery to the active muscles requires only a small heart rate increase, and vice versa with a relatively small stroke volume. *A step test provides a convenient means to use heart rate to evaluate efficiency of cardiovascular response to aerobic exercise.*

Figure 14.5 illustrates the heart rate response of three people performing 3 minutes of standard stepping exercise. Heart rate increases rapidly during the first minute and then levels off. Subject A, a varsity lacrosse player, attains a heart rate of 120 b · min^{-1} at the end of 4 minutes, whereas the heart rate of subject B, a physically active kinesiology major, equals 142 b · min^{-1}. For subject C, a sedentary college student, heart rate increases to 170 b · min^{-1}. Clearly, student C experiences considerably more cardiovascular stress (lower CR-F and smaller stroke volume) during bench stepping than the two other students, particularly student A, who has the smallest heart rate increase.

Figure 14.5 also illustrates the heart rate pattern for the three students during 2 minutes of recovery. Heart rate decreases rapidly during the first 30 seconds; it continues to decline, but at a much slower rate, to reach the resting level after about 2 minutes. The most noticeable differences emerge between students A, B, and C in the period immediately after exercise. *Thus, measuring heart rate soon after exercise stops provides a relatively simple means to distinguish heart rate response during exercise stress.*

Responders and Nonresponders

Not all people respond similarly to the same training regimen. Individual differences in

---

TABLE 14.2
Criterion standards for 1-mile run times and $\dot{V}O_{2max}$ for children between ages 10 to 17 years

AGE y	ONE MILE TIME min:s	$\dot{V}O_{2max}$ mL · kg^{-1} · min^{-1}
10	12:30	39
11	12:00	38
12	12:00	37
13	11:30	36
14	11:00	35
15	10:30	35
16	10:30	35
17	10:00	35

From Institute for Aerobic Research. The Prudential FITNESSGRAM Test Administration Manual. Dallas: Institute for Aerobics Research, 1992.

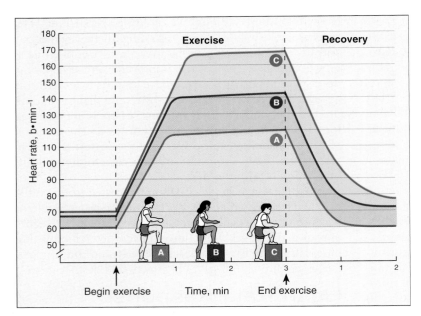

Figure 14.5
Heart rate response during stepping exercise and in recovery for three individuals with different levels of cardiorespiratory fitness.

43%. Noncompliance to the training protocol probably does not fully explain these results. Some individuals respond more readily than others to an identical training stimulus.

The concept of **responders** and **nonresponders** emerged from training data collected on identical twins. Ten pairs of identical twins, separated at birth and reared in different environments, completed the same 20-week endurance training program. The results showed a strong genetic component for improvements in CR-F. Both members of the twin pair showed nearly the same response; a large improvement in one twin mirrored similar improvement in the other, and vice versa. In the mid-1960s, the renowned Swedish physiologist Dr. Per-Olof Åstrand prophetically commented concerning the yet to be quantified role of genetics in exercise performance: "To be an Olympic-caliber performer, you must choose your parents wisely." Future research in molecular genetics may someday uncover a practical means to identify responders and nonresponders, and individualize conditioning programs to optimize CR-F improvements for each.

$\dot{V}O_{2max}$ improvement generally represents the rule rather than the exception, particularly among children and older adults. Among individuals in the same exercise training program, one person might show ten times more improvement than another. Figure 14.6 shows the large variations in $\dot{V}O_{2max}$ improvement with training in older men and women. Subjects trained similarly for 9 to 12 months, and aerobic capacity improvements ranged between 0 and

Exercise Adherence

Less than twenty percent of U.S. adults exercise regularly at sufficient intensity and duration to meet current guidelines to attain a minimal level of fitness. More than 60% of those who initiate or renew a personal exercise program do not maintain it at the intended level. Adherence rates range between 9 to 90% for worksite, commercial, and community-based exercise programs. Remarkably, the dropout rate for exercise programs duplicates that for other behavior-oriented programs like smoking, alcohol, and drug cessation, and weight loss and psychotherapy.

Figure 14.7 presents factors related to high and low adherence success to regular exercise. *Proper leadership exerts the greatest positive influence on exercise compliance.*

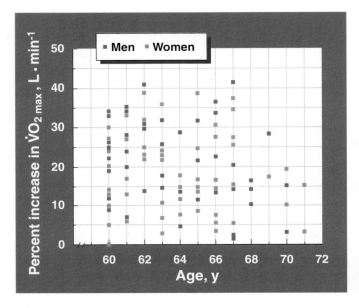

Figure 14.6
Variations in $\dot{V}O_{2max}$ improvement with training in older men and women. Note the extreme scatter in the data at any age. (From Kohrt, W.M., et al.: Effects of gender, age and fitness level on response of $\dot{V}O_{2max}$ to training in 60-71 yr olds. *J. Appl. Physiol.*, 71:2004, 1991.)

Improvement for the Average Person

As a broad guideline, individuals classified as average for $\dot{V}O_{2max}$ can improve aerobic power between 5 to 25% during a 12-week aerobic training program.

How to Perform the Tecumseh Step Test to Assess Cardiorespiratory Fitness

In the **Tecumseh step-test** the recovery heart rate from stepping exercise represents the criterion measure of CR-F. The test involves relatively moderate exercise on a stepping surface the approximate height of stairs found in the home. This test has proven useful for ranking CR-F among individuals (age 20 y and older), requires little time and equipment, and can be administered to almost anyone.

The Test

One performs the test alone or with a partner on a stair or stool 8 inches (20.3 cm) high. If necessary, adjust the stepping or floor surface with a board or similar hard, flat object to obtain the correct stepping height.

Perform the stepping cycle to a four-step cadence (up-up-down-down). Both men and women complete 24 step-ups per minute (up and down twice within a 5-s span). A partner can chant up-up, down-down, up-up, down, down within 5 seconds to establish proper cadence. Each new sequence starts at second 5, 10, 15, 20, and so on. For more precision, a metronome set at 96 b · min^{-1} gives the appropriate one footstep per beat cadence. Allow a brief practice period of 5 to 15 seconds to familiarize with the stepping cadence.

Begin the test and perform the step-ups for exactly 3 continuous minutes. On completion of the 3 minutes, remain standing, and take the heart rate (radial pulse) exactly 30 seconds into recovery for 30 seconds. The number of pulse beats in 30 seconds represents the CR-F score.

Tecumseh Step-Test CR-F Classification

The table provides the CR-F classifications based on the 30-second heart rate recovery for men and women. For example, a 25-year-old male with 38 beats in the 30-second recovery period achieves a CR-F ranking of very good.

CLASSIFICATION FOR TECUMSEH STEP TEST BASED ON A 30-SECOND HEART-RATE RECOVERY FOR MEN AND WOMEN

Classification	Age	20–29	30–39	40–49	50 & Older
			Number of Beats*		
Men					
Outstanding		34–36	35–38	37–39	37–40
Very Good		37–40	39–41	40–42	41–43
Good		41–42	42–43	43–44	44–45
Fair		43–47	44–47	45–49	46–49
Low		48–51	48–51	50–53	50–53
Poor		52–59	52–59	54–60	54–62
Women					
Outstanding		39–42	39–42	41–43	41–44
Very Good		43–44	43–45	44–45	45–47
Good		45–46	46–47	46–47	48–49
Fair		47–52	48–53	48–54	50–55
Low		53–56	54–56	55–57	56–58
Poor		57–66	57–66	58–67	59–66

*Thirty-second heart rate beginning 30 s after exercise stops.

From: Montoye, H.J.: *Physical Activity and Health: An Epidemiologic Study of an Entire Community*. Englewood Cliffs, N.J.: Prentice-Hall, 1975.

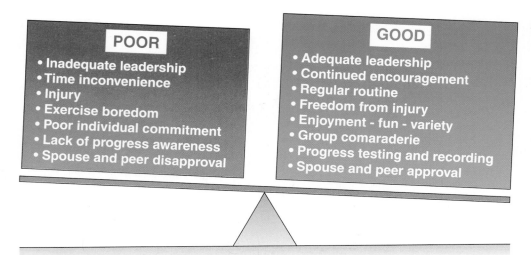

Figure 14.7
Variables related to good and poor adherence to regular exercise. (From Franklin, B.A.: Program factors that influence exercise adherence: Practical adherence skills for the clinical staff. In: *Exercise Adherence: Its Impact on Public Health*. Dishman, R.K., (ed.). Champaign, IL: Human Kinetics, 1988.)

Factors That Affect Aerobic Conditioning

Figure 14.8 illustrates the two major goals of aerobic conditioning:

1. Enhance central circulation's capacity to deliver oxygen
2. Develop the active muscles' capacity to consume oxygen

Several factors influence the outcome of aerobic conditioning, including initial level of cardiovascular fitness, training frequency, training duration, and training intensity.

Initial Level of Cardiorespiratory Fitness

As a general rule, a person's initial CR-F level affects the magnitude of training improvement. In simple terms, improvement occurs if one's initial fitness is low; conversely, an exceptionally high level of initial fitness leaves little room for improvement. Of course, a 5% improvement in physiologic function for an elite athlete can be more significant than a 25% increase in a sedentary person.

Frequency of Training

Exercising at least 3 days a week generally initiates adaptive changes in the aerobic system. Several research studies have reported significant improvements when training only 1 day a week. Those subjects, however, had been sedentary; for them, any form of overload would stimulate CR-F improvement. *The majority of studies of training frequency indicate that a training response occurs with exercise performed at least three times weekly for at least 6 weeks.*

Interestingly, several studies show training four or five times a week generated either no greater or only slightly greater improvements compared with thrice weekly exercise. For the average person, the small improvement in physiologic function (as measured by VO_{2max}) may not warrant the extra 1 or 2 day time investment in training. On the other hand, the extra caloric expenditure from daily exercise certainly becomes justified when using exercise primarily for weight control.

Duration of Training

A common inquiry about exercise participation concerns the duration of daily workouts. For example, does 10 minutes of jogging provide twice the benefits of 5 minutes? Would a 2- or 3-minute run repeated eight to ten times provide greater training benefits than a continuous 20- to 30-minute run at similar intensity? Precise answers to these questions remain elusive because of an incomplete understanding of the mechanisms underlying aerobic fitness improvements. We do know, however, that *both* continuous and more intense intermittent exercise overload improve aerobic capacity. In general, performing less exhaustive, moderate-paced exercise for 20 to 30 minutes each session sets a realistic exercise recommendation for the average person. In contrast, most competitive endurance athletes devote several hours each training session in activities that enhance the functional capacity of the aerobic system.

Intensity of Training

Exercise intensity is the most critical factor for successful aerobic training. Intensity reflects the activity's energy requirements per unit time and the specific energy systems activated. One can express exercise intensity in several ways:

- As calories expended per unit time
- As a particular exercise level or power output

Figure 14.8
Two major goals of aerobic training.

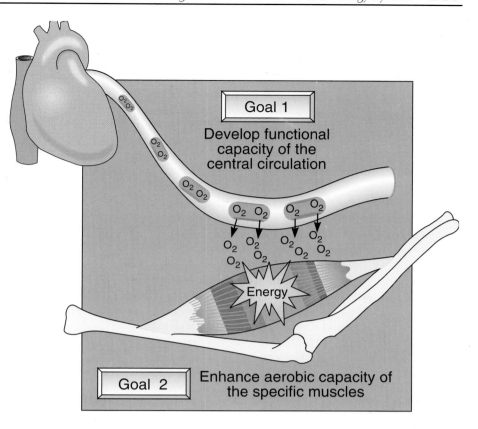

- As a level of exercise below, at, or above the lactate threshold
- As a percentage of $\dot{V}O_{2max}$
- As a particular heart rate or percentage of maximum heart rate
- As multiples of resting metabolic rate (METs)

By far, exercise heart rate is the most practical way to assess exercise strenuousness. Researchers frequently use exercise heart rate to structure a training program and evaluate the effectiveness of various training intensities. For college-age men and women, the exercise must reach sufficient intensity to raise heart rate to at least 130 to 140 b · min^{-1}. *This equals about 50 to 55% of $\dot{V}O_{2max}$, or 70% of HR_{max}.* As a general rule, this exercise intensity represents the minimal or **threshold stimulus** to cardiovascular improvement. However, more intense exercise proves even more effective. Conversely, extending the duration of the exercise session induces fitness improvement if intensity of effort falls below the threshold level.

An alternate, equally effective method to establish train-

ing threshold applies exercise at a heart rate of about 60% of the difference between resting and maximum. Use of the **heart rate reserve** to establish training heart rate (called the **Karvonen method** after the Finnish physiologist who first introduced this concept) provides a somewhat higher value compared to heart rate computed simply as 70% of HR_{max}. The Karvonen method computes training threshold heart rate as follows:

$$HR_{threshold} = HR_{rest} + 0.60 \, (HR_{max} - HR_{rest})$$

For example, the heart rate training threshold for a sedentary female with a HR_{rest} of 80 b · min^{-1} and HR_{max} of 180 b · min^{-1} would compute as:

$$HR_{threshold} = 80 + 0.60 \, (180 - 80)$$
$$= 140 \text{ b} \cdot \text{min}^{-1}$$

Overly Strenuous Exercise Not Necessary

An exercise heart rate at 70% HR_{max} (140 b · min^{-1} for young adults) represents only moderate exercise that can continue for a long duration with little or no physiologic discomfort. The term **conversational exercise** describes this training level (sufficiently intense to stimulate a training effect yet not so strenuous that it limits a person from talking during the workout).

A Regular Dose of Aerobic Exercise Combats Obesity

Sixty minutes of moderate daily exercise (low-impact walking or aerobic dancing, swimming, stationary cycling) reduces excess body fat. Exercise can be divided into 10-, 20-, or 30-minute sessions, as long as the daily total equals 60 minutes or more. For example, for an individual who weighs 216 pounds, the caloric expenditure during slow walking equals 7.8 kcal each minute (470 kcal per hour). Over 1 month, total exercise calories would accumulate to 14,100 kcal (470 kcal × 30 days), the equivalent of 4.0 pounds of body fat— 14,100 kcal ÷ 3500 kcal per pound of adipose tissue. In 1 year, as long as caloric intake remains constant, fat loss (without dieting) would amount to nearly 50 pounds.

Figure 14.9 shows that heart rate at a given level of submaximal exercise or oxygen uptake gradually decreases as aerobic fitness improves. Consequently, the absolute exercise level (e.g., running or swimming speed, power output on cycle ergometer) must increase accordingly to achieve the desired target heart rate. A person who began training by slow walking now walks more briskly, and periods of the workout would eventually include jogging. Ultimately, exercising at the training heart rate requires continuous running.

Although a minimal threshold intensity exists below which a training effect does not occur, a ceiling may also exist in which higher intensity exercise produces no further gains. The lower and upper limits of the training zone depend on the participant's age, initial fitness level, and state of training. For people with relatively poor aerobic fitness (including older men and women), the training threshold approaches 60-65% HR_{max}, which corresponds to about 45% VO_{2max}; more fit individuals generally require a higher threshold level. The ceiling for training intensity remains unknown, although 85% VO_{2max} (90% HR_{max}) probably represents an upper limit. Above this level, increases in intensity primarily overload the anaerobic system for energy transfer. We discuss more fully the use of heart rate to establish the appropriate exercise level for aerobic training on page 376.

How Long Before Improvement Occurs?

Measurable positive adaptations in CR-F and aerobic capacity with training generally occur within several weeks of beginning an exercise program. Figure 14.10 shows absolute and percentage improvements in VO_{2max} for men who trained 6 days a week for 10 weeks. Training consisted of 30-minutes of bicycling 3 days a week combined with running for up to 40 minutes on alternate days. This produced a continuous week-by-week improvement in aerobic capacity. Of course, adaptive responses to training eventually level off as a person reaches the genetically determined maximum. *Women and men show similar physiologic and metabolic adaptations to aerobic training.*

Adaptations to Exercise Training

Anaerobic System Changes

In accord with the concept of specificity of training, activities that demand a high level of anaerobic metabolism improve the immediate and short-term energy systems, with little impact on the aerobic system. Metabolic changes with sprint and power-type training include:

- Increased intramuscular levels of the anaerobic substrates ATP, PCr, and glycogen
- Increased quantity and activity of key enzymes (particularly in fast-twitch muscle fibers) that control the anaerobic (glycolytic) phase of glucose breakdown
- Increased capacity to generate high blood lactate levels during maximal exercise. This probably results from enhanced intramuscular glycogen and glycolytic enzyme levels, combined with improved motivation and discomfort tolerance for fatiguing exercise

Aerobic System Changes

Table 14.3 summarizes important metabolic and physiologic differences that emerge in comparison between healthy untrained individuals and endurance athletes.

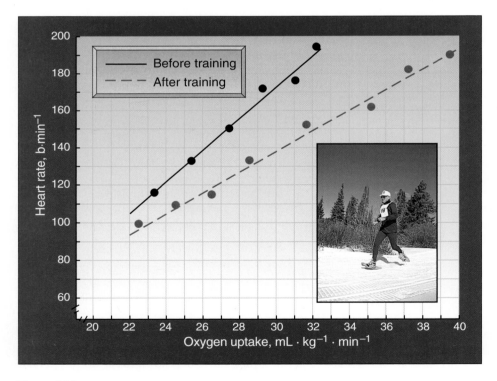

Figure 14.9
Improvements in heart rate response in relation to oxygen uptake with aerobic training. A reduction in submaximal exercise heart rate with training usually reflects an enhanced stroke volume of the heart.

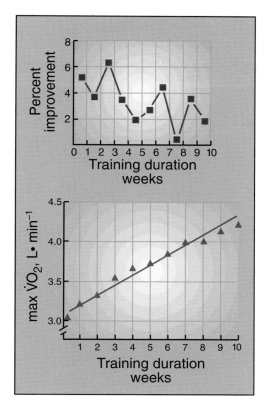

Figure 14.10
Continuous improvements in VO_{2max} during ten weeks of high-intensity, aerobic training. (From Hickson, R. C., et al.: Linear increases in aerobic power induced by a program of endurance exercise. *J. Appl. Physiol.*, 42: 373, 1977.)

Aerobic training adaptations generally occur independent of gender and age. They also take place in medically-cleared individuals with cancer, coronary heart disease, diabetes, hypertension, and obstructive lung disease (refer to Chapter 21).

Metabolic Adaptations
Aerobic exercise training induces intracellular changes that enhance a muscle fiber's capacity to generate ATP through aerobic metabolic pathways.

Metabolic Machinery. An increase in mitochondrial size and number in aerobically-trained skeletal muscle improves its capacity to generate ATP by oxidative phosphorylation.

Enzymes. A twofold increase in the level of aerobic system enzymes accompanies the increased mitochondrial size and number. These changes probably contribute to an athlete's ability to sustain a high percentage of aerobic capacity during prolonged exercise without accumulating blood lactate (higher lactate threshold). Enzymatic enhancement of metabolism does not result from an increase in enzyme activity per unit of mitochondrial protein, but rather from an increase in *total* mitochondrial material.

Fat Metabolism. *Regular aerobic exercise profoundly improves an individual's ability to oxidize fatty acids, particularly triglycerides stored within active muscle, during steady-rate exercise* (Fig. 14.11). Increased lipolysis results from greater blood flow within trained muscle, and a higher quantity of fat-mobilizing (from adipocytes) and fat-metabolizing (within muscle fibers) enzymes. This allows the endurance athlete to exercise at a higher absolute level of submaximal exercise before experiencing the fatiguing effects of glycogen depletion compared with an untrained person.

Carbohydrate Metabolism. *Aerobically trained muscle exhibits a greater capacity to oxidize carbohydrate.* Consequently, considerable pyruvate moves

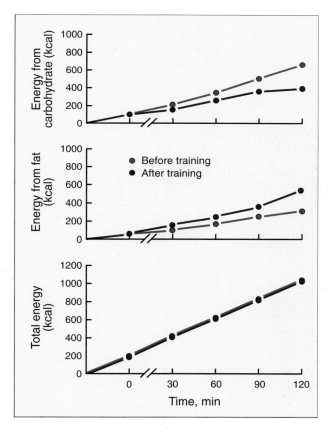

Figure 14.11.
Training enhances fat burning during submaximal exercise. This carbohydrate-sparing results from a facilitated release of fatty acids from adipose tissue depots, an increased intramuscular fat content, and enhanced mitochondrial fat oxidation capacity in endurance-trained muscle. (Data from Hurley, B.F., et al.: Muscle triglyceride utilization during exercise: effect of training. *J. Appl. Physiol.*, 5:62, 1986.)

TABLE 14.3
Typical metabolic and physiologic values for healthy endurance-trained and untrained men[a]

VARIABLE	UNTRAINED	TRAINED	PERCENT DIFFERENCE[b]
Glycogen, mmol · g wet muscle^{-1}	85.0	120	41
Number of mitochondria, mmol^3	0.59	1.20	103
Mitochondrial volume % muscle cell	2.15	8.00	272
Resting ATP, mmol · g wet muscle^{-1}	3.0	6.0	100
Resting CP, mmol · g wet muscle^{-1}	11.0	18.0	64
Resting creatine, mmol · g wet muscle^{-1}	10.7	14.5	35
Glycolytic enzymes			
Phosphofructokinase, mmol · g wet muscle^{-1}	50.0	50.0	0
Phosphorylase, mmol · g wet muscle^{-1}	4–6	6–9	60
Aerobic enzymes			
Succinate dehydrogenase, mmol · kg wet muscle^{-1}	5–10	15–20	133
Max lactate, mmol · kg wet muscle^{-1}	110	150	36
Muscle fibers			
Fast twitch, %	50	20–30	−50
Slow twitch, %	50	60	20
Max stroke volume, mL · beat^{-1}	120	180	50
Max cardiac output, L · min^{-1}	20	30–40	75
Resting heart rate, b · min^{-1}	70	40	−43
HR$_{max}$, b · min^{-1}	190	180	−5
Max a-$\bar{v}$O$_2$ diff, mL · 100 mL^{-1}	14.5	16.0	10
$\dot{V}$O$_{2max}$, mL · kg^{-1} · min^{-1}	30–40	65–80	107
Heart volume, L	7.5	9.5	27
Blood volume, L	4.7	6.0	28
$\dot{V}$E$_{max}$, L · min^{-1}	110	190	73
Percent body fat	15	11	−27

[a] In some cases, we list approximate values. In all cases, the trained values represent data from endurance athletes. We advise caution in assuming that the percent differences between trained and untrained necessarily result from training because genetic differences between individuals probably exert a strong influence on many of these factors.

[b] Computed as the percent that the value for the trained differs from the corresponding value for the untrained.

through the aerobic energy pathways during intense endurance exercise. A trained muscle's greater mitochondrial oxidative capacity and increased glycogen storage helps to explain enhanced capacity for carbohydrate breakdown. Increased carbohydrate catabolism during intense aerobic exercise serves two important functions:

1. Provides for a significantly faster aerobic energy transfer than from fat breakdown
2. Liberates about 6% more energy than fat per quantity of oxygen consumed

Muscle Fiber Type and Size.
Endurance training produces aerobic metabolic adaptations in *both* muscle fiber types, enhancing each fiber's existing aerobic capacity and lactate threshold level without likelihood of significantly changing fiber type. Specific overload training also selectively hypertrophies muscle fiber types. Highly trained endurance athletes have larger slow-twitch fibers than fast-twitch fibers in the same muscle. Conversely, for athletes trained in anaerobic-power activities, fast-twitch fibers occupy more of the muscle's cross-sectional area.

Cardiovascular Adaptations
Aerobic training produces significant changes to the cardiovascular and pulmonary systems.

Heart Size. Aerobic training normally enlarges the heart by increasing left ventricular cavity size and a slight thickening of its walls. Cardiac enlargement of this type, termed **eccentric hypertrophy**, improves stroke vol-

close up

Profile of "Super" Aerobic Athletes

The Ironman Triathlon, first organized in Hawaii in 1978 with 14 competitors, requires a marathon run (26.2 miles), a 112-mile bicycle ride, and a 2-mile endurance swim. In 1998, the number of participants swelled to 1520 from 46 countries (more than one-half from countries other than the U.S.). The age range spanned 19 years to 74 years (oldest female) and 80 years (oldest male), with an 89.8% finish rate. Since its inception, triathlon competitions continue to flourish worldwide with millions of competitors annually.

Studies of triathletes yield considerable insight concerning training specificity, particularly when compared with untrained subjects. In the untrained, the magnitude of $\dot{V}O_{2max}$ depends on the mode of testing, with the highest values attained during treadmill running. With cycle ergometry testing, $\dot{V}O_{2max}$ generally averages 8 to 12% below values running, and $\dot{V}O_{2max}$ falls 18 to 22% below treadmill values during tethered swimming. Among athletes who excel in single sports, elite cyclists often equal or exceed their treadmill $\dot{V}O_{2max}$ values when measured during cycle ergometry, and Olympic-caliber swimmers equal and even exceed their running $\dot{V}O_{2max}$ during swimming.

Because triathletes train specifically for three events, speculation arises whether these elite aerobic competitors attain equivalent values for aerobic capacity in each of the triathlon's three modes of exercise, or maintain the running-cycling-swimming differential in $\dot{V}O_{2max}$ observed for untrained persons.

The figure shows the results for aerobic capacity of 13 triathletes who averaged 2 years of competitive experience. The weekly training mileage averaged 32 miles of running, 156 miles of cycling, and 5.3 miles of swimming. Cycling $\dot{V}O_{2max}$ averaged 95.7% of the running value, while aerobic capacity swimming equaled 86.8% of the value running. These differences show remarkable similarity to values for single-sport athletes, and suggest that triathletes undergo highly specific adaptations that depend upon each of three training modes. Perhaps triathletes do not attain as high a cycling or swimming $\dot{V}O_{2max}$ compared with running because of difficulty equalizing training volume across each mode of exercise. While a triathlete spends considerable time training in each of three activities, total training volume per sport must necessarily be less than when training solely focuses on one sport. These data argue against a generalized cross-training effect in favor of a need for sport-specific aerobic training. Triathletes represent an exceptional group of aerobic athletes who attain world class physiology and performance in three distinct sport activities through arduous training in each activity.

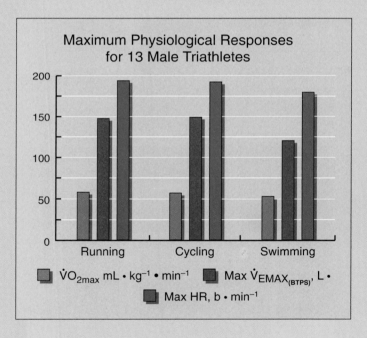

References

Kohrt, W. M., et al.: Physiological responses of triathletes to maximal swimming, cycling and running. *Med. Sci. Sports Exerc.*, 19:51, 1987.

Kohrt, W. M., et al.: Longitudinal assessment of responses of triathletes to swimming, cycling, and running. *Med. Sci. Sports Exerc.*, 21:569, 1989.

ume. With reduced training intensity, myocardial structure returns to control levels.

Plasma Volume. Increases in plasma volume of up to 20% occur within four training sessions. This adaptation enhances circulatory and thermoregulatory dynamics and facilitates oxygen delivery during exercise. The rapid increase in plasma volume with aerobic training also contributes to training-induced eccentric hypertrophy.

Stroke Volume. Figure 14.12 illustrates the stroke volume response for two groups of men during upright exercise of increasing intensity. One group of six highly trained endurance athletes had trained for several years; three sedentary college students comprised the other group. Graded exercise on a bicycle ergometer evaluated the students' responses before and after a 55-day training program designed to improve aerobic fitness.

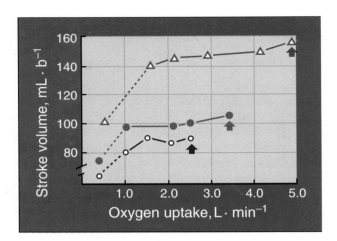

Figure 14.12
Stroke volume in relation to oxygen uptake during upright exercise in endurance athletes (△) and sedentary college students prior to (○) and following (●) 55 days of aerobic training; (◆ = maximal values). (From Saltin, B.: Physiological effects of physical conditioning. *Med. Sci. Sports.*, 1:50, 1969.)

These data reveal several important (and representative) findings concerning aerobic training adaptations:

- The endurance athlete's heart has a considerably larger stroke volume during rest and exercise than an untrained person of the same age.

- For trained and untrained individuals, the greatest increase in stroke volume in upright exercise occurs in the transition from rest to moderate exercise. Further increases in exercise intensity increase stroke volume only slightly.

- The heart's stroke volume achieves near-maximum values at 40 to 50% of $\dot{V}O_{2max}$; in young adults, this usually represents a heart rate between 120 and 140 beats per minute.

- For untrained individuals, only a small stroke volume increase occurs in the transition from rest to exercise. For them, acceleration in heart rate produces the major increase in cardiac output. For trained endurance athletes, increases in *both* heart rate and stroke volume augment cardiac output, with stroke volume increasing 50 to 60% above resting values.

- For previously sedentary subjects, 8 weeks of aerobic training substantially increases stroke volume, but these values remain well below those for elite athletes. The precise reason for this difference remains unknown. More than likely, prolonged, intense training, genetics, or a combination of both factors contribute to differences.

Heart Rate.   A proportionate reduction in heart rate during submaximal exercise usually accompanies the large stroke volume of elite endurance athletes and the stroke volume increase of sedentary subjects following aerobic training. Figure 14.13 illustrates this training effect on the relationship between heart rate and oxygen uptake (exercise intensity) for endurance athletes and sedentary students before and after training.

A linear relationship between heart rate and oxygen uptake exists for both groups throughout the major portion of the exercise range. As exercise intensity increases, the heart rates of the athletes accelerate to a lesser extent than untrained students; the slope (rate of change) of the lines differ considerably. Consequently, the athlete (or trained student) with an efficient cardiovascular response to exercise achieves a higher exercise intensity (oxygen uptake) before reaching a particular submaximal heart rate than a sedentary student. At an oxygen uptake of 2.0 L·min⁻¹, for example, the athletes' heart rate averages 70 b·min⁻¹ lower than the heart rate of the sedentary students. After 55 days of training, the difference in submaximal heart rate decreases to 40 b·min⁻¹. In each instance cardiac output remains about the same. This means that larger stroke volumes account for the lower exercise heart rates.

Cardiac Output.   *An increase in maximum cardiac output represents the most significant change in cardiovascular function with aerobic training.* Because maximum heart rate may decrease slightly with training, the heart's increased outflow capacity results directly from improved stroke volume.

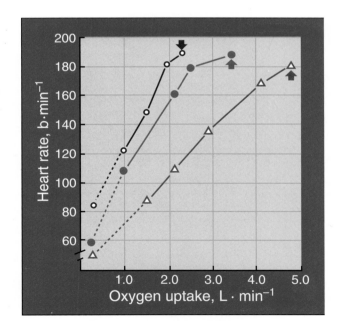

Figure 14.13
Heart rate in relation to oxygen uptake during upright exercise in endurance athletes (△) and sedentary college students prior to (○) and following (●) 55 days of aerobic training (◆ = maximal values). (From Saltin, B.: Physiological effects of physical conditioning. *Med. Sci. Sports.* 1:50, 1969.)

Oxygen Extraction. Aerobic training significantly increases the quantity of oxygen extracted from arterial blood during exercise. An increase in a-$\bar{v}$ O_2 difference results from more effective distribution of cardiac output to working muscles, and an enhanced capacity of muscle fibers to metabolize oxygen.

Blood Flow and Distribution. Aerobic training causes large increases in muscle blood flow during maximal exercise owing to:

- Improvements in maximal cardiac output
- Redistribution (shunting) of blood from non-active areas that temporarily compromise blood flow in all-out effort
- Increased capillarization within the trained muscle tissues

Blood Pressure. Systolic and diastolic blood pressures during rest and submaximal exercise decrease with aerobic exercise training. The most apparent effect occurs for systolic pressure, particularly for hypertensive subjects. Table 14.4 shows that the average resting systolic pressure of seven middle-aged male patients decreased from 139 to 133 mm Hg after 4 to 6 weeks of interval training. Systolic pressure in submaximal exercise declined from 173 to 155 mm Hg, while diastolic pressure decreased from 92 to 79 mm Hg. *Systolic and diastolic blood pressures generally decline approximately 6 to 10 mm Hg with regular aerobic exercise for previously sedentary men and women regardless of age.*

The exercise-lowering effect on blood pressure may result from reduced sympathetic nervous system hormones (catecholamines) with training. This response decreases peripheral vascular resistance to blood flow, causing blood pressure to decrease. Exercise training also facilitates sodium elimination by the kidneys; this subsequently reduces fluid volume and blood pressure. *Regular aerobic exercise represents a prudent first line of defense in most therapeutic programs to manage borderline hypertension.* More severe elevations in blood pressure require combinations of diet, weight loss, exercise, and pharmacologic therapy.

Pulmonary Adaptations

Aerobic training induces significant alterations in pulmonary dynamics during exercise, which contribute to a more effective response to the stress of physical activity.

Maximal Exercise. With training, maximal exercise minute ventilation increases with improvements in maximal oxygen uptake. This makes sense physiologically because improved aerobic capacity reflects larger oxygen utilization with greater carbon dioxide production, which requires elimination via increased alveolar ventilation.

Submaximal Exercise. Exercise training improves the ability to sustain high levels of submaximal ventilation. For example, 20 weeks of regular run training increased ventilatory muscle endurance by 16% in healthy adult men and women. Less lactate accumulated during submaximal breathing exercise, probably because of the increase in aerobic enzyme levels in the ventilatory muscles. Enhanced ventilatory endurance reduces the feeling of breathlessness and pulmonary discomfort frequently experienced by untrained persons who perform prolonged submaximal exercise.

TABLE 14.4
Measures of blood pressure during rest and submaximal exercise before and after 4 to 6 weeks of aerobic training in seven middle-aged patients with coronary heart disease[a]

MEASURE[b]	REST			SUBMAXIMAL EXERCISE		
	MEAN VALUE		DIFFERENCE (%)	MEAN VALUE		DIFFERENCE (%)
	BEFORE	AFTER		BEFORE	AFTER	
Systolic blood pressure (mm Hg)	139	133	−4.3	173	155	−10.4
Diastolic blood pressure (mm Hg)	78	73	−6.4	92	79	−14.1
Mean arterial blood pressure (mm Hg)	97	92	−5.2	127	109	−14.3

[a] Modified from Clausen, J. P., et al.: Physical training in the management of coronary artery disease. *Circulation*, 40:143, 1969.

[b] Blood pressure measured directly by a pressure transducer inserted into the brachial artery.

Even Cardiac Patients Benefit

Selected patients with coronary artery disease when trained at relatively intense exercise levels in supervised programs show physiologic adaptations much larger than previously believed. Particularly encouraging adaptations include favorable adjustments in myocardial oxygenation and enhanced left ventricular function.

Only 4 weeks of training considerably reduces the ventilation equivalent for oxygen ($V_E \div VO_2$) in submaximal exercise. Consequently, a particular level of submaximal oxygen uptake requires breathing less air; this reduces the percentage of the total oxygen cost of exercise attributable to breathing. Enhanced ventilatory economy contributes to endurance performance in two ways:

1. Reduces the fatiguing effects of exercise on the ventilatory musculature
2. Frees oxygen from the respiratory muscles for use by nonrespiratory active muscles

The precise mechanism for reduced ventilatory equivalent in submaximal exercise after training remains unresolved. The change has been consistently observed in adolescents and adults. In general, tidal volume increases, breathing frequency decreases, and air remains in the lungs for a longer time interval between breaths. This increases the amount of oxygen the alveoli captures (extracts) from the inspired air. For example, the exhaled air of trained individuals contains only 14 to 15% oxygen during submaximal exercise, whereas the untrained person's expired air contains about 17% oxygen at the same exercise intensity. This means the untrained person must ventilate proportionately more air to achieve the same submaximal oxygen uptake.

Specificity of Ventilatory Response. Ventilatory adaptations respond specifically to the form of exercise used in training. Figure 14.14 illustrates a significantly higher ventilation equivalent for arm exercise in subjects who performed arm and leg exercise at the same oxygen uptake. Exercise training decreased the ventilatory equivalent, but only during exercise requiring use of the specifically trained muscle groups. For the group trained by arm ergometry, the ventilation equivalent decreased *only* in arm exercise, and vice versa for the leg-trained group. This adaptation closely paralleled a less pronounced rise in blood lactate and heart rate in the specific training exercise. More than likely, the ventilatory adjustment to training results from neural and chemical adaptations in the specific muscles trained through aerobic exercise.

Other Adaptations

Other exercise-induced adaptations have also been documented.

Body Composition. For the obese and borderline obese person, regular aerobic exercise reduces body fat and often produces a slight increase in fat-free body

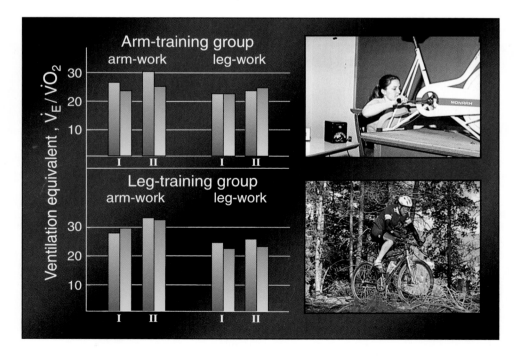

Figure 14.14
Ventilatory equivalents during light (I) and heavy (II) submaximal arm and leg exercise before and after arm training (top) and leg training (bottom). Yellow-green bars indicate post-training values. (From Rasmussen, B., et al.: Pulmonary ventilation, blood gases, and blood pH after training of the arms and legs. *J. Appl. Physiol.*, 38:250, 1975.)

mass. Because of exercise's conserving effect on the body's lean tissues, fat represents more of the weight lost with exercise (or exercise combined with prudent caloric restriction) compared with dieting only.

Body Heat Transfer. Well-hydrated, trained individuals exercise more comfortably in hot environments because of a larger plasma volume and more responsive heat regulatory mechanisms. Aerobically trained men and women dissipate metabolic heat faster and cool their bodies more effectively. This extends exercise capacity because heat generated by exercise causes less physiologic strain.

Figure 14.15 summarizes important adaptive changes that accompany aerobic training. Maximal oxygen uptake increases 15 to 30% in the first 3 months of intensive training, and may increase further to 40% over a 2-year period. When training stops, VO_{2max} returns toward the pretraining level. More impressive results occur for intramuscular aerobic enzymes that facilitate carbohydrate and fat breakdown; these enzymes increase rapidly and substantially throughout training in both muscle fiber types. Conversely, training cessation initiates rapid loss of this metabolic adaptation. The number of muscle capillaries increases throughout training; reversal of this favorable local circulatory adaptation probably occurs at a relatively slow rate when training ceases.

Intensive training lasting longer than 6 months substantially increases enzyme quantity and mitochondrial respiratory capacity in trained muscles. This local metabolic improvement exceeds the body's capacity to circulate, deliver, and use oxygen (as demonstrated by the relatively small further increase in VO_{2max}). In this phase of training, sub-

maximal blood lactate levels remain lower from reduced production and/or greater removal rate than in exercise of similar relative intensity before or earlier in training. These adjustments in cellular function contribute to a trained person's capacity to perform high intensities of steady-rate exercise.

Potential Psychologic Benefits of Regular Exercise

- Reduction in state anxiety
- Decrease in mild to moderate depression
- Reduction in neuroticism (long-term exercise)
- Adjunct to professional treatment of severe depression
- Improvement in mood, self esteem, and self concept
- Reduction in various indices of stress

Formulating an Aerobic Training Program

This section presents guidelines for initiating aerobic training, and describes a method to gauge and adjust training intensity. We also discuss advantages and possible limitations of aerobic conditioning through intermittent and continuous training procedures. Refer to Chapter 21 for guidelines for medical screening of adults for exercise.

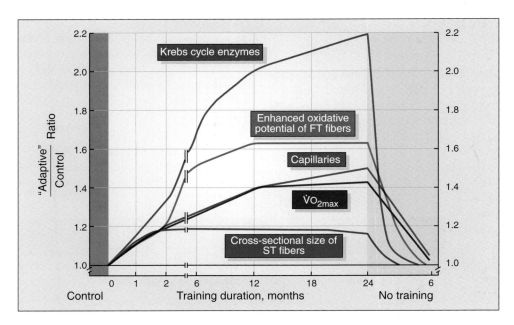

Figure 14.15
Generalized summary of adaptations in aerobic capacity and active muscle with endurance training based on longitudinal and cross-sectional studies of humans. FT = fast twitch; ST = slow twitch. (From Saltin, B., et al.: Fiber types and metabolic potentials of skeletal muscles in sedentary man and endurance runners. *Ann. N.Y. Acad. Sci.*, 301: 3, 1977.)

Guidelines

Regardless of a person's present physiologic fitness, some basic guidelines (based on both research and common sense) provide important structure when initiating an aerobic exercise training program:

- **Start slowly.** Injury can occur when initiating vigorous activity after years of sedentary living. Minor muscle aches and twinges of joint pain normally follow the start of an exercise program, particularly with eccentric muscle actions (see Chapter 15). Severe muscular discomfort and excessive cardiovascular strain offer no additional training benefits; excessive fatigue frequently discourages the beginner from continuing a regular exercise program.

- **Allow a warm-up period.** Mild stretching and aerobic exercise (running in place, jogging on a treadmill, skipping rope, rowing an ergometer, or stationary cycling) for several minutes provides adequate muscular and cardiovascular warm-up immediately before the aerobic workout phase. Rhythmic, moderate exercise at a heart rate between 50 to 60% of maximum also adjusts coronary blood flow for more favorable myocardial oxygenation.

- **Allow a cool-down period.** After the training phase of exercise, slow down gradually before stopping to allow metabolism to progress to resting levels. More importantly, a gradual cool-down prevents blood from pooling in the large veins of the previously exercised muscles. Venous pooling could decrease blood pressure and reduce blood flow to the heart and brain. This can produce dizziness, nausea, and even fainting. Reduced blood to the myocardium itself can precipitate a series of irregular heart beats that could trigger a catastrophic cardiac episode.

Guidelines for Children

Children are not small adults. Their physical activity programs should be general in nature compared with the rather specific formulations used to "train" adults. Guidelines from the National Association for Sport and Physical Education recommend the following:

- An accumulation of more than 60 minutes, and up to several hours per day, of age and developmentally appropriate activities for elementary school children
- Some of the child's physical activity each day should be in periods lasting 10 to 15 minutes or more and include moderate to vigorous activity. This activity will typically be intermittent in nature, involving alternating moderate to vigorous activity with brief rest and recovery periods.

- Extended periods of inactivity are *not* appropriate for normal, healthy children

- A variety of physical activities of various levels of intensity is recommended for elementary school children.

Establishing Training Intensity

What represents a considerable aerobic exercise stress for a sedentary person falls well below an elite athlete's threshold training intensity. Consequently, exercise intensity must be assessed relative to the stress it places on each person's aerobic system. Within this framework, one could justifiably maintain that three individuals performing their best marathon times of 2.5, 3.0, and 4.0 hours experience equivalent levels of physiological stress despite significant variations in running speed.

Two methods individualize exercise intensity for aerobic training:

Method 1. Train at Percentage of $\dot{V}O_{2max}$

In this method, an individual trains at a percentage of $\dot{V}O_{2max}$ (requires that $\dot{V}O_{2max}$ be determined directly or estimated from exercise intensity). For example, if running at 5.5 mph requires an oxygen uptake of 33 mL·kg^{-1}·min^{-1}, and the runner's $\dot{V}O_{2max}$ equals 60 mL·kg^{-1}·min^{-1}, the exercise represents a stress of 55% of aerobic capacity. For another individual with a lower $\dot{V}O_{2max}$ of 40 mL·kg^{-1}·min^{-1}, the oxygen cost of running at 5.5 mph still requires 33 mL·kg^{-1}·min^{-1}, yet this person must exercise at 83% of maximum. To provide a similar overload (intensity) of 83% of $\dot{V}O_{2max}$ for the first jogger, the pace must increase to a speed requiring 48 mL O$_2$ mL·kg^{-1}·min^{-1} or 8.6 mph.

Method 2. Train at Percentage of Maximum Heart Rate

Although highly accurate, assessing exercise intensity by direct measurement of oxygen uptake requires laboratory

Activity Recommendations for Children

Recommendations for general physical activity and fitness activities for children summarized from professional organizations and researchers:

Exercise Type	Frequency	Intensity	Duration
Large muscle, rhythmic, aerobic	3–5 days/wk	50–80% maximal functional capacity	30–60 min

Figure 14.16
Relationship between percent HR_{max} and percent $\dot{V}O_{2max}$.

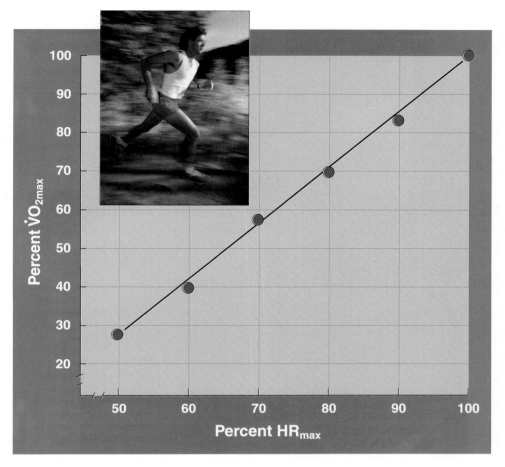

measurements. A more practical alternative uses heart rate to classify exercise by intensity (strenuousness) and individualizes aerobic training to keep pace with improving fitness. This approach applies the well-established relationship between percent $\dot{V}O_{2max}$ and percent HR_{max}. Figure 14.16 presents selected values for percent $\dot{V}O_{2max}$ and corresponding percentages of HR_{max}.

The error in estimating percent $\dot{V}O_{2max}$ from percent HR_{max}, or vice versa, averages about ±8%. Because of this intrinsic relationship, one need only monitor exercise heart rate to estimate percent $\dot{V}O_{2max}$. *The relationship between percent $\dot{V}O_{2max}$ and percent HR_{max} remains the same for arm or leg exercise among healthy subjects, normal weight and obese groups, cardiac patients, and people with spinal cord injury.* However, a significantly lower HR_{max} occurs in arm compared with leg exercise; one must consider this difference in formulating the exercise prescription for different exercise modes.

To train at a percentage of maximum heart rate requires knowledge of the heart rate in near-maximal exercise. Three or four minutes of all-out running or swimming elicits HR_{max}. Such intense exercise requires considerable motivation and endangers those predisposed to coronary heart disease. For this reason, people should consider themselves "average" and use the **age-predicted maximum heart rates** shown in Figure 14.17. Figure 14.17 also illustrates the **training-sensitive zone** that represents the lower threshold level of 70% and upper level of 90% of HR_{max} for each age group. *Maintaining exercise heart rates within this zone stimulates an aerobic training response.*

Example. If a 30-year-old woman wants to exercise at moderate intensity yet still achieve a training effect, the exercise heart rate should equal 70% of her age-predicted maximum (190 b · min^{-1}), or a target heart rate of 133 b · min^{-1} (0.70 × 190). For a 40-year-old man, on the other hand, the target heart rate equals 126 b · min^{-1} (0.70 × 180). By trial and error, using progressive increments of exercise, each person arrives at a walking, jogging, or cycling speed to produce the desired target heart rate.

In carrying out this procedure, the person should exercise moderately for 3 to 5 minutes and count the pulse rate for 10 seconds immediately afterward. If heart rate falls below the desired target, repeat the exercise at a higher intensity (jogging instead of walking, or cycling faster or against increased resistance). If the 30-year-old woman wants to train at 85% of HR_{max}, exercise intensity must increase to produce a heart rate of 161 b·min^{-1} (0.85 × 190).

Adjust for Swimming and Other Upper-Body Exercises. In trained and untrained subjects, maximum heart rate swimming averages about 13 b·min^{-1} lower than running. The smaller muscle mass of the arms primarily used during swimming exercise probably causes the difference. Consequently, estimated HR_{max} must be adjusted downward when selecting swimming or other forms of upper-body exercise as the training mode. We recommend subtracting 13 b·min^{-1} from the age-pre-

Estimating Maximum Heart Rate

$$HR_{max} \; (b{\cdot}min^{-1}) = 220 - age, \; y$$

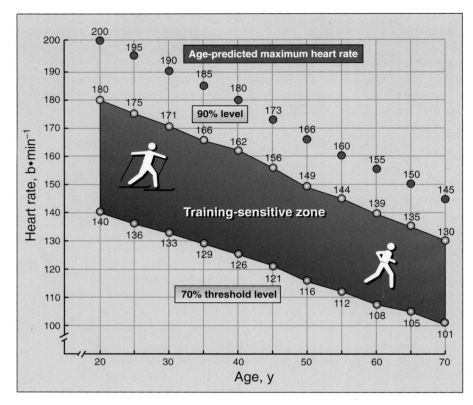

Figure 14.17
Maximal heart rates and training-sensitive zone for use in aerobic training for different ages.

sarily better because excessive exercise increases the chance for sustaining bone, joint, and muscle injuries. In Chapter 20, we point out that the health benefits from regular exercise do not require "heroic" levels of physical activity. Unfortunately, far too many people push themselves, adhering to the misleading slogan, "no pain, no gain."

Train at a Perception of Effort

In addition to oxygen uptake and heart rate, one can use a "Likert type" rating scale similar to that used in psychology to rate levels of perception. The most popular perceived effort rating scale used with exercise is the ratings of perceived exertion (RPE) scale. With this approach, a person rates how they feel (psychological perception) on a numerical scale (Fig. 14.18) Exercise intensities that produce greater energy expenditure and physiologic strain yield higher ratings of

dicted HR_{max} values in Figure 14.17. A 25 year-old person wanting to swim at 80% of HR_{max} should select a swimming speed that produces a heart rate of about 146 b·min^{-1} (0.80 × [195 − 13]). This more accurately represents the appropriate training heart rate for swimming.

Effectiveness of Less Intense Exercise

The recommendation for training at 70% of HR_{max} as the threshold for aerobic improvement represents a *general guideline* for establishing a comfortable, yet effective exercise intensity. Twenty to 30 minutes of continuous exercise at the 70% level stimulates a training effect; however, exercise at a lower intensity of 60 to 65% HR_{max} for 45 minutes also proves beneficial. *In general, longer exercise duration offsets lower exercise intensity, particularly for older and less fit subjects.* Regardless of exercise level, more is not neces-

Aerobic Training Reduces Submaximal Exercise Heart Rate

Submaximal exercise heart rate can decrease up to about 10 to 20 b·min^{-1} during a 12-week aerobic training program. For this reason, exercise intensity should be adjusted continually to maintain appropriate training intensity as training progresses.

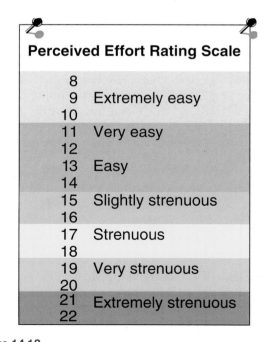

Perceived Effort Rating Scale

8	
9	Extremely easy
10	
11	Very easy
12	
13	Easy
14	
15	Slightly strenuous
16	
17	Strenuous
18	
19	Very strenuous
20	
21	Extremely strenuous
22	

Figure 14.18
Example showing a perceived effort rating scale ranging from # 8 – Extremely easy to # 22 – Extremely strenuous. The more popular RPE scale ranges from #6 to #20.

How to Determine 10,000-m Running Pace From Lactate Threshold

Physiologic measurements during exercise help to 1) pinpoint strengths and weaknesses about an individual's performance capacity and potential, and 2) optimize training intensity for the most effective outcome. For example, research indicates that athletes run 10,000 m at a pace approximately 5 m·min^{-1} faster than the running speed associated with their lactate threshold (LT). Knowledge of the exercise intensity associated with LT should provide the athlete and coach with a realistic performance expectation based on an individualized assessment of the aerobic metabolic response to exercise. This information puts into a biologic perspective (for both coach and athlete) an answer to the questions: "How fast can I perform this event?", and "What training pace is best for me?"

Testing

Step 1. Determine the LT (see *How to Measure Lactate Threshold*, Chapter 10; if you cannot directly measure blood lactate, use the ventilatory threshold method). Figure 1 shows the relationship between blood lactate and oxygen uptake ($\dot{V}O_2$) during graded treadmill exercise, with LT indicated by the arrow. In this example, LT occurred at a $\dot{V}O_2$ of 43.5 mL·kg^{-1}·min^{-1}.

Step 2. Determine the relationship between $\dot{V}O_2$ (mL·kg^{-1}·min^{-1}; either actual or estimated) and running speed (m·min^{-1}). The subject runs on a treadmill for 5 minutes at each of six different submaximal speeds. Construct a graph relating $\dot{V}O_2$ versus running speed (Fig. 2). Draw a best fit line through the plotted points.

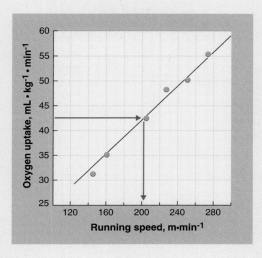

Figure 2
$\dot{V}O_2$ related to running speed during treadmill exercise at progressively faster running speeds.

Step 3. Convert the $\dot{V}O_2$ at LT (43.5 mL·kg^{-1}·min^{-1}; Fig. 1) to a running speed using the best-fit line presented in Figure 2. Draw a horizontal line from the oxygen uptake value on the Y-axis until it intersects the line of best fit; from this intersection, draw a perpendicular line to the X-axis that indicates running speed. The arrow shows the corresponding speed (m·min^{-1}) as 204 m·min^{-1}.

Computing Expected Performance

Assume an athlete exceeds by 5 m·min^{-1} his or her running speed at LT during training (and competition) for 10,000 m (and other endurance events); the projected average running speed for this person equals 209 m·min^{-1} (204 m·min^{-1} + 5 m·min^{-1}).

Determine the Projected Race Time for the 10,000-m Run

Use the data from Figures 1 and 2 to estimate the time for a 10,000-m race.

$$\text{Estimated time} = \text{Distance} \div \text{Speed}$$
$$= 10{,}000 \text{ m} \div 209 \text{ m·min}^{-1}$$
$$= 47.85 \text{ min } (47 \text{ min: } 51 \text{ s})$$

This analysis based on LT measurements indicates that the athlete should complete the 10,000-m run in 47 minutes and 51 seconds. It also represents a realistic estimate of an appropriate training intensity to achieve the performance goal.

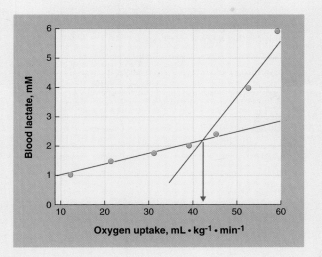

Figure 1
Determination of LT from measures of blood lactate and $\dot{V}O_2$ during graded treadmill exercise.

perceived effort. Ratings of physical effort can correspond with exercise heart rate, and individuals can readily learn to exercise at a specific rating level based on their subjective feeling of exertion. Within this framework, the axiom, "listen to your body," makes good sense.

Train at the Lactate Threshold

Research demonstrates the benefits of training at or slightly above an exercise level that represents the lactate threshold (LT). The accompanying *How to Determine 10,000-m Running Pace From Lactate Threshold* illustrates the use of the blood lactate-oxygen uptake relationship and oxygen uptake-running speed relationship to optimize exercise performance pace and training intensity. This approach determines exercise intensity at a level just slightly above the LT. As aerobic fitness improves, periodic re-evaluation should assess the LT-exercise intensity relationship.

One difference between the % HR_{max} and LT methods for setting training intensity lies in the physiologic systems overloaded. The heart rate method establishes an exercise stress for the central circulation (i.e., stroke volume, cardiac output), whereas adjusting training intensity to the lactate threshold considers the response and capability of the periphery (local vasculature and active muscle mass) for aerobic metabolism.

Continuous Versus Intermittent Aerobic Training

Two types of aerobic training include continuous and intermittent methods.

Continuous Training

Continuous or **long slow distance** (**LSD**) training requires sustained, steady-rate aerobic exercise. Because of its submaximal nature, exercise continues for considerable time in relative comfort. This makes LSD training ideal for people beginning an exercise program or wanting to reduce excess body weight.

The greatest health-related benefits of exercise emerge when a person moves from a sedentary lifestyle to one that incorporates only a moderate level of continuous aerobic exercise. LSD training generally progresses at the relatively comfortable threshold intensity of 70% HR_{max}, although it can increase to the 85 or 90% level.

Endurance athletes can overload the cardiovascular and energy transfer systems using continuous exercise training at nearly the same intensity as actual competition. This specifically activates slow-twitch muscle fibers in sustained exercise. A champion middle-distance runner may run five miles continuously in 25 minutes during workouts at a heart rate of 180 b·min^{-1}; this pace does not exhaust the athlete, but still nearly duplicates race conditions. By finishing each exercise session with several all-out sprints stopped 30 to 40 seconds before exhaustion, the athlete also trains the short-term anaerobic system (glycolysis) that contributes to race performance, particularly at the finish. A marathon runner trains at a slightly slower pace than a middle-distance athlete to simulate the intensity and distance of actual competition.

Interval Training

Periods of intense activity interspersed with moderate to low energy expenditure characterize many sport and life activities. **Interval exercise training** simulates this variation in energy transfer intensity through specific spacing of exercise and rest periods. With this approach, a person trains at an inordinately high exercise intensity with minimal fatigue that would normally prove exhausting if done continuously. Rest-to-exercise intervals vary from a few seconds to several minutes depending on the energy system(s) overloaded. Four factors help to formulate the interval training prescription:

1. Intensity of exercise
2. Duration of exercise interval
3. Duration of recovery interval
4. Repetitions of exercise-recovery interval

Running continuously at a 4-minute mile pace exhausts most people within a minute due to rapid lactate accumulation. However, running at this speed for only 15 seconds followed by a 30-second rest period enables a person to accomplish 4 minutes of running at this near-record pace. Of course, this does not equate to a 4-minute mile, but during 4 minutes of running, the person covers a one-mile distance even though the combined exercise and rest intervals require 11 minutes 30 seconds.

Rationale for Interval Training

A sound metabolic rationale forms the basis for interval training. In the example of a continuous run by an average person at a 4-minute mile pace, the predominant energy for exercise comes from the short-term anaerobic energy pathway with a rapid lactate accumulation. The individual becomes exhausted within 60 to 90 seconds. On the other hand, running at this speed for 15-second intervals or less places significant demands on the immediate energy system (intramuscular ATP and PCr) with little lactate accumulation. Recovery becomes predominantly "alactic" in nature and occurs rapidly. The subsequent exercise interval can begin after only a brief rest period. Repetitively linking specific exercise and rest intervals (interval training) eventually places considerable demand on aerobic energy metabolism.

In interval training, as with other forms of physiologic conditioning, exercise training intensity must overload the specific energy system(s) the person desires to improve. Table 14.5 outlines a practical method for determining exercise intensity for interval training in running and swimming.

Available evidence does *not* support superiority for either continuous or interval training to improve aerobic fitness. Both methods probably can be applied interchange-

ably. On the other hand, continuous LSD training gives the endurance athlete a more "task-specific" cardiovascular and metabolic overload that more closely mimics the duration and intensity of race conditions. Likewise, sprint and middle-distance athletes benefit from the intense metabolic demands and specific neuromuscular and fiber-type activation that interval training provides.

Formulating the Exercise:Relief Interval

Exercise Interval

- Add 1.5 to 5 s to the exerciser's "best time" for training distances between 60 and 220 yd for running and 15 and 55 yd for swimming. If a person covers 60 yd from a running start in 8 s, the exercise duration for each repeat equals 8 + 1.5 or 9.5 s. Add 3 s to the best running time for interval training distances of 110 yd and 5 s to a distance of 220 yd. This particular application of interval training most effectively trains the intramuscular high-energy phosphate component of the anaerobic energy system.

- For training distances of 440 yd running or 110 yd swimming, determine the exercise rate by subtracting 1 to 4 s from the average 440-yd portion of a mile run or 110-yd portion of a 440-yd swim. If a person runs a 7:00-minute mile (averaging 105 s per 440 yd), the interval time for each 440-yd repeat ranges between 104 s (105 − 1) and 101 s (105 − 4).

- For run training intervals beyond 440 yd (and swim intervals beyond 110 yd) add 3 to 4 s to the average

TABLE 14.5
Guidelines for determining interval-training exercise intensities for running and swimming different distances[a]

INTERVAL TRAINING DISTANCES (YARDS)		WORK RATE FOR EACH EXERCISE INTERVAL OR REPEAT	
Run	**Swim**		
55	15	1.5	seconds *slower* than best
110	25	3.0	times from a running
			(or swimming) start
220	55	5.0	for each distance
440	110	1 to 4 s *faster* than the average run or 110-yd swim time recorded during a 1-mile run or 440-yd swim	
660–1320	165–320	3 to 4 s *slower* than the average 440-yd run or 100-yard swim time recorded during a 1-mile run or 440-yd swim	

[a] From Fox, E. L., and Mathews, D. K.: *Interval Training.* Philadelphia: W. B. Saunders, 1974.

440-yard portion of a mile run or 110-yard portion of a 440-yard swim. In running an 880-yard interval, the 7:00-minute miler runs each interval in about 216 seconds ([105 + 3] × 2 = 216).

Relief Interval

- The relief (recovery) interval occurs either passively (rest-relief) or actively (exercise-relief). Recovery duration represents a multiple of the exercise interval. A 1:3 ratio overloads the immediate energy system. For a sprinter who runs 10-second intervals, the relief interval equals 30 seconds. For training the short-term glycolytic energy system, the relief interval doubles (ratio of 1:2). Thus, a 2-minute recovery follows a 1-minute run or swim. These specified ratios of exercise to relief for training provide for sufficient restoration of high-energy phosphates and lactate removal so subsequent exercise proceeds without undue fatigue.

- For training the long-term aerobic energy system, the exercise:relief interval usually equals 1:1 or 1:1.5. During a 60- to 90-second exercise interval, for example, oxygen uptake increases rapidly to a high level. Although some lactate accumulates during this relatively intense exercise, duration remains brief enough to prevent exhaustion. A one to two-minute recovery permits exercise to begin again before oxygen uptake returns to its pre-exercise level. Consecutive repeat exercise:relief intervals ensures that cardiovascular response and aerobic metabolism eventually maintain near-maximal levels throughout exercise and recovery. Performing continuously at this exercise intensity would exhaust the person within several minutes and training would cease.

Maintaining Aerobic Fitness

An intriguing question concerns the optimal frequency, duration, and intensity of exercise required to retain improved aerobic fitness. If exercise intensity remains at the training level, training frequency and duration can decrease by as much as two-thirds without decrements in aerobic power (e.g., 6-day a week training reduced to 2 days; 40-min a day reduced to 13 min). However, even a one-third reduction in exercise intensity, with training frequency and duration held constant causes $\dot{V}O_{2max}$ to significantly decline. *This indicates that exercise intensity represents the primary factor to maintain improved aerobic capacity with training.*

Fitness components other than $\dot{V}O_{2max}$ may more readily suffer adverse effects from reduced total training volume. In one study, $\dot{V}O_{2max}$ remained unchanged in endurance athletes who significantly reduced weekly training volume (decreased duration and frequency) from 6 to 10 hours weekly to one 35-minute weekly session over 4 weeks. Despite maintaining aerobic capacity, endurance running performance significantly decreased, as did glycogen reserves and the level of fat oxidization during high-intensity, aerobic exercise.

Exercise Training During Pregnancy

With a considerable numer of women involved in physically demanding occupations and active lifestyles, growing interest has emerged concerning exercise and pregnancy. Figure 14.19 shows that walking, swimming, and aerobics were the most popular physical activities during pregnancy among 9953 women from 48 states who gave birth during 1996. Forty-two percent of all women reported they exercised, with one-half exercising for longer than 6 months. Older mothers, women who delivered more than one child or had previous children, and women with unfavorable reproductive histories, were less likely to exercise during pregnancy. Areas of interest concerning exercise and pregnancy include:

- How pregnancy affects energy cost and physiologic demands of exercise
- Effects of exercise intensity on fetal blood supply
- Effects of regular exercise on pregnancy course and outcome

Energy Cost and Physiologic Demands of Exercise

Cardiovascular responses during exercise in pregnancy follow normal patterns. An uncomplicated pregnancy offers no greater physiologic strain to the mother during moderate exercise other than provided by the additional weight gain and possible encumbrance of fetal tissue. Increases in maternal body mass add significantly to exercise effort in weight-bearing activities like walking, jogging, and stair climbing.

Fetal Blood Supply

Any factor that might compromise fetal blood supply raises concern when counseling women about exercise during pregnancy. Studies of uterine blood flow during exercise in various mammalian species indicate that healthy animals maintain adequate oxygen supply to the developing fetus during moderate to intense maternal exercise. However, fetal oxygen supply decreased considerably with maternal exercise in animals with restricted placental circulation.

Exercise probably diverts some blood from the uterus and visceral organs for preferential redistribution to active muscles; thus, intense exercise could pose a hazard to a fetus with restricted placental blood flow. In addition, ele-

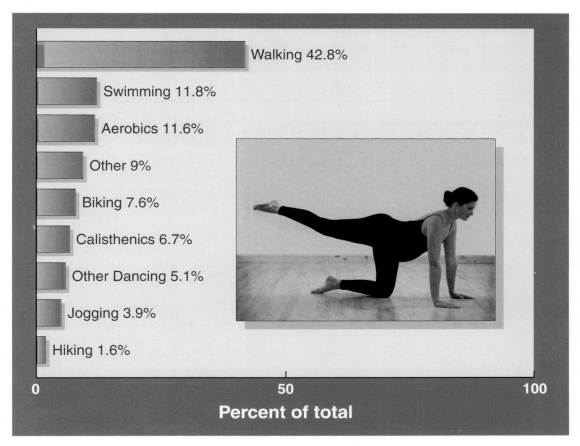

Figure 14.19
Pattern of exercise during pregnancy. (From Zhang, J. and Saultz, D.A.: Exercise during pregnancy among US women. *Ann. Epidemiol.*, 6:53, 1996.)

vated maternal core temperature hinders heat dissipation from the fetus through the placenta. Maternal hyperthermia negatively affects fetal development (e.g., increased risk for neural tube defect) early in pregnancy. During warm weather, pregnant women should exercise in the cool part of the day and for shorter intervals while maintaining regular fluid intake.

Current medical opinion maintains that 30 or 40 minutes of moderate aerobic exercise by a previously active, healthy, low-risk woman during an uncomplicated pregnancy does not compromise fetal oxygen supply, acid-base status, or produce other adverse effects to mother or fetus. Performed on a regular basis, moderate exercise not only maintains cardiovascular fitness but actually produces a training effect.

Pregnancy Course and Outcome

Until recently, no overall consensus existed on whether regular exercise enhanced the course of pregnancy, including labor, delivery, and outcome. We believe current data support a recommendation for regular, moderate physical activity during pregnancy, even after the first trimester. In many ways, maternal physiologic responses

and adaptations to exercise beneficially interact with physiologic changes in pregnancy.

Table 14.6 presents neonatal data from 77 babies whose mothers exercised at least 30 minutes, three or more times weekly before conception, and continued running and aerobic dancing at or above 50% of the preconception exercise level throughout pregnancy. Heart rate and daily duration of physical activity during field testing quantified exercise performance before and during pregnancy. The control group consisted of babies from mothers who, although physically active prior to pregnancy, chose not to continue exercising after confirmation of pregnancy (first trimester). Exercise and control groups were matched for general health, physical fitness, education, family income, age, parity, contraceptive use, pregravid weight, job type, dietary intake, sleep-activity cycles, smoking, and alcohol intake. All analyses included clinically normal pregnancies; delivery of all babies took place at term (between 266 and 294 days), and neonatal measurements occurred within 2 hours of birth.

The results indicated reductions in birth weight (-310 g), birth weight percentile (-20), two-site skinfold thickness (-1.5 mm), skinfold percentile (-30), calculated percent body fat (-5%), and fat mass (-220 g) for babies

TABLE 14.6
Effects of maternal exercise on neonatal parameters

PARAMETER	CONTROL N=55	EXERCISE N=77
Birth weight, g	3691	3381**
Birth weight percentile	65.0	45.0**
Length, cm	51.3	51.4
Sum triceps and subscapula skinfolds, mm	11.8	9.3**
Skinfold percentile	58.0	28.0**
%Body fat*	16.2	11.2**
Fat mass*, g	603	382**
Fat-free body mass*, g	3088	3000**
Head girth, cm	35.2	35.0

*Calculated from skinfolds

**Significantly different than control

From Clapp, I.F.: Neonatal morphometrics after endurance exercise during pregnancy. *Am. J. Obstet Gynecol.*, 163:1805, 1990.

in the maternal exercise group. These data confirm an asymmetric pattern of growth restriction, with approximately 70% of the difference in birth weight due to differences in neonatal fat mass. The researchers concluded that continuation of a regular aerobic exercise at or above a minimal training level during pregnancy impacts fetal size, primarily the quantity of body fat.

A 5-year follow-up of 20 of the original exercise and con-

trol babies provides insight into possible long-term effects of maternal exercise during the second and third trimesters of pregnancy. The researchers matched exercise and control children for gender, birth order, gestational age at delivery (±5 days), and the following post-natal events: clinically normal growth and development (between 10th and 90th percentiles throughout the first year and achievement of developmental milestones on schedule); absence of serious illness; type of child care in or outside the home; and new siblings. No child in either group had formal preschool academic experience outside the home. Also, parents of exercise and control children were matched for smoking behavior, socioeconomic status, education, marital stability, and maternal and paternal morphometry (stature, body mass, % body fat).

Table 14.7 shows the follow-up results at 5 years of age. The offspring of women who exercised maintained similar height and head girth, but weighed less (1.5 kg) and had a lower sum of five skinfolds (7 mm), and lower upper-arm fat (1.34 cm²) than control children. Surprisingly, the offspring of active mothers performed significantly better on the intelligence test (125 vs. 116) and oral language

TABLE 14.7
Effects of maternal exercise during pregnancy on different variables of the offspring at birth and 5 years

OFFSPRING CHARACTERISTIC	AT BIRTH		AT AGE 5 YEARS	
	EXERCISE N = 20	CONTROL N = 20	EXERCISE N = 20	CONTROL N = 20
Body mass, kg	3.4	3.6	18.0	19.5
Stature, cm	51.7	51.9	109.0	110.2
Sum 5 skinfolds, mm			37.0	44.0
Upper-arm fat, cm²			7.89	9.23
Body fat, %	10.5	15.1		
Fat-free body mass, kg	3.0	3.1		
Head girth, cm	35.2	35.4	51.8	51.4
Chest girth, cm	34.1	34.5	55.2	54.3
Abdominal girth, cm	30.9	33.6	50.9	51.9
General intelligence*			125	116
Oral language skill**			119	109

* Wechsler Preschool and Primary Scale of Intelligence

** Peabody Picture Vocabulary Test; Expressive One Word Picture Vocabulary Test; Clinical Evaluation of Language Fundamentals

From Clapp, J.F.: Morphometric and neurodevelopmental outcome at age 5 years of the offspring of women who continued to exercise regularly throughout pregnancy. *J. Pediatrics*, 129:856, 1996.

How to Prescribe Exercise During Pregnancy

Pregnancy places extraordinary demands on a women's physiology, necessitating some modification in exercise prescription. Pregnant women should consult a physician prior to initiating an exercise program (or to modify an existing program) to rule out possible complications. This pertains particularly to women of low fitness status and little exercise experience prior to pregnancy. The table lists 14 common contraindications to exercising during pregnancy.

Exercise during pregnancy should heighten awareness about heat dissipation, adequate calorie and nutrient intake, and knowing when to reduce exercise intensity. For a normal, uncomplicated pregnancy, light to moderate exercise does not negatively affect fetal development; the benefits of properly prescribed regular exercise during pregnancy generally outweigh potential risks.

EXERCISE GUIDELINES

Exercise Mode
Avoid exercise in the supine position, particularly after the first trimester. Supine exercise can impair venous return (mass of the fetus compresses the inferior vena cava), which could ultimately reduce cardiac output and uterine blood flow. Non-weight-bearing exercise (e.g., cycling, swimming) minimizes gravity's effects and the added mass associated with fetal development. Weight-bearing exercise in moderation should not pose a risk.

Exercise Frequency
Three days a week emphasizing continuous, steady-rate effort. With more frequent exercise, reduce the intensity.

Exercise Duration
Thirty to 40 minutes, depending on how the person feels.

Exercise Intensity
Pregnancy alters the relationship between heart rate and oxygen uptake, making it difficult to establish exercise guidelines from heart rate. An effective alternative establishes exercise intensity based on rating of perceived exertion (RPE), which should range between 11 ("fairly light") to 13 ("somewhat hard").

Rate of Progression
Perform exercise on a regular basis; moderate aerobic exercise maintains cardiovascular fitness and often produces a small training effect. For most women, exercise progression to induce training effects should not be a goal, but rather maintenance of cardiorespiratory fitness, muscle mass, and physician-recommended weight gain. The combined effects of pregnancy per se and regular exercise often produce improved fitness after delivery.

Other Issues
Hyperthermia can negatively affect fetal development (increased risk for neural tube defect) chiefly during the first trimester of pregnancy. Thus, exercise during hot weather should occur in the cool part of the day (for shorter intervals), while maintaining adequate fluid intake. Periodic rest intervals minimize excessive fatigue and thermal stress. *Using a sauna or hot tub immersion increases risk of fetal hyperthermia and impaired development.*

When to Stop Exercise and Seek Medical Advice
Exercise should be immediately discontinued under the following conditions:

- Any signs of vaginal bleeding
- Any gush of fluid from the vagina (premature rupture of membranes)
- Sudden swelling of ankles, hands, or face
- Persistent, severe headaches and/or disturbances in vision; unexplained lightheadedness or dizziness
- Elevated pulse rate or blood pressure that does not rapidly return to normal following exercise
- Excessive fatigue, palpitations, or chest pain
- Persistent uterine contractions (more than 6 to 8 per h)
- Unexplained or unusual abdominal pain
- Insufficient weight gain (less than 1.0 kg per month during the last two trimesters)

CONTRAINDICATIONS FOR EXERCISING DURING PREGNANCY

Pregnancy induced hypertension	Pre-term rupture of membranes
Pre-term labor during the prior or current pregnancy	Incompetent cervix
Persistent second to third trimester bleeding	Intrauterine growth retardation
Type 1 diabetes	History of two or more spontaneous abortions
Multiple pregnancy	Smoking
Excessive alcohol intake	History of premature labor
Anemia	Excessive obesity

skills (119 vs. 109). To explain the increased mental capacity of the exercise group, the researchers hypothesized that some stimulus associated with regular exercise during pregnancy (e.g., intermittent stress, vibration, sound, motion, accelerated heartbeat) benefits fetal neurological development. *The offspring of exercising women did not show evidence of a comparative deficit in any area examined.* These findings should reassure active women who chose to continue exercising during an uncomplicated pregnancy.

summary

1. Activation of a specific energy transfer system in exercise provides a means to classify diverse physical activities. Effective training allocates appropriate time to overload the energy system(s) involved in the activity.

2. Exercise intensity and duration largely contribute to anaerobic and aerobic energy transfer during physical activity. During sprint-power activities, primary energy transfer involves the immediate and short-term energy systems. The long-term aerobic system becomes progressively more important in activities longer than 2 minutes duration.

3. Proper exercise training recognizes four principles for producing and maintaining optimum improvements: overload, specificity, individual differences, and reversibility.

4. Anaerobic training increases resting intramuscular levels of anaerobic substrates and key glycolytic enzymes. This usually increases all-out, sprint-power exercise performance.

5. The step test uses heart rate to evaluate the efficiency of cardiovascular response to aerobic exercise and training.

6. Aerobic training must overload both circulatory function and metabolic capacity of specific muscles. Peripheral adaptations in active tissues exert a substantial effect on exercise performance.

7. Initial fitness level, frequency of training, duration of exercise, and exercise intensity constitute the major factors that affect aerobic training improvement. Of these, exercise intensity provides the most profound effect.

8. Aerobic training adaptations include increases in mitochondrial size and number, improved activity of aerobic enzymes, greater capillarization of trained muscle, and enhanced oxidation of fats during submaximal exercise. Each factor increases a muscle's potential to generate ATP aerobically.

9. Aerobic training induces functional and dimensional changes in the cardiovascular system. These include a decrease in resting and submaximal exercise heart rate, enlarged left ventricular cavity, enhanced stroke volume and cardiac output, and an expanded $a\text{-}\bar{v}O_2$ difference.

10. Two ways can establish training intensity: 1) on an absolute basis (standard exercise load or oxygen uptake), or 2) on a relative basis geared to an individual's physiologic response ($\%\dot{V}O_{2max}$ or $\%HR_{max}$).

11. Prescribing exercise based on a percent of HR_{max} (at least 65 to 70% age-predicted HR_{max}) or a rating of perceived exertion provide the most convenient yet effective methods.

12. Three days minimum per week represents an effective frequency for aerobic training. Optimal frequency levels have not been established.

13. When intensity, duration, and frequency remain constant, similar training improvements emerge regardless of training mode, provided the evaluation test utilizes the training exercise.

14. If exercise intensity remains at the training level, exercise frequency and duration can decrease by up to two-thirds without compromising gains in $\dot{V}O_{2max}$.

15. Moderate aerobic exercise by a previously active, healthy, low-risk women during an uncomplicated pregnancy does not compromise fetal well being or produce adverse affects to the mother.

thought questions

1. Discuss whether regular physical activity benefits a person, even if exercise remains insufficient to stimulate a training effect.

2. Your personal training client insists that a single mode of cross-training exercise improves aerobic fitness for all physical activities requiring a high level of aerobic fitness. Give your opinion regarding the effectiveness of single-mode cross-training exercise.

3. Respond to the question: "How long must I exercise to get in shape?"

4. What information do you need to know to develop a program to effectively improve and evaluate aerobic capacity for the specific physical job performance requirements for 1) firefighters, 2) police officers, and 3) oilfield workers.

5. As a personal trainer, outline your approach to establishing training guidelines and personalizing the exercise prescription for a fit male and unfit female.

selected references

Ahmaidi, S., et al.: Effects of interval training at the ventilatory threshold on clinical and cardiorespiratory responses in elderly humans. *Eur. J. Appl. Physiol.*, 78:170, 1998.

American College of Sports Medicine: Position stand on the recommended quantity and quality of exercise for developing and maintaining cardiorespiratory and muscular fitness, and flexibility in healthy adults. *Med. Sci. Sports Exerc.*, 30:975, 1998.

Anderson, R.E., et al.: Effects of lifestyle activity vs structured aerobic exercise in obese women. *JAMA*, 281:335, 1999.

Bassett, D.R., Jr., and Howley, E.T.: Maximal oxygen uptake: "classical" versus "contemporary" viewpoints. *Med. Sci. Sports Exerc.*, 29:591, 1997.

Belman, M. J., and Gaesser, G. A.: Exercise training below and above the lactate threshold in the elderly. *Med. Sci. Sports Exerc.*, 23 : 562, 1991.

Bouchard, C., and Pérusse, L.: Heredity, activity level, fitness, and health. In: *Physical Activity, Fitness, and Health*. Bouchard, C. et al. (eds.). Champaign, IL: Human Kinetics, 1994.

Carpenter, M.W.: Physical activity, fitness, and health of the pregnant mother and fetus. In: *Physical Activity, Fitness, and Health*. Bouchard, C. et al., (eds.). Champaign, IL: Human Kinetics, 1994.

Clapp, J.F., III, et al.: Neonatal behavior profile of the offspring of women who continue to exercise regularly throughout pregnancy. *Am. J. Obstet. Gynecol.*, 180:91, 1999.

Coggan, A.R.: Plasma glucose metabolism during exercise: effect of endurance training in humans. *Med. Sci. Sports Exerc.*, 29:620, 1997.

Cureton, K. J., et. al.: Generalized equation for prediction of $\dot{V}O_2$ peak from 1-mile run/walk performance. *Med. Sci. Sports Exerc.*, 27:445, 1995.

Donovan, C.M., and Sumida, D.D.: Training enhanced hepatic gluconeogenesis: the importance for glucose homeostasis during exercise. *Med. Sci. Sports Exerc.*, 29:628, 1997.

Dunn, A.L., et al.: Comparison of lifestyle and structured interventions to increase physical activity and cardiorespiratory fitness. *JAMA*, 281:327, 1999.

Foster, C., et al.: Stability of the blood lactate-heart rate relationship in competitive athletes. *Med. Sci. Sports Exerc.*, 31:578, 1999.

Hagberg, J.M., et al.: Expanded blood volumes contribute to increased cardiovascular performance of endurance-trained older men. *J. Appl. Physiol.*, 85:484, 1998.

Hatch, M., et al.: Maternal leisure-time exercise and timely delivery. *Am. J. Public Health*, 88:1528, 1998.

Hill, D.W., et al.: Temporal specificity in adaptations in high-intensity exercise training. *Med. Sci. Sports Exerc.*, 30:450, 1998.

Holloszy, J. O.: Metabolic consequences of endurance training. In: *Exercise, Nutrition, and Energy Metabolism*. Horton, E. S. and Terjung, R. L. (eds.). New York: Macmillan, 1988.

Jones, B. H., et al.: Epidemiology of injuries associated with physical training among young men in the army. *Med. Sci. Sports Exerc.*, 25: 197,1993.

Joyner, M. J.: Physiological limiting factors and distance running: influence of gender and age on record performances. In: *Exercise and Sport Sciences Reviews*. Vol. 21. Holloszy, J. O. (ed.). Baltimore, MD: Williams & Wilkins, 1993.

Kohrt, W. M., et al.: Longitudinal assessment of responses of triathletes to swimming, cycling, and running. *Med. Sci. Sports Exerc.*, 21:569, 1989.

Krieder, R.B., et al.: *Overtraining in Sport*. Champaign, IL: Human Kinetics, 1998.

Krip, B., et al.: Effect of alterations in blood volume on cardiac function during maximal exercise. *Med. Sci. Sports Exerc.*, 29:1469, 1997.

Kuipers, M.: How much is too much? Performance aspects of overtraining. *Res. Quart. Exerc. Sport*, 67:S65, 1996.

Londeree, B.R.: Effect of training on lactate/ventilatory thresholds: a meta-analysis. *Med. Sci. Sports Exerc.*, 29:837, 1997.

Londeree, B.R., et al.: %$\dot{V}O_{2max}$ versus %HR_{max} regressions for six modes of exercise. *Med. Sci. Sports Exerc.*, 27:458, 1995.

Lotgering, F.K., et al.: Respiratory and metabolic responses to endurance cycle exercise in pregnant and postpartum women. *Int. J. Sports Med.*, 19:193, 1998.

MacDougall, J.D., et al.: Muscle performance and enzymate adaptations to sprint interval training. *J. Appl. Physiol.*, 84:2138, 1998.

MacKinnon, L.T.: Effects of overtraining and overreaching on immune function. In: *Overtraining and Overreaching in Sport*. Kreider, R., et al. (eds.). Champaign, IL: Human Kinetics, 1997.

Martin, W.H: Effect of endurance training on fatty acid metabolism during whole body exercise. *Med. Sci. Sports Exerc.*, 29:635, 1997.

McAllister, R.M.: Adaptations in control of blood flow with training: splanchnic and renal blood flows. *Med. Sci. Sports Exerc.*, 30:375, 1998.

Minotti, J. R., et. al.: Training-induced skeletal muscle adaptations are independent of systemic adaptations. *J. Appl. Physiol.*, 68:289, 1990.

Moore, R.L., and Palmer, B.M.: Exercise training and cellular adaptations of normal and diseased hearts. *Exerc. Sport Sci. Revs.*, 27:285, 1999.

National Association for Sport and Physical Education. *Physical Activity for Children: A Statement of Guidelines*. Reston, VA: 1998.

Nieuwland, P., et al.: Training effects on peak $\dot{V}O_2$, specific of the mode of movement, in rehabilitation of patients with coronary artery disease. *Int. J. Sports Med.*, 19:358, 1998.

Pivarnick, J. M.: Potential effects of maternal physical activity on birth weight: a brief review. *Med. Sci. Sports Exerc.*, 30:400, 1998.

Pollock, M.L., et al.: The recommended quantity and quality of exercise for developing and maintaining cardiorespiratory and muscular fitness, and flexibility in healthy adults. *Med. Sci. Sports Exerc.*, 30:975, 1998.

Raglin, J., and Bardukas, A.: Overtraining in athletes: the challenge of prevention. A consensus statement. *ACSM's Health & Fitness J.*, 3(2)27: 1999.

Richardson, R.S.: Oxygen transport: air to muscle cell. *Med. Sci. Sports Exerc.*, 30:53, 1998.

Robertson, R.J., and Noble, B.J.: Perception of physical exertion: methods, mediators, and applications. *Exer. Sport Sci. Revs.*, 25:407, 1997.

Rowland, T.W.: The biological basis for physical activity. *Med. Sci. Sports Exerc.*, 30:392, 1998.

Shephard, R.J., and Shek, P.N.: Acute and chronic over-exertion: do depressed immune responses provide useful markers? *Int. J. Sports Med.*, 19:159, 1998.

Stepto, N.K., et al.: Effects of different interval-training programs on cycling time-trial performance. *Med. Sci. Sports Exerc.*, 31:736, 1999.

Stoudemire, N.M., et al.: The validity of regulating blood lactate concentration during running by rating perceived exertion, *Med. Sci. Sports Exerc.*, 28:490, 1996.

Swain, D.P., et al.: Target heart rates for the development of cardiorespiratory fitness. *Med. Sci. Sports Exerc.*, 26:112, 1994.

Symposium: Training/overtraining: the first Ulm symposium. *Med. Sci. Sports Exerc.*, 30:1137, 1998.

Tabata, I., et al.: Effects of moderate-intensity endurance and high-intensity intermittent training on anaerobic capacity and $\dot{V}O_{2max}$. *Med. Sci. Sports Exerc.*, 28:1327, 1996.

Tabata, I., et al.: Metabolic profile of high intensity intermittent exercises. *Med. Sci. Sports Exerc.*, 29:390, 1997.

Weltman, A., et al.: Repeated bouts of exercise alter the blood lactate-RPE relation. *Med. Sci. Sports Exerc.*, 30:1113, 1998.

Zhang, J., and Savitz, D.A.: Exercise during pregnancy among US women. *Ann. Epidemiol.*, 6:53, 1996.

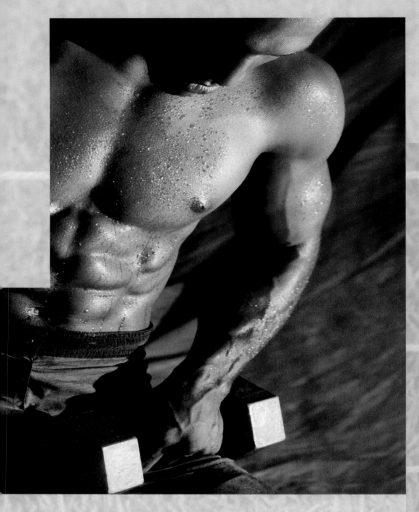

CHAPTER

15

Topics covered in this chapter

PART 1 Muscular Strength: Measurement and Improvement

Foundations for Studying Muscular Strength
Measurement of Muscular Strength
Strength Testing Considerations
Training Muscles to Become Stronger
Gender Differences in Muscular Strength
Resistance Training for Children
Systems of Resistance Training
Summary

PART 2 Adaptations To Resistance Training

Neural Adaptations
Muscle Adaptations
Connective Tissue and Bone Adaptations
Cardiovascular Adaptations
Metabolic Stress of Resistance Training
Body Composition Adaptations
Muscle Soreness and Stiffness
Summary
Thought Questions
Selected References

Training Muscles to Become Stronger

- Describe the following four methods to assess muscular strength: (a) cable tensiometry, (b) dynamometry, (c) one-repetition maximum (1-RM), and (d) computer-assisted isokinetic dynamometry.

- Outline the procedure to assess 1-RM for the bench press and leg press.

- Explain how to ensure test standardization and fairness when evaluating muscular strength.

- Compare absolute and relative upper- and lower-body muscular strength in men and women.

- Define concentric, eccentric, and isometric muscle actions, including examples of each.

- Recommend appropriate frequency, overload, and sets and repetitions for dynamic exercise resistance training.

- Explain the specificity of the training response for muscular strength relative to enhanced performance in sports and occupational tasks.

- Compare isokinetic resistance training with conventional dynamic and static resistance training.

- Describe the rationale for plyometric training to improve muscular strength and power, and give examples of exercises used for this purpose.

- Indicate how psychologic and muscular factors influence maximum strength capacity.

- Outline the major physiologic adaptations to resistance training.

- Develop a circuit resistance training program to improve muscular strength and aerobic fitness simultaneously.

- Describe tests to assess muscular endurance of the abdominals and chest-shoulder areas.

- Describe delayed-onset muscle soreness (DOMS) related to (a) type of exercise most frequently associated with DOMS, (b) best way to minimize DOMS effects when beginning a training program, and (c) significant cellular factors related to DOMS.

PART 1

Muscular Strength: Measurement and Improvement

Weightlifting began as a spectator sport in America in the early 1840s practiced by "strongmen" who showcased their prowess in traveling carnivals and sideshows. By the mid-1880s, measuring muscular strength was one way to evaluate an individual's fitness, particularly in schools and colleges. In 1897 at a meeting of College Gymnasium Directors, strength contests were established to determine overall body strength based on back, leg, arm, and chest strength. The first five colleges to rank in the 1898–1899 contest were Harvard, Columbia, Amherst, University of Minnesota, and Dickinson.

By the mid-1900s, physical culture specialists, body builders, competitive weight lifters, field-event athletes, and some wrestlers used weightlifting exercises. Most other athletes refrained from lifting weights because they feared they would lose joint flexibility and become muscle-bound and slow. Research in the late 1950s and early 1960s showed that muscle-strengthening exercises did not reduce movement speed or flexibility. In longitudinal experiments with untrained healthy subjects, heavy-resistance exercises actually *increased* speed and power of muscular effort.

In the following sections, we explore the underlying rationale for strength (resistance) training, including acute and chronic physiologic adjustments as muscles become stronger with training. The discussion centers on how to measure muscle strength, strength differences between men and women, different resistance training regimens, and longer-term adaptations to resistance training.

Foundations for Studying Muscular Strength

The inclusion of strength development programs as part of athletic training regimens is not new; it prepared men for warfare in ancient China, Greece, and Rome. When the ancient Olympic Games first began in 776 B.C., athletes trained nearly year-round and incorporated muscle-strengthening exercises into their training routines.

The scientific foundations for strength training for athletes began with the Chinese in 3600 B.C. In the Chou dynasty (1122-249 B.C.), conscripts had to pass weight-lifting tests before they became soldiers. Weight training also took place in ancient Egypt and India; sculptures and illustrations depict athletes training with heavy stone weights. Women also practiced weight training; wall mosaics recovered from Roman villas showed young girls exercising with hand-held weights. During the "Age of Strength" in the sixth century, weight lifting competitions often took place between soldiers and athletes. Galen, the famous early Greek physician (Chapter 1), refers to exercising with weights (halters) in his insightful treatise, *The Preservation of Health*.

The quest to develop muscular strength led to different systems of resistance training. The first modern text detailing a strength training system appears to be the 1561 text by Sir Thomas Elyot, *The Boke Named The Gouenour*. Elyot's treatise details a curriculum of study, including intellectual and artistic pursuits and physical education, about the role of gymnastics and strength development standards to which a governor should aspire. In the 1860s, Archibald MacLaren, a Scotsman, compiled the first system of physical training with dumbbells and barbells for the British army.

Objectives of Resistance Training

The study of strength development, besides having a theoretical basis, applies to six main areas:

1. Weight lifting and power lifting competition (who is strongest?)
2. Body building (maximize muscular hypertrophy for aesthetic goals)
3. General strength training (fitness and health enhancement)
4. Physical therapy (rehabilitation from injury or disease)
5. Sport-specific resistance training (maximize sport performance)
6. Muscle physiology (understanding muscle function and structure)

Definition of Terms in Resistance Training

Terms and jargon abound in the area of resistance training, yet certain terms consistently appear in the research literature and popular writings about resistance training methods and outcomes. Table 15.1 defines common resistance training terms.

Measurement of Muscular Strength

Four methods commonly assess **muscular strength**, i.e., the maximum force, tension, or torque generated by a muscle or muscle groups: cable tensiometry, dynamometry, one-repetition maximum, and computer-assisted electromechanical and isokinetic determinations.

Cable Tensiometry

Figure 15.1A shows a **cable tensiometer** measuring static muscular force during knee extension. Increased force on the cable depresses a riser over which the cable passes; this deflects the pointer and indicates the subject's strength score. The application of the tensiometer for strength measurements differs considerably from its original use for measuring tension on steel cables linking various parts of an airplane.

Cable tensiometry isolates a muscle at a specific joint angle to determine strength before and after training and rehabilitation. This strength assessment provides another advantage. Because it can be applied in different points of the movement phase, it clearly assesses strength (or weakness) of particular muscles at diverse joint angles throughout the range of motion (ROM). This cannot be done with standard weight-lifting tests.

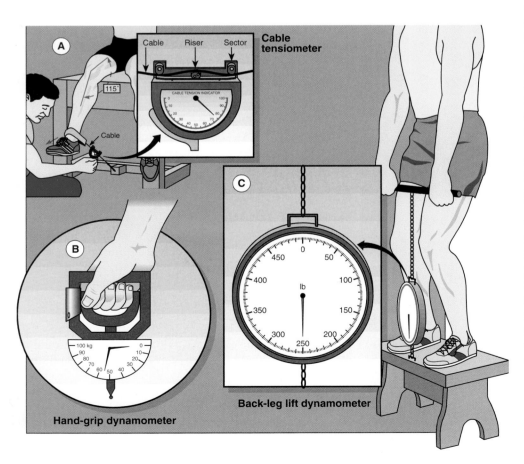

Figure 15.1
Measurement of static strength by (**A**) cable tensiometer, (**B**) hand-grip dynamometer, and (**C**) back-leg lift dynamometer.

TABLE 15.1
Definition of selected terms appearing in the resistance training literature

- **Cheating.** Breaking from strict form when performing an exercise (e.g., rather than maintaining an erect upper body when performing a standing arm curl, a slight body swing at the start the movement allows the person to lift a heavier weight or the same weight more times). Cheating increases injury risk if performed improperly.

- **Circuit Resistance Training (CRT).** Series of resistance training exercises performed in sequence with minimal rest between exercises. More frequent repetitions with less resistance (usually 40–50% of 1-RM) stimulate the cardiovascular system to produce an aerobic training effect.

- **Concentric Action.** Muscle shortening during force application.

- **Dynamic Constant External Resistance (DCER) Training.** Resistance training where external resistance or weight does not change; joint flexion and extension occurs with each repetition. Formerly (but incorrectly) referred to as "isotonic" exercise.

- **Eccentric Action.** Muscle lengthening occurs during force application.

- **Exercise Intensity.** Muscle force expressed as a percentage of muscle's maximum force-generating capacity or some level of maximum.

- **Isokinetic Action.** Muscle action performed at constant angular limb velocity.

- **Isometric Action.** Muscle action without noticeable change in muscle length.

- **Maximal Voluntary Muscle Action (MVMA).** Maximal force generated in one repetition (1-RM), or performing a series of submaximal actions to momentary failure.

- **Muscular Endurance.** Sustaining maximum (or submaximum) force; often determined by assessing maximum number of exercise repetitions at a percentage of maximum strength.

- **Overload.** A muscle acting against a resistance normally not encountered (unaccustomed stress).

- **Periodization.** Variation in training volume and intensity over a specified time period; goal to prevent staleness while peaking physiologically for competition.

- **Plyometrics.** Resistance training involving eccentric-to-concentric actions performed quickly so a muscle stretches slightly prior to the concentric action; utilizes stretch reflex to augment muscle's force-generating capacity.

- **Power.** Rate of performing work (Force × Distance ÷ Time, or Force × Velocity). Power applied to weightlifting relates to the mass lifted times the vertical distance it moves, divided by the time to complete the movement. If 100 pounds moves vertically three feet in one second, the power generated = 100 lb × 3 ft ÷ 1 s or 300 ft-lb · s^{-1}.

- **Progressive Overload.** Incrementally increasing the stress placed on a muscle to produce greater force or greater endurance.

- **Range of Motion (ROM).** Maximum movement through an arc of a body joint.

- **Repetition.** One complete exercise movement, usually consisting of concentric and eccentric muscle actions or one complete isometric muscle action.

- **Repetition Maximum (RM).** Greatest force generated for one repetition of a movement (1-RM), or predetermined number of repetitions (e.g., 5-RM or 10-RM).

- **Set.** Pre-established number of repetitions performed.

- **Sticking Point.** Region in an exercise movement (against a set resistance) that provides the greatest difficulty completing the movement.

- **Strength.** Maximum force-generating capacity of a muscle or group of muscles.

- **Torque.** Force that produces a turning, twisting, or rotary movement in any plane about an axis (e.g., movement of bones about a joint); commonly expressed in newton-meters (Nm).

- **Training Volume.** Total work performed in a single training session.

- **Variable Resistance Training.** Training with equipment that uses a lever arm, cam, hydraulic system, or pulley to alter the resistance to match increases and decreases in a muscle's capacity throughout a joint's ROM.

Objectives of Resistance Training for Overall Fitness and Sports Performance

- Increase maximal strength
- Increase explosive power (achieve maximum force rapidly)
- Improve repetitive rate of maximal power output
- Improve repetitive rate of submaximal power output (muscular endurance)
- Hypertrophy muscle fibers and connective tissue harness

Dynamometry

Figures 15.1B and C display hand-grip and back-lift **dynamometers** to assess static strength. Both devices operate on the principle of compression. Application of external force to the dynamometer compresses a steel spring and moves a pointer. By knowing how much force must move the pointer a given distance, one can determine how much external "static" force has been applied to the dynamometer.

One-Repetition Maximum

The **one-repetition maximum (1-RM)** technique refers to a dynamic method to assess muscular strength. To test **1-RM** for single or multiple muscle groups, the initial weight should be close to, but below maximum lifting capacity (see *How to Assess and Evaluate One-Repetition Maximum for Bench Press and Leg Press*). Depending on the muscle group, the weight increment usually ranges from 1 to 5 kg. The 1-RM maneuver requires concentric and eccentric muscle actions, but only the concentric phase of the action evaluates 1-RM.

Figure 15.2 illustrates two additional submaximal methods to evaluate a muscle's force-and power-generating capacity. In these tests, the greatest amount of weight lifted five or ten times becomes the repetition maximum to assess strength. The measurement procedure in these cases assesses 5-RM or 10-RM. The 5-RM and 10-RM methods are appropriate markers of muscular strength, particularly when testing children and older adults where maximal lifting may be contraindicated.

Computer-Assisted Electromechanical and Isokinetic Determinations

Microprocessor technology integrated with exercise equipment quantifies muscular force and power during a variety of movements. Modern instrumentation measures force, acceleration, and velocity of body segments in various movement patterns. Force platforms can measure the external application of muscular force by limbs during jumping. Other electromechanical devices measure forces generated dur-

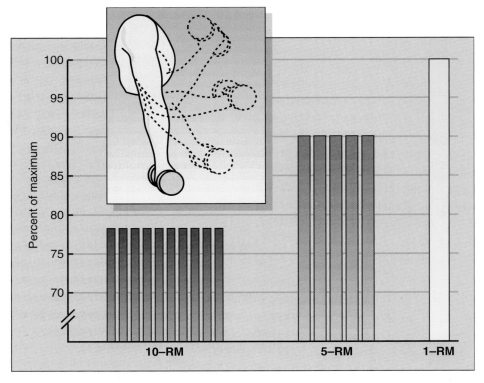

Figure 15.2
Three methods to assess force-generating capacity in a dynamic movement.

ing all movement phases of cycling, rowing, supine bench press, seated and upright leg press, and exercises for other trunk, arm, and leg movements.

An **isokinetic dynamometer**, an electromechanical instrument with a speed-controlling mechanism, accelerates to a preset, constant speed with applied force regardless of the force exerted on the movement arm. *Maximum force (or any percentage of maximum effort) can be applied during all phases of the movement at a constant velocity.* A load cell inside the dynamometer continuously records the applied force to calculate average force, power output, and total work throughout the ROM.

The interface of computer technology with mechanical devices provides valuable data for evaluating muscle function and prescribing exercise. Many devotees who still consider a maximum lift (1-RM) as the best criterion to assess overall muscular strength reject technologic advances that assess strength by computer. The argument for isokinetic methodology is that muscle strength dynamics involve considerably more than a final outcome from a 1-RM, 5-RM, or 10-RM lift. Even if two people have the same 1-RM score, the force-time curves could be considerably different. Differences in force dynamics (e.g., time to peak tension or rate of force development) reflect differences in how neuromuscular factors interact. The newer cyber-technologies assess many components of muscle dynamics, not *just* the maximum weight an individual can bench press or squat.

Strength Testing Considerations

The following factors affect strength testing, regardless of assessment method.

- Give standardized instructions.
- Allow a warm-up of uniform duration (e.g., 3 to 5 min) and intensity (e.g., 50% of previously established 1-RM).
- Provide adequate practice several days before testing to minimize a "learning" component that could compromise initial results or inflate evaluation of true training effects.
- Ensure constancy of limb position and/or measurement angle.
- Provide several trials (repetitions) to establish a criterion score for the strength measure.
- Administer strength tests with established high reliability (reproducibility) of scores (r >0.85).
- Consider individual differences in body size and composition when comparing strength scores among individuals and groups.

Physical Testing in the Occupational Setting

No one best measure of muscular strength exists. Each individual possesses an array of muscular strengths and powers. Often, these expressions of physiologic function and performance do not co-relate to each other. Likewise, a person has diverse capabilities for expressing aerobic capacity, depending on the muscle mass exercised. In the occupational setting, a 12-minute run to infer aerobic capacity for fire fighting or lumbering (both requiring significant upper-body aerobic function), or static grip or leg strength to evaluate the diverse dynamic strengths and powers required in such occupations, would be physiologically unwise in light of current knowledge about performance specificity. Measurement in the occupational setting should mimic specific job tasks and measure the physiologic demands of intensity, duration, and pace. For example, it would be unwise to assess ability to carry 20 kg of firehose by measuring leg press or squat strength. Even a bench press test would not be applicable. Instead, a functional test that assessed the ability to carry the 20-kg hose a distance of 30 m and then ascend 20 stairs, would more accurately reflect the requirements of performance specificity in the occupational setting.

Resistance Training Equipment

Speed of movement, amount of resistance, and ROM should be considered when training to improve muscle strength. To manipulate these factors, resistance training incorporates three types of equipment:

1. **Type I Resistance Equipment.** Standard weight lifting equipment (e.g., free weights or lifting machines) that does not control speed of movement or level of resistance through the full ROM.
2. **Type II Resistance Equipment.** Two subdivisions exist within this category: (a) constant speed (controlled by an isokinetic device), and (b) constant speed and variable resistance using a hydraulic or electromechanical device, but the individual controls the movement speed.
3. **Type III Resistance Equipment.** Variable movement speed and constant resistance provided by cam devices and concentric-eccentric machines. No currently available equipment allows muscles to exert maximum force at a muscle's maximum shortening velocity.

Training Muscles to Become Stronger

Strengthening muscles requires adherence to exercise training principles and specific guidelines.

How to Assess and Evaluate One-Repetition Maximum for Bench Press and Leg Press

Muscle strength refers to a muscle's maximum force-generating capacity. The maximum weight (resistance) lifted with proper form for one repetition (1-RM) for a particular muscle action measures dynamic muscular strength. A trial-and-error approach determines the 1-RM strength value. After each successful single lift, the weight increases by 5 to 10 pounds until the maximum weight is achieved. The individual rests 2 to 3 minutes between attempts.

The 1-RM bench press assesses maximum muscular strength of major muscle groups of the upper body; the leg press assesses maximum strength of major portions of the lower-body musculature. Dividing the 1-RM score by body weight (1-RM, lb ÷ body weight, lb) measures relative muscular strength and provides a frame of reference for evaluating different body weight comparisons (see table).

REFERENCE VALUES FOR 1-RM BENCH PRESS AND LEG PRESS EXPRESSED RELATIVE TO BODY WEIGHT*

	AGE, y			
RATING	**20–29**	**30–39**	**40–49**	**50–59**
		Men		
Excellent				
Bench Press	>1.26	>1.08	>0.97	>0.86
Leg Press	>2.08	>1.88	>1.76	>1.66
Good				
Bench Press	1.17–1.25	1.01–1.07	0.91–0.96	0.81–0.85
Leg Press	2.00–2.07	1.80–1.87	1.70–1.75	1.60–1.65
Average				
Bench Press	0.97–1.16	0.86–1.00	0.78–0.90	0.70–0.80
Leg Press	1.83–1.99	1.63–1.79	1.56–1.69	1.46–1.59
Fair				
Bench Press	0.88–0.96	0.79–0.85	0.72–0.77	0.65–0.69
Leg Press	1.65–1.82	1.55–1.62	1.50–1.55	1.40–1.45
Poor				
Bench Press	<0.87	<0.78	<0.71	<0.60
Leg Press	<1.64	<1.54	<1.49	<1.39
		Women		
Excellent				
Bench Press	>0.78	>0.66	>0.61	>0.54
Leg Press	>1.63	>1.42	>1.32	>1.26
Good				
Bench Press	0.72–0.77	0.62–0.65	0.57–0.60	0.51–0.53
Leg Press	1.54–1.62	1.35–1.41	1.26–1.31	1.13–1.25
Average				
Bench Press	0.59–0.71	0.53–0.61	0.48–0.56	0.43–0.50
Leg Press	1.35–1.53	1.20–1.34	1.12–1.25	0.99–1.12
Fair				
Bench Press	0.53–0.58	0.49–0.52	0.44–0.47	0.40–0.42
Leg Press	1.26–1.34	1.13–1.19	1.06–1.11	0.86–0.98
Poor				
Bench Press	<0.52	<0.48	<0.43	<0.39
Leg Press	<1.25	<1.12	<1.05	<0.85

Adapted from: Cooper Institute for Aerobics Research, 1997.

*Score = 1-RM, lb ÷ Body weight, lb.

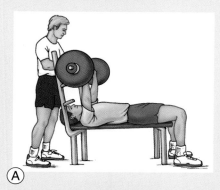
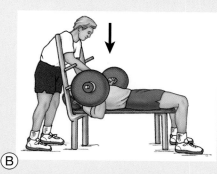
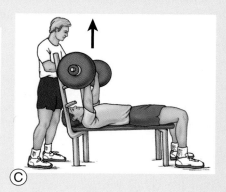

Beginning **(A)**, downward **(B)**, and upward **(C)** positions for the bench press.

Procedures for Bench Press Test

Muscle Groups
Shoulder flexors and adductors; elbow extensors.

Equipment
Barbell or bench press station on a single- or multi-station resistance machine.

Starting Position
1. Overhand (pronated) grip, slightly wider than shoulder-width apart.
2. Lay supine on a bench, feet on the floor straddling the bench.
3. Signal a spotter to position the bar at arms length above the chest with arms extended.

Movement
1. Downward movement: lower the bar until it touches the chest.
2. Upward movement: push the bar up to full elbow extension while maintaining body position without arching the back.

The spotter maintains grip on the bar throughout the movement without offering assistance; also helps to place the bar on the supports.

Procedures for Leg Press Test

Muscle groups
Knee extensors and hip extensors.

Equipment
Leg press on a single- or multi-station resistance machine.

Starting Position
1. Sit with the legs parallel and the feet on the machine's foot rests.
2. Grasp the seat's handle.

Movement
1. Forward movement: push the foot rests steadily forward; do not forcefully lock out the knees during extension.
2. Backward movement: move the footrests slowly back to the starting position.

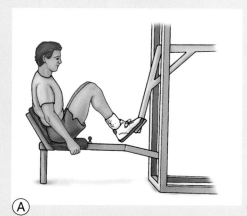
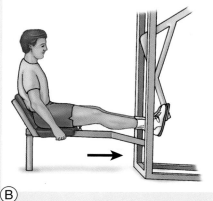
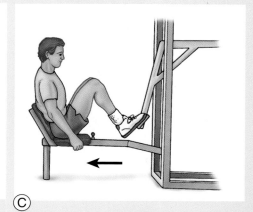

Beginning **(A)**, forward **(B)**, and return **(C)** positions for the seated leg press.

Overload and Intensity

Resistance training applies the **overload principle** with weights (dumbbells or barbells), immovable bars, straps, pulleys, or springs, and oil, air, and water hydraulic devices. *In each case, the muscle responds to the intensity of the overload rather than the form of overload.*

The amount of overload reflects a percent of maximum strength (1-RM) of a nonfatigued muscle or muscle group. Performing a **voluntary maximal muscle action** means the muscle must exert as much force as its *present* capacity allows. A partially fatigued muscle cannot generate the same force as a nonfatigued muscle. The last repetition to momentary failure in a set denotes a voluntary maximal muscle action. Muscular overload in resistance training usually requires such voluntary maximal muscle actions.

Three approaches (either singularly or in combination) apply muscular overload in resistance training:

1. Increase load or resistance
2. Increase number of repetitions
3. Increase speed of muscle action

Muscular overload, referred to as training intensity, is the most important concept in strength development; it relates to the necessity for training above a minimum threshold level to induce a training response. *Minimal intensity for muscular overload occurs between 60 to 70% of 1-RM.* This means that performing a large number of repetitions with a light resistance produces only minimal strength improvements.

Muscle Actions

- **Concentric action** (also called **miometric**) represents the most common form of muscle action; it occurs in dynamic activities where muscles shorten and produce tension through the ROM. Figure 15.3A illustrates a concentric muscle action by raising a dumb-

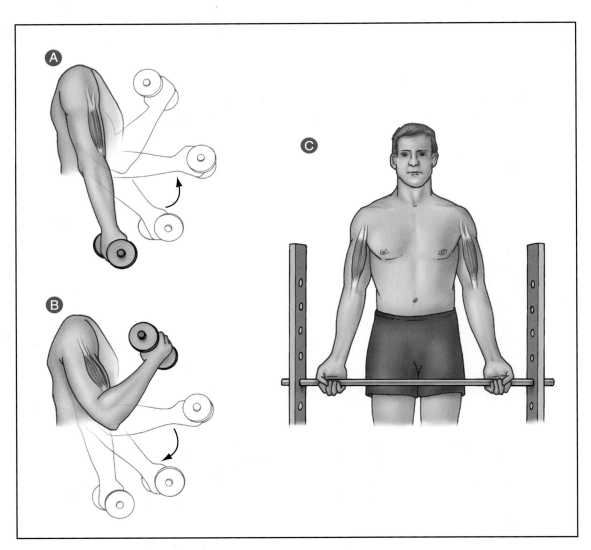

Figure 15.3
Muscular force during (**A**) concentric (shortening), (**B**) eccentric (lengthening), and (**C**) isometric (static) actions.

bell from the extended to flexed elbow position. Because a concentric muscle action actually shortens the muscle, the word "**contraction**" frequently describes this process.

- **Eccentric action** (also called **lengthening**, stretching, or plyometric) occurs when external resistance exceeds muscle force, and the muscle lengthens while tension develops. Figure 15.3B shows a weight slowly lowered against the force of gravity. The muscles of the upper arm increase in length as they brake to prevent the weight from crashing to the floor.

- **Isometric action** (also called **static** or stationary) occurs when a muscle attempts to shorten but cannot overcome the external resistance. Considerable force generates during an isometric action with no noticeable muscle lengthening or shortening or joint movement. Figure 15.3C illustrates an isometric muscular action against the immovable bar.

The term **isotonic** commonly describes concentric and eccentric muscle actions because movement occurs in both cases. This term comes from the Greek isotonos (*iso* meaning the same or equal; *tonos*, tension or strain). Actually this term should not be applied to most dynamic muscle actions that involve movement because the muscle's force-generating capacity varies as the joint angle changes; thus, force output does not remain constant at the same percent of maximum through the ROM.

Dynamic constant external resistance (DCER) refers to resistance training where external resistance or weight does not change, but lifting (concentric) and lowering (eccentric) phases occur during each repetition. *DCER implies that the external weight or resistance remains constant throughout the movement.*

Force:Velocity Relationship

Different physical activities require different amounts of strength (force) and power. Absolute or peak force generated in a movement depends on the speed of muscle lengthening and shortening. Figure 15.4 shows the **force:velocity relationship** for concentric and eccentric actions. Muscles shorten (and lengthen) at different velocities (horizontal axis of graph) depending on the load placed on them. *As the load increases, maximum shortening velocity decreases. Conversely, a muscle's force-generating capacity (vertical axis of graph) rapidly declines with increased shortening velocity.* This explains the difficulty in attempting to move a heavy weight rapidly.

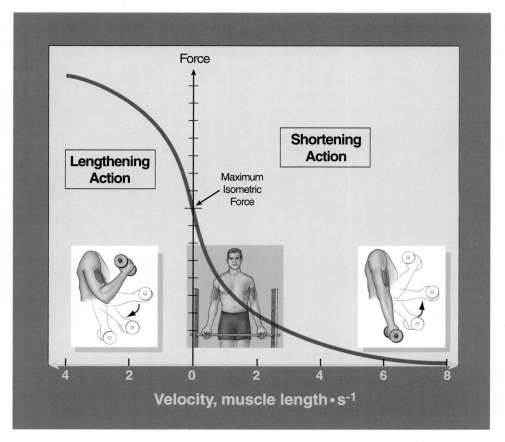

Figure 15.4
Maximum force-velocity relationship for shortening and lengthening muscle actions. Rapid shortening velocities generate the least maximum force. Shortening velocity becomes zero (maximum isometric force) when the curve crosses the y-axis. Force-generating capacity increases to its highest as the muscle lengthens at rapid velocities.

A concentric action becomes a lengthening (eccentric) action when the external load exceeds a muscle's maximum isometric force capacity (noted as point 0 on the horizontal axis.) In contrast to a concentric muscle action, rapid eccentric actions generate the greatest force. This may explain the relatively greater muscle damage and delayed muscle soreness that accompany a bout of eccentric exercise (see page 419). Force at zero velocity shortening (isometric action) exceeds all forces generated with concentric actions. Muscle fiber type also influences the force-velocity relationships; fast-twitch muscle fibers produce greater muscle force at fast movement speeds than slow-twitch fibers.

Power-Velocity Relationship

Figure 15.5 shows an inverted U relationship between a muscle's maximal power output and its speed of limb movement (concentric action). Peak power rapidly increases with increasing velocity to a **peak velocity region**. Thereafter, maximal power output decreases because of the reduction in maximum force at faster movement speeds (Fig. 15.4). *Each muscle group has an optimum movement speed to produce maximum power*. At any movement velocity, greater peak power occurs in fast-contracting fibers than slow-contracting fibers because of the biochemical differences between fibers.

Force: Power-Range of Motion Relationship

Figure 15.6 displays three different force:power-ROM curves based on movement mechanics. For ascending curve A, force:power output capacity increases propor-

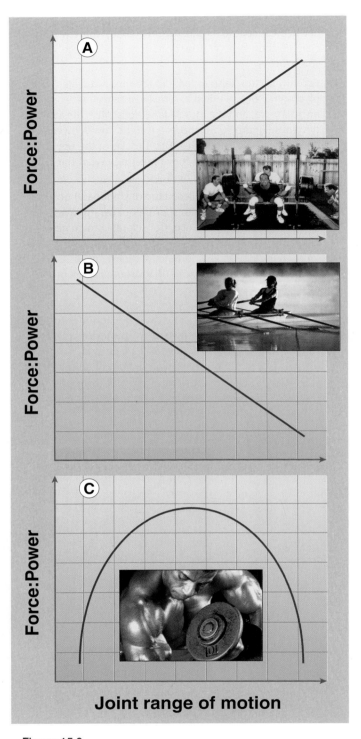

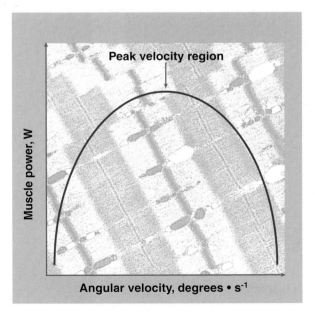

Figure 15.5
Power-velocity relationship. Power (work per unit time) increases as a function of movement velocity to a peak velocity region. Thereafter, power decreases with further increases in angular velocity.

Figure 15.6
Relationship between force:power and joint range of motion (ROM). Individuals exhibit different force:power relationships in different movements due to 1) individual differences in limb length, 2) point of attachment of a muscle to a bone, 3) bone dimensions, and 4) ROM for any segment.

tionately as the movement progresses from start to finish. A squat exercise exemplifies greater force-power generation towards the end of the ROM than at the beginning or middle. Descending curve B shows the opposite; the

All About Power

Power = [(force × distance) ÷ time)] represents the product of strength and speed of movement expressed in Watts (W; 1 W = 0.73756 ft-lb·s⁻¹, 6.12 kg-m·min⁻¹, or 0.01433 kcal·min⁻¹).

greatest force:power generation occurs during the initiation of movement and becomes progressively less toward the end of the movement. A rowing motion where the upper arms draw into the body produces a descending force:power-ROM curve. An inverted U for curve C shows that greater force:power occurs during the middle portion of the ROM with less force generated at either extreme. Elbow flexion (biceps curl) illustrates this kind of relationship.

Load:Repetition Relationship

The total work accomplished by muscle action depends on the load (resistance) placed on the muscle. One can perform high repetitions with light loads, but few repetitions with near-maximal loads. Figure 15.7A shows this relationship for the full range of percentages of 1-RM. Figure 15.7B expands the relationship for the 60 to 100% 1-RM range — the so-called **strength training zone**. From a practical standpoint, these graphs can be used to determine the (a) expected maximum repetition number for a given external load (as a percentage of 1-RM), and (b) load required to achieve a desired number of maximum repetitions.

These relationships apply to an average person; highly motivated, competitive athletes would need to establish their individual responses to different loading levels. Working at a particular percentage of 1-RM dictates the repetition number to failure. Apply the following equation to determine the expected number of repetitions to failure when lifting a percentage of 1-RM:

$$\text{Repetition number} = a_0 + [a_1 \times p] + [a_2 \times p^2] + [a_3 \times p^3] + [a_4 \times p^4]$$

where, p = percentage of 1-RM as a whole number, and $a_0 = 173.525$; $a_1 = -6.310$; $a_2 = 9.576 \times 10^{-2}$; $a_3 = -6.742 \times 10^{-4}$; and $a_4 = 1.750 \times 10^{-6}$.

For example, when lifting 70% of 1-RM, the expected maximum repetition number computes as follows:

$$\begin{aligned}
\text{Repetition number} &= 173.525 + [-6.310 \times 70] \\
&\quad + [(9.576 \times 0.01) \times 70^2] \\
&\quad + [(-6.742 \times 0.0001) \times 70^3] \\
&\quad + [(1.750 \times 0.000001) \times 70^4] \\
&= 173.525 + [-441.7] \\
&\quad + [469.224] + [-231.251] \\
&\quad + [42.02] \\
&= 11.82 \text{ (rounded to 12)}
\end{aligned}$$

Gender Differences in Muscular Strength

Two approaches can determine whether true gender differences exist in muscular strength.

1. Assess absolute strength (total force exerted)
2. Assess relative strength (force exerted related to body mass, fat-free body mass, or muscle cross-sectional area)

Absolute Strength

When comparing **absolute strength** (total force in pounds or kilograms), men score considerably higher in strength than women in all muscle groups, regardless of test mode. Gender differences in strength clearly emerge for upper-body strength evaluations; women exhibit about 50% less strength than men. In lower-body strength, females achieve 20 to 30% below the scores of male counterparts. Exceptions usually include strength-trained female track and field athletes and bodybuilders who train diligently with resistance exercise to increase the strength (and size) of specific muscle groups.

Table 15.2 shows the strength ratios for different muscle groups (female strength score ÷ male strength score). These data represent averages from the research literature based on strength scores of men and women for concentric:eccentric muscle actions. Overall, the typical woman's maximal total body strength represents 63.5% of the man's

TABLE 15.2
Ratio of female strength to male strength for different muscle groups[a]

MUSCLE GROUP	STRENGTH RATIO (FEMALE ÷ MALE)
Elbow flexors	0.55
Elbow extensors	0.48
Knee flexors	0.69
Knee extensors	0.68
Shoulder flexors	0.55
Trunk extensor and flexors	0.60
Hip extensors and flexors	0.80
Finger flexors	0.60

[a] Data represent an average of values in the literature that reported female–male data. The ratios were obtained by dividing the female mean strength for a given muscle(s) by the mean male strength score. These data can be used to 1) evaluate performance of women relative to men, 2) select first approximations of suitable loads for females based on male data, or 3) approximate male data if only female data are available.

strength; for upper-body strength, women average 56% of men's data, whereas lower-body strength averages 72% of men's scores.

Table 15.3 presents the female:male ratios for the top five weightlifting totals for male and female Olympic weight-lifters in the same body mass categories. The differences in strength at the same body mass indicate that factors in addition to body mass account for gender differences in muscular strength.

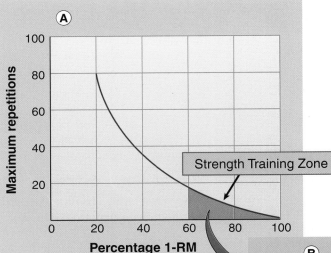

Figure 15.7
A, Relationship between maximum number of repetitions to failure and load at 20 to 100% 1-RM. **B,** Relationship between repetitions and load for the strength training zone (60 to 100% 1-RM). (Plots for the curves determined from the fourth order polynomial function equation. From Siff, M.C., and Verkhoshansky, Y.V.: *Supertraining: Special Strength Training for Sporting Excellence.* Perry, OH: Strength Coach, Inc., 1997.)

Relative Strength

Estimates indicate that human skeletal muscle fibers outside of the body (*in vitro*) have the capacity to generate 16 to 30 Newtons (N) force per square centimeter of **muscle cross-sectional area** (**MCSA**) regardless of gender. In the body (*in vivo*), force-output capacity varies depending on the bony lever's arrangement and muscle architecture. Figure 15.8 presents a comparison of arm flexor strength of men and women related to MCSA.

Individuals with the largest MCSA generate the greatest muscular force. The strong, linear relationship between strength and muscle size ($r = 0.95$) indicates little difference in arm flexor strength for the same size muscle in men and women. The inset graph shows the equality in strength (per unit MCSA) between men and women.

Maximum muscular force also can be expressed per unit of fat-free muscle mass. Ideally, this relative expression of muscle force output should consider the muscle groups evaluated. This requires estimating a particular muscle's fat-free mass using sophisticated imaging technology to determine its actual volume minus its fat component. The ratio 1-RM ÷ fat-free muscle mass can then be determined if one knows the 1-RM for the muscle (or muscle group.) It may be practical to use total fat-free body mass (FFM; determined by densitometry) for the strength ratio. The strength score in

---

Estimate 1-RM from Submaximal Effort

Estimate one-repetition maximum (1-RM) from 7- to 10-RM for untrained and trained persons with the following equations:

Untrained:
1-RM, kg = 1.554 (7- to 10-RM, kg) − 5.181

Trained:
1-RM, kg = 1.172 (7- to 10-RM, kg) + 7.704

For example, estimate 1-RM for an untrained person whose 10-RM equals 50 kg, as follows:

1-RM = 1.554 × 50-5.181 = 72.5 kg

Strength and Puberty

Until puberty, boys maintain about 10% greater muscle strength than girls. After age 12, boys continually increase in strength while strength plateaus in girls. Gender-related changes in body composition account for much of this difference.

TABLE 15.3
Strength ratios for top female and male Olympic weightlifters based on different body mass categories[a]

BODY MASS CATEGORY (KG)	STRENGTH RATIO (FEMALE ÷ MALE)
52.0	0.76
56.0	0.72
60.0	0.70
67.5	0.67
75.0	0.64
82.5	0.63
105.0	0.59

[a] Values based on average of five different lifts taken from different studies in literature.

FFM of 95 kg, his larger ratio of 2.983 (283.4 kg ÷ 95 kg) would indicate that he possessed greater strength relative to FFM.

This example illustrates the pitfall of reporting an absolute strength score without considering some aspect of body size and body composition. The following illustrates three ways to express **relative muscular strength** for a person weighing 93 kg (15.0% body fat), with upper-arm MCSA = 25.6 cm², and 1-RM bench press = 102 kg (225 lb):

1. **Body mass**
   Bench press ÷ Body mass
   102 kg ÷ 93 kg = 1.0968
2. **Fat-free body mass**
   Bench press ÷ FFM
   102 kg ÷ 79.05 kg = 1.2903
3. **Muscle cross-sectional area**
   Bench press ÷ MCSA
   102 kg ÷ 25.6 cm² = 3.984

The relative ratio scores to express bench press strength look strange because most people more readily relate to a 225-pound absolute bench press than a ratio expression. However, a relative score may ensure fairness in compar-

this case would represent a total strength score based on the sum (or average) of specific strength tests.

An example of **total strength score sum (TSSS)** would add bench press (e.g., 250 lb) and squat (e.g., 375 lb) to yield a TSSS of 625 pounds (283.4 kg). If FFM equaled 108 kg for a 120-kg football player, then relative maximum muscular strength per unit FFM would equal 283.4 kg ÷ 108 kg or 2.624. If a competitor of the same body mass and TSSS had a 13-kg lower

Figure 15.8
Plot of force (N) versus muscle cross-sectional area (MCSA, cm²). Data represent elbow flexion. Inset figure shows the strength per unit MCSA. (Data from Miller, J.D., et al.: Gender differences in strength and muscle fiber characteristics. *Eur. J. Appl. Physiol.*, 66: 254, 1992, and Ikai, M., and Fukunaga, R.: Calculation of muscle strength per unit cross-sectional area of human muscle by means of ultrasonic measurements. *Arbeitsphysiologie*, 26:26, 1968.)

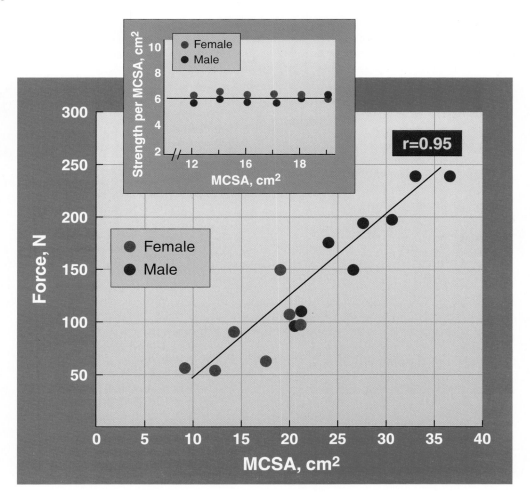

ing two individuals' strength performances (or the same person assessed before, during, and after a training regimen or weight-loss program).

Resistance Training for Children

Although resistance training for children has gained popularity, its benefits and possible risks remain relatively unknown. Because of incomplete skeletal development in young children and adolescents, obvious concern arises about the potential for bone and joint injury with heavy muscular overload. Furthermore, one might question whether resistance training improves strength at a relatively young age because the hormonal profile continues to develop (particularly for the tissue-building testosterone). *Limited evidence indicates that closely supervised resistance training programs using concentric-only muscle actions with high repetitions and low resistance significantly improve children's muscular strength with no adverse effect on bone or muscle.* Table 15.4 provides basic guidelines for resistance exercise progressions for children at different ages.

Systems of Resistance Training

Five fundamentally different but interrelated systems of training develop muscular strength:

1. Isometric training
2. Dynamic constant external resistance training
3. Variable resistance training
4. Isokinetic training
5. Plyometric training

Isometric Training (Static Exercise)

Isometric strength training gained popularity between 1955 and 1965. Research in Germany during this time showed a 5% per week increase in isometric strength from only a daily, single, two-thirds maximum isometric action for

Questions to Answer Before Initiating Resistance Training for Children

- Is the child psychologically and physically ready to participate?
- Does the child understand proper lifting techniques for each exercise?
- Does the child understand the safety needs?
- Does the equipment fit the child?
- Does the child have a balanced overall physical activity program?

6-seconds duration. Repeating this action 5 to 10 times increased isometric strength. Strength gains from this simple exercise seemed beyond belief, and subsequent research demonstrated that isometric strength gains progressed at a much slower rate. Research also showed that gains in strength from isometrics related to repetitions, duration of muscle action, and training frequency.

Research since 1965 has revealed the following information regarding isometric training:

- Maximal voluntary isometric actions (100% maximum) produce greater gains in isometric strength than submaximal isometric actions.
- Duration of muscle activation directly relates to increases in isometric strength.

TABLE 15.4
Guidelines for resistance exercise for children[a]

AGE, y	GUIDELINES
5–7	Introduce child to basic exercises with little or no weight; develop the concept of a training session; teach exercise techniques; progress from body weight calisthenics, partner exercises, and lightly resisted exercises; keep volume low.
8–10	Gradually increase exercise number; practice exercise techniques for all lifts; start gradual progressive loading of exercises; keep exercises simple; increase volume slowly; carefully monitor tolerance to exercise stress.
11–13	Teach all basic exercise techniques; continue progressive loading of each exercise; emphasize exercise technique; introduce more advanced exercises with little or no resistance.
14–15	Progress to more advanced resistance exercise programs; add sport-specific components; emphasize exercise techniques; increase volume.
16+	Entry level into adult programs after the person has mastered all background experience.

From: Kraemer W.J., and Fleck S.J.: *Designing Resistance Training Programs.* Champaign, IL: Human Kinetics, 1997.

[a]Note: If a child at a particular age level has no previous experience, progression must start at previous levels and move to more advanced levels as exercise tolerance, skill, and understanding permit.

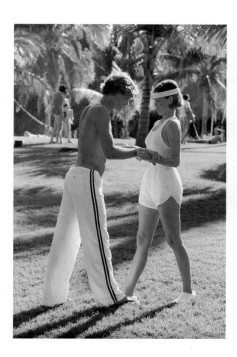

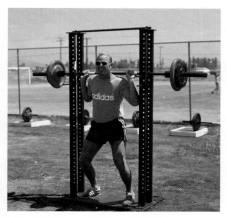

Figure 15.9
Examples of isometric muscle actions for resistance training. **Left**, Using opposing body movement to counter the attempted movement of a partner. **Right**, Fixing a dynamic squat exercise movement at a specific point (knee joint angle) in the ROM.

- One daily isometric action does not increase isometric strength as effectively as repeated actions.
- An optimal isometric training program consists of daily repeated isometric actions.
- Isometric training does not provide a consistent stimulus for muscular hypertrophy.
- Gains in isometric strength occur predominantly at the joint angle used in training.

Figure 15.9 shows examples of isometric muscle actions for resistance training.

Limitations of Isometrics

A drawback to isometric training involves difficulty in monitoring exercise intensity and training results. Because essentially no movement occurs, it is difficult to determine objectively if the person's strength actually improves and

Isometrics Not Ideal for Sports Training

Isometric training isolates, overloads, and strengthens muscles at precise points in the ROM. Although ideal for rehabilitation purposes, the specificity of the training response makes isometrics less optimal for most sports activities because they require dynamic rather than static muscle actions.

whether the person applies an appropriate overload force during training. Isometric force measurement requires specialized equipment (e.g., strain gauge or cable tensiometer) not readily available at most exercise facilities.

Benefits of Isometrics

Isometric exercise can effectively improve strength of a particular muscle or group of muscles when the applied isometric force covers four or five joint angles through the ROM. Isometric training works well in orthopedic applications that can isolate strength increases during rehabilitation. Isometric measurement can pinpoint an area of muscle weakness, and isometric training can strengthen muscles at the proper joint angle.

Dynamic Constant External Resistance (DCER) Training

This popular system of resistance training involves lifting (concentric) and lowering (eccentric) phases with each repetition using weight plates (barbells and dumbbells) or exercise machines that feature different applications of muscle overload.

Progressive Resistance Exercise

Researchers in rehabilitation medicine after World War II devised a method of resistance training to improve the force-generating capacity of previously injured limbs. Their method involved three sets of exercise, each consisting of 10 repetitions done consecutively without rest. The first set involved one-half the maximum weight lifted 10 times or one-half 10-RM; the second set used three-quarters 10-RM; the final set required maximum weight for 10 repetitions or 10-RM. As patients trained and became stronger, 10-RM resistance increased periodically to match strength improvements. The technique of **progressive resistance exercise** (**PRE**), a practical application of the overload principle, forms the basis for most resistance training programs.

Variations of PRE

Research has varied PRE to determine an optimal number of sets and repetitions and frequency and relative intensity of training to improve strength. The findings can be summarized as follows:

- Performing between 3-RM and 9-RM yields the most effective number of repetitions to increase muscular strength.
- PRE training once weekly with only 1-RM for one set

increases strength significantly after the first week of training, and each week up to at least the sixth week.

- No particular sequence of PRE training with different percentages of 10-RM improves strength more effectively, provided each training session consists of one set of 10-RM.

- Smaller strength increases occur when performing one set of an exercise rather than two or three sets, and three sets produce greater improvement than two sets.

- For beginners, significant strength increases occur with only one training day weekly, but the optimum number of training days per week with PRE remains unknown.

- When PRE training uses several different exercises, training four or five days a week may be less effective for increasing strength than training two or three times weekly. More frequent training may prevent sufficient recuperation between exercise sessions, which could minimize neuromuscular adaptations, energy replenishment, and strength development.

- A fast rate of movement for a given resistance may generate greater strength improvement than lifting at a slower rate. Neither free weights (barbells or dumbbells) nor concentric-eccentric-type weight machines produce inherently superior results compared with other strength development methods.

Responses of Men and Women to DCER Training

Figure 15.10 shows strength changes for men and women with DCER training. These data represent an average from 12 experiments. Women achieved higher percentage improvement than men, although considerable overlap existed among individuals. These findings indicate a relative equality in trainability between women and men, at least with short-duration resistance training.

Variable Resistance Training

A limitation of typical DCER weight-lifting exercise involves failure of muscles to generate maximum force through all movement phases. **Variable resistance training** equipment alters external resistance to movement by use of either a lever arm, irregularly shaped metal cam, hydraulics, or a pulley to match increases and decreases in force capacity related to joint angle (lever characteristics) throughout a ROM (Fig. 15.11). This adjustment, based on average physical dimensions of a population, theoretically should facilitate strength gains because it allows near-maximal force production throughout the full ROM.

Biomechanical research has shown that a single cam cannot possibly compensate fully for individual differences in mechanics and force applications at all phases of the particular movement. Variations in limb length, point of attachment of muscle tendons to bone, body size, and strength at different joint angles all affect maximum force generated throughout a ROM. In most cases, cams produce too much resistance during the first half and too little resistance during the second half of flexion and extension exercises. Despite these limitations, variable resistance devices improve strength comparable to other weight-lifting (resistance) equipment.

Special Consideration: The Lower Back

Approximately one-half of the work force in the United States suffers back problems at some time in their careers; this represents a primary cause for job-related disability. This translates into millions of lost hours in the work place,

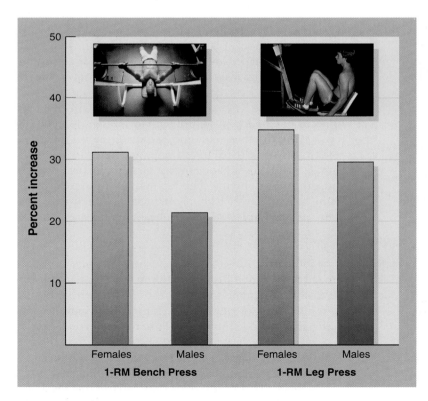

Figure 15.10
Percent increase in 1-RM bench press and leg press of women and men in response to resistance training. Values represent the average of 12 studies in the literature using dynamic constant external resistance (DCER) training for a minimum of nine weeks duration, three days per week, and two or more sets per training session.

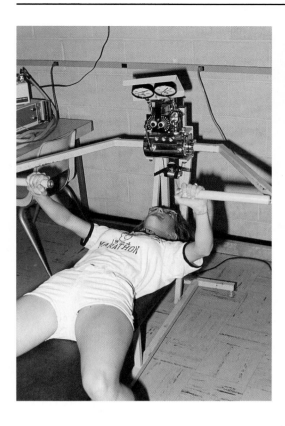

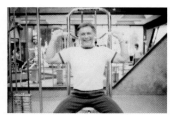

Figure 15.11
Examples of variable resistance training equipment. **Right**, Shoulder press on weight-stack machine with lever arm that alters resistance through ROM. **Left**, Bench press on hydraulic machine where resistance to movement changes to accomodate changing force capacity throughout the ROM.

stiff, back arched, and head thrown back, places unnecessary strain on the lower spine (sit-ups should always be done with the knees flexed and chin tucked to chest). Pressing and curling exercises with weights, performed with excessive hyperextension or back arch (another form of cheating) creates shearing forces that also produce undesirable muscle strain or spinal pressure.

Wearing a weightlifting belt during heavy lifts (squats, dead lifts, clean-and-jerk maneuvers) significantly reduces intra-abdominal pressure compared to lifting without a belt. A belt may reduce the potentially injurious compressive forces on spinal discs during heavy lifting as in most Olympic and power lifting events. The researchers recommend always wearing a belt for near-maximal or maximal lifts. In addition, a person who normally trains wearing a belt should generally refrain from lifting without one. Further recommendations include performing at least some submaximal resistance training without a belt to strengthen the deep abdominal muscles, and develop the proper pattern of muscle recruitment needed to generate high intra-abdominal pressures when not wearing a belt.

chronic physical discomfort, and billions of dollars spent on visits to orthopedists and chiropractors. The causes for this malady are not always apparent, and a cure remains elusive. Prime factors in **low back syndrome** include muscular weakness (particularly the abdominal region) and poor lower back and leg flexibility. Strengthening and flexibility exercises help alleviate and rehabilitate chronic low-back strain. Even continuing normal daily activities (within limits dictated by pain tolerance) leads to a more rapid recovery from an episode of acute back pain then bed rest.

Using resistance training exercises poses a dilemma. If done properly, resistance training strengthens the abdominal muscles and lumbar extensor muscles of the lower back that support and protect the spine. Unfortunately, the novice exerciser frequently performs exercises incorrectly while attempting to create too much force. This recruits additional muscle groups, improperly aligns the spinal column (especially with the back arching, a form of weightlifting cheating), and triggers lower-back strain. A seemingly simple sit-up exercise, if done improperly with legs

Isokinetic Training

Isokinetic resistance training differs markedly from isometric, DCER, and variable resistance methods. Isokinetic training employs a muscle action performed at constant angular limb velocity. Unlike dynamic resistance exercise, isokinetic exercise does not require a specified initial resistance; rather, the isokinetic device controls movement velocity. The muscles exert maximal forces throughout the ROM while shortening (concentric action) at a specific velocity. Advocates of isokinetic training argue that exerting maximal force throughout the full ROM optimizes strength development. Also, concentric-only actions minimize potential for muscle and joint injury and pain.

Figure 15.12 shows the differences in force curves, expressed as a percent of actual maximum force capacity at each point throughout the ROM, between a bench press performed with DCER (red line) and a bench press performed isokinetically (blue line). The green line illustrates the progression for absolute forces (actual values not given) against the electromechanical dynamometer throughout the bench press movement. This force curve indicates that the chest, shoulders, and upper arms can generate the greatest forces in the early phases of the bench press; thereafter, force-generating capacity dissipates as the movement progresses towards completion. As with all joints in the body, maximal muscle force exerted against an external resistance varies with the bony lever configuration as the joint moves through its normal ROM (see Figs. 15.6 and 15.15). *In the*

Hold That Stretch!

Stretching with fast, bouncing , jerky movement that uses the body's momentum can 1) strain or tear muscles, and 2) create a reflex action that actually resists the muscle stretch.

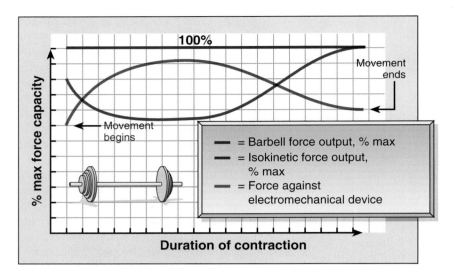

Figure 15.12
Differences in percent of maximum force-generating capacity between a bench press performed with weights (red line) and an isokinetic dynamometer (blue line). The green line represents changes in absolute force against the dynamometer (actual values not given) during progression of the bench press movement.

Experiments With Isokinetic Exercise and Training

Experiments using isokinetic exercise explored the force-velocity relationship in various exercises and related this to the muscle's fiber-type composition. Figure 15.13 displays the progressive decline in concentric peak torque output with increasing angular velocity of the knee extensor muscles in two groups that differed in sports training and muscle fiber composition. For movement at $180°·s^{-1}$ power athletes that included elite Swedish track and field sprinters and jumpers achieved significantly higher torque per kilogram of body mass than competition walkers and cross-country runners (endurance athletes). At this angular velocity, maximal torque equaled about 55% of maximal isometric force ($0°·s^{-1}$).

The athletes' muscle fiber composition distinguishes the two curves in Figure 15.13. At zero velocity shortening (isometric action), the same peak force (per unit body mass) occurred for athletes with relatively high (power athletes) or low (endurance athletes) percentages of fast-twitch muscle fibers; this indicated that maximal isometric knee extension activated both fast- and slow-twitch motor units. Increasing movement velocity produced greater torque by individuals with a higher percentage of fast-twitch fibers. Perhaps fast-twitch muscle fibers favor power

bench press with a conventional barbell, the weight lifted can not exceed the maximum force capacity of the muscles at the weakest point in the ROM; otherwise the complete movement could not take place. This means that the force generated during a dynamic weight-lifting action cannot reach maximum throughout all phases of the movement (red line).

With the isokinetic bench press, on the other hand, no change in the percentage of maximum force-generating capacity occurs during the progression of the lift (blue line), despite the significant decreases in *absolute force* against the dynamometer as the movement progresses (green line). In other words, the force exerted, although changing, remains maximal (100%) for every particular point in the ROM.

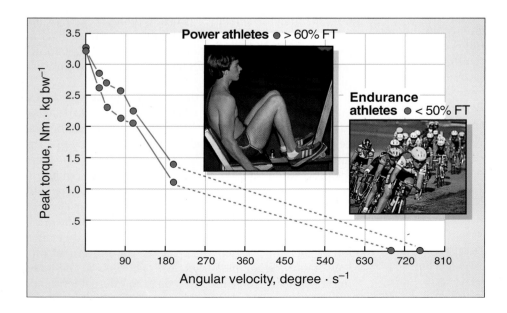

Figure 15.13
Peak torque output per unit body mass related to angular velocity in two groups of athletes with different muscle fiber compositions. The torque-velocity curves were extrapolated (dashed line) to an estimated maximal velocity for knee extension. (Data from Throstensson, A.: Muscle strength, fiber types, and enzyme activities in man. *Acta Physiol. Scand.*, Suppl. 443, 1976.)

activities where high torque generation at rapid movement velocities often dictates success.

Fast- Versus Slow-Speed Isokinetic Training

Strength and power improvements with isokinetic training at slow and fast limb speeds support the specificity principle for exercise performance and training responses. For example, power gained from slow-speed training becomes apparent at the relatively slow angular movement velocities used in training, with little improvement noted at fast velocities. In contrast, exercising at fast speeds of movement produces more general improvement because this form of training increases power output at *both* fast and slow movement velocities. Muscular hypertrophy results only during fast-speed training and only in the fast acting type II muscle fibers. Hypertrophy may explain the more general strength improvement with fast-speed isokinetic training. Despite the difference in training response with fast- and slow-speed training, the greatest improvement in muscular performance occurs at the specific angular velocity and movement pattern of training.

Isokinetic training proves useful because muscle overload occurs through a full ROM at speeds somewhat similar to, but considerably slower than, specific sport and physical activities. Although isokinetic-type training occurs at a constant, preselected angular movement velocity, few if any physical activities take place at a constant, relatively slow speed of joint motion. Furthermore, the current isokinetic dynamometers do not effectively overload eccentric muscular actions for limb deceleration and braking control of human movements. *Combined concentric-eccentric muscle actions during heavy resistance training facilitate optimal strength development compared with training that uses concentric-only muscle actions.* Adding an eccentric component may augment neural adaptations with training and thereby facilitate strength gains.

Plyometric Training

Athletes who require specific, powerful movements (e.g., in football, volleyball, sprinting, and basketball) often perform exercise training termed **plyometrics**. Plyometric training movements make use of the inherent stretch-recoil characteristics of skeletal muscle and neurological modulation via the stretch or myotatic reflex (see Chapter 12). Consider walking: When the foot first hits the ground, the quadriceps initially act eccentrically (stretch), then briefly isometrically, before the shortening phase of muscle action begins. The term **stretch-shortening cycle** describes the sequence of linked, eccentric-isometric-concentric muscle actions. When stretching occurs rapidly, stored elastic energy in muscle fibers, and initiation of the myotatic reflex combine to produce a powerful concentric action. Faster recruitment of muscle fibers and recruitment of more muscle fibers with prior stretching may also augment a muscle's response.

Vertical jumping provides an example of the stretch-short-ening cycle to enhance performance. During a normal vertical jump, the jumper bends at the knees and hips (eccentric action of extensors), pauses briefly (isometric action), and rapidly reverses direction (concentric action) to jump upward as high as possible. If this same movement stops for several seconds following the knee bend (just before reversing movement direction), the subsequent jump (concentric action) produces a lower jump height compared with a performance that uses the complete stretch-shortening cycle.

Practical Applications

A plyometric training drill incorporates body mass and the force of gravity to provide the all-important rapid prestretch or cocking phase, to activate the stretch reflex and the muscle's natural elastic recoil elements. Lower-body plyometric drills include a standing jump, multiple jumps, repetitive jumping in place, depth or drop jumps (from 1- to 4-ft heights), and various modifications of single- and double-leg jumps. Repeating these exercises regularly supposedly provides both neurological and muscular training to enhance power performance of the specific muscles. Figure 15.14 shows examples of plyometric exercises for strength-

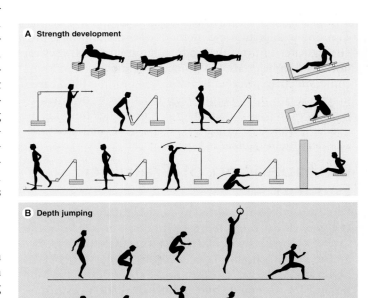

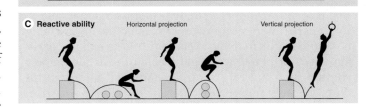

Figure 15.14
Examples of stretch-shortening cycle (plyometric) exercises. **A,** Strength devleopment. **B,** Depth jumping. **C,** Reactive ability.

power development using resistance and other apparatus, including general jumping exercises and depth jumps.

Research with Plyometric Exercises

Testimonials and opinions have promoted the beneficial effects of plyometric training, but carefully controlled scientific evaluations remain scarce. No consensus exists about optimal jump number with untrained subjects. Similarly, insufficient evidence makes it difficult to recommend optimal height for performing depth jumps (heights from 19 to 32 in have produced varying degrees of success).

Performing plyometric exercise while wearing a weighted vest or belt (up to 12% of body mass) reportedly augments the training effect. When individuals performed resistance training and plyometric exercises two to three times weekly for 4 to 10 weeks, vertical jump height increased between 1.2 to 4.2 inches. Plyometric training also improves standing long jump and sprint running performances. Concurrent resistance training with plyometrics improves performance to a greater extent than either method alone.

Injury and Other Considerations

Training with plyometric methods does not appear to produce greater injuries than other training modes, even in untrained individuals. Common sense dictates that to become effective, plyometric training should be introduced slowly into the total training regimen. Clearly, plyometrics should not serve as the main form of resistance training; instead, plyometrics can serve as an adjunct to a diverse muscle-strengthening program.

Comparison of Training Systems

Few research studies directly compare different training systems within the same experimental protocol. Some studies compare two different training systems (e.g., isometric versus variable resistance; isometric versus isokinetic; isometric versus eccentric). The results generally support the specificity and individual differences principles. When training and testing incorporate the same system, strength increases regardless of the training system. When testing uses a different system than in training, smaller training-induced strength increases occur, and in some experiments improvements become nonexistent. Difficulties arise in trying to compare different training systems because of methodologic problems equating training volume (sets and repetitions), total work, total training time, and most importantly, training intensity. This makes it almost impossible to directly prove one strength training system fares better than another. Moreover, for unknown reasons, some individuals simply respond more favorably to one system. More than likely, the specificity of training principle dictates the best training system for an individual based on desired outcomes and performance needs.

Specificity of resistance training makes sense because strength improvements result from (a) favorable adaptations within the muscle itself, and (b) enhanced neural organization for a particular movement pattern. When muscles train in a limited ROM, their greatest strength improvement occurs when evaluated in that specific ROM. This angle-specific training response occurs in both static and dynamic resistance training.

Practical Implications of Specificity

The complex interaction between the nervous and muscular systems partially explains why leg muscles strengthened using squats or deep knee bends do not show equivalent improvement in another leg movement such as jumping. Strengthening muscles for golf, rowing, swimming, or football requires more than just identifying and overloading the muscles involved in the movement. Newly acquired strength does not simply transfer to other patterns of movement, even when involving the same muscles. In a study of older men, a 227% increase in leg extension strength occurred through standard weight training. In contrast, when an isokinetic dynamometer evaluated peak leg extensor torque in the same subjects, only a 10 to 17% improvement occurred.

To emphasize the importance of angle-specific training, consider the "strength curves" for various muscle groups shown in Figure 15.15. Maximal force curves differ substantially for the flexor and extensor leg and arm muscles throughout the ROM. Two common factors affect the shape of a particular strength curve for a specific muscle group: (a) force developed at a given muscle length (less force at a shortened muscle length), and (b) perpendicular distance between the direction of the muscle's action and joint orientation (axis) during the action. A greater perpendicular distance produces a greater torque or rotational force.

Differences in the strength curves for arm and leg flexion and extension illustrate the effect of the perpendicular distance between the muscle's line of pull and resultant force. The coach and athlete should pay careful attention to the muscle group(s) involved in a particular movement. *Training should develop maximum force-generating capacity for that muscle group throughout its ROM at a movement pattern and speed that closely mimics the actual sports performance.* This goal cannot be accomplished with isometric actions because no limb movement takes place; isokinetic actions provide maximal overload potential and diverse movement velocities because movement speed with electromechanical dynamometers can approach $400°·s^{-1}$. Even moving at this relatively "fast" speed, however, does not mimic movement velocity during some sports where limb velocity approaches $2000°·s^{-1}$. Arm velocity measured about the elbow joint during a baseball pitch routinely exceeds $600-700°·s^{-1}$, and leg velocity during a football, rugby, or soccer kick nearly doubles the speed of the fastest electromechanical measuring and training devices.

Figure 15.15
Force-generating capacity of a muscle or muscle group varies with joint angle throughout the ROM in flexion and extension.

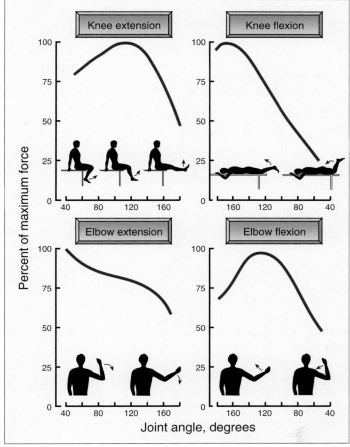

Periodization

Periodization refers to organizing resistance training into phases of different types of exercise done at varying intensities and volumes for a specific time period. In essence, the training model decreases training volume and increases training intensity as the program progresses. Fractionating the **macrocycle** (usually a one year time period) into component parts (**mesocycles**) enables manipulation of training intensity, volume, frequency, sets, repetitions, and rest periods (to prevent overtraining), and provides the means to alter the variety of workouts. This apparently reduces any negative effects from overtraining or "staleness" and enables the competitive athlete to achieve "peak" performance to coincide with competition. Figure 15.16 depicts the basic design for periodization, and a typical macrocycle with four distinct mesocycle phases. As competition approaches, periodization gradually decreases training volume while concurrently increases training intensity.

Periodization results in an inverse relation between training volume and training intensity up through the competition phase, and then decreases both aspects during the second transition, recuperation period. Note the increase in the time devoted to technique training as competition approaches, with training volume at the lowest point of the cycle.

Sport-specific principles of training usually apply in periodization as the coach designs the athlete's training based on the sport's particular strength, power, and endurance requirements. A detailed analysis of the metabolic and technical requirements of the sport also frames the training paradigm. While the concept of periodization makes intuitive sense, few if any studies present "conclusive" evidence for this training approach. This results from difficulty in controlling for differences in training intensity, training volume, and the participants' fitness capacities. One critical review of the relatively few stud-ies of periodized strength training concluded that this approach produced greater improvements in muscular strength, body mass, lean body mass, and percent body fat than nonperiodized multi-set and single-set training programs. Considerably more research must evaluate periodization, particularly relating to fitness status, age, gender, and specific sports (motor) performance. Studies must equate and then manipulate different training loads and intensities, and evaluate additional factors such as biome-

Figure 15.16
Basic periodization scheme comprising four transition phases. The periodization concept subdivides a macrocycle into distinct phases or mesocycles. These in turn usually separate into weekly microcycles.

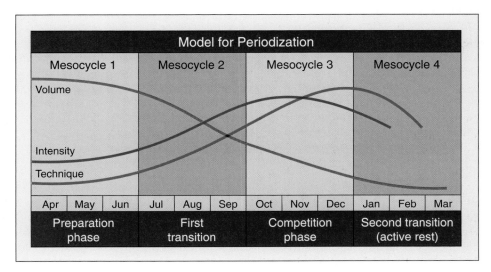

chanics and motor control in the actual sport skill, changes in segmental and whole-body composition, biochemical and ultrastructural tissue adaptations, and transfer of newly acquired fitness to subsequent performance measures.

summary

1. The four most common methods to measure muscular strength include: 1) tensiometry, 2) dynamometry, 3) 1-RM testing with weights, 4) computer-assisted force and work-output determinations including isokinetic measurement.

2. Substantial specificity of physiologic and performance measures and their response to training cast doubt on the appropriateness of using general fitness measures (including strength tests) to determine success in specific tasks or occupations.

3. Human skeletal muscle theoretically generates 16 to 30 N of maximum force per cm^2 of muscle cross section regardless of gender. On an absolute basis, men outperform women on tests of strength because of the male's larger quantity of muscle mass. These differences are greatest in upper-body strength measurements.

4. Muscles become stronger with overload training that 1) increases the load, 2) increases the speed of muscle action, or 3) combines both factors.

5. Strength gains occur when the overload represents at least 60 to 80% of a muscle's maximum force-generating capacity.

6. Based on limited data, closely supervised resistance training programs for children, using relatively moderate levels of concentric exercise, significantly improve muscular strength with no adverse effects on bone or muscle architecture.

7. Three major exercise systems develop muscular strength: 1) dynamic constant external resistance training, 2) isometric training, and 3) isokinetic training. Each system produces highly specific strength gains that relate directly to training mode.

8. Resistance training exercise, performed incorrectly with excessive hyperextension or back arch, creates shearing forces that can produce undesirable muscle strain or spinal pressure, and trigger low back pain.

9. Isokinetic-type training, because of the possibility for generating maximum force throughout the full range of motion (ROM) at different limb movement velocities, offers a unique method to apply resistance training to sports performance.

10. Plyometric training drills use the inherent stretch-recoil characteristics of the neuromuscular system to develop specific muscular power. Further research needs to determine risks, benefits, and proper applications of plyometric training.

11. Specificity of resistance training occurs because strength improvements result from favorable adaptations within the muscle itself, and enhanced neural organization for a particular movement pattern.

12. Training should be geared to develop maximum force-generating capacity for a muscle group throughout its ROM at a speed that closely mimics the actual sports performance.

PART 2
Adaptations to Resistance Training

Resistance training produces acute responses and chronic adaptations. An acute response refers to immediate changes (in muscle or other cells, tissues, or systems) that occur during or immediately after a single bout of exercise. For example, energy stores and cardiovascular dynamics change in response to specific muscle actions. Repeated exposure to the stimulus produces a longer lasting change that affects the acute response over time (e.g., less disruption in cellular integrity [muscle damage] with a given level of exercise). *Adaptation refers to how the body adjusts to repeated stimuli.*

Knowing the acute and chronic responses to resistance training facilitates exercise prescription and program design. Adaptations to repeated muscular overload ultimately determine a training program's effectiveness. The time-course of adaptations varies among individuals and depends on the nature and magnitude of prior adaptations. A resistance training program should consider the expression of individual differences in adaptation (training responsiveness).

Adaptations to resistance training occur in diverse body systems from the cellular to systemic levels. Figure 15.17 displays six factors that impact muscle mass development and maintenance. More than likely, genetic factors strongly influence the effect of each factor on the ultimate training outcome. Resistance training contributes little to tissue growth without appropriate nutrition. Similarly,

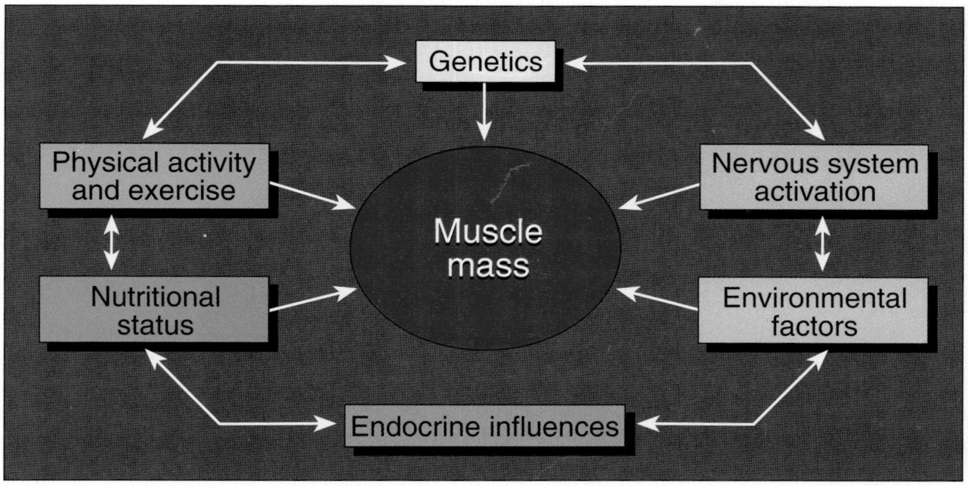

Figure 15.17
Six factors that impact the development and maintenance of muscle mass.

training outcome depends on specific hormones and patterns of nervous system activation. Without overload, however, each of the other factors cannot effectively increase muscle mass and muscle strength.

Neural Adaptations

Well-documented changes from overload training occur in the gross structural and microscopic architecture within muscle tissue. Figure 15.18 shows the adaptation of factors, broadly classified as neural and muscular, with regular resistance training.

A unique series of experiments clearly illustrated the importance of neural factors to express muscular strength. In one protocol, researchers measured upper-arm strength while intermittent gunshots were fired behind the subjects just before they performed a maximal voluntary contraction. At another time, subjects shouted or screamed loudly at the moment they exerted force. In addition to the "shoot and shout" series, the experimenters measured subjects' strength under the influence of two disinhibitory drugs, alcohol and amphetamines ("pep pills"). They also measured strength during hypnosis; subjects were told their strength would exceed their prior

strength and they should not fear injury. Arm strength significantly increased in almost all of the psychologic conditions. The greatest strength increases occurred under hypnosis, the most "mental" of all treatments.

To explain these observations, the researchers suggested that physical factors (size and type of muscle fibers and anatomic lever arrangement of bone and muscle) ultimately determine a person's muscular strength capacity. They claimed that psychologic or mental factors within the central nervous system exert neural influences that prevent most people from fully achieving their strength capacity. Neural inhibitions might result from social conditioning, unpleasant past experiences with physical activity, or an overprotective home environment. When performing under intense emotional conditions like athletic competition, emergency situations, or posthypnotic suggestion,

Figure 15.18
Relative roles of neural and muscular adaptations to strength training. Note that neural adaptation predominates in the early phase of training. This phase also encompasses most training studies. In intermediate and advanced training, progress becomes limited by the extent of muscular adaptation, notably hypertrophy; this increases the temptation to try anabolic steroids when hypertrophy by training alone becomes difficult. (Data from Sale, D. G.: Neural adaptation to resistance training. *Med. Sci. Sports Exerc.*, 20:135, 1988.)

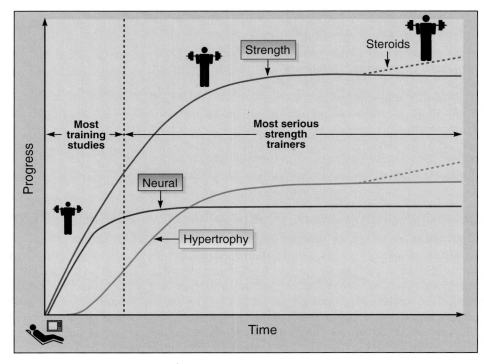

Neural Adaptations Important

Enhanced neural adaptations with resistance training may result from:
- Increased central nervous system activation
- Improved motor unit synchronization
- Lowered neural inhibitory reflexes

the inhibitory neural mechanisms decrease considerably, and the person achieves a "super performance" that more closely matches the physiologically determined capacity. Such observations help to explain the apparent beneficial effects of "psyching," or the almost self-induced hypnosis that athletes achieve immediately prior to competitive performance.

Excellent examples of disinhibition occur in weightlifters and powerlifters, high-jumpers, and other track and field competitors, and self-defense experts who perform nontraditional skills like smashing cement bricks with their hands, feet, or head. Great feats of strength during emergency situations also fit into this explanation. In addition, rapid improvements in muscular strength during the first few weeks of a strength training program may largely result from a learning phenomenon, or lessening of fear and psychologic inhibition, as the novice becomes familiar with the specific strength activity (e.g., proper form in bench press or squat exercise).

Motor Unit Activation: Size Principle

Recruitment of motor units occurs in sequence from low to high thresholds, and thus from low to high muscle force output. An increased rate of motor unit firing also increases a muscle's force output. These two factors, recruitment of motor units and an increase in their firing rate, produce a continuum of voluntary force output from muscle.

Type II motor units have a high twitch force; they become activated only in activities requiring significant force. On the other hand, Type I motor units become activated under lower force requirements and generate less twitch force. Individuals unaccustomed to high physical demands probably cannot voluntarily recruit all higher threshold, Type II motor units; thus, they cannot maximally tap their muscle's true strength capacity. An adaptation to resistance training develops the untrained person's ability to recruit more of their motor units to achieve a maximal muscle action. Increased synchronization of motor unit firing is another neural factor that increases force production with training. Greater synchronization causes more motor units to fire at one time.

Neural components also play a role in strength adaptations in advanced weight lifters. In one study, minimal changes took place in muscle fiber size in competitive

weight lifters, yet two years of training increased absolute strength and power. EMG analysis revealed enhanced voluntary activation of muscle over the training period, suggesting that the neural component contributed significantly to strength improvements.

Muscle Adaptations

Psychologic inhibitions and learning factors greatly modify muscular strength, but anatomic and physiologic factors within the muscle determine the ultimate limit of strength development. The gross and ultrastructural changes in muscle with chronic resistance training generally produce adaptations in the contractile apparatus, accompanied by substantial gains in muscular strength and power. An increase in the muscle's external size represents the most visible adaptation to resistance training. **Muscle fiber hypertrophy** (increase in size of individual fibers) usually explains increases in gross muscle size, although increased fiber number (**fiber hyperplasia**) provides a hotly debated complimentary hypothesis.

Muscle Fiber Hypertrophy

Increases in muscle size (hypertrophy) with resistance training for men and women can be viewed as a fundamental biologic adaptation. Weightlifters' and body builders' extraordinarily large muscle size and definition results from enlargement of individual muscle cells, mainly fast-twitch fibers. Growth takes place from one or more of the following adaptations:

- Increased contractile proteins (actin and myosin)
- Increased number and size of myofibrils per muscle fiber
- Increased amounts of connective, tendinous, and ligamentous tissues
- Increased enzymes and stored nutrients

Not all muscle fibers undergo the same degree of enlargement with resistance training. *Muscle growth depends on the muscle fiber type activated and the recruitment pattern.* With initiation of heavy resistance training, alterations in various muscle proteins begin within several workouts. As training continues, contractile proteins increase in conjunction with enlargement of muscle fiber cross-sectional area. Table 15.5 lists important cellular adaptations in muscle in response to resistance training.

Muscle Remodeling: Can Fiber Type Be Changed?

Fourteen men performed three sets of 6-RM leg squats three times per week to evaluate the effects of 8 weeks of resistance training on muscle fiber size and fiber composition in the leg extensor muscles. Biopsies from the vastus lateralis before and after training showed significant in-

c l o s e   u p

Muscular Strength and Age — Use It or Lose It!

The well-documented decline in muscular strength with age remains poorly understood. Contributing factors certainly include biological aging per se, the cumulative effects of disease, a sedentary lifestyle, and nutritional inadequacies. However, if the strength decline in the elderly results largely from a "disuse syndrome," an appropriate resistance training program should reverse or at least slow down loss of muscle function.

Resistance training by the elderly is rare, mainly because of safety considerations, but also because of the belief that "old" muscle does not respond to overload training. Fortunately, recent research has seriously challenged such tenents. In one study, 10 subjects who averaged 90.2 years of age participated in an 8-week resistance training program. Concentric and eccentric muscle actions during a seated leg extension/flexion movement trained the quadriceps and hamstring muscles. Training, conducted 3 days a week, consisted of three sets of eight repetitions (6 to 9 s per repetition) with a 1-to-2 minute rest between sets. During the first week of training, resistance equaled 50% 1-RM (measured every 2 wk); by the second week, the load increased to 80% 1-RM and remained the same for an additional 8 weeks.

The figure shows changes in 1-RM strength for the left leg from the pretraining baseline to after 8 weeks of training for each of the nine subjects. The changes averaged an impressive 174% (167% for the right leg.) The absolute weight lifted increased from 8.0 kg to 20.6 kg for the right leg, and 7.6 kg to 19.3 kg for the left leg. Strength increases progressed throughout the 8 weeks and did not plateau with continued training. Also, no differences in strength improvement occurred between women and men. Interestingly, each subject increased functional mobility, including rising out of a chair and increased walking speed, and two subjects no longer needed a cane to walk. After the resistance training program, subjects returned to their sedentary lifestyle. Within only 4 weeks of detraining, strength decreased 32%.

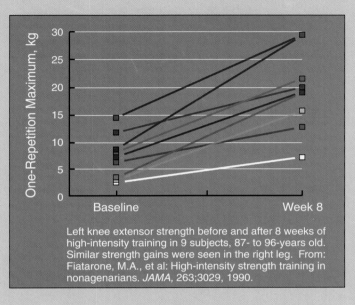

Left knee extensor strength before and after 8 weeks of high-intensity training in 9 subjects, 87- to 96-years old. Similar strength gains were seen in the right leg. From: Fiatarone, M.A., et al: High-intensity strength training in nonagenarians. *JAMA*, 263;3029, 1990.

The old adage, "use it or lose it," seems all too apropos. The study's remarkable results demonstrate the desirability of conventional resistance training for older-age adults; training profoundly reversed the effects of aging on muscular strength.

References

ACSM Position Stand on Exercise and Physical Activity for Older Adults. *Med. Sci. Sports Exerc.*, 30:992, 1998.

Exercise training guidelines for the elderly. *Med. Sci. Sports Exerc.*, 31:12, 1999.

Hurley, B.F., and Hagberg, J.M.: Optimizing health in older persons: Aerobic or strength training? *Exerc. Sport Sci. Revs.*, 26:61, 1998.

Wescott, W.L., and Baechle, T.R.: *Strength Training Past 50.* Champaign, IL: Human Kinetics, 1998.

creases in the volume of fast-twitch fibers. However, *no change* occurred in the percentage distribution of fast- and slow-twitch muscle fibers. This finding supported previous short-term studies of overload training and muscle fiber type. Several months of resistance training in adults does not alter basic skeletal muscle fiber composition. It remains unknown whether specific training early in life, or prolonged training such as engaged in by Olympic-caliber athletes, actually changes a muscle fiber's inherent twitch (speed of shortening) characteristics. Current consensus maintains that genetic factors determine an individual's predominant muscle fiber distribution. Significant muscle fiber type transformation (i.e., transforming Type I to Type II fibers) probably does not occur in healthy individuals.

Despite no change in fiber type with resistance training, metabolic characteristics of specific fibers and fiber subdivisions undergo significant change. The first study to document alterations in subdivisions of Type II muscle fibers evaluated men and women who performed high-intensity knee flexion/extension and squats twice weekly (6- to 8-RM on one day and 10- to 12-RM on the other) for 8 weeks. Type IIb muscle fiber percentage decreased significantly after just four workouts in 2 weeks of training in women, while men showed a decrease after eight workouts in 4 weeks. After 16 workouts (8 weeks), Type IIb muscle fibers decreased from 21% to about 7% of total muscle fibers for both sexes. Type II muscle fiber remodeling accompanied a significant strength increase over the training

TABLE 15.5
Physiologic adaptations to resistance training

SYSTEM/VARIABLE	RESPONSE
Muscle Fibers	
Number	Equivocal
Size	Increase
Type	Unknown
Capillary Density	
In bodybuilders	No change
In powerlifters	Decrease
Mitochondria	
Volume	Decrease
Density	Decrease
Twitch Contraction Time	Decrease
Enzymes	
Creatine phosphokinase	Increase
Myokinase	Increase
Enzymes of Glycolysis	
Phosphofructokinase	Increase
Lactate dehydrogenase	No change
Aerobic Metabolism Enzymes	
Carbohydrate	Increase
Triglyceride	Not known
Intramuscular Fuel Stores	
Adenosine triphosphate	Increase
Phosphocreatine	Increase
Glycogen	Increase
Triglycerides	Not known
$\dot{V}O_{2max}$	
Circuit resistance training	Increase
Heavy resistance training	No change
Connective Tissue	
Ligament strength	Increase
Tendon strength	Increase
Collagen content of muscle	No change
Bone	
Mineral content	Increase
Cross-sectional area	No change

Modified from Fleck, S.J., and Kramer, W.J.: Resistance training: physiological responses and adaptations (Part 2 of 4). *Phys. Sportsmed.*, 16:108, 1988.

Muscle Hypertrophy and Testosterone Levels

It is a popular belief that the male sex hormone testosterone facilitates muscle hypertrophy with resistance training. Testosterone, the chief male hormone, binds with special receptor sites on muscle and other tissues to contribute to male secondary sex characteristics. These include gender differences in muscle mass and strength that develop at puberty's onset. Variation in testosterone level would then explain individual differences in muscular enlargement with resistance training, and the alleged smaller hypertrophic response of women to muscular overload. Research to date, however, does not support such notions. Essentially no correlation exists between plasma testosterone levels and body composition and muscular strength in men and women. Individuals with significant muscle strength and/or FFM can have either high or low testosterone levels. While acute increases in sex hormone release follow a single bout of maximal resistance training (or any maximal effort exercise), the effect remains transient and probably of little consequence to training responsiveness.

Muscle Fiber Hypertrophy: Male Versus Female

Computed tomography scans to directly evaluate muscle cross-sectional area show that men and women experience a *similar* hypertrophic response to resistance training. Men achieve a greater absolute change in muscle size because of a larger initial total muscle mass, but no difference in muscle enlargement on a percentage basis compared to women of similar training status.

Other comparisons between elite male and female bodybuilders have verified these observations. *The limited data from short-term experiments suggest that women can use conventional resistance training and gain strength and size on a similar percentage basis as men without developing overly large muscles (i.e., significantly large absolute changes in girth).*

Muscle Fiber Hyperplasia

Do the actual number of muscle cells increase (hyperplasia) with resistance training? Research in the early 1980s showed that overload training of skeletal muscle of cats caused development of new muscle fibers. Hyperplasia occurred either through proliferation of satellite cells (cells between the basement layer and plasma membrane of muscle fibers) or longitudinal splitting (a relatively large muscle fiber splits into two or more smaller, individual daughter cells). However, species differences may influence a muscle's response to overload training; the massive cellular hypertrophy in humans with resistance training does not occur in many animal species. Thus, cellular proliferation represents their compensatory adjustment.

Cross-sectional studies of body builders with large limb circumferences and muscle mass failed to show significant hypertrophy of individual muscle fibers. While these ath-

period without significantly changing muscle fiber size or FFM. *Repeated stimulation of Type IIb muscle fibers initiates their rapid transformation toward a Type IIa profile for metabolic characteristics and fatigue resistance.* The slower process of muscle hypertrophy then follows.

letes could have inherited an initially large number of small muscle fibers (which then hypertrophied to normal size with training), the findings certainly raise the possibility of significant hyperplasia in humans under certain circumstances. Muscle fibers may adapt differentially to high-volume, high-intensity training that body builders employ compared with lower-repetition, heavy-load system favored by strength and power athletes. Under most conditions, hyperplasia does not represent the primary human skeletal muscle adaptation to overload. However, some hyperplasia may occur when Type II fibers reach their upper size limit.

Connective Tissue and Bone Adaptations

Supporting ligaments, tendons, and bone tissues strengthen as muscle strength and size increase. Changes in ligaments and tendons generally parallel the rate of muscle fiber adaptation, while bone changes more slowly, perhaps over a 6- to 12-month period. Connective tissue proliferates around individual muscle fibers; this thickens and strengthens the muscle's connective tissue harness. Such adaptations from resistance training protect joints and muscles from injury and justify resistance exercise for preventive and rehabilitative purposes. Resistance training also positively affects bone dynamics in young individuals. For example, elite 14-to-17-year-old junior Olympic weight lifters had significantly higher bone densities in the hip and femur regions than age-matched controls or adults (Table 15.6).

Cardiovascular Adaptations

Training volume and intensity influence the effect of resistance training on the cardiovascular system.

TABLE 15.7
Cardiovascular adaptations to resistance training

VARIABLE	ADAPTATION
Rest	
Heart rate	No change
Blood pressure	
Diastolic	Decrease or no change
Systolic	Decrease or no change
Rate-pressure product (HR $\times$ SBP)	Decrease or no change
Stroke volume	Increase or no change
Cardiac function	Increase or no change
Left ventricular wall thickness	Increase
Right ventricular wall thickness	No change
Left ventricular chamber volume	No change
Right ventricular chamber volume	No change
Left ventricular mass	Increase
Lipid profile	
Total cholesterol	Decrease
HDL-C	Increase or no change
LDL-C	Decrease or no change
During exercise	
Heart rate	No change
Blood pressure	
Diastolic	Decrease
Systolic	Decrease
Rate-pressure product	Decrease
Stroke volume	Increase or no change
Cardiac output	Increase or no change
$\dot{V}O_{2peak}$	Increase or no change

Table 15.7 lists chronic cardiovascular adaptations from resistance training.

Subtle yet important differences exist between myocardial enlargement from resistance training (**physiological**

TABLE 15.6
Bone mineral density values (g · mL^{-1}) for spine and proximal femur for elite junior weight lifters[a]

	BONE MINERAL DENSITY		
SITE	JUNIOR LIFTERS	AGE-MATCHED CONTROLS	ADULT REFERENCE VALUES
Spine	1.41 ± 0.20	1.06 ± 0.21	1.25
Femoral Neck	1.30 ± 0.15	1.05 ± 0.21	1.12
Trochanter	1.05 ± 0.13	0.89 ± 0.12	1.12
Ward's Triangle	1.26 ± 0.20	0.99 ± 0.16	1.24

[a] Values are mean ± SD

From Conroy, B.P., et al.: Bone mineral density in elite junior weightlifters. *Med. Sci. Sports Exerc.*, 25:1105, 1993.

hypertrophy) and enlargement from chronic hypertension (**pathological hypertrophy**). In pathologic conditions, ventricular wall thickness increases beyond normal limits regardless of assessment method and evaluative criteria. Dilation and weakening of the left ventricle, a frequent response to chronic hypertension (and subsequent congestive heart failure), do not accompany the compensatory increase in myocardial wall thickness with resistance training. The hearts of these athletes usually exceed the size of untrained counterparts, but heart size generally falls within the upper-range limits of normal in relation to various measures of body size or cardiac function.

Resistance exercise more acutely increases blood pressure than lower-intensity dynamic movements, but does *not* produce any long-term increase in resting blood pressure. Weight lifters and body builders with hypertension probably have existing essential hypertension, experience chronic overtraining syndrome, use steroids, or possess an undesirable level of body fat or other hypertension risks established for the general population.

Metabolic Stress of Resistance Training

Metabolic and cardiovascular evaluations indicate that traditional resistance training methods offer little benefit for aerobic fitness or weight control, or for significantly modifying risk factors related to cardiovascular disease.

Isometric and Weight-Lifting Exercise

A series of experiments in one of our laboratories studied the immediate physiologic effects of isometric and resistance exercise. Subjects performed the two-arm curl, two-arm press, bench press, and squat with resistance that allowed them to complete eight repetitions of a particular movement. Isometric exercise involved a 6-second maximal action against a bar placed in a position mid-way through the ROM of the corresponding weightlifting exercise.

Results for oxygen uptake showed that both exercise methods would classify as "light to moderate" for energy expenditure, even though subjects reported considerable muscular stress. A person can perform 15 or 20 different resistance exercises during a 1-hour training session, yet the total time devoted to actual exercise does not usually last longer than 6 or 7 minutes. This relatively brief activity period (with only moderate energy expenditure) shows that traditional resistance training programs would not improve endurance capacity for running, cycling, or swimming. Resistance training exercises also would be of only limited value as major activities in weight-loss programs because of the typically low total energy expenditure during a training session.

Circuit Resistance Training

Modifying standard resistance training by de-emphasizing heavy overload can increase exercise caloric expenditure and workout volume, thus improving more than one aspect of physical fitness. Research has focused on the energy cost and cardiorespiratory demands of **circuit resistance training** (**CRT**). In CRT, a pre-established exercise-rest sequence usually consists of eight to 15 different exercise stations, with 15 to 20 repetitions performed for each exercise. *Exercise resistance requires between 40 and 50% of 1-RM.* After a 15- to 30-second rest interval, participants move to succeeding exercise stations to complete the circuit. Figure 15.19 outlines the sequence of progression through a multilevel, 5- to 12-station circuit.

In one experiment, 20 men and 20 women performed three exercise circuits (10 stations per circuit using weight machines) with a 15-second rest between exercises (22.5 min to perform the three circuits; Table 15.8). Net energy expended each minute (excluding resting

---

Low Energy Expenditure

Standard resistance training with weights and barbells generates a relatively small number of calories "burned" during a workout. The total energy expended during this exercise equals about the same number of calories as walking on level ground at 4 mph, gardening, or swimming slowly for the equivalent time period.

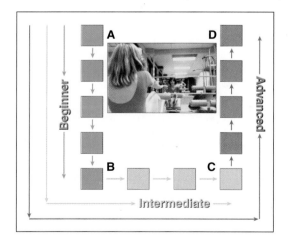

Figure 15.19
A basic multi-level circuit. Beginners can work twice through the circuit from A to B; after several weeks, they progress three times through this portion of the circuit; finally, they increase the number of circuit revolutions up to six, depending on the number of stations. At the intermediate level, add several stations; participants proceed three to six times through circuit A to C. Build progression into each circuit by increasing the number of stations (A to D), and/or exercise load, repetitions, and duration.

How to Assess Muscular Endurance

Muscular endurance represents how well a muscle (or muscle group) exerts submaximum force repeatedly within a given time period, or the duration a given muscle action can sustain a percentage of its 1-RM either dynamically or isometrically. The number of total repetitions of a muscle action in a given time (e.g., number of curl-ups, sit-ups, or push-ups within one minute) provides a common yardstick for expressing muscular endurance. Muscular endurance depends somewhat on a muscle's maximum strength, but little on cardiorespiratory fitness because components of aerobic fitness represent separate physiological (and fitness) entities. To test muscular endurance using weights, the weight lifted should coincide with either a percentage of body weight (Table 1) or a percentage of 1-RM so total repetition number averages between 15 and 20.

TABLE 1. RECOMMENDED PERCENT OF BODY WEIGHT LIFTED IN DIFFERENT RESISTANCE EXERCISE MOVEMENTS TO ASSESS MUSCULAR ENDURANCE

	PERCENT OF BODY WEIGHT	
EXERCISE	**MEN**	**WOMEN**
Arm curl	0.33	0.25
Bench press	0.66	0.50
Lateral pull down	0.66	0.50
Triceps extension	0.33	0.33
Leg extension	0.50	0.50
Leg curl	0.33	0.33

Two of the more popular muscular endurance tests do not require weights to assess endurance of the abdominal (curl-up) and upper-body (push-up) musculatures.

Curl-Up Muscular Endurance Test

Initial Position

The individual lies supine with knees flexed and feet about one foot from the buttocks. The arms extend forward with fingers palm-down on the thighs pointing towards the knees (Fig. 1A). The tester kneels behind the person with hands cupped (about 2 in off the floor) under the individual's head.

Movement

The person curls up slowly, sliding the fingers up the legs until the fingertips touch the patellae (knee caps; Fig. 1B), followed by slowly returning to the starting position with the back of the head touching the tester's hands. To reduce lower back strain, minimize rectus femoris involvement, and emphasize abdominal muscle action, no assistance should anchor or support the feet.

The Test and Standards

Required curl-up rate equals 20 repetitions per minute (3 s per curl-up; metronome set at 40 b · min^{-1}, or 2 beats per curl-up and recovery). Individuals perform as many curl-ups as possible at cadence, up to a maximum of 75. Table 2 presents standards for evaluating scores on the curl-up test.

TABLE 2. TEST STANDARDS TO ASSESS CURL-UP PERFORMANCE

	NUMBER CURL-UPS COMPLETED		
	AGE, y		
RATING	**<35**	**35–44**	**>45**
Excellent			
Men	60	50	40
Women	50	40	30
Good			
Men	45	40	25
Women	40	25	15
Fair			
Men	30	25	15
Women	25	15	10
Poor			
Men	15	10	5
Women	10	6	4

From Faulkner, R.A., et al.: A partial curl-up protocol for adults based on an analysis of two procedures. *Can. J. Sport Sci.*, 14:135, 1989; Sparling, P.B., et al.: Development of a cadence curl-up for college students. *Res. Q. Exerc. Sport.*, 68:309, 1997.

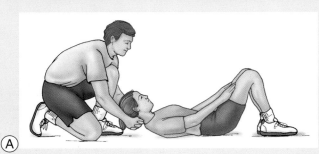
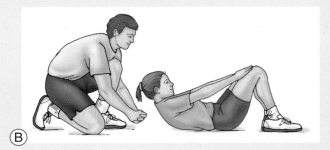

Figure 1.
Start **(A)** and finish **(B)** positions for the curl-up test.

Continued

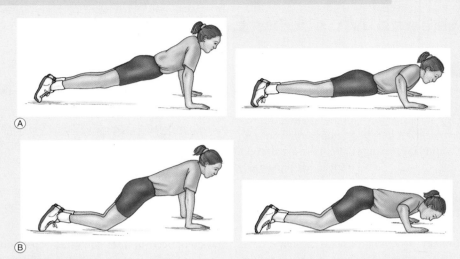

Figure 2.
Start and finish positions for **(A)** full body push-up and **(B)** modified push-up.

Push-Up Muscular Endurance Test

The push-up muscular endurance test can be performed in one of two ways: 1) full body push-up, and 2) modified push-up, which reduces the body mass above the arms, chest, and shoulders. Because females possess considerably less relative strength in upper-body musculature compared with males, the modified push-up serves as an alternative to assess individual differences in upper-body strength for females.

Initial Position

Full Body Push-Up: The person assumes a relatively stiff prone position from head to ankles, keeping the hands shoulder width apart and arms fully extended (Fig. 2A).

Modified Push-Up: The person assumes the bent-knee position with hips and buttocks pressing downward in line with the neck and shoulders (Fig. 2B).

Movement

Full Body Push-Up and Modified Push-Up: The body lowers until the elbows reach 90° of flexion; the return action requires pushing up until the arms fully extend. The push-up action should proceed in a continuous motion without rest pauses between flexion-extension movements.

Standards

Table 3 presents standards for scoring the full body push-up and modified push-up test.

TABLE 3. TEST STANDARDS TO ASSESS PUSH-UP PERFORMANCE OF MEN (FULL BODY PUSH-UP) AND WOMEN (MODIFIED PUSH-UP)

	NUMBER PUSH-UPS COMPLETED				
	AGE, y				
RATING	20–29	30–39	40–49	50–59	60+
Full body push-up					
Excellent	>54	>44	>39	>34	>29
Good	45–54	35–44	30–39	25–34	20–29
Average	35–44	25–34	20–29	15–24	10–19
Fair	20–34	15–24	12–19	8–14	5–9
Poor	<20	<15	<12	<8	<5
Modified push-up					
Excellent	>48	>39	>34	>29	>19
Good	34–48	25–39	20–34	15–29	5–19
Average	17–33	12–24	8–19	6–14	3–4
Fair	6–16	4–11	3–7	2–5	1–2
Poor	<6	<4	<3	<2	<1

From Pollock, M.L., et al.: *Health and Fitness Through Physical Activity*. New York: John Wiley & Sons, 1984.

TABLE 15.8
Net energy expenditure during circuit resistance training for men and women

BODY WEIGHT, lb	KCAL EXPENDED PER MINUTE[a]											
	100	110	120	130	140	150	160	170	180	190	200	210
Men			4.1	4.4	4.8	5.1	5.4	5.7	6.0	6.4	6.7	7.0
Women	3.4	3.6	3.7	3.9	4.1	4.3	4.4	4.6	4.8			

[a] Calculated from data of Wilmore, J.H., et al.: Energy cost of circuit weight training. *Med. Sci. Sports*, 10:75, 1978. To determine the total number of calories expended above rest during workouts, multiply the value in the column that corresponds to body weight by the duration of the circuit. For example, a 160-pound man who exercises for 43 minutes expends 232 kcal (5.4 kcal · min^{-1} × 43), excluding resting metabolism.

metabolism) equaled 129 kcal for men and 95 kcal for women over the total exercise period. Heart rate averaged 142 b · min^{-1} (72% HR$_{max}$; 40% VO$_{2max}$) for men and 158 b · min^{-1} (82% HR$_{max}$; 45% VO$_{2max}$) for women.

Because energy expended during the circuit related to the participant's body mass, Table 15.8 expresses the results in terms of body mass. On average, the continuous level of energy expended in CRT equaled that of a slow jog, hiking in the hills at a moderate pace, playing basketball or tennis, or leisurely swimming the crawl stroke.

CRT provides an alternative for fitness enthusiasts who desire a general conditioning program that improves both muscular strength and aerobic capacity. It can also supplement an off-season fitness program for sports requiring a high level of strength, power, and muscular endurance.

Body Composition Adaptations

Table 15.9 shows changes in body composition with DCER training from different experiments. For the most part, small decreases occur in body fat, with minimal increases in total body mass and FFM. The largest FFM increases amount to about 3 kg (6.6 lb) over 10 weeks, or about 0.3 kg weekly, with results about the same for men and women. Body composition data for other dynamic strength training systems show similar results. Thus, no one resistance training system proved superior for changing body composition.

Muscle Soreness and Stiffness

Following an extended layoff from exercise, most people experience pain, aches, soreness, tenderness, stiffness, or an uncomfortable feeling in exercised muscles and joints. Temporary soreness can persist several hours immediately following unaccustomed exercise, whereas residual **delayed-onset muscle soreness (DOMS)** may appear 24-hours later and last up to 2 weeks, depending on its severity. DOMS can range from mild (24 h post-exercise) to severe (5 d post-exercise.) Any one of at least six factors may cause DOMS:

1. Minute tears in muscle tissue damage cells, which release chemical substances (e.g., histamines, prostaglandins, bradykinin, proteolytic enzymes, potassium ions, anaerobic metabolites) that stimulate free nerve endings.
2. Osmotic pressure changes cause fluid retention (swelling) in surrounding tissues.
3. Muscle spasms or cramps (sudden, involuntary, severe contraction in a shortened position).
4. Overstretching and tearing of portions of the muscle's connective tissue harness (muscle-tendon junction) or the muscle's external surface. Structural damage to the internal myofibrils occurs in the region of the Z-line. Damage to this region, called Z-line streaming, may involve mechanical factors induced by high-force, eccentric muscle actions.
5. Alterations in the cell's mechanism for calcium regulation.
6. Inflammation responses (increases in white blood cells and interleukin-1 beta, and monocyte and leukocyte accumulation).

DOMS and Eccentric Muscle Action

Although the precise cause of muscle soreness remains unknown, the degree of discomfort largely depends on intensity and duration of effort and, most importantly, the type of exercise performed. *High-force/high-tension eccentric muscle actions (actively resisting muscle lengthening) generally produce the greatest postexercise damage and discom-*

TABLE 15.9
Body composition changes with resistance training[a]

GENDER	TRAINING DURATION	# OF EXERCISES	BODY COMPOSITION CHANGES		
			BODY MASS, kg	FFM, kg	%BODY FAT
F	10	10	0.1	1.3	−1.8
M	20	10	0.7	1.7	−1.5
M	9	5	0.5	1.4	−1.0
F	24	4	−0.04	1.0	−2.1
F	9	11	0.4	1.5	−1.3
M	8	10	1.0	3.1	−2.9
M	10	11	1.7	2.4	−9.1
F	10	8	−0.1	1.1	−1.9
M	10	8	0.3	1.2	−1.3
M	20	10	0.5	1.8	−1.7
F	7	7	−0.9	0.3	−1.5
M	7	7	0.6	0.5	−0.2
F	20	3	2.0	6.0	−4.0
F	18	4	0	1.0	−1.0
M	8	10	1.0	1.0	−4.0
M	8	3	0.7	1.8	−2.1
F	8	3	1.3	2.4	−2.9

[a] Data from different studies in the literature.

fort. This effect does not relate to lactate buildup because level running (primarily concentric actions) produces no residual soreness despite significant elevations in blood lactate. In contrast, downhill running (primarily eccentric actions) causes moderate-to-severe DOMS without significantly elevating lactate during or following exercise.

Cell Damage

Significant DOMS develops 42 hours following downhill running. Corresponding increases occur for serum levels of the muscle-specific enzyme creatine kinase (CK) and myoglobin (Mb) — both common markers of muscle damage. Subjects were retested on the same exercise after three, six, and nine weeks. Figure 15.20 shows the perceived soreness rating for the leg muscles as a function of time postexercise for the three study durations. For the three- and six-week comparisons, the differences between bouts were significant, with diminished DOMS for the second trial (open squares).

A similar pattern occurred for CK and Mb in relation to perception of muscle soreness. Interestingly, peak soreness ratings achieved at 48 hours did not correlate with absolute or relative changes in CK or Mb. Individuals reporting the greatest soreness did not necessarily have the highest CK and Mb values.

The first bout of repetitive, unaccustomed physical activity disrupts the integrity of the cells' internal environ-

ment. This can produce microlesions and subsequent temporary ultrastructural muscle damage in a pool of stress-susceptible or degenerating muscle fibers. Damage becomes more extensive several days after exercise than in the immediate postexercise period. *A single bout of moderate concentric exercise provides a significant prophylactic effect on muscle soreness in subsequent high-force eccentric exercise, with the effect persisting up to 6 weeks. Such results support the wisdom of initiating a training program with repetitive, moderate concentric exercise to protect against the muscle soreness that occurs following exercise with an eccentric component.*

Vitamin E Helps Reduce DOMS

As discussed in Chapter 3, vitamin E, an important antioxidant, thwarts free radical damage from lipid peroxidation, a process that increases the vulnerability of the cell and its constituents. Supplements of 800 IU of vitamin E taken every day for 7 days before 45 minutes of downhill running minimized muscle damage and reduced inflammation and soreness compared with a control group that received a placebo. In a subsequent experiment, subjects matched for prior training status and body size received either a placebo or vitamin E supplement (120 IU) for 2 weeks prior to resistance training. The acute exercise protocol, described as heavy or intense, consisted of a three-circuit workout using bench press, shoulder press, calf both groups equally rated the exercise as intense. The vitamin E-supplemented group had significantly lower 24-hour post-exercise CK levels than the placebo group. While plasma malondialdehyde concentration significantly increased in both groups compared to the pre-exercise conditions, no statistical difference existed between the groups. This study demonstrates that heavy resistance exercise increases free radical formation, and that supplementing with vitamin E minimizes damage to muscle fiber membranes as reflected by CK levels.

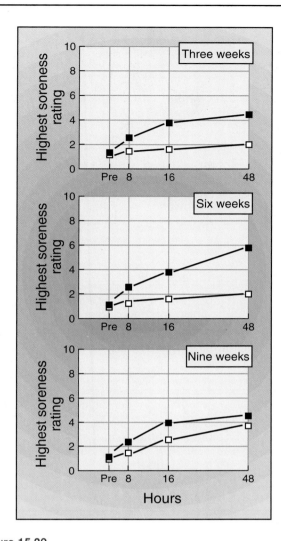

Figure 15.20
Highest soreness rating prior to and 8, 16, and 48 hours following bout 1 (closed square) and bout 2 (open square) performed three, six, and nine weeks later. Similar results were obtained for creatine kinase and myoglobin. (Data from Byrnes, W. C., et al.: Delayed onset muscle soreness following repeated bouts of downhill running. *J. Appl. Physiol.*, 59: 710, 1985.)

raise, and leg press exercises (Universal Gym apparatus), bent-over rows and arm curls (free weights), and squats (Tru-Squat machine). Following a warm-up set of 8-to-10 repetitions at 50% 1-RM, subjects performed three sets of 10-RM with a 2-minute rest following set 1, 1.5-minute rest after set 2, and 1-minute rest after set 3. Markers for tissue damage were assessed from blood sampled before and immediately after exercise, and for 6, 24, and 48 hours post exercise.

Figure 15.21 illustrates the effects of vitamin E supplementation on CK (upper panel) and plasma malondialdehyde (marker for free radical interaction with cell membranes; lower panel). Resistance exercise significantly increased blood lactate concentration in both groups, and

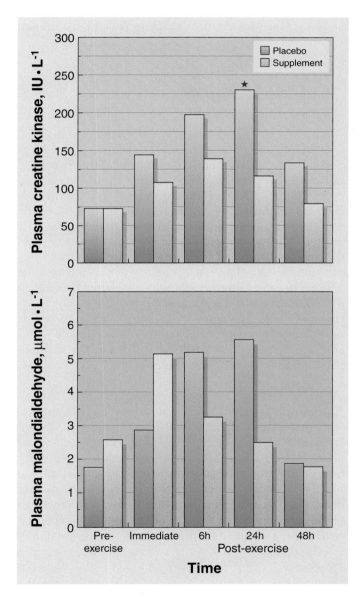

Figure 15.21
Time course of changes in plasma creatine kinase (top) and plasma malondialdehyde (bottom) following acute, intense circuit resistance training to evaluate the effects of vitamin E on free radical production and tissue damage. * indicates statistically significant between-group differences. (Adapted from McBride, J.M., et al.: Effect of resistance exercise on free radical production. *Med. Sci. Sports Exerc.*, 30:67, 1998.)

The proposed mechanism remains unknown concerning why intensive exercise increases free radical formation. Research suggests that mitochondrial hyperoxia may increase free radical formation during aerobic exercise. For intense muscular activities that emphasize high force production, reperfusion of blood at the muscle site following exercise may also trigger increased free radical formation as oxygen becomes available for recovery metabolisms. Additional research should focus on different modes of high-force exercise, including variations in intensity, duration, and frequency, and vitamin E supplementation on muscle remodeling.

Several theories attempt to explain DOMS, including:

* Spasm
* Tear
* Excess metabolite
* Connective tissue damage

Spasm Theory

Several early experiments support the **spasm theory** of muscle soreness. In one study, repeated wrist hyperextensions against a 4.3-kg resistance produced soreness in both arms. The muscles of one arm were then statically stretched. This proved beneficial because significantly greater soreness occurred 24 and 48 hours after exercise in the arm not stretched following exercise. Another study evaluated resting electromyographic (EMG) activity of the anterior lower leg muscles after static stretching in subjects with shin splints (musculoskeletal disorder involving severe pain along the anterior lower leg). Static stretching provided symptomatic relief and markedly reduced EMG activity. Despite these positive results, DOMS still persisted after postexercise stretching.

Tear Theory

The **tear theory** of muscle soreness proposes that minute tears or ruptures of individual fibers cause the delayed soreness. Because rapid, high-force eccentric actions place greater strain on connective tissue and muscle fibers compared with concentric muscle action (refer to Fig. 15.4), eccentric actions structurally change muscle fibers (with resulting enzyme efflux). In addition, white blood cells move into the area of damaged muscle fibers in response to acute inflammation and release chemicals like histamines and prostaglandins that activate pain receptors.

Excess Metabolite Theory

The **excess metabolite theory** proposes that prolonged exercise that follows a layoff causes metabolite accumulation in muscle. Fluid retention occurs because the metabolites trigger osmotic changes in the cellular environment. Edema caused by increased osmotic pressure excites sensory nerve endings and causes pain. Edema does not fully explain muscle soreness because greater soreness occurs

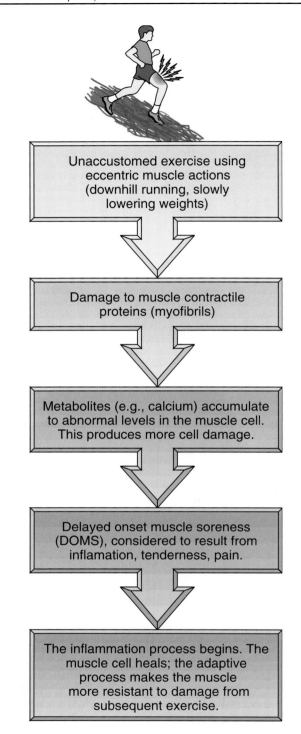

Figure 15.22
Proposed sequence for developing DOMS following unaccustomed exercise. Cellular recuperation from previous exercise provides enhanced resistance to subsequent damage and pain.

following eccentric exercise than after static or concentric actions. However, the metabolic stress of concentric (positive) work exceeds eccentric work by about five to seven times. Consequently, one would expect greater metabolite buildup and accompanying soreness in concentric and not eccentric exercise. This is not the case.

Connective Tissue Damage Theory

Research has evaluated the effects of connective tissue damage (**connective tissue damage theory**) from repeated bouts of arm-curl, weight-lifting exercise, and bench stepping to shed light on possible causative mechanisms for DOMS. Surface electrodes recorded EMG activity for up to 48 hours post exercise. Urine sampled at selected intervals evaluated myoglobinuria because myoglobin in the urine indicates trauma to muscle fibers. Urinary levels of hydroxyproline also evaluated connective tissue damage. This assay determines specific breakdown products of connective tissue and evaluates collagen metabolism. Subjects also rated muscle soreness using a subjective rating scale. No relationship emerged between muscle pain and EMG activity in sore muscles. Static stretching alleviated soreness somewhat for several minutes with no change in EMG activity. In fact, slowly flexing and extending the arm relieved pain to the same extent as static stretching.

Interesting results occurred for hydroxyproline excretion rates related to muscle soreness from bench stepping. All subjects reported soreness in the concentric (quadriceps) and eccentric (gastrocnemius) active muscles. Statistically significant increases occurred in 48-hour postexercise hydroxyproline levels, and in the total 4-day average excretion levels for the exercise compared with nonexercise conditions. The significant postexercise hydroxyproline increase, coupled with pain in the tendons of the eccentrically exercised muscles, suggests that connective tissue damage within muscle or an imbalance of collagen

metabolism (a degradation process) contributes to DOMS. Figure 15.22 outlines probable steps in DOMS development and recuperation.

Reducing DOMS

One strategy to help reduce DOMS (and muscle damage) uses fatiguing concentric exercise prior to initiating high-force eccentric muscle actions. Figure 15.23 displays changes in rating of DOMS for 5 days following either (a) fatiguing concentric elbow flexor exercise (100 maximal isokinetic, concentric actions at 1.05 rad·s^{-1}) that resulted in a 60% work decrement, followed by 12 fast, high-force eccentric actions with the same muscles, or (b) only the eccentric actions. Two weeks separated each of the experimental sessions. While both exercise conditions significantly increased perceived muscle soreness (based on rating scale from "no pain" to "very sore"), the eccentric only condition produced significantly more soreness. The same pattern of recovery from soreness occurred between exercise conditions. Changes in post-exercise plasma CK were also significantly greater when the eccentric exercise took place without prior concentric exercise. In other words, performing fatiguing concentric exercise before eccentric exercise diminished DOMS and an associated chemical marker of muscle damage. The beneficial effects of using concentric only exercise prior to a heavy bout of exercise with an eccentric component can be applied by initiating heavy resistance training when a significant episode of DOMS might profoundly affect optimal training ability.

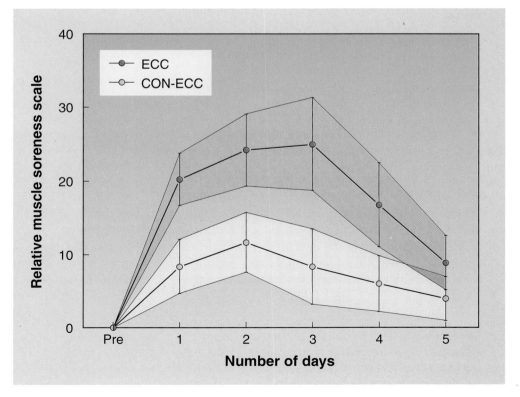

Figure 15.23
Changes in rating of muscle soreness before (Pre) and for five days following high-force, elbow flexor eccentric exercise. The shaded areas represent inter-individual variability. The experimental conditions represent eccentric only exercise (ECC) and concentric exercise (CON) preceding eccentric exercise (CON-ECC). (Data from Nosakia, K., and Clarkson, P.M.: Influence of previous concentric exercise on eccentric exercise-induced muscle damage. *J. Sports Sci.*, 15:477, 1997.)

summary

1. Genetic, exercise, nutritional, hormonal, environmental, and neural factors interact to regulate skeletal muscle mass and corresponding strength development.

2. Physiologic factors (e.g., size and type of muscle fibers, and anatomic-lever arrangement of bone and muscle) largely determine an individual's muscular strength. Neural influences from the central nervous system that activate prime movers in a specific movement greatly affect strength capacity.

3. Muscular strength increases with resistance training result from (a) improved capacity for neuromuscular activation, and (b) significant alterations in a muscle fiber's contractile elements.

4. As overloaded muscles become stronger, individual fibers normally grow larger (hypertrophy). Total muscle enlargement involves (a) increased protein synthesis within the fiber's contractile elements, and (b) proliferation of connective tissue cells that thicken and strengthen the muscle's connective tissue harness.

5. Muscle fiber hypertrophy involves (a) structural changes within the contractile mechanism of individual fibers (particularly fast-twitch fibers), and (b) increases in intramuscular anaerobic energy stores. If new muscle fibers actually develop, their contribution to muscular enlargement remains unknown.

6. Heavy resistance training does not induce cellular component adaptations that enhance aerobic energy transfer.

7. Women and men improve strength and muscle size to about the same relative extent (percentage) with resistance training.

8. Conventional resistance-training exercises contribute little to cardiovascular-aerobic fitness. Because of the relatively low caloric cost, most resistance training programs would not reduce body fat significantly.

9. Circuit resistance training using lower resistance and higher repetitions offers an effective alternative to heavy muscular overload by combining the muscle-training benefits of resistance exercise with cardiovascular, calorie-burning benefits of continuous exercise.

10. Eccentric muscle actions produce significantly more delayed-onset muscle soreness (DOMS) compared with concentric only and isometric exercise.

11. A single bout of exercise provides a significant protective effect from muscle damage and soreness in subsequent exercise. This supports the wisdom of gradual progression when beginning an exercise program.

12. Experimental evidence supports the argument for muscle tears and connective tissue damage causing DOMS. Disruption of the sarcoplasmic reticulum and associated changes in calcium regulation may damage cells.

thought questions

1. For a football lineman, how would you apply the principle of specificity to (a) evaluate current muscular strength and power, and (b) improve muscular performance for football?

2. If women respond to resistance training essentially the same as men, why doesn't the upper arm girth of female body builders equal their male counterparts?

3. Outline how you would design a resistance training program for sedentary, middle-age men and women.

4. Discuss the statement: No one best system of resistance training exists.

5. Describe the ideal resistance training equipment for a competitive sprint swimmer.

6. Outline tests to evaluate muscular performance to best reflect the force-power requirements for firefighters.

selected references

Abernethy, P.J., and Quigley, B. M.: Concurrent strength and endurance training of the elbow flexors. *J. Strength and Cond. Res.*, 7 : 234, 1993.

Adams, G.R., et al.: Skeletal muscle myosin heavy chain composition and resistance training. *J. Appl. Physiol.*, 74:911, 1993.

Allerheiligen, W.B.: Speed development and plyometric training. In: *Essentials of Strength Training and Conditioning.* Baechle T.R. (ed.). Champaign, IL: Human Kinetics, 1994.

Alway, S.E., et al.: Contrasts in muscle and myofibers of elite male and female body builders. *J. Appl. Physiol.*, 67:24, 1989.

Baker, D., et al: Periodization: the effect on strength of manipulating volume and intensity. *J. Strength and Cond. Res.*, 8: 235, 1994.

Bentsen, H., et al.: The effect of dynamic strength back exercise and/or home training program in 57-year-old women with chronic low back pain: results of a prospective randomized study with a 3-year follow-up period. *Spine*, 2:1494, 1997.

Braith, R.W., et al.: Effect of training on the relationship between maximal and submaximal strength. *Med. Sci. Sports Exerc.*, 25 : 132, 1993.

Carpenter, D.M., and Nelson, B.W.: Low back strengthening for the prevention and treatment of low back pain. *Med. Sci. Sports Exerc.*, 31:18, 1999.

Carson, J.A.: The regulation of gene expression in hypertrophying skeletal muscle. *Exer. Sport Sci. Revs.*, 25:301, 1997.

Clarkson, P.M.: Oh, those aching muscles: Causes and consequences of delayed onset muscle soreness. *ACSM's Health & Fitness J.*, 1(3):12, 1997.

Clarkson, P.M., et al.: Muscle function after exercise-induced muscle damage and rapid adaptation. *Med. Sci. Sports Exerc.*, 24:512, 1992.

Cureton, K. J., et al.: Muscle hypertrophy in men and women. *Med. Sci. Sports Exerc.*, 20 : 338, 1988.

DeLorme, T.L., and Watkins, A.L.: *Progressive Resistance Exercise.* New York: Appleton-Century-Crofts, 1951.

Duarte, J.A., et al.: Exercise-induced signs of muscle overuse in children. *Int. J. Sports Med.*, 20:103, 1999.

Evans, W.J., and Cannon, J.G.: The metabolic effects of exercise-induced muscle damage. In: *Exercise and Sport Sciences Reviews.* Vol. 19. Holloszy J.O. (ed.). Baltimore: Williams & Wilkins, 1991.

Feigenbaum, M.S., and Pollock, M.L.: Prescription of resistance training for health and disease. *Med. Sci. Sports Exerc.*, 31:38, 1999.

Fleck, S.J.: Periodized strength training: A critical review. *J. Strength and Cond. Res.*, 13:82, 1999.

Fleck, S.J., and Kraemer, W.J.: *Designing Resistance Training Programs.* 2nd Ed. Champaign, IL: Human Kinetics, 1997.

Fletcher, G.F., et al.: Statement on exercise: benefits and recommendations for physical activity programs for all Americans: a statement for health professionals by the committee on exercise and cardiac rehabilitation of the Council on clinical cardiology. American Heart Association. *Circulation*, 94:857, 1996.

Frontera, W.R., et al.: Strength conditioning in older men: skeletal muscle hypertrophy and improved function. *J. Appl. Physiol.*, 64:1038, 1988.

Graves, J.E., et al.: Specificity of limited range of motion variable resistance training. *Med. Sci. Sports Exerc.*, 21:84, 1989.

Harmon, E: Resistive torque analysis of 5 Nautilus exercise machines. *Med. Sci. Sports Exerc.*, 15: 113, 1983.

Hather, B.M., et al.: Influence of eccentric actions on skeletal muscle adaptations to resistance training. *Acta Physiol. Scand.*, 143:177, 1992.

Heyward, V. H., et al.: Gender differences in strength. *Res. Q. Exerc. Sport*, 57:154, 1986.

Housh, D.J., et al.: Effects of unilateral concentric-only dynamic constant external resistance training on quadriceps femoris cross-sectional area. *J. Strength and Cond. Res.*, 12:185, 1998.

Ikai, M., and Steinhaus, A.H.: Some factors modifying the expression of human strength. *J. Appl. Physiol.*, 16:157, 1961.

Katch, F.I., et al.: Evaluation of acute cardiorespiratory responses to hydraulic resistance exercise. *Med. Sci. Sports Exerc.*, 17:168, 1985.

Kellis, E., and Blatzopoulos, V.: Muscle activation differences between eccentric and concentric isokinetic exercise. *Med. Sci. Sports Exerc.*, 30:1616, 1998.

Kyröläinen, H., et al.: Muscle damage induced by stretch-shortening cycle exercise. *Med. Sci. Sports Exerc.*, 30: 415, 1998.

Layne, J.E., and Nelson, M.E.: The effects of progressive resistance training on bone density: a review. *Med. Sci. Sports Exerc.*, 31:25, 1999.

Lieber, R.L.: *Skeletal Muscle Structure and Function.* Baltimore: Williams & Wilkins, 1992.

Lyttle, A.D., et al.: Enhancing performance: Maximal power versus combined weights and plyometric training. *J. Strength and Cond. Res.*, 10:173, 1996.

McBride, J.M., et al.: Effect of resistance exercise on free radical production. *Med. Sci. Sports Exerc.*, 30:67, 1998.

Narici, M., et al.: Human quadriceps cross-sectional area, torque, and neural activation during 6 months strength training. *Acta Physiol. Scand.*, 1547:175, 1996.

Newton, R.U., et al.: Effects of ballistic training on preseason preparation of elite volleyball players. *Med. Sci. Sports Exerc.*, 31:323, 1999.

Ozmun, J.C., et al.: Neuromuscular adaptations following prepubescent strength training. *Med. Sci. Sports Exerc.*, 26: 510, 1994.

Payne, V.G., et al.: Endurance training in children and youth: a meta-analysis. *Res. Q. Exerc. Sport*, 68:80, 1997.

Pollock, M.L., et al.: The recommended quantity and quality of exercise for developing and maintaining cardiorespiratory fitness, strength, and flexibility in healthy adults. *Med. Sci. Sports Exerc.*, 30:975, 1998.

Prevost, M.C., et al.: The effect of two days of velocity-specific isokinetic training on torque production. *J. Strength and Cond. Res.*, 13:35, 1999.

Rantanen, T., et al.: Midlife hand grip strength as a predictor of old age disability. *JAMA*, 281:558, 1999.

Sale, D.G.: Influence of exercise and training on motor unit activation. In: *Exercise and Sport Sciences Reviews.* Vol. 15. Pandolf K.B. (ed.). New York: Macmillan, 1987.

Seger, J.Y., et al.: Specific effects of eccentric and concentric training on muscle strength and morphology in humans. *Eur. J. Appl. Physiol.*, 79:49, 1998.

Sipalä, S., and Suominen, H.: Effects of strength and endurance training on thigh and leg muscle mass and composition in elderly women. *J. Appl. Physiol.*, 78: 334, 1995.

Sjöström, M., et al.: Evidence of fiber hyperplasia in human skeletal muscles from healthy young men. *Eur. J. Appl. Physiol.*, 62: 301, 1992.

Staron, R.S., et al.: Skeletal muscle adaptations during the early phase of heavy-resistance training in men and women. *J. Appl. Physiol.*, 76: 1247, 1994.

Takarada, Y., et al.: Stretch-induced enhancement of mechanical power output in human multi-joint exercise with countermovement. *J. Appl. Physiol.*, 83:1749, 1997.

Walshe, J.P., et al.: Stretch-shorten cycle compared with isometric preload: contributions to enhanced muscular performance. *J. Appl. Physiol.*, 84:97, 1998.

Wathan, D.: Periodization: concepts and applications. In: *Essentials of Strength Training and Conditioning.* Baechle T.R. (ed.). Champaign, IL: Human Kinetics, 1994.

Weir, J.P., et al.: Electromyographic evaluation of joint angle specificity and cross-training after isometric training. *J. Appl. Physiol.*, 77: 1927, 1994.

Weltman, A.W., et al.: The effects of hydraulic resistance strength training in pre-pubertal males. *Med. Sci. Sports Exerc.*, 18:629, 1986.

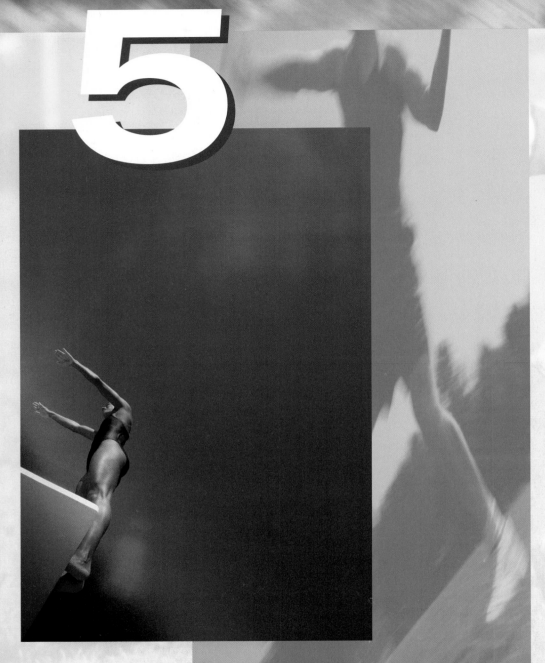

SECTION 5

Factors Affecting Physiological Function, Energy Transfer, and Exercise Performance

In many instances, the environment influences the body's physiology in a way that augments the stress of exercise and reduces performance. For example, sport competitions held at altitudes can impair the normal oxygenation of blood flowing through the lungs. Above a certain elevation, the capacity to generate energy aerobically becomes severely compromised. Exercise in a hot humid environment or under conditions of extreme cold can impose a severe thermal stress that dramatically affects not only exercise performance but also the participant's health and safety. The degree to which an environmental stressor deviates from neutral conditions as well as the duration of the exposure determines its total effect. In addition, several environmental stressors operating at the same time (e.g., extreme cold exposure at high altitude) may exceed and override the simple additive effects of each stressor imposed singularly.

In addition to attempting to blunt the adverse effects of environmental stress, coaches and athletes continually search for additional ways to gain the competitive "edge" and improve athletic performance. It should come as no suprise, therefore, that a variety of substances and procedures are used routinely at almost all competitive levels, often without regard for potential health dangers or lack of scientific evidence to support their effectiveness. College and professional athletes most frequently use drugs, whereas nutrition supplementation and warm-up procedures are common among the general population who train for fitness and sports activities.

Chapter 16 presents a discussion of the specific problems encountered at altitude and during exercise in hot and cold environments. We present this information within the framework of the immediate physiological adjustments and longer-term adaptations as the body strives to maintain internal consistency despite an environmental challenge. In Chapter 17, we explore a variety of substances and "treatments" alleged to improve physiologic function, exercise capacity, or athletic performance.

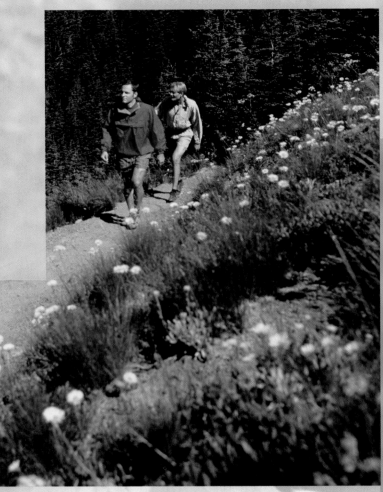

CHAPTER

16

Topics covered in this chapter

PART 1 Mechanisms of Thermoregulation

Thermoregulation
Thermal Balance
Hypothalamic Regulation of Body Temperature
Thermoregulation in Cold Stress
Thermoregulation in Heat Stress
Integration of Heat Dissipating Mechanisms
Effects of Clothing on Thermoregulation
Nutritional Aspects of Exercise in Extreme Environments
Summary

PART 2 Thermoregulation and Environmental Stress During Exercise

Exercise in the Heat
Circulatory Adjustments
Core Temperature During Exercise
Water Loss in the Heat
Factors That Improve Heat Tolerance
Evaluating Environmental Heat Stress
Exercise in the Cold
Evaluating Environmental Cold Stress
Summary

PART 3 Exercise at Altitude

Stress of Altitude
Acclimatization
Altitude-Related Medical Problems
Exercise Capacity at Altitude
Altitude Training and Sea Level Performance
Summary
Thought Questions
Selected References

Environment and Exercise

- Explain the statement: The hypothalamus plays the most important role in regulating the body's thermal balance.

- Name four physical factors contributing to heat exchange during rest and exercise.

- Describe how the circulatory system serves as a "workhorse" for thermoregulation.

- List desirable clothing characteristics for exercising in cold and warm weather.

- Describe how cardiac output, heart rate, and stroke volume respond during submaximal and maximal exercise in the heat.

- Describe circulatory adjustments that maintain blood pressure during exercise in the heat.

- Quantify fluid loss during hot-weather exercise.

- Identify the physiologic consequences resulting from dehydration.

- Explain how acclimatization, training, age, gender, and body fat modify heat tolerance during exercise.

- Identify factors comprising the Heat Stress Index.

- Explain the purpose of the Wind Chill Index.

- Describe the physiologic adjustments to cold stress.

- Outline the effects of increasingly higher altitudes on (a) partial pressure of oxygen in ambient air, (b) saturation of hemoglobin with oxygen in pulmonary capillaries, and (c) $\dot{V}O_{2max}$.

- Describe a plausible scenario for the occurrence of blackout during attempts to extend the duration of a breath-hold dive.

- Describe the immediate and long-term physiologic adjustments to altitude exposure.

- Outline three approaches for creating an altitude environment at sea level so an athlete can spend sufficient time to stimulate an acclimatization response.

PART 1

Mechanisms of Thermoregulation

Thermoregulation

Normal body temperature fluctuates several degrees during the day in response to physical activity, emotions, and ambient temperature variations (Fig. 16.1)—with oral temperature averaging about 1.0°F (0.56°C) less than rectal temperature. Body temperature also exhibits diurnal fluctuations; lowest temperatures occur during sleep, and slightly higher temperatures persist when awake, even when the person remains relaxed in bed.

Thermoregulation plays such an important role in the body's homeostatic balance that the price of failure can be death. A person can tolerate a drop in deep body temperature of 18°F (10°C) but only an increase of 5°C (9°F). More than 100 times over the past 20 years, football players have died from excessive heat stress during practice or competition. Hypothermia and dehydration have been linked to the deaths of three collegiate wrestlers in the latter part of 1997. Heat injury also commonly occurs during military operations and longer-duration athletic events. Athletes who illegally use erythropoietin, a hormone that boosts production of red blood cells, have an even greater risk of heat injury because blood viscosity increases (from an increased hematocrit) as dehydration progresses while exercising in the heat.

Understanding thermoregulation and the most effective ways to support temperature control mechanisms can significantly reduce heat-related tragedies. Coaches, athletes, and race and event organizers must reduce factors that foster heat gain and dehydration. Concern should also focus on the most effective behavioral approaches (e.g., prudent scheduling of events, acclimatization, proper clothing, and fluid and electrolyte replacement before, during, and after exercise) to blunt the potential for negative effects on performance and safety.

Thermal Balance

Figure 16.2 lists factors that contribute to heat gain and loss as the body attempts to maintain thermal neutrality. This balance results from integrative mechanisms that:

- Alter heat transfer to the periphery (**shell**)
- Regulate evaporative cooling
- Vary the body's rate of heat production

Core temperature rises quickly when heat gain exceeds heat loss during vigorous exercise in a warm environment.

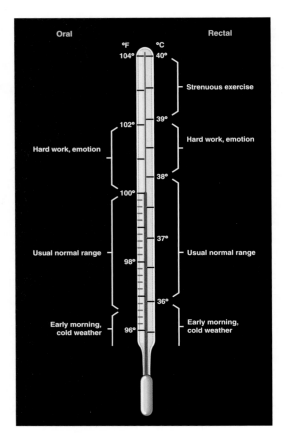

Figure 16.1
Normal range of body temperature in humans.

In the cold, on the other hand, heat loss often exceeds heat production, and core temperature falls.

Body Temperature Measurement

A thermal gradient exists within the body, with core body temperature (T_{core}) being the highest and surface temper-

ature (T_{skin}) the lowest. Mean body temperature ($\overline{T}_{body}$) represents an average of skin and internal temperatures. Common sites to estimate average core temperature ($\overline{T}_{core}$) include the rectum, eardrum (tympanic temperature), and esophagus (esophageal temperature). Although variations among these measures exist, the values estimate brain temperature that controls thermoregulation. Temperature sensors (thermistors) placed at various skin locations estimate T_{skin}. Mean skin temperature ($\overline{T}_{skin}$) denotes the weighted average of different skin temperatures, taking into account the portion of the body's surface each site encompasses (e.g., arm, trunk, leg, head). $\overline{T}_{body}$ computes as follows:

$$\overline{T}_{body} = (0.6 \times \overline{T}_{core}) + (0.4 \times \overline{T}_{skin})$$

where the relative proportion of the body's average temperature represented by the core equals 0.6 (60%) and 0.4 (40%) for the skin.

Hypothalamic Regulation of Temperature

The **hypothalamus** *contains the central coordinating center for temperature regulation.* This group of specialized neurons at the floor of the brain serves as a thermostat to carefully regulate temperature within a narrow range of 37°C ±1°C (98.6°F ±1.8°F). Unlike a home thermostat, however,

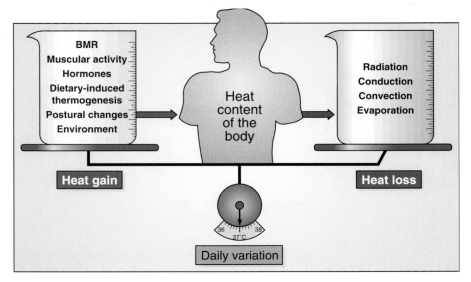

Figure 16.2
Factors that contribute to heat gain and heat loss as the body regulates core temperature at approximately 98.6°F (37°C).

the hypothalamus cannot turn off the heat; it only initiates responses to protect the body when core temperature changes from its "norm" because of heat gain or heat loss. Heat-regulating mechanisms become activated in two ways:

1. Thermal receptors in the skin provide peripheral input to the hypothalamic central control center
2. Temperature changes in blood perfusing the hypothalamus directly stimulate the hypothalamic central control center

Free nerve endings in the skin serve primarily as peripheral thermal receptors (i.e., sensors responsive to rapid changes in heat and cold). The receptors relay sensory information to the hypothalamus and cerebral cortex to conserve or dissipate heat. This also causes the individual to consciously seek relief from the thermal challenge.

The central hypothalamic regulatory center plays the most important role in maintaining thermal balance. Cells in the anterior hypothalamus directly detect changes in blood temperature, in addition to receiving peripheral input. The cells then activate either the posterior hypothalamus to initiate coordinated responses for heat conservation or the anterior hypothalamus for heat loss. Peripheral receptors primarily detect cold, but the hypothalamus monitors body warmth via the temperature of the blood perfusing this area. Table 16.1 summarizes the mechanisms for regulating body temperature; each responds in graded manner, increasing or decreasing as required.

Thermoregulation in Cold Stress

Heat normally transfers from the body to the environment, and core temperature regulates without excessive physiologic strain. In extreme cold, however, excessive heat loss can occur especially at rest. This increases the body's heat production and slows heat loss as physiologic adjustments combat a decrease in core temperature.

Vascular Adjustments

Circulatory adjustments "fine tune" temperature regulation. Stimulation of cutaneous cold receptors constricts peripheral blood vessels. Vasoconstriction immediately reduces the flow of warm blood to the body's cooler surface and redirects it to the warmer core (cranial, thoracic, and abdominal cavities and portions of the muscle mass). Consequently, skin temperature decreases toward ambient temperature, which optimizes the insulatory benefits of skin and subcutaneous fat.

Muscular Activity

The greatest contribution of muscle in defending against cold occurs during physical activity, although shivering generates significant metabolic heat (maximum of 3 to 5 times resting metabolism). Exercise energy metabolism can sustain a constant core temperature in air temperatures as low as $-30°C$ ($-22°F$) without the need for heavy clothing.

Hormonal Output

The action of the two adrenal medulla hormones, epinephrine and norepinephrine, partially accounts for increased basal heat production during cold exposure. Prolonged cold stress also increases the release of thyroxine, the thyroid hormone, which elevates resting metabolism.

Thermoregulation in Heat Stress

The body's thermoregulatory mechanisms primarily protect against overheating. Thwarting excessive body heat buildup becomes important during intense exercise where metabolic rate often increases 20 to 25 times the resting level—heat production that could increase core temperature by 1.8°F (1°C) every 5 minutes. Here, competition exists between mechanisms that maintain a large muscle blood flow and mechanisms that regulate body temperature. Figure 16.3 illustrates potential avenues for heat exchange in an exercising human. Body heat loss occurs in four ways:

1. Radiation
2. Conduction
3. Convection
4. Evaporation

Heat Loss by Radiation

Objects continually emit electromagnetic heat waves. Because our bodies are usually warmer than the environ-

TABLE 16.1
Mechanisms for temperature regulation

STIMULATED BY COLD

Decreases heat loss	Vasoconstriction of skin vessels; postural reduction of surface area (curling up)
Increases heat production	Shivering and increased voluntary activity; increased thyroxine and epinephrine secretion

STIMULATED BY HEAT

Increases heat loss	Vasodilation of subcutaneous skin vessels; sweating
Decreases heat production	Decreased muscle tone and voluntary activity; decreased secretion of thyroxine and epinephrine

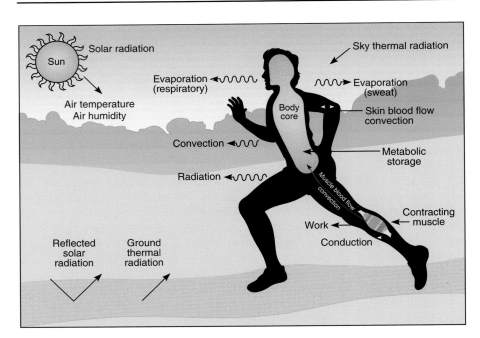

Figure 16.3
Heat production within active muscle and its subsequent transfer to the core and skin. Under appropriate environmental conditions, excess body heat dissipates to the environment and core temperature regulates within a narrow range.

(as it does on a breezy day, in a room with a fan, or during running), heat loss increases because convective currents carry the heat away. For example, air currents at 4 mph cool twice as effectively as air moving at 1 mph.

ment, the net exchange of **radiant heat energy** occurs from the body through the air to solid, cooler objects in the environment. This form of heat transfer, similar to how the sun's rays warm the earth, does not require molecular contact between objects. Despite subfreezing temperatures, a person can remain warm by absorbing sufficient radiant heat energy from direct sunlight (or reflected from the snow, sand, or water). The body absorbs radiant heat energy when the temperature of objects in the environment exceeds skin temperature, making evaporative cooling the only avenue for heat loss.

Heat Loss by Conduction

Heat loss by **conduction** involves the direct transfer of heat through a liquid, solid, or gas from one molecule to another. Although circulation transports most of the body heat to the shell, a small amount continually moves by conduction directly through the deep tissues to the cooler surface. Conductive heat loss then involves the warming of air molecules and cooler surfaces that contact the skin.

The rate of conductive heat loss depends on the temperature gradient between the skin and surrounding surfaces and their thermal qualities. Warm-weather hikers gain considerable body heat from physical activity and the environment. Some relief comes from lying on a cool rock shielded from the sun. Conductance between the rock's cold surface and the hiker's warmer surface facilitates body heat loss until the rock warms to body temperature.

Heat Loss by Convection

The effectiveness of heat loss by conduction depends on how rapidly air near the body exchanges once it becomes warmed. With little or no air movement (**convection**), air next to the skin warms and acts as a zone of insulation, minimizing further conductive heat loss. Conversely, if cooler air continuously replaces warmer air surrounding the body

Heat Loss by Evaporation

Evaporation provides the major physiologic defense against overheating. Water vaporization from the respiratory passages and skin surface continually transfers heat to the environment. For each liter of water vaporized, 580 kcal of heat energy transfer from the body to the environment.

In response to heat stress, the body's two to four million sweat (eccrine) glands secrete large quantities of hypotonic saline solution (0.2 to 0.4% NaCl). Cooling occurs when sweat reaches the skin and fluid evaporates. The cooled skin then cools the blood shunted from the interior to the surface. Along with heat loss through sweating, approximately 350 mL of water seeps through the skin (**insensible perspiration**) each day and evaporates to the environment. Also, approximately 300 mL of water vaporizes daily from respiratory passages' moist mucous membranes. In cold weather, respiratory tract evaporation appears as "foggy breath."

Evaporative Heat Loss at High Ambient Temperatures

Increased ambient temperature reduces the effectiveness of heat loss by conduction, convection, and radiation. When ambient temperature exceeds body temperature, these three mechanisms of thermal transfer actually contribute to heat gain. When this occurs (or when conduction, convection, and radiation cannot adequately dissipate a large metabolic heat load), sweat evaporation and water vaporization from the respiratory tract provide the only avenue for dissipating heat. For someone relaxing in a hot, humid environment, the normal 2-L daily fluid requirement doubles or even triples because of evaporative fluid loss.

Heat Loss in High Humidity

Sweat evaporation from the skin depends on three factors:

1. Surface exposed to the environment
2. Temperature and relative humidity of ambient air
3. Convective air currents around the body

How to Estimate the Evaporative Cooling Required to Maintain Constant Core Temperature During Exercise

Evaporation describes the conversion of a substance from liquid form into a gaseous state. The process requires heat energy to overcome the cohesive forces that hold molecules together so as to form the vapor. Heat loss from water evaporation accounts for nearly 25% of all heat loss at rest, and at least 75% during exercise. Heat transfers from the body to water on the skin and pulmonary surfaces. Evaporation results from a vapor pressure gradient (the pressure exerted by water molecules as they convert to a gas, or water vapor) between the skin and ambient air (see figure). A large vapor pressure gradient between water molecules on the skin and in ambient air facilitates evaporation and subsequent body cooling. An increase in ambient air's relative humidity increases its vapor pressure, thwarting evaporative skin cooling because of a diminished vapor pressure gradient between skin and air. This explains the difficulty in dissipating body heat during vigorous exercise in a humid environment.

Each one liter of water evaporated from the skin and pulmonary airways transfers 580 kcal of heat energy (0.58 kcal per mL) to the environment. Consequently, if evaporative cooling represented the *only* mechanism for heat dissipation, one can estimate the magnitude of evaporation required to maintain a constant core temperature during exercise.

Problem

An individual walks at 3.5 mph for 60 minutes on the level at an oxygen uptake of 0.8 L·min^{-1}. Estimate the following:

1. Heat production during exercise
2. Magnitude of evaporative cooling required to prevent a core temperature increase

Solution

A. Determine total energy expenditure during exercise

1. Compute total $\dot{V}O_2$ during exercise.

Total $\dot{V}O_2$ = $\dot{V}O_2$, L·min^{-1} × minutes of exercise
= 0.8 L·min^{-1} × 60 min
= 48.0 L

2. Convert total $\dot{V}O_2$ to enegy expenditure (assume 1 L O_2 = 5.05 kcal)

Total energy expenditure = 48.0 L × 5.05 kcal
= 242.4 kcal

B. Determine total heat produced during exercise

Computation of total heat production must consider mechanical efficiency for exercise (i.e., % total energy converted to mechanical work versus % total energy dissipated as heat); assume 22% mechanical efficiency for walking. Consequently, of the total energy required for exercise, 78% appears as heat (100% − 22%).

Total heat produced, kcal = total energy expenditure, kcal × percent lost as heat
= 242.4 kcal × 0.78
= 189.1 kcal

C. Calculate total fluid evaporation required to prevent an increase in core temperature

Total evaporation = total heat produced, kcal ÷
required   kcal heat loss per L evaporation
= 189.1 kcal ÷ 580 kcal·L^{-1}
= 0.326 L or 326 mL or 11 oz

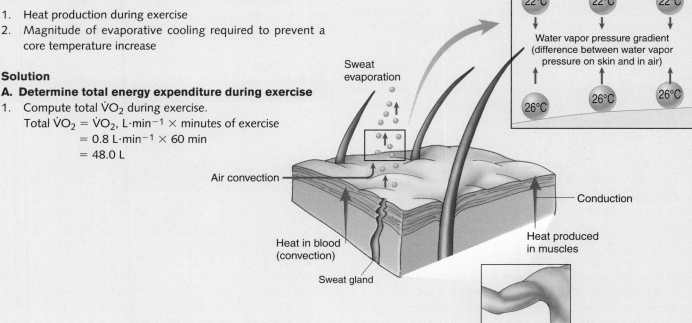

*By far, **relative humidity** exerts the greatest impact on the effectiveness of evaporative heat loss.*

With high humidity, ambient air's vapor pressure approaches that of moist skin (approximately 40 mm Hg), and evaporation decreases substantially, even though large quantities of sweat bead on the skin and eventually roll off. This represents a useless water loss that can lead to dehydration and overheating.

Continually drying the skin with a towel before sweat evaporates also hinders evaporative cooling. *Sweat does not cool the skin; rather, skin cooling occurs when sweat evaporates.* Individuals can tolerate relatively high environmental temperatures when humidity remains low. For this reason, people prefer the comfort of hot, dry desert climates over cooler but more humid tropical climates.

Integration of Heat-Dissipating Mechanisms

Heat dissipation involves the integration of several factors, including circulation, evaporation, and hormonal adjustments.

Circulation

The circulatory system serves as the "workhorse" to maintain thermal balance. At rest in hot weather, heart rate and cardiac output increase while superficial arterial and venous blood vessels dilate to divert warm blood to the body's shell. Peripheral vasodilation causes a flushed or reddened face on a hot day or during vigorous exercise. With extreme heat stress, 15 to 25% of the cardiac output passes through the skin, greatly increasing thermal conductance of peripheral tissues. This favors radiative heat loss to the environment, mostly from the hands, forehead, forearms, ears, and tibial region.

Evaporation

Sweating begins several seconds after initiation of vigorous exercise, and after about 30 minutes reaches an equilibrium directly related to exercise load. A large cutaneous blood flow coupled with evaporative cooling usually produces an effective thermal defense. The cooled peripheral blood then returns to deeper tissues and picks up additional heat on its return to the heart.

Hormonal Adjustments

Heat stress initiates hormonal adjustments to conserve salts and fluid lost in sweat. The pituitary gland releases **vasopressin (antidiuretic hormone or ADH)** in response to a thermal challenge. *ADH increases water reabsorption from kidney tubules, causing more concentrated urine during heat stress.* Concurrently, with even a single bout of exercise or repeated days of exercise in hot weather, the adrenal cortex releases the sodium-conserving hormone **aldosterone** to increase the renal tubules' reabsorption of sodium. Aldosterone also acts on the sweat glands to reduce sweat's osmolality, further conserving electrolytes.

Figure 16.4 shows the major temperature-regulating mechanisms. The dashed lines represent hormonal pathways, which probably serve a minor role in humans. The major input provided by thermoreceptors in the skin and the temperature of blood flowing through the hypothalamus initiates a series of conscious (behavioral) and subconscious (physiologic, metabolic) responses to reduce thermal stress.

Effects of Clothing On Thermoregulation

Clothing insulates the body from its surroundings. It can reduce radiant heat gain in a hot environment, or retard conductive and convective heat loss in the cold.

Cold-Weather Clothing

The mesh of the clothing's fibers traps air and warms it to provide insulation from the cold. This establishes a barrier to heat loss because cloth and air both conduct heat

Air Contains Water

Relative humidity describes the ratio of water in ambient air to its total capacity for moisture at a particular ambient temperature, expressed as a percentage. For example, 40% relative humidity means that ambient air contains only 40% of the air's moisture-carrying capacity at a specific temperature.

Football Uniforms Impede Thermoregulation

Football uniforms present a significant barrier to heat dissipation. Even with loose-fitting porous jerseys, the wrappings, padding (with plastic covering), helmet, and other objects of "armor" effectively seal off 50% of the body's surface from evaporative cooling. The players' large body size further magnifies heat load, particularly for offensive and defensive linemen. They possess a relatively small body surface area-to-body mass ratio and a higher percentage of body fat than players at other positions, which makes them subject to greater risk for heat illness.

poorly. A thicker zone of trapped air next to the skin provides more effective insulation. For this reason, several layers of light clothing, or garments lined with animal fur, feathers, or synthetic fabrics (with numerous layers of trapped air), insulate better than a single bulky layer of winter clothing.

The clothing layer against the skin must transport moisture away from the body's surface to the next clothing layer (the insulating layer) for subsequent evaporation. Wool or synthetics (e.g., polypropylene) that insulate well and dry quickly serve this purpose. When clothing becomes wet, either through external moisture or condensation from sweating, it loses nearly 90% of its insulating properties. Wet clothing actually facilitates heat transfer from the body because water conducts heat much faster than air.

When working or exercising in cold air, adequacy of in-

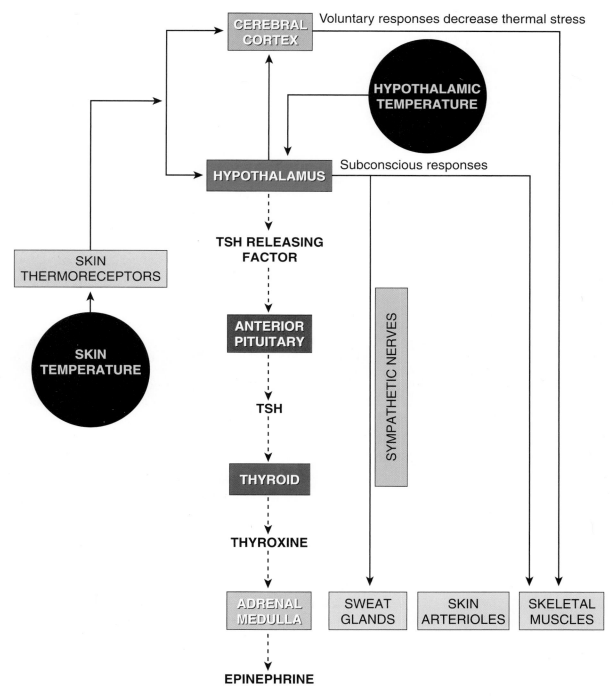

Figure 16.4
Summary of major temperature regulating mechanisms to reduce thermal stress (TSH = Thyroid stimulating hormone). (Modified from Vander, A., et al.: *Human Physiology: The Mechanisms of Body Function.* New York: McGraw-Hill, 1993).

The Modern Cycling Helmet Does Not Thwart Heat Dissipation

To evaluate the physiologic and perceptual responses of wearing one of the new modern aerodynamic and lightweight cycling helmets, ten male and four female competitive cyclists pedaled for 90 minutes at 60% $\dot{V}O_{2peak}$ in both hot-dry (95°F [35°C], 20% RH) and hot-humid (95°F, 70% RH) environments with and without a protective helmet. Oxygen uptake, heart rate, and core, skin, and head skin temperatures, rating of perceived exertion, and perceived thermal sensations of the head and body were measured. The results showed that exercising in a hot-humid environment produced significantly greater thermal stress (as expected), yet wearing the helmet during exercise did *not* increase the riders' level of heat strain or perceived heat sensation of the head or body.

sulation does not usually present a problem; rather the key factor involves dissipation of metabolic heat (and sweat) through a thick air-clothing barrier. Cross-country skiers alleviate this problem by removing layers of clothing as the body warms. This maintains core temperature without reliance on evaporative cooling.

Warm-Weather Clothing

Dry clothing, no matter how lightweight, retards heat exchange more than the same clothing soaking wet. The common practice of switching to a dry tennis, basketball, or football uniform in hot weather makes little sense for temperature regulation because evaporative heat loss occurs only when clothing becomes wet throughout. A dry uniform simply prolongs the time between sweating and cooling.

Different materials absorb water at different rates. Cottons and linens, for example, readily absorb moisture. In contrast, heavy sweat shirts and rubber or plastic garments produce high relative humidity close to the skin, thus retarding sweat evaporation and cooling. Individuals should wear loose-fitting clothing to permit free convection of air between the skin and environment to promote evaporation from the skin. Color also plays an important role; dark colors absorb light rays and add to radiant heat gain, whereas lighter color clothing reflects heat rays.

TABLE 16.2
Practical guidelines for recreational and expedition meal planning when anticipating environmental stress

DO	DON'T
Do provide group hot meals whenever possible. People eat more when warm meals are consumed "socially."	**Don't** assume that everyone eats adequately in group feeding situations.
Do schedule breaks for meals and snacks even when individual food will be consumed for the meal or snack. Left to their own initiative, people frequently skip or shorten meals to accomplish tasks they believe are more important.	**Don't** allow snack food to substitute for meals. Snacks should augment or supplement daily meals, primarily to increase total daily energy or carbohydrate intake. Snacks should be a morale and performance booster, not an obsession.
Do observe what food items are being consumed. Picky dietary habits can lead to imbalances of vitamins, minerals, or energy. Vitamin and mineral supplements are usually not needed; a multivitamin supplement provides some nutritional "insurance" for finicky eaters.	**Don't** permit individuals to use the expedition as a "crash" weight loss program. Dehydrated, ketotic, and weak team members jeopardize the safety of others and themselves.
Do encourage water consumption with meals. Meal time is often a major fluid consumption point due to the opportunity to prepare beverages, soups, and other water containing food items. Encourage drinking during prolonged periods of strenuous work and during breaks.	**Don't** permit food and personal hygiene to slip due to field conditions. Safe food preparation, especially in temperate or hot environments or during breaks requires clean hands, clean utensils, and disinfected water.

From Askew, E.W.: Nutrition and performance in hot, cold, and high altitude environments. In: *Nutrition in Exercise and Sport.* 3rd Ed., Wolinsky, I., (ed.). Boca Raton, FL: CRC Press, 1997.

Nutritional Aspects of Exercise in Extreme Environments

Proper nutrition plays an important but often overlooked role in planning work, exercise, or recreation in extremes of heat, cold, and/or altitude. Mountaineering, cross-country skiing, snow-boarding, snow-shoeing, sledding, and backpacking can be as physically demanding as most conventional sport activities. In addition, these activities often take place under stressful environmental conditions. Figure 16.5 illustrates that in environmental extremes, factors such as 1) increased energy and water requirements, 2) physiologic effects (depressed appetite and thirst), and 3) practical considerations (limited food and fluid availability) often make it difficult to achieve energy and fluid balance. The combination of physical activity and extreme environmental stress creates a cascade of events that ultimately impair physiologic functions and exercise capacity. In addition to energy (carbohydrate) and water, environmental extremes can also affect the need for vitamins and minerals. Table 16.2 provides practical dietary recommendations for recreational or expedition meal planning in environmental extremes.

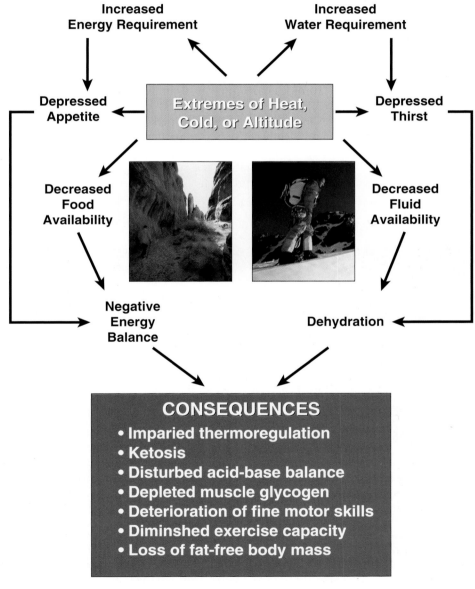

Figure 16.5
Effects of environmental extremes on energy balance, hydration status, physiologic functions, and exercise capacity. (Adapted from Askew, E.W.: In: *Nutrition in Exercise and Sport*, 2nd Ed., Boca Raton, FL: CRC Press, 1994.)

summary

1. Humans tolerate only relatively small variations in internal (core) temperature. Exposure to heat or cold stress initiates thermoregulatory mechanisms that either generate or conserve heat at low ambient temperatures and dissipate heat at high temperatures.

2. Oral temperature does not accurately measure core temperature after strenuous excercise. This discrepancy partly results from evaporative cooling of the mouth and airways during high-level pulmonary ventilation.

3. The hypothalamus serves as the "thermostat" for temperature regulation. This coordination center initiates adjustments from peripheral thermal receptors in skin and changes in hypothalamic blood temperature.

4. Heat conservation in cold stress occurs by vascular adjustments that shunt blood from the cooler periphery to the warmer deep tissues of the body's core. If this proves ineffective, shivering significantly increases metabolic heat. Thermogenic hormones initiate an additional small but prolonged increase in resting metabolism.

5. Heat stress causes warm blood to divert from the body's core to the shell. The body loses heat by radiation, conduction, convection, and evaporation. Evaporation provides the major physiologic defense against overheating at high ambient temperatures and during exercise.

6. Humid environments dramatically decrease effectiveness of evaporative heat loss. This makes a physically active person particularly vulnerable to a dangerous state of dehydration and spiraling core temperature.

7. Ideal warm-weather clothing consists of lightweight, loose-fitting, and light-color clothes. Even when wearing ideal clothing, heat loss slows until evaporative cooling achieves optimal levels.

8. Several layers of light clothing provide a thick zone of trapped air near the skin, insulating better than a single thick layer of clothing. Wet clothing decreases insulation, and heat flows readily from the body.

9. Metabolic heat generated during vigorous exercise generally maintains core temperature in cold air environments, even if the person wears little clothing.

10. Environmental extremes can influence nutritional requirements (primarily, carbohydrates and water), and pose adverse physiologic and exercise performance implications for people who live, work, and recreate under these conditions.

PART 2

Thermoregulation and Environmental Stress During Exercise

Exercise in the Heat

Cardiovascular adjustments and evaporative cooling control metabolic heat dissipation during exercise, particularly in hot weather. A trade-off occurs, however, because fluids lost in thermoregulation often create a relative state of dehydration. Excessive sweating leads to more serious fluid loss that reduces plasma volume. The extreme end result involves circulatory failure as core temperature increases to lethal levels.

Circulatory Adjustments

The body faces two competitive cardiovascular demands when exercising in hot weather:

1. Oxygen delivery to muscles must increase to sustain energy metabolism.
2. Peripheral blood flow to the skin must increase to transport metabolic heat from exercise for dissipation at the body's surface; this blood no longer remains available for oxygen delivery to active muscles

Cardiac output remains the same during submaximal exercise in hot and cold environments. However, the heart's stroke volume becomes smaller when exercising in the heat. In fact, stroke volume decreases in proportion to the fluid deficit created during exercise, producing *higher* heart rates at all submaximal exercise levels. Maximal cardiac output and aerobic capacity decrease during exercise in the heat because the compensatory increase in heart rate does not offset the heart's stroke volume decrease.

Vascular Constriction and Dilation

Adequate skin and muscle blood flow during heat stress take place at the expense of other tissues that temporarily compromise their blood supply. For example, compensatory constriction of the splanchnic vascular bed and renal tissues rapidly counters vasodilation of the subcutaneous vessels. A prolonged reduction in blood flow to visceral tissues probably contributes to liver and renal complications sometimes noted with exertional heat stress.

Maintaining Blood Pressure

In the heat, arterial blood pressure remains stable during exercise because visceral vasoconstriction increases total vascular resistance, redirecting blood to areas in need. During near maximal exercise, with accompanying dehydration, relatively less blood diverts to peripheral areas for heat dissipation. This reflects the body's attempt to maintain cardiac output despite sweat-induced decreases in plasma volume. *Circulatory regulation and maintenance of muscle blood flow take precedence over temperature regulation, often at the expense of a spiraling core temperature.*

Core Temperature During Exercise

Heat generated by active muscles can increase core temperature to fever levels that would incapacitate a person if caused by external heat stress alone. However, champion distance runners show no ill effects from rectal temperatures as high as 105.8°F (41°C) recorded at the end of a 3-mile race.

Within limits, the increased core temperature with exercise does not reflect heat-dissipation failure. To the contrary, this well-regulated response occurs even during exercise in the cold. Figure 16.6A illustrates the relationship between esophageal (core) temperature and oxygen uptake during exercise of increasing severity for five men and two women of varying fitness levels. Core temperature increased as exercise became more intense, with considerable variability in temperature response among subjects. Plotting core temperature in relation to exercise oxygen uptake, expressed as a percentage of each person's $\dot{V}O_{2max}$ (Fig. 16.6B), moves the lines closer together. This indicates that relative workload (i.e., percentage of one's capacity) determines the change in core temperature with exercise. *More than likely, a modest increase in core temperature reflects favorable internal adjustments that create an optimal thermal environment for physiologic and metabolic function.*

Water Loss in the Heat

Dehydration induced by a few hours of heavy exercise in the heat can reach levels that impede heat dissipation and severely compromise cardiovascular function and exercise capacity. Figure 16.7 shows average water loss per hour from sweating at various air temperatures during rest, and light and moderate activity for a typical adult.

Magnitude of Fluid Loss in Exercise

For an acclimatized person, sweat loss peaks at about 3 $L \cdot hr^{-1}$ during intense exercise in the heat, and averages nearly 12 L (26 lb) on a daily basis. Intense sweating for several hours can induce sweat-gland fatigue, which impairs core temperature regulation. Elite marathon runners frequently sweat in excess of 5 L of fluid during competition; this represents 6 to 10% of body mass. For slower-paced marathons or ultramarathons, average fluid loss rarely exceeds 500 mL $\cdot$ hr^{-1}. For more intense exercise, even in a temperate climate, soccer players averaged a fluid loss of 2 L during a 90-minute game played at about 50°F (10°C).

A large sweat output and subsequent fluid loss occur in sports other than distance running; football, basketball, and hockey players also deplete large quantities of fluid during competition. High school wrestlers can lose 9 to 13% of their preseason body mass before certification, the greatest portion of weight loss coming from voluntarily water restriction and excessive sweating before weigh-in. Collegiate wrestlers, excluding heavyweights, regained an average of 3.7 kg (8.1 lb) during the 20-hour period between weigh-in and competition. *This means that high school and collegiate wrestlers usually compete in a dehydrated state to make weight.*

Hot, humid environments impede the effectiveness of evaporative cooling (because of the high vapor pressure of ambient air) and promote large fluid losses. Figure 16.8 illustrates a linear relationship between sweat rate during rest and exercise and the air's moisture content (expressed as wet bulb temperature; see p. 446). Ironically, excessive sweat output in high humidity contributes little to cooling

Figure 16.6
Relationship between esophageal temperature and (**A**) oxygen uptake (exercise intensity expressed as power output), and (**B**) oxygen uptake as percent of $\dot{V}O_{2max}$. (Data from Saltin, B., and Hermansen, L.: Esophageal, rectal, and muscle temperature during exercise. *J. Appl. Physiol.*, 21: 1757, 1966.)

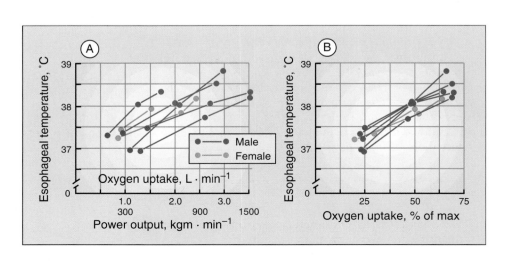

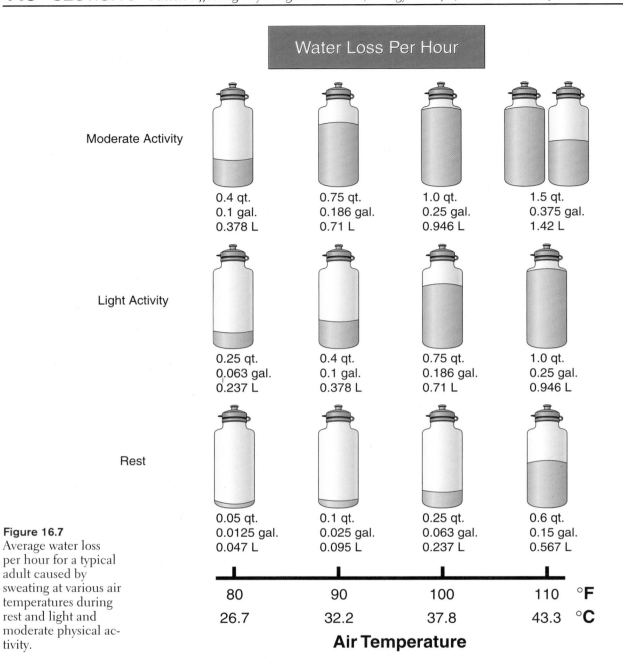

Figure 16.7
Average water loss per hour for a typical adult caused by sweating at various air temperatures during rest and light and moderate physical activity.

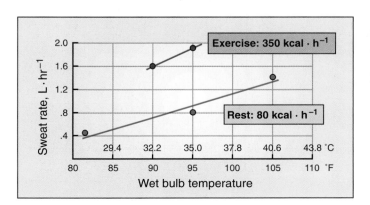

Figure 16.8
Effects of humidity (wet-bulb temperature) on sweat rate during rest and exercise in the heat. Ambient temperature (dry-bulb) equaled 43.3°C (110°F). (Data from Iampietro, P.F.: Exercise in hot environments. In: *Frontiers of Fitness.* Shephard, R.J., (ed.). Springfield, IL: Charles C. Thomas, 1971.)

because minimal evaporation takes place. In this regard, clothing that retards rapid evaporation of sweat creates an extremely humid microclimate at the skin's surface and encourages dehydration and overheating.

Consequences of Dehydration

Just about any degree of dehydration impairs physiologic function and thermoregulation. When plasma volume decreases as dehydration progresses, peripheral blood flow and sweating rate diminish, making thermoregulation progressively more difficult. Compared with normal hydration, a reduced plasma volume increases heart rate, perception of effort, and core temperature, and causes premature fatigue. A fluid loss equivalent to only 1% of body mass significantly increases rectal temperature compared with the same exercise performed fully hydrated. Pre-exercise dehydration equivalent to 5% of body mass (common among high school wrestlers) significantly increases rectal temperature and heart rate, while decreasing sweating rate, $\dot{V}O_{2max}$, and exercise capacity compared with the normally hydrated condition. *The 5 hours available to wrestlers between weigh-in and match time does not adequately ensure complete rehydration and electrolyte balance.*

Blood plasma supplies most of the water lost through sweating; thus, maintaining cardiac output becomes problematic as sweat loss progresses. Loss of plasma volume initiates increases in systemic vascular resistance to maintain blood pressure and reduces skin blood flow. Reduced cutaneous blood flow thwarts a major avenue for heat dissipation. *Dehydration reduces circulatory and temperature-regulating capacity to meet metabolic and thermal demands of exercise.*

Factors that affect sweat-loss dehydration include exercise intensity and duration, environmental temperature, solar load, wind speed, relative humidity, and clothing. Table 16.3 shows theoretical water requirements at different ambient temperatures and relative humidities with and without a solar load. Just 100°F (37.8°C) ambient air temperature increases the resting water requirement by 50 to 60%. Adding physical activity and radiant heat increases the requirement even more. Eight hours of heavy work outdoors at temperatures of 96°F or higher (relative humidity 20% or greater) could increase total water requirements to 15 L. Replacing this much fluid requires drinking water at regular intervals throughout the day. During the 1990–1991 Desert War in Iraq and Kuwait, the US military imposed forced water intake through a planned drinking program before, during, and after job tasks. The Army attributed the relatively low incidence of heat casualties to the discipline of planned hydration.

Fluid Loss in Winter Environments

Dehydration also becomes a risk during vigorous cold-weather exercise. For example, colder air contains less moisture than air at warmer temperature, particularly at higher elevations. Fluid volume loss increases from the respiratory passages as incoming cold, dry air fully humidifies and warms to body temperature. Up to 1 L of fluid can be lost daily. In addition, cold stress increases urine production, which adds to total body fluid loss. Ironically, many people overdress for outdoor winter activities. Sweating begins as exercise progresses because body heat production exceeds heat loss. These factors become magnified because many individuals consider it unimportant to consume fluids before, during, and flowing strenuous exercise in cold weather. Figure 16.9 illustrates a back-mounted hydration system that provides ready access to water *during* winter activities like Nordic or alpine skiing, hiking, distance cycling, and running. The system can be purchased at sporting goods or cycling shops, or through sports mail-order catalogs.

Diuretic Use

Athletes who take diuretics to lose body water rapidly reduce plasma volume, which negatively affects thermoregulation and cardiovascular function. Diuretic drugs can

TABLE 16.3
Water requirements (L · h⁻¹) for rest and work in the heat indoors and outdoors

AIR TEMP (°F) AND RH*	INDOORS (NO SOLAR LOAD)				OUTDOORS (CLEAR SKY)			
	REST	LIGHT	MEDIUM	HEAVY	REST	LIGHT	MEDIUM	HEAVY
85° @ 50%	0.2	0.5	1.0	1.5	0.5	0.9	1.3	1.8
96° @ 30%	0.3	0.9	1.3	1.9	0.8	1.2	1.7	2.0
105° @ 30%	0.6	1.0	1.5	2.0	0.9	1.3	1.9	2.0
115° @ 20%	0.8	1.2	1.7	2.0	1.1	1.5	2.0	2.0
120° @ 20%	0.9	1.3	1.9	2.0	1.3	1.7	2.0	2.0

*RH = relative humidity
From Askew, E.W.: Nutrition and performance in hot, cold, and high altitude environments. In: *Nutrition in Exercise and Sport*. 3rd Ed., Wolinsky, I., (ed.). Boca Raton, FL: CRC Press, 1997.

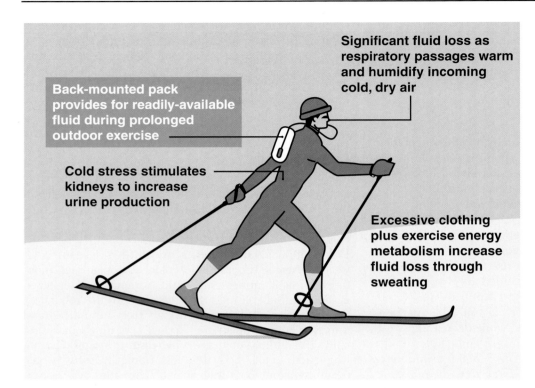

Back-mounted pack provides for readily-available fluid during prolonged outdoor exercise

Significant fluid loss as respiratory passages warm and humidify incoming cold, dry air

Cold stress stimulates kidneys to increase urine production

Excessive clothing plus exercise energy metabolism increase fluid loss through sweating

Figure 16.9
Factors that increase potential for dehydration during cold-weather exercise. A back-mounted hydration system provides ready water access during continuous exercise in outdoor environments.

also significantly impair neuromuscular function not noted when comparable fluid loss occurs by exercise. Athletes who vomit and take laxatives to lose weight not only become dehydrated, but also lose minerals, which weakens muscle and impairs motor function. This clearly gives the opponent the competitive "edge"—an entirely opposite result than anticipated.

Water Replacement – Rehydration

Adequate fluid replacement sustains evaporative cooling of acclimatized humans. Properly scheduling fluid replacement maintains plasma volume so that circulation and sweating progress optimally. This, however, may be "easier said than done" because some coaches and athletes still believe water consumption hinders performance. When left on their own, most athletes voluntarily replace only about one-half of water lost during exercise (< 500 mL·h^{-1}).

For wrestlers, dehydration to lose weight becomes a "way of life" so they can compete in a lower-weight category. This also may occur with ballet dancers who strive to maintain a thin appearance, and power athletes who try to make weight to compete in lighter-weight category. The enlightened coach and exercise specialist must remain vigilant about an athlete's hydration and its impact on exercise performance and safety. The competitive wrestler (and others who dehydrate to compete in a specific weight class) and athletes engaged in more than one event or training session on a given day must replenish fluids regularly.

Cold treatments (periodic application of cold towels to the forehead and abdomen during exercise, or taking a cold shower before exercising in a hot environment) do not facilitate heat transfer at the body's surface compared with the same exercise without skin wetting. Adequate hydration provides the most effective defense against heat stress by balancing water loss with water intake, not by pouring water over the head or body. A *well-hydrated athlete always functions at a higher physiologic and performance level than a dehydrated one.*

Model for Rehydration

Table 16.4 shows sample computations for determining the quantity and rate of fluid loss in exercise. The estimated hourly fluid loss from a workout or competition should be partitioned into 10- or 15-minute periods, and that amount of fluid should be ingested at those intervals. This will optimize stomach volume and properly match fluid loss with fluid intake. For example, consume 250 mL of fluid every 15 minutes for hourly losses up to 1000 mL, whereas larger fluid ingestion at 10-minute intervals optimizes replenishing a greater fluid loss. Allow for unrestricted access to water at any time the athlete wants to consume fluids during practice or competition. *Athletes must rehydrate themselves on a schedule because the thirst mechanism imprecisely gauges water needs.*

Electrolyte Replacement

The athlete's primary concern should focus on replacing fluids rather than ions because sweat remains less concentrated (hypotonic) in relation to body fluids. Adding a slight amount of salt to foods readily replenishes NaCl for a fluid loss less than 2.7 kg (6 lb) in adults. Sodium-conservation mechanisms by the kidneys contribute to balancing sodium losses in sweat during endurance exercise.

A small amount of electrolytes added to a rehydration fluid contributes to a more complete rehydration than water alone. Pure water absorbed from the gut rapidly dilutes the plasma's sodium concentration. This stimulates urine production and blunts stimulation of thirst by the hypothalamus. Adding a small amount of an electrolyte to the rehydration fluid maintains plasma sodium concentration, sustains the thirst drive, promotes retention of ingested fluid (less urine output), and more rapidly restores lost plasma volume during rehydration.

With prolonged exercise in the heat, sweat loss may de-

TABLE 16.4
Computing the magnitude of sweat loss and rate of sweating in exercise

A	B	C	D	E	F	G	H
BM Before Exercise	BM After Exercise	DBM (A−B)	Drink Volume	Urine Volume Output	Sweat Loss (C+D−E)	Exercise Time	Sweat Rate (F÷G)
61.7 kg	60.3 kg	1400 g	420 mL	90 mL*	1730 mL	90 min	19.2 mL · min^{-1}** (1152 mL · h^{-1})

Sweat rate mL·h^{-1}	Fluid intake mL	oz	Rehydration intervals, min
500	125	4	15
750	190	6.5	15
1000	250	8.5	15
1500	250	8.5	10
2000	330	11	10
2500	415	14	10
3000	500	17	10

*Weight of uirne should be subtracted if urine was excreted prior to to postexercise body weight measurement

**1152 mL · h^{-1}; in this example, Mackinzie should drink about 1000 mL (32 oz) of fluid during each hour of activity (250 mL every 15 min) to remain well hydrated.

The top data show calculations of sweat rate (column H) for a person who exercises for 90 min (column G) and who consumes 420 mL of fluid (column D); BM = body mass; DBM = difference in body mass before and after exercise (column C); urine volume (in mL; column E) measured prior to post-exercise body mass measurement. The bottom data show the recommended rehydration intervals based on the determined sweat rate in mL · h^{-1} (column H). For example, with a sweat rate of 1152 mL · h^{-1} the person would need to consume about 1000 mL (32 oz) during each hour to match total fluid loss during activity at a rate of 250 mL (8.5 oz) at 15-minute intervals. (Modified from: Gatorade Sports Science Institute, Vol. 9, No. 4 (suppl 63), 1996.)

plete the body of up to 17 g of salt daily (2.3 to 3.4 g NaCl per L sweat). This represents about 8 g more than the salt in the daily diet. As a preventive measure on the day before exercise, consuming extra salt may be desirable (about one-third tsp. table salt per L water). Except in these unusual cases, dietary modifications and electrolyte conservation by the kidneys adequately compensate for electrolyte loss through sweating.

Factors That Improve Heat Tolerance

Numerous factors improve heat tolerance of individuals.

Acclimatization
Relatively light exercise performed easily in cool weather becomes taxing if attempted on the first hot day of spring.

The early stages of spring training often represent a hazard for sustaining heat injury because thermoregulatory mechanisms have not adjusted to the dual challenge of exercise and environmental heat. *Repeated exposure to hot environments, particularly when combined with exercise, improves capacity for exercise with less discomfort during heat stress.*

Heat acclimatization *refers to the physiologic adaptive changes that improve heat tolerance.* Figure 16.10 shows that 2 to 4 hours daily of heat exposure produce essentially complete acclimatization after 10 days. In practical terms, the first several exercise sessions in a hot environment should be light in intensity, and last about 15 to 20 minutes in duration. Thereafter, exercise sessions can increase systematically to reach normal training duration and intensity.

Table 16.5 summarizes the main physiologic adjustments during heat acclimatization. Optimal acclimatization necessitates adequate hydration. As acclimatization progresses, proportionately larger quantities of blood flow to cutaneous vessels to facilitate heat transfer from the core

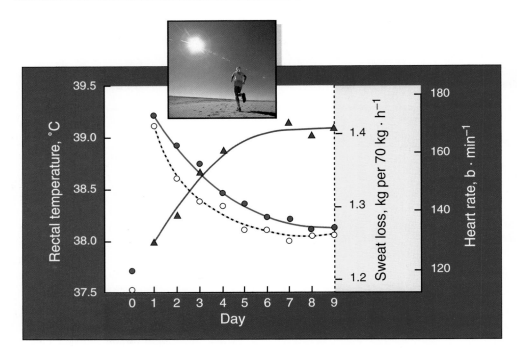

Figure 16.10
Average rectal temperature (○), heart rate (●), and sweat loss (▲) during 100 minutes of daily heat-exercise exposure for 9 consecutive days. On day 0, the men walked on a treadmill at an exercise intensity of 300 kcal·h^{-1} in a cool climate. Thereafter, they performed the same daily exercise in the heat at 48.9°C (26.7°C wet-bulb). (Data from Lind, A. R., and Bass, D. E.: Optimal exposure time for development of acclimatization to heat. *Fed. Proc.*, 22: 704, 1963.)

to the periphery. More effective cardiac output distribution maintains blood pressure during exercise; a lowered threshold (earlier onset) for sweating complements this circulatory acclimatization. These responses initiate cooling before internal temperature increases substantially. After 10 days of heat exposure, sweating capacity nearly doubles, and sweat dilutes (less salt lost) and more evenly distributes on the skin surface. In an acclimatized individual, increased sweat loss creates a greater need to rehydrate during and following exercise. A heat-acclimatized person exercises with a lower skin and core temperature and heart rate than an unacclimatized individual. This occurs due to adjustments in circulatory function and evaporative cooling. Unfortunately, the major benefits of acclimatization to hot environments dissipate within 2 to 3 weeks after return to a more temperate environment.

Exercise Training

The normal exercise-induced "internal" heat stress from strenuous physical activity in a cool environment adjusts peripheral circulation and evaporative cooling in a manner qualitatively similar to hot ambient temperature acclimatization. This enables well-conditioned men and women to respond more effectively to severe heat stress than sedentary counterparts.

Exercise training increases sweating response sensitivity and capacity so sweating begins at a lower core temperature. It also produces larger volumes of more dilute sweat. These beneficial responses relate to the significant increase in plasma volume that occurs early in endurance training. Increased plasma volume supports sweat gland function during heat stress and maintains adequate plasma volume for the cardiovascular (skin and muscle blood flow) demands of exercise. A trained person, therefore, stores less heat early during exercise, reaching a thermal steady state sooner and at a lower core temperature than an untrained person. The training advantage for thermoregulation occurs *only* if the individual fully hydrates during exercise.

As might be expected, exercise "heat conditioning" in cool weather proves less effective than acclimatization from similar exercise train-

TABLE 16.5
Physiologic adjustments during heat acclimatization

ACCLIMATIZATION RESPONSE	EFFECT
• Improved cutaneous blood flow	• Transports metabolic heat from deep tissues to the body's shell
• Effective distribution of cardiac output	• Appropriate circulation to skin and muscles to meet demands of metabolism and thermoregulation; greater stability in blood pressure during exercise
• Lowered threshold for start of sweating	• Evaporative cooling begins early in exercise
• More effective distribution of sweat over skin surface	• Optimum use of effective surface for evaporative cooling
• Increased sweat output	• Maximizes evaporative cooling
• Lowered salt concentration of sweat	• Dilute sweat preserves electrolytes in extracellular fluid

ing in the heat. *Full heat acclimatization does not occur without exposure to environmental heat stress.* Athletes who train and compete in hot weather have a distinct thermoregulatory advantage over athletes who train in cooler climates, yet periodically compete in hot weather.

Age

Studies that consider body size and composition, aerobic fitness level, hydration level, and degree of acclimatization show little or no age-related effects on thermoregulatory capacity or acclimatization to heat stress. For example, in comparing young and middle-aged competitive runners, no age-related decrements emerged in thermoregulatory ability during marathon running. Likewise, temperature regulation was not impaired in physically trained 50-year-old men compared with young men. For men 58 to 84 years of age who walked in the desert, sweating capacity adequately regulated body temperature.

Children

Prepubescent children have a lower sweating rate and exhibit a higher core temperature during heat stress than adolescents and adults, despite their larger number of heat-activated sweat glands per unit skin area. Thermoregulatory differences probably last through puberty without limiting exercise capacity except during extreme environmental heat stress. Sweat composition also differs between children and adults; children have higher concentrations of sodium and chlorine, but lower lactate, H^+, and potassium concentrations. Also, children may take longer to acclimatize to heat compared with adolescents and young adults. *From a practical and health standpoint, children exposed to environmental heat stress should exercise at a reduced intensity and receive additional time to acclimatize compared with more mature competitors.*

Gender

Comparisons of thermoregulation between men and women initially showed that men had greater tolerance to environmental heat stress during exercise. However, the research had deficiencies; the comparison group of women consistently exercised at higher metabolic intensities in relation to their aerobic capacity than men. Gender differences in thermoregulation became much less pronounced when no difference existed in the fitness level between women and men. *Generally, women tolerate the physiologic and thermal stress of exercise as well as men of comparable fitness and acclimatization levels; both genders acclimatize to a similar degree.*

Sweating

A distinct gender difference in thermoregulation exists for sweating. Compared with men, women possess more heat-activated sweat glands per unit skin area than men. Women begin sweating at higher skin and core temperatures; they also produce less sweat for a similar heat-exercise load, even when acclimatized comparably to men.

Evaporative Versus Circulatory Cooling

Despite a lower sweat output, women show heat tolerance similar to men of equal aerobic fitness at the same exercise level. Women probably rely more on circulatory mechanisms for heat dissipation, whereas men exhibit greater evaporative cooling. Women who sweat less to maintain thermal balance have less chance of suffering dehydration during exercise at high ambient temperatures.

Body Surface Area-to-Mass Ratio

Women possess a relatively large **body surface area-to-mass ratio**, a favorable dimensional characteristic to dissipate heat. Stated differently, the smaller female has a larger external surface per unit of body mass exposed to the environment. Under identical conditions of heat exposure, women cool at a rate faster than men through a smaller body mass across a relatively large surface area. In this regard, children also possess a "geometric" advantage during heat stress because boys and girls have larger surface areas per unit body mass compared with adults.

Menstruation

Initiation of sweating requires a higher core temperature threshold during the luteal phase of menstruation. This change in thermoregulatory sensitivity during the menstrual cycle does *not* affect ability to exercise or perform hard physical work.

Body Fat Level

Excess body fat negatively impacts work performance in hot environments. Because fat's specific heat exceeds that of

American College of Sports Medicine Recommendations for Continuous Activities Like Endurance Running and Cycling		
Temperature	**Category**	**Recommendation**
Above 28°C (82°F)	Very high risk	Postpone competitive activity
23 to 28°C (73–82°F)	High risk	Heat-sensitive individuals (e.g., obese, low physical fitness, unacclimatized, dehydrated, previous history of heat injury) should not compete
18 to 23°C (65–73°F)	Moderate risk	
Below 18°C (65°F)	Low risk	

muscle tissue, fat insulates the body's shell, retarding heat conduction to the periphery. The relatively large, overfat person also has a small body surface area-to-mass ratio for sweat evaporation compared with a leaner, smaller person.

Excess body fat directly adds to the metabolic cost of weight-bearing activities in addition to retarding effective heat exchange. When these effects compound by the additional demands of the evaporation-retarding characteristics and weight of equipment (e.g., football and lacrosse gear), intense competition, and a hot, humid environment, the overfat person experiences considerable difficulty with temperature regulation and exercise performance. Fatal heat stroke occurs 3.5 times more frequently in obese young adults than nonobese counterparts.

Evaluating Environmental Heat Stress

Besides air temperature, other factors determine the physiologic strain imposed by heat. These include:

- Individual variations in body size and fatness
- State of training
- Degree of acclimatization
- Level of hydration
- External factors such as convective air currents, radiant heat gain, intensity of exercise, amount, type, and color of clothing, and most importantly relative humidity (several football deaths from heat injury occurred when air temperature dipped below 75°F [23.9°C] but relative humidity exceeded 95%)

Prevention is the most effective way to control heat-stress injuries. Acclimatization minimizes the chances for heat injury. Another defense involves evaluating the environment for its potential thermal challenge with the **wet bulb-globe temperature (WB-GT)** guide. This index of environmental heat stress, developed by the United States military, relies on ambient temperature, relative humidity, and radiant heat to calculate WB-GT as follows:

$$WB\text{-}GT = 0.1 \times DBT + 0.7 \times WBT + 0.2 \times GT$$

where: **DBT** = dry-bulb (air) temperature in the shade recorded by an ordinary mercury thermometer.

WBT = wet-bulb temperature (accounts for 70% of the index) recorded by a similar thermometer, except that a wet wick surrounds the mercury bulb exposed to rapid air movement in direct sunlight. With relative humidity high, little evaporative cooling occurs from the wetted bulb so the temperature of this thermometer remains similar to the dry-bulb. On a dry day, however, significant evaporation occurs from the wetted bulb, maximizing the difference between the two thermometer readings. A small difference between readings indicates a high relative humidity, whereas a large difference indicates little air moisture and a high evaporation rate.

GT = globe temperature in direct sunlight recorded by a thermometer with a black metal sphere around the bulb. The black globe absorbs radiant energy from the surroundings to provide a measure of this important source of heat gain.

Figure 16.11 presents WB-GT guidelines to reduce the chance of heat injury during athletic activities. These standards apply to lightly clothed humans; they do not consider the specific heat load imposed by football uniforms or other types of equipment. For football, the lower end of each temperature range serves as a more prudent guide.

An indication of ambient heat load also comes from the **wet-bulb temperature** because this reading reflects air temperature and relative humidity. Most industrial supply companies sell inexpensive wet-bulb thermometers. Figure 16.11 (bottom) presents heat stress recommendations based on the WBT. Without the WBT, but knowing relative humidity (local meteorological stations or media reports), the **Heat Stress Index** evaluates the relative degree of heat stress (Fig. 16.12). To eliminate potential error from using meteorologic data some distance

WB-GT Range		Recommendations
°F	°C	
80–84	26.5–28.8	• Use discretion, especially if unconditioned or unacclimatized
85–87	29.5–30.5	• Avoid strenuous activity in the sun
88	31.2	• Avoid exercise training

WBT Range		Recommendations
°F	°C	
60	15.5	• No prevention necessary
61–65	16.2–18.4	• Alert all participants to problems of heat stress and importance of adequate hydration
66–70	18.8–21.1	• Insist that appropriate quantity of fluid be ingested
71–75	21.6–23.8	• Rest periods and water breaks every 20 to 30 minutes; limits placed on intense activity
76–79	24.5–26.1	• Practice curtailed and modified considerably
80	26.5	• Practice cancelled

Figure 16.11
Wet Bulb-Globe Temperature (WB-GT) and Wet-Bulb Temperature (WBT) guide, including recommendations for physical activity.

Heat Stress Index

Air temperature (°F)

	70°	75°	80°	85°	90°	95°	100°	105°	110°	115°	120°
					Heat sensation						
0%	64°	69°	73°	78°	83°	87°	91°	95°	99°	103°	107°
10%	65°	70°	75°	80°	85°	90°	95°	100°	105°	111°	116°
20%	66°	72°	77°	82°	87°	93°	99°	105°	112°	120°	130°
30%	67°	73°	78°	84°	90°	96°	104°	113°	123°	135°	148°
40%	68°	74°	79°	86°	93°	101°	110°	123°	137°	151°	
50%	69°	75°	81°	88°	96°	107°	120°	135°	150°		
60%	70°	76°	82°	90°	100°	114°	132°	149°			
70%	70°	77°	85°	93°	106°	124°	144°				
80%	71°	78°	86°	97°	113°	136°					
90%	71°	79°	88°	102°	122°						
100%	72°	80°	91°	108°							

(Relative humidity — left axis)

Heat sensation	Risk of heat injury
90°–105°	Possibility of heat cramps
105°–130°	Heat cramps or heat exhaustion likely Heat stroke possible
130°+	Heat stroke a definite risk

Figure 16.12
Heat Stress Index. Stress on the body relates directly to air temperature and relative humidity.

greatly increases effective insulation because blood in the periphery moves centrally to the body's core in cold water. These athletes often swim in ocean waters with almost no decrease in core temperature. For leaner swimmers, however, the heat generated during exercise cannot counter the heat drain to the water and the body core cools.

Acclimatization to Cold

Humans adapt more successfully to chronic heat exposure than regular cold exposure. Avoiding the cold or minimizing its effects represents the basic response of Eskimos and LapLanders. The clothing of these cold-weather inhabitants provides a near-tropical microclimate, and the temperature inside an igloo averages about 70°F (21°C).

Some indication of cold adaptation comes from studies of the Ama, the women divers of Korea and southern Japan. These women tolerate daily prolonged exposure to diving for food in water as cold as 50°F (10°C). In addition to an apparent psychologic toughness, a 25% increase in resting metabolism probably contributes to their cold tolerance. Interestingly, the Ama have similar body fat levels as nondiving female counterparts. Perhaps circulatory adaptations retard heat transfer from the core to the skin.

A type of general cold adaptation occurs following regular and prolonged cold-air exposure. As a result, increased heat production does not accompany body heat loss, and individuals regulate at a lower core temperature in response to cold. Some peripheral adaptations also reflect a form of acclimation with severe localized cold stress. Repeated cold exposure of the hands or feet brings about blood flow increases through these areas when subjected to cold stress. This becomes readily apparent in fishermen who handle nets and fish in extreme cold. Although such local adaptations actually facilitate regional heat loss, they provide a form of self-defense because vigorous circulation in exposed areas defends against tissue damage from localized hypothermia (frostbite).

from the event site, determine the index close to the actual competition site. Data collected on the 24-hour trend for ambient temperature and relative humidity justified the change in race time for the 1996 Olympic Marathon run in Atlanta from 6:30 PM to 7:00 AM to reduce risk of heat injury.

Exercise in the Cold

The physiologic strain imposed by the cold depends largely on three factors:

1. Specific environmental temperature
2. Level of energy metabolism
3. Resistance to heat flow provided by body fat

Water represents an excellent medium to study physiologic adjustment to cold; the body loses heat about two to four times as fast in cool water as in air at the same temperature. Metabolic heat generated by muscular activity contributes to thermoregulation during cold stress. Shivering frequently results if people remain inactive in a pool or ocean environment because of a large conductive heat loss. Swimming at a submaximal pace at 18°C (64°F) water requires about 500 mL more oxygen each minute than similar swimming at 26°C (79°F). The extra oxygen directly relates to the added energy cost of shivering as the body attempts to combat heat loss. Often, additional metabolic heat cannot counter the large thermal drain and core temperature falls.

Individual differences in body fat content exert a significant effect on physiologic function in a cold environment during rest and exercise. Successful distance swimmers have more subcutaneous fat than other endurance athletes. This

Evaluating Environmental Cold Stress

Heightened participation in outdoor winter activities has increased cold injuries from overexposure. Pronounced peripheral vasoconstriction during severe

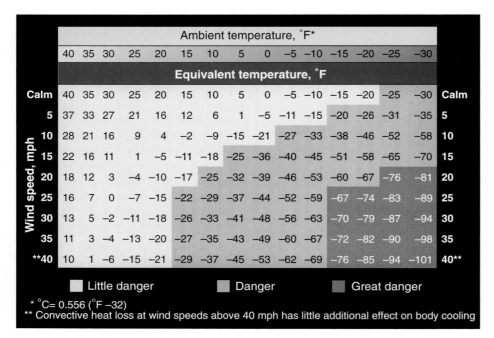

Ambient temperature, °F*															
	40	35	30	25	20	15	10	5	0	−5	−10	−15	−20	−25	−30
Equivalent temperature, °F															
Calm	40	35	30	25	20	15	10	5	0	−5	−10	−15	−20	−25	−30
5	37	33	27	21	16	12	6	1	−5	−11	−15	−20	−26	−31	−35
10	28	21	16	9	4	−2	−9	−15	−21	−27	−33	−38	−46	−52	−58
15	22	16	11	1	−5	−11	−18	−25	−36	−40	−45	−51	−58	−65	−70
20	18	12	3	−4	−10	−17	−25	−32	−39	−46	−53	−60	−67	−76	−81
25	16	7	0	−7	−15	−22	−29	−37	−44	−52	−59	−67	−74	−83	−89
30	13	5	−2	−11	−18	−26	−33	−41	−48	−56	−63	−70	−79	−87	−94
35	11	3	−4	−13	−20	−27	−35	−43	−49	−60	−67	−72	−82	−90	−98
**40	10	1	−6	−15	−21	−29	−37	−45	−53	−62	−69	−76	−85	−94	−101

Wind speed, mph

■ Little danger   ■ Danger   ■ Great danger

* °C= 0.556 (°F −32)
** Convective heat loss at wind speeds above 40 mph has little additional effect on body cooling

Figure 16.13
Wind Chill Index.

0°F (−17.8°C) in calm air; a 25-mph wind at 10°F (−12.2°C) causes the same effect as calm air at −29°F (−34°C). When a person runs, skis, or skates into the wind the effective cooling from the wind increases directly with the exerciser's velocity. Thus, running at 8 mph into a 12- mph headwind produces the effect of a 20-mph headwind. Conversely, running at 8 mph with a 12-mph tailwind creates a relative wind speed of only 4 mph. The yellow-shaded zone on the left of the figure indicates relatively little danger from cold exposure for a person properly clothed. In contrast, in the orange-shaded zone (which generally begins at an ambiant air temperature of about 22°F [−5.6°C]), increasing danger exists to exposed flesh, particularly ears, nose, and fingers. In the red zone on the right, the equivalent temperatures pose serious danger of exposed flesh freezing within minutes.

cold exposure causes skin temperature in the extremities to fall to dangerous levels. Early warning signs of cold injury include a tingling and numbness in the fingers and toes, or burning sensation in the nose and ears. Disregarding these signs of overexposure can lead to tissue damage (**frostbite**); irreversible damage occurs in extreme cases and tissue must be removed surgically.

Wind Chill Index

A dilemma arises in evaluating the environment's thermal quality because ambient temperature alone does not always indicate coldness. All too often we have experienced the chilling winds of a spring day with air temperature well above freezing. In contrast, a calm subfreezing day can feel comfortable. The wind differentiates the two environments; on a windy day, air currents magnify convective heat loss as cooler ambient air continually replaces the warmer insulating air layer around the body.

The **Wind Chill Index** (Fig. 16.13) illustrates the cooling effects of increased wind velocity on bare skin for different air temperatures. For example, 30°F (−1°C) with wind speed at 25 mph produces the same chilling effect as

Respiratory Tract During Cold-Weather Exercise

Cold ambient air does not damage respiratory passages. Even in extreme cold, incoming air warms to between 80°F (27°C) and 90°F (32°C) as it reaches the bronchi. Warming an incoming breath of cold air greatly increases its capacity to hold moisture. Thus, humidification of inspired cold air causes a significant loss of water and heat from the respiratory tract, especially with large ventilatory volumes during exercise. This contributes to dryness of mouth, a burning sensation in the throat, irritation of the respiratory passages, and general dehydration. Wearing a scarf or mask-type "baklava" that covers the nose and mouth and traps the water in exhaled air (and warms and moistens the next incoming breath) reduces uncomfortable respiratory symptoms.

summary

1. Cutaneous and muscle blood flow increase during exercise in the heat, whereas other tissues temporally compromise their blood supply.

2. Core temperature normally increases during exercise; the relative stress of exercise determines the magnitude of increase. A well-regulated temperature response creates a more favorable environment for physiologic and metabolic function.

3. Sweating strains fluid reserves, creating a relative state of dehydration. Excessive sweating without fluid replacement decreases plasma volume and causes a precipitous, dangerous increase in core temperature.

4. Exercise in a hot, humid environment poses a thermoregulatory challenge because the large sweat loss contributes little to evaporative cooling.

5. Relatively small degrees of dehydration impede heat dissipation, com-

promise cardiovascular function, and diminish exercise capacity.

6. Adequate fluid replacement preserves plasma volume to maintain circulation and sweating at optimal levels. The ideal replacement schedule during exercise matches fluid intake with fluid loss, a process effectively monitored by changes in body weight.

7. A small amount of electrolytes added to a rehydration beverage replenishes fluid more quickly than drinking plain water.

8. Repeated heat stress initiates thermoregulatory adjustments that improve exercise capacity and reduce discomfort on subsequent heat exposure. Heat acclimatization favorably redistributes cardiac output and increases sweating capacity. Full acclimatization generally requires about 10 days of heat exposure.

9. Studies that consider body size and composition, aerobic fitness, level of hydration, and degree of acclimatization show little or no age-related decrement in thermoregulatory capacity during moderate heat-exercise stress, or ability to acclimatize to heat stress.

10. When equated for level of fitness and acclimatization, women and men thermoregulate equally well during exercise. However, women sweat less than men at the same core temperature.

11. The Heat Stress Index uses ambient temperature and relative humidity to evaluate the environment's potential heat challenge to an exercising person.

12. Water conducts heat about 25 times greater than air; thus, immersion in water of only 28 to 30°C provides considerable thermal stress. This initiates thermoregulatory adjustments in a relatively short period.

13. Subcutaneous fat provides excellent insulation against cold stress. It enhances the effectiveness of vasomotor adjustments and helps to maintain a large percentage of metabolic heat. This becomes apparent in cold water when individuals with greater body fat show proportionately smaller thermal and cardiovascular adjustments and greater exercise tolerance compared with leaner counterparts.

14. The body adapts better physiologically to prolonged heat stress than prolonged cold exposure. In most instances, appropriate clothing enables humans to tolerate the coldest climates on earth.

15. Ambient temperature and wind speed determine the "coldness" of an environment. The Wind Chill Index describes the interacting effects of ambient temperature and wind speed on exposed flesh.

16. The temperature of inspired ambient air does not pose a danger to the respiratory tract. Considerable water evaporation from the respiratory passages during cold-weather exercise magnifies body fluid loss.

PART 3
Exercise at Altitude

Some high-altitude natives live in permanent settlements in the Andes and Himalayan mountains as high as 5486 m (18,000 ft). Prolonged exposure of an unacclimatized person to such a high altitude can cause death from subnormal levels of oxygen in air (**hypoxia**) even if the person remains physically inactive. The physiologic challenge of even medium altitude becomes readily apparent during physical activity, particularly for newcomers who have not acclimatized to the decreased partial pressure of oxygen (Po_2) at higher elevations.

Stress of Altitude

Figure 16.14 illustrates the barometric pressure, the pressures of the respired gases, and the percent saturation of hemoglobin at various terrestrial elevations. The density of air decreases progressively with ascents above sea level. For example, the barometric pressure at sea level averages 760 mm Hg whereas at 3048 m the barometer reads 510 mm Hg; at an elevation of 5486 m, the pressure of a column of air at the earth's surface represents about one-half its pressure at sea level. Dry ambient air, whether at sea level or altitude, contains 20.9% oxygen. However, the Po_2 (density of oxygen molecules) decreases in direct proportion to the decrease in barometric pressure upon ascending to higher elevations ($Po_2 = 0.209 \times$ barometric pressure). Ambient Po_2 at sea level averages 150 mm Hg, but only 107 mm Hg at 3048 m. *Reduced Po_2 (and accompanying arterial hypoxia) precipitates the immediate physiologic adjustments to altitude and longer-term acclimatization.*

Oxygen Loading at Altitude

The inherent nature of the oxyhemoglobin dissociation curve (Chapter 11) shows that only a small change in hemoglobin's percent saturation occurs with decreasing Po_2 until about 3048 m. At 1981 m (6500 ft), for example, the alveolar Po_2 lowers from its sea level value of 100 mm Hg to 78 mm Hg, yet hemoglobin still remains 90% saturated with oxygen. This relatively small decrease in oxygen carried by blood has little effect on a resting or mildly active individual. Nevertheless, the small reduction in oxygen transport (due to arterial desaturation) at the 1968 Mexico

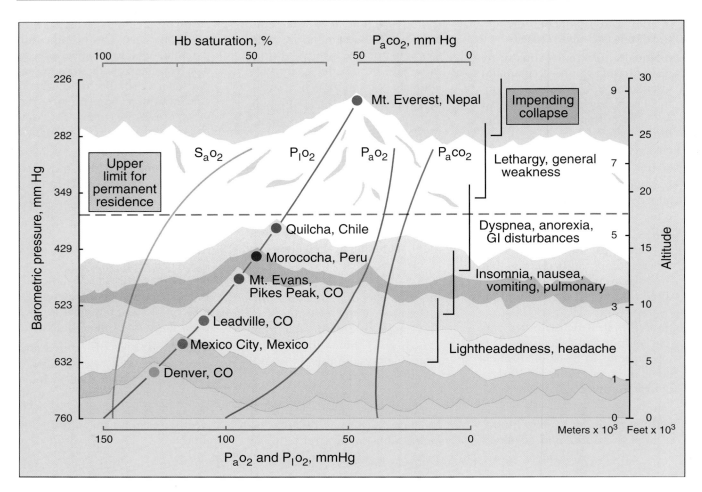

Figure 16.14

Changes in environmental and physiologic variables with progressive elevations in altitude (P_aO_2 = partial pressure of arterial oxygen; P_aCO_2 = partial pressure of arterial carbon dioxide; P_IO_2 = partial pressure of oxygen in inspired air; S_aO_2 = oxygen saturation of hemoglobin).

City Olympics (altitude 2300 m; 7546 ft) contributed to the relatively poor performance of athletes in diverse endurance competitions.

In the transition from moderate to higher elevations, values for alveolar (arterial) oxygen partial pressure exist on the steep part of the oxyhemoglobin dissociation curve. This dramatically reduces hemoglobin oxygenation and negatively impacts even moderate aerobic activities. An acute exposure to 4300 m, for example, reduces aerobic capacity 32% compared with sea level. Above 5182 m (17,000 ft), permanent living becomes nearly impossible, and mountain climbing usually progresses with the aid of oxygen equipment. However, acclimatized mountaineers have lived for weeks at 6706 m (22,002 ft) breathing only ambient air. Members of two Swiss expeditions to Mt. Everest remained at the summit for 2 hours without using oxygen equipment (an impressive feat considering arterial P_{O_2} equals 28 mm Hg with a corresponding 58% oxygen saturation of arterial blood). An unacclimatized person under these conditions becomes unconscious within 30 seconds. Although such performances clearly represent an exception, they demonstrate the enor-

mous adaptive capability of humans to work and survive without external support at extreme altitudes.

Acclimatization

A *ltitude acclimatization broadly describes the adaptive responses that improve one's tolerance to altitude hypoxia.* Acclimatization adjustments occur progressively to each higher elevation, and full acclimatization requires time. As a broad guideline, it takes about 2 weeks to adapt to 2300 m. Thereafter, for each 610-m increase in altitude, it requires an additional week for full adaptation up to 4572 m. As summarized in Table 16.6, certain compensatory responses to altitude occur almost immediately, whereas others take weeks or even months.

Immediate Adjustments

At elevations above 2300 m, rapid physiologic adjustments compensate for the thinner air and reduced alveolar oxygen pressure. The most important of these responses include:

Not Much Oxygen at the Top

At the summit of Mt. Everest (8848 m, 28,028 ft), the pressure of ambient air averages 250 mm Hg with a concomitant alveolar oxygen pressure of 25 mm Hg, or about 30% of the oxygen available at sea level. At this altitude, $\dot{V}O_{2max}$ decreases to the sea-level value of an average 70- to 80-year old man. Concerning the importance of conserving oxygen in the assault on Mt. Everest, one experienced mountaineer commented: "This is a place where people will cut their toothbrushes in half to save weight."

- Hyperventilation triggered by increased respiratory drive
- Increased blood flow (cardiac output) during rest and submaximal exercise

Hyperventilation

Hyperventilation represents the immediate first line of defense to altitude exposure. Chemoreceptors located in the aortic arch and branching of the carotid arteries in the neck detect reductions in arterial P_{O_2}. Chemoreceptor stimulation increases ventilation, increasing alveolar oxygen concentration toward the level in ambient air. Any increase in alveolar P_{O_2} with hyperventilation facilitates oxygen loading in the lungs.

Fluid Loss.   A decreased thirst sensation at altitude negatively affects the body's fluid balance. In addition, owing to the cool and dry air in mountainous regions, considerable body water evaporates as air warms and moistens in the respiratory passages. Respiratory fluid loss often leads to moderate dehydration and accompanying symptoms of dryness of the lips, mouth, and throat, particularly for active people with relatively large daily pulmonary ventilations (and exercise sweat loss). For these active people, body weight should be checked frequently (to ensure against dehydration), augmented with unlimited fluid availability.

Accelerated Circulatory Response

In the early stages of altitude acclimatization, submaximal heart rate and cardiac output can increase 50% above sea-level values, whereas the heart's stroke volume remains essentially unchanged. Because sea level and altitude exercise oxygen uptake remain similar, increased submaximal exercise blood flow at altitude compensates for the reduced arterial oxygen content. In contrast, the circulatory adjustments to acute altitude exposure with maximal exercise cannot compensate for the lower oxygen content of arterial blood. This causes dramatic decreases in $\dot{V}O_{2max}$ and exercise capacity.

Longer-Term Adjustments

Hyperventilation and increased submaximal cardiac output provide a rapid, effective counter to the acute chal-

TABLE 16.6
Immediate and longer-term adjustments to altitude hypoxia

SYSTEM	IMMEDIATE	LONGER-TERM
Pulmonary Acid-Base	Hyperventilation Body fluids become more alkaline due to reduction in CO_2 (H_2CO_3) with hyperventilation	Hyperventilation Excretion of base (HCO_3^-) via the kidneys and concommitant reduction in alkaline reserve
Cardiovascular	Increase in submaximal heart rate Increase in submaximal cardiac output Stroke volume remains the same or lowers slightly Maximum cardiac output remains the same or lowers slightly	Submaximal heart rate remains elevated Submaximal cardiac output falls to or below sea-level values Stroke volume lowers Maximum cradiac output lowers
Hematologic		Decrease in plasma volume Increased hematocrit Increased hemoglobin concentration Increased total number of red blood cells Possible increased capillarization of skeletal muscle
Local		Increased red-blood-cell 2,3-DPG Increased mitochondria Increased aerobic enzymes

lenge of altitude. Other slower acting physiologic adjustments commence during a prolonged altitude stay. These three adjustments include:

- Acid-base adjustment
- Hematological changes
- Cellular adaptations

Acid-Base Adjustment

Hyperventilation at altitude favorably increases alveolar oxygen concentration, while the opposite effect occurs for carbon dioxide. Because ambient air contains essentially no carbon dioxide, increased ventilation at altitude tends to wash out (dilute) carbon dioxide in the alveoli. This creates a larger than normal gradient for carbon dioxide diffusion from blood into the lungs, reducing arterial carbon dioxide considerably. During prolonged high-altitude exposure, alveolar carbon dioxide pressure often decreases to 10 mm Hg compared with the sea-level value of 40 mm Hg.

Carbon dioxide loss from body fluids causes pH to increase as the blood becomes more alkaline. (Recall from Chapter 10 that carbonic acid transports the largest amount of the body s carbon dioxide.) Control of respiratory alkalosis produced by hyperventilation occurs through the kidneys, which slowly excrete base (HCO_3^-) through the renal tubules.

The establishment of acid-base equilibrium with acclimatization occurs with a loss of alkaline reserve. Although altitude does not affect the anaerobic metabolic pathways per se, the blood's buffering capacity for acids gradually decreases, reducing the critical level for accumulation of acid metabolites like lactate.

Hematological Changes

An increase in the blood's oxygen-carrying capacity is the most important long-term adaptation to altitude. This takes place through a decrease in plasma volume and an increase in red blood cell mass.

- *Decrease in plasma volume.* A rapid decrease in plasma volume increases red blood cell concentration during the first few days at altitude. This causes arterial blood's oxygen content to increase significantly above values observed on immediate ascent to altitude.

- *Increase in red cell mass.* Reduced arterial Po_2 increases the total number of red blood cells. This response, termed **polycythemia**, directly increases the blood's capacity to transport oxygen.

The kidneys release the erythrocyte-stimulating hormone **erythropoietin** within 15 hours after altitude ascent. This hormone mediates the polycythemic response to a lowered arterial Po_2. In the weeks that follow, red blood cell production in the marrow of the long bones increases considerably and remains elevated. For example, oxygen-carrying capacity of blood for high-altitude residents of Peru averages 28% above sea-level values. For well-acclimatized mountaineers, oxygen transport capacity for each 100 mL of blood (at sea-level Po_2) ranges between 25 and 31 mL compared to about 20 mL for lowland residents. Even with hemoglobin's reduced oxygen saturation at altitude, the actual *quantity* of oxygen in arterial blood of elite mountaineers nearly equals sea-level values.

Figure 16.15 illustrates the general trend for increased hemoglobin and hematocrit during altitude acclimatization for eight young women at the University of Missouri (altitude 213 m) who lived and worked for ten weeks at the 4267-m summit of Pikes Peak. Upon reaching Pikes Peak, red blood cell concentration increased rapidly from a reduced plasma volume during the first 24 hours. Over the following month, hemoglobin concentration and hematocrit continued to rise and then stabilized for the remainder of the stay. Two weeks after the women returned to Missouri, hemoglobin and hematocrit recovered to prealtitude values. Part B of the figure shows that women who supplemented with iron improved their hematocrit closer to nonsupplemented male values.

The Lactate Paradox

On ascent to high altitude, lactate production to a given submaximal exercise load increases compared with sea level. Presumably, this results from altitude hypoxia with added reliance on anaerobic glycolysis. Surprisingly, the lactate response to the same exercise (and in maximal exercise) after acclimatization results in *lower* lactate production, despite failure of either $\dot{V}O_{2max}$ or regional blood flow to increase. Thus, the question arises concerning this apparent physiologic contradiction, called the **lactate paradox**: "How does reduced lactate accumulation occur without a concomitant increase in tissue oxygenation"? Research points to reduced output of the glucose-mobilizing hormone epinephrine during chronic altitude exposure. Because glucose and glycogen are the only macronutrient sources of anaerobic energy (and lactate formation), reduced glucose mobilization blunts the capacity for lactate formation. Reductions in intracellular ADP during chronic altitude exposure may also inhibit glycolytic pathway activation. In addition, reduction in lactate levels during maximal exercise has been partly attributed to a reduced central nervous system drive, which diminishes capacity for all-out effort

Figure 16.15
A, Effects of altitude on
hemoglobin and hematocrit levels
of eight young women prior to, during, and two weeks after exposure to
4267 m. (From Hannon, J. P., et al.:
Effects of altitude acclimatization
on blood composition of women. *J.
Appl. Physiol.*, 26: 540, 1968.) **B,**
Hematocrit response of young
women receiving supplemental iron
(+Fe) prior to and during altitude
exposure compared to groups of
male and female subjects receiving
no supplemental iron. (Courtesy of
Dr. J. T. Hannon.)

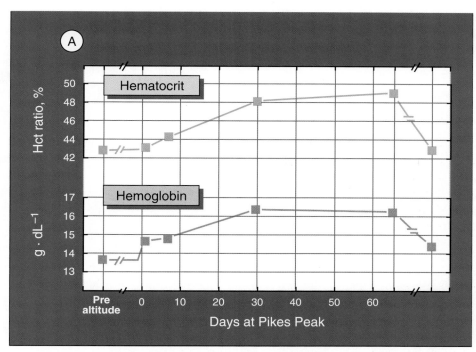

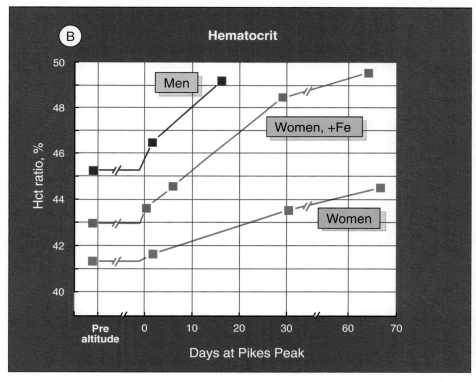

Cellular Adaptations.

Long-term acclimatization initiates peripheral changes that facilitate aerobic metabolism including:

- Capillaries become more concentrated in skeletal muscle, reducing the distance for oxygen
diffusion between blood and
tissues.

- An increase in mitochondria
number and aerobic enzyme
concentration complements a
nearly 16% increase in myoglobin. This increases oxygen
storage within specific muscle
fibers and facilitates intracellular
oxygen delivery and utilization,
particularly at low tissue P_{O_2}.

- Increased concentration of the
metabolic intermediate, 2,3-
diphosphoglycerate (2,3-DPG)
within red blood cells augments
release of available oxygen for
a given decrease in cellular P_{O_2}.

Altitude-Related Medical Problems

Natives who live and work at high altitudes, and newcomers to altitude, encounter medical problems associated with reduced ambient P_{O_2}. Some mild problems

dissipate within hours or several days, depending on the rapidity of ascent and degree of exposure; other medical
complications become severe and significantly compromise overall health and safety. Three medical conditions
pose potential problems: (a) acute mountain sickness, (b)
high-altitude pulmonary edema, and (c) high-altitude
cerebral edema.

c l o s e   u p

Breath-Hold Diving: Not Without Its Dangers

Underwater exploration offers discoveries of new and colorful species of plants and fish, old-world relics, and a feeling of self-awareness unknown to most. But the lure of the deep is not without hazards.

Many individuals swim at the surface of the water with fins, mask, and snorkel. If a person takes a full inspiration of ambient air, about 600–1000 mL of oxygen (depending on vital capacity) enters the lungs. If breath-hold begins, the oxygen in the lungs can sustain metabolism until arterial Po_2 and Pco_2 signal the need to renew breathing. With some training, individuals can readily breath-hold for 1 minute or longer. During this time, arterial Po_2 drops to about 60 mm Hg while arterial Pco_2 rises towards 50 mm Hg. Exercise greatly reduces breath-hold time because oxygen utilization and carbon dioxide production increase with exercise intensity. Hyperventilating prior to a dive significantly extends breath-hold, but substantial risks accompany this maneuver.

A sudden loss of consciousness (**blackout**) can occur in novice and skilled divers during attempts to extend breath-hold underwater. Most reports of blackout involve men (97% of all incidents) between the ages of 16 and 20 years, all known to be good or excellent swimmers. In most cases, the person competed with himself or others for underwater swimming distance or duration. Surprisingly, in about 80% of the cases, the accident occurred in a swimming pool with a lifeguard on duty. For the survivors of underwater blackout, most reported that they had an urge to breathe, but still lost consciousness without recognizable warning signs. In several cases, the victim did not remember any feelings associated with reaching the " breaking point" before becoming unconscious.

The break point for breath-hold usually corresponds to an increase in arterial Pco_2 to about 50 mm Hg. Some people still ignore this stimulus and continue to breath-hold until Pco_2 reaches levels that cause severe disorientation and blackout. With hyperventilation prior to breath-hold, arterial Pco_2 may decrease from its normal value of 40 mm Hg to 15 mm Hg or lower. Eliminating carbon dioxide from body fluids significantly extends breath-hold duration until arterial Pco_2 increases to the level that triggers the urge to breathe. Two-hundred and seventy seconds (4.5 min) represents the longest breath-hold recorded while breathing air without prior hyperventilation. Breath-holds of 15 to 20 minutes have been reported with hyperventilation followed by several breaths of pure oxygen immediately before breath-holding.

Consider the risks of this procedure during a dive. Alveolar oxygen continually moves into the blood for delivery to working muscles. With prior hyperventilation, arterial carbon dioxide remains low. The diver, free from the urge to breathe, continues in the activity. As diving depth increases, external water pressure compresses the thorax (see table) maintaining a relatively high Po_2 within the alveoli. Thus, even though the absolute quantity of oxygen in the lungs decreases (as oxygen diffuses into the blood), adequate oxygen pressure continues to load hemoglobin as the prolonged dive progresses. As the diver senses the need to breathe and begins to ascend, significant pressure reversals occur. Alveolar Po_2 decreases proportionately as water pressure on the thorax decreases and lung volume expands. When the diver nears the surface, alveolar Po_2 may be so low that dissolved oxygen leaves the blood and flows into the alveoli! This can trigger sudden loss of consciousness before the diver reaches the surface.

RELATIONSHIP OF DEPTH IN WATER TO EXTERNAL PRESSURE AGAINST THORAX AND A 6-L VOLUME OF A GAS WITHIN LUNGS[a]

Depth Feet (M)	Atmosphere	Pressure (mm Hg)	Lung Volume (mL)
Sea level	1	760	6000
33 (10)	2	1520	3000
66 (20)	2	2280	2000
99 (30)	3	3040	1500
133 (40)	5	3800	1200
166 (50)	6	4560	1000
200 (60)	7	5320	875

[a] If divers fill their lungs with 6 L of air at sea level and descend to a depth of 33 feet, the lung volume compresses to 3 L; diving an additional 33 feet, the original 6-L lung volume reduces one third to 2 L. When the diver returns to the surface, the air volume re-expands to its original 6-L volume.

References

Craig, A. B.: Summary of 58 cases of loss of consciousness during underwater swimming and diving. *Med. Sci. Sports*, 8 : 171, 1976.

Craig, A.B.: Principles and problems of underwater diving. *Phys. Sportsmed.*, 8:72, 1980.

Acute Mountain Sickness

Despite the body's rapid defense against the challenge of altitude, many people experience the discomfort of **acute mountain sickness (AMS)** during the first few days at altitudes of about 3048 m (10,000 ft) or higher. Symptoms usually include headache (most frequent, probably from dilation of cerebral blood vessels), dizziness, nausea, vomiting, dimness of vision, insomnia, and generalized weakness. For people suffering AMS, even moderate exercise becomes intolerable. With acclimatization, symptoms subside and many disappear. Acclimatizing gradually to moderate altitudes, followed by a slow progression to higher altitudes usually prevents mountain sickness.

Appetite may be suppressed during the early stages of a high-altitude stay, reducing energy intake and body mass by 40%; decreased thirst sensations contribute to a relative state of hypohydration (refer to Fig. 16.5). Individuals prefer low-salt, high-carbohydrate diets during the initial phase of a high-altitude stay. Adequate availability and utilization of carbohydrate at altitude liberates greater energy per unit oxygen consumed compared with fat (5.0 kcal versus 4.7 kcal per L O_2). Also, high levels of circulating lipids following a high-fat meal may reduce arterial oxygen saturation. In general, a high-carbohydrate diet tends to:

- Enhance altitude tolerance
- Reduce severity of mountain sickness
- Lessen decrements in physical performance during early stage of altitude exposure

High-Altitude Pulmonary Edema

For unknown reasons, approximately 2% of sojourners to altitudes above 3048 m experience a severe complication from acute mountain sickness termed **high-altitude pulmonary edema** or **HAPE**. Symptoms usually manifest within 12 to 96 hours after rapidly ascending to high altitudes. The brain and lungs accumulate fluid in this life-threatening condition. At first, symptoms appear mild (general fatigue, dyspnea upon exertion, pain or pressure in the substernal area, headache, nausea, and persistent dry, irritating cough without phlegm and pulmonary infection). Eventually, pulmonary edema and fluid retention by the kidneys set in. Chest examination reveals wheezy and raspy sounds known as rales. Immediate descent to lower altitude prevents severe disability or even death from HAPE.

High-Altitude Cerebral Edema

If left untreated, increased intracranial pressure associated with **high-altitude cerebral edema (HACE)** leads to coma and ultimately death. The early manifestations of HACE mirror acute mountain sickness and HAPE, but symptoms eventually increase in severity. HACE occurs in approximately 1% of people exposed to altitudes above 2700 m (9000 ft). In addition to debilitating headache and severe fatigue, HACE also disrupts vision, bladder and bowl dysfunction, loss of coordination involving the trunk muscles, paralysis on one side of the body, generally poor reflexes, and mental confusion. Cerebral edema probably results from cerebral vasodilation and elevated capillary hydrostatic pressure. The additional cerebral fluid then distorts brain structures, which intensifies mountain sickness symptoms and increases sympathetic nervous system activity. Because of the difficulty diagnosing and treating HACE at high altitude, immediate descent to a lower elevation becomes crucial for effectively treating this condition.

Exercise Capacity at Altitude

The stress of high altitude imposes significant limitations on exercise capacity and physiologic function. Even at lower altitudes, the body's adjustments do not fully compensate for reduced oxygen pressure and diminishing exercise performance.

Aerobic Capacity

Aerobic capacity progressively and somewhat linearly decreases due to arterial oxygen desaturation as altitude increases. Trained and untrained men and women can generally expect a 1.5 to 3.5% reduction in $\dot{V}O_{2max}$ for every 305 m (1000 ft) increase above 1524 m (5000 ft), with a slightly greater rate of decrease for elite athletes. The aerobic capacity of a relatively fit man atop Mt. Everest would only equal about 1000 mL of oxygen per minute (14 to 18 $mL \cdot kg^{-1} \cdot min^{-1}$).

Circulatory Factors

Aerobic capacity still remains significantly below sea-level values even after several months of acclimatization. This occurs because of reduced circulatory efficiency in moderate and strenuous exercise that offsets the benefits of acclimatization. During submaximal exercise the immediate altitude response involves an increase in submaximal exercise blood flow; cardiac output decreases in the days that follow and does not improve with longer altitude exposure. A decrease in stroke volume as the altitude stay progresses accounts for diminished cardiac output. At maximal exercise, a decrease in maximum cardiac output occurs after about a week above 3048 m and persists throughout the altitude stay. *Reduced maximal exercise blood flow results from the combined effect of decreased maximum heart rate and stroke volume.*

Fit subjects experience a 2 to 13% decrement in 1- and 3-mile running performance at medium altitude (2300 m). The effects become more pronounced at higher elevations. Even after 4 weeks of acclimatization, endurance performance at altitude remains significantly below sea-level values. The small improvements in endurance at altitude during acclimatization probably relate to increases in (1) minute ventilation (ventilatory acclimatization), and (2) arterial oxygen saturation.

Altitude Training and Sea-Level Performance

Unquestionably, altitude acclimatization improves one's capacity to exercise at altitude. However, the effect of altitude exposure and altitude training on $\dot{V}O_{2max}$ and endurance performance immediately on return to sea level remains equivocal. Altitude adaptations in local circulation and cellular function, and compensatory increases in the blood's oxygen-carrying capacity should enhance sea-level performance. Unfortunately, much of the previous altitude research has not adequately evaluated this possibility. Often, poor control exists over the subjects' physical activity level, making it difficult to determine whether any improved sea-level $\dot{V}O_{2max}$ or performance score on return from altitude represents a training effect, an altitude effect, or synergism between altitude and training.

$\dot{V}O_{2max}$ on Return to Sea Level

When aerobic capacity serves as the criterion, sea-level performance does not significantly improve after living at altitude. Compared to the prealtitude measures, no significant change in $\dot{V}O_{2max}$ occurred for young runners on return to sea level after 18 days at an altitude of 3100 m. In addition, training in chambers designed to simulate altitude provided no additional benefit to sea-level performance compared to similar training at sea level. As expected, the altitude-trained group showed superior physical performance in the altitude experiments compared to sea-level counterparts.

Some physiologic changes produced during prolonged altitude exposure actually *negate* adaptations that could improve exercise performance upon return to sea level. The residual effects of muscle mass loss and reduced maximum heart rate and stroke volume observed with prolonged altitude exposure would not enhance immediate performance on return to sea level. Any reduction in maximum cardiac output during a stay at altitude offsets benefits derived from the blood's greater oxygen-carrying capacity.

Can Altitude Training Be Maintained?

Exposure to altitudes of 2300 m and higher makes it nearly impossible for athletes to train at the same intensity as sea level. At 4000 m, for example, runners can only train at 40% of their sea level $\dot{V}O_{2max}$ compared to 80% of this value at sea level. This altitude-related reduction in absolute training intensity makes it difficult for athletes to maintain peak condition for sea-level competition.

Altitude Training Versus Sea Level Training

To evaluate the effectiveness of exercise training at altitude, middle-distance runners trained at sea level for three weeks at 75% of sea level $\dot{V}O_{2max}$; another group of six runners trained an equivalent distance at the same $\dot{V}O_{2max}$ percentage at 2300 m. The groups then exchanged training sites and continued three weeks of similar training. Initially, 2-mile run times decreased by 7.2% at altitude compared to sea level. The times improved about 2.0% for both groups after altitude training, but postaltitude performance at sea level remained unchanged compared to prealtitude sea-level runs. Figure 16.16 shows that $\dot{V}O_{2max}$ for both groups at altitude decreased initially by about 17%, and improved only slightly after 20 days of altitude training. When the runners returned to sea level, aerobic capacity averaged 2.8% below prealtitude sea level values! Clearly, for these well-conditioned runners, no synergistic effect occurred with hard aerobic training at medium altitude compared with equally severe training at sea level.

"Live High-Train Low"
Failure to maintain the muscular power outputs of sea-level training at altitude may actually initiate a detraining effect.

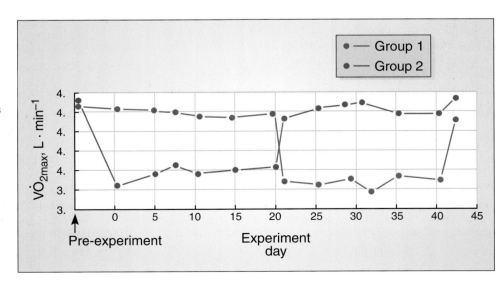

Figure 16.16
Maximal oxygen uptakes of two equivalent groups during training for three weeks at altitude and three weeks at sea level. Group 1 trained first at sea level and then continued training for three weeks at altitude. For Group 2, the procedure reversed as they trained first at altitude and then at sea level. (Data from Adams, W. C., et al.: Effects of equivalent sea-level and altitude training on $\dot{V}O_{2max}$ and running performance. *J. Appl. Physiol.*, 39:262, 1975.)

For these reasons, elite endurance athletes have resorted to the banned (and dangerous) practices of blood doping and erythropoeitin injections (see Chapter 17) to increase hematocrit and hemoglobin concentration, without the bother and potential negative effects of an altitude stay.

Athletes who lived at 2500 m but returned regularly to 1250 m to train showed greater performance increases in the 5000-m run than athletes who lived and trained at 2500 m, or athletes who lived and trained at sea level. These findings indicate that altitude acclimatization, and ability to maintain sea-level training intensity, provide important additive benefits to endurance at sea level. Alternatives exist to combining altitude living with regular returns to sea level for training. Three approaches can create an altitude environment so an athlete, mountaineer, or hot air balloonist at sea level spends a portion of the day at an "altitude" sufficient to stimulate an acclimatization response:

1. **Gamow Hypobaric Chamber** (named after its inventor, Professor Igar Gamow). A person rests and sleeps in a small chamber; the chamber's total air pressure can be reduced to simulate the barometric pressure of a given altitude. Reductions in barometric pressure bring about proportionate reductions in inspired air's Po_2.
2. **Increasing air's nitrogen concentration.** To eliminate the necessity of constructing an enclosure to withstand differentials between ambient sea-level air and reduced pressure within the hypobaric chamber, altitude has been simulated at sea-level by increasing the nitrogen percentage of the air within an enclosure. Increased nitrogen percentage reduces the air's oxygen percentage, thus decreasing the Po_2 of inspired air. Nordic skiers have applied this technique by living for 3 to 4 weeks in a specially constructed house that provides air with only 15.3% oxygen compared with the normal concentration of 20.9%. However, this system requires nitrogen gas and careful monitoring of the breathing mixture.
3. **Wallace Altitude Tent**—a suitcase-sized unit (Fig. 16.17), developed by British Olympic cyclist Shaun Wallace, continuously supplies air with an oxygen

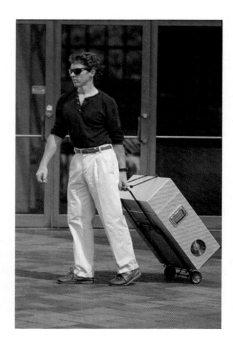

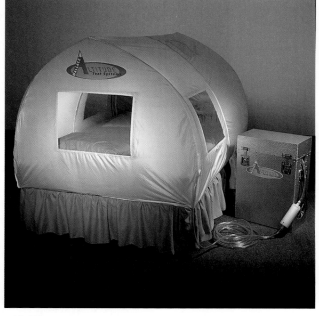

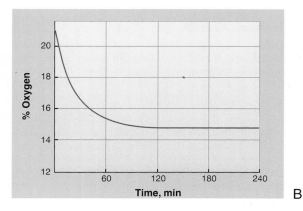

Figure 16.17
Wallace altitude tent. **A,** Easily transportable hypoxic generator and specially designed tent to fit over double or queen size bed. Patches of breathable nylon permit diffusion of ambient oxygen (at higher Po_2) into the tent (at lower Po_2) to maintain percentage of oxygen within tent air at approximately 15%. Hypoxic generator continuously supplies air with an oxygen content that equilibrates within the tent at 15%. **B,** Time course for equilibration of oxygen in air within the tent to reach the 15% level. Photos courtesy of Shaun Wallace.

content that eventually equilibrates at 15% to simulate an altitude of 2500 m (8200 ft). The 70-pound unit consists of a portable tent that fits over a normal bed; an hypoxic generator (housed in an airline suitcase) continually feeds altitude-simulating hypoxic air into the tent. The porosity of the tent's material limits the diffusion rate of outside oxygen into the tent to maintain the 15% value for oxygen within the tent. Equilibration of the tent's environment at the 15% oxygen level requires about 90 minutes.

summary

1. Inadequate oxygenation of hemoglobin occurs from the progressive reduction in ambient P_{O_2} upon altitude ascent. This produces noticeable performance decrements in aerobic activities at 2000 m and higher.

2. Reduced arterial P_{O_2} and accompanying tissue hypoxia at altitude stimulate physiologic responses that improve one's tolerance during rest and exercise. Hyperventilation and increased submaximal cardiac output via an elevated heart rate represent the primary immediate responses.

3. Longer-term acclimatization involves physiologic adjustments that greatly improve tolerance to altitude hypoxia. The main adjustments involve (a) re-establishing acid-base balance of body fluids, (b) increased hemoglobin and red blood cell synthesis, and (c) enhanced local circulation and cellular metabolic functions. Adjustments (b) and (c) significantly facilitate oxygen transport, delivery, and utilization.

4. Level of altitude dictates the rate and magnitude of acclimatization. Noticeable improvements occur within several days, but major adjustments require about two weeks. Acclimatization to high altitudes takes 4 to 6 weeks.

5. For acclimatized men at a simulated altitude that approaches the summit of Mt. Everest, alveolar P_{O_2} equals about 25 mm Hg. This reduces $\dot{V}O_{2max}$ by 70%. Unacclimatized individuals at this altitude would become unconscious within 30 seconds.

6. Acclimatization does not fully compensate for altitude stress. Even after acclimatization, $\dot{V}O_{2max}$ decreases about 2% for every 300 m above 1500 m. Impaired performance in endurance-related activities generally parallels the reduction in aerobic capacity.

7. Altitude-related decrements in maximum heart rate and stroke volume offset the beneficial effects of acclimatization. This partially explains the inability to achieve sea-level $\dot{V}O_{2max}$ values at altitude.

8. Research does not show enhanced sea-level $\dot{V}O_{2max}$ and endurance performance following altitude acclimatization. More than likely, reduced circulatory efficiency in moderate and strenuous exercise (and possible detraining and a decrease in muscle mass) offsets the benefits of acclimatization.

9. Training at altitude provides no additional benefit to sea-level performance compared with equivalent training only at sea level.

thought questions

1. How should a person dress who wants to play 90 minutes of outdoor paddle tennis at 20°F (−6.7°C)?

2. Suppose you had to run across a desert for 8 hours (sea level, 115°F [46.1°C], 20% relative humidity) while carrying only a backpack. What items would you take? Why?

3. What track and field events would be (a) hindered, and (b) enhanced by competition at moderate altitude? Why?

4. Your Vermont-based soccer team is scheduled for a tournament in Hawaii in early spring. Discuss how you would prepare the team to compete in this hot, humid environment (a) if all preparations had to be done at your school, and (b) if time, money, and travel were not considerations.

5. Explain the greater chance for resuscitation and survival from cold-water drowning compared with drowning in warmer water.

6. For their assault on Mt. Everest, elite mountaineers take 3 months to establish base camps at 16,600 ft (4216 m), 19,500 ft (4953 m), 21,300 ft (5410 m), 24,000 ft (6096 m), and 26,000 ft (6604 m) before their final ascent. Explain the physiological rational for a stage ascent approach to mountaineering.

7. Describe ideal personal physical and physiological characteristics that minimize heat injury risk during environmental heat stress.

selected references

American College of Sports Medicine: American College of Sports Medicine position stand on Heat and Cold Illnesses During Distance Running. *Med. Sci. Sports Exerc.*, 28:1, 1996.

Armstrong, L.E., and Maresh, C.M.: Effects of training, environment, and host factors on the sweating response to exercise. *Int. J. Sports Med.*, 19 (Suppl. 2):s103, 1998.

Ashenden, M.J., et al.: "Live high, train low" does not change the total haemoglobin mass of male endurance athletes sleeping at a simulated altitude of 3000 m for 23 nights. *Eur. J. Appl. Physiol.*, 80:479, 1999.

Bailey, D.M., et al.: Implications of moderate altitude training for sea-level endurance in elite distance runners. *Eur. J. Appl. Physiol.*, 78:360, 1998.

Bärtsh, P.: High altitude pulmonary edema. *Med. Sci. Sports Exerc.*, 31, No. 1 (Suppl.):S23, 1999.

Beidleman, B.A., et al.: Exercise responses after altitude acclimatization are retained during reintroduction to altitude. *Med. Sci. Sports Exerc.*, 29:1588, 1997.

Boero, J.A., et al.: Increased brain capillaries in chronic hypoxia. *J. Appl. Physiol.*, 86:2111, 1999.

Brooks, G.A., et al.: Muscle accounts for glucose disposal but not blood lactate appearance during exercise after acclimatization to 4,300 m. *J. Appl. Physiol.*, 72:2435, 1992.

Butterfield, G.E.: Nutrient requirements at high altitude. *Clin. Sports Med.*, 18:607, 1999.

Chapman, R.F., et al.: Individual variation in responses to altitude training. *J. Appl. Physiol.*, 85:1448, 1998.

Cheung, S.S., and Mclellan, T.M.: Heat acclimation, aerobic fitness, and hydration effects on tolerance during uncompensable heat stress. *J. Appl. Physiol.*, 84:1731, 1998.

Cymerman, A., et al.: Operation Everest II: maximal oxygen uptake at extreme altitude. *J. Appl. Physiol.*, 66:2446, 1989.

Dematte, J.E., et al.: Near-fatal heat stroke during the 1995 heat wave in Chicago. *Arch., Intern. Med.*, 129:173, 1998.

Emonson, D.L., et al.: Training-induced increases in sea level $\dot{V}O_{2max}$ and endurance training are not enhanced by acute hypobaric exposure. *Eur. J. Appl. Physiol.*, 76:8, 1997.

Epstein, Y., et al.: Exertional heat stroke: a case series. *Med. Sci. Sports Exerc.*, 31:224, 1999.

Falk, B.: Exercise in the pediatric population — effects of thermal stress. In: *Environmental and Exercise Physiology*. Doubt, T. (ed.). Champaign, IL: Human Kinetics, 1997.

Fulco, C.S., et al.: Maximal and submaximal exercise performance at altitude. *Aviat. Space Environ. Med.*, 69:793, 1998.

Gardner, J.W., et al.: Risk factors predicting exertional heat illness in male Marine Corps recruits. *Med. Sci. Sports Exerc.*, 28:939, 1996.

Gonzalez-Alonso, J.R., et al.: Influence of body temperature on the development of fatigue during prolonged exercise in the heat. *J. Appl. Physiol.*, 86:1032, 1999.

Greiwe, J.S., et al.: Effects of dehydration on isometric muscular strength and endurance. *Med. Sci. Sports Exerc.*, 30:284, 1998.

Hackett, P.H., et al.: High-altitude cerebral edema evaluated with magnetic resonance imaging. Clinical correlation and pathophysiology. *JAMA*, 280:1920, 1998.

Hales, J.R.S.: Hyperthermia and heat illness: pathological implications for avoidance and treatment. *Ann. N.Y. Acad. Sci.*, 813:534, 1997.

Inoue, Y., et al.: Mechanisms underlying the age-related decrement in the human sweating response. *Eur. J. Appl. Physiol.*, 79:121, 1999.

Jacobs, I., et al.: Thermoregulatory thermogenesis in humans during cold stress. *Exerc. Sport Sci. Rev.*, 22: 221, 1994.

Jansen, G.F., et al.: Cerebral vasomotor reactivity at high altitude in humans. *J. Appl. Physiol.*, 86:681, 1999.

Johnson, J.M.: Physical training and the control of skin blood flow. *Med. Sci. Sports Exerc.*, 30:382, 1998.

Kenney, W.L.: Thermoregulation at rest and during exercise in healthy older adults. *Exerc. Sport Sci. Rev.*, 25:41, 1997.

Levine, B.D., and Stray-Gunderson, J.: "Living high-training low": effect of moderate-altitude acclimatization with low-altitude training on performance. *J. Appl. Physiol.*, 83:102, 1997.

Liu, Y., et al.: Effect of "living high-training low" on the cardiac functions at sea level. *Int. J. Sports Med.*, 19:380, 1998.

Maxwell, N.S., et al.: Intermittent running: muscle metabolism in the heat and effect of hypohydration. *Med. Sci. Sports Exerc.*, 31:675, 1999.

McArdle, W.D., et al.: Thermal responses of men and women during cold-water immersion: influences of exercise intensity. *Eur. J. Appl. Physiol.*, 65: 265, 1992.

McCann, D.J., and Adams, W.C.: Wet bulb globe temperature index and performance in competitive distance runners. *Med. Sci. Sports Exerc.*, 29:955, 1997.

Montain, S.J., et al.: Hypohydration effects on skeletal muscle performance and metabolism: a ^{31}P-MRS study. *J. Appl. Physiol.*, 84:1889, 1998.

Nielsen, R.: Olympics in Atlanta: a fight against physics. *Med. Sci. Sports Exerc.*, 28:665, 1996.

Nielsen, B.: Heat acclimatization—Mechanisms of adaptation to exercise in the heat. *Int. J. Sports Med.*, 19(Suppl. 2):s1534, 1998.

Pandolf, K.B., et al.: Does erythrocyte infusion improve 3.2-km run performance at high altitude? *Eur. J. Appl. Physiol.*, 79:1, 1998.

Pilmanis, A.A., et al.: Exercise-induced altitude decompression sickness. *Aviat. Space Environ. Med.*, 70:22, 1999.

Ray, M.L., et al.: Effect of sodium in a rehydration beverage when consumed as a fluid or meal. *J. Appl. Physiol.*, 85:1329, 1998.

Rehrer, N.J.: The maintenance of fluid balance during exercise. *Int. J. Sports Nutr.*, 15 : 122, 1996.

Rennie, D. W.: Tissue heat transfer in water: lessons from the Korean divers. *Med. Sci. Sports Exerc.*, 20:S177, 1988.

Rico-Sanz, J., et al.: Effects of hyperhydration on total body water, temperature regulation and performance of elite young soccer players in a warm climate. *Int. J. Sports Med.*, 17:85, 1996.

Robergs, R.A., et al.: Multiple variables explain the variability in the decrement in $\dot{V}O_{2max}$ during acute hypobaric hypoxia. *Med. Sci. Sports Exerc.*, 30:869, 1998.

Rodriguez, F.A., et al.: Intermittent hypobaric hypoxic stimulates erythropoiesis and improves aerobic capacity. *Med. Sci. Sports Exerc.*, 31:264, 1999.

Saltin, B.: Exercise and the environment: Focus on altitude. *Res. Q. Exerc. Sport*, 67:1, 1996.

Sawka, M.N., and Coyle, E.F.: Influence of body water and blood volume on thermoregulation and exercise performance in the heat. *Exerc. Sport Sci. Rev.*, 27:167, 1999.

Sheffield-Moore, M., et al.: Thermoregulatory responses to cycling with and without a helmet. *Med. Sci. Sports Exerc.*, 29:755, 1997.

Shibasaki, M., et al.: Mechanisms of underdeveloped sweating responses in prepubertal boys. *Eur. J. Appl. Physiol.*, 76:340, 1997.

Stray-Gundersen, J., et al.: "Living high and training low" can improve sea level performance in endurance athletes. *Br. J. Sports Med.*, 33:150, 1999.

Tikuisis, P., et al.: Physiological responses of exercise-fatigued individuals exposed to wet-cold conditions. *J. Appl. Physiol.*, 86:1319, 1999.

Toner, M.M., and McArdle, W.D.: Human thermoregulatory responses to acute cold stress with special reference to water immersion. In: *Handbook of Physiology*. Section 4: Environmental Physiology, vol. 1. Fregly, M.J., and Blatteis, C.M., (eds.). New York: Oxford University Press, 1996.

U.S. Department of Health and Human Services. Hyperthermia and dehydration-related deaths associated with intentional weight loss in three collegiate wrestlers—North Carolina, Wisconsin, and Michigan, November-December, 1997, *Morbidity and Mortality Weekly Report*, 47:105, 1998.

West, J.B.: *High Life: A History of High Altitude Physiology and Medicine*. Oxford, England: Oxford University Press, 1998.

Westerterp-Plantenga, M.S., et al.: Appetite at "high altitude" [Operation Everest III (Comex-'97)]: a simulated ascent of Mount Everest. *J. Appl. Physiol.*, 87:391, 1999.

Young, A.J., et al.: Exertional fatigue, sleep loss, and negative energy balance increase susceptibility to hypothermia. *J. Appl. Physiol.*, 85:1210, 1998.

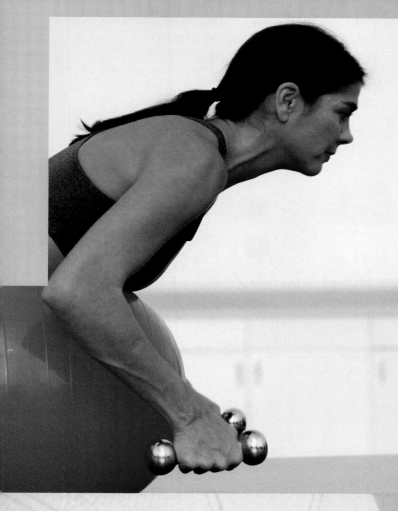

CHAPTER 17

Ergogenic Aids

Topics covered in this chapter

PART 1 Pharmacologic and Nutritional Agents

Anabolic Steroids
Androstenedione: A Legal Supplement in Some Sports
Clenbuterol: Anabolic Steroid Substitute
Growth Hormone: The Next Magic Pill?
DHEA: New Drug On the Circuit
Amphetamines
Caffeine
Alcohol
Pangamic Acid
Buffering Solutions
Phosphate Loading
Anti-Cortisol Producing Compounds
Chromium
Creatine
Summary

PART 2 Physiologic Agents

Red Blood Cell Reinfusion
Warm-Up
Breathing Hyperoxic Gas
Summary
Thought Questions
Selected References

- Define the term ergogenic aid.
- List four examples of substances and procedures alleged to provide ergogenic benefits.
- Advise an athlete about anabolic steroid use to increase muscle mass and sports performance.
- Describe the mode of action of anabolic steroids, their effectiveness, and risks involved for males and females.
- Give the proposed ergogenic action of androstenedione, its potential risks, and the objective evidence concerning its effectiveness.
- Describe the medical use of human growth hormone, including its potential dangers from use by healthy athletes.
- Describe the rationale for DHEA use as an ergogenic aid, including potential risks from supplementing with this hormone.
- Describe research that shows the possible ergogenic benefits and risks of taking clenbuterol, amphetamines, caffeine, chromium picolinate, beta-hydroxy-beta-methylbutyrate, and buffering solutions.
- Describe the theoretical role of creatine supplements for ergogenic effects, including physical activities that can benefit from supplementation.
- Describe the typical time course for red blood cell reinfusion and the mechanism for its ergogenic effect on endurance performance and aerobic capacity.
- Define "general warm-up" and "specific warm-up."
- Identify potential cardiovascular benefits of moderate warm-up before extreme physical effort.
- Provide a rationale for breathing a hyperoxic gas mixture to enhance exercise performance, and quantify its potential to increase tissue oxygen availability.

Ergogenic aids consist of substances and procedures believed to improve physical work capacity, physiologic function, or athletic performance. Part 1 of this chapter discusses the possible ergogenic role of some popular pharmacologic and nutritional agents, while Part 2 explores physiologic procedures purported to enhance exercise performance. In addition to their proposed role in augmenting one's capacity for exercise, many nutritional and pharmacologic compounds are believed to increase the quality and quantity of training.

PART 1
Pharmacologic and Nutritional Agents

Considerable literature exists concerning the effects of different nutritional and pharmacologic aids on exercise performance and training. Product promotional materials often include testimonials and endorsements for untested products from sports professionals and organizations, media publicity, television infomercials, and Internet home pages. Frequently touted are research studies concerning potential performance benefits from alcohol, amphetamines, hormones, carbohydrates, amino acids (either consumed singularly or in combination), fatty acids, caffeine, buffering compounds, wheat-germ oil, vitamins, minerals, catecholamine agonists, and even marijuana and cocaine. Athletes routinely use many of these substances because they believe they enhance acute exercise performance or improve training effectiveness. The general population believes supplements improve physical appearance; in this regard, products marketed to reduce body fat and increase muscle mass become overnight best sellers.

Five mechanisms explain how nutritional and pharmacologic agents might enhance exercise performance.

1. By acting as a central or peripheral stimulant to the nervous system (e.g., caffeine, choline, amphetamines, alcohol)
2. By increasing the storage and/or availability of a limiting substrate (e.g., carbohydrate, creatine, carnitine, chromium)
3. By acting as a supplemental fuel source (e.g., glucose, medium-chain triglycerides)
4. By reducing or neutralizing performance-inhibiting metabolic byproducts (e.g., sodium bicarbonate, citrate, pangamic acid, phosphate)
5. By facilitating recovery from strenuous exercise (e.g., high-glycemic carbohydrates, water)

The International Olympic Committee's (IOC) banned drugs

The IOC initiated drug testing in 1968 after a Tour de France British cyclist died from an amphetamine overdose a year earlier. Testing has consistently expanded; random unannounced drug testing began in track and field in 1989. The following categories comprise substances currently banned by the IOC:

- Stimulants
- Narcotic Analgesics
- Androgenic-Anabolic Steroids
- Beta Blockers
- Diuretics
- Peptide Hormones and Analogues
- Substances that Alter the Integrity of Urine Samples

<http://test.olympic-usa.org/inside/in_1_3_7_1.html#TOC>

In our drug-oriented, competitive culture, using drugs for ergogenic purposes continues on the upswing among high school and even junior high school athletes. Before the 1996 Atlanta Olympic Games, only two sports, women's field hockey and gymnastics, remained free from anabolic steroid detection. When winning becomes all important, cheating to win becomes pervasive. The use and abuse of drugs by male and female athletes increases yearly, despite scant scientific evidence indicating a performance-enhancing effect from many of these chemicals. Ironically, athletes usually go to great lengths to promote all aspects of their health (they train hard, eat well-balanced meals, receive medical attention even for minor injuries) yet they purposely ingest synthetic agents, many of which trigger negative health effects ranging from nausea, hair loss, itching, and nervous irritability, to severe consequences of sterility, liver dysfunction, drug addiction, and even death from liver and blood cancer.

Anabolic Steroids

Anabolic steroids for therapeutic use became prominent in the early 1950s to treat patients deficient in natural androgens or with muscle-wasting diseases. Other legitimate steroid uses include treatment for osteoporosis and severe breast cancer in women, and to counter the excessive decline in lean body mass and increase in body fat often observed among elderly men.

Anabolic steroids have become an integral part of the high-technology scene of competitive American sports, beginning with the 1955 U.S. weightlifting team's use of Dianabol (modified, synthetic testosterone molecule, methandrostenolone). A new era of "drugging" competi-

tive athletes ushered in with the formulation of other anabolic steroids. An estimated one to three million athletes (e.g., 90% of male and 80% of female professional body builders) currently use androgens, often combined with stimulants, diuretics, and other drugs.

Structure and Action

An anabolic steroid functions in a manner similar to testosterone. By binding with special receptor sites on muscle and other tissues, testosterone contributes to male secondary sex characteristics, including gender differences in muscle mass and strength that develop at the onset of puberty. The hormone's androgenic (masculinizing) effects become minimized by synthetically manipulating the anabolic steroid's chemical structure to increase muscle growth from anabolic tissue building and nitrogen retention. Nevertheless, the masculinizing effect of synthetically derived steroids still occurs despite chemical alteration, particularly in females.

Athletes who take these drugs do so typically during the active years of their athletic careers. They combine multiple steroid preparations in oral and injectable form (combined because they believe various androgens differ in their physiologic action), a practice called "**stacking**," progressively increasing the drug dosage (**pyramiding**) during 6- to 12-week cycles. The drug quantity far exceeds the recommended medical dose. The athlete then alters drug dosage and/or combines it with other drugs before competition to minimize chances of detection.

The difference between dosages used in research studies and the excess typically abused by athletes has contributed to a credibility gap between scientific findings (often, no effect of steroids) and what most in the athletic community believe to be true. Table 17.1 lists examples of oral and injectable anabolic steroids, including typical retail cost and estimated range of black market prices. The latter vary considerably in different domestic regions and internationally. A conservative estimate would be at least twice the retail cost, and up to 100 times more.

Estimates of Steroid Use

Male and female athletes usually combine anabolic steroid use with resistance training and augmented protein intake because they believe this combination improves sports performance that requires strength, speed, and power. The steroid abuser often has an image of a massively developed body builder; however, abuse also occurs frequently in competitive athletes participating in road cycling, tennis, track and field, and swimming. A survey of U.S. Powerlifting Team (60% response rate) revealed that two-thirds used androgenic-anabolic steroids.

Federal authorities conservatively estimate that the emerging business of illegal trafficking in steroids exceeds $150 million yearly—a figure likely to increase through the turn of the century. Because many competitive and recreational athletes obtain steroids on the black market, misinformed individuals take massive and prolonged

TABLE 17.1
Examples of oral and injectable anabolic steroids, including typical retail cost and black market prices[a]

GENERIC	COMMERCIAL	FORM[b]	RETAIL COST	BLACK MARKET
Oxymetholone	Anadrol-50	Oral; 50 mg	$116/100 tabs	$200–500
Oxandrolone	Oxandrin	Oral; 2.5 mg	$421/100 tabs	$600–1500
Stanazolol	Winstrol V	Oral; 2 mg	$97/100 tabs	$200–450
Nandrolone Phenpropionate	Durabolin Nandrobolic	Injectable; $25 mg \cdot mL^{-1}$	$28/5 mL vial	$200–450
Nadrolone Deconate Androlone-D 200	Deca-Durabolin Neo-durabolic	Injectable; $50 mg \cdot mL^{-1}$	$12/2 mL vial	$400–750

[a] 1999 typical retail prices in the Amherst/Boston area. Prices vary depending on country and local conditions. The black market price reflects a range of prices from various sources.

[b] Anabolic steroids taken by mouth or injected into a muscle. Tablets or capsules taken by mouth are often called "orals." Oral androgens do not metabolize into testosterone but act directly on androgen receptors. The injectable forms, known as "oils" or "waters," usually have longer-lasting effects than orals. Injectables release slowly into the body once the injection enters a muscle (usually the buttocks). One injection (at normal concentrations prescribed medically) maintains normal serum testosterone levels for 10-14 days. Oral androgens are not as biologically active as the injectable forms.

dosages without medical monitoring, which often adversely alters physiologic functions. Particularly worrisome is steroid abuse among young boys and girls and its accompanying risks, including extreme masculinization and premature cessation of bone growth. Children as young as 11 years of age use anabolic-androgenic steroids. Approximately 1 in 15 high school students or about one-half million adolescents (250,000 high school seniors) have used steroids; the same youngsters are likely to abuse other illicit drugs and share needles. The teenagers cite improved athletic performance as the most common reason for taking steroids, although 25% acknowledged enhanced appearance as the main reason. In this regard, a disturbance in body image (dissatisfaction/unhappiness with upper and lower body parts, facial features) can lead to anabolic steroid abuse among teenagers and young men.

Effectiveness of Anabolic Steroids

Much of the confusion about the ergogenic effectiveness of anabolic steroids comes from variations in experimental design, poor controls, differences in specific drugs, and dosages (50 to >200 mg per day versus the usual medical dosage of 5 to 20 mg), treatment duration, training intensity, measurement techniques, previous experience as subjects, individual variation in response, and nutritional supplementation. Also, the relatively small residual androgenic effect of the steroid can make the athlete more aggressive (so-called "roid rage"), competitive, and fatigue resistant. Such disinhibitory central nervous system effects

allow the athlete to train harder for a longer time, or believe that augmented training effects actually occurred. Abnormal alterations in mood, including psychiatric dysfunction, have been attributed to androgen use.

Research with animals suggests that anabolic steroid treatment, when combined with exercise and adequate protein intake, stimulates protein synthesis and increases a muscle's protein content. In contrast, other research shows no benefit from steroid treatment on the leg muscle weight of rats subjected to functional overload by surgically removing the synergistic muscle. The researchers concluded that anabolic steroid treatment did not complement functional overload to augment muscle development. The effects on humans, however, remains difficult to interpret. Some studies show augmented body mass gains and reduced body fat with steroid use in men who train, whereas other studies show no effects on strength and power or body composition, even with sufficient energy and protein intake to support an anabolic effect. When steroid use pro-

It's Against the Law

A federal law makes it illegal to prescribe, distribute, or possess anabolic steroids for any purpose other than treatment of disease or other medical conditions. First offenders face up to 5 years in prison and a fine up to $250,000.

Figure 17.1
Changes from baseline in mean fat-free body mass, triceps and quadriceps cross-sectional areas, and muscle strength in the bench-press and squatting exercises over ten weeks of testosterone treatment (Data from Bhasin, S., et al.: The effects of supraphysiological doses of testosterone on muscle size and strength in normal men. *N. Engl. J. Med.*, 335:1, 1996.)

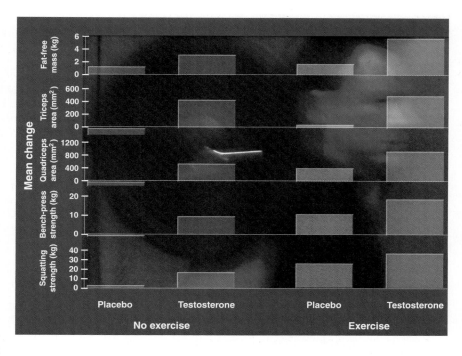

duced body mass gains, the compositional nature of these gains (water, muscle, fat) remained unclear.

Dosage An Important Factor

Variations in drug dosage contribute to the confusion (and credibility gap between scientist and steroid abuser) about the true effectiveness of anabolic steroids. Recent research with anabolic steroids studied 43 healthy men with some resistance training experience. Diet (energy and protein intake) and exercise (standard weight lifting, three times weekly) were controlled, with steroid dosage exceeding previous human studies (600 mg testosterone enanthate injected weekly or placebo).

Figure 17.1 illustrates changes from baseline average values for fat-free body mass (FFM; hydrostatic weighing), triceps and quadriceps cross-sectional muscle areas (magnetic resonance imaging), and muscle strength (1-RM) after ten weeks of testosterone treatment. The men who received the hormone and continued to weight train gained about 0.5 kg (1 lb) of lean tissue weekly, with no increase in body fat over the relatively brief treatment period. Even the group that received the drug, but did not train, significantly increased muscle mass and strength compared with the group receiving the placebo, although their increases were less than the group that trained while taking testosterone. The researchers emphasized that they did not design the study to justify or endorse steroid use for athletic purposes because significant health risks occur from steroid abuse. These data did show the potential for medically supervised anabolic steroid treatment to restore muscle mass in tissue-wasting diseases.

Risks of Steroid Use

The infrequent but distinct possibility of harmful side effects from anabolic steroid treatment, particularly orally administered steroids, likely outweighs any potential ergogenic effect. Prolonged high dosages of steroids (often at levels 10 to 200 times the therapeutic recommendation) can impair normal testosterone-endocrine function. A study of five male power athletes showed that 26 weeks of steroid administration reduced serum testosterone to less

than one-half the level measured when the study began, with the effect lasting throughout a 12- to 16-week follow-up. Infertility, reduced sperm concentrations (azoospermia), and decreased testicular volume pose additional problems for the male steroid user.

Other accompanying hormonal alterations during steroid use in males include a seven-fold increase in the concentration of estradiol, the major female hormone. The higher estradiol level represents an average value for normal females, and possibly explains the **gynecomastia** (excessive development of the male mammary glands, sometimes secreting milk) often reported among males who take anabolic steroids. Furthermore, steroids can cause:

1. Chronic stimulation of the prostate gland (may increase prostate size)
2. Injury and functional alterations in cardiovascular function and myocardial cell cultures
3. Possible pathologic ventricular growth and dysfunction when combined with resistance training
4. Increased blood platelet aggregation, which can compromise cardiovascular health and function, and possibly increase risk of stroke and acute myocardial infarction (from blood clots)

Steroid Use and Life-Threatening Disease

Table 17.2 lists detrimental side effects of anabolic steroid use. Concern regarding risks centers on evidence about possible links between androgen abuse and abnormal liver function. Because the liver almost exclusively metabolizes androgens, it becomes susceptible to damage from long-term steroid use and toxic excess. One of the serious effects of androgens on the liver occurs when it (and sometimes splenic tissue) develops localized blood-filled lesions (cysts), a condition called **peliosis hepatis**. In extreme cases, the liver eventually fails or intra-abdominal hemorrhage develops and the patient dies. These data emphasize the potentially serious side effects even when a physician prescribes the drug in the recommended dosage. Although patients often take steroids for a longer duration than athletes, some athletes take steroids on and off for years, with dosage exceeding typical therapeutic levels.

Preliminary data also suggest that anabolic steroids interfere with the responsiveness of the body's immune system. A type of withdrawal syndrome can occur (similar to alcohol and narcotic withdrawal), as well as an addiction syndrome that makes it difficult to discontinue steroid use.

Steroid Use and Plasma Lipoproteins

Anabolic steroid use (particularly the orally active 17-alkylated androgens) in healthy men and women rapidly lowers high-density lipoprotein cholesterol (HDL-C), elevates both low-density lipoprotein cholesterol (LDL-C) and total cholesterol, and lowers the HDL-C:LDL-C ratio. Weight lifters who took anabolic steroids averaged an HDL-C of 26 mg·dL^{-1} compared with 50 mg·dL^{-1} for weight lifters not taking these drug. Reduction of HDL-C to this level significantly increases a steroid user's risk of coronary artery disease. Even after abstaining from steroids

for at least 8 weeks between consecutive cycles, the reduced HDL-C remained low.

Steroid Use by Females

Females have additional concerns from anabolic steroid use besides the range of side effects discussed. These include masculinization (more apparent than in men), disruption of normal growth pattern by premature closure of the plates for bone growth (also for boys), deepened voice, altered menstrual function, dramatic increase in sebaceous gland size, acne, hirsutism (excessive body and facial hair), decreased breast size, and enlarged clitoris. The long-term effects of steroid use on reproductive function remain unknown.

Androstenedione: A Legal Supplement in Some Sports

Many athletes take an over-the-counter nutritional supplement, androstenedione, because they believe it produces endogenous testosterone, which enables them to train harder, build muscle mass, and repair injury more rapidly. Found naturally in meat and extracts of some plants, androstenedione is touted on the web as "a metabo-

TABLE 17.2
Oral adrenergic-anabolic steroids associated with detrimental side affects[a]

CHEMICAL NAME	TRADE NAME	DAILY DOSAGE (MG)	DURATION IN AFFECTED PATIENTS (MONTHS)	COMPLICATIONS
Oxymetholone	Ora-Testryl Adroyd Anapolon Anadrol 50	10–250	10–51	Pellosis hepatis[b]
Methyltestosterone	Oreton Methyl Metandren Android	20–50	1–165	Hepatoma[c]
Stanazolol	Winstrol	15	18	Hepatoma[c]
Methandrostenolone	Dianabol	10–15	12–18	Hepatoma[c]
Fluoxymesterone	Halotestin	15–80	4–16	Pellosis hepatis[b]
Norethandrolone	Nilevar	20–30	1.5–9	Pellosis hepatis[b]

[a] Data from Johnson, F.L.: The association of oral androgenic-anabolic steroids and life threatening disease. *Med. Sci. Sports*, 7:284, 1975.

[b] Severe liver malfunction.

[c] Liver cancer.

American College of Sports Medicine (ACSM) Position Statement on Anabolic Steroids

Based on the world literature and a careful analysis of claims about anabolic-androgenic steroids, ACSM issued the following statement:

1. Anabolic-androgenic steroids in the presence of an adequate diet and training can contribute to increases in body weight, often in the lean mass compartment.

2. The gains in muscular strength achieved through high-intensity exercise and proper diet can occur by the increased use of anabolic-androgenic steroids in some individuals.

3. Anabolic-androgenic steroids do not increase aerobic power or capacity for muscular exercise.

4. Anabolic-androgenic steroids have been associated with adverse effects on the liver, cardiovascular, reproductive system, and psychologic status in therapeutic trials and in limited research on athletes. Until further research is completed, the potential hazards of the use of the anabolic-androgenic steroids in athletes must include those found in therapeutic trials.

5. The use of anabolic-androgenic steroids by athletes is contrary to the rules and ethical principles of athletic competition as set forth by many of the sports governing bodies. The American College of Sports Medicine supports these ethical principles and deplores the use of anabolic-androgenic steroids by athletes.

lite that is only one step away from the biosynthesis of testosterone." The National Football League, the National Collegiate Athletic Association, the Men's Tennis Association, and the IOC ban its use because they believe it provides an unfair competitive advantage and may endanger health, similar to anabolic steroids. The IOC banned for life the 1996 Olympic shot-put gold medalist because he used androstenedione. As of December, 1999 Major League Baseball, the National Basketball Association, and the National Hockey League do not forbid its use.

Originally developed by East Germany in the 1970s to enhance performance of their elite athletes, androstenedione was first commercially manufactured and sold in the U.S. in 1996. By calling the substance a supplement and avoiding any claims that it offers medical benefits, the 1994 Food and Drug Administration rules enable androstenedione to be marketed as a food. Because many countries consider androstenedione a controlled substance, athletes travel to this country to purchase the compound, which contributes to the supplement industry's $12 billion yearly sales. Currently available products include androstenedione-containing chewing gum and a steroid lozenge that dissolves under the tongue.

Action and Effectiveness

Androstenedione, an intermediate or precursor hormone between DHEA and testosterone, aids the liver to synthesize other biologically active steroid hormones. It is normally produced by the adrenal glands and gonads, and converts to testosterone through enzymatic action in diverse tissues of the body. Androstenedione also converts into estrogens.

Little scientific evidence supports claims about this supplement's effectiveness or anabolic qualities. At this time, only one study has systematically evaluated whether short- and long-term oral androstenedione supplementation elevated blood testosterone concentrations and enhanced gains in muscle size and strength during resistance training. In one phase of the investigation 10 young adult men received a single 100-mg dose of androstenedione or a placebo containing 250 mg of rice flour. Serum androstenedione rose 175% during the first 60 minutes following ingestion, and then rose further by about 350% above baseline values between minutes 90 and 270. However, no effect emerged for androstenedione supplementation and serum concentrations of either free or total testosterone.

In the experiment's second phase, 20 young, untrained men received either 300 mg of androstenedione daily (N = 10) or 250 mg of rice flour placebo daily during weeks 1, 2, 4, 5, 7, and 8 of an 8-week total body resistance training program. Serum androstenedione increased 100% in the androstenedione-supplemented group and remained elevated throughout training. Although serum testosterone levels were significantly higher in the androstenedione-supplemented group than the placebo group before and following supplementation, serum free and total testosterone remained unaltered for both groups during the supplementation-training period. However, serum estradiol and estrone concentrations increased significantly during the training period only for the group receiving the supplement, suggesting an increased aromatization of the ingested androstenedione to estrogens. Furthermore, although resistance training significantly increased muscle strength and lean body mass, and reduced body fat for both groups, *no synergistic effect* emerged for the group supplemented with androstenedione. The supplement did, however, cause a 12% significant reduction in HDL-cholesterol after only 2 weeks, which remained lower for the 8 weeks of training and supplementation. Serum concentrations of liver function enzymes remained within normal limits for both groups throughout the experimental period.

Taken together, these findings indicate *no effect* of androstenedione supplementation on (1) basal serum concentrations of testosterone, or (2) training responsiveness in terms of muscle size and strength and body composition. A worrisome outcome relates to the potential significant negative effect of the reduction of HDL on overall heart disease risk and the elevated serum estrogen levels on risk of gynecomastia and possibly pancreatic and other cancers. These findings must be viewed within the context of this specific study because test subjects took dosages of androstenedione far smaller than routinely taken by body builders.

Concern has been raised over the legal use of androstenedione by professional baseball players to break the home run records of Babe Ruth and Roger Maris during the 1998 season. The sport-related issues focus on 1) whether supplementation significantly increases muscular strength and power, and 2) whether any fitness increases actually improve performance in the diverse, precise motor skills required in baseball, basketball, ice and field hockey, soccer, and golf. If the answer is yes, then scientists should be able to objectively assess any improvements in such tasks. As far as we know, no such credible scientific evidence exists concerning skill acquisition.

Clenbuterol: Anabolic Steroid Substitute

Extensive random testing of competitive athletes for anabolic steroid use has resulted in a number of steroid substitutes appearing on the illicit health food, mail order, and "black market" drug network. One such drug, the sympathomimetic amine **clenbuterol** (trade names Clenasma, Monores, Novegan, Prontovent, and Spiropent), has become popular among athletes because of its purported tissue-building, fat-reducing benefits. Typically, when a body builder discontinues steroid use before competition to avoid detection and possible disqualification, he or she substitutes clenbuterol to retard muscle loss and facilitate fat burning to achieve the "cut" look.

Clenbuterol, one of a group of chemical compounds classified as a beta-adrenergic agonist (albuterol, clenbuterol, salbutamol, salmeterol, terbutaline), is not approved for human use in the United States, but is commonly prescribed abroad as an inhaled bronchodilator for treating obstructive pulmonary disorders. Clenbuterol facilitates responsiveness of adrenergic receptors to circulating epinephrine, norepinephrine, and other adrenergic amines. A review of available animal studies (no human studies exist) indicates that when sedentary, growing livestock receive clenbuterol in dosages in excess of those prescribed in Europe for human use for bronchial asthma, clenbuterol increases skeletal and cardiac muscle protein deposition and slows fat gain by enhancing lipolysis. Clenbuterol has also been used experimentally in animals with

some success to counter the wasting effects on muscle of aging, immobilization, malnutrition, and pathologic conditions. The enlarged muscle size from clenbuterol treatment resulted from a decrease in protein breakdown and increase in protein synthesis.

Potential Negative Effect On Muscle Function

Female rats treated with clenbuterol ($2 \text{ mg} \cdot \text{kg}^{-1}$ injected subcutaneously) or injected with the same volume of fluid carrier (placebo) each day for 14 days significantly increased (a) muscle mass, (b) absolute maximal force-generating capacity, and (c) hypertrophy of fast- and slow-twitch muscle fibers. However, hastened fatigue during short-term, intense muscle actions also occurred. Similar positive and negative effects have been noted by other studies. For example, regular exercise, and regular exercise combined with clenbuterol decreased muscular dystrophy progression in mice. On the other hand, the group receiving clenbuterol experienced increased muscle fatigability and cellular deformities not apparent in the exercise only group. Reported short-term side effects in humans accidentally "overdosing" from eating animals that were treated with clenbuterol include muscle tremor, agitation, palpitations, muscle cramps, rapid heart rate, and headache. Despite such negative side effects, supervised use of clenbuterol may prove beneficial for humans with muscle wasting from disease, forced immobilization, and aging. Unfortunately, no data exist for its potential toxicity level in humans, or its efficacy and safety in long-term use. Clearly, clenbuterol cannot be justified or recommended as an ergogenic aid at the present time.

Amino Acid Supplements Do Not Augment Training Responsiveness

Research on healthy subjects does not provide convincing evidence for an ergogenic effect of oral amino acid supplements on hormone secretion, training responsiveness, or exercise performance. For example, in studies with appropriate design and statistical analysis, supplements of arginine, lysine, ornithine, tyrosine, and other amino acids, either singularly or in combination, did not affect human growth hormone (hGH) levels, insulin secretion, diverse measures of anaerobic power, or all-out running performance at $\dot{V}O_{2max}$. Furthermore, elite junior weight liters who supplemented with all 20 amino acids, showed no improvement in physical performance or resting or exercise-induced responses for testosterone, cortisol, or hGH.

Growth Hormone: The Next Magic Pill?

Physicians and pharmacologists predict that **human growth hormone** (**hGH**), also known as somatotropic hormone, will replace anabolic steroids as a training aid. This hormone, produced by the adenohypophysis of the pituitary gland, facilitates tissue-building processes and normal human growth. Specifically, hGH stimulates bone and cartilage growth, enhances fatty acid oxidation, and inhibits glucose and amino acid breakdown. Reduced hGH secretion accounts for some of the decrease in FFM and increase in fat mass that accompany aging; reversal occurs with exogenous hGH supplements produced by genetically engineered bacteria. However, hGH supplementation does not reverse the negative effects of aging on functional measures of muscular strength and aerobic capacity. Furthermore, men receiving the supplement experienced hand stiffness, malaise, joint pain, and lower-extremity edema.

Medically, children who suffer from kidney failure or hGH-deficient children take this hormone to help them achieve near-normal size. hGH use appeals to the strength and power athlete because at physiologic levels it stimulates amino acid uptake and protein synthesis by muscle, while enhancing fat breakdown and conserving glycogen reserves. However, few well-controlled studies have examined how hGH supplements affect healthy subjects who undergo exercise training.

In a double-blind study, six well-trained men received either biosynthetic hGH or a placebo while maintaining a high-protein diet. During 6 weeks of standard resistance training with hGH, percent body fat decreased and FFM increased significantly. No changes in body composition occurred for the group who trained with the placebo. These findings, however, have not been supported by more recent investigations. Sixteen previously sedentary young men who participated in a 12-week resistance training program received recombinant hGH (40 μg·kg^{-1}·d^{-1}) or a placebo. FFM, total body water, and whole body protein synthesis increased more in the hGH recipients, with no significant differences between groups in (a) fractional rate of protein synthesis in skeletal muscle, (b) torso and limb circumferences, or (c) muscle function in dynamic and static strength measures. The researchers attributed the greater increase in whole body protein synthesis in the GH group to a possible increase in nitrogen retention in lean tissue other than skeletal muscle (e.g., connective tissue, fluid, and noncontractile protein).

Because hGH occurs naturally in the body, no foolproof way currently exists to detect its use as an ergogenic substance. However, drug-testing experts believe an effective test using blood markers will be available for the year 2000 Olympic Games in Sydney, Australia. Such testing would require a change in current Olympic policy, which just permits urine testing. Healthy people can only obtain hGH on the black market, often in adulterated form. The use of human cadaver-derived GH (discontinued by U.S. physicians, May, 1985) to treat children of short stature greatly increases the risk for contracting Creutzfeldt-Jakob Disease, an infectious, incurable fatal brain-deteriorating disorder. A synthetic form of hGH (Protoropin and Humantrope), produced by genetic engineering, currently treats hGH-deficient children (cost $20,000 to $40,000 per year). Undoubtedly, child athletes who take hGH believing they gain a competitive edge will suffer increased incidence of gigantism, while adults can develop acromegalic syndrome. Additional less visual side effects include insulin resistance leading to type 2 diabetes, water retention, and carpal tunnel compression.

DHEA: New Drug on the Circuit

Synthetic **dehydroepiandrosterone** (**DHEA**) use among athletes and the general population concerns sports medicine personnel and the medical community because of issues related to safety and effectiveness. DHEA and its sulfated ester, DHEAS, are relatively weak steroid hormones synthesized primarily by primates in the adrenal cortex from cholesterol. The quantity of DHEA (commonly referred to as mother hormone) produced by the body surpasses all other known steroids; its chemical structure closely resembles the sex hormones testosterone and estrogen, with a small amount of DHEA serving as a precursor for these hormones for men and women.

Because DHEA occurs naturally, the Food and Drug Administration has no control over its distribution or claims for its action and effectiveness. The lay press, mail order catalogs, and health food industry describe DHEA as a "superhormone" (even available as a chewing gum, each piece containing 25 mg of the hormone) to increase testosterone production, preserve youth, protect against heart disease, cancer, diabetes, and osteoporosis, invigorate sex drive, facilitate lean tissue gain and body fat loss, enhance mood and memory, extend life, and boost immunity to a variety of infectious diseases, including AIDS. The International Olympic Committee and United States Olympic Committee have placed DHEA on their banned substance lists at zero tolerance levels.

Figure 17.2 illustrates the generalized trend for plasma DHEA levels during a lifetime, plus six common claims made by manufacturers for DHEA supplements. For boys and girls, DHEA levels are substantial at birth and then decline sharply. A steady increase in DHEA production occurs from age six to ten years (an occurrence that some researchers feel contributes to the actual beginning of puberty and sexuality), followed by a rapid rise with peak

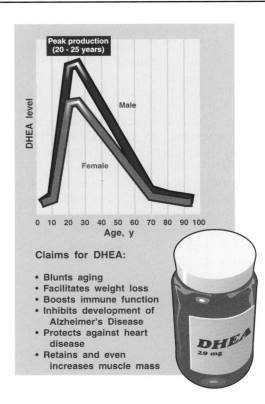

Figure 17.2
Generalized trend for plasma levels of DHEA for men and women during a lifetime.

production (higher in males than females) reached between ages 20 to 25 years.

In contrast to the glucocorticoid and mineralocorticoid adrenal steroids whose plasma levels remain relatively high with aging, a long, steady decline in DHEA occurs after age 30. By age 75, plasma levels decrease to only about 20% of the value in young adulthood. This has led to speculation that plasma levels of DHEA might serve as a bio-

An Amazing Amount of Money

Under the 1994 Dietary Supplement Health and Education Act, unless the Food and Drug Administration can prove a dietary supplement (e.g., vitamins, minerals, herbs, botanicals, meal supplements, enzymes, hormones) unsafe, manufacturers can say what they wish so long as they do not claim their products can prevent, treat, or cure a disease. Since the Act's passage, dietary supplements in the United States have skyrocketed, jumping to nearly $12 billion in 1997 from more than $8 billion in 1994. Of this total amount, consumers spend nearly $1 billion on dietary supplements related to "sports nutrition."

chemical marker of biologic aging and disease susceptibility. Popular reasoning concludes that supplementing with DHEA blunts the negative effects of aging by raising plasma levels to more youthful concentrations. In fact, many people supplement with this hormone "just in case" it turns out to be beneficial—without considering the potential for biologic harm. DHEA and its potential benefit for aging are further explored in Chapter 20.

DHEA Safety

In 1994, the Food and Drug Administration reclassified DHEA from the category of unapproved new drug (prescription required for use) to a dietary supplement for sale over the counter without a prescription. Despite its quantitative significance as a hormone, researchers know little about DHEA's (a) relation to health and aging, (b) cellular or molecular mechanisms of action, (c) possible receptor sites, or (d) the potential for negative side effects from exogenous dosage, particularly among young adults with normal DHEA levels. Appropriate DHEA dosage for humans also has not been determined. Concern exists about possible harmful effects on blood lipids, glucose tolerance, and prostate gland health, particularly because medical problems associated with hormone supplementation often do not appear until years after their first use. The National Institute on Aging has mounted a media blitz to caution Americans about taking such miracle compounds which can easily be purchased through mainstream grocery chains, drug and nutrition stores, health clubs, mail-order catalogs, and the Internet.

Early support for DHEA came from studies of rodents fed daily supplements of this hormone. Treatment indicated beneficial effects in preventing cancer, atherosclerosis, viral infections, obesity, and diabetes, enhancing immune function, and even extending life span. Scientists have argued, however, that the findings of research on rats and mice (who produce little if any DHEA) do not necessarily apply to healthy humans. Cross-sectional observations relating low levels of DHEA to risk of death from heart disease provided the early indirect evidence for a beneficial effect in humans. A high DHEA level conferred protection in men, while a high DHEA level in women represented increased heart disease risk. Subsequent research showed only a moderate protective association for men and no association for women. Studies also suggest that DHEA supplements may provide a cardioprotective effect with aging (more beneficial in men than women), boost immune function in disease, and perhaps provide antioxidant protection during aging.

In recent human research, eight men and eight women (ages 50 to 65 years) received either 100 mg of DHEA or a placebo daily for 3 months; treatment then reversed for another 3 months. A slight increase of 1.2% occurred in FFM in men and women during DHEA supplementation compared with the placebo. Fat mass decreased in the men but a small increase resulted for the women. Chemical markers also indicated improved immune function. These findings suggest some possible positive effects of exogenous DHEA on muscle mass and immune function in middle-aged adults, but no data exist for young adults.

Concern centers on the effect of unregulated, long-term DHEA supplementation (particularly in daily dosages greater than 50 mg). Converting DHEA into potent androgens like testosterone in females promotes facial hair growth and alters normal menstrual function. As with exogenous anabolic steroids, DHEA lowers HDL-cholesterol levels, which increases heart disease risk. Limited but conflicting data exist concerning its effects on breast cancer risk. Clinicians have expressed fear that elevated plasma DHEA through supplementation may stimulate the growth of otherwise dormant prostate gland tumors or cause benign hypertrophy of the prostate gland itself. With an existing cancer, DHEA may accelerate its growth. *Despite its popularity among exercise enthusiasts, no data exist concerning the ergogenic effects of DHEA supplements on young adult men and women.*

Amphetamines

Amphetamines, or pep pills, consist of pharmacologic compounds that exert a powerful stimulating effect on central nervous system function. Athletes most frequently use amphetamine (Benzedrine) and dextroamphetamine sulfate (Dexedrine). These compounds, referred to as **sympathomimetic,** mimic the actions of the sympathetic hormones epinephrine and norepinephrine, which trigger increases in blood pressure, heart rate, cardiac output, breathing rate, metabolism, and blood glucose. Taking five to 20 mg of amphetamine usually produces an effect for 30 to 90 minutes after ingestion, although the drug's influence persist much longer. Aside from causing an aroused level of sympathetic function, amphetamines supposedly increase alertness, wakefulness, and augment work capacity by depressing sensations of muscle fatigue. The deaths of two famed cyclists in the 1960s during competitive road racing were attributed to amphetamine use for just such purposes. In one of these deaths in 1967, British Tour de France rider Tom Simpson, overheated and suffered a fatal heart attack during the ascent of Mont Ventoux. Soldiers in World War II commonly used amphetamines to increase alertness and reduce fatigue. Athletes frequently use amphetamines to gain an ergogenic edge; ironically, they do not.

Dangers of Amphetamines

Dangers of amphetamine use include the following:

- Continual use can lead to physiological or emotional drug dependency. This often causes cyclical dependency on "uppers" (amphetamines) or "downers" (barbiturates) — the barbiturates blunt or tranquilize the "hyper" state brought on by amphetamines.
- General side effects include headache, tremulousness, agitation, insomnia, nausea, dizziness, and confusion, all of which negatively impact sports performance.

- Prolonged use eventually requires more drug to achieve the same effect because drug tolerance increases; this may aggravate and even precipitate cardiovascular and psychological disorders. Medical risks include hypertension, stroke, sudden death, and glucose intolerance.
- Amphetamines inhibit or suppress the body's normal mechanisms for perceiving and responding to pain, fatigue, or heat stress, severely jeopardizing health and safety.
- Prolonged intake of high doses of amphetamines can produce weight loss, paranoia, psychosis, repetitive compulsive behavior, and nerve damage.

Amphetamine Use and Athletic Performance

Athletes take amphetamines to get "up" psychologically for competition. On the day or evening before a contest, competitors often feel nervous, irritable, and have difficulty relaxing. Under these circumstances, a barbiturate induces sleep. The athlete then regains the "hyper" condition by taking an "upper." This undesirable cycle of depressant-to-stimulant becomes dangerous because the stimulant acts abnormally after barbiturate intake. Knowledgeable and prudent sports professionals urge banning amphetamines from athletic competition. Most athletic governing groups have rules regarding athletes who use amphetamines. Ironically, the majority of research indicates that amphetamines do not enhance physical performance. Perhaps their greatest influence pertains to the psychologic realm, where naive athletes believe that taking any supplement contributes to superior performance. A placebo containing an inert substance often produces identical results.

Caffeine

Caffeine, a possible exception to the general rule against taking stimulants, remains a controlled/restricted drug in athletic competition. Caffeine belongs to a group of compounds called methylxanthines found naturally in coffee beans, tea leaves, chocolate, cocoa beans, and cola nuts, and added to carbonated beverages and nonprescription medicines (Table 17.3). Sixty-three plant species contain caffeine in their leaves, seeds, or fruit. In the United States, 75% (14 million kg) of caffeine intake comes from coffee and 15% from tea. Depending on preparation, one cup of brewed coffee contains between 60 to 150 mg of caffeine, instant coffee about 100 mg, brewed tea between 20 and 50 mg, and caffeinated soft drinks about 50 mg. As a frame of reference, 2.5 cups of percolated coffee contain 250 to 400 mg, or generally between three and six mg per kg of body mass. This produces urinary caffeine concentrations below the IOC acceptable limit of 12 $\mu g \cdot mL^{-1}$ and the National Collegiate Athletic Association limit of 15 $\mu g \cdot mL^{-1}$. Caffeine absorption by the small intestine occurs rapidly, reaching peak plasma concentrations between 30 and 120 minutes after inges-

TABLE 17.3
Caffeine content of some common foods, beverages, and over-the-counter and prescription medications

BEVERAGES AND FOOD		OVER-THE-COUNTER PRODUCTS	
SUBSTANCE	CAFFEINE CONTENT, mg	SUBSTANCE	CAFFEINE CONTENT, mg
Coffee[a]		**Cold Remedies**	
Coffee, Starbucks, grande, 16 oz	550	Dristan, Coryban-D, Triaminicin, Sinarest	30-31
Coffee, Starbucks, tall, 12 oz	375	Excedrin	65
Coffee, Starbucks, short, 8 oz	250	Actifed, Contac, Comtrex, Sudafed	0
Coffee, Starbucks, Americano, tall, 12 oz	70		
Coffee, Starbucks, Latte or Cappucinno, grande 16 oz	70	**Diuretics**	
Brewed, drip method	110-150	Aqua-ban	200
Brewed, percolator	64-124	Pre-Mens Forte	100
Instant	40-108		
Expresso	100	**Pain Remedies**	
Decaffeinated, brewed or instant; Sanka	2-5	Vanquish	33
		Anacin; Midol	32
Tea, 5 oz cup[a]		Aspirin, any brand; Bufferin, Tylenol, Excedrin P.M.	0
Brewed, 1 min	9-33		
Brewed, 3 min	20-46	**Stimulants**	
Brewed, 5 min	20-50	Vivarin tablet, NoDoz maximum strength caplet, Caffedrine	200
Iced tea, 12 oz; instant tea	12-36	NoDoz tablet	100
		Energets lozenges	75
Chocolate			
Baker's semi-sweet, 1 oz; Baker's chocolate chips, amt 5 1/4 cup	13	**Weight Control Aids**	
Cocoa, 5 oz cup, made from mix	6-10	Dexatrim, Dietac	200
Milk chocolate candy, 1 oz	6	Prolamine	140
Sweet/dark chocolate, 1 oz	20		
Baking chocolate, 1 oz	35	**Pain Drugs[b]**	
Chocolate bar, 3.5 oz	12-15	Cafergot	100
Jello chocolate fudge mousse	12	Migrol	50
Ovaltine	0	Fiornal	40
		Darvon compound	32
Soft Drinks			
Jolt	100		
Sugar Free Mr. Pibb	59		
Mellow Yellow, Mountain Dew	53-54		
Tab	47		
Coca Cola, Diet Coke, 7-Up Gold	46		
Shasta-Cola, Cherry Cola, Diet Cola	44		
Dr. Pepper, Mr. Pibb	40-41		
Dr. Pepper, sugar free	40		
Pepsi Cola	38		
Diet Pepsi, Pepsi Light, Diet RC, RC Cola, Diet Rite	36		

[a] Brewing tea or coffee for longer periods slightly increases the caffeine content.

[b] Prescription required.

Data from product labels and manufacturers, and National Soft Drink Association, 1997. **Caffeinism** refers to caffeine intoxication characterized by restlessness, tremulousness, nervousness, excitement, insomnia, flushed face, diuresis, gastrointestinal complaints, rambling flow of thought and speech, tachycardia or cardiac arrhythmia, periods of inexhaustibility, and/or psychomotor agitation.

tion to exert an influence on the nervous, cardiovascular, and muscular systems. Caffeine's metabolic half-life of 3 hours means that it clears from the body fairly rapidly, certainly following a night's sleep.

Ergogenic Effects

All studies do not support caffeine's ergogenic benefits. Ingesting the amount of caffeine (330 mg) commonly found in 2.5 cups of regularly percolated coffee (a caffeine dose legal under current IOC guidelines) 1 hour before exercising significantly extends endurance in moderately strenuous exercise. Subjects who drank caffeine exercised for an average of 90.2 minutes compared with 75.5 minutes during an exercise session without caffeine. Even though similar values occurred for heart rate and oxygen uptake during the two trials, the caffeine made the work seem easier.

Caffeine also provides an ergogenic benefit during maximal swimming performances completed in less than 25 minutes. In a double-blind, cross-over research study, seven male and four female experienced distance swimmers (<25 min for 1500 m) consumed caffeine (6 mg·kg body mass^{-1}) 2.5 hours before swimming 1500 m. Figure 17.3 illustrates that the split times improved significantly with caffeine for each 500-m of the swim. Total swim time averaged 1.9% faster with caffeine than without it (20 min, 58.6 s vs 21 min, 21.8 s). Lower plasma potassium concentration prior to exercise and higher blood glucose levels at the end of the trial accompanied enhanced performance with caffeine. This suggested that electrolyte balance and glucose availability may be key factors in caffeine's ergogenic effect.

Proposed Mechanism For Ergogenic Action

A precise explanation for the exercise-enhancing boost from caffeine remains elusive. *In all likelihood, the ergogenic effect of caffeine (or other related methylxanthine compounds) in high-intensity, endurance exercise results*

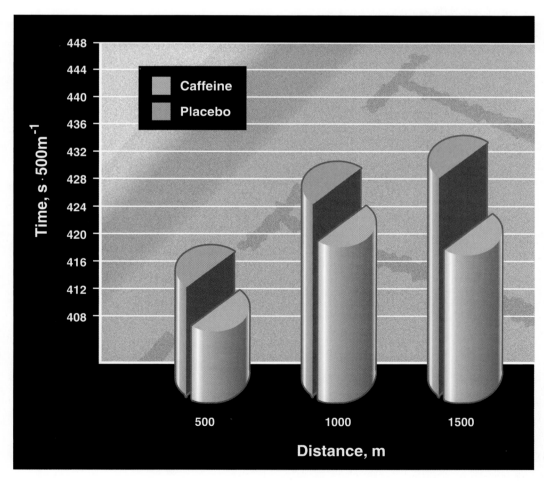

Figure 17.3
Split times for each 500-m of a 1500-m time trial for caffeine (*light purple*) and placebo (*dark purple*) trials. Caffeine produced significantly faster split times. (From MacIntosh, B.R., and Wright, B.M.: Caffeine ingestion and performance of a 1,500-metre swim. *Can. J. Appl. Physiol.*, 20:168, 1995.)

How to Recognize Warning Signs Of Alcohol Abuse and Addictive Behaviors

Alcohol consumption has been a socially acceptable behavior for centuries. Consumed at parties, religious ceremonies, dinners, sport contests, it has also been used as a mild sedative or as a pain killer for surgery. Some athletes possess a negative attitude about drinking, but they as a group are not immune from alcohol abuse.

Addiction to alcohol develops slowly. Most people believe they can control their drinking habits and do not realize they have a problem until they become alcoholic; they develop a physical and emotional dependence on the drug, characterized by excessive use and constant preoccupation with drinking. Alcohol abuse, in turn, leads to mental, emotional, physical, and social problems.

Alcohol Abuse: Are You Drinking Too Much?

The top table can help identify problem behaviors with alcohol. Two or more "Yes" answers on this questionnaire indicate a potential for jeopardizing health through excessive alcohol consumption.

Addictive Behaviors

The bottom table presents a questionnaire that can help identify possible addictive behaviors. If the answers to more than half of these questions are positive, the respondent may have a problem and should seek professional help.

IDENTIFYING ALCOHOL ABUSE[a]

Yes	No	Question
☐	☐	When you are holding an empty glass at a party do you always actively look for a refill instead of waiting to be offered one?
☐	☐	If given the chance, do you frequently pour out a more generous drink for yourself than seems to be the "going" amount for others?
☐	☐	Do you often have a drink or two when you are alone, either at home or in a bar?
☐	☐	Is your drinking ever the direct cause of a family quarrel, or do quarrels often seem to occur, if only by coincidence, after you have had a drink or two?
☐	☐	Do you feel that you must have a drink at a specific time every day (e.g., right after work, for your nerves)?
☐	☐	When worried or under unusual stress do you almost automatically take a stiff drink to "settle your nerves?"
☐	☐	Are you untruthful about how much you have had to drink when questioned on the subject?
☐	☐	Does drinking ever cause you to take time off work, or to miss scheduled meetings or appointments?
☐	☐	Do you feel physically deprived if you cannot have at least one drink every day?
☐	☐	Do you sometimes crave a drink in the morning?
☐	☐	Do you sometimes have "mornings after" when you cannot remember what happened the night before?

[a] Answer "Yes" or "No" to each question. **Evaluation:** One "Yes" answer should be viewed as a warning sign. Two "Yes" answers suggests an alcohol dependency. Three or more "Yes" answers indicates serious problems that requires immediate professional help.

ADDICTIVE BEHAVIOR QUESTIONNAIRE[a]

Yes	No	Question
☐	☐	I am a person of excesses. I can't regulate what I do for pleasure, and often use a substance or indulge in activity heavily, in order to get high.
☐	☐	I am an extremely self-involved person. People tell me that I am into myself too much.
☐	☐	I am compulsive. I must have what I want when I want it, regardless of the consequences.
☐	☐	I am excessively dependent on or independent of others.
☐	☐	I am preoccupied. I spend a lot of time thinking or fantasizing about a particular activity or substance. Also, I will work my day around doing it or go to pains to make sure it's available.
☐	☐	I deny that I do this and lie about it to others who ask me.
☐	☐	I have been involved in this behavior for at least one year.
☐	☐	I've told myself I could easily stop, even though I've shown no signs of slowing down.
☐	☐	Once I start indulging in this behavior or substance, I find I have trouble stopping.
☐	☐	One or more members of my family are also involved in some kind of excessive behavior or substance abuse.
☐	☐	I find I gravitate mostly toward people who have the same behavior or take the same substance as I do.
☐	☐	I seem to be developing a tolerance to the behavior or substance. I have had a need to steadily increase the amount I take or the time I spend doing it.

ADDICTIVE BEHAVIOR QUESTIONNAIRE (continued)

Yes	No	Question
☐	☐	I have found that my excessive use of highs has, in fact, only made my problems worse.
☐	☐	If someone tries to keep me from obtaining the substance or practicing the activity, I get angry and reject or abuse them.
☐	☐	I experience withdrawal symptoms if I cannot indulge in the substance or activity.
☐	☐	This has gotten in the way of my functioning. I have missed days at work, time with friends, family, children.
☐	☐	The substance/activity is destroying my home life. I know I am hurting those closest to me.
☐	☐	I have failed in many goals in life, lost money, given up many social and occupational contacts, all because of my excessive behavior.
☐	☐	I have tried to stop or cut down on my excesses but have been unsuccessful.
☐	☐	I have physically endangered myself or others in accidents that were a direct result of my excessive behavior.

[a] Answer "Yes" or "No" to each question. This questionnaire is aimed at helping individuals understand addictive behavior; it should not be used for diagnostic purposes. **Evaluation:** A "yes" to 10 or more of the questions suggests a problem with addictive disease and a need to seek professional help.

[From: *Family Medical Guide by the American Medical Association.* New York: Random House, 1982.]

from the facilitated use of fat as a fuel for exercise, thus sparing the body's limited carbohydrate reserves. In the quantities usually administered to humans, caffeine probably acts in one of two ways:

- Directly by stimulating adipose tissues to release fatty acids
- Indirectly by stimulating epinephrine release from the adrenal medulla; epinephrine then facilitates fatty acid release from adipocytes into plasma

Increased plasma free-fatty acid levels, in turn, increase fat oxidation, thus conserving liver and muscle glycogen. Caffeine also produces analgesic effects on the central nervous system and enhances motoneuronal excitability, facilitating motor unit recruitment.

Endurance Effects Often Inconsistent

Prior nutrition may partly account for variation in response to exercise after individuals consume caffeine. Although group improvements in endurance occur with taking caffeine, individuals who maintain a high-carbohydrate intake show a blunted effect on free fatty acid mobilization. Individual differences in caffeine sensitivity, tolerance, and hormonal response from short- and long-term patterns of caffeine consumption also affect this drug's ergogenic qualities. *Beneficial effects do not consistently occur among habitual caffeine users; thus, a caffeine-using athlete should omit caffeine-containing foods and beverages 4 to 6 days before competition to optimize caffeine's potential for ergogenic benefits.*

Effects on Muscle

Caffeine may act directly on muscle to enhance its capacity for exercise. A double-blind research design evaluated voluntary and electrically stimulated muscle actions under "caffeine free" conditions and after oral administration of 500 mg of caffeine. Electrically stimulating the motor nerve enabled researchers to remove central nervous system control and quantify caffeine's direct effects on skeletal muscle. Caffeine produced no effect on maximal muscle force during voluntary or electrically stimulated muscle actions. For submaximal effort, however, caffeine increased force output for low frequency electrical stimulation before and after muscle fatigue. This suggests that caffeine exerts a direct and specific ergogenic effect on skeletal muscle during repetitive low-frequency stimulation. Perhaps caffeine increases the sarcoplasmic reticulum's permeability to Ca^{++}, thus making this mineral readily available for contraction. Caffeine could also influence the myofibril's sensitivity to Ca^{++}.

Warning

Individuals who normally avoid caffeine may experience undesirable side effects when they consume it. Caffeine stimulates the central nervous system and can produce restlessness, headaches, insomnia and nervous irritability, muscle twitching, tremulousness, psychomotor agitation, and trigger premature left ventricular contractions. From the standpoint of temperature regulation, caffeine acts as a potent diuretic. This could cause an unnecessary pre-exercise fluid loss, negatively affecting thermal balance and exercise performance in a hot environment.

Alcohol

Alcohol, more specifically ethyl alcohol or ethanol (a form of carbohydrate), classifies as a depressant drug. Alcohol provides about seven kcal of energy per gram (mL) of pure substance (100% or 200 proof). Adolescents and adults, both athletes and non-athletes, abuse alcohol more than any other drug in the United States. Estimates indicate between 25% and 30% of males and 5% and 10% of females abuse alcohol. About 16% of alcohol abusers report a family history of alcoholism in first-, second-, or third-degree relatives.

Perhaps the depressing statistics about alcoholism reflect, in part, the tremendous amount of money spent to advertise alcoholic beverages on television and other media. For the first 8 months of 1996, The National Clearinghouse for Alcohol and Drug Information (http://www.health.org) reports that total dollars spent to advertise alcoholic beverages equaled $630 million ($520 million to advertise beer and wine; $110 million for liquor). In 1998, Americans spent over $105 billion on alcoholic beverages; beer accounted for more than 60% market share of retail sales compared with more than 28% for spirits and more than 11% for wine.

Use Among Athletes

Statistics remain equivocal about alcohol use among athletes compared with the general population. In a study of athletes in Italy, 330 male high school, non-athletes consumed more beer, wine, and hard liquor and had greater episodes of heavy drinking (including greater cigarette smoking rates) than 336 young athletes. Interestingly, the strongest predictor of a participant's alcohol consumption related to the drinking habits of his or her best friend and boyfriend or girlfriend. In other research, physically active men drank less alcohol than sedentary counterparts. Some athletes may possess a more negative attitude about drinking than the general population, but collegiate athletes drink more heavily and drive while intoxicated more often than non-athletes.

Table 17.4 compares serious male and female recreational runners and matched controls on responses to the Michigan Alcoholism Screening Test (MAST). Male runners drank more than nonexercising controls (14.2 vs. 5.4 drinks per week) and felt more guilty about their drinking (26.6%) controls (13.8%). Male and female runners drank more frequently than controls (2.8 vs. 2.3 times per week), while runners with MAST scores suggesting a history of problem drinking drank significantly less than nonathletic controls with a similar score. Men also consumed more alcohol and drank more frequently (including binge drinking) than women. Control subjects reported that drinking alcohol did not interfere with sports participation and performance, but runners reported they were unsure of alcohol's effect on training and race performance. This study illustrates that problems associated with alcohol consumption do not exclude adult runners.

Level in Beverages and the Body

One alcoholic drink contains 1.0 ounce (28.4 g or 28.4 mL) of 100 proof (50%) alcohol. This translates into 12 ounces of regular beer (about 4% alcohol by volume) or five ounces of wine (11-14% alcohol by volume). The stomach absorbs between 15 to 25% of the alcohol ingested; the small intestine rapidly takes up the remainder for distribution throughout the body's water compartments (particularly the water-rich tissues of the central nervous system). The absence of food in the digestive tract facilitates alcohol absorption. The liver, the major organ for alcohol metabolism, removes alcohol at a rate of about 10 g per hour, equivalent to the alcohol content of one drink.

Consuming two alcoholic drinks in 1 hour produces a blood alcohol concentration of between 0.04 and 0.05 $g \cdot dL^{-1}$. Age, body mass, body fat content, and gender influence blood alcohol level. The legal state limit for alcohol intoxication ranges between a blood alcohol concentration of 0.11 and 0.16 $g \cdot dL^{-1}$. Blood alcohol concentration greater than 0.40 (19 drinks or more in 2 hours) can lead to coma, respiratory depression, and eventual death.

Psychological and Physiological Effects

Some athletes use alcohol to enhance performance due to its supposed psychological and physiological effects. In the psychological realm, some have argued that alcohol before competition reduces tension and anxiety (**anxiolytic effect**), enhances self-confidence, and promotes aggressiveness. It also facilitates neurologic "disinhibition" due to its initial, though transitory, stimulatory effect. Thus, the athlete may believe that alcohol facilitates physical performance at or close to one's physiologic capacity, particularly for maximal strength and power activities. *Research does not substantiate any ergogenic effect of alcohol on muscular strength, short-term maximal anaerobic power, or longer-term aerobic exercise performance.*

Although initially acting as a stimulant, alcohol ultimately depresses neurologic function (impaired memory, visual perception, speech, motor coordination) in direct relation to blood alcohol concentration. Damping of psychomotor function causes the anti-tremor effect of alcohol ingestion. Consequently, alcohol use has been particularly prevalent in sports that require extreme steadiness and accuracy such as rifle and pistol shooting and archery. (Achieving an anti-tremor effect has also been the primary rationale for using beta-blockers such as propranolol, which blunt the arousal effect of sympathetic stimulation.) Despite this specific potential for performance enhancement, the majority of research indicates that alcohol at best provides no ergogenic benefit; at worst, it can precipitate dangerous side effects that significantly impair performance (**ergolytic effect**). For example, alcohol's depression of nervous system function profoundly impairs almost all sports performances that require balance, hand-eye coordination, reaction time, and overall need to process information rapidly. Although

TABLE 17.4

Responses from male and female recreational runners and matched controls to the shortened[1] and brief[2] versions of the Michigan Alcholism Screening Test (MAST)

	MEN (N = 536)		WOMEN (N = 262)	
MAST ITEM	RUNNERS % (N)	CONTROLS % (N)	RUNNERS % (N)	CONTROLS % (N)
1. I am not a normal drinker.[1,2]	19.1 (75)	22.8 (31)	12.1 (17)	13.9 (16)
2. My friends and relatives think I'm not a normal drinker.[1,2]	14.5 (56)	22.8 (31)	10.1 (14)	13.0 (15)
3. Attended Alcoholics Anonymous for drinking.[1,2]	4.5 (18)	8.9 (12)	2.1 (3)	4.3 (5)
4. Lost friends because of drinking.[1]	6.1 (24)	7.9 (11)	1.4 (2)	4.3 (5)
5. Trouble at work because of drinking.[1,2]	3.8 (15)	5.0 (7)	0.7 (1)	3.4 (4)
6. Feel guilty about drinking.[2]	26.6 (105)	13.8 (19)	16.7 (24)	15.5 (18)
7. Neglected obligations, family, work for 2 or more days in a row due to drinking.[1,2]	4.8 (19)	5.0 (7)	1.4 (2)	0.9 (1)
8. Experienced delirium tremens.[1]	4.3 (17)	2.9 (4)	0.7 (1)	3.4 (4)
9. Unable to stop drinking when desired.[2]	5.4 (21)	7.2 (10)	4.3 (6)	3.4 (4)
10. Sought help for drinking.[1,2]	5.3 (21)	7.2 (10)	2.1 (3)	6.0 (7)
11. Hospitalized for drinking.[1,2]	1.5 (6)	4.3 (6)	0.7 (1)	3.4 (4)
12. Drinking caused problems with spouse, parent, or other relative.[2]	20.6 (81)	21.0 (29)	2.8 (4)	8.5 (10)
13. Arrested for drunk driving.[1,2]	9.4 (37)	11.5 (16)	2.8 (4)	2.6 (3)
14. Arrested for drunken behavior.[2]	5.5 (22)	5.8 (8)	0.7 (1)	1.7 (2)

Adapted from Gutgesell, M., et al.: Reported alcohol use and behavior in long-distance runners. *Med. Sci. Sports. Exerc.*, 28:1063, 1996.

[1] Shortened MAST: From Binokur, A., and VanRooijen, I.: A self-administered short Michigan Alcoholism Screening Test (SMAST). *J. Studies Alcohol*, 36:117, 1975.

[2] Brief MAST: From Pokorny, A.D., et al.: The Brief MAST: a shortened version of the Michigan Alcoholism Screening Test. *Am. J. Psychiatry*, 129:342, 1972.

these effects may vary among individuals, they become apparent in a dose-response relationship at blood alcohol levels above 0.05 g·dL^{-1}. In the extreme, a legally intoxicated person could not perform optimally in competitive sports such as ping pong, volleyball, baseball, tennis, gymnastics, diving, figure skating, basketball, or soccer.

From a physiological perspective, alcohol impairs cardiac function. In one study, ingesting 1 g of alcohol per kg of body mass during 1 hour raised the blood alcohol level to just over 0.10 g·dL^{-1}. This level, often observed among social drinkers, acutely depressed myocardial contractility. For metabolism, alcohol blunts the liver's capacity to synthesize glucose from non-carbohydrate sources via gluconeogenesis. These effects could significantly impair performance in high-intensity aerobic activities that rely heavily on cardiovascular capacity and energy from carbohydrate catabolism. Alcohol provides no benefit as an energy substrate and does not favorably alter the metabolic mixture in endurance exercise.

Alcohol and Fluid Replacement

Alcohol exaggerates the dehydrating effect of exercise in a warm environment. It acts as a potent diuretic by (a) depressing anti-diuretic hormone release from the posterior pituitary, and (b) blunting the arginine-vasopressin response. These effects could impair thermoregulation during heat stress, placing the athlete at greater risk for heat injury. Many athletes consume alcohol-containing beverages after exercising and/or sports competition; thus, one question concerns whether alcohol impairs rehydration in recovery.

Alcohol's effect on rehydration has been studied after exercise-induced dehydration equal to approximately 2% of body mass. The subjects consumed a rehydration fluid volume equivalent to 150% of fluid lost and containing either 0, 1, 2, 3, or 4% alcohol. Urine volume produced during the 6-hour study period directly related to the beverage's alcohol concentration; greater alcohol consumed produced more urine. The increase in plasma volume in recovery compared with the dehydrated state averaged 8.1% when the rehydration fluid contained no alcohol, but only 5.3% for the beverage with 4% alcohol content. *The bottom line—alcohol-containing beverages impede rehydration.*

Because of alcohol's action as a peripheral vasodilator, it should not be consumed during extreme cold exposure or to facilitate recovery from hypothermia. A good "stiff drink" won't warm you up. Current debate exists as to whether moderate alcohol intake exacerbates body cooling during mild cold exposure.

The major conclusions of a position statement of the American College of Sports Medicine on alcohol use in sports are as germane today as when first published in 1982:

1. Acute alcohol ingestion impairs psychomotor skill, including reaction time, balance, accuracy, hand-eye coordination, and complex coordination.

2. Alcohol does not improve and may even decrease strength, power, speed, local muscular endurance, and cardiovascular endurance.

Pangamic Acid

A thletes often tout pangamic acid, commonly known as "vitamin" **B₁₅**, for its alleged ergogenic benefits in aerobic exercise. Confusion exists as to the exact chemical structure of B_{15}. The products sold as pangamic acid contain a variety of different chemicals, although the original compound consisted of a mixture of calcium gluconate and N,N-dimethylglycine in a 60:40 ratio.

The proponents of pangamic acid argue that studies conducted in Russia showed this compound increased blood cellular efficiency to use oxygen, reduced blood lactate buildup, and thus enhanced endurance. As with many proposed ergogenic aids, testimonials from athletes abound as to its effectiveness as a training aid and performance enhancer. On careful scrutiny of the early studies of pangamic acid, one cannot interpret the validity of the findings in light of the significant limitations in research design. Research in the United States has not shown any benefit of pangamic acid on $\dot{V}O_{2max}$, endurance performance, or circulating levels of blood glucose and blood lactate. *From a nutritional perspective, pangamic acid has no vitamin or provitamin properties; it apparently serves no particular purpose in the body.* Concern has been expressed that synthetic mixtures sold as B_{15} may be harmful. The Food and Drug Administration guidelines prohibit the sale of this compound as a dietary supplement or drug.

Buffering Solutions

D ramatic alterations take place in the chemical balance of intracellular and extracellular fluids during all-out exercise between 30 and 120 seconds duration. This occurs because muscle fibers rely predominantly on anaerobic energy transfer, which significantly increases lactate formation and decreases intracellular pH. An increase in acidity inhibits the energy-transfer and contractile qualities of active muscle fibers. In the blood, acidosis results from increases in the concentrations of H$^+$ and lactate.

The bicarbonate aspect of the body's buffering system defends against an increase in intracellular H$^+$ concentration (refer to Chapter 10). Maintaining high levels of extracellular bicarbonate causes rapid H$^+$ efflux from cells and reduces intracellular acidosis. This fact has fueled speculation that increasing the body's bicarbonate (alkaline) reserve might enhance subsequent anaerobic performance by delaying the decrease in intracellular pH. Research in this area, however, has produced conflicting results owing to: (a) variations in pre-exercise doses of sodium bicarbonate, and (b) type of exercise to evaluate the ergogenic effects of **pre-exercise alkalosis**.

One study, attempting to correct previous limitations, evaluated the effects of acute induced metabolic alkalosis on short-term fatiguing exercise that generated significant lactate accumulation. Six trained middle-distance runners consumed a sodium bicarbonate solution (300 mg per kg body mass) or a similar quantity of calcium carbonate placebo prior to running an 800-m race or under control conditions (no exogenous substance). Table 17.5 shows that ingesting the alkaline drink increased pH and standard bicarbonate levels before exercise. Subjects ran an average 2.9 seconds faster under alkalosis, and achieved higher post-exercise blood lactate, pH, and extracellular H^+ concentration compared with the placebo or control conditions. Similar ergogenic benefits of induced alkalosis occur in short-term anaerobic performance using exogenous **sodium citrate** as the alkalinizing agent.

The ergogenic effect of induced alkalosis, either with sodium bicarbonate or sodium citrate, taken prior to high-intensity, short-term exercise probably results from increased anaerobic energy transfer during exercise. Increases in extracellular buffering provided by exogenous buffers may facilitate coupled transport of lactate and H^+ across muscle cell membranes into extracellular fluid during anaerobic exercise. This would delay decreases in intracellular pH and its subsequent negative effects on muscle function. A 2.9-second faster 800-m race time represents a dramatic improvement; it transposes to a distance of about 19 m at race pace, bringing a last place finisher to first place in most 800-m races.

Effects Relate to Dosage and Degree of Exercise Anaerobiosis

The interaction of bicarbonate dosage and cumulative, anaerobic nature of exercise influences potential ergogenic effects of pre-exercise bicarbonate loading. *For men and women, dosages of at least 0.3 g per kg body mass (ingested 1 to 2 hours before competition) facilitate H^+ efflux from cells.* This significantly enhances a single maximal effort of 1 to 2 minutes, or longer-term arm or leg exercise that leads to exhaustion within 6 to 8 minutes. No ergogenic effect occurs for typical resistance training exercises (e.g., squat, bench press). All-out effort lasting less than 1 minute may improve only for repetitive exercise bouts. This form of intermittent anaerobic exercise produces high intracellular H^+ concentrations; consequently, buffering and power output capacity benefit from a higher pre-exercise bicarbonate level in extracellular fluids.

The IOC currently does not ban alkalinizing agents, but more research must clarify the ergogenic benefits and possible dangers of acute induced alkalosis. Individuals who bicarbonate-load often experience abdominal cramping and diarrhea about 1 hour after ingestion. These negative side effects would surely minimize any potential ergogenic benefit. Substituting 0.4 to 0.5 g per kg body mass of the buffering agent sodium citrate for sodium bicarbonate can reduce or eliminate adverse gastrointestinal effects.

TABLE 17.5
Performance time and acid-base profiles for subjects under control, placebo, and induced pre-exercise alkalosis conditions prior to and following an 800-m race

VARIABLE	CONDITION	PRE-TREATMENT	PRE-EXERCISE	POST-EXERCISE
pH	Control	7.40	7.39	7.07
	Placebo	7.39	7.40	7.09
	Alkalosis	7.40	7.49**	7.18*
Lactate ($mmol \cdot L^{-1}$)	Control	1.21	1.15	12.62
	Placebo	1.38	1.23	13.62
	Alkalosis	1.29	1.31	14.29*
Standard HCO_3^{-1} ($mEq \cdot L^{-1}$)	Control	25.8	24.5	9.90
	Placebo	25.6	26.2	11.0
	Alkalosis	25.2	33.5**	14.30*

	Control	Placebo	Alkalosis
Performance time (min:s)	2:05.8	2:05.1	2:02.9***

* Alkalosis values significantly higher than placebo and control values post exercise.

** Pre-exercise values significantly higher than pre-treatment values.

*** Alkalosis time significantly faster than control and placebo times.

(From Wilkes, D., et al.: Effects of induced metabolic alkalosis on 800-m racing time. *Med. Sci. Sports Exerc.*, 15:277, 1983.)

Phosphate Loading

The rationale concerning pre-exercise phosphate supplementation (**phosphate loading**) focuses on increasing extracellular and intracellular phosphate levels. This may in turn:

- Increase ATP phosphorylation
- Increase aerobic exercise performance and myocardial functional capacity
- Augment peripheral oxygen extraction in muscle tissue by stimulating red blood cell glycolysis and subsequent elevation of erythrocyte 2,3-diphosphoglycerate (2,3-DPG)

The compound 2,3-DPG, produced within the red blood cell during anaerobic glycolytic reactions, binds loosely with subunits of hemoglobin reducing its affinity for oxygen. This releases additional oxygen to the tissues for a given decrease in cellular oxygen pressure.

Despite the proposed theoretical rationale for ergogenic effects with phosphate loading, benefits have not been consistently observed. Some studies show improvement in $\dot{V}O_{2max}$ and arteriovenous oxygen difference following phosphate loading, whereas other studies report no effects on aerobic capacity and cardiovascular performance.

One reason for inconsistencies in research findings concerns variations in exercise mode and intensity, dosage and duration of supplementation, standardization of pre-testing diets, and subjects' fitness level. *Presently, little reliable scientific evidence exists to recommend exogenous phosphate as an ergogenic aid.* On the negative side, excess plasma phosphate stimulates secretion of parathormone, the parathyroid hormone. Excessive parathormone production accelerates the kidneys' excretion of phosphate, and facilitates reabsorption of calcium salts from bones to cause loss of bone mass. Research has not yet determined whether short-term phosphate supplementation jeopardizes normal bone dynamics.

Anti-Cortisol Producing Compounds

The anterior pituitary gland secretes adrenocorticotropic hormone (ACTH), which induces adrenal cortex release of the glucocorticoid hormone **cortisol** (hydrocortisone). Cortisol decreases amino acid transport into cells; this blunts anabolism and stimulates protein breakdown to its building-block amino acids in all cells except the liver. The liberated amino acids circulate to the liver for synthesis to glucose (gluconeogenesis) for energy. Cortisol also serves as an insulin antagonist by inhibiting cellular glucose uptake and oxidation.

Prolonged, elevated serum concentrations of cortisol (usually resulting from exogenous intake) ultimately lead to excessive protein breakdown, tissue wasting, and negative nitrogen balance. The potential catabolic effect of exogenous cortisol has convinced bodybuilders and other strength and power athletes to use supplements believed to inhibit the body's normal cortisol release. Some believe that blunting cortisol's normal increase after exercise in healthy, highly fit individuals augments muscular development with resistance training because muscle tissue synthesis progresses unimpeded in recovery. Athletes use the supplements glutamine and phosphatidylserine to produce an anti-cortisol effect.

Glutamine

Glutamine, a non-essential amino acid, exhibits many regulatory functions in the body, one of which provides an anticatabolic effect to augment protein synthesis. The rationale for glutamine's use as an ergogenic aid comes from findings that glutamine supplementation effectively counteracted protein breakdown and muscle wasting from repeated use of exogenous glucocorticoids. In one study with female rats, infusing a glutamine supplement for 7 days blunted the normal depressed protein synthesis and atrophy in skeletal muscle with chronic glucocorticoid administration. However, no research exists concerning the efficacy excess glutamine in altering the normal hormonal milieu and training responsiveness in healthy men and women. Thus, any objective decision about glutamine supplements for ergogenic purposes must await the results of further research.

Interestingly, infusing glutamine to increase its availability after exercise promotes muscle glycogen accumulation in human muscle in recovery. The practical application of these findings to promote glycogen replenishment after exercise, or to enhance glycogen accumulation in the pre-exercise period through oral glutamine supplementation, also requires further study.

Phosphatidylserine

Phosphatidylserine (PS) represents a glycerophospholipid typical of a class of natural lipids that comprise the

Skip the Carnitine

Vital to normal metabolism, carnitine facilitates influx of long-chain fatty acids into the mitochondrial matrix where they enter β-oxidation during energy metabolism. Patients with progressive muscle weakness benefit from carnitine administration, but healthy adults do not require carnitine supplements above that contained in a well-balanced diet. No research supports ergogenic benefits, positive metabolic alterations (aerobic or anaerobic), or body fat-reducing effects from carnitine supplementation.

structural components of biological membranes, particularly the internal layer of the plasma membrane surrounding all cells. Speculation exists that PS, through its potential for modulating functional events in cell membranes (e.g., number and affinity of membrane receptor sites), modifies the body's neuroendocrine response to stress.

In one study, nine healthy men received 800 mg of PS derived from bovine cerebral cortex in oral form daily for 10 days. Three, six-minute intervals of cycle ergometer exercise of increasing intensity induced physical stress. Compared with the placebo condition, the PS treatment significantly diminished ACTH and cortisol release without affecting growth hormone release. These results confirmed earlier findings by the same researchers showing that a single intravenous PS injection counteracted hypothalamic-pituitary-adrenal axis activation with exercise. Soybean lecithin provides the majority of PS used for supplementation by athletes, yet research showing physiologic effects used bovine-derived PS. Subtle differences in the chemical structure of these two forms of PS may create differences in physiologic action, including the potential ergogenic effects of this compound.

Normal Cortisol Release: A Bad Response?

Research must determine if the normal release and rise in serum cortisol with heavy training actually counteracts optimal muscle growth and development, and recovery and repair. One could argue that cortisol release in response to exercise stress represents an appropriate and beneficial response to bodily function and overall good health. Also, it remains unclear whether a supplement-induced inhibition of cortisol output with resistance training translates into greater training improvements.

Chromium

The trace mineral **chromium** serves as a cofactor for potentiating insulin function, although its precise mechanism of action remains unclear. Recall that insulin promotes carbohydrate transport into cells, augments fatty acid metabolism, and triggers cellular enzyme activity to facilitate protein synthesis. Chronic chromium deficiency may trigger a rise in blood cholesterol and decrease the body's sensitivity to insulin, thus increasing the risk of type 2 diabetes. In all likelihood, some adult Americans consume less than the 50 to 200 μg of chromium, considered the estimated safe and adequate daily dietary intake. This occurs largely because chromium-rich foods (brewer's yeast, broccoli, wheat germ, nuts, liver, prunes, egg yolks, apples with skins, asparagus, mushrooms, wine, and cheese) do not usually constitute part of the regular daily diet. Food processing also removes significant chromium from foods in natural form. In addition, strenuous exercise and associated high carbohydrate intake promote urinary chromium losses, thus increasing the potential for chromium deficiency. For athletes with chromium-deficient diets, dietary modifications to increase chromium intake or prudent use of chromium supplements seem appropriate.

Alleged Benefits

Chromium, touted as a "fat burner" and "muscle builder," represents one of the most hyped minerals in the health food/fitness literature. Supplement intake of chromium, usually as **chromium picolinate**, often reaches 600 μg daily. This picolinic acid combination supposedly improves chromium absorption compared with the inorganic salt chromium chloride. Millions of Americans believe the claims of health food faddists, television infomercials, and exercise zealots that additional chromium promotes muscle growth, curbs appetite, fosters body fat loss, and even lengthens life. Advertising targets chromium to body builders and other resistance-trained athletes as a safe alternative to anabolic steroids. Chromium supplements supposedly potentiate insulin's action, thus increasing skeletal muscle's amino acid anabolism.

Generally, studies suggesting beneficial effects of chromium supplements on body fat and muscle mass inferred body composition changes from changes in body weight (or unvalidated anthropometric measurements), instead of a more appropriate assessment by hydrostatic weighing. One study observed that supplementing daily with 200 μg (3.85 μmol) chromium picolinate for 40 days produced a small increase in FFM (estimated from skinfold thickness) and decrease in body fat in young men who resistance trained for 6 weeks. No data were presented, however, to show muscular strength increased.

Another study reported increases in body mass without change in strength or body composition in previously untrained female college students (no change in males) receiving daily chromium supplements of 200 μg during a 12-week resistance training program compared to unsupplemented controls. Other research evaluated the effects of 200 μg daily chromium supplementation on muscle strength, body composition, and chromium excretion in 16 untrained males who trained for 12 weeks with resistance exercises. Muscular strength improved significantly for supplemented (24%) and placebo (33%) groups during the training period. No changes occurred in any of the body composition variables. The group receiving the supplement did show significantly higher chromium excretion than controls after six weeks of training. The researchers concluded that chromium supplements provided *no ergogenic benefits* on any of the measured variables. Supplementing with 800 μg of chromium picolinate (plus 6 mg of boron) proved no more effective than a placebo to enhance lean tissue gain or promote fat loss during resistance training.

For sedentary obese women, supplementing with 400 μg chromium picolinate daily for nine weeks did not promote weight loss; instead, it actually caused significant

Beta-hydroxy-beta-methylbutyrate

Beta-hydroxy-beta-methylbutyrate (HMB), a bioactive metabolite generated from the breakdown of the essential branched-chain amino acid leucine, may decrease protein loss during stress by inhibiting protein catabolism. Protein breakdown markedly decreased and protein synthesis increased slightly in muscle tissue samples (in vitro) of rats and chicks exposed to HMB. Data also suggest an HMB-induced increase in cellular fatty acid oxidation in vitro in mammalian muscle cells exposed to HMB. Depending on the amount of HMB contained within foods (relatively rich sources include catfish, grapefruit, and breast milk), the body synthesizes 0.3 to 1.0 g of HMB daily, of which about 5% comes from dietary leucine catabolism. Because of its possible nitrogen-retaining effects, many resistance-trained athletes supplement directly with HMB to prevent or slow muscle damage and blunt muscle breakdown (proteolysis) associated with intense physical effort.

To determine the effect of exogenous HMB on skeletal muscle's response to resistance training, young adult men partici-

pated in two randomized trials. In Study 1, 41 subjects received either 0, 1.5, or 3.0 g of HMB (calcium salt of HMB mixed with orange juice) daily at two protein levels of either 117 g or 175 g per day for 3 weeks. The men lifted weights during this time for 1.5 hours, three days a week for 3 weeks. In Study 2, 28 subjects consumed either 0 or 3.0 g of HMB per day and weight lifted for 2 to 3 hours, 6 days weekly for 7 weeks.

The results from the first study showed that HMB supplementation significantly blunted the exercise-induced increase in muscle proteolysis (reflected by urine 3-methylhistidine and plasma creatine phosphokinase) during the first 2 weeks of exercise training. These biochemical indices of muscle damage ranged between 20 and 60% lower in the HMB-supplemented group.

In addition, the total weight lifted by this group significantly exceeded the unsupplemented group during each training week (Part A of figure), with the greatest effect in the group receiving the largest HMB supplement. Muscular strength increased 8% for the unsupplemented group, whereas the increase was larger for the HMB-supplemented groups (13% for the $1.5 \text{ g} \cdot \text{d}^{-1}$ and 18.4% for the $3.0 \text{ g} \cdot \text{d}^{-1}$ groups). The added protein (not indicated in graph) provided no augmenting effect on any of the measurements. The lack of effect with additional protein should be viewed in proper context because the group consuming the "lower" protein quantity received an amount equivalent to twice the RDA ($117 \text{ g} \cdot \text{d}^{-1}$).

The results of Study 2 showed that FFM increased with HMB supplementation to a significantly greater extent than the unsupplemented group at 2 and 4 to 6 weeks of training (Part B of figure). However, at the last measurement during training, the difference between groups in FFM decreased to the point where statistical significance between pretraining baseline values could not be demonstrated.

The exact mechanism for HMB's action on muscle metabolism, strength improvement, and body composition remains unknown. The researchers speculated that taking this metabolite during resistance training inhibits normal proteolytic processes that accompany intense muscular overload. Such results appear to demonstrate an ergogenic effect of HMB supplementation. What component of the FFM (protein, bone, water) HMB actually alters remains unknown. Furthermore, the data in Part B of the figure indicate that the potential body composition benefits of supplementation may be transient, tending to revert towards the unsupplemented state as training progresses. Additional, longer-term studies by other laboratories need to verify these findings, and assess the long-term effects of HMB supplements on body composition, training responsiveness, and overall health and safety.

Reference

Nissen, S., et al.: Effect of leucine metabolite β-hydroxy-β-methylbutyrate on muscle metabolism during resistance-exercise training. *J. Appl. Physiol.*, 81:2095, 1996.

weight gain during the treatment period. When collegiate football players received daily supplements of 200 μg of chromium picolinate for nine weeks, no changes occurred in body composition and muscular strength from intense weight-lifting training compared with a control group receiving a placebo. Among obese personnel enrolled in the U.S. Navy's mandatory remedial physical conditioning program, consuming 400 μg additional chromium picolinate daily caused no greater loss in body weight or percent body fat, or increase in FFM, compared with a group receiving a placebo.

A comprehensive double-blind research design studied the effect of a daily chromium supplement (3.3-3.5 μmol either as chromium chloride or chromium picolinate) or a placebo for 8 weeks during resistance training in 36 young men. For each group, dietary intakes of protein, magnesium, zinc, copper, and iron equaled or exceeded recommended levels during training; subjects also had adequate baseline dietary chromium intakes. Chromium supplementation increased serum chromium concentration and urinary chromium excretion equally, regardless of its ingested form. Table 17.6 shows that compared with a placebo treatment, chromium supplementation did not affect training-related changes in muscular strength, physique, FFM, or muscle mass.

Not Without a Potential Down Side

Chromium competes with iron to bind with transferrin, a plasma protein that transports iron from ingested food and damaged red blood cells to tissues in need. The chromium picolinate supplement for the group whose data appear in Table 17.6 significantly reduced serum transferrin (a measure of the adequacy of current iron intake) compared with chromium chloride or placebo treatments. However, in other research with men ages 56 to 69 years, supplementing with 924 μg of chromium daily as chromium picolinate for 12 weeks did not influence hematologic indices or indices of iron metabolism or status. Thus, more research must determine whether chromium supplementation above recommended values adversely affects iron transport and distribution within the body. No studies have evaluated the safety of long-term supplementation with chromium picolinate, nor ergogenic efficacy of supplementation in individuals with suboptimal chromium status. Concerning the bioavailability of trace minerals in the diet, excessive dietary chromium inhibits zinc and iron absorption. At the extreme, this could induce a state of iron-deficiency anemia, blunt ability to train intensely, and negatively affect exercise performance requiring a high level of aerobic metabolism.

TABLE 17.6
Effects of two different forms of chromium supplementation on average values for anthropometric, bone, and soft tissue composition measurements before and after weight training

	PLACEBO		CHROMIUM CHLORIDE		CHROMIUM PICOLINATE	
	PRE	POST	PRE	POST	PRE	POST
Age (y)	21.1	21.5	23.3	23.5	22.3	22.5
Stature (cm)	179.3	179.2	177.3	177.3	178.0	178.2
Weight (kg)	79.9	80.5[a]	79.3	81.1[a]	79.2	80.5
Σ4 skinfold thickness (mm)[b]	42.0	41.5	42.6	42.2	43.3	43.1
Upper arm (cm)	30.9	31.6[a]	31.3	32.0[a]	31.1	31.4[a]
Lower leg (cm)	38.2	37.9	37.4	37.5	37.1	37.0
Endomorphy	3.68	3.73	3.58	3.54	3.71	3.72
Mesomorphy	4.09	4.36[a]	4.25	4.42[a]	4.21	4.33[a]
Ectomorphy	2.09	1.94[a]	1.79	1.63[a]	2.00	1.88[a]
FFMFM (kg)[c]	62.9	64.3[a]	61.1	63.1[a]	61.3	62.7[a]
Bone mineral (g)	2952	2968	2860	2878	2918	2940
Fat-free body mass (kg)	65.9	67.3[a]	64.0	65.9[a]	64.2	66.1[a]
Fat (kg)	13.4	13.1	14.7	15.1	14.7	14.5
Body fat (%)	16.4	15.7	18.4	18.2	18.4	17.9

From Lukaski, H.C., et al.: Chromium supplementation and resistance training: effects on body composition, strength, and trace element status of men. *Am. J. Clin. Nutr.*, 63:954, 1996.

[a] Significantly different from pretraining value.

[b] Measured at biceps, triceps, subscapular, and suprailiac sites.

[c] Fat-free, mineral-free mass.

CoQ₁₀ Supplements Not Needed

Coenzyme Q_{10} (CoQ_{10}, ubiquinone in oxidized form and ubiquinol when reduced) functions as an integral component of the mitochondrion's electron transport system of oxidative phosphorylation. Based on the belief that supplementation could increase the rate of flux of electrons through the respiratory chain, and thus augment aerobic ATP resynthesis, popular literature touts CoQ_{10} supplements to improve stamina and enhance cardiovascular function. CoQ_{10} supplementation does increase serum CoQ_{10} levels; however, no improvements take place for aerobic capacity, cardiovascular dynamics, endurance performance, plasma glucose or lactate levels in submaximal exercise compared to a placebo.

Moreover, laboratory cultures of human tissue that received extreme doses of chromium picolinate showed eventual chromosomal damage. Critics contend that such high laboratory dosages would not occur with supplement use in humans. Nonetheless, an argument could be made that cells continually exposed to excessive chromium could accumulate this mineral and retain it for years. The possible ill effects of long-term chromium supplementation of the considerable excess ingested by some athletes requires further research.

In November 1996, the Federal Trade Commission ordered three makers of chromium supplements to cease promoting unsubstantiated weight loss and health claims (reduced body fat, increased muscle mass, increased energy level) for chromium picolinate. Under the settlement, the companies could no longer make statements of benefit unless credible research data validated such claims.

Creatine

Meat, poultry, and fish provide rich sources of **creatine**; they contain approximately 4 to 5 g of creatine per kg of food weight. The body synthesizes only about 1 g of this nitrogen-containing organic compound daily, primarily in the kidneys, liver, and pancreas from the nonessential amino acids arginine, glycine, and methionine. Thus, adequate dietary creatine becomes important. The richest creatine-containing foods occur in animal meats; this places vegetarians at a distinct disadvantage for obtaining ready sources of exogenous creatine. Approximately 95% of the body's total creatine exists in skeletal muscle.

Creatine, sold in its supplemental form (**creatine monohydrate** or C_rH_2O), comes in powder, tablet, capsule, and stabilized liquid form. Creatine can be purchased over-the-counter or via mail order as a nutritional supplement (without guarantee of purity). Ingesting a liquid suspension of creatine monohydrate at the relatively high dose of 20 to 30 g a day for up to 2 weeks increases intramuscular concentrations of free creatine and phosphocreatine up to 30%. This level remains high for weeks after only a few days of supplementation. To date, international sport's governing bodies do not consider creatine an illegal chemical substance.

Important Component of High-Energy Phosphates

Creatine passes through the digestive tract unaltered for absorption by the intestinal mucosa. Just about all ingested creatine becomes incorporated within skeletal muscle (average concentration 125 mmol [range 90 to 160 mmol] per kg dry muscle). About 40% exists as free creatine, the remainder combining readily with phosphate (in the creatine kinase reaction shown below) to form phosphocreatine (PCr). Type II, fast-twitch muscle fibers store about four to six times more PCr than ATP. As emphasized in Chapter 4, PCr serves as the cells energy reservoir to provide rapid phosphate-bond energy to resynthesize ATP (more rapid than ATP resynthesis in glycogenolysis) in the reaction:

$$PCr + ADP \xrightarrow{\text{creatine kinase}} Cr + ATP$$

PCr may also "shuttle" intramuscular high-energy phosphate between the mitochondria and cross-bridge sites that initiate muscle action. *Maintaining a high sarcoplasmic ATP/ADP ratio by energy transfer from PCr becomes important in all-out effort lasting up to ten seconds, which places significant demands on ATP resynthesis.* The energy requirements of such short-term power activities greatly exceed the energy available from the aerobic hydrolysis of intracellular macronutrients. Improved capacity from PCr energy transfer also lessens reliance on energy transfer from anaerobic glycolysis, which increases intramuscular H^+ concentration and decreases intracellular pH because of lactate accumulation.

Documented Benefits

Creatine supplementation received notoriety as an ergogenic aid from its use by British sprinters and hurdlers in the 1992 Barcelona Olympic Games. Impressive ergogenic effects of exogenous creatine at the recommended intake occur without producing harmful side effects (Table 17.7). However, anecdotal reports indicate a possible association between creatine intake and cramping in multiple muscle areas during competition or lengthy practice in football players. This effect may result from (a) altered intracellular dynamics due to increased levels of free

TABLE 17.7
Selected studies showing an increase in exercise performance following creatine monhydrate supplementation

REFERENCE	EXERCISE	PROTOCOL	EXERCISE PERFORMANCE
d	Isokinetic, unilat. knee extensions ($180° \cdot s^{-1}$)	5 bouts of 30 ext. w/ 1-min est periods	Reduction in decline of peak torque production during bouts 2, 3, and 4.
e	Running	4 - 300 m w/ 4-min rest periods 4 - 300 m w/3-min rest periods	Improved time for final 300- and 100-m runs. Improved total time for 4 - 1000-m runs. Reduction in best time for 300- and 1000-m runs.
a	Cycle ergometry (140 rev·min^{-1})	Ten 6-s bouts w/ 1 min rest periods	Better able to maintain pedal frequency during s 4–6 of each bout.
f	Cycle ergometry (140 rev·min^{-1})	Five 6-s bouts w/ 30-s recovery followed by one 10-s bout	Better able to maintain pedal frequency near end of 10-s bout.
b	Cycle ergometry (80 rev·min^{-1})	Three 30-s bouts w/ 4-min rest periods	Increase in peak power during bout 1 and increase in mean power and total work during bouts 1 and 2.
c	Bench press	1-RM bench press and total reps at 70% 1-RM	Increase in 1-RM. Increase in reps at 70% of 1-RM.
g	Bench press	5 sets bench press w/ 2-min rest periods	Increase in reps completed during all 5 sets.
g	Jump squat	5 sets jump squat w/ 2-min rest periods	Increase in peak power during all 5 sets
h	Bench press, squats, power clean	1-RM strength	Increase in 1-RM

From Volek, J.S., and Kraemer, W.J.: Creatine supplementation: Its effect on human muscular performance and body composition. *J. Strength and Cond. Res.*, 10:200, 1996.

[a] Balsom, P.D., et al.: Creatine supplementation and dynamic high-intensity intermittent exercise. *Scand. J. Med. Sci. Sports*, 3:143, 1993.

[b] Birch, R., et al.: The influence of dietary creatine supplementation on performance during repeated bouts of maximal isokinetic cycling in man. *Eur. J. Appl. Physiol.*, 69:268, 1994.

[c] Earnest, C.P., et al.: The effect of creatine monohydrate ingestion on anaerobic power indices, muscular strength and body composition. *Acta Physiol. Scand.*, 153:207, 1995.

[d] Greenhaff, P.L., et al.: Influence of oral creatine supplementation on muscle torque during repeated bouts on maximal voluntary exercise in man. *Clin. Sci.*, 84:565, 1993.

[e] Harris, R.C., et al.: The effect of oral creatine supplementation on running performance during maximal short-term exercise in man. *J. Physiol.* 467:74P, 1993.

[f] Soderlund, K., et al.: Creatine supplementation and high-intensity exercise: Influence on performance and muscle metabolism. *Clin. Sci.*, 87 (Suppl.):120, 1994.

[g] Volek, J.S., et al.: Creatine supplementation enhances muscular performance during high-intensity resistance exercise. *J. Am. Diet. Assoc.*, 97:765, 1997.

[h] Pearson, D.R., et al.: Long-term effects of creatine monohydrate on strength and power. *J. Strength and Cond. Res.*, 13:187, 1999.

creatine and PCr, or (b) an osmotically induced enlarged cell volume due to greater cellular hydration caused by the muscle fibers' increased creatine content.

Oral supplements (20 to 25 g · d^{-1}) of creatine monohydrate significantly increase intramuscular creatine and performance in high-intensity exercise, particularly repeated muscular effort. Even daily doses as low as 6 g daily for five days induce significant improvements in interval power performance. In other research, a creatine dose of 30 g daily was given to trained runners for six days to evaluate effects under two conditions: (a) four repeated 300-m runs with four-minute recovery, and (b) four 1000-m runs with three-minute recovery. Compared with the placebo treatment, creatine supplementation significantly improved both running events, with the most impressive improvements in repeated 1000-m runs. Supplementing with

Possible Benefits of Increased Intramuscular PCr Through Creatine Supplementation

- Contribute to faster ATP turnover rate to maintain power output during short-term muscular effort
- Delay PCr depletion
- Delay excessive dependence on anaerobic glycolysis with subsequent lactate formation
- Facilitate recovery from repeated bouts of an intense, brief effort by increasing rate of ATP and PCr resynthesis (thus allowing for higher-level power output, i.e., quality training)

20 g of creatine per day for 4 days also benefited anaerobic capacity on three 30-second bicycle ergometer Wingate tests with a 5-minute rest between trials. Creatine supplementation does *not* improve performance requiring a high level of aerobic energy transfer.

Taking a high dose of creatine helps to replenish muscle creatine following heavy exercise. *This metabolic reloading should facilitate recovery of a muscle's contractile capacity after exercising, enabling athletes to maintain repeated efforts of high-intensity exercise.* Whether this potential to maintain quality workouts produces an enhanced training response for strength and power athletes has recently been studied. The research evaluated the effect of creatine supplementation in conjunction with resistance training on body composition, muscle fiber hypertrophy, and exercise performance adaptations. Nineteen resistance-trained men were matched on physical characteristics and maximal strength and then randomly assigned to either a placebo (N = 9) or creatine supplemented (N = 10) group. Supplementation consisted of 25 g daily followed by maintenance with 5 g daily. Both groups engaged in heavy resistance training for the 12-week study period. There occured significantly greater increases in body mass (6.3%) and FFM (6.3%) for the creatine-supplemented group compared to controls (3.6% increase body mass and 3.1% increase FFM) at the end of training. Maximum bench press (+24%) and squat strength (+32%) increases were also significantly greater in the creatine group compared to controls (+16% bench press and +24% squat). Creatine supplementation also induced a greater hypertrophy of muscle fibers in response to resistance training as indicated by significantly greater enlargement in Type I (35% vs. 11%), IIA (36% vs. 15%), and Type IIAB (35% vs. 6%) muscle fiber cross-sectional areas. A significantly larger average volume of weight lifted in the bench press during weeks 5 to 8 for the group receiving the supplement suggests that the higher quality of the training sessions mediated the augmented adaptations in FFM, muscle morphology, and strength performance in response to resistance training plus creatine supplementation.

Only limited information exists about the effects of long-term creatine supplementation, particularly effects on cardiac muscle and kidney function (creatine degrades to creatinine before excretion in urine). For healthy subjects, no differences emerged in plasma contents and urine excretion rates for creatinine, urea, and albumin between control subjects and individuals who consumed creatine for between 10 months and 5 years. In addition, glomerular filtration rate, tubular reabsorption, and glomerular membrane permeability remained normal in creatine users. A word of caution: individuals with suspected renal malfunction should refrain from creatine supplementation because of the potential for aggravating the disorder. As a nutritional supplement, creatine requires less stringent regulations governing its manufacturing standards, purity, and reporting of adverse side effects than if it classified as a drug.

The benefical effects of creatine supplementation may be influenced by age. When older-aged men (60–80 y) supplemented with creatine in different doses (20 g for 10 days and 4 g for 20 days), no significant improvements occurred between the groups that supplemented and a control group on body composition or upper-arm strength. Reduced muscle fatigue occurred with 30 days of creatine supplementation, however. More research in this age group will help to further document the effects of this supplement's role on physical performance.

Figure 17.4 outlines possible mechanisms of how creatine supplementation and elevated intramuscular free creatine and PCr enhance exercise performance and training response.

Effects on Body Mass

Body mass increases of 0.5 to 5.2 kg often accompany the ergogenic benefits of creatine supplementation. Research needs to uncover the relative degree that compositional changes in body mass result from (a) anabolic effect of creatine on muscle tissue synthesis, (b) retention of intracellular water from increased creatine stores, or (c) other factors. Recent findings indicate that the body mass gains associated with creatine supplementation *plus* resistance training, relate to increases in muscle cross-sectional area, not just to increases in total body water.

Creatine Loading

Many creatine users pursue a loading phase by ingesting 20 to 30 g of creatine daily (usually in tablet form or powder added to liquid) for 5 to 7 days. Individuals who consume vegetarian-type diets show the greatest increase in muscle creatine levels because of the already low creatine content of their diets. Large increases also characterize individuals with normally low basal levels of intramuscular creatine. A maintenance phase follows the loading phase during which the athlete supplements with as little as 2 to 5 g of creatine daily.

Practical questions for the athlete desiring to elevate intramuscular creatine levels concern the (a) magnitude and time course of intramuscular creatine increase with supplementation, (b) dosage necessary to maintain creatine

Figure 17.4
Possible mechanisms how elevating intracellular creatine (Cr) and phosphocreatine (PCr) might enhance intense, short-term exercise performance and the exercise-training response. (Modified from Volek, J.S., and Kraemer, W.J.: Creatine supplementation: its effect on human muscular performance and body composition. *J. Strength and Cond. Res.*, 10:200, 1996.)

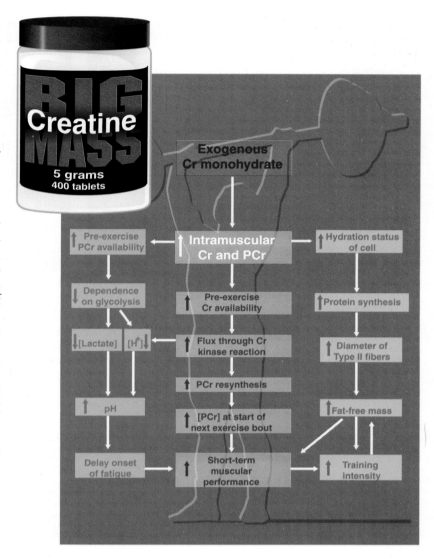

increase, and (c) rate of creatine loss or washout following cessation of supplementation. To provide insight into these questions, two groups of men were studied. In one experiment, six men ingested 20 g of creatine monohydrate (approximately 0.3 g per kg of body mass) for 6 consecutive days, at which time the supplements stopped. Muscle biopsies were taken before supplement ingestion and at days 7, 21, and 35. Similarly, nine men took 20 g of creatine monohydrate daily for 6 consecutive days. Instead of discontinuing supplementation, they reduced dosage to 2 g daily (approximately 0.03 g per kg body mass) for 28 additional days. Figure 17.5A illustrates that total muscle creatine concentration increased by approximately 20% after six days. Without continued supplementation, muscle creatine content gradually declined to baseline in 35 days. The group that continued to supplement with reduced creatine intake for an additional 28 days maintained muscle creatine content at the increased level (Fig. 17.5B).

For both groups, the increase in total muscle creatine content during the initial 6-day supplement period averaged about 23 mmol per kg of dry muscle, which represented about 20 g (17%) of the total creatine ingested. Interestingly, a similar 20% increase in total muscle creatine concentration occurred with only a 3-g daily supplement. However, this increase took place more gradually and required 28 days instead of only 6 days with the 6-g supplement.

*A rapid way to "**creatine load**" human skeletal muscle requires 20 g of creatine monohydrate daily for 6 days; by switching to a reduced dosage of 2 g per day, these levels remain elevated for up to 28 days.* If rapidity of loading does not matter, supplementing 3 g daily for 28 days achieves the same high levels.

Caffeine Blunts Creatine's Effect

Caffeine blunts the ergogenic effect of creatine supplementation. To evaluate the effect of pre-exercise caffeine on intramuscular creatine stores and high-intensity exercise performance, subjects consumed either a placebo, a daily creatine supplement (0.5 g per kg body mass), or the same daily creatine supplement plus caffeine (5 mg per kg body mass) for six days. Under each condition, subjects performed maximal intermittent knee extension exercise isokinetic dynamometer to fatigue. Creatine supplementation, with or without caffeine, significantly increased intramuscular PCr by 4 to 6%. Dynamic torque production also increased 10 to 23% with creatine compared to the placebo. Taking caffeine, however, completely negated creatine's ergogenic effect.

The researchers initially speculated that caffeine, through its action as a sympathomimetic agent, might assist skeletal muscle's uptake and trapping of exogenous creatine. However, no enhanced retention occurred. From a practical standpoint, caffeine supplements *totally counteracted* the ergogenic effect of muscle creatine loading. *Thus, athletes who creatine load should refrain from caffeine-containing foods and beverages for several days before competition.*

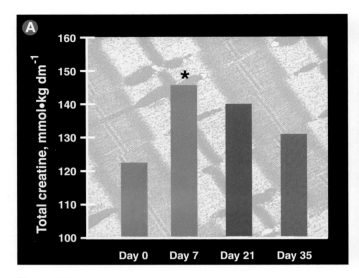
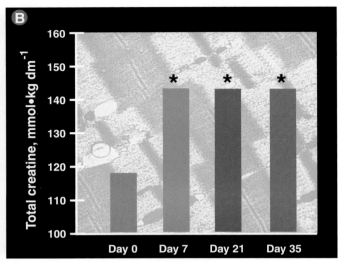

Figure 17.5

A, Muscle total creatine concentration in six men who ingested 20 g of creatine for 6 consecutive days. **B,** Muscle total creatine concentration in nine men who ingested 20 g of creatine for 6 consecutive days and thereafter ingested 2 g of creatine per day for the next 28 days. In both A and B, muscle biopsy samples taken before ingestion (day 0) and on days 7, 21, 35. Values refer to averages per kg dry muscle mass (dm). *Significantly different from day 0. (From Hultman, E., et al.: Muscle creatine loading in men. *J. Appl. Physiol.*, 81:232, 1996.)

summary

1. Ergogenic aids are substances or procedures believed to improve physical work capacity, physiologic function, or athletic performance.

2. Anabolic steroids function similarly to the hormone testosterone. Although inconsistent research findings often emerge, the precise mechanism(s) of steroid action remains unclear, yet some individuals benefit from steroids to increase muscle size, strength, and power.

3. Beta-adrenergic agonists (e.g., clenbuterol and albuterol) increase skeletal muscle mass and slow fat gain in certain experimental animals to counter the effects of aging, immobilization, malnutrition, and tissue-wasting pathology. Untrained muscle appears more responsive to these effects, perhaps from down-regulation of beta-receptors in the trained state.

4. Conflicting evidence exists as to whether exogenous growth hormone taken by normal, healthy people facilitates muscle mass increases when combined with resistance training. As with anabolic steroids, significant health risks exist for those who abuse this chemical.

5. Little credible evidence exists that amphetamines (pep pills) aid exercise performance or psychomotor skills any better than an inert placebo. Side effects of amphetamines include drug dependency, headache, dizziness, confusion, and upset stomach.

6. In some individuals, caffeine exerts an ergogenic effect to prolong high-intensity aerobic exercise by increasing fat utilization for energy, thus conserving glycogen reserves. These effects become less apparent in individuals who (a) maintain a high-carbohydrate diet, or (b) habitually use caffeine.

7. Consuming ethyl alcohol produces an acute anxiolytic effect because it temporarily reduces tension and anxiety, enhances self-confidence, and promotes aggression. It ultimately acts as a generalized neurologic depressant; this helps to explain alcohol's antitremor effect. Alcohol does not convey ergogenic benefits and impairs overall athletic performance (ergolytic effect).

8. Increasing the body's alkaline reserve before exercising by ingesting concentrated buffering solutions (sodium bicarbonate or sodium citrate) significantly improves anaerobic performance. Buffer dosage and cumulative anaerobic nature of exercise interact to influence the ergogenic effect of pre-exercise bicarbonate (or citrate) loading.

9. Presently, little scientific evidence exists to recommend exogenous phosphates or pangamic acid as ergogenic aids.

10. Glutamine and phosphatidylserine supplements allegedly shift the balance between protein degradation and synthesis to provide a natural anabolic boost when coupled with resistance training. Some competitors believe that supplements of beta-hydroxyl-beta-methyl butyrate decrease protein loss by inhibiting protein catabolism. An objective decision about the potential benefits and risks of these compounds for ergogenic purposes among healthy individuals requires further research.

11. Chromium potentiates insulin function in the body. Athletes tout chromium supplements (usually as chromium picolinate) for fat burning and muscle building properties.

12. For individuals with adequate dietary chromium intakes, well-designed research fails to show any beneficial effect of chromium supplements on training-related changes in muscular strength, physique, fat-free body mass, or muscle mass. In fact, excess chromium in picolinate form may adversely affect iron transport and distribution in the body. Prolonged excess may even damage chromosomes.

13. Due to its role in electron transport-oxidative phosphorylation, athletes supplement with coenzyme Q_{10} to improve endurance performance, Available data indicate that CoQ_{10} supplements in healthy individuals provide no ergogenic effect on aerobic capacity, endurance, submaximal exercise lactate levels, or cardiovascular dynamics.

14. In supplement form, phosphocreatine (PCr) significantly increases intramuscular levels of creatine and PCr, enhances short-term anaerobic power output capacity, and facilitates recovery from repeated bouts of intense effort. Effective creatine loading takes place by ingesting 20 g of creatine monohydrate for six consecutive days. Reducing intake to 2 g daily maintains elevated intramuscular levels of this supplement.

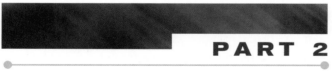

PART 2
Physiologic Agents

Red blood cell reinfusion, pre-exercise warm-up, and breathing hyperoxic gas mixtures represent three commonly used procedures to enhance the physiologic responses to exercise.

Red Blood Cell Reinfusion

Red blood cell reinfusion, often called **induced erythrocythemia, blood boosting,** or **blood doping,** came into public prominence as a possible ergogenic technique during the 1972 Munich Olympics, when a gold-medal winner endurance athlete allegedly used this technique to prepare for his endurance runs in the 5000- and 10,000-m events.

How It Works
Red blood cell reinfusion requires withdrawal of between one and four units (1 unit = 450 mL) of a person's blood. The plasma is removed and immediately reinfused, and the packed red cells frozen for storage. To prevent dramatic reductions in blood cell concentration, removal of each unit of blood occurs over 3- to 8-weeks because it takes this long to reestablish normal red blood cell levels. Reinfusion of stored red blood cells (referred to as **autologous transfusion**), occurs up to seven days before endurance competition. (Homologous transfusion infuses a type-matched donor's blood.) This increases the hematocrit and hemoglobin levels by 8 to 20%, and represents an average hemoglobin increase for men from a normal of 15 g per 100 mL of blood to 19 g per 100 mL (hematocrit increases from a normal value of 40% up to 60%). Theoretically, the added blood volume increases maximal cardiac output while the increased hematocrit augments the blood's oxygen-carrying capacity (increasing the quantity of oxygen available to working muscles). This increase benefits the endurance athlete, especially long distance runners, for whom oxygen transport often limits exercise capacity.

Infusing 900 to 1800 mL of freeze-preserved autologous blood usually provides ergogenic benefits. Each 500 mL infusion of whole blood, or its equivalent of 275 mL packed red cells, theoretically adds about 100 mL of oxygen to the blood's total oxygen-carrying capacity. This occurs because each 100 mL of whole blood normally carries about 20 mL of oxygen. An endurance athlete's total blood volume circulates five times each minute in high-intensity exercise. This makes the potential "extra" oxygen available to the tissues from each unit of reinfused blood (or its packed red cell component) equal to 0.5 liters (5×100 mL extra O_2).

Blood doping may also have effects opposite to those intended. A large infusion of packed red blood cells (and resulting inordinate large increase in cellular concentration or polycythemia) could increase blood viscosity and decrease

On July 16, 1998, the international govern-ing body of bicycle racing suspended the coach of the top-ranked Festina team of France in a drug scandal that threatened to overwhelm the 85th Tour de France, bicy-cle racing's most prestigious and financially rewarding competition. The suspension re-sulted after the team car was found to con-tain large quantities of illicit drugs including amphetamines, steroids, masking drugs (usually diuretics to prevent steroid detec-tion), and the blood-boosting erythropoietin, a genetically engineered copy of a kidney hormone linked to more than a dozen heart attacks among competitive cyclists. The following day, after the sixth stage of the Tour, all nine members of Festina were suspended after its coach admitted supply-ing illegal drugs to his riders. One week later, four Chinese swimmers were sus-pended from all meets for two years for us-ing triamterene, a banned diuretic that can mask anabolic steroids, during the world championships in January.

cardiac output, which would reduce aerobic capacity. Cer-tainly any significant increase in blood viscosity or thickness would compromise blood flow through atherosclerotic ves-sels of individuals with coronary artery disease.

Does It Work?

Research generally confirms physiologic and performance improvements with red blood cell re-infusion. The differences among the various research studies origi-nate largely from blood storage methods. Frozen red blood cells store in excess of six weeks without significant loss of cells compared to conventional storage at 4°C (used in earlier studies); substantial

Figure 17.6
Time course of hematologic changes after removal and reinfu-sion of 900 mL of freeze-preserved blood. (Data from Gledhill, N.: Blood doping and related issues: a brief review. *Med. Sci. Sports Ex-erc.*, 14: 183, 1982.)

hemolysis (destruction) occurs at 4°C after only 3 weeks. This is important because it usually takes a person about 6 weeks to replenish blood cells after withdrawal of two units of whole blood (Fig. 17.6).

Red blood cell reinfusion significantly elevates hemato-logic characteristics in men and women. This translates to a 5 to 13% increase in aerobic capacity, reduced submaxi-mal heart rate and blood lactate for a standard exercise task, and improved endurance performance at sea level and altitude. Table 17.8 illustrates hematologic, physio-logic, and performance responses for five adult men dur-ing submaximal and maximal exercise before and 24 hours after a comparatively large 750 mL infusion of packed red blood cells. These response patterns generally reflect the results of more recent research in this area.

A New Twist – Hormonal Blood Boosting

To eliminate the somewhat cumbersome and lengthy pro-cess of blood doping, endurance athletes now experiment with **erythropoietin**, a hormone normally produced by the kidneys. This hormone stimulates bone marrow to produce red blood cells. From a medical standpoint, erythropoietin combats anemia in patients with severe kidney disease. Normally, with low hematocrit or when arterial oxygen pressure decreases (as in severe lung disease or ascent to high altitude), erythropoietin release stimulates red blood cell production. Unfortunately, if administered exoge-nously in an unregulated and unmonitored fashion (simply injecting the hormone requires much less sophistication than blood doping procedures), hematocrit can exceed dangerous levels in excess of 60%. Hemoconcentration in-creases blood viscosity and greatly augments the exercise-induced increase in systolic blood pressure. This potenti-ates the likelihood for stroke, heart attack, heart failure, pulmonary embolism, and even death.

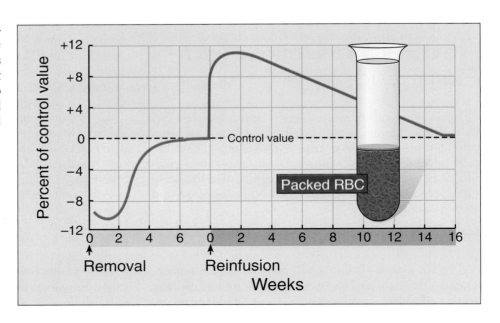

TABLE 17.8
Physiologic, performance, and hematologic characteristics prior to and 24 hours after the reinfusion of 750 mL of packed red blood cells

VARIABLE	PRE-INFUSION	POST-INFUSION	DIFFERENCE	DIFFERENCE, %
Hemoglobin, $g \cdot 100$ mL blood^{-1}	13.8	17.6	3.8*	+27.5*
Hematocrit, %	43.3	54.8	11.5*	+26.5*
Submaximal $\dot{V}O_2$, $L \cdot min^{-1}$	1.60	1.59	−0.01	−0.6
Submaximal HR, $b \cdot min^{-1}$	127.4	109.2	18.2	−14.3*
$\dot{V}O_{2max}$, $L \cdot min^{-1}$	3.28	3.70	0.42*	+12.8*
HR_{max}, $b \cdot min^{-1}$	181.6	180.0	−1.6	−0.9
Treadmill run time, s	793	918	125*	+15.8

[a] Hematocrit presented as the percent (%) of 100 mL of whole blood occupied by red blood cells.

[b] Statistically significant difference.

From Robertson, R.J., et al.: Effect of induced erythrocytemia on hypoxia tolerance during exercise. *J. Appl. Physiol.*, 53:490, 1982.

Warm-Up

Coaches, trainers, and athletes at all levels of competition believe in the benefit of some type of mild physical activity or **warm-up** before vigorous exercise. They believe that preliminary exercise enables the performer to (a) prepare either physiologically or psychologically for an event, and (b) reduce chances of joint and muscle injury. In animal studies, it required greater forces and increases in muscle length to injure a "warmed-up" muscle compared with a muscle in a "cold" condition. The explanation maintained that warming-up stretches the muscle-tendon unit to allow for greater length and less tension at any given load on the unit.

Two categories classify warm-up, although considerable overlap exists:

1. **General warm-up** involves calisthenics, stretching, and general body movements or "loosening-up" exercises usually *unrelated* to the specific neuromuscular actions of the anticipated performance.
2. **Specific warm-up** provides *a skill rehearsal* for the actual activity. Swinging a golf club, throwing a baseball or football, practicing tennis or basketball, and preliminary lead-up in the high jump or pole vault are examples of specific warm-up.

Psychologic Considerations

Competitors at all levels believe that some prior activity prepares them mentally for their event so they can concentrate on the upcoming performance. *Evidence supports the contention that a specific warm-up related to the activity itself improves the skill and coordination required by the activity.* Sports that require accuracy, timing, and precise movements benefit from specific or formal preliminary practice.

Competitors also believe that prior exercise, particularly before strenuous effort, gradually prepares them to go "all out" with less fear of injury. The ritual warm-up of baseball pitchers provides a case in point. A starting or relief pitcher would never enter a game throwing at competitive speeds without previously warming up. Would any elite athlete begin competition without first engaging in a particular form, intensity, or duration of warm-up? Because topflight athletes believe in warming up, it becomes nearly impossible to design an experiment to resolve whether or not warm-up actually improves subsequent performance and reduces injury potential.

Consider Psychological Factors

Psychologic factors (e.g., athlete's ingrained belief in the importance of warming up) establish a definite bias in comparing performance in the no warm-up and warm-up conditions. It becomes difficult to obtain maximum effort with no warm-up if a subject believes in the importance of warm-up. In this regard, some researchers have hypnotized subjects to neutralize preconceived notions about this time-honored practice.

In certain situations, peak performance occurs as soon as play begins, with no time for warming up. For example, when a reserve player goes in a game the last few minutes no time exists for preliminary stretching, vigorous calisthenics, or taking practice shots; the player must go all out with no warm-up, except that done before the game or at intermission. Do more injuries occur in such cases? Does poorer basketball defense or rebounding, or football line play take place during the first few minutes of an "unwarmed" condition than following a performance preceded by a warm-up or later in the game?

Physiologic Considerations

On purely physiologic grounds, the following mechanisms suggest how warm-up may improve performance:

- Increased speed of contraction and relaxation of warmed muscles
- Greater economy of movement because of lowered viscous resistance within warmed muscles
- Facilitated oxygen utilization by warmed muscles because hemoglobin releases oxygen more readily at higher muscle temperatures
- Facilitated nerve transmission and muscle metabolism at higher temperatures; a specific warm-up can facilitate motor unit recruitment required in subsequent all-out activity
- Increased blood flow through active tissues as local vascular beds dilate, increasing metabolism and muscle temperatures

Effects on Performance

Little concrete evidence exists that warm-up per se directly affects subsequent exercise performance. This lack of scientific justification does not necessarily mean that warm-up should be disregarded. Because of the strong psychologic component and possible physical benefits of warming up, whether passive (massage, heat applications, and diathermy), general (calisthenics, jogging), or specific (practice of the actual movements), we recommend that such procedures be continued. Until substantial evidence justifies its elimination, a brief warm-up provides a comfortable way to lead into more vigorous exercise. A gradual warm-up should increase muscle and core temperature without causing fatigue or reducing energy stores. This consideration makes the warm-up highly individualized; the duration and intensity of an adequate warm-up for an Olympic swimmer would totally exhaust a recreational swimmer. To reap the possible benefits from increased core temperature, the actual event or activity should begin within several minutes from the end of the warm-up. In warming up, the specific muscles should be engaged in a way that mimics the anticipated activity and brings about a full range of joint motion.

Warm-up and Sudden Strenuous Exercise

Several studies have evaluated the effects of preliminary exercise on cardiovascular responses to sudden, strenuous exercise. The findings provide an essentially different physiologic framework for justifying warm-up for those involved in adult fitness and cardiac rehabilitation, and occupations and sports requiring a sudden burst of high-intensity exercise.

In one study, 44 men free from overt symptoms of coronary heart disease performed high-intensity treadmill exercise for ten to 15 seconds without prior warm-up. Evaluation of the post-exercise electrocardiogram (ECG) revealed that 70% of subjects displayed abnormal ECG changes attributed to inadequate myocardial oxygen supply. These changes did not relate to age or fitness level. To evaluate the effect of warm-up, 22 of the men jogged in place at moderate intensity (heart rate about 145 b·min^{-1}) for two minutes before the treadmill run. With warm-up, ten men with previously abnormal ECG responses to the treadmill run now showed normal tracings and ten men improved their ECGs; only two subjects still showed significant ischemic changes (poor oxygen supply) after the warm-up. Warm up also improved the blood pressure response. For seven subjects with no warm-up, systolic blood pressure averaged 168 mm Hg immediately after the treadmill run. This decreased to 140 mm Hg with the two-minute warm-up.

These observations show that coronary blood flow adaptation to sudden, intense exercise does not take place instantaneously, and that transient myocardial ischemia can occur in apparently healthy and fit individuals. The positive effect of prior warm-up (at least 2 min of easy jogging) on the ECG and blood pressure response indicates a more favorable relationship between myocardial oxygen supply and demand.

Warm-up preceding strenuous exercise probably benefits all people, yet the greatest effect occurs for those with compromised myocardial oxygen supply. A brief pre-exercise warm-up provides more optimal blood pressure and hormonal adjustment at the onset of subsequent strenuous exercise. The warm-up serves two purposes: (a) reduces myocardial workload and thus myocardial oxygen requirement, and (b) enhances coronary blood flow to augment myocardial oxygen supply.

Breathing Hyperoxic Gas

Athletes often breathe oxygen-enriched or **hyperoxic gas mixtures** during times out, at half-time, or following strenuous exercise. They believe that this procedure significantly enhances the blood's oxygen-carrying capacity, thus facilitating recovery from prior exercise. In actuality, when healthy people breathe ambient air at sea level, the hemoglobin in arterial blood leaving the lungs contains 95 to 98% of its full oxygen complement. Consequently:

- Breathing higher than normal concentrations of oxygen (hyperoxic mixtures) would increase hemoglobin's oxygen transport by only about 10 mL of extra oxygen for every 1000 mL of blood.
- Oxygen dissolved in plasma when breathing a hyperoxic mixture would increase slightly from its normal quantity of 3 mL to about 7 mL per 1000 mL of blood.

This means that breathing hyperoxic gas increases the blood's oxygen-carrying capacity by 14 mL of oxygen for every 1000 mL of blood—10 mL extra attached to hemoglobin and 4 mL extra dissolved in plasma.

Pre-Exercise

The blood volume of a 70-kg person equals approximately 5000 mL. A hyperoxic breathing mixture could therefore potentially add about 70 mL of oxygen in the total blood volume (5000 mL blood × 14.0 mL extra O_2 per 1000 mL blood = 70 mL O_2). Thus, despite any potential psychological benefit to the athlete believing that pre-exercise oxygen breathing helps performance, only a slight performance advantage exists from the small amount of extra oxygen (70 mL) per se. In addition, any advantage occurs only if the subsequent exercise took place *immediately* after hyperoxic breathing. This means the athlete cannot breathe ambient air in the interval between hyperoxic breathing and exercise. Breathing ambient air (considerably lower Po_2 than the previously inspired hyperoxic mixture) actually facilitates oxygen's movement from the body back into the environment. The halfback who breathes oxygen on the sideline before returning to the game, or the swimmer who takes a few breaths of oxygen before moving to the blocks for starting instructions (while breathing ambient air), gains no competitive edge because of physiologic benefits. This becomes particularly ironic in football, because the energy to power each play generates almost totally from metabolic reactions that do not require oxygen!

During Exercise

Breathing hyperoxic gas during submaximal and maximal aerobic exercise enhances endurance performance. Oxygen breathing during submaximal aerobic exercise reduces blood lactate, heart rate, and ventilation volume, and significantly increases maximal oxygen uptake.

In one study, subjects performed a 6.5-minute endurance ride on a bicycle ergometer at an exercise level equivalent to 115% of $\dot{V}O_{2max}$ while breathing either room air or 100% oxygen. Subjects breathed both air and oxygen from identical tanks of compressed gas to mask knowledge of the breathing mixture.

Figure 17.7 A gives the details of the endurance ride showing superiority in endurance (with less drop-off in pedal revolutions) during the hyperoxic trials. Figure 17.7 B shows the oxygen uptake curves during the endurance ride while subjects breathed oxygen and room air. The results indicated a higher oxygen uptake breathing 100% oxygen with a correspondingly faster increase in oxygen uptake early in exercise. The small increase in hemoglobin saturation with hyperoxic breathing, and the additional oxygen dissolved in plasma, significantly increase total oxygen availability during maximal exercise where total blood volume circulates up to seven times each minute in an elite endurance athlete. Quantitatively, the 70 mL of extra oxygen in the total blood volume with hyperoxic breathing (circulated 7 times each min) represents an additional 490 mL oxygen available during intense aerobic exercise. The increased partial pressure of oxygen in solution while breathing hyperoxic gas facilitates its diffusion across the tissue-capillary membrane to the mitochondria. This accounts for a more rapid rate of oxygen utilization early in exercise. Although of physiologic benefit during exercise, the practical sports application of breathing hyperoxic mixtures seems limited. The added weight of an appropriate breathing system would negate any ergogenic benefit. Plus, the legality of the system's use during competition seems unlikely.

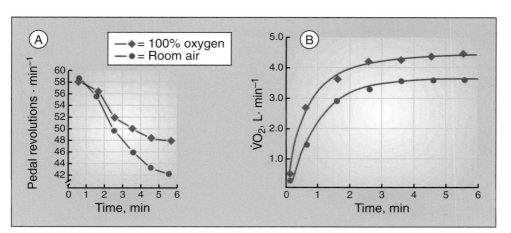

Figure 17.7
A, Superiority of endurance (measured by pedal revolutions each minute) breathing pure oxygen versus breathing ambient air. **B,** Oxygen uptake curves during the endurance rides show enhanced oxygen uptake while breathing pure oxygen. (Data from Weltman, A., et al.: Effects of increasing oxygen availability on bicycle ergometer endurance performance. *Ergonomics*, 21: 427, 1978.)

In Recovery

Figure 17.8 illustrates the effects of breathing hyperoxic gas during recovery from strenuous exercise on subsequent exercise performance. After 1 minute of all-out bicycle ergometer exercise, subjects recovered passively (quiet sitting) or actively (light pedaling) while breathing room air or 100% oxygen for either 10 or 20 minutes. They then repeated the all-out bicycle ride. No significant differences emerged in the six-second revolutions and cumulative revolutions (top graph) for the 1-minute ride after breathing either room air or pure oxygen during recovery. Also, no difference resulted between the trials breathing room air or oxygen when comparing blood lactates during the 10- and 20-minute recovery periods. This indicated that oxygen inhalation did not preferentially alter lactate removal. These findings do not support the use of hyperoxic breathing mixtures to facilitate recovery, or as an adjuvant to improved performance following different durations of recovery from prior exercise.

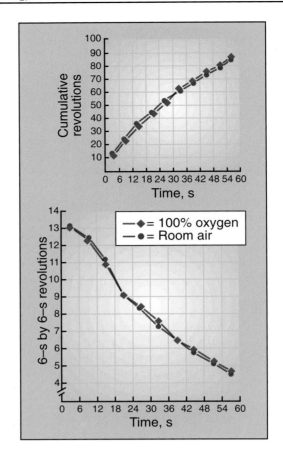

Figure 17.8
Cumulative (**top**) and absolute (**bottom**) pedal revolutions on a bicycle ergometer during one-minute of maximal exercise subsequent to breathing either oxygen or ambient air during recovery from a previous maximal exercise bout. (Data from Weltman, A., et al.: Exercise recovery, lactate removal, and subsequent high intensity exercise performance. *Res. Q.*, 48:786, 1977.)

summary

1. Red blood cell reinfusion (blood doping) involves drawing, storing, and reinfusing concentrated red blood cells several weeks later. Physiologic rationale maintains that added blood volume and red blood cell concentration create a larger maximum cardiac output and an increase in the blood's oxygen-carrying capacity, both of which increase VO_{2max}.

2. Studies applying appropriate methods of blood storage and research design support the ergogenic benefits of red blood cell reinfusion for aerobic exercise and thermoregulation.

3. Diverse physiologic reasons justify warm-up for ergogenic purposes and injury prevention. These include potential benefits for muscular speed and efficiency, tissue compliance, enhanced oxygen delivery and utilization, and facilitated nerve impulse transmission. Only limited research supports the performance benefits of warm-up, other than its positive effect on psychological factors in some individuals. Likewise, little evidence justifies its elimination if the performer feels that warm-up provides benefits.

4. A moderate cardiovascular warm-up before sudden strenuous exercise reduces cardiac work load and may enhance coronary blood flow. This form of warming-up could prevent transient myocardial ischemia at the onset of intense physical activity.

5. Breathing 100% oxygen during exercise extends endurance by increasing oxygen uptake, reducing blood lactate, and lowering pulmonary ventilation. Breathing hyperoxic mixtures before or after exercise provides no ergogenic benefit.

thought questions

1. A student claims that a chemical compound added to the diet profoundly improved weight-lifting performance. Your review of the research literature indicates no ergogenic benefits for this compound. How would you reconcile the discrepancy?

2. Outline the points you would make in a talk to a high school football team concerning whether they should consider using performance-enhancing chemicals and hormones.

3. If hormones like testosterone, growth hormone, and DHEA occur naturally in the body, how could supplementing with these "natural" compounds cause harm?

4. Discuss the importance of the psychologic or placebo effect in evaluating the effectiveness of a particular nutrient, chemical, or procedure as an ergogenic aid.

selected references

American Academy of Pediatrics. Adolescents and anabolic steroids: a subject review. *Pediatrics*, 99:904, 1997.

American College of Sports Medicine. The use of alcohol in sports. *Med. Sci. Sports Exerc.*, 14: 481, 1982.

American College of Sports Medicine. The use of anabolic-androgenic steroids in sports. *Sports Med. Bull.*, 19:13, 1984.

Anderson, R.A.: Effects of chromium on body composition and weight loss. *Nutr Rev.*, 56:266, 1998.

Angell, M., and Kassirer, J.P.: Alternative medicine—the risks of untested and unregulated remedies. *N. Engl. J. Med.*, 339:831, 1998.

Anshel, M.H., and Russel, K.G.: Examining athletes' attitudes toward using anabolic steroids and their knowledge of the possible effects. *J. Drug Education*, 27:121, 1997.

Barnard, R. J., et al.: Ischemic response to sudden strenuous exercise in healthy men. *Circulation*, 48:936, 1973.

Bhasin, S., et al.: The effects of supraphysiological doses of testosterone on muscle size and strength in normal men. *N. Engl. J. Med.*, 335: 1, 1996.

Birkeland, F.I., et al.: The future of doping control in athletes. Issues related to blood sampling. *Sports Med.*, 28:25, 1999.

Bogandis, G.C., et al.: Contribution of phosphocreatine and aerobic metabolism to energy supply during repeated sprint exercise. *J. Appl. Physiol.*, 80:876, 1996.

Bowers, L.D.: Analytical advances in detection of performance-enhancing compounds. *Clin. Chem.*, 43:1299, 1997.

Bredle, D.L., et al. Phosphate supplementation, cardiovascular function, and exercise performance in humans. *J. Appl. Physiol.*, 65:1821, 1988.

Brien, A. J., and Simon, T. L.: The effects of red blood cell infusion on 10-km race time. *JAMA*, 257:2761, 1987.

Campbell, W.W., et al.: Chromium picolinate supplementation and resistive training by older men: effects on iron-status and hematologic indexes. *Am. J. Clin. Nutr.*, 66: 220, 1997.

Castell, L.M. et al.: Does glutamine have a role in reducing infections in athletes? *Eur J Appl Physiol.*, 73:488, 1996.

Catlin,, D.H., and Murray, T.H.: Performance-enhancing drugs, fair competition, and Olympic sport. *JAMA*, 276, 231, 1996.

Chandler, J. V., and Blair, S. N.: The effect of amphetamines on selected physiological components related to athletic success. *Med. Sci. Sports*, 12:65, 1980.

Cheng, W., et al.: Beta-hydroxy-beta-methyl butyrate increases fatty acid oxidation by muscle cells. *FASEB J.*, 11(3):A381, 1997.

Clarkson P.M., et al.: Nutritional supplements to increase muscle mass. *Crit. Rev. Food. Sci. Nutr.*, 39:317, 1999.

Cohen, B.S., et al.: Effects of caffeine ingestion on endurance racing in heat and humidity. *Eur. J. Appl. Physiol.*, 73:358, 1996.

Colombani, P., et al.: Effects of L-carnitine supplementation on physical performance and energy metabolism of endurance-trained athletes—a double-blind crossover field study. *Eur. J. Appl. Physiol.*, 783:434, 1996.

Corrigan, A.B.: Dehydroepiandrosterone and sport. *Med. J Aust.*, 16;171:206, 1999.

Curry, L.A., et al.: Qualitative description of the prevalence and use of anabolic androgenic steroids by United States powerlifters. *Percept. Mot. Skills*, 88: 224, 1999.

Dawson, R.T.: Drug testing. *Br. J. Sports Med.*, 33: 219, 1999.

De Cree, C.: Androstenedione and dehydroepiandrosterone for athletes. *Lancet.*, 354: 779, 1999.

Delbeke, F.T., et al.: The abuse of doping agents in competing body builders in Flanders (1988—1993). *Int. J. Sports Med.*, 16: 60, 1995.

Dodd, S.L., et al.: Effects of clenbuterol on contractile and biochemical properties of skeletal muscle. *Med. Sci. Sports Exerc.*, 28:669, 1996.

Durant, R.H., et al: Use of multiple drugs among adolescents who use anabolic steroids. *N. Engl, J. Med.*, 328: 922, 1993.

Eiken, O., et al.: Human skeletal muscle function and metabolism during intense exercise at high O_2 and N_2 pressures. *J. Appl. Physiol.*, 63: 571, 1987.

Evans, N.A.: Gym and tonic: a profile of 100 male steroid users. *Br. J. Sports Med.*, 31:54, 1997.

Forman, E.S., et al.: High-risk behaviors in teenage male athletes. *Clin. J. Sports Med.*, 5:36, 1995.

Franke, W.W., and Berendonk, B.: Hormonal doping and androgenization of athletes: a secret program of the German Democratic Republic government. *Clin. Chem.*, 43 : 1262, 1997.

Galloway, S.D.R., et al.: The effects of acute phosphate supplementation in subjects of different aerobic fitness levels. *Eur. J. Appl. Physiol.*, 72: 224, 1996.

Girandola, R. N., et al.: Effects of pangamic acid (B_{15}) ingestion on metabolic response to exercise. *Biochem. Med.*, 24:218, 1980.

Goldberg, L., et al.: Effects of a multidimensional anabolic steroid prevention intervention: The Adolescents Training and Learning to Avoid Steroids (ATLAS) program. *JAMA*, 276:1555, 1996.

Graham, T.E., et al.: Metabolic and exercise endurance effects of coffee and caffeine ingestion. *J. Appl. Physiol.*, 85:883, 1998.

Grandjean, A.: Nutritional requirements to increase lean mass. *Clin. Sports Med.*, 18: 623, 1999.

Granier, P.L., et al.: Effect of $NaHCO_3$ on lactate kinetics in forearm muscles during leg exercise in man. *Med. Sci. Sports Exerc.*, 28:692, 1996.

Grant, K.E., et al.: Chromium and exercise training: effect on obese women. *Med. Sci. Sports Exerc.*, 29:992, 1997.

Greenhauf, P.L.: Creatine and its application as an ergogenic aid. *Int. J. Sports Nutr.*, 5:S100, 1995.

Gutgesell, M., et al.: Reported alcohol use and behavior in long-distance runners. *Med. Sci. Sports Exerc.*, 28:1063, 1996.

Hallmark, M.A., et al.: Effects of chromium and resistive training on muscle strength and body composition. *Med. Sci. Sports Exerc.*, 28:139, 1996.

Heinonen, O.J.: Carnitine and physical exercise. *Sports Med.*, 22:109, 1996.

Hornsby, P.J.: Biosynthesis of DHEAS by the human adrenal cortex and its age-related decline, *Ann. N.Y. Acad. Sci.*, 774:29, 1995.

Houston, M.E.: Gaining weight: the scientific basis of increasing skeletal muscle mass. *Can. J. Appl. Physiol.*, 24: 305, 1999.

Hultman, E., et al.: Muscle creatine loading in men. *J. Appl. Physiol.*, 81:232, 1996.

Johnson, C.E., et al.: Alcohol lowers the vasoconstriction threshold in humans without affecting core cooling rate during mild cold exposure. *Eur. J. Appl. Physiol.*, 74:293, 1996.

Juhn, M.S.: Oral creatine supplementation. Separating fact from hype. *Phys. Sportsmed.*, 27:47, 1999.

King, D.S., et al.: Effect of oral androstenedione on serum testosterone and adaptations to resistance training in young men, *JAMA*, 281:2020, 1999.

Kreider, R.B.: Dietary supplements and the promotion of muscle growth with resistance exercise. *Sports Med.*, 27: 97, 1999.

Kreider, R.B., et al.: Effects of creatine supplementation on body composition, strength, and sprint performance. *Med. Sci. Sports Exerc.*, 30: 73, 1998.

Lukaski, H.C., et al.: Chromium supplementation and resistance training effects on whole body and regional composition, strength, and trace element status of men. *Am. J. Clin. Nutr.*, 63: 954, 1996.

Magnani, M., et al.: Monitoring erythropoietin abuse in athletes. *Br. J. Haematol.*, 106: 260, 1999.

McNaughton, L.R., et al.: Effect of sodium bicarbonate ingestion on high intensity exercise in moderately trained women. *J. Strength and Cond. Res.*, 11:98, 1997.

Metzl, J.D.: Strength training and nutritional supplement use in adolescents. *Curr. Opin. Pediatr.*, 11:292, 1999.

Moskowitz, H., et al.: Skills performance at low blood alcohol levels. *J. Studies Alcohol*, 46:482, 1995.

Murphy, R.J.L., et al.: Clenbuterol has a greater influence on untrained than previously trained skeletal muscle in rats. *Eur. J. Appl. Physiol.*, 73: 304, 1996.

Papadakis, M.A., et al.: Growth hormone replacement in healthy older men improves body composition but not functional ability. *Ann. Intern. Med.*, 124:708, 1996.

Philen, R.M., et al.: Survey of advertising for nutritional supplements in health and bodybuilding magazines. *JAMA*, 268:1008, 1992.

Poortmans, J.R., and Francaux, M.: Long-term oral creatine supplementation does not impair renal function in healthy athletes. *Med. Sci. Sports Exerc.*, 31:1108, 1999.

Potteiger, J.A., et al.: The effects of buffer ingestion on metabolic factors related to distance running. *Eur. J. Appl. Physiol.*, 72:365, 1996.

Portington, K.J., et al.: Effect of induced alkalosis on exhaustive leg press performance. *Med. Sci. Sports Exerc.*, 30:523, 1998.

Prather, I.D., et al.: Clenbuterol: a substitute for anabolic steroids? *Med. Sci. Sports Exerc.*, 27 : 1118, 1995.

President's Council on Physical Fitness and Sports: Nutritional ergogenics and sports performance. *Research Digest*, 3 (No. 2):June, 1998.

Rawson, E.S. et al.: Effects of 30 days of creatine ingestion in older men. *Eur. J. Appl. Physiol.*, 80: 139, 1999.

Rhode, T., et al.: Effect of glutamine supplementation on changes in the immune system induced by repeated exercise. *Med. Sci. Sports Exerc.*, 30:856, 1998.

Rogol, A. D.: Growth hormone: physiology, therapeutic use, and potential for abuse. In: *Exercise and Sport Sciences Reviews*. Vol 17. Pandolf K. B.: (ed.). Baltimore, MD: Williams & Wilkins, 1989.

Sachtleben, T.R., et al.: Serum lipoprotein patterns in long-term anabolic steroid users. *Res. Q. Exerc. Sport*, 68:110, 1997.

Safran, M. R., et al.: The role of warm up in muscular injury prevention. *Am. J. Sports Med.*, 16: 123, 1988.

Shirreffs, S.M., and Maughan, R.J.: The effect of alcohol consumption on the restoration of blood and plasma volume following exercise-induced dehydration in man. *J. Physiol.*, 491:64P, 1996.

Street, C., et al.: Androgen use by athletes: A reevaluation of the health risks. *Can. J. Appl. Physiol.*, 21:421, 1996.

Tricker, R., and Connolly, D.: Drugs and the college athlete: an analysis of the attitudes of student athletes at risk. *J. Drug Education*, 27:105, 1997.

Vandenberghe, K., et al.: Caffeine counteracts the ergogenic action of creatine loading. *J. Appl. Physiol.*, 80:452, 1996.

Volek, J.S., et al.: Testosterone and cortisol in relationship to dietary nutrients and resistance exercise. *J. Appl. Physiol.*, 82:49, 1997.

Volek, J.S., et al.: Performance and muscle fiber adaptations to creatine supplementation and heavy resistance training. *Med. Sci. Sports Exerc.*, 31:1147, 1999.

Welsh, H. G.: Hyperoxia and human performance: a brief review. *Med. Sci. Sports Exerc.* 14:253, 1982.

Wemple, R.D., et al.: Caffeine vs caffeine-free sports drinks: effects on urine production at rest and during prolonged exercise. *Int. J. Sports Med.*, 18:40, 1997.

Williams, M.H.: *The Ergogenics Edge: Pushing the Limits of Sports Performance*. Champaign, IL: Human Kinetics, 1998.

Yarasheski, K.E.: Growth hormone effects on metabolism, body composition, muscle mass, and strength. *Exerc. Sport Sci. Rev.*, 22: 285, 1994.

SECTION
6

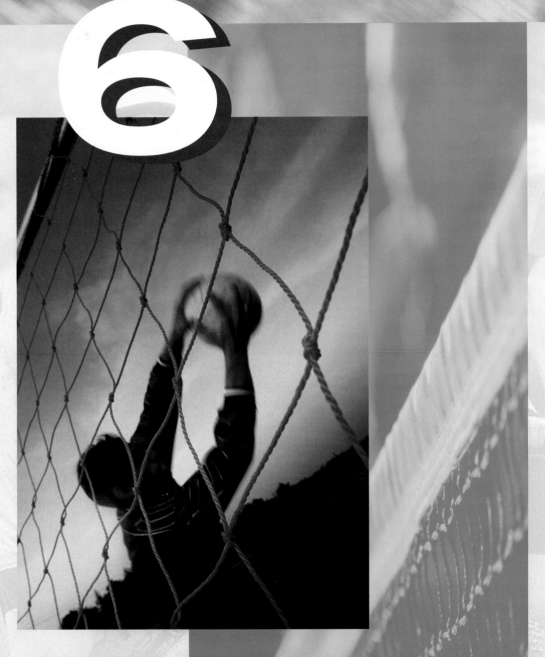

Optimizing Body Composition, Aging, and Health-Related Exercise Benefits

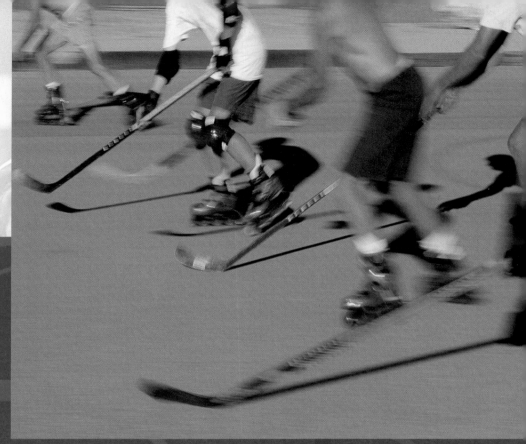

Accurate body composition appraisal provides an important component in a comprehensive program of total physical fitness and its assessment. Athletes clearly illustrate this point since many exceed the average weight for their height and gender but otherwise have less body fat compared with non-athletic counterparts. These individuals do not require a weight-loss program. In contrast, a prudent weight loss regimen would benefit the 97 million Americans currently classified as overweight, and the one in four of these men and women classified as obese. Effective weight control programs (that include regular physical activity) would also benefit the millions of children and adults who suffer the insidious consequences of physical inactivity.

Elderly persons make up the fastest growing segment of the American population. Thirty years ago, age 65 represented the onset of old age. Now gerontologists mark 85 as a demarcation of "oldest-old" and age 75 as the "young old." Demographers estimate that nearly one-half of the children born in 1996 will survive to age 95 or 100 years. Within this framework, the "new gerontology" addresses areas beyond age-related diseases, and recognizes that *successful aging* requires enhanced physiologic func-

tion and improved physical fitness. To a large extent, physiologic deterioration previously considered "normal aging" is now viewed as largely dependent on lifestyle and environmental influences and subject to significant modification through proper diet and exercise.

With regard to the effects of aging, the physiologic and exercise capacities of older people generally rate below those of younger counterparts. One can question whether such differences reflect true biologic aging, or simply the effect of disuse (brought on by alterations in lifestyle as people age). A meaningful upswing has occurred in participation of "senior citizens" in a range of physical activities. Research clearly demonstrates that an active lifestyle retains a relatively high level of functional capacity. This enables older men and women to safely engage in more vigorous sports and physical activities. In addition, maintaining an active lifestyle throughout life offers significant protection against many diseases, particularly those related to skeletal and cardiovascular health.

Carefully prescribed physical activity contributes significantly to overall good health and quality of life, not only for healthy individuals but also for those who fall within the broad spectrum of

disease to handicap. Clinical exercise physiologists have become part of a team approach to health care; they make significant contributions to total patient care. In the clinical setting, the exercise physiologist primarily focuses on restoring the patient's mobility and functional capacity while working closely with the physical therapist, occupational therapist, and physician. To this end, exercise physiologists assume an increasingly more important clinical role in sports medicine to evaluate and recondition individuals with diseases and physical disabilities.

In this section, Chapter 18 focuses on body composition—its components and assessment, and differences that exist between men and women and trained and untrained, Chapter 19 deals with topics relevant to obesity, and the role of diet and exercise for weight loss and weight maintenance. In Chapters 20 and 21, we explore aspects of the aging process. We emphasize regular physical activity as a health-related behavior with important implications for disease prevention and rehabilitation.

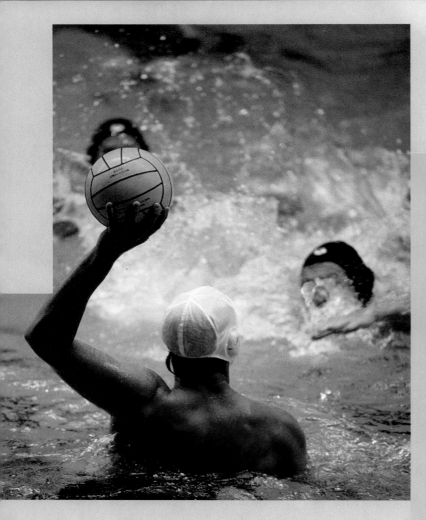

Topics covered in this chapter

Gross Composition of the Human Body

Leaness, Exercise, and Menstrual Irregularities

Methods to Assess Body Size and Composition

Body Mass Index

Average Values For Body Composition

Body Composition of Champion Athletes

Summary

Thought Questions

Selected References

Body Composition: Components, Assessment, and Human Variability

- Summarize early research about the inadequacies of "height–weight" tables.
- Outline characteristics of the "reference man" and "reference woman," including specific values for storage fat, essential fat, and sex-specific essential fat.
- Define (a) lean body mass, (b) fat-free body mass, and (c) minimal weight.
- Identify factors that trigger menstrual irregularities among some female athletes.
- Describe Archimedes' principle applied to human body volume measurement.
- List three assumptions for computing percent body fat from body density.
- Outline specific procedures for hydrostatic weighing, and explain the importance of computing residual lung volume.
- Describe the anatomic location for six frequently measured skinfold and girth sites.
- Describe how skinfold and girth measurements provide information about body fat and its distribution.
- Explain how population-specific skinfold and girth equations predict body fat.
- Give the strengths and weaknesses of the body mass index for assessing excess weight and excess fat, and overall disease risk
- Compare the body composition values of average young men and women with elite competitors in endurance running, wrestling, weight lifting, and body building.
- Outline steps for predicting minimal wrestling weight from skinfolds.

Height–weight tables assess the extent of "overweightness." The tables use the average ranges of body mass related to stature, in which men and women ages 25 to 59 years have the lowest mortality rate. Height–weight tables do not consider composition of the body or specific causes of death or quality of health before death. Different versions of the tables recommend different "desirable" weight ranges, with some considering frame-size, age, and gender. Table 18.1A and B present examples of two height–weight standards; the top table suggests body weights for adults adjusted for age. Table 18.1B, proposed by the Metropolitan Life Insurance Company, presents gender-specific weight standards for body frame size, while Table 18.1C shows how to estimate gender-specific frame size using elbow breadth and height.

In the early 1940s, Dr. Albert Behnke, a U.S. Navy physician and foremost authority on body composition, made detailed size, shape, and structural measurements of 25 professional football players. According to military standards of that time, a person whose body mass exceeded the average "weight-for-height" by 15% or more, was rejected for military service as "overweight." Applying these standards to the football players—whose body mass ranged from 72.3 to 118.2 kg (159 to 261 lb)—caused the military to reject 17 of them as too fat and unfit for service. However, when Behnke carefully evaluated each player's body composition, 11 of the 17 players classified as "overweight" actually had relatively low percentages of body fat compared to normal, non-athletic counterparts. Behnke concluded that their "excess weight" primarily came from excessive muscular development, not excess body fat. These data clearly highlighted limitations of height-weight tables concerning body composition. Most football players exceed an "average," "ideal," or "desirable" body weight based on height-weight tables; in many instances; however, an "overweight" athlete does not possess excessive body fat or need to reduce body weight.

This chapter analyzes the gross composition of the human body, and presents the rationale of direct and indirect methods to partition the body into two basic compartments, body fat and fat-free body mass. It also presents simple, noninvasive methods to analyze an individual's body composition.

Gross Composition of the Human Body

A full understanding of human body composition requires consideration of complex interrelationships among its chemical, structural, and anatomical components. Figure 18.1 displays a five-level, multicomponent model for quantifying body composition. Each level of the model becomes progressively more complex as biological organization increases (atoms → molecules → cells → tissue systems → whole body.) The model's essential feature views each level as distinct, with measurable characteris-

TABLE 18.1
Suggested body weights for adults

A. NATIONAL INSTITUTES OF HEALTH RECOMMENDATIONS

	WEIGHT IN POUNDS[2]	
HEIGHT[1]	19 TO 34 y	35 y+
5'0"	97–128	108–138
5'1"	101–132	111–143
5'2"	104–137	115–148
5'3"	107–141	119–152
5'4"	111–146	122–157
5'5"	114–150	126–162
5'6"	118–155	130–167
5'7"	121–160	134–172
5'8"	125–164	138–178
5'9"	129–169	142–183
5'10"	132–174	146–188
5'11"	136–179	151–194
6'0"	140–184	155–199
6'1"	144–189	159–205
6'2"	148–195	164–210
6'3"	152–200	168–216
6'4"	156–205	173–222
6'5"	160–211	177–228
6'6"	164–216	182–234

[1]Without shoes

[2]Without clothes

(From *Understanding Adult Obesity*, National Institute of Diabetes and Digestive and Kidney Diseases. National Institutes of Health, U.S. Department of Health and Human Services.)

C. HOW TO DETERMINE FRAME SIZE.

The person's right arm extends forward perpendicular to the body, with the arm bent so the angle at the elbow forms 90° with the fingers pointing up and the palm turned away from the body. The greatest breadth across the elbow joint is measured with a sliding caliper along the axis of the upper arm, on the two prominent bones on either side of the elbow. This breadth represents elbow breadth. The following give the elbow breadth measurements for medium-framed men and women of various heights. Measurements lower than those listed indicate a small frame size; higher measurements indicate a large frame size.

MEN		WOMEN	
HEIGHT 1" HEELS	ELBOW BREADTH	HEIGHT 2" HEELS	ELBOW BREADTH
5'2"-5'3"	2 1/2'–2 7/8"	4'10"–4'11"	2 1/4'–2 1/2"
5'4"–5'7"	2 5/8'–2 7/8"	5'0"–5'3"	2 1/4'–2 1/2"
5'8"–5'11"	2 3/4'–3"	5'4"–5'7"	2 3/8'–2 5/8"
6'0"–6'3"	2 3/4'–3 1/8"	5'8'–5'11"	2 3/8'–2 5/8"
> 6'4"	2 7/8'–3 1/4"	≥ 6'0"	2 1/2'–2 3/4"

From Metropolitan Life Insurance Company, 1983.

B. 1983 METROPOLITAN LIFE INSURANCE HEIGHT-WEIGHT TABLE*

	MEN				WOMEN		
HEIGHT FT. IN.	SMALL FRAME	MEDIUM FRAME	LARGE FRAME	HEIGHT FT. IN.	SMALL FRAME	MEDIUM FRAME	LARGE FRAME
5' 2"	128–134	131–141	138–150	4' 10"	102–111	109–121	118–131
5' 3"	130–136	133–143	140–153	4' 11"	103–113	111–123	120–134
5' 4"	132–138	135–145	142–156	5' 0"	104–115	113–126	122–137
5' 5"	134–140	137–148	144–160	5' 1"	106–118	115–129	125–140
5' 6"	136–142	139–151	146–164	5' 2"	108–121	118–132	128–143
5' 7"	138–145	142–154	149–168	5' 3"	111–124	121–135	131–147
5' 8"	140–148	145–157	152–172	5' 4"	114–127	124–138	134–151
5' 9"	142–151	148–160	155–176	5' 5"	117–130	127–141	137–155
5' 10"	144–154	151–163	158–180	5' 6"	120–133	130–144	140–159
5' 11"	146–157	154–166	161–184	5' 7"	123–136	133–147	143–163
6' 0"	149–160	157–170	164–188	5' 8"	126–139	136–150	146–167
6' 1"	152–164	160–174	168–192	5' 9"	129–142	139–153	149–170
6' 2"	155–168	164–178	172–197	5' 10"	132–145	142–156	152–173
6' 3"	158–172	167–182	176–202	5' 11"	135–148	145–159	155–176
6' 4"	162–176	171–187	181–207	6' 0"	138–151	148–162	158–179

*Weights at ages 25-59 y based on lowest comparative mortality. Weight in lb according to frame size for men wearing indoor clothing weighing 5 lb, shoes with 1-in. heels; for women, indoor clothing, shoes 2-in. heels.

(From *Statistical Bulletin*, Metropolitan Life Insurance Company, New York City.)

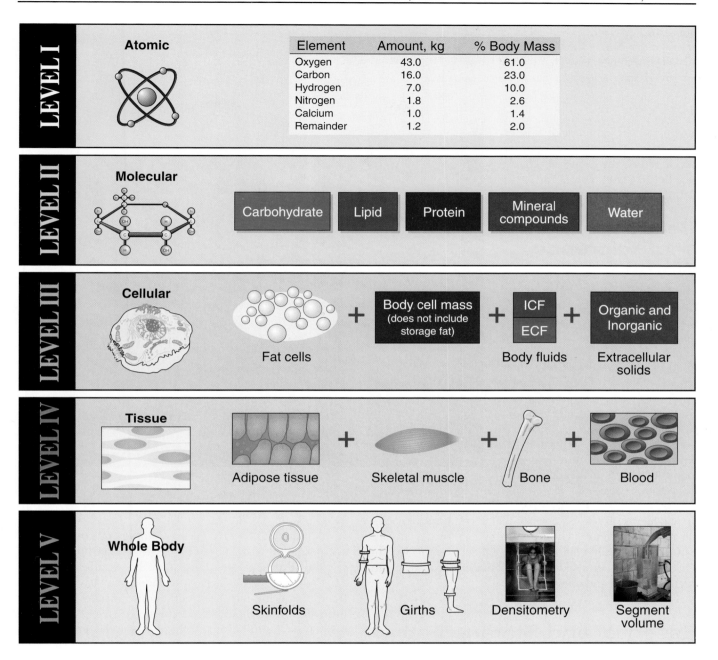

Figure 18.1

Five-level, multicomponent model to assess and interpret body composition. Each component within a level becomes more complex with an increase in the body's level of biological organization. A key feature of the model utilizes appropriate measurement within each level, particularly Level V. ICF = intracellular fluid; ECF = extracellular fluid. (Modified from Wang, Z. M., et al.: The five-level model: A new approach to organizing body composition research. *Am. J. Clin. Nutr.*, 56:19, 1992).

Frame Size and Body Fat

Do individuals with a large frame size possess more body fat than persons with a small or medium bony frame? Many people justify their large body mass (and extra fat) on the basis of a large skeletal structure. Limited research indicates that when properly classified by frame size and body composition, bony structure and body fatness do not relate.

tics or subdivisions. This allows the researcher to focus on a particular aspect of body composition related to a specific or general biological effect, including changes in molecular, cellular, or tissue composition from body weight gain or loss, or diverse forms of exercise training.

Body composition analysis most often focuses on the tissue and whole body levels, primarily because of methodologic and practical limitations. Gender differences in several of the body's compositional components provide a convenient framework for understanding body composi-

Figure 18.2
Body composition of the reference man and reference woman.

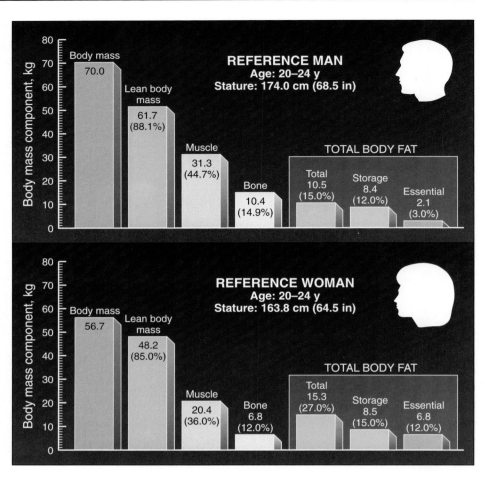

tion using the concept of a **reference man** and **reference woman** developed in the 1960s by Dr. Albert Behnke (Fig. 18.2).

Reference Man and Reference Woman

The reference man is taller by 10.2 cm and heavier by 13.3 kg than the reference woman, his skeleton weighs more (10.4 vs. 6.8 kg), and he possesses a larger muscle mass (31.3 vs. 20.4 kg) and lower total fat content (10.5 vs. 15.3 kg). These differences exist even when expressing the amount of fat, muscle, and bone as a percentage of body mass. This holds true, particularly for body fat, which represents 15% of the reference man's total body mass and 27% for the reference women. The concept of reference standards does not mean that men and women should strive to achieve these body composition values, or that reference values actually represent "average." Instead, the model provides a useful frame of reference to interpret statistical comparisons of athletes, individuals involved in physical training programs, and the underweight and obese.

Essential and Storage Fat

According to the reference model, total body fat exists in two storage sites or depots: essential fat and storage fat.

Essential Fat

The **essential fat** depot (equivalent to approximately 3% of body mass) consists of fat stored in the marrow of bones, heart, lungs, liver, spleen, kidneys, intestines, muscles, and lipid-rich tissues of the central nervous system (brain and spinal cord.) *Normal physiologic functioning requires this fat.* In females, essential fat also includes additional **sex-specific essential fat** (equivalent to approximately 9% of body mass). More than likely, this additional fat depot is important to childbearing and other hormone-related functions. Essential body fat probably represents a biologically established limit, beyond which encroachment could impair health status as in prolonged semistarvation from famine, malnutrition, and disordered eating behaviors.

Storage Fat

In addition to essential fat depots, **storage fat** consists of fat accumulation in adipose tissue. Storage fat includes the **visceral adipose tissues** that protect the various internal organs within the thoracic and abdominal cavities from trauma, and the larger **subcutaneous adipose tissue** volume deposited beneath the skin's surface. Men and women have similar quantities of storage fat—on average about 12% of body mass in males and 15% in females. For the reference standards, this amounts to 8.4 kg for the reference man and 8.5 kg for the reference woman (e.g., 70 kg body mass × 0.12 = 8.4 kg for males).

Sex-Specific Essential Fat

Breast fat probably contributes no more than 4% of body mass among women whose total body fat content varies from 14 to 35%. Sites other than the breasts (perhaps the lower body region that includes pelvis, hips, and thighs) furnish a large proportion of sex-specific essential fat.

Fat-Free Body Mass and Lean Body Mass

The terms **fat-free body mass** (**FFM**) and **lean body mass** (**LBM**) refer to specific entities. LBM (a theoretical entity) contains the small percentage of essential fat stores; in contrast, FFM represents the body mass devoid of *all* extractable fat. *In normally-hydrated, healthy male adults, the FFM and LBM differ only in terms of organ-related essential fat.* Thus, LBM calculations include the small quantity of essential fat, whereas FFM computations exclude total body fat (FFM = Body mass − Fat mass). Many researchers use the terms interchangeably; technically, however, the differences are subtle but real.

Minimal Body Mass

In contrast to the lower limit of body mass for the reference man which includes 3% essential fat, the lower body mass limit for females, termed **minimal body mass,** includes about 12% essential fat (3% essential fat + 9% sex-specific essential fat). Generally, the leanest women in the population do not have body fat levels below 10 to 12% of body mass, a value that probably represents the lower limit of fatness for most women in good health. *The theoretical minimal body mass concept developed by Behnke, incorporating about 12% essential fat, corresponds to a man's lean body mass with about 3% essential fat.* Information from popular magazines and health clubs not withstanding, females cannot achieve the same low body fat content as males. Therefore, women should not expect to "sculpt" their bodies below 12% body fat. Even world-class female body builders, triathletes, and gymnasts *rarely* have body fat levels lower than 12 to 14%.

Table 18.2 presents body fat data for selected groups of male and female athletes. Striking differences exist among these groups in percent body fat

Underweight and Thin

The terms underweight and thin are not necessarily synonymous. Measurements in our laboratories have focused on the structural characteristics of apparently "thin" looking females. Subjects were initially categorized subjectively as appearing thin or "skinny." Each of the 26 women then underwent a thorough anthropometric evaluation that included skinfolds, circumferences, and bone diameters, and percent body fat and FFM from hydrostatic weighing.

The results were unexpected because the women's percent body fat averaged 18.2%, about 7 percentage points below the average 25 to 27% body fat typically reported for young adult women. Another striking finding included equivalence in four trunk and four extremity bone-diameter measurements among the 26 thin-appearing women, 174 women who averaged 25.6% body fat, and 31 women who averaged 31.4% body fat. Appearing thin or skinny did not necessarily correspond to a diminutive frame-size or an excessively low body fat content using lower limits of minimal body mass and essential body fat proposed in Behnke's model.

TABLE 18.2
Percent body fat of male and female athletes

SPORT	PERCENT BODY FAT	
	MALE	FEMALE
Ballet dancing	8–14	13–20
Baseball/softball	12–15	12–18
Basketball	6–12	20–27
Body building	5–8	10–15
Canoe/Kayak	6–12	10–16
Cycling	5–15	15–20
Football		
Backs	9–12	
Linebackers	13–14	
Lineman	15–19	
Quarterbacks	12–14	
Gymnastics	5–12	10–16
Horse racing	8–12	10–16
Ice/field hockey	8–15	12–18
Orienteering	5–12	12–24
Racquetball	8–13	15–22
Rock climbing	5–10	13–18
Rowing	6–14	12–18
Rugby		10–17
Skiing		
Alpine	7–14	18–24
Cross-country	7–12	16–22
Jumping	10–15	12–18
Speed skating	10–14	15–24
Synchronized swimming		12–24
Swimming	9–12	14–24
Tennis	12–16	16–24
Track and field		
Discus throwers	14–18	22–27
Jumpers	7–12	10–18
Long distance	6–13	12–20
Shot putters	16–20	20–28
Sprinters	8–10	12–20
Decathletes	8–10	
Triathlon	5–12	10–15
Volleyball	11–14	16–25
Weightlifters	9–16	
Wrestling	5–16	

Data compiled from the research literature.

Leanness, Exercise, and Menstrual Irregularity

Physically active women in general, and participants in "low weight" or "appearance" sports like distance running, body building, figure skating, diving, ballet, and gymnastics in particular, increase their chances of menstrual cycle disturbances. These include delayed onset of menstruation, an irregular menstrual cycle (**oligomenorrhea**), or complete cessation of menses (**amenorrhea**). Amenorrhea in the general population occurs in 2 to 5% of women of reproductive age, whereas it can reach as much as 40% in women participating in sports.

Studies of female ballet dancers support this position; as a group, ballet dancers are quite lean and have a greater incidence of menstrual dysfunction, eating disorders, and a higher mean age at menarche compared with age-matched, female non-dancers. One-third to one-half of female athletes in endurance-type sports probably have some menstrual irregularity. In premenopausal women, irregularity or absence of menstrual function increases bone loss and their risk of musculoskeletal injury in vigorous exercise.

In some way, the body seems to "sense" high physical stress and inadequate energy reserves to sustain a pregnancy; in such cases, ovulation ceases. Some researchers have argued that at least 17% body fat represents a "critical level" for onset of menstruation and 22% fat as a level required to sustain normal menstrual cycles. They argue that body fat below these levels triggers hormonal and metabolic disturbances that affect the menses.

Leanness Not the Only Factor

The lean-to-fat ratio may play a key role in normal menstrual function (perhaps through peripheral fat's role in converting androgens to estrogens, or through production of the hormone leptin in adipose tissue), but so may other factors. *Many physically active females fall significantly below the supposed critical level of 17% body fat, but have normal menstrual cycles and maintain a high level of physiologic function and performance capacity.* Conversely, some amenorrheic athletes have average levels of body fat. In a study from one of our laboratories, we compared menstrual cycle regularity for 30 athletes and 30 nonathletes, all with less than 20% body fat. Four of the athletes and three nonathletes ranging from 11 to 15% body fat had regular cycles, whereas seven athletes and two nonathletes had irregular cycles or were amenorrheic. For the total sample, 14 athletes and 21 nonathletes had regular menstrual cycles. These data corroborate other research and disprove a once prevailing hypothesis that normal menstrual function requires a critical body fat level of 17 to 22%.

Potential causes of menstrual dysfunction include the complex interplay of physical, nutritional, genetic, hormonal, regional fat distribution, psychological, and environmental factors. An intense exercise bout releases an array of hormones, some of which have antireproductive properties. Further research needs to determine whether regular heavy exercise affects cumulative hormone release enough to disrupt normal menses. In this regard, when injuries prevent young amenorrheic ballet dancers from exercising regularly, normal menstruation resumes, even though body weight remains stable. Additional predisposing factors for reproductive endocrine dysfunction among athletes in-

When a Model Is Not Ideal

In 1967, only an 8% difference existed in body weight between professional fashion models and the average American woman. Today, a model's body weight averages 23% lower than the national average. Twenty years ago, gymnasts weighed about 20 pounds more than present day counterparts. Thus, it should come as no surprise that disordered eating patterns and unrealistic weight goals (and general dissatisfaction with one's body) remain so common among females of all ages.

clude nutritional inadequacy and an exercise-induced energy deficit with heavy training.

Based on current research, approximately 13 to 17% body fat should be regarded as an estimate of a minimal body fat level associated with regular menstrual function. The effects and risks of sustained amenorrhea on the reproductive system remain unknown. A gynecologist/endocrinologist should evaluate failure to menstruate or cessation of the normal cycle because it may reflect a significant medical condition (e.g., pituitary or thyroid gland malfunction or premature menopause). As explained in Chapter 3, prolonged menstrual dysfunction can negatively affect the density of the body's bone mass.

Delayed Onset of Menstruation and Cancer Risk

Some researchers claim that the delayed onset of menarche noted in active young females provides a positive health benefit. Compared with nonathletic counterparts, female athletes who started training in high school or earlier showed a lower lifetime occurrence of breast cancer and cervical and ovarian cancers. A lower cancer risk with delayed menstruation may be linked to less total estrogen production or a less potent form of estrogen over a lifetime. Lower body fat levels among athletes also may play a role because fatty tissues convert androgens to estrogen.

Methods to Assess Body Size and Composition

Two general approaches determine the fat and fat-free components of the human body:

1. Direct measurement by chemical analysis
2. Indirect estimation by hydrostatic weighing, anthropometric measurements, and other simple procedures including body stature and mass

Direct Assessment

Two approaches directly assess body composition. In one technique, a chemical solution literally dissolves the body into its fat and non-fat (fat-free) components. The other technique requires physical dissection of fat, fat-free adipose tissue, muscle, and bone. Such analyses require extensive time, meticulous attention to detail, and specialized laboratory equipment, and pose ethical questions and legal problems in obtaining cadavers for research purposes.

Figure 18.3 presents the chemical analyses data from five disease-free human cadavers. Water content equaled 60%, ranging between 50 to 70%. Nearly identical averages emerged for protein (17%) and fat (18%), although twice the range in individual values existed for body fat. Ash (total major and trace mineral content) represented 5% of body mass. These data exhibit variation in total body fatness, yet the composition of skeletal mass and fat-free tissues remain relatively stable. Compositional consistency of various tissues provides a theoretical basis to formulate mathematical equations to estimate body fat percentage from noninvasive, indirect measures.

Indirect Assessment

Many indirect procedures assess body composition including Archimedes' principle applied to **hydrostatic weighing** (also known as **underwater weighing**). This method computes percent body fat from **body density** (the ratio of body mass to body volume). Other procedures to predict body fat use skinfold thickness and girth measurements, x-ray, total body electrical conductivity or impedance, near-infrared interactance, ultrasound, computed tomography, air plethysmography, magnetic resonance imaging, and dual energy x-ray absorptiometry.

Hydrostatic Weighing (Archimedes' Principle)

The Greek mathematician and inventor Archimedes (287–212 BC) discovered a fundamental principle still applied to evaluate human body composition. An itinerant scholar of that time described the interesting circumstances surrounding the event:

"King Hieron of Syracuse suspected that his pure gold crown had been altered by substitution of silver for gold. The King directed Archimedes to devise a method for testing the crown for its gold content without dismantling it. Archimedes pondered over this problem for many weeks without succeeding, until one day, he stepped into a bath filled to the top with water and observed the overflow. He thought about this for a moment, and then, wild with joy, jumped from the bath and ran naked through the streets of Syracuse shouting, 'Eureka! Eureka!' I have discovered a way to solve the mystery of the King's crown."

Archimedes reasoned that gold must have a volume in proportion to its mass, and to measure the volume of an irregularly shaped object required submersion in water with collection of the overflow. Archimedes took lumps of gold and silver, each having the same mass as the crown, and submerged each in a container full of water. To his delight, he discovered the crown displaced more water than the lump of gold and less than the lump of silver. This could only mean the crown consisted of *both* silver and gold as the King suspected.

Essentially, Archimedes evaluated the **specific gravity** of the crown (i.e., the ratio of the crown's mass to the mass of an equal volume of water) compared with the specific gravities for gold and silver. Archimedes probably also reasoned that an object submerged or floating in water becomes buoyed up by a counterforce equaling the weight of the volume of water it displaces. This buoyant force supports an immersed object against the downward pull of gravity. Thus, an object "loses weight in water." *Because the object's loss of weight in water equals the weight of the volume of water it displaces, the specific gravity refers to the ratio of the weight of an object in air divided by its loss of weight in water.* The loss of weight

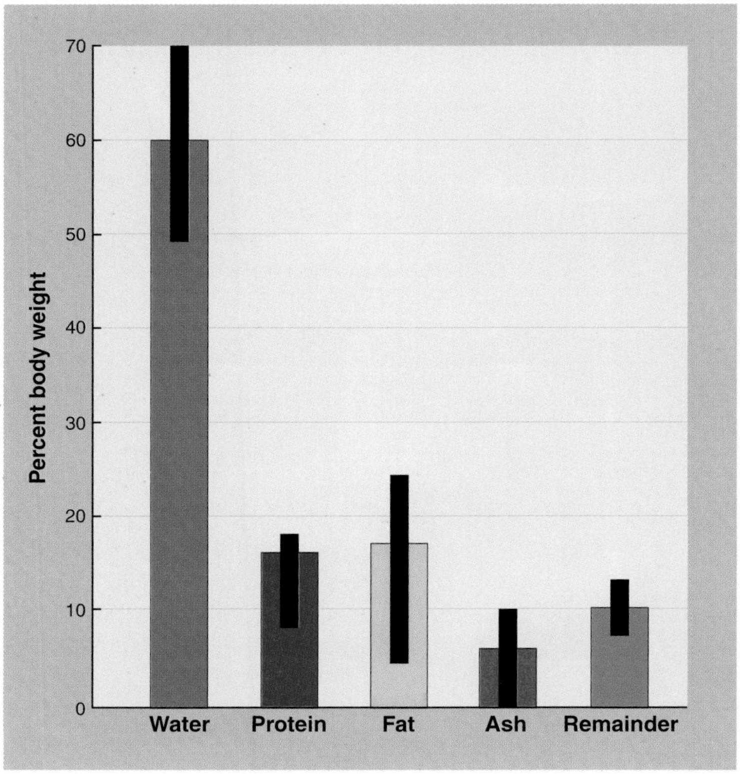

Figure 18.3
Body composition of five cadavers determined by direct chemical analysis. The height of the individual bars indicates the arithmetic mean for the five cadavers, and the black vertical bars represent the range. [Data From Widdowson, E.M. In: *Human Body Composition: Approaches and Applications.* Brožek, J., (ed.). London: Pergamon Press, 1965.]

in water equals the weight in air minus the weight in water.

$$\text{Specific gravity} = \frac{\text{Weight in air}}{\text{Loss of weight in water}}$$

In practical terms, suppose a crown weighed 2.27 kg in air and 0.13-kg less (2.14 kg) when weighed underwater (Fig. 18.4). Dividing the weight of the crown (2.27 kg) by its loss of weight in water (0.13 kg) results in a specific gravity of 17.5. Because this ratio differs considerably from the specific gravity of gold (19.3), we too can conclude: "Eureka, the crown must be fraudulent!"

Archimedes' principle allows us to apply water submersion or hydrodensitometry to determine the body's volume. Dividing a person's body mass by body volume yields body density (Density = Mass ÷ Volume), and from this an estimate of percent body fat.

Determining Body Density

For illustrative purposes, suppose a 50-kg woman weighs 2 kg when submerged in water. According to Archimedes' principle, a 48-kg loss of weight in water equals the weight of the displaced water. The volume of water displaced can be computed easily because researchers know the density of water at any temperature. In the example, 48 kg of water equals 48 L, or 48,000 cm³ (1 g of water = 1 cm³ by volume at 39.2°F). If the woman were measured at the cold-water temperature of 39.2°F, no density correction for water would be necessary. In practice, researchers use warmer water and apply the density value for water at the particular temperature. The body density of this person, computed as mass ÷ volume, would equal 50,000 g (50 kg) ÷ 48,000 cm³, or 1.0417 g·cm⁻³.

Computing Percent Body Fat, Fat Mass, and Fat-Free Body Mass

The equation that incorporates whole body density to estimate the body's fat percentage derives from the following three premises:

1. Densities of fat mass (all extractable lipid from adipose and other body tissues) and FFM (remaining lipid-free tissues and chemicals, including water) remain relatively constant (fat tissue = 0.90 g·cm⁻³; fat-free tissue = 1.10 g·cm⁻³), even with variations in total body fat and the FFM components of bone and muscle.

2. Densities for the components of the FFM at a body temperature of 37°C remain constant within and among individuals: water, 0.9937 g·cm⁻³ (73.8% of FFM); mineral, 3.038 g·cm⁻³ (6.8% of FFM); protein, 1.340 g·cm⁻³ (19.4% of FFM).

3. The person measured differs from the reference body only in fat content (reference body assumed to possess 73.8% water, 19.4% protein, 6.8% mineral).

The following equation, derived by Berkeley scientist Dr. William Siri, computes percent body fat from estimates of whole body density:

Siri Equation

$$\text{Percent body fat} = 495 \div \text{Body density} - 450$$

Based on the previous three assumptions, the following example incorporates the body density value of 1.0417 g·cm⁻³ (determined for the woman in the previous example) in the **Siri equation** to estimate percent body fat:

$$\begin{aligned}\text{Percent body fat} &= 495 \div \text{Body density} - 450 \\ &= 495 \div 1.0417 - 450 \\ &= 25.2\%\end{aligned}$$

The mass of body fat can be calculated by multiplying body mass by percent fat:

$$\begin{aligned}\textbf{Fat mass (kg)} &= \textbf{Body mass (kg)} \times (\textbf{Percent fat} \div \textbf{100}) \\ &= 50 \text{ kg} \times 0.252 \\ &= 12.6 \text{ kg}\end{aligned}$$

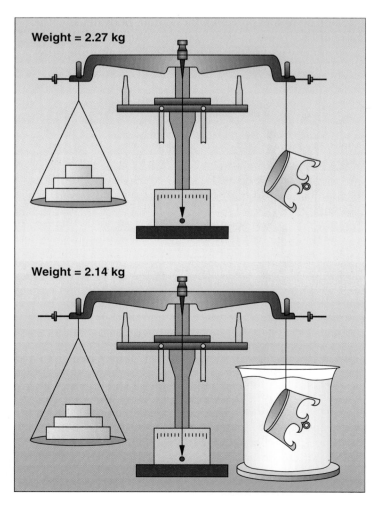

Weight = 2.27 kg

Weight = 2.14 kg

Figure 18.4
Archimedes' principle for determining the volume and subsequently the specific gravity of the king's crown.

Subtracting mass of fat from body mass yields FFM:

$$\text{FFM (kg)} = \text{Body mass (kg)} - \text{Fat mass (kg)}$$
$$= 50\,\text{kg} - 12.6\,\text{kg}$$
$$= 37.4\,\text{kg}$$

In this example, 25.2% or 12.6 kg of the 50-kg body mass consists of fat, with the remaining 37.4 kg representing the FFM.

Limitations and Errors in Hydrostatic Weighing

The generalized density values for fat-free ($1.10\ \text{g·cm}^{-3}$) and fat ($0.90\ \text{g·cm}^{-3}$) tissues represent average values for young and middle-age adults. However, these constants vary among individuals and groups—particularly the density and chemical composition of the FFM. This variation limits the accuracy of predicting percent body fat from whole body density. For example, blacks and Hispanics have significantly larger densities for FFM than whites ($1.113\ \text{g·cm}^{-3}$ for blacks, $1.105\ \text{g·cm}^{-3}$ for Hispanics, and $1.100\ \text{g·cm}^{-3}$ for whites). Consequently, using the existing density-to-fat equations (based on assumptions for whites) to calculate body composition from body density in blacks or Hispanics *overestimates* FFM and *underestimates* percent body fat. The following proposed modification of the Siri equation computes percent body fat from body density for blacks:

Modification for Blacks

Percent body fat = 437.4 ÷ Body density − 392.8

Applying constant density values for the various tissues for children (who are growing) or for aging adults also introduces errors in predicting body composition. For example, the water and mineral contents of the FFM continually change during the growth period, and demineralization from osteoporosis occurs with aging. Reduced bone density makes actual density of the fat-free tissues of young children and the elderly lower than the assumed constant of $1.10\ \text{g·cm}^{-3}$, thus *overestimating* percent body fat. In trained amateur and professional football players, distance runners, and body builders, the density of the fat-free component could also be altered, thus affecting the hydrostatic weighing estimate of body fat.

Table 18.3 presents density estimates of FFM for different male and female population subgroups, and equations to predict percent body fat from whole body density based on assumptions regarding the densities and proportions of the body's protein, mineral, and water content. Obviously, different equations to convert body density to percent body fat yield different values, depending on their underlying assumptions. This variation (depending on the equation applied) does not reflect an inherent error in the underwater weighing method; rather, careful use of hydrostatic weighing to assess body volume generates a technical error of less than 1 percent.

TABLE 18.3
Equations to predict percent body fat from body density (Db) based on different estimates of the fat-free body density (FFBD)

AGE, Y	EQUATION	FFBD[a]
Male		
White		
7–12	%fat = 5.03/Db − 4.89	1.084
13–16	%fat = 5.07/Db − 4.64	1.094
17–19	%fat = 4.99/Db − 4.55	1.098
20–80	%fat = 4.95/Db − 4.50	1.100
African American		
18–32	%fat = 4.37/Db − 3.93	1.113
Japanese		
18–48	%fat = 4.97/Db − 4.52	1.099
61–78	%fat = 4.87/Db − 4.41	1.105
Female		
White		
7–12	%fat = 5.35/Db − 4.95	1.082
13–16	%fat = 5.10/Db − 4.66	1.093
17–19	%fat = 5.05/Db − 4.62	1.095
20–80	%fat = 5.01/Db − 4.57	1.097
Native American		
18–60	%fat = 4.81/Db − 4.34	1.108
African American		
24–79	%fat = 4.85/Db − 4.39	1.106
Hispanic		
20–40	%fat = 4.87/Db − 4.41	1.105
Japanese		
18–48	%fat = 4.76/Db − 4.28	1.111
61–78	%fat = 4.95/Db − 4.50	1.100
Anorexic		
15–30	%fat = 5.26/Db − 4.83	1.087
Obese		
17–62	%fat = 5.00/Db − 4.56	1.098

Equations from the research literature

[a] Each estimate of the fat-free body density (FFBD) uses slightly different values for the proportions of the body's protein, mineral, and water content.

Residual Lung Volume Affects Computed Body Density

Not accounting for residual lung volume causes the computed body density value to decrease because the lungs' air volume contributes to buoyancy (lighter underwater weight) without affecting body mass. A lower body density makes a person "fatter" when converting body density to percent body fat.

How to Predict Residual Lung Volume

ydrostatic weighing represents a valid and reliable laboratory technique to assess body composition. The procedure accurately assesses body volume in the course of determining whole body density (body mass ÷ body volume). Body volume equals the difference between body mass measured in air minus body weight measured underwater (subtracting residual lung volume [RLV] and air in the GI tract) and corrected for water density at the weighing temperature. The small volume of air trapped in the GI tract (<100 mL), can be disregarded. In contrast, RLV represents a large and variable gas volume that must be subtracted to accurately determine body volume.

Laboratory techniques of helium dilution, nitrogen washout, or oxygen dilution routinely measure RLV. Each procedure requires complicated and expensive laboratory equipment. An alternate, although less valid, approach estimates RLV using gender-specific prediction equations based on age, stature, and body mass. The standard error of estimate for predicting RLV ranges between ±325 to 500 mL; this can correspond to errors in predicting percent body fat of up to about ±2.5% or more body fat units.

RLV Prediction Equations

Variables: age, y; stature (St), cm; body mass (BM), kg
Normal-weight males:

$$RLV, L = (0.022 \times Age) + (0.0198 \times St) - (0.015 \times BM) - 1.54$$

Normal-weight females (uses only age and stature):

$$RLV, L = (0.007 \times Age) + (0.0268 \times St) - 3.42$$

Overfat males (%fat ≥ 25) and females (%fat ≥ 30):

$$RLV, L = (0.0167 \times Age) + (0.0130 \times BM) + (0.0185 \times St) - 3.3413$$

Examples

1. Male: age, 21 y; body mass; 80 kg (176.4 lb); stature, 182.9 cm (72 in)

$$
\begin{aligned}
RLV (L) &= (0.022 \times 21) + (0.0198 \times 182.9) - \\
&\quad (0.015 \times 80) - 1.54 \\
&= 0.462 + 3.621 - 1.2 - 1.54 \\
&= 1.34 \ L
\end{aligned}
$$

2. Female: age, 19 y; stature, 160.0 cm (63 in)

$$
\begin{aligned}
RLV (L) &= (0.007 \times 19) + (0.0268 \times 160.0) - 3.42 \\
&= 0.133 + 4.288 - 3.42 \\
&= 1.00 \ L
\end{aligned}
$$

3. Overfat male: age, 35 y; body mass, 104 kg (229.3 lb); stature, 179.5 cm (70.7 in)

$$
\begin{aligned}
RLV (L) &= (0.0167 \times 35) + (0.0130 \times 104) + \\
&\quad (0.0185 \times 179.5) - 3.3413 \\
&= 0.5845 + 1.352 + 3.321 - 3.3413 \\
&= 1.39 \ L
\end{aligned}
$$

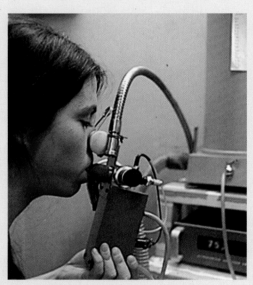

Measuring residual lung volume by oxygen dilution. First, the nitrogen concentration in the subject's lungs is determined at the end point of a forced, maximal expiration. This represents the residual volume's initial alveolar nitrogen concentration. The subject then inspires and expires (rebreathes) at approximately two-thirds vital capacity at a rate of one complete ventilation cycle every three seconds from a spirometer containing a known volume (about 4 to 6 L) of 100% oxygen. After 5 to 8 breaths, nitrogen concentration decreases dramatically and equilibrates between the spirometer gas and the subject's residual volume. This occurs because pure oxygen in the spirometer mixes and dilutes the nitrogen in the subject's unknown residual lung volume. A mathematical formula computes the subject's residual volume from the initial and final alveolar nitrogen concentrations, and initial volume and concentration of oxygen. The residual lung volume normally occupies 20 to 25% of vital capacity in healthy males and females.

References

Grimby, G., and Söderholm, B.: Spirometric studies in normal subjects, III: static lung volumes and maximum ventilatory ventilation in adults with a note on physical fitness. *Acta Med Scand.*, 2: 199, 1963.

Miller, W.C.T., et al.: Derivation of prediction equations for RV in overweight men and women. *Med. Sci. Sports Exerc.*, 30: 322, 1998.

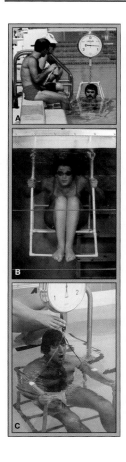

Figure 18.5
Measuring body volume by underwater weighing. **A,** In a swimming pool. **B,** In a stainless steel pool with plexiglas front in the laboratory. **C,** Seated in a therapy pool.

Body Volume Measurement

Figure 18.5 illustrates measurement of body volume by hydrostatic weighing. First the subject's body mass in air is accurately assessed, usually to the nearest ±50 g. A diver's belt secured around the waist prevents less dense (more fat) subjects from floating to the surface during submersion. Seated with the head out of water, the subject then makes a forced maximal exhalation while lowering the head beneath the water. The breath is held for several seconds while the underwater weight is recorded. The subject repeats this procedure 8 to 12 times to obtain a dependable underwater weight score. Even when achieving a full exhalation, a small volume of air, the **residual lung volume**, remains in the lungs. The calculation of body volume requires subtraction of the buoyant effect of the residual lung volume, measured immediately before, during, or after the underwater weighing.

A Word About Residual Volume. The greatest source of error in calculating body volume by hydrostatic weighing results from errors in measuring residual lung volume (RLV). The techniques for measuring RLV require specialized equipment and trained personnel. In situations that do not demand research-level accuracy (general screening, teaching laboratories), RLV predictions based on age, stature, body mass, or vital capacity provide an appropriate estimate (see *How to Estimate Residual Lung Volume*).

Body Volume Measurement by Air Displacement

Techniques other than hydrodensitometry can measure body volume. Figure 18.6 illustrates the **BOD POD,** a plethysmographic device for determining body volume. The technology applies the gas law, which states that a volume of air compressed under isothermal conditions decreases in proportion to a pressure change. Essentially, body volume equals the chamber's reduced air volume when the subject enters the chamber. The subject sits in a structure comprised of two chambers, each of known volume. A molded fiberglass seat forms a common wall separating the front (test) and rear (reference) chambers. A volume-perturbing element (a moving diaphragm) connects the two chambers. Changes in pressure between the two chambers

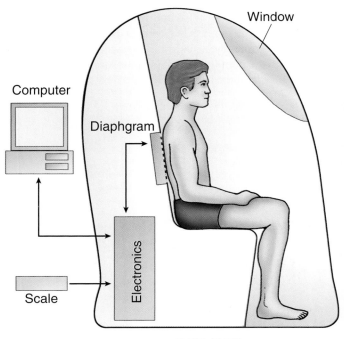

BOD POD

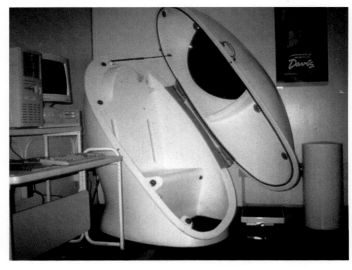

Figure 18.6
Right, BOD POD for measuring total body volume by air displacement. **Left,** Diagrammatic representation of the major system components of the air displacement chamber. Photo courtesy of Life Sciences Instruments. Concord, CA.

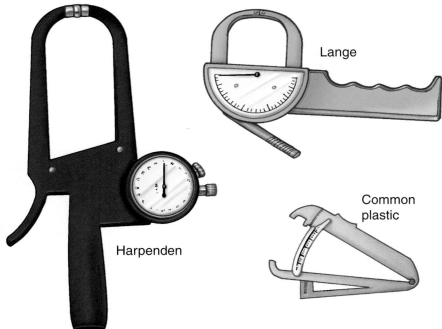

Figure 18.7
Three types of skinfold calipers to measure subcutaneous fat for body composition assessment.

oscillate the diaphragm, which directly reflects any change in chamber volume. The subject makes several breaths into an air circuit to assess thoracic gas volume (which when subtracted from measured body volume yields true body volume). Body density computes as body mass (measured in air) ÷ body volume (measured by BOD POD). The Siri equation converts body density to percent body fat.

Research has confirmed the accuracy and reproducibility of air displacement determinations of total body volume. Specific advantages include rapidity of testing (measurement requires only 5 min), good subject compliance (does not require water submersion with maximal air exhalation and residual volume determina-

tions), device mobility, and minimal technician training. Negative aspects include cost, and further need to document biological and technical error sources with the methodology. BOD POD technology holds great promise to assess body composition for a broad segment of the population.

Skinfold Measurements

Simple anthropometric procedures can successfully predict body fatness. The most common of these procedures uses **skinfolds**. The rationale for using skinfolds to estimate total body fat comes from the close relationships among three factors: (a) fat in adipose tissue deposits directly beneath the skin (**subcutaneous fat**), (b) internal fat, and (c) whole body density.

The Caliper

By 1930, a special pincer-type caliper accurately measured subcutaneous fat at selected body sites. The **skinfold caliper** (Figure 18.7) works on the same principle as a micrometer used to measure distance between two points. The pincer jaws exert a constant tension of 10 g·mm^{-2} at the point of contact with the double layer of skin plus subcutaneous tissue. The caliper dial indicates skinfold thickness in millimeters.

Example of Body Composition Calculations

Data for a professional football player (offensive guard) illustrates the computations for (1) body volume, (2) body density, (3) % body fat, (4) fat mass, and (5) fat-free body mass.

Data
Body mass = 110 kg; underwater weight = 3.5 kg; residual lung volume (RLV) = 1.2 L; water temperature correction (WTC) = 0.996 kg · L^{-1}

Computations
1. Body volume = Loss of body weight in water
   ÷ WTC − RLV
   = (110 kg − 3.5 kg)
   ÷ 0.996 − 1.2 L
   = 106.9 − 1.2
   = 105.7 L

2. Body density = Body mass ÷ Body volume
   = 110 kg ÷ 105.7 L
   = 110 kg · L^{-1}
   = 1.0407 g · cm^{-3}

3. % Body fat (Siri eq) = 495 ÷ Body density − 450
   = 495 ÷ 1.0407 − 450
   = 475.6 − 450
   = 25.6%

4. Fat mass = Body mass × (% Body fat ÷ 100)
   = 110 kg × 0.256
   = 28.2 kg

5. Fat-free body mass = Body mass − Fat mass
   = 110 kg − 28.2 kg
   = 81.8 kg

c l o s e   u p

When Should Skinfold Readings Be Taken?

A frequently asked question about skinfold measurements concerns when to read the caliper value. Should you leave the caliper on the site for 1, 3, or 5 seconds, or until the pointer stops moving? The body composition literature has rarely addressed this question.

Research-quality skinfold calipers exert an average compression force of 10 g per mm^2 at all jaw openings. This means that, regardless of skin-plus-fat thickness, the caliper always exerts the same pressure. Once applied to the skinfold site, the caliper continues to displace subcutaneous interstitial water, connective tissue, and fat throughout the measurement period until the skinfold's rebound force counteracts the caliper pressure. One study has investigated the extent of this skin-plus-fat compression in males and females, recommending optimal timing of the caliper readings.

The inset shows the compression data for triceps skinfold for 18 males and 18 females. Modification of the caliper provided for an instantaneous record of skinfold thickness throughout the measurement period. The data indicate that more than 70% of the total compression of skin and underlying fat takes place within the first 4 seconds after applying the caliper. Thus, to record the uncompressed skin-plus-fat measurement, the reading should be made when applying the caliper to the skin (as it exerts its full pressure), and certainly within 4 seconds. Any prolonged delay in reading the caliper *significantly underestimates* the actual skinfold value.

The absolute change in skinfold thickness among subjects over 60 seconds ranged between 0.3 mm and 4.5 mm. Although not a dramatic absolute change, this error can affect the accuracy of percent body fat when using skinfold prediction equa-

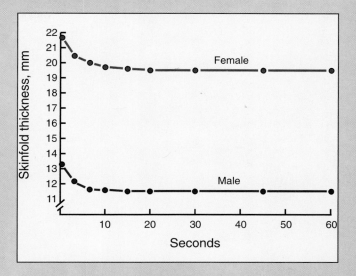

tions. In the present data, for example, using the initial uncompressed versus the final compressed skinfold value (after 60 s) produced differences in predicted percent body fat that ranged between 2 and 8 fat percentage units (a 10 to 50% error). When considered with other errors in using skinfold measurements, this large error should not be ignored. Almost all of the research studies using skinfolds have not specified when they recorded their readings. One can only surmise that it occurred immediately after placing the calipers on the skin (uncompressed value).

Reference

Becque, D.M., et al.: Time course of skin-plus-fat compression in males and females. *Hum. Biol.*, 58:33, 1986.

Figure 18.7 shows three different types of calipers. Compared with the most costly calipers (Harpenden and Lange), the less expensive models are less precise, exert nonconstant jaw tension throughout the range of measurement, have a smaller measurement scale (<40 mm), and produce less consistent scores when used by inexperienced testers.

Measuring skinfold thickness requires grasping a fold of skin and subcutaneous fat firmly with the thumb and forefingers, pulling it away from the underlying muscle tissue following the natural contour of the skinfold. The skinfold is recorded within 2 seconds after applying the full force of the caliper. This time limitation avoids skinfold compression when taking the measurement (see Close up: *When Should Skinfold Readings Be Taken?*). For research purposes, the investigator should have considerable experience in taking measurements and demonstrate consistency in duplicating values for the same subject made on the same day, consecutive days, or even

weeks apart. A good rule of thumb to achieve consistency requires taking duplicate or triplicate practice measurements on approximately 50 individuals who vary in body fat. Careful attention to details usually ensures high reproducibility of measurement.

Sites

The most common skinfold sites are the triceps, subscapular, suprailiac, abdominal, and upper thigh. An average of two or three measurements made at each site on the right side of the body with the subject standing represents the skinfold score. Figure 18.8 shows the anatomic location for five of the most frequently measured skinfold sites:

1. **Triceps:** Vertical fold at the posterior midline of the upper arm, halfway between the tip of the shoulder and tip of the elbow; elbow remains in an extended, relaxed position.

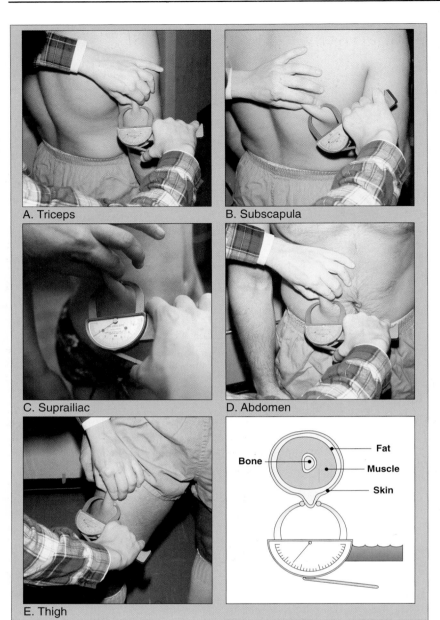

A. Triceps

B. Subscapula

C. Suprailiac

D. Abdomen

E. Thigh

Figure 18.8
Anatomic location of five common skinfold sites: **A**, Triceps. **B**, Subscapular. **C**, Suprailiac. **D**, Abdomen. **E**, Thigh. The lower right schematic shows a skinfold caliper and the compression of a double layer of skin and underlying tissue during the measurement. Except for the subscapular and suprailiac sites, which are measured diagonally, measurements are taken in the vertical plane.

Use of Skinfold Data

Skinfolds provide meaningful information about body fat and its distribution. There are basically two ways to use skinfolds. The first adds the scores as an indication of relative fatness among individuals. The "sum of skinfolds" (and individual skinfold values) also reflect absolute or percentage changes in fatness before and after physical conditioning or diet regimens.

The following observations come from the skinfold data shown in Table 18.4 for a 22-year-old female college student before and after a 16-week exercise program:

- The largest absolute decreases in skinfold thickness occurred at suprailiac and abdominal sites.

- The triceps showed the largest percentage decrease and subscapular the smallest percentage decrease.

- Skinfold thickness decreased 16.6 mm (12.6%) at the five sites compared with the pretraining condition.

2. **Subscapular:** Oblique fold just below the bottom tip of the scapula.
3. **Suprailiac (iliac crest):** Slightly oblique fold just above the hip bone (crest of ileum); the fold follows the natural diagonal line.
4. **Abdomen:** Vertical fold 1 inch to the right of the umbilicus.
5. **Thigh:** Vertical fold at the midline of the thigh, two-thirds the distance from the middle of the patella (knee cap) to the hip.

Other sites include:

6. **Chest:** Diagonal fold (with its long axis directed towards the nipple) on the anterior axillary fold as high as possible.
7. **Biceps:** Vertical fold at the posterior midline of the upper arm.

A second way applies skinfolds with mathematical equations to predict body density or percent body fat. These equations apply to specific populations because they predict fatness fairly accurately for subjects similar in age, gender, state of training, fatness, and race to those on whom the equations were derived. In young adults, approximately one-half of the body's total fat consists of subcutaneous fat, with the remainder visceral and organ fat. With advancing age, a proportionately greater quantity of fat deposits internally compared to subcutaneous fat. Thus, the same skinfold score reflects *greater* total percent body fat as one ages. *For this reason, one should use age-adjusted, generalized equations to predict body fat from skinfolds for a broad age range of adult men and women (see How to Choose Appropriate Skinfold Equations to Predict Body Fat in Diverse Populations).*

TABLE 18.4
Changes in selected skinfolds for a young woman during a 16-week exercise program

SKINFOLDS, mm	BEFORE	AFTER	ABSOLUTE CHANGE	PERCENT CHANGE
Triceps	22.5	19.4	−3.1	−13.8
Subscapular	19.0	17.0	−2.0	−10.5
Suprailiac	34.5	30.2	−4.3	−12.8
Abdomen	33.7	29.4	−4.3	−12.8
Thigh	21.6	18.7	−2.9	−13.4
Sum	131.3	114.7	−16.6	−12.6

A person can become a skilled skinfold technician by adhering to the following guidelines:

- Take great care in locating (and marking) anatomical landmarks for each site prior to measurement.
- Read the caliper dial to the nearest one-half marking (e.g., 0.5 mm).
- Take a minimum of two measurements at each site, and use the average in subsequent calculations.
- Take duplicate (or triplicate) measurements in rotational order rather than consecutive readings at each site to avoid a compression effect.
- Do not take measurements immediately after exercise; the shift in body fluid to the skin spuriously increases the reading.
- Practice on at least 50 subjects to gain experience with the technique.
- Avoid using inexpensive plastic calipers (they lack jaw-tension control).
- Train with skilled technicians and compare your results.
- Take measurements on dry, lotion-free skin.

Girth Measurements

Girth measurements offer an easily administered, valid, and attractive alternative to skinfolds. Apply a linen or plastic measuring tape lightly to the skin surface so the tape remains taut but not tight. This avoids skin compression that lowers the value. Take duplicate measurements at each site and average the scores. Figure 18.9 displays the six anatomic landmarks for taking girths:

1. **Right upper arm (biceps):** Palm up, arm straight, and extended in front of the body; taken at the midpoint between shoulder and elbow
2. **Right forearm:** Maximum girth with arm extended in front of the body with palm up
3. **Abdomen:** 1 inch above the umbilicus
4. **Hips (buttocks):** Maximum protrusion with heels together
5. **Right thigh:** Upper thigh just below the buttocks
6. **Right calf:** Widest girth midway between ankle and knee

Usefulness of Girth Measurements. The equations and constants presented in Appendix F for young and older men and women predict an individual's percent body fat within ±2.5 to 4.0% body fat units of the actual value, provided the individual's physical characteristics resemble the original validation group. Relatively small prediction errors make population-specific girth equations useful to those without access to laboratory facilities. The equations should not be used to predict fatness in individuals who appear excessively thin or fat, or who participate regularly in strenuous sports or resistance training that often increases girth without changing in subcutaneous fat. Along with predicting percent body fat, girths can also analyze patterns of body fat distribution (**fat patterning**), including changes in fat distribution during weight loss and gain.

Predicting Body Fat from Girths. From the appropriate tables in Appendix F, substitute the corresponding constants A, B, and C in the formula shown at the bottom of each table. This requires one addition and two subtraction steps. The following five-step example shows how to compute percent fat, fat mass, and FFM for a 21-year-old man who weighs 79.1 kg:

Step 1. Measure the upper arm, abdomen, and right forearm girths with a cloth tape to the nearest 0.25 in (0.6 cm): upper arm = 11.5 in (29.21 cm); abdomen = 31.0 in (78.74 cm); right forearm = 10.75 in (27.30 cm).

Step 2. Determine the three constants A, B, and C corresponding to the three girths from Appendix F: Constant A corresponding to 11.5 in = 42.56; Constant B corresponding to 31.0 in = 40.68; Constant C corresponding to 10.75 in = 58.37.

Step 3. Compute percent body fat by substituting the appropriate constants in the formula for young men shown at the bottom of Chart 1 in Appendix F as:

$$\text{Percent fat} = \text{Constant A} + \text{Constant B} - \text{Constant C} - 10.2$$
$$= 42.56 + 40.68 - 58.37 - 10.2$$
$$= 83.24 - 58.37 - 10.2$$
$$= 24.87 - 10.2$$
$$= 14.7\%$$

How to Choose Appropriate Skinfold Equations to Predict Body Fat in Diverse Populations

More than 100 different equations exist to predict body density and percent body fat from skinfolds. The equations, often formulated from homogeneous groups, incorporate between two and seven measurement sites to predict body density, which then converts to percent body fat using an appropriate equation for the specific population. The different equations yield predicted values that (at best) usually fall within ±3 to 5% body fat units assessed by hydrostatic weighing.

Different Equations

The table presents examples of skinfold equations for different populations. The following abbreviations apply (all skinfolds in mm): Skf = skinfolds; Σ = sum; tri = tricep; calf = calf; scap = subscapular; midax = midaxillary; iliac = suprailiac; abdo = abdomen; thigh = thigh; Db = body density, $g \cdot cm^{-3}$ BF = body fat; age in years (y).

EQUATIONS TO PREDICT PERCENT BODY FAT FROM SKINFOLDS

Population	Age, y	Variables	Equation	Comments
Children				
Boys	6–10	tri + calf	%BF = 0.735 (Σ2Skf) + 1.0	
		tri + scap	%BF = 0.783 (Σ2Skf) + 1.6	Use when ΣSkf > 35 mm
Girls	6–10	tri + calf	%BF = 0.610 (Σ2Skf) + 5.1	
		tri + scap	%BF = 0.546 (Σ2Skf) + 9.7	Use when ΣSkf > 35 mm
Native Americans				
Women	18–60	tri + midax + iliac	Db = 1.061 − 0.000385 (Σ3Skf) − 0.000204 (age)	%BF = [(4.81 ÷ Db) − 4.34]100
African Americans				
Women	18–55	chest + abdo + thigh + tri + scap + iliac + midax	Db = 1.0970 − 0.00046971 (Σ7Skf) + 0.00000056(Σ7Skf)^2 − 0.00012828 (age)	%BF = [(4.85 ÷ Db) − 4.39]100
Men	18–61	chest + abdo + thigh + tri + scap + iliac + midax	Db = 1.1120 − 0.00043499 (Σ7Skf) + 0.00000055 (Σ7Skf)^2 − 0.00028826 (age)	%BF = [(4.37 ÷ Db) − 3.93]100
Hispanics				
Women	20–40	chest + abdo + thigh + tri + scap + iliac + midax	Db = 1.10970 − 0.00046971 (Σ7Skf) + 0.00000056 (Σ7Skf)^2 − 0.00012828 (age)	%BF = [(4.87 ÷ Db) − 4.41]100
Native Japanese				
Women	18–23	tri + scap	Db = 1.0897 − 0.00133 (Σ2Skf)	%BF = [(4.76 ÷ Db) − 4.28]100
Men	18–27	tri + scap	Db = 1.0913 − 0.00116 (Σ2Skf)	%BF = [(4.97 ÷ Db) − 4.52]100
White Americans				
Women	18–55	tri + iliac + thigh	Db = 1.0994921 − 0.0009929 (Σ3Skf) + 0.0000023 (Σ3Skf)^2 − 0.0001392 (age)	%BF = [(5.01 ÷ Db) − 4.57]100
Men	18–55	chest + abdo + thigh	Db = 1.109380 − 0.0008267 (Σ3Skf) + 0.0000016 (Σ3Skf)^2 − 0.0002574 (age)	%BF = [(4.95 ÷ Db) − 4.50]100
Athletes (all sports)				
Women	18–29	tri + iliac + abdo + thigh	Db = 1.096095 − 0.0006952 (Σ4Skf) + 0.0000011 (Σ4Skf)^2 − 0.0000714 (age)	%BF = [(5.01 ÷ Db) − 4.57]100
Men	18–29	chest + midax + tri + scap + abdo + iliac + thigh	Db = 1.112 − 0.00043499 (Σ7Skf) + 0.00000055 (Σ7Skf)^2 − 0.00028826 (age)	%BF = [(4.95 ÷ Db) − 4.50]100

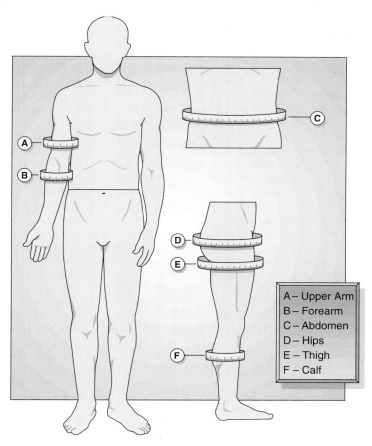

| A – Upper Arm |
| B – Forearm |
| C – Abdomen |
| D – Hips |
| E – Thigh |
| F – Calf |

Figure 18.9
Anatomic landmarks for measuring various girths.

Bioelectrical Impedance Analysis

A small, alternating current flowing between two electrodes passes more rapidly through hydrated fat-free body tissues and extracellular water compared with fat or bone tissue because of the greater electrolyte content (lower electrical resistance) of the fat-free component. Consequently, impedance to electric current flow relates to the quantity of total body water, which in turn relates to FFM, body density, and percent body fat.

Bioelectrical Impedence Analysis (**BIA**) *requires measurement by experienced personnel under strictly standardized conditions, particularly for electrode placement and subject's body position, hydration status, previous food and beverage intake, skin temperature, and recent physical activity.* Using this technique, the subject lies on a flat, nonconducting surface. Injector (source) electrodes attach on the dorsal surfaces of the foot and wrist, and detector (sink) electrodes attach between the radius and ulna (styloid process) and at the ankle between the medial and lateral malleoli (Fig. 18.10).

The person receives a painless, localized electrical current with impedance (resistance) to current flow between the source and detector electrodes determined. Conversion of the impedance value to body density—adding body mass and stature, gender, age, and sometimes race, level of fatness, and several girths to the equation—computes percent body fat from the Siri or other similar density conversion equation.

Step 4. Calculate the mass of body fat as:

$$\text{Fat mass} = \text{Body mass} \times (\% \text{ fat} \div 100)$$
$$= 79.1\,\text{kg} \times (14.7 \div 100)$$
$$= 79.1\,\text{kg} \times 0.147$$
$$= 11.6\,\text{kg}$$

Step 5. Determine FFM as:

$$\text{FFM} = \text{Body mass} - \text{Fat mass}$$
$$= 79.1\,\text{kg} - 11.63\,\text{kg}$$
$$= 67.5\,\text{kg}$$

Consider Level of Hydration and Ambient Temperature.

Hydration level affects BIA accuracy. Either hypohydration or hyperhydration alters the body's normal electrolyte concentrations, which modifies current flow independent of a real change in body composition. For example, impedance decreases from body water loss through sweating in prior exercise or voluntary fluid restriction. This produces a lower percent body fat estimate, whereas hyperhydration produces the opposite effect (higher fat estimate).

Skinfold Equations for Use With College-age Women and Men

Young women, ages 17 to 26 y

% Body fat = 0.55 (A) + 0.31(B) + 6.13

A = triceps skinfold (mm); B = subscapular skinfold (mm)

Example

Triceps = 22.5 mm; subscapular = 19.0 mm

% Body fat = 0.55 (22.5) + 0.31 (19.0) + 6.13

= 12.38 + 5.89 + 6.13

= 24.4%

Young men, ages 17 to 26 y

% Body fat = 0.43 (A) + 0.58 (B) + 1.47

A = triceps skinfold (mm); B = subscapular skinfold (mm)

Example

Triceps = 12.0 mm; subscapular = 9.0 mm

% Body fat = 0.43 (12) + 0.58 (9) + 1.47

= 5.16 + 5.22 + 1.47

= 11.8%

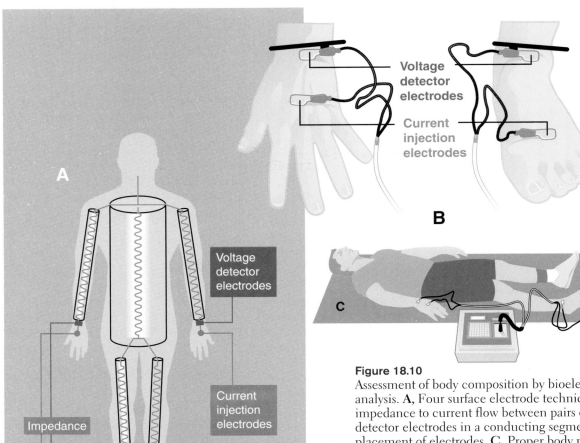

Figure 18.10
Assessment of body composition by bioelectrical impedance
analysis. **A,** Four surface electrode technique that measures
impedance to current flow between pairs of injection and
detector electrodes in a conducting segment. **B,** Standard
placement of electrodes. **C,** Proper body position.

Skin temperature (influenced by ambient conditions)
also affects whole-body resistance, and thus the BIA prediction of body fat. A significantly lower predicted body fat
occurs in a warm (less impedance to electrical flow) than
a cold environment.

Even under normal hydration and environmental temperature, body fat predictions may be questionable compared with hydrostatic weighing. BIA tends to overpredict
body fat in lean and athletic subjects and underpredict
body fat in the obese. BIA may be no more accurate than
the various anthropometric methods that use girths and
skinfolds to predict body fat. Also, conflicting evidence exists whether BIA can detect small changes in body composition during weight loss.

Dual-Energy X-ray Absorptiometry

Dual-energy x-ray absorptiometry (DXA), a high-technology procedure routinely used to assess bone mineral density in osteoporosis screening, permits quantification of fat
and muscle around bony areas of the body, including regions without bone present. DXA has become an accepted
clinical tool for assessing spinal osteoporosis and related

bone disorders. The method does not require assumptions
about the biological constancy of the fat and fat-free components as does hydrostatic weighing.

With DXA, two distinct x-ray energies (short exposure
with low-radiation dosage) penetrate into bone and soft tissue areas to a depth of about 30 cm. Specialized computer
software reconstructs an image of the underlying tissues.
The computer-generated report quantifies bone mineral
content, total fat mass, and FFM. Selected body regions can
also be pinpointed for more in-depth analysis (Fig. 18.11).

Body Mass Index

Clinicians and researchers frequently use the **body mass index (BMI),** derived from body mass related to stature, to evaluate the "normalcy" of one's body weight. The BMI has a
somewhat higher association with body fat than estimates
based simply on stature and mass (e.g., height-weight tables).

$$BMI = Body\ mass,\ kg \div Stature,\ m^2$$

Example:

Male: Stature = 175.3 cm, 1.753 m, (69 in); body
mass = 97.1 kg (214.1 lb)

$$BMI = 97.1\ kg \div (1.753\ m \times 1.753\ m)$$
$$= 97.1 \div 3.073$$
$$= 31.6$$

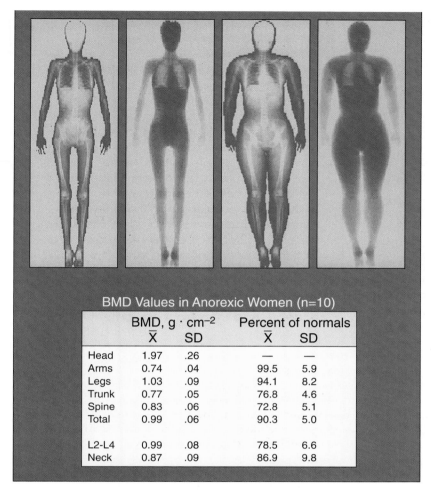

BMD Values in Anorexic Women (n=10)

| | BMD, g · cm⁻² | | Percent of normals | |
	X̄	SD	X̄	SD
Head	1.97	.26	—	—
Arms	0.74	.04	99.5	5.9
Legs	1.03	.09	94.1	8.2
Trunk	0.77	.05	76.8	4.6
Spine	0.83	.06	72.8	5.1
Total	0.99	.06	90.3	5.0
L2-L4	0.99	.08	78.5	6.6
Neck	0.87	.09	86.9	9.8

Figure 18.11
Dual-energy X-ray absorptiometry. Example of an anorexic female (two left images) and a typical female (two right images) whose body fat percentage averages 25% of her total body mass of 56.7 kg (125 lb). The average anorexic subject weighed 44.4 kg (97.9 lb) with DXA-estimated 7.5% body fat from the fat percentages at the arms, legs, and trunk regions. The values in the right column of the inset table present the average percentage values for bone mineral density (BMD) for different regional body areas in the anorexic group compared with a group of 287 normal females aged 20 to 40 years. (Photo courtesy of R.B. Mazess, Department of Medical Physics, University of Wisconsin, Madison, WI, and the Lunar Radiation Corporation, Madison, WI. Data from Mazess, R.B., et al.: Skeletal and body composition effects of anorexia nervosa. Paper presented at the international Symposium on In Vivo Body Composition Studies, June 20–23, Toronto, Ontario, Canada, 1989.)

The importance of this easy-to-obtain index is its curvilinear relationship to all-cause mortality ratio: as BMI becomes larger, risk increases for cardiovascular complications (including hypertension), diabetes, and renal disease (Fig. 18.12). The disease risk levels along the bottom of the figure represent the degree of risk with each 5-unit change in BMI. The lowest health risk category occurs for BMIs in the range 20 to 25, with the highest risk for BMIs exceeding 40. For women, 21.3 to 22.1 is the suggested desirable BMI range; the corresponding range for men equals 21.9 to 22.4. An increased incidence of high blood pressure, diabetes, and coronary heart disease occurs when BMI exceeds 27.8 for men and 27.3 for women.

Based on new classifications established on June 18, 1998 by the 24-member expert panel convened by the National Heart, Lung and Blood Institute, "overweight" classifies as a BMI of 25 to 29.9 and "obesity" represents a BMI ≥ 30 (see *How to Calculate and Interpret Body Mass Index*, Chapter 19). Under these classifications nearly 55% of Americans (an estimated 97 million adults) now classify as overweight and one in four classifies as obese.

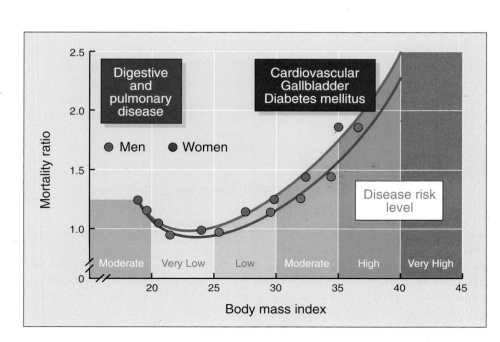

Figure 18.12
Curvilinear relationship based on American Cancer Society data between all-cause mortality and body mass index. At extremely low BMIs, the risk for digestive and pulmonary diseases increases, while cardiovascular, gallbladder, and type 2 diabetes risk increases with higher BMIs. (Modified from Bray, G.A.: Pathophysiology of obesity. *Am. J. Clin. Nutr.*, 55:488S, 1992).

Resarchers maintain that if this trend continues, the entire population could be overweight within a few generations. Particularly disturbing is that 15 to 20% of American children and 12% of adolescents (up from 7.6% in 1976-1980) classify as overweight. Obesity represents their most common chronic disorder, particularly prevalent among poor and minority children. Childhood obesity has increased by about 45% over the last 30 years (20% in the past decade)— and excessive fatness in one's youth may represent even more of an adult health risk than obesity that begins in adulthood. Regardless of their final body weight as adults, overweight children and adolescents exhibit a significantly greater risk of a broad range of illnesses as adults compared to adults who are of normal weight during their youth.

Limitations of BMI for Athletes

As with height-weight tables, BMI does not consider the body's proportional composition. Specifically, factors other than excess body fat (bone and muscle mass, and even the increased plasma volume induced by exercise training) affect the numerator of the BMI equation. A high BMI could lead to an incorrect interpretation of overweightness in lean individuals with excessive muscle mass, when in fact genetic makeup or exercise training caused the high BMI.

The possibility of misclassifying someone as overweight using BMI standards applies particularly to large-size, field-event athletes, bodybuilders, weightlifters, upperweight class wrestlers, and professional football players. For example, the BMI for seven defensive linemen from a former NFL Super Bowl team averaged 31.9 (team BMI averaged 28.7), clearly signaling these professional athletes as overweight and placing them in the moderate category for mortality risk. However, their body fat content, 18.0% for lineman and 12.1% for the team, misclassified them for fatness using BMI as the overweight standard.

In contrast to the professional football players, the average player in the National Basketball Association for the 1993–1994 season had a BMI of only 24.5. This relatively low BMI places them at low risk and keeps them out of the overweight category, although they would be classified overweight by height-weight standards.

Average Values for Body Composition

Table 18.5 lists average values for percent body fat in men and women in different areas of the United States. The column headed "68% Variation Limits" indicates the range for percent body fat that includes ±1 standard deviation, or about 68 of every 100 persons measured. As an example, the average percent body fat of 15.0% for young men from the New York sample includes the 68% variation limits from 8.9 to 21.1% body fat. Interpreting this statistically, for 68 of every 100 young men measured,

---

Questionable Validity for Near-Infrared Interactance

Near-infrared interactance (NIR) employs principles of light absorption and reflection. A fiber optic probe (light "wand") emits a low-energy beam of near-infrared light into the single measuring site at the anterior midline surface of the biceps of the dominant arm. A detector within the same probe measures the intensity of the reemitted light, expressed as optical density. Shifts in the wavelength of the reflected beam as it interacts with organic material in the arm, added to the manufacturer's prediction equation (including subject's body mass and stature, estimated frame size, gender, and physical activity level) computes percent body fat and FFM. The safe, portable, and lightweight equipment (commercial versions include the Futrex-5000 and 1000 and children's model 5000A) requires minimal training and necessitates little physical contact with the subject. These aspects of test administration make the technique popular for body composition assessment in health clubs, hospitals, and weight-loss centers. Unfortunately, available objective data do not support NIR as a valid means to assess human body composition compared to hydrostatic weighing. Less accuracy exists for NIR than skinfold measures. NIR overestimates body fat in lean men and women and underestimates body fat in fatter subjects. Furthermore, NIR produces large errors when estimating percent body fat for children and youth wrestlers. It also significantly underestimates body fat in college football players.

---

percent fat ranges between 8.9 and 21.1%. Of the remaining 32 young men, 16 would possess more than 21.1% body fat, whereas the 16 other men would have a body fat percentage less than 8.9. *Percent body fat for young adult men averages between 12 and 15%, whereas the average fat value for women ranges between 25 and 28%.*

Representative Samples Lacking

Considerable data exist for average body composition for many groups of males and females who differ in age and fitness level. However, no systematic evaluation of the body composition of a representative sample of the general population exists to warrant setting up precise normative stan-

TABLE 18.5
Average percent body fat for younger and older women and men from selected studies

STUDY	AGE RANGE, y	STATURE, cm	MASS, kg	% FAT	68% VARIATION LIMITS
Younger Women					
North Carolina, 1962	17–25	165.0	55.5	22.9	17.5–28.5
New York, 1962	16–30	167.5	59.0	28.7	24.6–32.9
California, 1968	19–23	165.9	58.4	21.9	17.0–26.9
California, 1970	17–29	164.9	58.6	25.5	21.0–30.1
Air Force, 1972	17–22	164.1	55.8	28.7	22.3–35.3
New York, 1973	17–26	160.4	59.0	26.2	23.4–33.3
North Carolina, 1975		166.1	57.5	24.6	—
Army recruits, 1986	17–25	162.0	58.6	28.4	23.9–32.9
Massachusetts, 1994	17–30	165.3	57.7	21.8	16.7–27.8
Older Women					
Minnesota, 1953	31–45	163.3	60.7	28.9	25.1–32.8
	43–68	160.0	60.9	34.2	28.0–40.5
New York, 1963	30–40	164.9	59.6	28.6	22.1–35.3
	40–50	163.1	56.4	34.4	29.5–39.5
North Carolina, 1975	33–50	—	—	29.7	23.1–36.5
Massachusetts, 1993	31–50	165.2	58.9	25.2	19.2–31.2
Younger Men					
Minnesota, 1951	17–26	177.8	69.1	11.8	5.9–11.8
Colorado, 1956	17–25	172.4	68.3	13.5	8.3–18.8
Indiana, 1966	18–23	180.1	75.5	12.6	8.7–16.5
California, 1968	16–31	175.7	74.1	15.2	6.3–24.2
New York, 1973	17–26	176.4	71.4	15.0	8.9–21.1
Texas, 1977	18–24	179.9	74.6	13.4	7.4–19.4
Army recruits, 1986	17–25	174.7	70.5	15.6	10.0–21.2
Massachusetts, 1994	17–30	178.2	76.3	12.9	7.8–18.9
Older Men					
Indiana, 1966	24–38	179.0	76.6	17.8	11.3–24.3
	40–48	177.0	80.5	22.3	16.3–28.3
North Carolina, 1976	27–50	—	—	23.7	17.9–30.1
Texas, 1977	27–59	180.0	85.3	27.1	23.7–30.5
Massachusetts, 1993	31–50	177.1	77.5	19.9	13.2–26.5

dards for body composition. At this time, the best approach presents average values from diverse studies of different age groups.

Body fat percentage usually increases in adult men and women as they age. In contrast, individuals who maintain a vigorous physical activity profile throughout life blunt "average" or "normal" fat increases with aging. Body composition changes with age likely occur because the aging skeleton demineralizes and becomes porous, reducing body density due to decreased bone density. Sedentary living provides another reason for the typical increase in body fat with age. As adults reduce physical activity (and thus energy expenditure), fat storage increases and muscle mass decreases, even without marked changes in daily caloric intake. Regular physical activity, on the other hand, maintains or even increases bone mass and muscle tissue.

Determining Goal Body Weight

Excess body fat detracts from good health, physical fitness, and athletic performance. However, no one really knows the optimum body fat or body weight for a particular individual. Inherited genetic factors greatly influence body fat distribution, and impact long-term programming of body size. Average values for percent body fat for young adults approximate 15% for men and 25% for women. Women and men who exercise regularly or train for athletic competition typically have lower body fat than age-matched sedentary counterparts. In contact sports and activities requiring muscular power, successful performance usually requires a large body mass with average to low body fat. In contrast, weight-bearing endurance activities require a lighter body mass and a minimal level of body fat. *Proper assessment of body composition, not body weight, should determine an athlete's ideal body weight.* Establishing an athlete's goal body weight should coincide with optimizing sport-specific measures of physiologic functional capacity and exercise performance. A "goal" body weight target that uses a desired (and prudent) percentage of body fat can be computed as follows:

Goal body weight = Fat-free body mass ÷ (1.00 − % fat desired)

Suppose a 120-kg (265-lb) shot-put athlete, currently with 24% body fat, wants to know how much fat weight to lose to attain a body fat composition of 15%. The following computations provide this information:

Fat mass = Body mass, kg × Decimal %body fat
$$= 120 \text{ kg} \times 0.24$$
$$= 28.8 \text{ kg}$$

Fat-free body mass = Body mass, kg − Fat mass, kg
$$= 120 \text{ kg} - 28.8 \text{ kg}$$
$$= 91.2 \text{ kg}$$

Goal body weight = Fat-free body mass, kg ÷ (1.00 − Decimal % fat desired)
$$= 91.2 \text{ kg} \div (1.00 - 0.15)$$
$$= 91.2 \text{ kg} \div 0.85$$
$$= 107.3 \text{ kg (236.6 lb)}$$

Desirable fat loss = Present body weight, kg − Goal body weight, kg
$$= 120 \text{ kg} - 107.3 \text{ kg}$$
$$= 12.7 \text{ kg (28.0 lb)}$$

If this athlete lost 12.7 kg of body fat, his new body mass of 91.2 kg would have a fat content equal to 15% of body mass. These calculations assume no change in FFM during weight loss. Moderate caloric restriction plus increased daily energy expenditure reduces body fat (and conserves lean tissue.) Chapter 19 discusses prudent yet effective approaches to reducing body fat.

Body Composition of Champion Athletes

Athletes often weigh more than average weight-for-height standards of life insurance company statistics; the "extra" weight is due to additional muscle mass. According to Table 18.1A, the desirable body weight for a 24-year old professional football player 6′2″ (188 cm) and 255 pounds (116 kg) ranges between 148 pounds (67.3 kg) and 195 pounds (88.6 kg). This means that the "overweight" player should reduce body mass at least 60 pounds (27 kg) just to reach the upper limit of the desirable weight range for a man of his stature.

If the player followed these guidelines, he would jeopardize his football career and maybe his overall health. Al-

---

A Desirable Range for Goal Weight

For practical purposes, recommend a "desirable body weight range" rather than a single goal weight. This range should lie within 2 pounds of the computed "goal body weight." For example, if goal body weight equals 135 pounds, the person should strive for a weight between 133 and 137 pounds.

---

though some larger-sized persons may be "overweight," they may also fall within a normal range for body fat without need to reduce body weight. The following sections highlight examples of the body composition of male and female elite athletes in specific sports.

Long-Distance Runners

Table 18.6 presents data for body mass, stature, and body composition (determined by underwater weighing) for male and female distance runners of national and international caliber. For comparative purposes, data include a typical sample of untrained young adult men and women. The female runners averaged 15.2% body fat, similar to high school cross-country runners, but considerably lower than 26% reported for sedentary females of the same age, stature, and body mass. Compared with other female athletes, runners have a lower average fat value than collegiate basketball players (20.9%), competitive gymnasts (15.5%), swimmers (20.1%), and tennis players (22.8%). Interestingly, the average body fat for the female runners equaled the 15% average reported for non-athletic males, and close to the essential fat content proposed by Behnke's model for the reference woman.

Male endurance runners had extremely low body fat values, considering that essential fat constitutes about 3% of body mass in the reference man. These endurance runners represent the lower end of the fat-to-lean continuum for topflight athletes. Apparently, this physique characteristic influences success in distance running. This makes sense for two reasons. First, effective heat dissipation during running maintains thermal balance (excess fat hinders heat loss). Second, excess body fat serves as "dead weight" that adds directly to running's energy cost without providing corresponding propulsive energy.

High School Wrestlers

Table 18.7 presents anthropometric characteristics for three groups of high school wrestlers. The "certified" Iowa and Minnesota wrestlers competed at one of 12 different weight categories; the "champion" wrestlers competed in state or conference finals. Except for age and skinfolds, little difference exists in the wrestlers' physical characteristics. From skinfolds, the champions were leaner than less successful teammates. Because of small differences in body mass

TABLE 18.6
Body composition of male and female elite endurance runners

GROUP	N	STATURE cm	BODY MASS kg	FFM kg	BODY FAT %
Runners					
Male[a]	19	176.4	62.6	60.7	3.0
Female[b]	11	169.4	57.2	48.5	15.2
Untrained[c]					
Male	54	176.4	71.4	60.5	15.3
Female	69	160.4	59.0	43.5	26.2

[a] Computed from data in Pollock, M.L., et al.: Body composition of elite class distance runners. *Ann. N.Y. Acad. Sci.*, 301:361, 1977.

[b] Computed from data in Wilmore, J.H., and Brown, C.H.: Psychological profiles of women distance runners. *Med. Sci. Sports*, 6:178, 1974.

[c] Data from Katch, F.I., and McArdle, W.D.: Prediction of body density from simple anthropometric measurements in college-age men and women. *Hum. Biol.*, 45:445, 1973.

Minnesota certified wrestlers. The percent body fat of the Nebraska wrestlers, determined by hydrostatic weighing averaged 11.0 ±4.0% (range from 1.5 to 26.0%). Minimal wrestling weight at 5% body fat averaged 59.1 kg (see *How to Determine Minimal Wrestling Weight from Two Skinfolds in High School Wrestler*).

Male and Female Weight Lifters and Body Builders

among groups, elite wrestlers actually competed at a heavier FFM, which may have contributed to their success in a particular weight class. The last column in Table 18.7 presents additional data on 409 Nebraska high school wrestlers. Their anthropometric characteristics most resemble the Iowa and Minnesota certified wrestlers.

Resistance-trained male athletes, particularly body builders, Olympic weight lifters, and power weight lifters, exhibit remarkable muscular development and FFM. Values for percent body fat average 9.3% in body builders, 9.1% in power weight lifters, and 10.8% in Olympic weight

TABLE 18.7
Anthropometric comparisons between certified and champion Iowa and Minnesota high school wrestlers and comparison to Nebraska wrestlers

MEASUREMENT	CERTIFIED WRESTLERS IOWA (N = 484)	MINN (N = 245)	CHAMPION WRESTLERS IOWA (N = 382)	MINN (N = 164)	NEBRASKA WRESTLERS (N = 409)
Age, y	15.9	16.8	17.8	17.4	16.4
Stature, cm	169.9	172.0	171.7	172.5	171.0
Body mass, kg	64.3	65.3	64.6	64.7	63.2
Chest diameter, cm	26.8	26.5	27.7	26.6	27.9
Chest depth, cm	19.0	16.8	19.2	17.3	18.9
Bitrochanteric diameter, cm	31.0	31.4	31.1	31.5	31.0
Ankles diameter, cm	14.3	14.3	14.0	14.3	13.8
Skinfolds, mm					
Scapular	8.4	7.9	6.4	6.8	8.8
Triceps	8.6	9.1	6.0	5.6	8.9
Suprailiac	13.3	12.3	9.1	7.5	11.8
Abdomen	13.1	12.2	8.6	8.3	11.6
Thigh	10.8	13.6	7.7	8.3	9.4
Sum of 5 skinfolds	54.2	55.1	37.8	36.5	50.5

[a] From Clarke, K.S.: Predicting certified weight of young wrestlers; a field study of the Tcheng-Tipton methods. *Med Sci. Sports*, 6:52, 1974.

[b] From Housh, T.J., et al.: Validity of anthropometric estimations of body compositions in high school wrestlers, *Res. Q. Exec. Sport*, 60:239, 1989.

How to Determine Minimal Wrestling Weight from Two Skinfolds in High School Wrestlers

Minimal Wrestling Weight

The lowest acceptable level for safe wrestling competition equals body weight at 5% body fat (determined by hydrostatic weighing or population-specific regression equations with anthropometry). For wrestlers below age 16, 7% body fat represents the recommended lower limit (5% for ages > 16 y). If the wrestler's body weight exceeds the "**minimal wrestling weight**" based on this percent body fat level, a gradual fat loss program through diet and exercise sets a realistic and prudent weekly weight loss of 1 to 2 pounds.

Equations to Predict Percent Body Fat and Minimal Wrestling Weight

Triceps and abdominal skinfolds can accurately predict percent body fat and minimal wrestling weight for interscholastic wrestlers.

1. **Body density (Db)**, $g \cdot cm^{-3} = 1.0982 - (0.000815 \times [triceps + abdomen skinfolds]) + (0.00000084 \times [triceps + abdomen skinfolds]^2)$
2. **% Body fat** $= ([4.570 \div Body density] - 4.142) \times 100$
3. **Fat weight (FW)**, $lb = Body weight \times Decimal \%body fat$
4. **Fat-free body weight (FFW)**, $lb = Body weight - Fat weight$
5. **Minimal wrestling weight (MWW)**, $lb = FFW \div (1.00 - Desired decimal \%body fat)$

Example

Problem

An 18-year-old high school wrestler wants to compete in the lowest possible weight category compatible with good health and exercise performance. He weighs 154 pounds and has the following skinfolds: triceps = 8 mm; abdomen = 13 mm. He desires to wrestle at the lowest permissible percent body fat (5%).

Solution

1. $Db, g \cdot cm^{-3} = 1.0982 - (0.000815 \times [8 + 13]) + (0.00000084 \times [8 + 13]^2)$
   $= 1.0982 - (.017115) + (.0003704)$
   $= 1.08146 \ g \cdot cm^{-3}$
2. $\% \ Body \ Fat = ([4.570 \div 1.08146] - 4.142) \times 100$
   $= 8.3\%$
3. $FW, lb = 154 \times 0.083$
   $= 12.8 \ lb$
4. $FFW, lb = 154 - 12.8$
   $= 141.2 \ lb$
5. $MWW, lb = 141.2 \div (1.00 - 0.05)$
   $= 141.2 \div 0.95$
   $= 148.6 \ lb$

In this example, minimal wrestling weight would equal 149 pounds. With increased training and moderate caloric restriction, a weight loss of two pounds per week becomes a prudent objective. In about three weeks, the desired six-pound weight loss should be achieved.

Reference

Thorland, W., et al.: New equations for prediction of a minimal weight in high school wrestlers. *Med. Sci. Sports Exerc.*, 21:S72, 1989.

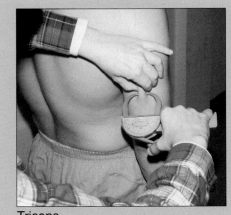

Triceps

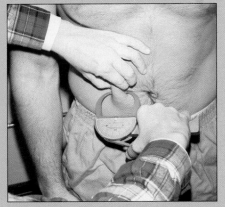

Abdomen

lifters. This similar but considerable degree of leanness occurs for each group of athletes, even though "height-weight" tables would classify between 14% and 19% of these men as "overweight." In one study, no differences among groups occurred in skeletal frame size, FFM, skinfolds, and bone diameter measurements. Differences only emerged for shoulders, chest, biceps (both relaxed and flexed), and forearm girths, with body builders larger at each site. For excess muscle (i.e., muscle mass in excess of that predicted from skeletal dimensions), the body builders had nearly 16 kg of excess muscle, power weight lifters 15 kg, and Olympic weight lifters 13 kg (see Close up: *Excess Muscle*, Chapter 12).

Female body building gained widespread popularity throughout the United States during the late 1970s. As women aggressively undertook the vigorous demands of resistance training, competition became more intense, and achievement level increased markedly. Because success in bodybuilding depends on a lean appearance, com-plemented by a well-defined yet enlarged musculature, interesting questions arise with regard to body composition. How lean do these competitors become? Does a low level of body fat accompany their relatively large muscle mass?

A study of the body composition of 10 competitive female body builders revealed these athletes averaged 13.2% body fat (range from 8.0 to 18.3%) and 46.6 kg of FFM. Except for champion gymnasts, who also average about 13% body fat, body builders were 3 to 4% shorter in stature, 4 to 5% lighter in body mass, and possessed 7 to 10% less total mass of body fat compared with other top female athletes. Female body builders' most striking compositional characteristic, a dramatically large FFM/fat mass ratio of 7:1, nearly doubles the 4.3:1 ratio for other female athletic groups. This difference presumably occurred without using steroids (as reported by questionnaire). Interestingly, 8 of 10 body builders reported normal menstrual function despite their relatively low levels of body fat.

summary

1. Total body fat consists of essential fat and storage fat. Essential fat contains fat in bone marrow, nerve tissue, and organs; it does not represent an energy reserve, but an important component for normal biologic function. Storage fat, the energy reserve, accumulates mainly as adipose tissue beneath the skin and in visceral depots.

2. Storage fat averages 12% of body mass for young adult men and 15% of body mass for women.

3. True sex differences exist for essential fat. It averages 3% body mass for men and 12% for women. The greater essential fat for females probably relates to child-bearing and hormonal functions (sex-specific essential fat).

4. A person probably cannot reduce body fat below the essential fat level and still maintain good health.

5. Menstrual dysfunction occurs among female athletes who train hard and maintain low levels of body fat. The precise interaction among menstrual dysfunction and the physiological and psychological stress of intense, regular training and competition, hormonal balance, energy and nutrient intake, and body fat requires further study.

6. A positive aspect may exist between the delayed onset of menarche observed in chronically active young females and health because of a lower lifetime occurrence of reproductive organ and other types of cancer.

7. The most popular indirect methods of body composition assessment include hydrostatic weighing and prediction methods based on skinfolds and girths. Hydrostatic weighing determines body density with subsequent estimation of percent body fat. The computation assumes a constant density for the body's components of fat and fat-free tissues. Subtracting fat mass from body mass yields fat-free body mass (FFM).

8. Part of the error inherent in predicting body fat from whole-body density lies in the assumptions concerning the densities of the body's fat and fat-free components. These densities, principally FFM, differ from assumed constants due to race, age, and athletic experience.

9. An air displacement method (BOD POD) offers promise for body composition assessment due to ease of administration, and high reproducibility of body volume scores and high validity compared with densitometry.

10. Common field methods to assess body composition use prediction equations developed from relationships among selected skinfolds and girths and body density and percent body fat. These equations are "population specific"; they predict most accurately with subjects similar to those who participated in the equations' original derivation.

11. Body mass index (BMI) relates more highly to body fat content and health risk then simply body mass and stature. As with height-weight tables, BMI does not consider the body's proportional composition.

12. The concept of bioelectrical impedance analysis (BIA) states that hydrated, fat-free body tissues and extracellular water facilitate electrical flow compared to fat tissue because of greater electrolyte content of the fat-free component. This makes impedance to electric

current flow relate directly to the body's fat content. BIA represents a noninvasive, indirect general assessment of body composition, provided users observe strict standardized conditions.

13. Based on data from healthy young adults, average males possess a body fat content of about 15% and women 25%. These values furnish a yardstick to evaluate deviations from "average" for the body fat of individual athletes and specific athletic groups.

14. Standard "height-weight" tables reveal little about an individual's body composition. Studies of athletes show that overweight does not coincide with overfat.

15. Physique characteristics combined with highly developed physiologic support systems provide important ingredients for a champion performance. Pronounced differences in physique exist among same gender participants in diverse sports.

16. Topflight male and female endurance runners represent the lower end of the fat-to-lean continuum.

17. Wrestlers, a unique group of lean athletes, undergo severe training and repeated bouts of acute weight loss. They generally loose 2 to 6 kg of body mass, usually combining food restriction with dehydration in an attempt to "make weight."

18. Female body builders can probably alter muscle size to almost the same relative extent as males. Female body builders' most striking compositional characteristic, a dramatically large FFM/fat mass ratio of 7:1, nearly doubles the 4.3:1 ratio for other female athletic groups.

thought questions

1. Explain if and why different body fat standards should apply to people of different ages.

2. How would you use anthropometric data to estimate optimal body composition?

3. Do established differences in body composition between men and women justify using gender-specific normative standards when evaluating diverse components of physical fitness and motor performance? Why?

4. What arguments counter the position that no true gender difference exists in body fat, only a difference from regular physical activity and caloric intake.

5. A friend complains that three different fitness centers determined her percent body fat from skinfolds as follows: 21%, 25%, and 31%. How can you reconcile the discrepancies?

selected references

Ainsworth, B. E., et al.: Predictive accuracy of bioimpedance in estimating fat-free mass of African-American women. *Med. Sci. Sports Exerc.*, 29:781, 1997.

Behnke, A. R., and Wilmore, J. H.: *Evaluation and Regulation of Body Build and Composition.* Englewood Cliffs, NJ: Prentice-Hall, 1974.

Bioelectrical impedance analysis in body composition measurement: National Institutes of Health Technology Assessment Conference Statement. *Am. J. Clin. Nutr.*, 64(suppl): 524S, 1996.

Broeder, C. E., et al: Assessing body composition before and after resistance or endurance training. *Med. Sci. Sports Exerc.*, 29:705, 1997.

Brožek, J., et al.: Densitometric analysis of body composition: revision of some quantitative assumptions. *Ann. N. Y. Acad. Sci.*, 110:113, 1963.

Calle, E. E. et al.: Body-mass index and mortality rate in a prospective cohort of U.S. adults. *N. Engl. J. Med.*, 341:1097, 1999.

Clark, R. R., et al.: A comparison of methods to predict minimal weight in high school wrestlers. *Med. Sci. Sports Exerc.*, 25:1541, 1993.

Constantine, N. W., and Warren, M. P.: Physical activity, fitness, and reproductive health in women: Clinical observations. In: *Physical Activity, Fitness, and Health.* Bouchard C., et al., (eds.). Champaign, IL: Human Kinetics, 1994.

Coté, K. D., and Adams, W. C.: Effect of bone density on body composition estimates in young adult black and white women. *Med. Sci. Sports Exerc.*, 25:290, 1993.

Dempster, P., and Aitkens, S., A new air displacement method for the determination of human body composition. *Med. Sci. Sports. Exerc.*, 27:1692, 1995.

Drinkwater, B. L.: Amenorrhea, body weight, and osteoporosis. In: *Eating, Body Weight and Performance in Athletes.* Brownell, K. D., et al., (eds.). Philadelphia: Lea & Febiger, 1992.

Ellis, K. J., et al.: Body composition of a young, multiethnic female population. *Am. J. Clin. Nutr.*, 65:724, 1997.

Freedson, P. A., et al.: Physique, body composition, and psychological characteristics of competitive female body builders. *Phys. Sportsmed.*, 11:85, 1983.

Forbes, G. B., Body composition. In: *Present Knowledge in Nutrition*, 7th Ed. Aiegler, E. and Filer, L., (eds.). Washington, D.C.: International Life Sciences Institute, 1996.

Frisch, R. E., et al.: Delayed menarche and amenorrhea in ballet dancers. *N. Engl. J. Med.*, 303:17, 1980.

Frisch, R. E., et al.: Lower lifetime occurrence of breast cancer and cancers of the reproductive system among former college athletes. *Am. J. Clin. Nutr.*, 45:328, 1987.

Going, S., et al.: Aging and body composition: biological changes and methodological issues. *Exerc. Sport Sci. Rev.*, 23:459, 1995.

Guo, S.S., et al.: Aging, body composition and lifestyle: the Fels Longitudinal Study. *Am. J. Clin. Nutr.* 70:405, 1999.

Heyward, V. H., and Stolarczyk, L. M.: *Applied Body Composition Assessment*. Champaign, IL: Human Kinetics, 1996.

Housh, T. J., et al.: Validity of near-infrared interactance instruments for estimating percent body fat in youth wrestlers. *Pediatric Exerc. Sci.*, 8:69, 1996.

Katch, F. I., et al.: The underweight female. *Phys. Sportsmed.*, 8:55, 1980.

Katch, F. I., and Katch, V. L.: Measurement and prediction errors in body composition assessment and the search for the perfect prediction equation. *Res. Q. Exerc. Sport*, 51:249, 1980.

Katch, F. I., and McArdle, W. D.: Validity of body composition prediction equations for college men and women. *Am. J. Clin. Nutr.*, 28:105, 1975.

Katch, V. L., et al.: Contribution of breast volume and weight to body fat distribution in females. *Am. J. Phys. Anthropol.*, 53:93, 1980.

Kohrt, W. M.: Body composition by DXA: tried and true? *Med. Sci. Sports Exerc.*, 27:1359, 1995.

Kushner, R. F., et al.: Clinical characteristics influencing bioelectrical impedance analysis measurements. *Am. J. Clin. Nutr.*, 64 (suppl):423S, 1996.

Lohman, T. G., et al.: Body fat measurement goes high-tech: Not all equations are created equal. *ACSM's Health & Fitness J.*, 1:30, 1997.

Lukaski, H. C., Body composition in Exercise and Sport. In: *Nutrition in Exercise and Sport, 3rd Ed.* Wolinsky, I., (ed.). Boca Raton, FL: CRC Press, 1997.

McCrory, M. A., et al.: Evaluation of a new air displacement plethysmograph for measuring human body composition. *Med. Sci. Sports Exerc.*, 27:1686, 1995.

McKee, J. E., and Cameron, N.: Bioelectrical impedance changes during the menstrual cycle. *Am. J. Hum. Biol.*, 9:155, 1997.

Mokdad, A. H., et al.: The spread of the obesity epidemic in the United States, 1991–1998. *JAMA*, 282:1519, 1999.

Must, A., et al.: The disease burden associated with overweight and obesity. *JAMA*, 282:1523, 1999.

Opplinger, R. A., et al.: Wisconsin minimum weight rule curtails weight cutting practices in high school wrestlers. *Med. Sci. Sports. Med.*, 27:S12, 1995.

Penn, I-W., et al.: Body composition and two-compartment model assumptions in male long distance runners. *Med. Sci. Sports Exerc.*, 26:392, 1994.

Roche, L. F., et al. (eds.). *Human Body Composition*. Champaign, IL: Human Kinetics, 1996.

Roemmich, J. N., and Sinning, W. E.: Weight-loss and wrestling training: effects of nutrition, growth, maturation, body composition, and strength. *J. Appl. Physiol.*, 82:1751, 1997.

Ross, R.: Effects of diet- and exercise-induced weight loss on visceral adipose tissue in men and women. *Sports Med.* 24:55, 1997.

Schutte, J. E., et al.: Density of lean body mass is greater in Blacks than Whites. *J. Appl. Physiol.*, 56:1647, 1984.

Segal, K. R. Use of bioelectrical impedance analysis measurements as an evaluation for participating in sports, *Am. J. Clin. Nutr.*, 64 (suppl):469S, 1996.

Shangold, M. M., et al.: Evaluation and management of menstrual dysfunction in athletes. *JAMA*, 262:1665, 1990.

Thorland, W. G., et al.: Estimation of body composition in black adolescent male athletes. *Pediatric Exerc. Sci.*, 5:116, 1993.

Tran, Z. V., and Weltman, A.: Predicting body composition of men from girth measurements. *Hum. Biol.*, 60:167, 1988.

Tran, Z. V., and Weltman, A.: Generalized equation for predicting body density of women from girth measurements. *Med. Sci. Sports Exerc.*, 21:101, 1989.

Vogel, J. A., and Kasper, M. J.: Body fat assessment in women: special considerations. *Sports. Med.*, 13:245, 1992.

Wang, J., et al.: Bio-impedance analysis for estimation of total body potassium, total body water, and fat-free mass in white, black, and Asian adults. *Am. J. Hum. Biol.* 7:33, 1995.

Wang, Z. M., et al.: The five-level model: a new approach to organizing body composition research. *Am. J. Clin. Nutr.* 56:19, 1992.

Williams, M.J., et al.: Regional fat distribution in women and risk of cardiovascular disease. *Am. J. Clin. Nutr.*, 65:855, 1997.

Wilmore, J. H., et al.: Alterations in body weight and composition consequent to 20 wk of endurance training: the HERITAGE Family Study. *Am. J. Clin. Nutr.* 70:346, 1999.

CHAPTER

19

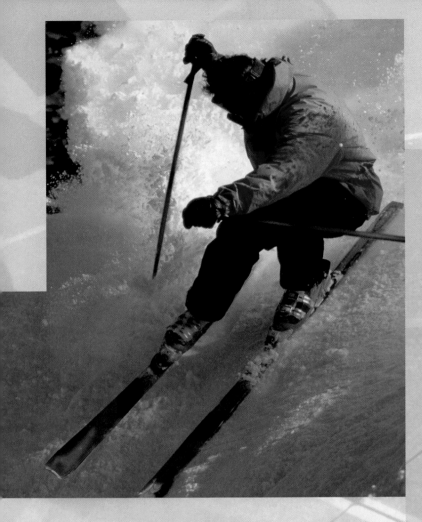

Topics covered in this chapter

PART 1 Obesity

Obesity: A Long-Term Process
Not Necessarily Overeating
Health Risks of Obesity
How Fat is Too Fat?
Summary

PART 2 Achieving Optimal Body Composition Through Diet and Exercise

The Energy Balance Equation
Dieting to Tip the Energy Balance Equation
Exercising to Tip the Energy Balance Equation
Diet Plus Exercise: The Ideal Combination
Gaining Weight
Summary
Thought Questions
Selected References

Obesity, Exercise, and Weight Control

- Describe the current status of overweight and obesity among American adults and children.

- List ten significant health risks of obesity.

- Describe each of the following as a criterion for obesity: (a) percent body fat, (b) body fat distribution, and (c) fat cell size and number.

- Define fat cell hypertrophy and fat cell hyperplasia. Explain how each contributes to obesity, and how each becomes modified with changes in body weight.

- Compare fat cell size and fat cell number for individuals with average body fat and those classified as massively obese.

- Outline how "unbalancing" the energy balance equation affects body weight.

- Summarize why proponents of the "setpoint theory" argue that dieting offers little benefit for long-term weight loss.

- Explain the meaning and implications of weight cycling.

- Present the rationale for including regular physical activity in a prudent weight loss program.

- Explain how a moderate increase in physical activity for a previously sedentary, overweight person affects: (a) daily food intake, and (b) overall energy expenditure on a short- and long-term basis.

- Explain the rationale for and effectiveness of specific exercise for localized fat loss.

- Give diet and exercise advice to a person who wants to gain weight to improve appearance or enhance sports performance.

Americans consume more fat per capita than any other nation. They also consume more than 90% of foods high in saturated fatty acids and processed, high-glycemic carbohydrates. A national preoccupation with food and effortless living caused 55% of American men and women to become overweight and almost 50 million to classify as obese. Equally disturbing is the fact that 15 to 20% of American children and 12% of adolescents (up from 7.6% in 1976–1980) classify as overweight. Obesity represents this age group's most chronic disorder, particularly prevalent among poor and minority children.

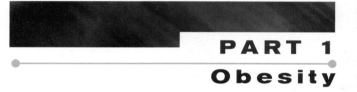

PART 1
Obesity

Obesity: A Long-Term Process

Obesity frequently begins in childhood. For these children, the chances of becoming obese adults increase three-fold compared with children of normal body mass. Simply stated, a child usually does not grow out of obesity. Tracking body weight through generations indicates that obese parents likely give birth to children who become overweight and whose offspring also often become overweight.

Excessive fatness also develops slowly through adulthood, most weight gain occurring between the ages of 25 to 44 years. In one longitudinal study, fat content of 27 adult men increased an average of 6.5 kg over a 12-year period from age 32 to 44 years. Women gained the most weight; about 14% gained 13.6 kg (30 lb) between ages 25 and 34. The typical American man (beginning at age 30) and woman (beginning at age 27) gains between 0.2 to 0.8 kg (0.5 to 1.8 lb) of body weight each year until age 60, despite a progressive decrease in total food intake. Whether this **creeping obesity** during adulthood reflects a normal biologic pattern of aging remains unknown.

Not Necessarily Overeating

If obesity existed as a singular disorder, with gluttony and overindulgence as causative factors, decreasing food intake would provide the most effective means to permanently reduce weight. Obviously, other influences, such as genetic, environmental, social, and perhaps racial interact. Proposed factors that predispose a person to excessive weight gain include eating patterns, eating environment, food packaging, body image, biochemical differences related to resting metabolic rate, basal body temperature, dietary-induced thermogenesis, spontaneous activity or fidgeting, quantity of and sensitivity to satiety hormones, levels of cellular adenosine triphosphatase, lipoprotein lipase and other enzymes, presence of metabolically active brown adipose tissue, and physical inactivity.

Regardless of the specific causes of obesity and their interactions, common treatment procedures — diets, surgery, drugs, psychologic methods, and exercise, either alone or in combination — have not succeeded on a long-term basis. Nonetheless, researchers continue to strive to devise effective strategies to prevent and treat this national health affliction.

Genetics Play a Role

Genetic makeup does not necessarily cause obesity, but it does lower the threshold for its development; it contributes significantly to differences in weight gain for individuals fed an identical daily caloric excess. Figure 19.1 summarizes findings from a large number of individuals representing nine different types of relations. Genetic factors determined about 25% of the transmissible variation among people in percent body fat and total fat mass, whereas the largest transmissible variation related to a cultural effect. *In an obesity-producing environment (sedentary and stressful,*

The Supersizing of America

Despite all of the recent discoveries in obesity research, including the identification of obesity genes, and appetite- and satiety-regulating hormones, substantial changes in genetic makeup cannot account for the rapid increase in obesity among Americans over the last 20 years. More than one-half of the United States population are now overweight, and 25% classify as obese. Researchers maintain that if this trend continues, the entire population could be overweight within a few generations. More than likely, the culprits in the fattening of America are a sedentary lifestyle and the ready availability of tasty, lipid- and calorie-rich foods, currently served in increasingly larger portions. Despite an outright obesity epidemic (with notable associated health implications), weight control remains low on the list of national public health priorities.

with easy access to calorie-dense food), the genetically susceptible individual gains weight. Athletes with a genetic propensity for obesity often battle to achieve and maintain an optimal body size and composition for competitive performance.

A Mutant Gene?

Research with a strain of mice that enlarge to five times normal size provides evidence to support the important genetic contribution to body weight and body fat deposition. The mutation of a gene, called *obese* or simply *ob*, probably disrupts hormonal signals that regulate the animal's appetite, metabolism, and fat storage, causing energy balance to tip towards fat accumulation.

Figure 19.2 proposes that the *ob* gene, normally activated in adi-

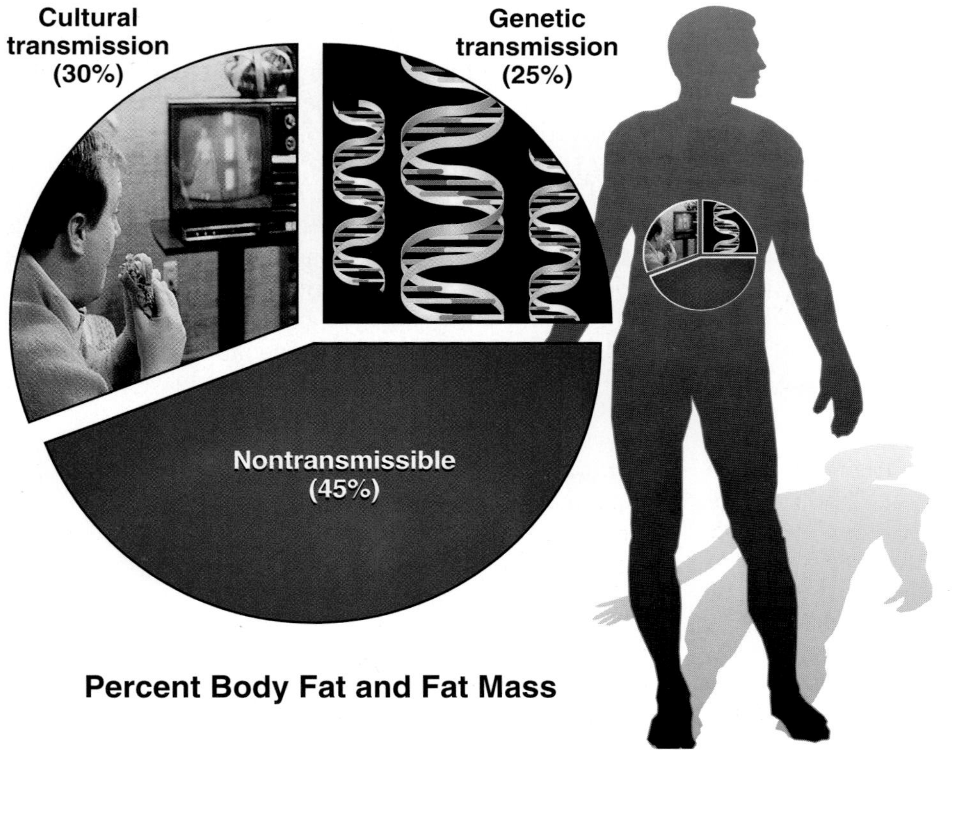

Cultural transmission (30%)

Genetic transmission (25%)

Nontransmissible (45%)

Percent Body Fat and Fat Mass

Figure 19.1
Total transmissible variance for body fat. Total body fat and percent body fat determined by hydrostatic weighing. (Data from Bouchard, C., et al.: Inheritance of the amount and distribution of human body fat. *Int. J. Obes.*, 12:205, 1988.)

close up

Television and Childhood Obesity

The prevalence and persistence of childhood obesity represents a bona fide national health calamity. As many as 25–30% of American children can be classified as overweight, and the number of extremely obese children has increased steadily in the last 10 years. As with adults, obesity prevention and treatment in the young remains extremely difficult, regardless of the strategy applied. As many as 90% of children who lose weight revert rapidly to their initial body weight percentile ranking, a process complicated by normal growth and development.

Although the precise contribution of exercise and diet to childhood obesity remains unclear, an interesting line of research has focused on obesity's relationship to television watching. Children in the U.S. spend as much time in front of the TV each year as they do attending school. Estimates indicate that children ages 6 to 11 years watch TV an average of 26 hours weekly, whereas adolescents spend about 22 hours each week in front of the television.

Television viewing also links to obesity; each hourly increment of weekly TV watching by adolescents reflects a 2% increase in obesity prevalence. (A similar pattern emerges for adults; men who view more than 3 hours of daily TV increase their likelihood for obesity to twice that of men who view TV less than 1 hour daily.) The question remains: Does the sedentary nature of TV-watching causally contribute to obesity, or does the TV-obesity association merely reflect the fact that the obese condition causes one to become sedentary, and watching TV provides a pleasant sedentary pastime.

To answer this question, researchers assessed energy metabolism in 15 obese and 16 normal-weight girls (average age 10.2 y) for 25 minutes during rest and during rest when viewing TV. The inset figure illustrates that watching television depressed the resting metabolism by 15% in obese girls and 17% in nonobese girls. Because obese children watch more daily TV than normal-weight peers, the cumulative effect of a depressed metabolic rate while viewing TV exerts greater impact on the obese. Children who watch excessive television increase their risk for obesity; their resting energy expenditure drops below the value obtained if they did nothing at all!

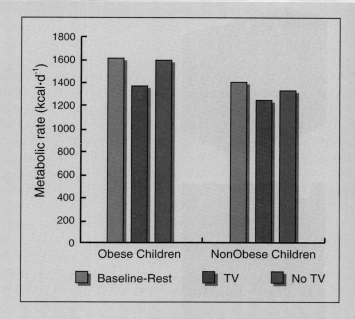

The acute decrease in energy expenditure during TV viewing supports a causal relationship between time spent watching television and excessive weight gain. A vicious cycle develops because children also tend to snack with high-calorie foods while watching television. These findings become worrisome when coupled with the fact that 30% of American children average less than 30 minutes of daily physical activity.

The authors of this text believe that parents, teachers, and school administrators should encourage children to exercise 1 hour per day during the elementary school years. Eliminating required physical education in the elementary school curriculum contributes to the national obesity epidemic. Avocating regular exercise is one way to help.

References

Anderson, R. E., et al.: Relationship of physical activity and television watching with body weight and level of fatness among children. *JAMA*, 279:938, 1998.

Kliegs, R. C. et al.: Effects of television on metabolic rate: potential implications for childhood obesity. *Pediatrics*, 91 : 281, 1993.

pose tissue, produces **leptin**, a satiety hormone that influences the appetite control center in the hypothalamus. Normally, leptin blunts the urge to eat when caloric intake maintains sufficient fat stores. In this way, body fat level and the brain intimately connect through a physiologic pathway that regulates caloric intake. A defective gene causes inadequate leptin production. As a result, the brain receives an under assessment of the body's adipose status, and the urge to eat outstrips the energy needed to maintain a desirable body fat level. This biological control mecha-

nism compliments the setpoint theory (refer to Part 2) to explain excessive body fat accumulation. It also clarifies why obese individuals find it extremely difficult to sustain significant losses in body fat.

The genetic connection to obesity provides a sound rationale for viewing the overfat condition as a disease, rather than some psychological flaw or personality weakness that one could correct with sufficient willpower. The discovery of the *ob* gene does not herald an instant "cure" for the obese condition. Human obesity results from a complex interac-

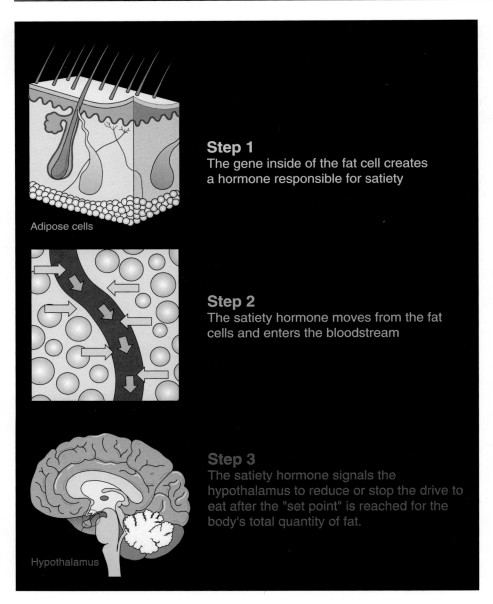

Step 1
The gene inside of the fat cell creates a hormone responsible for satiety

Adipose cells

Step 2
The satiety hormone moves from the fat cells and enters the bloodstream

Step 3
The satiety hormone signals the hypothalamus to reduce or stop the drive to eat after the "set point" is reached for the body's total quantity of fat.

Hypothalamus

Figure 19.2
Genetic model for obesity. A malfunction of the satiety gene affects production of the satiety hormone leptin. Underproduction of leptin disrupts proper function of the hypothalamus (Step #3), the center responsible for regulating the body's fat level. (Model based on research conducted at Rockefeller University, New York).

feelings of hunger and deprivation that often accompany conventional diet plans. Identifying a genetic predisposition toward obesity early in life may someday provide a way to curtail obesity before it becomes firmly established.

Physical Activity: An Important Component

Maintaining a physically active lifestyle blunts the "normal" tendency to gain fat during adulthood. For young and middle-age men who exercised regularly, time spent in physical activity related inversely to body fat level – the more exercise, the less body fat. Surprisingly, *no relationship* emerged between body fat and caloric intake. This suggests that less demanding activity, not greater food intake, produced the greater body fat levels observed among the active middle-age men compared with younger, more active counterparts.

tion of factors and influences. However, scientists continue to research drugs that mimic satiety proteins or affect the sensitivity of the brain's receptors to such chemicals. This would produce satiety with a smaller caloric intake and less

Health Risks of Obesity

In 1998, *obesity joined cigarette smoking, hypertension, elevated serum cholesterol, and physical inactivity in the American Heart Association's list of primary coronary heart disease risk factors.* Clear associations exist between obesity and hypertension, type 2 diabetes, and various lipid abnormalities (**dyslipidemia**), in addition to increased risk of cerebrovascular disease, alterations in fatty acid metabolism, and atherosclerosis. However, health risks do not confront every obese person. *Indeed, evidence accumulated over the last 15 years confirms the heterogeneous nature of obesity, not only its cause(s) but also its complications.* Nevertheless, obesity should be viewed as a chronic

Leptin Plus Other Factors

Leptin alone does not determine obesity or explain why some people eat what they want and gain little weight, while others become obese for the same caloric intake. In addition to deficient leptin production, scientists also propose the possibility of defective receptor action (via a leptin receptor molecule on brain cells), which increases an individual's resistance to satiety chemicals produced by the body.

Potent Heart Disease Risk

An 8-year study of nearly 116,000 female nurses concluded that all but the thinnest women showed increased risk for heart attack and chest pains. Women of average body mass had 30% more heart attacks than women of low body mass, while the risk for moderately overweight nurses averaged 80% higher than for the lightest women. Women who gained just 9 kg (20 lb) from their late teens to middle age doubled their heart attack risk.

medical condition because multiple biologic hazards of premature illness and death exist at surprisingly low levels of excess body fat. Staggering economic expenses arise from obesity-related medical complications; in the year 2000, 12% of the cost of illness in the US will relate to excessive body fatness.

How Fat Is Too Fat?

Although the body mass index currently provides the most popular surrogate measure to infer body fat (see *How to Calculate and Intrepret Body Mass Index*), three criteria can directly evaluate a person's body fat status:

1. Percent body fat
2. Fat patterning
3. Fat cell size and number

Percent Body Fat

The demarcation between normal body fat levels and obesity often becomes arbitrary. In Chapter 18, we identified the normal range of body fat in adult men and women as at least plus or minus one unit of variation (standard deviation) from the average population value. That variation unit equals 5% body fat for men and women between ages 17 and 50 years. Within this statistical boundary, overfatness corresponds to any percent body fat value above the average value for age and gender, plus 5 percentage points. For young men, whose fat mass averages 15% of body mass, borderline obesity equals 20% body fat. For older men, average percent fat equals about 25%. Consequently, a body fat content in excess of 30% represents overfatness for this group. For young women, obesity corresponds to a body fat content above 30%, while for older women borderline obesity begins at 37% body fat.

The use of age-specific demarcations for obesity assumes that men and women normally become fatter with age. However, this does not necessarily occur for physically active older men and women. If lifestyle actually accounts for the greatest portion of body fat increase during adulthood,

then the criterion for overfatness could justifiably represent the standard for younger men and women:

Men: >20% body fat
Women: >30% body fat

Gradations of obesity progress from the upper limit of normal to as high as 50 to 70% of body mass. Common terms for gradations in obesity include pleasantly plump for those just above the cut-off, to the more clinical demarcations of moderately obese, massively obese, and morbidly obese. The last category includes people who weigh in the range of 170 to 275 kg (385 to 600 lb) and whose fat content exceeds 55%. In such cases, body fat can exceed fat-free body mass (FFM), and obesity becomes life threatening.

Fat Patterning

Fat cells (**adipocytes**) display remarkable diversity depending on their anatomic location. Some cells efficiently "capture" excess nutrient calories from the bloodstream and synthesize them into triglycerides for storage, while others accumulate triglycerides but also readily release this stored energy for use by other tissues. This explains why certain fat deposits resist reduction while others change readily in response to the body's energy balance. *Patterning of adipose tissue distribution, independent of total body fat and body mass, alters the health risk from obesity.*

Studies using MRI and CT-scanning to (refer to Chapter 18) precisely discriminate subcutaneous from visceral (intra-abdominal) adipose tissue (V-AT) show that V-AT accumulation relates to an altered metabolic profile that includes:

- Hyperinsulinemia
- Insulin resistance and glucose intolerance
- Hypertriglyceridemia
- Reduced high-density lipoprotein (HDL) cholesterol concentrations
- Increased apolipoprotein B, the regulatory protein constituent of the harmful low-density lipoprotein (LDL) cholesterol

Proposed Types of Obesity

Type	Location of Excess Fat
I	Total body (most common)
II	Subcutaneous fat on the trunk (android)
III	Subcutaneous fat in the lower body (gynoid)
IV	Visceral fat in abdomen (intra-abdominal fat)

(Proposed by Dr. Claude Bouchard, Executive Director, Pennington Biomedical Research Center, Baton Rouge, LA)

Excessive insulin production and depressed insulin sensitivity that characterize V-AT obesity not only increase risk for type 2 diabetes, but also risk for ischemic heart disease. *Thus, visceral obesity constitutes an additional component of the insulin-resistant, **dyslipidemic syndrome**, which represents the most prevalent cause of coronary artery disease in industrialized countries.*

The importance of body fat distribution in the clinical assessment of obese patients first emerged in 1947, and has been confirmed in subsequent epidemiological studies. A preferential abdominal fat accumulation, first described as **android obesity** (male-pattern or central obesity), exists largely among overweight patients with hypertension, type 2 diabetes, and coronary heart disease. This contrasts to the lower health risks of **gynoid obesity** (female-pattern or peripheral obesity), where the majority of excess fat deposits in the body's gluteal and femoral regions.

The **waist-to-hip girth ratio (WHR)** provides an initial clinical assessment of V-AT. In general, ratios exceeding 0.80 for women and 0.95 for men indicate excessive visceral fat accumulation, which predicts increased risk of

Waist Girth —The Second Dimension of Obesity

The following presents gender-neutral guidelines for abdominal girth measurements corresponding to visceral adipose tissue equal to and exceeding the "risky" internal quantity of 130 cm².

Age	Waist Girth
<40 years	≥100 cm (39.4 in)
40–60 years	≥ 90 cm (35.4 in)

death from coronary artery disease and other illnesses with greater accuracy than the popular measurement of BMI.

The accompanying *How to Calculate and Interpret the Waist-to-Hip Girth Ratio* (page 537) describes measurement procedures and health implications of this important measure.

As a substitute for WHR, waist circumference by itself gives a good anthropometric indication of V-AT. For this reason, we recommend that either WHR or waist girth be used as the **second dimension of obesity** (% body fat being the first dimension) in comprehensive assessment of body composition and health risk profile.

To some extent, people inherit their unique pattern of fat distribution. Variations in regional activity of lipoprotein lipase (LPL), the rate-limiting enzyme for triglyceride uptake by adipocytes, probably govern one's patterning of fat on the body. Changes in LPL activity level also may explain changes in fat distribution that occur during pregnancy and in middle age.

Fat Cell Size and Number

The size and number of fat cells provide a view of the structure, form, and dimensions of normal and abnormal levels of body fatness. Increased in adipose tissue mass occurs in two ways:

1. Enlarging (filling) of existing fat cells with more fat — **fat cell hypertrophy**
2. Increasing the total number of fat cells — **fat cell hyperplasia**

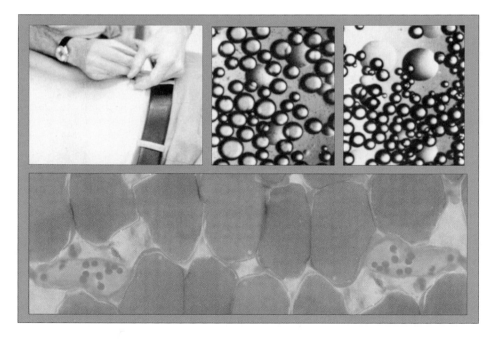

Figure 19.3
Upper panel: Needle biopsy procedure to extract fat cells of the upper buttocks region. The area is sterilized, anesthetized, and the biopsy needle placed beneath the skin surface. The syringe sucks small tissue fragments from the site. The two photomicrographs at right indicate that fat cells biopsied from the buttocks of a physically active professor prior to and after 6-months of marathon training. The average fat cell diameter averaged 8.6% smaller following training. The volume of fat in each cell decreased by 18.2%. The large spherical structures in the background represent intracellular lipid droplets. (Photomicrographs courtesy of P.M. Clarkson, Muscle Biochemistry Laboratory, University of Massachusetts, Amherst, MA.) **Bottom panel:** Cross-section of human fat cells magnified × 440. (From Geneser, F.: *Color Atlas of Histology*. Philadelphia, Lea & Febiger, 1985.)

The technique for assessing adipocyte size and number involves sucking small fragments of subcutaneous tissue, usually from the upper back, buttocks, abdomen, and back of the upper arm, into a syringe through a needle inserted directly into the fat depot (Fig. 19.3). Chemical treatment of the biopsy sample enables the researcher to separate and count the fat cells. Dividing the amount of fat in the sample by the total number of cells it contains determines the average quantity of fat per cell. The body's quantity of total fat divided by the average fat content per cell reasonably estimates total fat cell number.

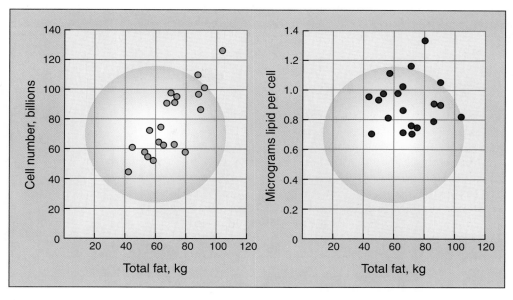

Figure 19.4
Adipose cell number (**left**) and size (**right**) related to the body's total fat mass.

Fat Cell Size and Number in Normal and Obese Adults

The data in the left side of Figure 19.4 demonstrate the strong association between total fat mass in obese individuals and their number of fat cells. The person with the lowest body fat content had the fewest number of fat cells, while the fattest subject had considerably more adipocytes. On the other hand, the data displayed in the right panel of Figure 19.4 show little relationship between total body fat and average fat cell size in the obese. This suggests that a biologic upper limit exists for fat cell size. After reaching this size, cell number probably becomes the key factor that determines the extent of extreme obesity. Even if the size of normal fat cells doubled, this would not account for the tremendous difference in the fat content between obese and nonobese people. The excessive adipose tissue mass in severe obesity, therefore, must occur by fat cell hyperplasia. As a frame of reference, an average person has about 25 to 30 billion fat cells. For the moderately obese this number ranges between 60 and 100 billion, whereas fat cell number for the massively obese may increase to 310 billion or more.

Fat Cell Size and Number After Weight Loss

Figure 19.5 shows that when obese adults reduce body mass and total fat to normal levels, individual fat cells shrink to a size actually smaller than the adipocytes of people who have never been obese. In this study, 19 obese subjects who initially weighed 149 kg reduced body mass by 45.8 kg, weighing 103 kg at the end of the first part of the experiment. Prior to weight reduction the number of fat

cells averaged 75 billion. This number remained essentially unchanged with weight reduction. The average size of the fat cells, on the other hand, decreased by 33% from 0.9 μg to a normal value of 0.6 μg of fat per cell. Subjects attained a normal body mass when they lost an additional 28 kg. Cell number again remained unchanged, while cell size continued to shrink to about one-third the size of the fat cells in normal, nonobese subjects. Other experiments have confirmed these findings in young children and adults.

The formerly obese person who reduces body mass and body fat to near average values still does not become "cured" of obesity, at least in terms of adipocyte number. Clinical evidence reveals that formerly obese individuals find it difficult to maintain their new body size. Perhaps the large number of relatively small fat cells in the reduced obese somehow relate to appetite control, and the person craves food, overeats, and regains lost weight (fat). This certainly makes sense within the framework of the body fat-hormone (leptin)-satiety interaction discussed previously (page 530).

Three general periods relate to significant increases in the number of fat cells:

1. Last trimester of pregnancy
2. First year of life
3. Adolescent growth spurt

The total number of fat cells probably cannot be altered to any significant degree during adulthood; an exception occurs in extreme adult obesity, in which further cell proliferation takes place. A fundamental question remains:

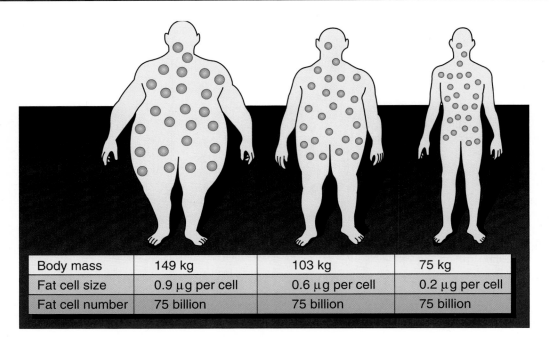

Body mass	149 kg	103 kg	75 kg
Fat cell size	0.9 µg per cell	0.6 µg per cell	0.2 µg per cell
Fat cell number	75 billion	75 billion	75 billion

Figure 19.5
Changes in adipose cellularity with weight reduction in obese subjects (Data from Hirsch, J.: Adipose cellularity in relation to human obesity. In: *Advances in Internal Medicine*, Vol. 17. Stollerman, G. H. (ed.). Chicago: Year Book, 1971.)

Can fat cell number be altered before adulthood, or do certain genes code for hypercellularity and extreme obesity?

Fat Cell Size and Number After Weight Gain

Nonobese subjects with no prior personal or family history of obesity, increased body mass an average of 16.4 kg from voluntary overeating. In comparisons of cell size and number before and after the 4-month weight gain, average adipocyte size increased substantially with *no change* in cell number. When subjects reduced to normal weight through caloric restriction, total body fat decreased and the adipocytes returned to their original size. Thus, fat acquisition in adults who overeat occurs primarily by filling existing adipocytes with more lipid, rather than from an increase in new fat cells.

New Fat Cells Can Develop In adult-onset, severe obesity, if the person becomes even fatter, new adipocytes develop in addition to the hypertrophy of existing cells. This probably occurs because fat cells have an upper-size limit of about 1.0 µg of lipid per cell. In the massively obese (60% body fat; 170% of normal weight), almost all adipocytes achieve a hypertrophic limit; for the person to become fatter, new cells must proliferate from a preadipocyte cell pool.

How to Calculate and Interpret Body Mass Index

The body mass index (BMI) represents the ratio of body mass (weight, Wt) to stature (height, Ht) squared.

$$BMI = Body\ mass \div Stature^2$$

BMI and Overweightness

In June, 1998, the National Institutes of Health, National Heart, Lung, and Blood Institute, and National Institute of Diabetes and Digestive and Kidney Diseases, released the first Federal Guidelines for identifying, evaluating, and treating overweight and obesity. The new classifications based on BMI are as follows:

Classification	BMI Score
Underweight	<18.5
Normal	18.5–24.9
Overweight	25.0–29.9
Obesity Class I	30.0–34.9
Obesity Class II	35.0–39.9
Extreme obesity	>40.0

The Guidelines have fueled controversy among health professionals because previous guidelines established overweight at a BMI of 27 (not 25). The lowering of the demarcation that differentiates overweight propels an additional 30 million Americans into the overweight category. This now means that 55% of the U.S. population qualifies as overweight. In contrast to these new guidelines, others recommend a transitional BMI range of 25 to 26 as a *Caution Zone* for overweight.

BMI and Health Risk

The BMI predicts body fat and disease risk better than the popular height-weight tables. A high BMI links to increased risk of death from all causes, hypertension, cardiovascular disease, dyslipidemia, diabetes, sleep apnea, osteoarthritis, and female infertility. Competitive athletes and body builders with a high BMI due to increased muscle mass, and pregnant or lactating women, should not use BMI to infer overweightness or relative disease risk. Also, the BMI does not apply to growing children or frail and sedentary elderly adults.

BMI Score	Health Risk
>25	Minimal
25–27	Low
27–30	Moderate
30–<35	High
35–<40	Very High
>40	Extremely High

Calculations

Male: Wt, 149 lb (67.6 kg); Ht, 5 feet 5 inches (65 in; 1.651 m)

$BMI = Body\ mass\ (kg) \div (Stature\ [m] \times Stature\ [m])$
$= 67.6\ kg \div (1.651\ m \times 1.651\ m)$
$= 67.6\ kg \div 2.726\ m^2$
$= 24.8\ kg \cdot m^{-2}$ or 24.8

To calculate BMI with non-metric data, apply the following formula:

$BMI = Wt\ (lb) \times 703 \div (Ht\ [in] \times Ht\ [in])$
$= 149\ lb \times 703 \div (65\ in \times 65\ in)$
$= 104,747\ lb \div 4225\ in^2$
$= 24.8\ lb \cdot in^{-2}$ or 24.8

Reference

Calle, E.E., et al.: Body-mass index and mortality in a prospective cohort of U.S. Adults. N. Engl. J. Med., 341:1097, 1999.

BODY MASS INDEX

Weight, lbs / Height	100	105	110	115	120	125	130	135	140	145	150	155	160	165	170	175	180	185	190	195	200	205
5'0"	20	21	21	22	23	24	25	26	27	28	29	30	31	32	33	34	35	36	37	38	39	40
5'1"	19	20	21	22	23	24	25	26	26	27	28	29	30	31	32	33	34	35	36	37	38	39
5'2"	18	19	20	21	22	23	24	25	26	27	27	28	29	30	31	32	33	34	35	36	37	37
5'3"	18	19	19	20	21	22	23	24	25	26	27	27	28	29	30	31	32	33	34	35	35	36
5'4"	17	18	19	20	21	21	22	23	24	25	26	27	27	28	29	30	31	32	33	33	34	35
5'5"	17	17	18	19	20	21	22	22	23	24	25	26	27	27	28	29	30	31	32	32	33	34
5'6"	16	17	18	19	19	20	21	22	23	23	24	25	26	27	27	28	29	30	31	31	32	33
5'7"	16	16	17	18	19	20	20	21	22	23	23	24	25	26	27	27	28	29	30	31	31	32
5'8"	15	16	17	17	18	19	20	21	21	22	23	24	24	25	26	27	27	28	29	30	30	31
5'9"	15	16	16	17	18	18	19	20	21	21	22	23	24	24	25	26	27	27	28	29	30	30
5'10"	14	15	16	17	17	18	19	19	20	21	22	22	23	24	24	25	26	27	27	28	29	29
5'11"	14	15	15	16	17	17	18	19	20	20	21	22	22	23	24	24	25	26	26	27	28	29
6'0"	14	14	15	16	16	17	18	18	19	20	20	21	22	22	23	24	24	25	26	26	27	28
6'1"	13	14	15	15	16	16	17	18	18	19	20	20	21	22	22	23	24	24	25	26	26	27
6'2"	13	13	14	15	15	16	17	17	18	19	19	20	21	21	22	22	23	24	24	25	26	26
6'3"	12	13	14	14	15	16	16	17	17	18	19	19	20	21	21	22	23	23	24	24	25	26
6'4"	12	12	13	14	15	15	16	16	17	18	18	19	19	20	21	21	22	23	23	24	24	25

How to Calculate and Interpret the Waist-to-Hip Girth Ratio

Waist-to-hip girth ratio (WHR) indicates relative fat distribution in adults and risk of disease (see table). A higher ratio reflects a greater proportion of abdominal fat with greater risk for hyperinsulinemia, insulin resistance, type 2 diabetes, endometrial cancer, hypercholesterolemia, hypertension, and atherosclerosis.

WHR computes as abdominal girth (cm or in) ÷ hip girth (cm or in); waist girth represents the smallest girth around the abdomen (the natural waist), and hip girth reflects the largest girth measured around the buttocks (see figure).

WAIST–HIP RATIO AND RELATIVE DISEASE RISK

| | Age, y | \multicolumn{4}{c}{Risk Level} | | | |
		Low	Moderate	High	Very High
Men	20–29	<0.83	0.83–0.88	0.89–0.94	>0.94
	30–39	<0.84	0.84–0.91	0.92–0.96	>0.96
	40–49	<0.88	0.88–0.95	0.96–1.00	>1.00
	50–59	<0.90	0.90–0.96	0.97–1.02	>1.02
	60–69	<0.91	0.91–0.98	0.99–1.03	>1.03
Women	20–29	<0.71	0.71–0.77	0.78–0.82	>0.82
	30–39	<0.72	0.72–0.78	0.79–0.84	>0.84
	40–49	<0.73	0.73–0.79	0.80–0.87	>0.87
	50–59	<0.74	0.74–0.81	0.82–0.88	>0.88
	60–69	<0.76	0.76–0.83	0.84–0.90	>0.90

Calculating WHR

Example #1

Male: age, 21 y; abdominal girth, 101.6 cm; hip girth, 93.5 cm.

WHR = abdominal girth (cm) ÷ hip girth (cm)

= 101.6 ÷ 93.5

= 1.08 (very high relative disease risk)

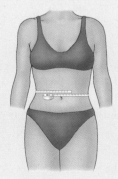 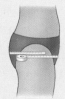

Abdomen: Minimum girth; standing, feet together

Hips: Maximum girth around buttocks; standing, feet together

Example #2

Female: age 41 y; abdominal girth, 83.2 cm; hip girth, 101 cm.

WHR = abdomen girth (cm) ÷ hip girth (cm)

= 83.2 ÷ 101

= 0.82 (high relative disease risk)

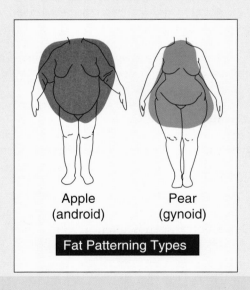

Apple (android)   Pear (gynoid)

Fat Patterning Types

summary

1. Obesity, defined as an excessive quantity of body fat, represents a complex disorder in which interrelated factors tip energy balance in favor of weight gain. Physical inactivity (and accompanying reduced energy expenditure) plays a significant contributory role in the dynamics of gaining weight.

2. Numerous health risks accompany relatively low levels of excess body fat. These include increased risk for hypertension, coronary heart disease, type 2 diabetes, renal disease, abnormal blood lipids, gallbladder and pulmonary disease, and various types of cancer.

3. Probably no biologic reason fully accounts for the typical body fat increases observed for American

men and women with aging. Therefore, body fat standards for borderline overfatness in adult men and women could justifiably be the values for younger adults: 20% body fat for men and 30% for women.

4. Adipose tissue patterning on the body provides important health-related information. Fat distributed in the abdominal-visceral region (android-type obesity) poses a greater health risk compared to fat deposited at the thigh, hips, and buttocks (gynoid-type obesity).

5. Either the waist-to-hip ratio or abdominal girth provides a second dimension of obesity and should be included in assessing the obesity health-risk profile. Abdominal girth in excess of 100 cm for men and women less than 40 years of age, and 90 cm for ages 40 to 60 years, increases the risk for heart disease, hypertension, and type II diabetes.

6. Another obesity classification evaluates the size and number of adipocytes. Before adulthood, body fat increases by (a) enlargement of individual fat cells (fat cell hypertrophy), and (b) increases in total number of fat cells (fat cell hyperplasia). Because cell size probably reaches some biologic upper limit, cell number plays the key role determining the ultimate extent of obesity.

7. Increases in fat cell number generally involve three broad time periods: last trimester of pregnancy, first year of life, and adolescent growth spurt before adulthood.

8. Adipocyte number stabilizes sometime before adulthood; any weight gain or loss thereafter usually relates to a change in fat cell size. In extreme obesity, cell number can increase once adipocytes reach their hypertrophic limit.

PART 2
Achieving Optimal Body Composition Through Diet and Exercise

The following statement by renowned University of Pennsylvania obesity specialist Dr. Albert Stunkard presents a realistic view about the possibility of long-term weight loss for the obese: "Most obese persons will not stay in treatment. Of those who stay in treatment, most will not lose weight, and of those who do lose weight, most will regain it."

This bleak outlook delivered three decades ago buttresses the majority of subsequent research showing that initial modifications in body composition have little relation to long-term success. Participants who remain in supervised weight-loss programs lose about 10% of their original body mass. Unfortunately, individuals typically regain one- to two-thirds of the lost weight within 1 year, and almost all of it within 5 years. Figure 19.6 illustrates that over a 7.3-year follow-up of 121 patients, the tendency to regain lost weight occurred independent of length of fasting (up to 2 months), extent of weight loss (up to 41.4 kg), or age at obesity onset. One-half of the subjects returned to their original weight within 3 years, and only 7 patients remained at their reduced body weight. Such discouraging statistics indicate the difficulty in sustaining long-term weight loss, particularly in the relaxed atmosphere of one's home, which often provides ready access to food and little emotional support. While prognosis for long-term success remains poor, some individuals achieve success. These men and women frequently lose one-third of their original weight and keep it off for a lifetime (see Masters of Weight Loss, page 543).

The annual intake of food in the United States averages

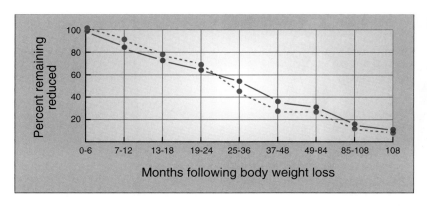

Figure 19.6
Percent of patients remaining at reduced body weights at various time intervals following accomplished weight loss. The red line represents 60 subjects with obesity onset before age 21; green line indicates 42 subjects with obesity onset after age 21. (Data from Johnson, D, and Drenick, E.J.: Therapeutic fasting in morbid obesity. *Arch. Intern. Med.*, 137: 1381, 1977.)

nearly 1985 pounds (900 kg) and includes 280 eggs, 15 pounds (7 kg) of breakfast cereal, 185 pounds (84 kg) of meat, 200 pounds (91 kg) of fruit, 251 pounds (114 kg) of vegetables, 68 pounds (31 kg) of bread, 429 soft drinks, 2 gallons (8 L) of wine, 25 gallons (96 L) of beer, and 2 gallons (8 L) of liquor! The fact that many adults' body mass fluctuates only slightly during the year illustrates the body's exquisite potential for regulatory control in balancing energy intake with energy expenditure. Only when calories from food exceed the daily energy requirement do calories accumulate as fat in adipose tissue. An effective weight control program must establish a chronic balance between energy input and energy output.

The Energy Balance Equation

The rationale underlying the **energy balance equation** forms the basis for a weight-loss program. Figure 19.7 (top) shows the ideal situation where energy input (calories in food) balances energy output (calories expended in daily physical activities) to maintain a desirable body mass. The middle part of the figure depicts what happens all too frequently when energy input exceeds energy output. Under such conditions, calories store as fat in adipose tissue. Thirty-five hundred "extra" kcal through either increased

> **Excess Calories Accumulate Fat**
>
> Each 0.45 kg (1 lb) of adipose tissue contains about 87% pure lipid or 3500 kcal (395 g × 9 kcal · g^{-1}). An excess of 3500 kcals consumed accumulates 0.45 kg of extra fat. This cannot be undone by magic potions, trick diets, or special formula foods.

energy intake or decreased energy output equals the energy equivalent of 1 pound (0.45 kg) of stored body fat (adipose tissue). The bottom of the figure illustrates what occurs when energy intake falls below energy output. In this case, the body obtains required calories from its energy stores, with a reduction in body mass and body fat.

Three ways "unbalance" the energy balance equation to cause weight loss:

1. Maintain caloric output and decrease caloric intake below daily energy requirements
2. Maintain caloric intake and increase caloric output above daily requirements through additional physical activity
3. Combine methods 1 and 2 by decreasing daily food intake and increasing daily energy expenditure

To appreciate the sensitivity of the energy balance equation for weight control, consider what happens when daily calorie intake exceeds output by only 100 kcal. This could occur by eating just one banana extra each day. Annually, the "extra" number of ingested calories equals 36,500 kcal (365 days × 100 kcal). Because 0.45 kg (1 lb) of body fat contains about 3500 kcal, the small daily increase in caloric intake would cause a yearly gain of 4.7 kg (10.4 lb) of body fat. If this energy imbalance continued, then theoretically fat mass would increase by 23.6 kg (52 lb) over 5 years. On the other hand, reducing daily food intake by only 100 kcal and increasing energy expenditure a similar amount by walking one extra mile each day would reduce total body fat by 9.5 kg (21 lb) in a year!

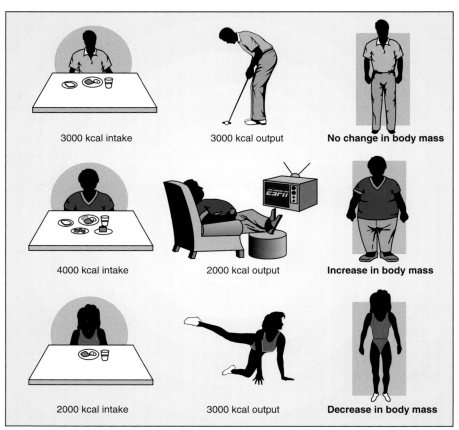

3000 kcal intake	3000 kcal output	**No change in body mass**
4000 kcal intake	2000 kcal output	**Increase in body mass**
2000 kcal intake	3000 kcal output	**Decrease in body mass**

Figure 19.7
The energy balance equation.

Personal Assessment

An objective assessment of food intake and energy expenditure provides the frame of reference for unbalancing the energy balance equation to favorably modify body mass and body composition.

Energy Intake

Estimates of caloric intake from daily food intake records (refer to Section II of the Student Study Guide and Workbook) usually fall within 10% of the number of calories actually consumed. For example, suppose the energy value of a person's daily food intake (directly measured in the bomb calorimeter) averaged 2130 kcal. By use of a careful 3-day dietary history to estimate caloric intake, the daily value would fall between 1920 and 2350 kcal.

Careful record keeping of food intake also provides the dieter with an objective list of foods actually consumed (rather than a "guesstimate") and triggers an important behavioral aspect of the weight control process — awareness of current food habits and preferences.

Energy Output

In addition to caloric restriction through dieting, a physically active lifestyle becomes crucial to long-term success at weight loss. This does not mean playing a token game of tennis twice a year, going for a swim on weekends during the summer, or walking to the store when the car needs repair. Modifying personal exercise habits entails a serious commitment to changing daily routines to include regular periods of moderate to vigorous physical activity. Section III of the Student Study Guide and Workbook outlines a method to assess daily energy expenditure.

Diet Composition Makes a Difference in Gaining Weight

The composition of the diet influences the body's efficiency for converting and storing excess calories as body fat. Only about 3% of the calories in an ingested lipid excess goes to convert these calories to stored body fat, whereas 25% of the calories in a carbohydrate excess "burns" in the conversion process. Simply stated, the body synthesizes fat from dietary lipid more economically than from an equivalent caloric excess as carbohydrate. Consequently, shifting the diet's composition toward higher carbohydrate would result in less body fat gain should a caloric excess occur.

Dieting to Tip the Energy Balance Equation

Many believe that *only* calories from dietary lipids have the potential to increase body fat. Thus, individuals reduce fat intake to achieve body fat loss (generally a good idea) but often disproportionately increase carbohydrate and protein intakes so total caloric intake remains unchanged or even increases. In contrast, the prudent dietary approach to weight loss unbalances the energy balance equation by reducing daily energy intake 500 to 1000 kcal below the daily energy expenditure while consuming well-balanced meals. Compared with more severe energy restriction, which augments lean tissue loss, a moderate reduction in food intake produces a greater fat loss in relation to energy deficit. Total energy intake, not the mixture of macronutrients, determines the effectiveness of weight loss with low-energy diets. Most people do not tolerate prolonged daily caloric restriction of more than 1000 kcal; more extreme semi-starvation also increases the likelihood for malnourishment, depletion of glycogen reserves, and loss of lean tissue.

Practical Illustration

Suppose a wrestler who consumes 3800 kcal daily and maintains body mass at 80 kg (176 lb) wants to lose 5 kg (11 lb). He decides to maintain his activity level but decrease food intake to create a daily caloric deficit of 1000 kcal. Thus, instead of consuming 3800 kcal, he takes in only 2800 kcal daily. In 7 days, the accumulated deficit equals 7000 kcal (1000 kcal · d^{-1} × 7 d), or the energy equivalent of 0.9 kg (2 lb) of body fat. Actually, during the first week of caloric restriction, considerably more than 0.9 kg would be lost because the body's energy deficit initially comes mainly from glycogen stores. This stored nutrient contains fewer calories per gram and more water than stored fat. For this reason, short periods of caloric restriction often encourage the dieter, but result in large percentages of water and carbohydrate loss per unit weight loss with only a small decrease in body fat. As weight loss continues, the energy deficit created by food restriction requires a larger proportion of body fat breakdown. By adhering to the 2800 kcal diet, the wrestler reduces body fat at the rate of 0.45 kg of

Prudent Weight Loss Advice

- Set realistic weight loss goals
- Consume more fruits and vegetables
- Reduce total fat intake
- Exercise regularly

fat every 3.5 days, provided daily energy output remains unchanged.

Results Not Always Predictable

The mathematics of weight loss through caloric restriction seems straightforward, but results do not always follow. First, one assumes that daily energy expenditure remains relatively unchanged throughout the dieting period. Some people experience lethargy (because caloric restriction depletes the body's glycogen stores), which actually decreases daily energy expenditure. Second, the energy cost of physical activity decreases in proportion to the weight lost. This also shrinks the energy output side of the energy balance equation. If weight loss indeed progressed in proportion to caloric restriction, a progressive decrease in body mass would depend solely on the extent of caloric deprivation. However, metabolic changes also take place during caloric restriction that further blunt the weight loss effort.

Setpoint Theory: A Case Against Dieting

One can lose large amounts of weight in a relatively short time simply by not eating, but success remains short-lived; eventually the urge to eat wins out and the lost weight returns. The reason for this failure may lie in a "setpoint" that differs from that desired by the dieter. The proponents of a **setpoint theory** argue that all people, fat or thin, have a well-regulated internal control mechanism or setpoint. This controller, probably located deep within the brain's lateral hypothalamus, drives the body to preserve a particular level of body weight and/or body fat. *In a practical sense, this would be the body weight one achieves if not counting calories.* Various factors, like the drugs fenfluramine, amphetamine, and nicotine, and regular exercise may lower an individual's setpoint, whereas dieting does not. Each time the level of body fat decreases below one's natural setpoint, the body makes internal adjustments to resist this change and conserve or replenish body fat. In fact, even when a person overeats to gain weight above their normal level, resting metabolism increases to resist this change.

Resting Metabolism Lowered

A *dramatic and sustained reduction in resting metabolism often occurs when dieting produces weight loss.* The decrease in resting metabolism exceeds the decrease attributable to loss of either body mass or FFM; severe caloric restriction can depress resting metabolic rate by 45%! A blunted metabolism characterizes individuals attempting to lose weight, regardless if they dieted previously or were fat or lean. Reduced metabolism conserves energy, causing the diet to become progressively less effective despite a low caloric intake. Weight loss stabilizes (plateaus), and further weight losses diminish relative to weight loss predicted from the mathematics of the restricted energy intake.

Figure 19.8 displays the results for body mass and resting oxygen uptake (minimal energy requirement) during 31 days of carefully monitored caloric intakes for six obese men. During the pre-diet period, body mass and resting oxygen uptake stabilized on an average daily food intake of 3500 kcal. When subjects switched to a 450 kcal low-calorie diet, body mass and resting metabolism decreased, but the percentage decline in metabolism exceeded the decrease in body mass. The dashed line represents the expected weight loss from the 450-kcal diet. *The decline in resting metabolism actually conserved energy, causing a progressively less effective diet.* More than one-half of the total weight loss occurred over the first 8 days of dieting, with the remaining weight loss during the final 16 days. The dieter often becomes frustrated and discouraged when a plateau occurs in their anticipated weight-loss curve.

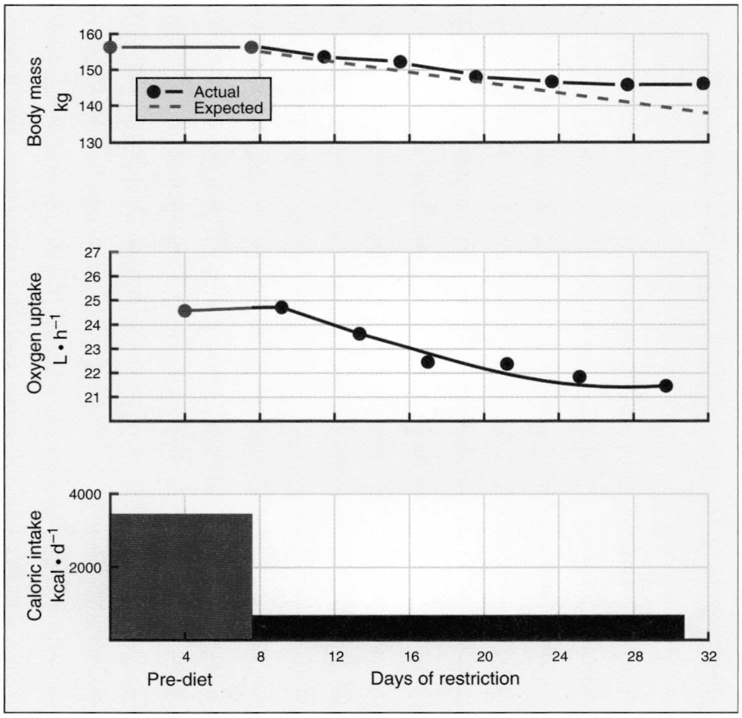

Weight Cycling: Going No Place Fast

The futility of repeated cycles of weight loss and weight gain — the off-and-on or "yo-yo" effect — oc-

Figure 19.8
Effects of two levels of caloric intake on changes in body mass and resting oxygen uptake. Often the failure of the actual weight loss to keep pace with predictions based on food restriction leaves the dieter frustrated and discouraged. (Adapted from Bray, G.: Effect of caloric restriction on energy expenditure in obese subjects. *Lancet*, 2: 397, 1969.)

curs with animals in food efficiency studies that evaluate weight loss and weight gain in relation to ingested calories. Although considerable debate exists on the subject, weight gain may occur more readily with repeated cycles of weight loss. Animals required twice the time to lose the same weight during a second period of caloric restriction and only one-third the time to regain it.

While obesity raises the risk of heart disease, the failure to keep lost weight off may pose an additional risk. Although a highly controversial topic, some epidemiological studies suggest that repeated bouts of weight loss-weight gain increase risk of dying from a heart attack. If it does turn out that weight cycling poses an additional health risk, one can only speculate about long-term negative effects from repeated weight cycling so common among high school and collegiate wrestlers and others who compete in sports requiring a lean and/or low body mass. At this point, however, the health risks from obesity are far more definitive than from weight cycling. *Overfat people (including competitive athletes) should not consider the potential hazards of* **yo-yo dieting** *as an excuse to abandon efforts to achieve a more desirable body composition.*

Although the setpoint theory may be unwelcome news to those with a setpoint tuned too high, the good news indicates that regular exercise can lower the setpoint to a more desirable level. Concurrently, regular exercise augments the weight loss effort in the following three ways:

1. Conserves and even increases FFM
2. Raises resting metabolism (if FFM increases)
3. Induces metabolic changes that facilitate fat breakdown

Overfat men and women who begin regular exercise often experience an initial decline in food intake despite increased caloric output. Eventually, maintaining an active lifestyle decreases body fat reserves, and daily energy intake balances the higher energy requirements so body mass stabilizes at a new, lower level.

How to Select a Diet Plan

The most difficult aspect of dieting involves deciding exactly what foods to include in the daily menu. One can choose from literally hundreds of diet plans: water diets, drinker's diets, zone diets, fruit or vegetable diets, fast-food diets, eat to win diets, and diets named for cities (e.g., New York City or Beverly Hills diets), not to mention the potentially dangerous varieties of high-fat, low-carbohydrate, and liquid-protein diets. Some authors have even stated that total caloric intake should not be considered, but rather the order of eating foods. For individuals desperate to shed excess weight, such misinformation reinforces negative eating behaviors, causing another repeat cycle of failure. Table 19.1 summarizes the principles and the main advantages and disadvantages of some popular dietary approaches to weight loss.

Well Balanced, But Less of It

A calorie-counting approach to weight loss should provide a well-balanced diet containing all the essential nutrients. As long as one maintains a caloric deficit, diet composition has little effect on the magnitude of weight loss. Reducing diets should contain the RDA for the micronutrients and protein, with reduced cholesterol and saturated fatty acids; for the physically active person, the remainder should consist predominantly of unrefined, fiber-rich, complex carbohydrates. *Calories do count; the trick necessitates keeping within the daily limit specified by the rate of fat loss desired.*

Maintenance of Goal Weight

Relatively little information exists concerning individual attempts to maintain body weight on a long-term basis. Figure 19.9 presents data on the body weights of two women who recorded their weight weekly. Subject 1 gained about 30 pounds over a 16-year period, while subject 2 gained 22 pounds over 10 years.

Subject 1 participated in six weight loss programs during her recording period. Each of the three formal programs lasted about 5 months, while the three self-directed efforts lasted 2 months. Weight loss for all programs averaged 9.2 pounds; the woman regained an average of 12 pounds within 1 year after each weight loss attempt.

Subject 2 attempted weight loss eight times during the 10 years of recording body weight. The attempts lasted be-

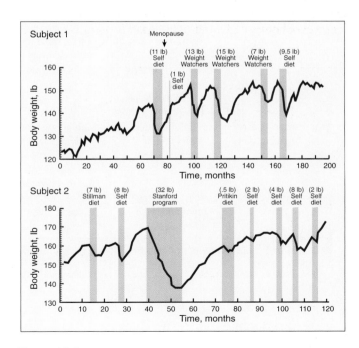

Figure 19.9
Tracking of weekly body weights of two women over a prolonged time. Subject 1 gained 30 pounds over a 16-year period; subject 2 gained 22 lb over 10 years. (Data from Black, D.R. et al.: A time series analysis of longitudinal weight changes in two adult women. *Int. J. Obes.*, 15:623, 1991.)

TABLE 19.1
Principles and main advantages and disadvantages of some popular weight loss methods

METHOD	PRINCIPLE	ADVANTAGES	DISADVANTAGES	COMMENTS
Surgical procedures	Alteration of the gastrointestinal tract changes capacity or amount of absorptive surface	Caloric restriction is less necessary	Risks of surgery and post-surgical complications can include death	Radical procedures include stapling of the stomach and removal of a section of the small intestine (a jejunoileal bypass)
Fasting	No energy input assures negative energy balance	Weight loss is rapid (which may be a disadvantage) Exposure to temptation is reduced	Ketogenic A large portion of weight lost is from lean body mass Nutrients are lacking	Medical supervision mandatory and hospitalization recommended
Protein-sparing modified fast	Same as fasting except protein or protein with carbohydrate intake assumedly helps preserve lean body mass	Same as in fasting	Ketogenic Nutrients are lacking Some unconfirmed deaths have been reported, possibly from electrolyte depletion	Medical supervision mandatory Popular presentation was made in Linn's *The Last Chance Diet*
One–food-centered diets	Low-caloric intake favors negative energy balance	Being easy to follow has initial psychologic appeal	Being too restrictive means that nutrients are probably lacking Repetitious nature may cause boredom	No food or food combination is known to "burn off" fat Examples include the grapefruit diet and the egg diet
Low-carbohydrate/ high-fat diets	Increased ketone excretion removes energy-containing substances from the body Fat intake is often voluntarily decreased; results in a low caloric intake	Inclusion of rich foods may have psychologic appeal Initial rapid loss of water may be an incentive	Ketogenic High-fat intake is contraindicated for heart and diabetes patients Nutrients are lacking	Popular versions have been offered by Taller and Atkins; some have been called the "Mayo", "Drinking Man's", and "Air Force" diets
Low-carbohydrate/ high-protein diets	Low caloric intake favors negative energy balance	Initial rapid loss of water weight may be an incentive Increased thermic effect of protein	Expense and repetitious nature may make it difficult to sustain	If meat emphasized, the diet becomes high in fat The Pennington diet The Pritikin diet
High-carbohydrate/ low-fat diets	Low caloric intake favors negative energy balance	Wise food selections can make the diet nutritionally sound	Initial water retention (from glycogen storage) may be discouraging	

Modified and reprinted by permission from Reed, P.B.: *Nutrition: An Applied Science.* Copyright © 1980 by West Publishing Co. All Rights Reserved.

tween 2 to 16 months, with weight loss averaging 8 pounds for all attempts. Similar to subject 1, she regained all lost weight (average gain of 9.9 lb over 9 months).

For both women, significant gains in body weight occurred over time despite interruptions from dieting; these gains could not be attributed to menopause, alterations in exercise patterns, pregnancy, changes in smoking status, or seasonal variation. Following each period of weight loss, body weight increased to the original prediet level or higher. The trend of steady weight gain for both women when not dieting counters the idea of a fixed setpoint, but rather supports the hypothesis that physiologic changes occur that facilitate weight gain (and perhaps reset the setpoint) with aging.

Masters of Weight Control

While the outlook for long-term weight loss maintenance remains poor, success stories have been documented. A recent project recruited 784 individuals (629 women; 155 men) in the National Weight Control Registry (NWCR), the largest database assembled of individuals who successfully achieved prolonged weight loss. Criteria for NWCR membership included: (a) 18 years of age or older, and (b) weight loss of at least 30 pounds (13.6 kg) maintained for one year or longer. Participants had lost on average 66 pounds (30 kg), and 14% had lost more than 100 pounds (45.4 kg). Members maintained the required minimum 30-pound weight loss for a 5.5-year average, while 16% of the group maintained this loss for 10 years or longer! Most of the participants had been overweight since childhood; nearly one-half had one overweight parent, and more than 25% had both parents overweight. *While genetic background may have predisposed these men and women to obesity, their impressive ability to take weight off and keep it off proves that heredity alone need not destine a person to a lifetime of obesity.*

About 55% of the NWCR members used either a formal program or professional assistance to lose weight, while the rest achieved success on their own. In response to questions about weight loss methods, 89% modified both food intake and physical activity to achieve their goal weight. Only 10% relied singularly on diet and 1% used exercise exclusively. The diet strategy practiced by nearly 90% of participants restricted intake of certain types and/or amounts of foods (43% counted calories, 33% limited lipid intake, and 25% restricted actual grams of lipid). More than 44% ate the same foods they normally ate, but in reduced amounts (Table 19.2).

The registry members belief in the importance of physical activity for weight maintenance represents a significant finding. Nearly all of the men and women used exercise in their weight control strategy. Ninety-two percent exercised at home, and about one-third exercised regularly with friends. Women primarily walked and did aerobic dancing, while men chose competitive sports and resistance training.

The data in Table 19.3 show that successful weight loss had far reaching, positive effects on diverse aspects of the lives of these masters of weight loss. At least 85% of the group improved quality of life, level of energy, physical mobility, general mood, self confidence, and physical health. Only 13 (1.6%) worsened in any

of these areas. Such observations offer hope that weight loss through diet and exercise can override genetic predisposition for those dedicated to controlling this aspect of their lives.

Exercising to Tip the Energy Balance Equation

The precise contributions of sedentary living and excessive caloric intake to the development of obesity remain poorly defined. Undoubtedly, an increased level of regular physical activity impacts significantly on energy balance.

Not Simply a Problem of Gluttony

Conventional wisdom considers excess body fat the culmination of excessive food intake. Most people believe the only way to reduce unwanted body fat entails caloric restriction by dieting. This simplistic view of combating excess body fat negates the key role increased energy expenditure from exercise plays in regulating body weight. Among active young and middle-aged endurance-trained men, body fat related inversely to energy expenditure (low body fat, high energy expenditure and vice versa); no relationship existed between body fat and food intake. Among physically active people, those who eat the most often weigh the least and exhibit the highest levels of physical fit-

TABLE 19.2
Dietary strategies to achieve weight loss of participants of the National Weight Control Registry

STRATEGY	PERCENTAGE		
	WOMEN	MEN	TOTAL
Restricted intake of certain types or classes of foods	87.8	86.7	87.6
Ate all foods but limited quantity	47.2	32.0	44.2
Counted calories	44.8	39.3	43.7
Limited % lipid intake	31.1	36.7	33.1
Counted lipid grams	25.7	21.3	25.2
Followed exchange diet	25.2	11.3	22.5
Used liquid formula	19.1	26.0	20.4
Ate only 1 or 2 foods types	5.1	6.7	5.5

From Klem, M.L. et al.: A descriptive study of individuals successful at long-term maintenance of substantial weight loss. *Am. J. Clin. Nutr.*, 66:239, 1997.

TABLE 19.3
Effect of weight loss on various dimensions of life as reported by the NWCR participants

AREA OF LIFE	IMPROVED	NO DIFFERENCE	WORSENED
Quality of life	95.3	4.3	0.4
Level of energy	92.4	6.7	0.9
Mobility	92.3	7.1	0.6
General mood	91.4	6.9	1.6
Self-confidence	90.9	9.0	0.1
Physical health	85.8	12.9	1.3
Interactions with			
Opposite sex	65.2	32.9	0.9
Same sex	5.0	46.8	0.4
Strangers	69.5	30.4	0.1
Job performance	54.5	45.0	0.6
Hobbies	49.1	36.7	0.4
Spouse interactions	56.3	37.3	5.9

From Klem, M.L. et al.: A descriptive study of individuals successful at long-term maintenance of substantial weight loss. *Am. J. Clin. Nutr.*, 66:239, 1997.

ness. In the United States, per capita caloric intake has not increased enough to account for the steady increase in the national body mass. Americans now eat 5 to 10% fewer calories than they did 20 years ago, yet they weigh an average of 2 to 4 kg more. Certainly, if food intake were the sole culprit in weight gain, the reduced caloric intake should bring the national body mass to a lower not higher level.

Pattern Also Holds for Children

Obese infants do not characteristically consume more calories than the recommended dietary standards. Children age 6 to 17 years have consumed 4% fewer calories over the past 20 years, yet the prevalence of childhood obesity continues to increase (currently more than 10 million children and teenagers are overfat). In contrast, physically active children tend to be leaner than less active counterparts. Time-in-motion photography that documented activity patterns of elementary school students clearly showed less physical activity among overweight children than normal-weight peers; their excess weight did not relate to food intake. Overfat high school girls and boys actually consumed fewer calories than nonobese peers. The observation that fat people often eat the same or even less than thinner people holds true for adults over a broad age range as they become less active and their weight slowly begins to increase. Reducing caloric intake

does not by itself effectively combat the overfat condition on a permanent basis.

Increasing Energy Output

A physically active lifestyle at all ages contributes to a desirable level of body weight and body composition. Increased exercise energy expenditure provides a significant option for unbalancing the energy balance equation toward weight loss. Two arguments generally have been raised against the exercise option: One position maintains that exercise inevitably increases appetite so that proportionately greater food intake cancels any caloric deficit. The second argument posits that typical exercise generates such small calorie-burning effects that a sensible use of exercise barely dents the body's fat reserves compared with significant food restriction.

Exercise Effects on Food Intake

Overweight, sedentary people do not always balance food intake with energy expenditure. A lack of precision in regulating food intake at the low end of the physical activity spectrum may account for creeping obesity common in highly mechanized and technically advanced societies. On the other hand, for individuals who regularly exercise, appetite control operates in a *reactive zone* where food intake more precisely matches energy expenditure.

No compelling evidence exists that exercise-induced energy expenditure automatically triggers compensatory food intake in previously sedentary, overweight individuals. Rather, only a weak coupling exists between a moderate increase in physical activity and altered eating behavior and energy intake. For this reason, regular physical activity serves as a vital link in producing weight loss and subsequent weight maintenance.

Exercise Effects on Energy Expenditure

The second misconception concerns the number of calories generated by regular exercise, i.e., the idea that only an extraordinary amount of exercise leads to a loss in body fat. Examples include chopping wood for 10 hours, golfing for 20 hours, performing mild calisthenics for 22 hours, playing ping-pong for 28 hours or volleyball for 32 hours, or running 35 miles just to reduce body fat by 0.45 kg (1 lb).

In contrast, if a person played golf only two hours (about 350 kcal) 2 days a week (700 kcal), then in about 5 weeks (10 golfing days) the golfer would reduce 0.45 kg of fat (3500 kcal). Assuming the person played year-round, golfing just twice weekly would translate to a 4.5-kg yearly fat-loss provided food intake remained fairly constant. While most of us would not play golf this frequently (nor would we golf for 20 consecutive hours), the calorie-expending effects of exercise become *cumulative*: a caloric deficit of 3500 kcal equals a 0.45-kg body fat loss whether it occurs rapidly or systematically over time.

The caloric expenditure values for the physical activities presented in Section IV of the Student Study Guide and Workbook should not be considered absolute. They represent average values, applicable under average conditions when applied to the average person of a given body mass. However, the values do provide a good approximation of energy expenditure and serve a useful purpose in selecting higher caloric yield physical activities for a weight loss program.

Exercise Alters Body Composition

Increasing regular exercise, with or without dietary restriction, favorably changes body mass and body composition. As a general rule, persons with the largest amounts of excess fat lose weight and body fat more readily with exercise than leaner counterparts. Even without dietary restriction, exercise provides a significant positive spin-off; it reduces body fat and maintains or even increases FFM. Even exercise regimens that involve less energy-demanding, conventional resistance training positively affect the fat-free body mass during weight loss compared with programs relying solely on food restriction. Conserving or increasing lean tissue maintains a high level of resting metabolism because FFM remains metabolically more active than body fat. This reduces the body's tendency to store calories, augmenting the potential effectiveness of the weight loss program. *For an athlete, maintaining FFM during weight reduction becomes crucial to counter potential negative effects of weight loss on exercise performance.*

A person planning to exercise for weight control should consider the frequency, intensity, duration, and mode of physical activity. Ideal activities consist of continuous, big muscle aerobic exercises that have a moderate to high caloric cost like brisk walking, running, rope skipping, cycling, and swimming. Many recreational sports and games also positively affect body weight, although precise quantification of energy expenditure becomes difficult. Aerobic exercises burn considerable calories, stimulate fat catabolism, reduce body fat, establish a favorable blood pressure response, and generally promote cardiovascular health and fitness. An extra 300 kcal expended with moderate jogging daily for 30 to 45 minutes causes a 0.45 kg fat loss in about 12 days. Over a year's time, this theoretically represents a total caloric deficit equivalent to about 13.6 kg (30 lb) of body fat!

Dose-Response Relationship

A larger *total quantity* of fat combustion occurs in higher-intensity aerobic exercise compared to less intense physical activity performed for equivalent time periods (refer to Chapter 5.) *More importantly, the total number of calories expended in creating the caloric deficit, not the percentage mixture of macronutrients oxidized, determines the effectiveness of exercise in weight loss. A direct dose-response relationship exists between weight loss and calories expended exercising.* The person who adds additional daily exercise by walking accrues a considerable caloric expenditure simply by extending exercise duration. Also, a proportional relationship exists between the energy cost of weight-bearing exercise like walking and body mass; thus, the overfat person expends more calories walking than someone of average body mass.

A study of three groups of men who exercised for 20 weeks by walking and running either 15, 30, or 45 minutes per session illustrates the importance of exercise duration (total calories burned) in weight loss. Compared with a sedentary control group, the three exercise groups significantly decreased total body fat, skinfolds, and waist girth. Comparisons among the three groups showed the 45-minute training group lost more body fat than either the 30- or 15-minute groups. Greater fat loss occurred because of greater caloric expenditure from longer duration exercise.

Maximize Total Energy Expenditure

The person wishing to lose weight and alter the diabetogenic and atherogenic complications of obesity must choose between activities that improve cardiorespiratory fitness (higher intensity) and those that induce a large total energy expenditure (lower intensity, longer duration). Research shows that losses in body fat with regular exercise relate more to exercise volume (and related increase in energy expenditure) than improved cardiovascular (aerobic) fitness. If weight loss and improved heart disease risk profile represent the primary goals for the obese person, the exercise program should substantially increase total energy expenditure rather than focus on improving physical fitness.

No One "Best" Aerobic Exercise

No selective effect on weight loss occurs for diverse big muscle activities like running, walking, swimming, or bicycling; each produces similar effects in altering body composition, provided equivalence exists for exercise duration, frequency, and intensity.

How to Calculate Upper-Arm Muscle and Fat Area

A girth measurement around the upper arm includes bone surrounded by a mass of muscle tissue ringed by a layer of subcutaneous fat. Because muscle represents the largest component of the girth (except in the obese and elderly), a girth can indicate relative muscularity. The procedure for estimating limb muscle area assumes similarity between a limb and a cylinder, and that the cylinder represents the limb with evenly distributed subcutaneous fat.

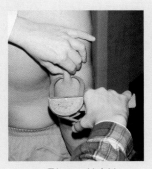

Bone
Fat
Muscle

$$A = \frac{c^2}{4\pi}$$

Measurements
Take the following measurements:

1. Arm girth (relaxed triceps): measured with the arm extended relaxed at the side (or parallel to the ground in an abducted position). Measure the girth at the point midway between the acromial and olecranon process (see bottom left figure).

2. Triceps skinfold (Sf_{tri}): measured on the back of the arm over the triceps muscle as a vertical fold at the same level as the relaxed, arm girth (see bottom right figure).

Example

Data
Upper-arm girth, (C_{arm}) in cm = 30.0; triceps skinfold (Sf_{tri}) in cm = 2.5 cm (25 mm).

Formulae and Solutions

1. **Arm muscle girth, cm = $C_{arm} - (\pi Sf_{tri})$**
   $= 30.0 \text{ cm} - (\pi 2.5 \text{ cm})$
   $= 30.0 \text{ cm} - 7.854$
   $= 22.1 \text{ cm}$

2. **Arm muscle area (A), cm² = $[C_{arm} - (\pi Sf_{tri})]^2 \div 4\pi$**
   $= [30.0 \text{ cm} -$
   $(\pi 2.5 \text{ cm})]^2 \div 4\pi$
   $= 488.4 \div 12.566$
   $= 38.9 \text{ cm}^2$

3. **Arm area, cm² = $(C_{arm})^2 \div 4\pi$**
   $= (30.0 \text{ cm})^2 \div 4\pi$
   $= 900 \div 12.566$
   $= 71.6 \text{ cm}^2$

4. **Arm fat area, cm² = arm area − arm muscle area**
   $= 71.6 \text{ cm}^2 - 38.9 \text{ cm}^2$
   $= 32.7 \text{ cm}^2$

5. **Arm fat index, % fat area = (arm fat area $\div$ arm area) ×100**
   $= (32.7 \text{ cm}^2 \div 71.6 \text{ cm}^2) \times 100$
   $= 45.7\%$

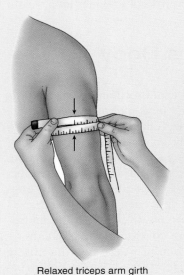

Relaxed triceps arm girth

Triceps skinfold

A standard exercise prescription generally consists of 30 minutes of aerobic exercise performed at 50 to 60% of $\dot{V}O_{2max}$ three days weekly. While this regimen of exercise training improves aerobic fitness, the total exercise volume generates a relatively modest added increase in weekly energy expenditure (unlikely to induce substantial weight loss). In contrast, performing lower-intensity exercise 60 to 90 minutes daily expends a considerable extra energy each week. This considerably large dose of exercise positively influences body fat, insulin sensitivity, and the plasma lipoprotein profile, all important benefits for the overfat person.

Start Slowly

A person beginning an exercise program for weight loss should adopt long-term goals, exert personal discipline, and restructure their eating and exercise behaviors. It is of-ten counterproductive to include unduly rapid training progressions because many obese men and women initially are psychologically resistant to physical training. It takes at least 6 to 8 weeks for changes to occur.

Table 19.4 shows the effectiveness of regular exercise for weight loss. Six sedentary, obese young men exercised 5 days a week for 16 weeks by walking for 90 minutes at each session. The men lost nearly 6 kg of body fat; this represented a percent body fat decrease from 23.5% to 18.6%. In addition, physical fitness and work capacity improved, as did the level of high-density lipoprotein cholesterol (15.6%) and the high- to low-density lipoprotein cholesterol ratio (25.9%).

Diet Plus Exercise: The Ideal Combination

Combining exercise with diet offers considerably more flexibility for achieving a negative caloric balance than either exercise or diet alone. Including regular exercise in a weight control program also facilitates longer-term maintenance of fat loss than does total reliance on food restriction. *Most nutrition experts agree that body fat losses up to 2 pounds (0.9 kg) each week fall within acceptable limits, although a steady 0.5- to 1.0-pound a week loss may be even more desirable.*

Setting a Target Time

Suppose 20 weeks represents the target time to achieve a 9-kg (20-lb) fat loss. Based on this goal, the weekly deficit would have to average 3500 kcal, or a daily average of 500 kcal ($3500 \div 7$). To achieve this deficit by dieting, daily caloric intake must decrease by 500 kcal for 20 weeks to achieve the desired 9-kg fat loss. However, if the dieter performed an additional 45 minutes of moderate exercise equivalent to 350 extra kcal 3 days a week, then the weekly caloric deficit would increase by 1050 kcal (3 days per week × 350 kcal per exercise session). Consequently, to achieve the weekly desired 0.45-kg fat loss, the weekly caloric intake needs to decrease by only 2400 kcal (about 350 kcal a day) instead of 3500 kcal. If the number of exercise days increases from three to five, daily food intake need only decrease by 250 kcal. If duration of the 5-day per week extra exercise lengthens from 45 minutes to 90 minutes, then the

TABLE 19.4
The effects of a 16-week walking program on changes in body composition and blood lipids in six obese young adult men walking program[a]

VARIABLE	PRE-TRAINING[a]	POST-TRAINING[a]	DIFFERENCE
Body mass, kg	99.1	93.4	−5.7[b]
Body density, g · mL^{-1}	1.044	1.056	+0.012[b]
Body fat, %	23.5	18.6	−4.9[b]
Fat mass, kg	23.3	17.4	−5.9[b]
Fat-free body mass, kg	75.8	76.0	+0.2
Sum of skinfolds, mm	142.9	104.8	−38.1[b]
HDL cholesterol, mg · 100 mL^{-1}	32	37	−5.0[b]
HDL/LDL cholesterol	0.27	0.34	+0.07[b]

From Leon, A.S., et al.: Effects of a vigorous walking program on body composition, and carbohydrate and lipid metabolism of obese young men. *Am. J. Clin. Nutr.*, 33:1776, 1979.

[a] Values are means

[b] Statistically significant

desired weight loss occurs without reducing food intake because the required deficit of 3500 kcal comes entirely from additional physical activity.

If the intensity of the 90-minute exercise performed 5 days a week increased by only 10% (cycling at 22 instead of 20 mph; running one mile in 9 min instead of 10 min; swimming each 50 yd in 54 s instead of 60 s), the number of calories burned each week through exercise increases by 350 kcal (3500 kcal · wk^{-1}× 10%). This new weekly deficit of 3850 kcal (550 kcal · d^{-1}) then permits the dieter to increase daily food intake by 50 kcal yet still lose a pound of fat each week.

The effective use of physical activity by itself, or combined with mild dietary restriction, readily unbalances the energy balance equation in the direction of weight loss. This dual approach reduces feelings of intense hunger and psychological stress compared to weight loss exclusively by caloric restriction. In addition, prolonged dieting increases the chances of developing a variety of nutritional deficiencies, which obviously hinders exercise training and competitive performance.

Adding aerobic and resistance exercise to a weight loss effort protects against the loss of FFM usually observed when relying solely on diet to achieve weight loss. This occurs partly because exercise training enhances fat mobilization from the body s adipose depots and fat catabolism by the active muscles. In addition, exercise protects against loss of protein in skeletal muscle (maintains nitrogen balance). *The protein-sparing effects of regular exercise explains, in part, why weight loss occurs more readily from fat in a weight-reduction program that employs regular exercise.*

General Observations on Weight Loss

The following summarizes research results on exercise and diet for weight loss:

- Exercise combined with food restriction proves more effective for achieving long-term negative caloric balance compared with exercise or diet alone.

- Initial, rapid weight loss results from body water loss and depletion of glycogen reserves; longer periods of weight reduction result in a substantially greater loss of fat per unit weight lost.

- Water intake should not be restricted during weight reduction because this can precipitate dehydration without additional fat loss.

- Prolonged caloric restriction at levels significantly below minimal energy requirements can produce undesirable psychological stress and medically-related problems.

- Weight loss by diet alone causes loss of muscle mass. Exercise protects against lean tissue losses; thus, fat represents more of the lost weight.

- Exercise, particularly if combined with an increase in the lean tissue mass, blunts the decline in resting metabolism often observed with weight loss through food restriction only.

Spot Reduction: Does It Work?

The notion of **spot reduction** *maintains that exercising a specific muscle facilitates relatively greater fat mobilization from the adipose tissue in close proximity to the muscle.* Therefore, exercising a specific body area should selectively reduce more fat from that area than if different muscle groups performed exercise of the same caloric value. Advocates of spot reduction recommend performing excessive sit ups or side bends to reduce abdominal fat, while push ups and bench presses would be advocated to selectively remove fat from the chest area. The promise of spot reduction conveys not only aesthetic benefits but also an improved health profile (e.g., selective reduction of "risky" abdominal fat). Unfortunately, research evidence does not support the use of spot reducing, nor the use of topical creams, heat, massage, wraps, magnet therapy, and electrical stimulation for localized fat reduction.

To examine the claims for spot reduction critically, comparisons were made of the girths and subcutaneous fat stores of the right and left forearms of high-caliber tennis players. As expected, the girth of the dominant or playing arm exceeded the nondominant arm because of modest muscular hypertrophy from years of playing tennis. Measurements of skinfold thickness, however, indicated *no difference* in the quantity of subcutaneous fat on the two forearms. Clearly, regular and prolonged exercise did not reduce fat deposits in the playing arm.

No one doubts that a negative caloric balance created through regular exercise can significantly reduce total body fat. However, exercise mobilizes fatty acids through hormones that target fat depots throughout the body. Areas of greatest body fat concentration and/or lipid-mobilizing enzyme activity supply the major portion of this energy. No evidence exists for a preferential release of fatty acids from the fat pads directly over the active muscle.

Gaining Weight

For most people, weight loss to reduce body fat and improve overall health and aesthetic appearance becomes the primary focus of any attempt to alter body composition. However, certain individuals desire to gain weight to improve the body composition profile and/or performance in sport or exercise requiring muscular strength and power. This goal poses a unique dilemma that is not easily resolved. Gaining weight per se occurs easily by tilting the body's energy balance to favor greater caloric intake. In a sedentary person, an accumulated excess intake of 3500 kcal produces a body fat gain of about 0.5 kg because adipocytes store the excess calories. Weight gain for athletes, however, should ideally occur in lean tissue, specifically muscle mass and accompanying connective tissue. Generally, this form of weight gain takes place if an increased caloric intake (adequate carbohydrate for energy and protein sparing, and enough protein for tissue synthesis) accompanies the proper exercise regimen.

Increase Lean, Not Fat

Heavy muscular overload (resistance training) supported by adequate energy and protein intake, with sufficient recovery, increases muscle mass and strength. Adequate energy intake assures that protein available for muscle growth does not catabolize for any energy deficit created by training. *Consequently, intense aerobic training should not coincide with resistance training when trying to achieve maximal increases in muscle mass.* More than likely, the added energy (and perhaps protein) demands of concurrent resistance and aerobic exercise training impose a limit on muscle growth and responsiveness to resistance training. A safe (although not proven in effectiveness) recommendation would increase daily protein intake to about 1.5 g per kg of body mass during the resistance training period. The individual should obtain diverse sources of plant and animal proteins; relying totally on animal sources for increased dietary protein (high in saturated fatty acids and cholesterol) potentially increases risk for heart disease.

If all the calories consumed in excess of energy requirements during resistance training go towards muscle growth, then 2000 to 2500 extra kcal from a well-balanced diet would support each 0.5 kg (1.1 lb) increase in lean tissue. In practical terms, 700 to 1000 kcal added to the daily diet supports a weekly 0.5- to 1.0-kg (1.1- to 2.2-lb) gain in lean tissue and additional energy for training. This ideal situation presupposes that all extra calories synthesize lean tissue.

How Much Gain to Expect

Experience indicates that a one-year, heavy resistance training regimen for young, athletic-type men produces about a 20% increase in body mass, the major portion consisting of lean tissue mass. The rate of lean tissue gain then rapidly plateaus as training progresses beyond the first year. For athletic women, first year gains in lean tissue mass average 50 to 75% of absolute values for men, probably due to women's smaller initial lean body mass. Individual differences in the amount of nitrogen incorporated into body protein (and protein incorporated into muscle) each day may explain variations in lean tissue gains with resistance training. Regularly monitoring body mass and body fat by hydrostatic weighing or other validated indirect techniques verifies whether the combination of training and additional food intake increases lean tissue and not body fat.

summary

1. Most participants in programs of weight loss through dietary restriction achieve little success in long-term maintenance of a reduced body mass.

2. Three ways unbalance the energy balance equation to bring about weight loss: 1) reduce caloric intake below daily energy expenditure, 2) maintain regular food intake and increase energy output, and 3) combine both methods and decrease food intake and increase energy expenditure.

3. A caloric deficit of 3500 kcal created through either diet or exercise equals the calories in one pound (0.45 kg) of body fat (adipose tissue).

4. Dieting for weight loss can be effective if done in a prudent and proper manner. The significant disadvantages of semistarvation include loss of lean body tissue, lethargy, possible malnutrition and metabolic disorders, and a decrease in the basal energy expenditure. Some of these factors actually conserve energy and blunt the diet's effectiveness.

5. Repeated cycles of weight loss and weight gain may increase the body's efficiency to conserve energy. This could ultimately cause greater difficulty achieving weight loss with subsequent dieting attempts, and facilitate regaining the lost weight.

6. The calories expended in exercise accumulate; a modest amount of extra exercise performed routinely creates a dramatic calorie-burning effect over time.

7. For previously sedentary, overfat men and women, moderate increases in physical activity do not necessarily increase food intake proportionately. Eventually, most individuals consume enough calories to counterbalance caloric expenditure, but many athletes maintain an exceptionally lean body composition.

8. Combining exercise and diet offers a flexible yet effective approach to weight control. Exercise enhances fat mobilization, and utilization for energy, im-

proves insulin sensitivity, and retards lean tissue loss.

9. Rapid weight loss during the first few days of caloric deficit comes mainly from body water loss and glycogen depletion. Continued weight reduction occurs at the expense of greater fat loss per unit weight loss.

10. Selective fat reduction at specific body areas by spot exercise does not work. Exercise stimulates fatty acid mobilization through hormones and enzyme action that target fat depots throughout the body. The areas of greatest body fat concentration and/or lipid-mobilizing enzyme activity supply the greatest amount of energy.

11. Resistance training complemented by a well-balanced diet increases muscle mass. Intense aerobic training should not coincide with resistance training when trying to achieve maximal increases in muscle mass.

thought questions

1. What strategy, advice, and words of encouragement can you offer to a person who has attempted several diets yet never achieved long-term weight loss?

2. Respond to this comment. "The only way to lose weight is to stop eating. It's that simple!"

3. Outline your response to a student who asks: Why am I considered overweight by some criteria, but with other measures, my body fat assessment falls within normal limits?

4. Outline a prudent, yet effective plan for losing weight for a middle-age woman whose physician has advised her to shed 20 pounds of excess weight. Provide the rationale for each of your recommendations.

5. Respond to a colleague who comments that the obesity war would easily be won if the overfat could just learn to apply greater willpower and self control.

selected references

American College of Sports Medicine: Position statement on proper and improper weight loss programs. *Med. Sci. Sports Exerc.*, 15(1):ix, 1983.

Anderson, R.E., et al.: Relationship of physical activity and television watching with body weight and level of fatness among children. *JAMA*, 279:938, 1998.

Anderson, R.E.: Effects of lifestyle activity vs structured aerobic exercise in obese women. *JAMA*, 281:335, 1999.

Bar-Or, O., et al.: Physical activity, genetic, and nutritional considerations in childhood weight management. *Med. Sci. Sports Exerc.*, 30:2, 1998.

Bahr, R., et al.: Effect of supramaximal exercise on excess postexercise O_2 consumption. *Med. Sci. Sport Exerc.*, 24:66, 1992.

Ballor, D. L., and Poehlman, E. T.: Exercise training enhances fat-free mass preservation during diet-induced weight loss: a meta-analytical finding. *Int. J. Obes.*, 18: 35, 1994.

Bender, R., et al.: Effect of age on excess mortality in obesity. *JAMA*, 281:1498, 1999.

Bouchard, C.: Genetics of obesity: overview and research directions. In *The Genetics of Obesity*. Bouchard, C., (ed.). Boca Raton, FL: CRC Press, 1994.

Bouchard C.: Human variation in body mass: evidence for a role of the genes. *Nutr. Rev.*, 55:S21, 1997.

Bouchard, C., et al.: The response to long term feeding in identical twins. *N. Engl. J. Med.*, 322: 1477, 1990.

Broeder, C.E., et al.: Assessing body composition before and after resistance or endurance training. *Med. Sci. Sports Exerc.*, 29:705, 1997.

Brownell, K. D., et al. (eds.).: *Eating, Body Weight and Performance in Athletes*. Philadelphia: Lea & Fegiber, 1992.

Bungard, L.B., et al.: Energy requirements of middle-aged men are modifiable by physical activity. *Am. J. Clin. Nutr.*, 69:1136, 1998

Caro, J.R., et al.: Leptin: the tale of an obesity gene. *Diabetes*, 45:1455, 1996.

Centers for Disease Control and Prevention: Update: prevalence of overweight among children, adolescents, and adults: United States, 1988–1994. *MMWR*, 46:199, 1997.

Daniel, S.R., et al.: Body fat distribution and cardiovascular risk factors in children. *Circulation*, 99:541, 1999.

Després, J-P.: Visceral obesity, insulin resistance, and dyslipidemia: Contribution of endurance exercise training to the treatment of the plurimetabolic syndrome. *Exerc. Sport Sci. Rev.*, 25:271:1997.

Dietz, W.H.: Health consequences of obesity in youth: childhood predictors of adult disease. *Pediatrics*, 101:518, 1998.

DiPietro, L.: Physical activity, body weight, and adiposity: an epidemiologic perspective. *Exerc. Sport Sci. Rev.*, 23:275, 1995.

Dolezal, B.A., and Potteiger, J.A.: Concurrent resistance and endurance training influence basal metabolic rate in nondieting individuals. *J. Appl. Physiol.*, 85:695, 1998.

Dullo, A. G., and Girardier, L.: Adaptive changes in energy expenditure during refeeding following low-calorie intake: evidence for a specific metabolic component favoring fat storage. *Am. J. Clin. Nutr.*, 52:415, 1990.

Dunn, A.I., et al.: Comparison of lifestyle and structured interventions to increase physical activity and cardiorespiratory fitness. *JAMA*, 281:327, 1999.

Executive summary of the clinical guidelines on the identification, evaluation, and treatment of overweight and obesity in adults. *Arch. Intern. Med.*, 158:1855, 1998.

Grundy, S.M.: Multifactorial causation of obesity: implications for prevention. *Am. J. Clin. Nutr.*, 67(suppl.):563S, 1998.

Gunnell, D.J., et al.: Childhood obesity and adult cardiovascular mortality: a 57-y follow-up study based on the Boyd Orr cohort. *Am. J. Clin. Nutr.*, 67:1111, 1998.

Heymsfield, S.B., et al.: The calorie: myth, measurement and reality. *Am. J. Clin. Nutr.*, 62 (suppl.):1034S, 1995.

Hill, J. O., et al.: Exercise and moderate obesity. In: *Physical Activity, Fitness, and Health.* Bouchard C., et al., (eds.). Champaign, IL: Human Kinetics, 1994.

Hill, J.O., and Peters, J.C.: Environmental contributions to the obesity epidemic. *Science*, 280:1371, 1998.

Hill, J.O. et al.: Racial differences in amounts of visceral adipose tissue in young adults: the CARDIA (Coronary Artery Risk Development in Young Adults) Study. *Am. J. Clin. Nutr.*, 69:381, 1999.

Hirsch, J., et al.: Diet composition and energy balance in humans. *Am. J. Clin. Nutr.*, 67(suppl.):551S, 1998.

Horswill, C. R.: Weight loss and weight cycling in amateur wrestlers: implications for performance and resting metabolic rate. *Int. J. Sport Nutr.*, 3:245, 1993.

Hu, G.B., et al.: Walking compared with vigorous physical activity and the risk of type 2 diabetes. *JAMA*, 282:1433, 1999.

Hunter, G.R., et al.: Fat distribution, physical activity, and cardiovascular risk factors. *Med. Sci. Sports Exerc.*, 29:362, 1997.

Jakicic, J.M., et al.: Effects of intermittent exercise and use of home exercise equipment on adherence, weight loss, and fitness in overweight women. A randomized trial. *JAMA*, 282:1554, 1999.

Jeffery, R.W.: Does weight cycling present a risk? *Am. J. Clin. Nutr.*, 63(suppl.):452S, 1996.

Kessey, R.E.: A set-point theory of obesity. In: *Handbook of Eating Disorders.* Brownell, K.D., and Foreyt, J.P. New York: Basic Books, 1986.

King, M. A., and Katch, F. I.: Changes in body density, fatfolds, and girths at 2.3 kg increments of weight loss. *Hum. Biol.*, 58:709, 1986.

Lee, C.D., et al.: Cardiorespiratory fitness, body composition, and all-cause and cardiovascular disease mortality in men. *Am. J. Clin. Nutr.*, 69:373, 1999.

Leibel, R.L, et al.: Changes in energy expenditure resulting from altered body weight. *N. Engl. J. Med.*, 332:621, 1995.

Mayer, J., et al.: Relation between calorie intake,

body weight and physical work: studies in an industrial male population in West Bengal. *Am. J. Clin. Nutr.*, 4:169, 1956.

McArdle, W. D., and Toner, M. M.: Application of exercise for weight control: the exercise prescription. In: *Eating Disorders Handbook: Complete Guide to Understanding and Treatment.* Frankle, R., and Yang, M-U., (eds). Rockville, MD: Aspen Publishers, 1988.

Mokdad, A.H., et al.: The spread of the obesity epidemic in the United States, 1991–1998. *JAMA*, 282:1519, 1999.

Molé, P., et al.: Exercise versus depressed metabolic rate produced by severe caloric restriction. *Med. Sci. Sports Exerc.*, 21:29, 1989.

Montague, C.T., et al.: Congenital leptin deficiency is associated with severe early-onset obesity in humans. *Nature*, 387:903, 1997.

Must, A., et al.: The disease burden of obesity. *JAMA*, 282:1523, 1999.

National Task Force on the Prevention and Treatment of Obesity: Weight cycling. *JAMA*, 272:1196, 1994.

Ogden, C.L., et al.: Prevalence of overweight among preschool children in the United States, 1971–1994. *Peadiatrics*, 99:1, 1997.

Pérusse, L., et al.: Acute and chronic effects of exercise on leptin levels in humans. *J. Appl. Physiol.*, 83:5, 1997.

Pescatello, L.S., and Murphy, D.: Lower intensity physical activity is advantageous for fat distribution and blood glucose among viscerally obese older adults. *Med. Sci. Sports Exerc.*, 30:1408, 1998.

Pollock, M.L.: Twenty-year follow-up of aerobic power and body composition of older track athletes. *J. Appl. Physiol.*, 82:1508, 1997.

Pi-Sunyer, F. X.: Medical hazards of obesity. *Ann. Intern. Med.*, 119: 655, 1993.

Pouliot, M. C., et al.: Waist circumference and abdominal sagittal diameter: best simple anthropometric indexes of abdominal visceral adipose tissue accumulation and related cardiovascular risk in men and women. *Am. J. Cardiol.*, 73:460, 1994.

Rexrode, K.M., et al.: Abdominal adiposity and coronary heart disease in women. *JAMA*, 280:1843, 1998.

Roemmich, J.N., and Sinning, W.E.: Weight loss and wrestling training: effects of nutrition, growth, maturation, body composition, and strength. *J. Appl. Physiol.*, 82:1751, 1997.

Rosengren, A., et al.: Body weight and weight gain

during adult life in men in relation to coronary heart disease and mortality. *Eur. Heart J.*, 20:269, 1999.

Ryan, S.S., et al.: Resistive training increases fat-free mass and maintains RMR despite weight loss in postmenopausal women. *J. Appl. Physiol.*, 79:818, 1995.

Schoeller, D.A.: Balancing energy expenditure and body weight. *Am. J. Clin. Nutr.*, 68(Suppl): 956S, 1998.

Skender, M.I., et al.: Comparison of 2-year weight loss trends in behavioral treatments of obesity: Diet, exercise, and combination interventions. *J. Am. Diet. Assoc.*, 96:342, 1996.

Stefanick, M. L.: Exercise and weight control. *Exerc. Sport Sci. Rev.*, 21: 363, 1993.

Sweeney, M. E., et al.: Severe versus moderate energy restriction with and without exercise in the treatment of obesity. *Am. J. Clin. Nutr.*, 5:491, 1993.

Taubes, G.: As obesity rates rise, experts struggle to explain why. *Science*, 280:1367, 1998.

Tremblay, A., et al.: Exercise-training, macronutrient balance and body weight control. *Int. J. Obes.*, 19:79, 1995.

VanEtten, L.M.L.A., et al.: Effect of an 18-wk weight-training program on energy expenditure and physical activity. *J. Appl. Physiol.*, 82:298, 1997.

Wadden, T.A.: Characteristics of successful weight loss maintenance. In: *Obesity Treatment: Establishing Goals, Improving Outcomes, and Establishing the Research Agenda.* Pi-Sunyer, F.X., and Allison, D.B. (eds). New York: Plenum Press, 1995.

Westerterp, K.R.: Alterations in energy balance with exercise. *Am. J. Clin. Nutr.*, 970S, 1998.

Willett, W.C.: Is dietary fat a major determinant of body fat? *Am. J. Clin. Nutr.*, 67(suppl.):556S, 1998.

Wilmore, J.H.: Increasing physical activity: alterations in body mass and composition. *Am. J. Clin. Nutr.*, 63: (suppl.):456S, 1996.

Whitaker, R.C., et al.: Predicting obesity in young adulthood from childhood and parental obesity. *N. Engl. J. Med.*, 337:869, 1997.

Wickelgren, I.: Obesity: How big a problem? *Science*, 280:1364, 1998.

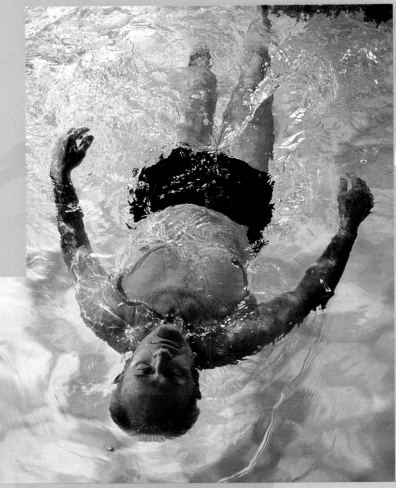

CHAPTER

20

Topics covered in this chapter

Surgeon General's Report on Physical
    Activity and Health
Safety of Exercising
The New Gerontology
Concept of Successful Aging
Aging and Bodily Function
Regular Exercise: A Fountain Of Youth?
Coronary Heart Disease
Risk Factors for Coronary Heart Disease
Behavioral Changes Improve Overall
    Health Profile
Summary
Thought Questions
Selected References

Exercise, Aging, and Cardiovascular Health

- Describe the physical activity level of typical American men and women.

- Outline the major findings of the 1996 Surgeon General's Report on physical activity and health.

- Answer the question: "How safe is exercise?"

- Outline the major differences in physiologic response to exercise between children and adults.

- List important age-related changes in: (a) muscular strength, (b) joint flexibility, (c) nervous system function, (d) cardiovascular function, (e) pulmonary function, and (f) body composition.

- Describe five field tests to assess flexibility of major body areas.

- Explain the following statement: "An impressive plasticity exists in physiologic function and exercise performance, and marked training-induced improvements occur into the eighth decade of life."

- Describe research that shows that regular physical activity protects against disease and may even extend life.

- Describe the age-related progression of heart disease risk for women.

- List major risk factors for coronary heart disease, and describe how regular exercise affects each.

- List the specific components of the blood lipid profile and give values considered normal or desirable for each.

- Discuss factors that affect the levels of cholesterol and lipoprotein.

- Outline the proposed role of homocysteine in the development of coronary heart disease.

- Explain how regular physical activity reduces the risk of coronary heart disease.

Aside from the positive effects of exercise in maintaining physiologic function, regular physical activity protects against this nation's greatest killer, **coronary heart disease (CHD)**. Individuals in physically active occupations have a two- to threefold lower risk of heart attack than individuals in sedentary jobs. Furthermore, chances of surviving a heart attack increase substantially for those with a physically demanding job or lifestyle. Physical activity also favorably modifies important CHD risk factors. Regular aerobic exercise lowers elevated blood pressure, reduces excess body fat, and improves the blood lipid profile. The blood clotting mechanism can normalize with exercise training, which reduces the chances of a blood clot forming on the roughened surface of a coronary artery. Regular exercise may also improve myocardial blood flow, and retard the progression of heart disease, or at least maintains adequate blood supply to the heart muscle to compensate for coronary arteries narrowed by fatty deposits within their walls.

Surgeon General's Report on Physical Activity and Health

The Surgeon General of the United States acknowledged the importance of physical activity in 1996 in a report that summarized the benefits of regular exercise in disease prevention. The conclusions and recommendations of this report apply to all individuals trying to improve their health. Hopefully this document will generate as great an impact as the 1964 Surgeon General's Report on the hazards of cigarette smoking.

The report focuses on three objectives:

1. Summarize existing literature relating regular physical activity to disease prevention
2. Evaluate current status of physical activity in the population
3. Stimulate increased physical activity among Americans of all ages

Concerning the benefits of regular physical activity, the report concludes:

- Almost everyone derives health benefits from participation in regular physical activity.

- Significant health and quality of life benefits emerge with only moderate, daily physical activity (e.g., 30 min brisk walking or raking leaves, 15 min running, or 45 min playing volleyball).

- People who maintain a regular regimen of vigorous activity of relatively longer duration obtain the greatest health-related benefits.

Adults

- 15% engage in regular vigorous physical activity during leisure time (3 times a wk for at least 20 min)
- More than 60% do not engage in physical activity regularly; 25% lead sedentary lives
- Walking, gardening, and yard work represent the most popular leisure-time activities for adults
- 22% engage in light-to-moderate physical activity regularly during leisure time (5 times a wk for at least 30 min)
- Physical inactivity occurs more among women than men, blacks and Hispanics than whites, older than younger adults, and less affluent than wealthier persons
- Participation in fitness activities declines with age. A large number of older citizens have such poor functional capacity that they cannot raise from a chair or bed, walk to the bathroom, or climb even a single stair without assistance

Children and Teenagers

- Nearly one-half between ages 12 and 21 years do not exercise vigorously on a regular basis; a sharp decline in physical activity occurs during adolescence
- 14% report no recent physical activity (more prevalent among females, particularly black females)
- 25% engage in light to moderate physical activity (e.g., walk or bicycle) nearly every day
- Participation in all types of physical activity declines strikingly as age and school grade increase
- More males participate in vigorous physical activity, strengthening activities, and walking or bicycling than females
- Daily attendance in school physical education programs declined from 42% in early 1990 to only 25% in 1996
- 19% of high school students report being physically active for at least 20 minutes in daily physical education classes

- Regular physical activity reduces premature mortality risk, and specific risks of coronary heart disease, hypertension, osteoporosis, colon cancer, and type 2 diabetes. It also enhances overall mental well being and contributes to optimal neuromuscular-skeletal functioning.

Physical Activity and Specific Health Concerns

The Surgeon General's Report detailed the effects of physical activity on different diseases and health conditions. Many of the studies reviewed in this report formed the basis for: (a) the American Heart Association (1992; www.americanheart.org/) to identify *physical inactivity* as the fourth major coronary heart disease risk factor, (b) the National Institutes of Health Consensus Development Conference on Physical Activity and Cardiovascular Health (1995; www.americanheart.org/) to confirm the importance of physical activity for cardiovascular health, and (c) the American College of Sports Medicine; www.acsm.org/ and Centers of Disease Control and Prevention (1995; www.cdc.gov/) to jointly recommend that all Americans accumulate *at least* 30 minutes of daily moderate-intensity physical activity.

Table 20.1 summarizes conclusions concerning the effects of regular exercise on health and disease. These findings emerged from research strategies that compared physical activity levels of healthy individuals and people with pre-existing disease conditions (or who develop a disease); assessed the association between physical activity and disease at a single point in time (**cross-sectional studies**); followed a group of individuals forward in time (**longitudinal studies**) to observe how physical activity habits relate to disease occurrence or death; intentionally altered physical activity patterns and assessed subsequent modification of disease occurrence or severity (**clinical trials**). Clearly, the findings indicate that regular physical activity has wide-ranging effects on diverse aspects of a person's overall health, well being, and quality of life.

Safety of Exercising

People have questioned the safety of exercising because of several well-publicized reports of sudden death during physical activity. Actually, sudden death rates during exercise have declined over the past 20 years despite an increase in exercise participation. In one report of cardiovascular episodes over a 5-year period, 2935 exercisers recorded 374,798 exercise hours that included 2,726,272 km (1.7 million miles) of running and walking; equivalent of running 65,000 marathons. No deaths occurred during this time (with only two nonfatal cardiovascular complications). *Certainly, a small increased risk of a cardiovascular episode during exercise exists compared with resting. However, the total reduction in heart disease risk from regular physical activity (compared with remaining sedentary) far outweighs any slight increase in risk during actual exercise.*

TABLE 20.1
Effects of regular physical activity on health and disease

VARIABLE	EFFECT
Overall mortality	1. Higher levels of regular physical activity (PA) associate with lower mortality rates for both older and younger adults. 2. Even those moderately active on a regular basis have lower mortality rates than those who are least active.
Cardiovascular diseases	1. Regular PA decreases the risk of cardiovascular disease mortality in general and of CHD in particular. 2. The level of decreased risk of CHD attributable to regular PA is similar to that of other healthful lifestyle behaviors, such as obstaining from cigarette smoking. 3. Regular PA prevents or delays the development of high blood pressure, and reduces blood pressure in people with hypertension.
Cancer	1. Regular PA associates with decreased risk of colon cancer. 2. No association exists between physical activity and rectal cancer. Conclusions regarding the relationship between PA and other cancers require further research. 3. Inconsistent data exist regarding the association between PA and breast or prostate cancer.
Type 2 Diabetes mellitus	1. PA lowers the risk of developing type 2 diabetes mellitus.
Osteoarthritis	1. PA maintains normal muscle strength and joint function. PA does not relate to joint damage or development of osteoarthritis and may benefit people with arthritis. 2. Sports-related injuries most likely cause development of osteoarthritis later in life.
Osteoporosis	1. Weight-bearing PA is essential for normal skeletal development during childhood and adolescence. 2. It remains controversial the degree to which resistance- or endurance-type PA reduces the accelerated rate of bone loss in postmenopausal women in the absence of estrogen replacement therapy.
Falling	1. Promising evidence indicates that resistance training and other forms of exercise in older adults preserve the ability to maintain independent living and reduce the risk of falling.
Obesity	1. Low levels PA, resulting in fewer kcal used than consumed, contribute to the high prevalence of obesity. 2. PA may favorably affect body fat distribution.
Mental heath	1. PA appears to relieve symptoms of depression and anxiety and improve mood.
Health-related quality of life	1. PA appears to improve health-related quality of life by enhancing psychological well-being and by improving physical functioning in persons compromised by poor health.

Modified from U.S. Department of Health and Human Services: *Surgeon General's Report: Physical Activity and Health.* Washington, D.C., 1996.

Perhaps not surprisingly, musculoskeletal injury represents the most prevalent exercise complication. For 351 participants and 60 instructors at six aerobic dance facilities, 327 medical complaints were reported during nearly 30,000 hours of activity. Eighty-four of the injuries caused disability (2.8 per 1000 person-hours of participation), and only 2.1% of the injuries required medical attention. Orthopedic injuries are more common in those who run or jog for extended durations. In this sense, more is definitely *not* better.

The New Gerontology

Genes influence life span, patterns of aging, and susceptibility to disease. Yet scientists know little about why humans live five times longer than cats, cats five times longer than mice, mice outlive fruit flies by a factor of 25, or why the onset of different diseases (e.g., Alzheimer's disease) often differ by many years in identical twins.

The contribution of genetics to the unprecedented increase in human life expectancy remains unanswered. In the early 1900s, for example, 4% of the U.S. population exceeded 65 years of age. By 1998, that percentage increased to 13%. A citizen's average life expectancy has increased from 47 years in 1900 to 76 years today, and should reach 83 years by the year 2050. Sixty-three percent of today's 65-year-olds will achieve their 85th birthday, and 24% will celebrate age 95. Researchers now believe that the average child born today may live healthfully to age 95 or 100, with the limit of human life span currently estimated at 130 years. Interestingly, there are more people above age 80 in China than the entire United States population, in which

Current Life Expectancy for People Who Have Attained a Given Age

Age	Years Remaining	Age	Years Remaining
30	55.1	70	18.7
35	50.3	75	15.0
40	45.4	80	11.6
45	40.6	85	8.8
50	36.0	90	6.5
55	31.4	95	4.8
60	27.0	100	3.5
65	22.8		

only 15% of the total population exceed age 61. Future research needs to consider a multidisciplinary life-span approach for the health and well-being of individuals who possess a mosaic of abilities.*

Improved overall health accompanies the extended life span. The prevalence of chronic disorders (e.g., arthritis, dementia, hypertension, stroke, and emphysema) continues to decline. Eighty-nine percent of Americans age 65 to 74 years report no disability; even after 85 years of age, 4% remain fully functional. A decline in the population of elders living in nursing homes (6.3% in 1982 to 5.2% in 1998) accompanies the upgraded functional status of the elderly. Concurrently, a **"new gerontology"** expands the focus on aging from the previous focus on preoccupation with disease and frailty to a more positive, dynamic notion of **"successful aging."**

---

*Personal communication. C.A. Tate, University of Illinois at Chicago.

Concept of Successful Aging

The aging process, including physical frailty in the last decade of life, traditionally was viewed as physiologically inevitable. The typical "aging syndrome" included a broad array of age-related and/or lifestyle-dependent deleterious changes in blood pressure, bone mass, body composition and body fat distribution, insulin sensitivity, and homocysteine levels that convey increased health risk, dysfunction, or actual disease. This traditional view has changed dramatically; now chronologic aging does not conform to the grim notion that loss of body structure and functional capacity cannot be altered. *As more people reach that "ripe old age," successful aging encompasses more than just preventing or delaying disease. Many gerontologists consider that successful aging includes four main components: 1), physical health, 2), spirituality, 3), emotional and educational health, and 4), social satisfaction. Successful aging involves maintaining, and even enhancing, physical and cognitive functions, and fully engaging in life, including productive activities and interpersonal relations.*

Lifestyle changes that include sound nutrition and diverse forms of exercise substantially blunt the decline in function and increased disease risk with aging. Lack of muscle strength often limits a healthy elderly person's chance to live a full, independent, and productive life into the ninth and tenth decades. In a study of 100 frail nursing home residents (average age: 87 years), resistance training for only 45 minutes, three times weekly for 10 weeks *doubled* muscular strength and improved gait and stairclimbing ability. Such findings demonstrate that the healthy human body can respond and adapt favorably to regular exercise at *any* age. However, consideration must be paid to what types of exercise professionals prescribe for the older population with documented risk factors for osteoporosis, particularly reduced bone mineral density. More research relating to the factor of risk requires elucidation. Specifically, cross-disciplinary studies in the exercise sciences and engineering should evaluate the forces involved during falling (especially falling sidewards that causes about 80% of hip fractures), and the efficacy of different exercises typically prescribed and engaged in by the elderly.

Aging and Bodily Function

Figure 20.1 shows that bodily functions improve rapidly during childhood

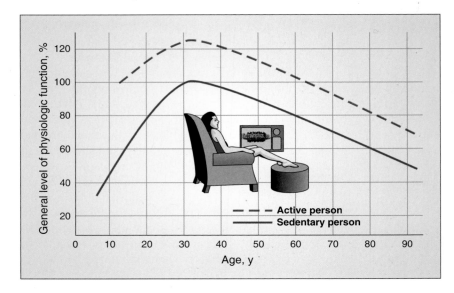

Figure 20.1
Generalized curve to illustrate age-related changes in physiologic function. All comparisons made against the 100% value achieved by the 20- to 30-year-old sedentary person.

and reach a maximum at about age 30 years; thereafter, a decline in functional capacity occurs with age. Although a similar age trend exists for physically active persons, physiologic function averages about 25% higher compared with sedentary counterparts at each age category (an active 50-year-old man or woman often maintains the functional level of a 30-year-old). All physiologic measures eventually decline with age, but not all decrease at the same rate.

Nerve conduction velocity, for example, declines only 10 to 15% from 30 to 80 years of age, whereas resting cardiac index (ratio of cardiac output to surface area) and joint flexibility decline 20 to 30%; maximum breathing capacity at age 80 averages 40% of values for a 30-year-old. Brain cells die at a fairly constant rate until age 60, whereas liver and kidneys lose 40 to 50% of their function between ages 30 and 70. By the seventh decade, the average female has lost 30% of her bone mass, whereas men lose only 15%. Gerontologists often considered these aging patterns "normal" and "expected" decreases in structure and function.

Aging and Muscular Strength

Men and women achieve maximum strength between ages 20 to 30 years, when muscle cross-sectional area achieves maximum size. Thereafter, strength progressively declines for most muscle groups; by age 70, overall strength decreases by 30%.

Decrease in Muscle Mass

Strength decreases with age because of a reduction in muscle mass. The smaller muscle mass in older adults reflects a loss of total muscle protein induced by inactivity, aging, or the combined effects of both. Some loss in muscle fiber number also takes place with aging. For example, the biceps of a newborn contains about 500,000 individual fibers, whereas the same muscle for an 80-year-old man has 300,000 fibers or 40% less.

Muscle Trainability Among the Elderly

Regular exercise training retains body protein and blunts the loss of muscle mass and strength with aging. Healthy men between age 60 and 72 years participated in a 12-week standard resistance training program (similar to that outlined in Chapter 15). Figure 20.2 shows that the men's muscle strength increased progressively throughout the program, averaging about 5% each exercise session—a training response similar to young adults. Many exercise specialists who work with the elderly believe that improving strength effectively maintains muscle mass, increases mobility, and reduces injury incidence.

Aging and Joint Flexibility

With advancing age, connective tissue (cartilage, ligaments, and tendons) becomes stiffer and more rigid, which reduces joint flexibility. It is unclear whether these changes result from biologic aging or reflect the impact of chronic disuse through sedentary living and/or degenerative tissue diseases of specific joints. Regardless of the cause, appropriate exercises that regularly move joints through their full range of motion increase flexibility 20 to 50% in men and women at all ages.

Endocrine Changes with Aging

Endocrine function, particularly the pituitary, pancreas, adrenal, and thyroid glands, changes with age. About 40% of individuals between ages 65 and 75 years, and 50% of those older than age 80, have impaired glucose tolerance, which leads to type 2 diabetes. This represents the most common form of diabetes and afflicts 1 in 17 Americans; nearly one-half of these cases remain undiagnosed. Impaired glucose metabolism leading to high blood glucose levels in type 2 diabetes results from:

- Decreased effect of insulin on peripheral tissue (**insulin resistance**)
  - Inadequate insulin production by the pancreas to control blood sugar (**relative insulin deficiency**)
  - Combined effect of insulin resistance and relative insulin deficiency

Figure 20.2
Weekly measurement of dynamic muscle strength (1-RM) in left knee extension (yellow) and flexion (red). (Data from Frontera, W.R., et al.: Strength conditioning in older men: skeletal muscle hypertrophy and improved function. *J. Appl. Physiol.*, 64:1038, 1988.)

How to Assess Joint Flexibility in Common Body Areas

Two types of flexibility: (1) **static**—full range of motion (ROM) of a specific joint, and (2) **dynamic**—torque or resistance encountered as the joint moves through its ROM. Improper alignment of the vertebral column account for more than 80% of all lower back ailments and pelvic girdle; this often results from poor flexibility in regions of the lower back, trunk, hip, and posterior thigh (common in runners) and weak abdominal and erector spinae muscles.

dons, ligaments, and skin constitute major factors influencing static and dynamic flexibility. Other influences include a well-developed musculature and excess fatty tissue of adjacent body segments. Flexibility progressively decreases with advancing age, due mainly to decreased soft tissue extensibility. How decrements in flexibility reflect true aging or rather result from a "disuse" effect of an increasingly sedentary lifestyle remains unclear. On average, women remain more flexible than men at any age.

Specificity and Flexibility

Significant specificity exists for joint ROM depending on joint structure. Triaxial joints (ball and socket) of the hip and shoulder afford a greater degree of movement than either uniaxial or biaxial joints (wrist, knee, elbow, ankle). "Tightness" of the soft tissue structures of the joint capsule, muscle and its fascia, ten-

Five Common Field Tests of Static Flexibility

Field tests assess static flexibility indirectly through linear measurement of ROM. Administer a minimum of three trials after a warm-up.

Test 1: Hip and Trunk Flexibility (Modified Sit-and-Reach Test)

Starting Position

A
Sit on the floor with the back and head against a wall, legs fully extended with the bottom of the feet against the sit-and-reach box. Place the hands on top of each other, stretching the arms forward while keeping the head and back against the wall. Measure the distance from the finger tips to the box edge with a yardstick. This becomes zero or starting point.

Movement
Slowly bend and reach forward as far as possible (head and back move away from the wall), sliding the fingers along the yardstick; hold the final position for 2 seconds.

B

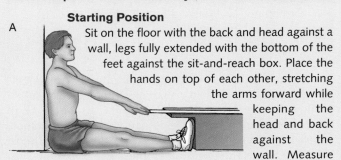

Score
Total distance reached to the nearest one-tenth inch.

Test 2: Shoulder-Wrist Flexibility (Shoulder and Wrist Elevation Test)

Starting Position
Lay prone on the floor with the arms fully extended overhead; grasp a yardstick with the hands shoulder width apart.

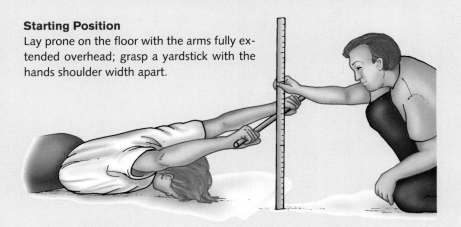

Movement
Raise the stick at high as possible.

- Measure the vertical distance (nearest 1/2 in) the yardstick rises from the floor.
- Measure arm length from the acromial process to the tip of longest finger.
- Subtract the best vertical score from arm length.

Score
- Arm length − Best vertical score (nearest 1/4 in).

Test 3: Trunk and Neck Flexibility (Trunk and Neck Extension Test)

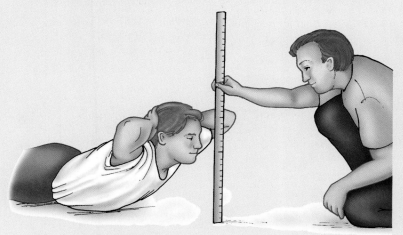

Starting Position
Lay prone on the floor with the hands clasped together behind the head.

Movement
Raise the trunk as high as possible while keeping the hips in contact with the floor. An assistant can hold the legs down.

Score
- Vertical distance (nearest 1/4 in) from the tip of the nose to the floor.

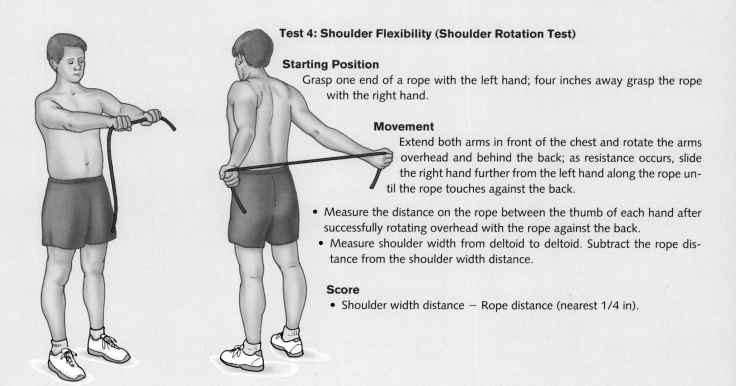

Test 4: Shoulder Flexibility (Shoulder Rotation Test)

Starting Position
Grasp one end of a rope with the left hand; four inches away grasp the rope with the right hand.

Movement
Extend both arms in front of the chest and rotate the arms overhead and behind the back; as resistance occurs, slide the right hand further from the left hand along the rope until the rope touches against the back.

- Measure the distance on the rope between the thumb of each hand after successfully rotating overhead with the rope against the back.
- Measure shoulder width from deltoid to deltoid. Subtract the rope distance from the shoulder width distance.

Score
- Shoulder width distance − Rope distance (nearest 1/4 in).

Test 5: Ankle Flexibility (Ankle Flexion Test)

Starting Position
Stand facing a wall. With feet flat on the floor, lean into the wall.

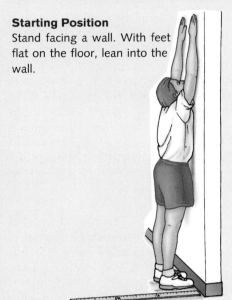

Movement
Slowly slide back from the wall as far as possible, while keeping the feet flat on the floor, body and knees fully extended, and chest in contact with the wall.

Score
1. Distance between the toe line and the wall (nearest 1/4 in).

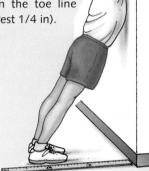

Static Flexibility Classifications

Test Item	Men		Performance Rating	Women	
Shoulder and wrist elevation	6.00 or less		Excellent	5.50 or less	
	8.25–6.25		Good	7.50–5.75	
	11.50–8.50		Average	10.75–7.75	
	12.50–11.75		Fair	11.75–11.0	
	12.75 or more		Poor	12.00 or more	
Trunk and neck extension	3.00 or less		Excellent	2.00 or less	
	6.00–3.25		Good	5.75–2.25	
	8.00–6.25		Average	7.75–6.00	
	10.00–8.25		Fair	9.75–8.00	
	10.25 or more		Poor	10.00 or more	
Shoulder rotation	7.00 or less		Excellent	5.00 or less	
	11.50–7.25		Good	9.75–5.25	
	14.50–11.75		Average	13.00–10.00	
	19.75–14.75		Fair	17.75–13.25	
	20.00 or more		Poor	18.00 or more	
Ankle flexion	26.50 or less		Excellent	24.25 or less	
	29.50–26.75		Good	26.50–24.50	
	32.50–29.75		Average	30.25–26.75	
	35.25–32.75		Fair	31.75–30.50	
	35.50 or more		Poor	32.00 or more	

Modified sit-and-reach					
Age range	<35 y	36–49 y		<35 y	36–49 y
	>17.9	>16.1	Excellent	>17.9	>17.4
	17.0–17.9	14.6–16.1	Good	16.7–17.9	16.2–17.4
	15.8–17.0	13.9–14.6	Average	16.2–16.7	15.2–16.2
	15.0–15.8	13.4–13.9	Fair	15.8–16.2	14.5–15.2
	<15.0	<13.4	Poor	<15.4	<14.5

Adapted from Johnson B.L., and Nelson J.K.: *Practical Measurements for Evaluation in Physical Education. 4th Ed*. N.Y.: Macmillan Publishing, 1986.

Exercise Prescription for Type 2 Diabetes

Screening	Cardiovascular risk factor analysis; medical clearance plus stress ECG for patients over 35 years of age
Frequency	**Exercise Program**
Intensity	5 to 7 days per week
Time	50 to 70% $\dot{V}O_{2max}$; heart rate 120 to 150 b · min^{-1}
Type	20 to 40 minutes per session
Precautions	Aerobic; rhythmic activities involving large muscle mass
Compliance	Warm-up and cool-down periods if necessary; avoid high-impact activities; emphasize good footwear and proper foot hygiene; blood glucose monitoring

Young, J.C.: Exercise for clients with Type 2 diabetes. *ACSM's Health & Fitness J.*, 2(3):24, 1998.

With the exception of a genetic predisposition, increased disease prevalence largely relates to "controllable" factors like poor diet, inadequate physical activity, and increased body fat, particularly in the visceral-abdominal region.

Thyroid dysfunction, resulting from a lowered pituitary gland release of thyroid-stimulating hormone thyrotropin (and reduced output of thyroxine from the thyroid gland), commonly occurs among the elderly. This affects metabolic function, including decreased glucose metabolism and protein synthesis.

Figure 20.3 depicts changes in three other hormonal systems associated with aging: the hypothalamic-pituitary-gonadal axis, adrenal cortex, and growth hormone/insulin-like growth factor axis.

Hypothalamic-Pituitary-Gonadal Axis

Alteration in the interaction between stimulating hormones from the hypothalamus and the anterior pituitary gland and gonads decreases estradiol output from the ovaries, which probably initiates permanent cessation of the menses (**menopause**) in the aging female. Changes in hypothalamic-pituitary-gonadal axis activity in males occur more slowly and subtly. For example, serum total and free testosterone decline with aging in males. Age-related decreases in gonadotropic secretions from the anterior pituitary gland characterize male **andropause.**

Adrenal Cortex

Adrenopause refers to the significant decrease in output from the adrenal cortex of dehydroepiandrosterone (DHEA) and its sulfated ester (DHEAS). In contrast to the glucocorticoid and mineralocorticoid adrenal steroids whose plasma levels remain relatively high with aging, a long, progressive but slow decline in DHEA occurs after age 30. This has led to speculation concerning DHEA's role in aging and has produced a dramatic increase in unregulated supplementation of this hormone by the general public. Chapter 17 provides a more detailed discussion of DHEA, its uses, risks, and alleged role as an ergogenic aid.

Growth Hormone/Insulin-Like Growth Factor 1 Axis

Mean pulse amplitude, duration, and fraction of secreted growth hormone (GH) gradually decrease with aging, a condition termed **somatopause.** A parallel decrease in circulating insulin-like growth factor (IGF-1) levels also takes place. IGF-1, produced by the liver and other cells, stimulates tissue growth and protein synthesis. The trigger for the age-related GH decrease probably lies in the interaction between the hypothalamus and anterior pituitary gland.

To what extent changes in gonadal function (menopause and andropause) contribute to adrenopause and somatopause (present in both sexes) remains unknown. A growing body of evidence indicates that functional correlates, such as muscle size and strength, body composition, and bone mass alterations, and progression of atherosclerosis, directly relate to hormonal changes with aging. Hormonal replacement therapy, nutritional supplementation, and regular exercise may delay or even prevent aspects of hormone-related aging dysfunction.

Aging and Nervous System Function

A 37% decline in the number of spinal cord axons, and 10% decline in nerve conduction velocity reflect cumulative effects of aging on central nervous system function. Such changes partially explain age-related decrements in neuromuscular performance. Partitioning reaction time into central processing time and muscle contraction time indicates that aging exerts the greatest effect on stimulus detection and information processing to produce a response. For example, the knee jerk reflex does not require central nervous system processing, instead, it becomes less affected by aging than voluntary responses and movement patterns.

Despite the real effects of aging on reaction and movement time, physically active young or old groups move significantly faster than a corresponding less active age group. These observations fuel speculation that regular participation in physical activity may thwart the biologic aging of certain neuromuscular functions.

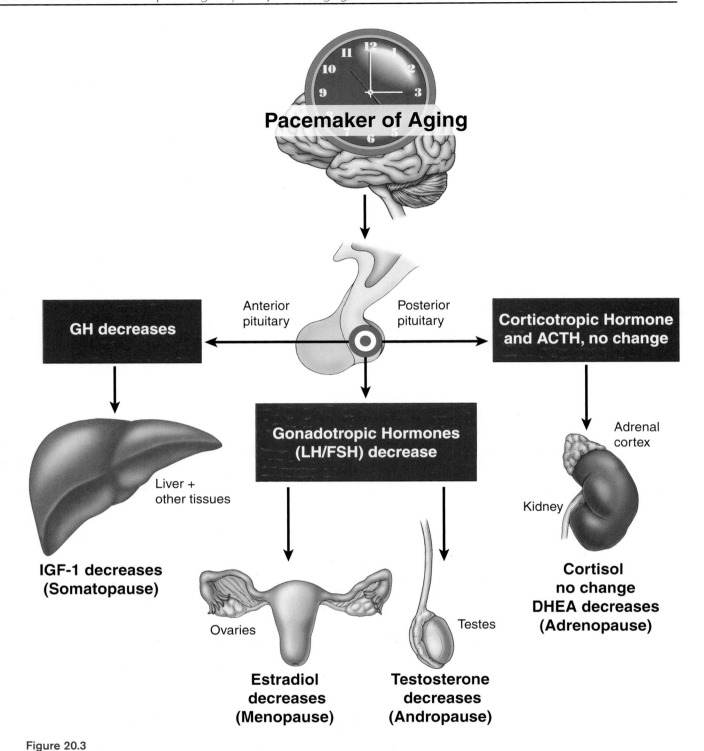

Figure 20.3
Age-related decline in three hormone systems that profoundly affect the rate of biological aging. **Left,** Decreased growth hormone (GH) release by the anterior pituitary depresses production of IGF-1 by the liver and other tissues, which inhibits cellular growth (a condition of aging termed somatopause). (**Middle**) Decreased output of the gonadotropic luteinizing hormones, (LH) and follicle-stimulating hormone (FSH), by the anterior pituitary, coupled with reduced estradiol secretion from the ovaries and testosterone from the testes, causes menopause (females) and andropause (males). **Right,** Adrenocortical cells responsible for DHEA production decrease their activity (termed adrenopause) without clinically evident changes in this gland's corticotrophin (ACTH) and cortisol secretion. A central "pacemaker" in the hypothalamus and/or higher brain areas probably mediates these processes to produce aging related changes in peripheral organs (ovaries, testicles, and adrenal cortex).

Aging and Pulmonary Function

Whether regular exercise throughout one's life overrides pulmonary system "aging" remains unknown. Cross-sectional studies indicate that dynamic pulmonary capacity of older endurance-trained athletes exceeds that of sedentary peers. Although longitudinal studies will provide a definitive answer, available data suggests that regular physical activity retards pulmonary function deterioration associated with aging. Much of this affect probably relates to maintenance of power and endurance of the ventilatory musculature with regular exercise.

Aging and Cardiovascular Function

Different indices of cardiovascular function and exercise endurance decline with age, yet regular physical activity can exert a profound influence on age-related decrements.

Maximal Oxygen Uptake

Maximal oxygen uptake ($\dot{V}O_{2max}$) declines steadily after age 20, decreasing by 35 to 40% at age 65 (slightly less than 1% per year). A slower rate of decline occurs for individuals who maintain an active lifestyle that includes regular aerobic training, without a decline in fat-free body mass (FFM). *Physical activity, however, does not entirely prevent aging's effect on $\dot{V}O_{2max}$, even when adjusting for a person's quantity of muscle mass.*

Figure 20.4 shows the relationship between $\dot{V}O_{2max}$ and active appendicular (legs and arms) muscle mass for young (average age 25 y) and old (average age 63 y) aerobically-trained men and women. Young subjects had trained 9 consecutive years, and older subjects trained 20 consecutive years. Older men and women exhibited about a 14% lower $\dot{V}O_{2max}$ than younger counterparts throughout the broad range of variation in muscle mass among subjects. In other words, despite an equivalence in appendicular muscle mass between a young and older subject, the young subject exhibited a *higher* $\dot{V}O_{2max}$.

Deterioration in $\dot{V}O_{2max}$ with aging probably results from age-associated loss of muscle mass, increase in body fat, and altered cardiovascular and pulmonary functions. The reductions in aerobic power per kg of active muscle mass with aging displayed in Figure 20.4 can reflect only age-associated reduced oxygen delivery and/or reduced oxygen extraction at the active muscle. However, skeletal muscle oxidative capacity and capillarization (important components of oxygen extraction) remain similar in older and younger individuals with comparable physiologic characteristics and training histories. Consequently, the well-documented reduction in cardiac output (decreases in both maximum heart rate and stroke volume) represents the most likely explanation for the decrease in $\dot{V}O_{2max}$ per kg of active muscle accompanying aging.

Aging Response to Exercise Training

Among the healthy elderly, exercise training enhances the heart's capacity to pump blood and increases aerobic capacity to the same relative degree as in younger adults. Nine to 12 months of endurance training in healthy older adults increased $\dot{V}O_{2max}$ 19% in men and 22% in women. These values represent the high end of the typical training response for young adults. Regular aerobic training for middle-age men over a 20-year period significantly delayed the usual 10 to 15% decline in exercise capacity and aerobic fitness. At age 55, these active men maintained nearly

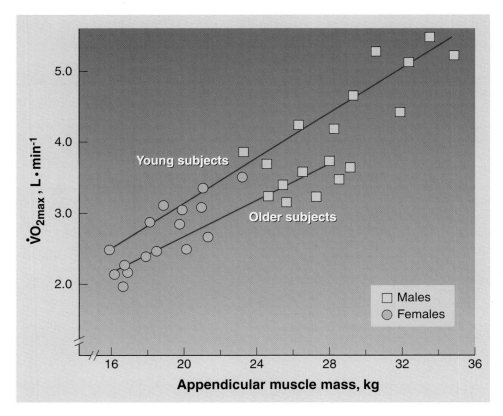

Figure 20.4
Maximal oxygen uptake ($\dot{V}O_{2max}$) related to appendicular muscle mass in young and older endurance-trained men and women. $\dot{V}O_{2max}$ per kg of active muscle mass decreases with age, independent of training status. (Modified from: Proctor, D.N., and Joyner, M.J.: Skeletal muscle mass and the reduction of $\dot{V}O_{2max}$ in trained older subjects. *J. Appl. Physiol.*, 82: 1411, 1997).

close up

Differences in Exercise Physiology Between Children and Adults

Considerable physiologic and exercise performance differences exist between children and adults. For example, in weight-bearing walking and running, children's oxygen uptake ($mL \cdot kg^{-1} \cdot min^{-1}$) averages 10 to 30% higher than adults at a designated submaximal pace. This lower running economy, likely results from the shorter stride length and greater stride frequency of children. This makes a standard walking or running pace physiologically more stressful (and performance score poorer) for children than adults, even though children average equal or slightly higher aerobic capacities than adults.

Because of a smaller body size, children have lower absolute ($L \cdot min^{-1}$) aerobic capacities than larger adults. Thus, exercising against a standard absolute external resistance not adjusted to body size (e.g., stationary cycling, arm cranking) disadvantages children. This occurs because the fixed oxygen cost in $L \cdot min^{-1}$ of exercise represents a greater percentage of the child's smaller absolute aerobic capacity. In weight-bearing exercise, energy cost directly relates to body mass; thus, children do not become disadvantaged by a small body size.

Children do less well than adults on tests of anaerobic power. This probably results from their inability to generate a high level of blood lactate (a marker for glycolysis) during exhaustive anaerobic exercise. Also, the significantly lower levels of the glycolytic enzyme phosphofructokinase in children compared with adults contribute to poor anaerobic capacity.

During submaximal exercise, children exhibit larger ventilation volumes at any oxygen uptake (larger ventilatory equivalent) than adults.

Children, like adults, significantly increase muscular strength in response to resistance training. Unlike pubescent children and adults, prepubescent children show limited muscle mass increases with local muscle overload. This probably results from their relatively low androgen levels.

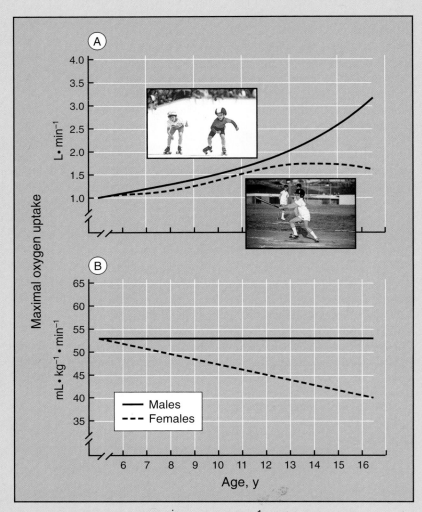

A, Boys and girls display a similar $\dot{V}O_{2max}$ ($L \cdot min^{-1}$) to about age 12. By age 14, the boys average 25% higher, and by age 16 the difference exceeds 50%. The development of a greater muscle mass in boys and more daily physical activity largely explains this sex-related difference in aerobic capacity. **B,** $\dot{V}O_{2max}$ ($mL \cdot kg^{-1} \cdot min^{-1}$) for boys stabilizes at about 52 $mL \cdot kg^{-1} \cdot min^{-1}$ from age 6 to 16; for females, the line slopes downward with age reaching about 40 $mL \cdot kg^{-1} \cdot min^{-1}$ at age 16, a value 32% below male counterparts. This difference probably reflects females' greater accumulation of body fat; extra fat must be transported but does not contribute to enhanced aerobic capacity. (Data from Krahenbuhl, G.S., et al.: Developmental aspects of maximal aerobic power in children. In: *Exercise and Sport Sciences Reviews, Vol. 13.* Terjung, R. L. (ed.). New York: Macmillan, 1985).

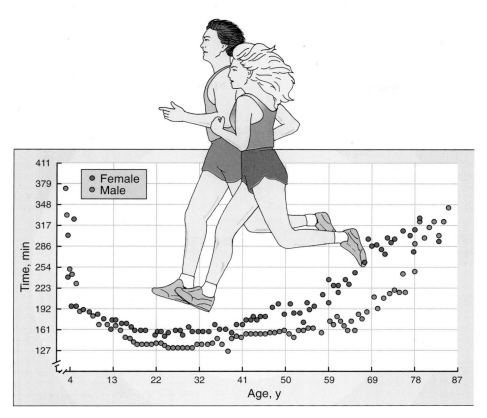

Figure 20.5
World record marathon times for men and women of different ages.

Other Age-Related Variables

Figure 20.6 shows longitudinal changes for maximum heart rate, minute pulmonary ventilation, and oxygen pulse (mL O_2 per heart beat; used to estimate stroke volume) of 21 men tested at ages 50 (T1), 60 (T2), and again at age 70 years (T3). The men trained continuously throughout the 20-year period; each had placed either first, second, or third in regional, national, or international competition in running events during a 10-year measurement interval. With the exception of pulmonary ventilation (small increase at T2), each variable decreased over time. Maximum heart rate decreased by five to seven beats per minute at each measurement over the 20 years (a smaller decrease than generally reported for nonathletes as expressed by the equation: $HR_{max} = 220 - age, y$. Age-related decrements in maximum heart rate have been attributed to:

- Alterations in the innate activity of the sinoatrial (S-A) node
- Reduced output of sympathetic activity from the medulla
- Reluctance of researchers to encourage older, nonathletic individuals to go "all-out" to attain a maximal effort during testing

Reduction in the heart's stroke volume (indicated by the change in the oxygen pulse measurements), most likely reflects changes in myocardial contractility with aging. Other age-related cardiovascular changes include reduced blood flow capacity to peripheral tissues, narrowing of the coronary arteries (30% obstruction by middle age), and decreased elasticity of major blood vessels.

the same values for blood pressure, body mass, and $\dot{V}O_{2max}$ as at age 35; by age 70, their $\dot{V}O_{2max}$ equaled values for individuals 25 years younger. These remarkable findings attest to the adaptability of the aerobic system to training at any age.

Aging and Endurance Performance

Comparing endurance performance times among individuals of different ages points out the dramatic effects of exercise training on preserving cardiovascular function throughout life. Figure 20.5 shows the world-record marathon times for males and females of different ages, starting at about age 4 and into the mid-80s. The world record time of 340.2 minutes for a 86-year-old male corresponds to a 12.9 min per mile pace; for the 80-year-old female, the world record time equals 328.6 minutes (12.5-min per mile pace). This represents a remarkable 26.2-mile average running speed for men and women in their eighth decade of life. Performances of this quality attest to the tremendous cardiovascular capabilities of the healthy elderly who continue to train regularly as they grow older.

Aging and Body Composition

Excess body fat accumulation usually begins in childhood or develops slowly during adulthood. Middle-age men and women invariably weigh more than their college-age counterparts of the same stature (with differences in body fat accounting for the weight difference). Scientists do not know if gains in body fat during adulthood represent a normal biologic pattern. Observations of physically active older individuals suggest that, while the typical individual grows fatter with age, those who remain physically active counter the

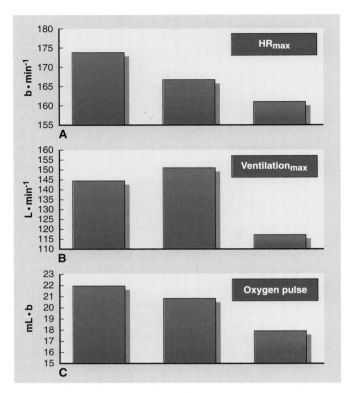

Figure 20.6

Changes in maximum (**A**) heart rate, (**B**) minute ventilation, and (**C**) oxygen pulse for 21 endurance athletes who continued to train over a 20-year period, beginning at age 50. Modified from Pollock, M.L. et al.: Twenty-year follow-up of aerobic power and body composition of older track athletes. *J. Appl. Physiol.*, 82: 1508, 1997.

"normal loss" in FFM while blunting the typical increase body fat percentage. In addition to preservation of FFM, the very real concern about the lack of weight-bearing (mechanical loading) deserves concern because it impacts on osteoporosis with aging. Longitudinal research of bone mineral content assessed every 6 months in children from age 6 to 12 years showed that 26% of adult total body bone mineral accrued during just 2 years of peak bone mineral deposition. Such direct evidence seems self evident for it's long range implications. From our perspective, we strongly endorse the position that increased physical activity should play an increasingly more important role as children grow into adolescence and adulthood. In this scenario, daily, required classroom physical education begun in kindergarten seems worthwhile and entirely justified.

Perhaps the eventual "cure" for osteoporosis and its attendant medical and societal costs really should be viewed as a problem of young age (pediatric medicine) and not older age (geriatric medicine).

We believe that more research emphasis should focus on "bone health" and physical activity status of the very young in our societies worldwide.

Figure 20.7 shows body composition changes over a 20-

year period for the same 21 elite master's runners depicted in Figure 20.6. Despite maintaining a relatively constant body mass during the prolonged period of exercise training (T1 = 70.1 kg; T2 = 69.4 kg; T3 = 70.8 kg), gains occurred

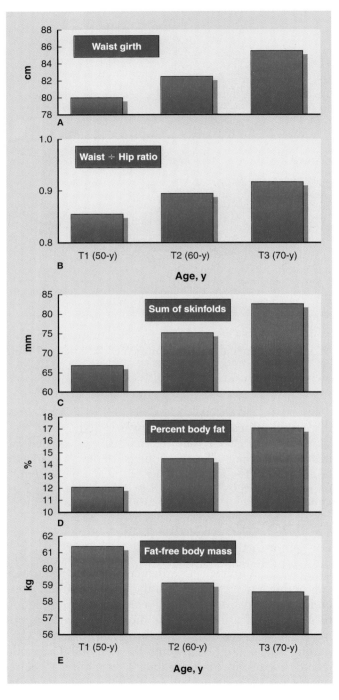

Figure 20.7

Changes in (**A**) waist girth, (**B**) waist:hip girth ratio, (**C**) sum of skinfolds, (**D**) percent body fat, and (**E**) fat-free body mass, for 21 endurance athletes who continued to train over a 20-year period, starting at age 50. (Modified from Pollock, M.L. et al.: Twenty-year follow-up of aerobic power and body composition of older track athletes. *J. Appl. Physiol.*, 82: 1508, 1997.)

in body fat while FFM declined. The roughly 3% body fat unit increase per decade paralleled similar increases in waist girth. These data support an argument that some alterations in body composition and body fat distribution represent a normal aging response.

Regular Exercise: A Fountain of Youth?

Although exercise may not necessarily represent a "fountain of youth," regular physical activity not only retards the decline in functional capacity associated with aging and disuse, but often reverses the loss of function regardless of when a person becomes active.

Does Exercise Improve Health and Extend Life?

Medical experts have debated if a lifetime of regular exercise contributes to good health and perhaps longevity compared with a sedentary "good life." Because older, fit individuals exhibit many functional characteristics of younger people, one could argue that improved physical fitness and a vigorous lifestyle retard biological aging and confer health benefits later in life.

Nearly 45 years ago, one group of researchers investigated the diseases and longevity of former college athletes. This seemed like an excellent group to study possible links between exercise and longevity, because collegiate athletes usually have longer involvement in habitual physical activity prior to entering college than nonathletes, and they *may* remain more physically active after graduation.

Figure 20.8 shows essentially *no difference* in the longevity of ex-athletes compared with nonathletes. Some degree of equality in genetic background existed between the groups because of similarities in average age at death of grandparents, parents, and siblings of ex-athletes and nonathletes. *These and more recent findings suggest that participation in athletics as a young adult does not assure significant longevity.*

Enhanced Quality to a Longer Life: A Study of Harvard Alumni

Research concerning current lifestyles and exercise habits of 17,000 Harvard alumni who entered college between 1916 and 1950 indicates that only moderate aerobic exercise, equivalent to jogging three miles a day, promotes good health and actually adds time to life. Men who expended 2000 kcal in weekly exercise had up to one-third lower death rates than classmates who did little or no exercise. To achieve a 2000 kcal energy output weekly requires moderate additional physical activity such as a daily 30 to 45-minute brisk walk, or a moderate run, cycle, swim, cross-country ski, or aerobic dance. The following summarizes the results of the long-term study of alumni:

- Regular exercise counters the life-shortening effects of cigarette smoking and excess body weight
- Even for people with high blood pressure (a primary heart disease risk), those who exercised regularly reduced their death rate by one-half
- Regular exercise countered genetic tendencies toward an early death. For individuals who had one or both parents die before age 65 (another significant but non-modifiable risk), a lifestyle that included regular exercise reduced the risk of death by 25%
- A 50% reduction in mortality rate occurred for those whose parents lived beyond 65 years

Figure 20.9 shows that among physically active people, a person who exercises more has a greater reduced risk of death. For example, men who walked 9 or more miles a week had a 21% lower mortality rate than men who walked 3 miles or less. Exercising in light sports activities increased life expectancy 24% over men who remained sedentary. From a perspective of energy expenditure, the life expectancy of Harvard alumni increased steadily from a weekly exercise energy

Figure 20.8
Age at death of athletes and nonathletes. None of the differences between the groups achieved statistical significance. (Data from Montoye, H.J., et al.: *The Longevity and Morbidity of College Athletes.* Indianapolis, IN: Phi Epsilon Kappa, 1957.)

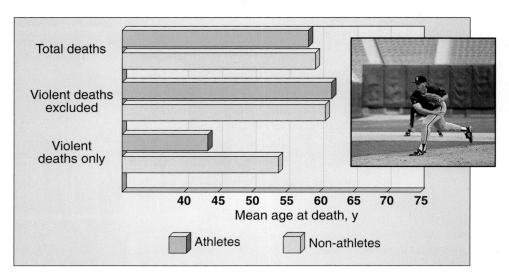

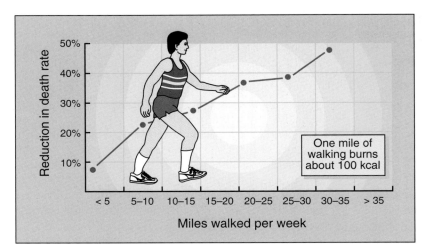

Figure 20.9
Reduced risk of death with regular exercise. (Data from Paffenbarger, R.S., Jr., et al.: Physical activity, all-cause mortality, and longevity of college alumni. N. *Engl. J. Med.*, 314: 605, 1986.)

lustrates that the least fit group died at a three-times greater rate than the most fit subjects.

The most striking finding was that the group rated just above the most sedentary category derived the greatest change in health benefits. The decrease in death rate for men from the least fit to the next category equaled 38 (64.0 vs. 25.5 deaths per 10,000 person-year), whereas the decline from the second group to the most fit category equaled only seven. Women obtained similar benefits as men. The amount of exercise required to move from the most sedentary category to the next more fit category (the jump showing the greatest increase in health benefits) occurred for moderate-intensity exercise like walking briskly for 30 minutes several times weekly. *According to available evidence, if life-extending benefits of exercise exist, they are associated more with preventing early mortality than improving overall life span.* While the maximum life span may not extend greatly, only moderate exercise enables many men and women to live a more productive and healthy life.

output of 500 kcal to 3500 kcal, the equivalent of six to eight hours of strenuous weekly exercise. In addition, active men lived an average of 1 to 2 years longer than sedentary classmates. (Other research estimates a life expectancy increase of about 10 months with regular exercise.)

No additional health or longevity benefits accrued beyond weekly exercise of 3500 kcal. Men who performed extreme exercise actually had higher death rates than less active colleagues (another example of why more does not necessarily indicate better exercise benefits).

Improved Fitness: A Little Goes a Long Way

A study of more than 13,000 men and women over an 8-year interval indicates that even modest amounts of exercise substantially reduce the risk of death from heart disease, cancer, and other causes. The study evaluated fitness performance directly rather than by relying on verbal or written reports of physical activity habits. To isolate the effect of physical fitness per se, the researchers considered factors of smoking, cholesterol and blood sugar levels, blood pressure, and family history of coronary heart disease. Figure 20.10, based on age-adjusted death rates per 10,000 person-years, il-

Coronary Heart Disease

Figure 20.11 illustrates that diseases of the heart and blood vessels cause 50% of total deaths in the United States. This means 1.5 million Americans will have a heart attack this year and about one-third of them will die.

Figure 20.10
Physical fitness and longevity. The greatest reduction in death rate risk occurs when going from the most sedentary category to a moderate fitness level. (Data from Blair, S.N., et al.: Physical fitness and all-cause mortality: a prospective study of healthy men and women. *JAMA*, 262: 2395, 1989.)

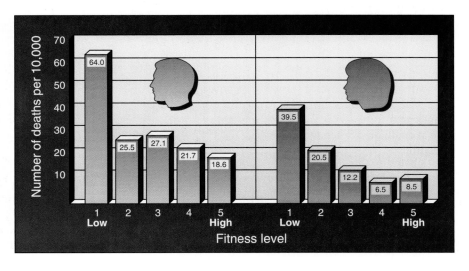

Vigorous Exercisers

People who expend 200 to 300 kcal daily (walk, jog, or run at least 10 miles weekly or the equivalent energy expenditure in swimming, cycling, racquet sports, or other "big muscle" activities) qualify as vigorous exercisers. This represents a reasonable exercise standard associated with beneficial health and health-related changes.

While deaths from CHD have declined more than 35% since 1970, heart disease still remains the leading cause of death in the Western world. Although death rates for women lag about 10 years behind men, the gap has closed fast, particularly for women who smoke. For every American who dies of cancer, about two die of heart-related diseases. This health disaster produces staggering economic losses—$130 billion in 1996 from medical costs, loss of earnings, and lost productivity. This does not include the emotional impact of losing a loved one in the prime of life.

Women at Risk

Women have increased their risk for developing CHD. Since 1910, more American women have died of heart disease than any other cause. Because women develop heart disease 10 to 15 years later in life than men, they more likely have heart attacks when past middle age. Only 1% of women under age 45 develop CHD, whereas 13% above age 75 show clinical heart disease manifestations. This gender-age difference in heart disease episodes makes

Heart Attack Versus Cardiac Arrest

- *Heart attack:* Caused by (a) blockage in one or more arteries supplying the heart, thus cutting off myocardial blood supply, or (b) sudden spasms (constrictions) of a coronary vessel, causing part of the heart muscle to die (necrosis) from lack of oxygen.

- *Cardiac arrest:* Caused by irregular neural-electrical transmission within the myocardium, resulting in chaotic, unregulated beating in the heart's upper chambers (atrial fibrillation) or lower chambers (ventricular fibrillation).

CHD appear as a more pervasive and dramatic problem in men; a heart attack for a 75-year-old woman seems less shocking than for a male "wage earner" who suffers an attack in the prime of life. Increased CHD for women in later years partly relates to loss of protection offered by estrogen, which declines markedly after menopause. Despite limited heart disease research on women, available evidence indicates that disease symptoms, progression, and outcome differ in women and men. Some interesting gender-related heart disease differences include:

- After a heart attack, women usually die sooner
- Women who survive a heart attack frequently experience a second episode
- Women become more incapacitated by heart disease-related pain and disability
- Women are less likely to survive coronary artery bypass surgery

Several factors seem clear: A similar process probably exists for CHD development in men and women, i.e., fatty deposits narrow coronary arteries and reduce blood flow to the myocardium. Gender-related hormonal differences may also affect blood clot formation, coronary artery smooth muscle cell proliferation, and the tendency of coronary vascular walls to spasm in the final stages preceding a heart attack. Moreover, CHD diagnosis may differ in women and men. Diagnostic tests, like the treadmill stress test and ECG response, have limited use with women because men have provided the subject pool for test validation. A diagnostic gap also exists because some physicians do not treat heart disease signs in women as aggressively as in men. Consequently, they do not prescribe coronary angiography (a valid way to diagnose CHD) as often following a positive stress test.

Despite a lower CHD risk, premenopausal women are not immune from heart disease, particularly if they smoke. Cigarette smoking accounts for almost one-half of all heart attacks in women before age 55. Smoking as few as four cigarettes daily doubles a women's CHD risk. Hypertension also exists in more than 50% of women over age 55 who suffer a heart attack; after age 65 it affects two-thirds of female victims. Elevated blood sugar afflicts women more often than men. The presence of either type 1 or type 2 diabetes raises a woman's CHD risk to equal that for a non-diabetic man of the same age, and elevates her risk of dying from a heart attack even more than the man's risk. Use of birth-control pills also raises CHD risk.

A Life-Long Process

Almost all people show some evidence of CHD, which can be severe in seemingly healthy young adults. This degenerative process probably begins early in life, as fatty streaks emerge in the coronary arteries of children as young as age five. Little harm exists for most people until the coronary

	Age groups, y					
Rank	**<1**	**1-4**	**5-9**	**10-14**	**15-24**	**25-34**
1	Congenital Anomalies 20,537	Unintentional Injuries 7387	Unintentional Injuries 4806	Unintentional Injuries 5712	Unintentional Injuries 41,706	Unintentional Injuries 40,909
2	Short Gestation 12,497	Congenital Anomalies 2213	Malignant Neoplasms 1648	Malignant Neoplasms 1520	Homicide 23,824	HIV 35,310
3	SIDS 12,139	Malignant Neoplasms 1528	Congenital Anomalies 757	Homicide 1283	Suicide 14,589	Homicide 20,328
4	Respiratory Distress Syndrome 4836	Homicide 1,389	Homicide 407	Suicide 963	Malignant Neoplasms 5120	Suicide 18,953
5	Maternal Complications 3948	Heart Disease 832	Heart Disease 388	Congenital Anomalies 611	Heart Disease 3012	Malignant Neoplasms 15,010
6	Placenta Cord Membranes 2904	HIV 613	HIV 333	Heart Disease 536	HIV 1879	Heart Disease 10,520
7	Unintentional Injuries 2574	Pneumonia Influenza 517	Pneumonia Influenza 202	Bronchitis Emphysema Asthma 286	Congenital Anomalies 1387	Cerebro-vascular 2319
8	Perinatal Infections 2388	Perinatal Period 301	Benign Neoplasms 142	HIV 193	Bronchitis Emphysema Asthma 684	Liver Disease 2058
9	Pneumonia Influenza 1581	Septicemia 267	Bronchitis Emphysema Asthma 122	Pneumonia Influenza 164	Pneumonia Influenza 679	Pneumonia Influenza 1993
10	Intrauterine Hypoxia 1561	Benign Neoplasms 210	Septicemia 92	Benign Neoplasms 136	Cerebro-vascular 563	Diabetes 1898

Figure 20.11
Leading causes of death in the United States.

arteries become markedly narrowed. Figure 20.12 shows that atherosclerosis involves degenerative changes in the inner lining of the arteries that supply the heart muscle.

The action and chemical modification of various com-
pounds, including oxidation of cholesterol in low-density lipoproteins, initiates a complex process that ultimately causes bulging lesions in the arterial wall. The lesions initially take the form of fatty streaks. With further damage

Age groups, y					
Rank	35-44	45-54	55-64	65+	TOTAL
1	HIV 53,148	Malignant Neoplasms 130,146	Malignant Neoplasms 267,834	Heart Disease 1,845,511	Heart Disease 2,213,432
2	Malignant Neoplasms 50,708	Heart Disease 100,798	Heart Disease 209,618	Malignant Neoplasms 1,128,877	Malignant Neoplasms 1,602,699
3	Unintentional Injuries 41,040	Unintentional Injuries 26,058	Bronchitis Emphysema Asthma 30,994	Cerebro-vascular 404,653	Cerebro-vascular 461,405
4	Heart Disease 39,967	HIV 22,302	Cerebro-vascular 28,937	Bronchitis Emphysema Asthma 261,951	Bronchitis Emphysema Asthma 305,604
5	Suicide 19,012	Cerebro-vascular 15,885	Diabetes 23,450	Pneumonia Influenza 220,912	Unintentional Injuries 275,280
6	Homicide 12,189	Liver Disease 14,993	Unintentional Injuries 19,580	Diabetes 127,554	Pneumonia Influenza 247,216
7	Liver Disease 11,159	Suicide 12,996	Liver Disease 16,499	Unintentional Injuries 85,197	Diabetes 169,840
8	Cerebro-vascular 8008	Diabetes 11,134	Pneumonia Influenza 10,667	Nephritis 59,591	HIV 122,496
9	Diabetes 5326	Bronchitis Emphysema Asthma 7926	Suicide 8677	Alzheimer's Disease 54,869	Suicide 93,528
10	Pneumonia Influenza 4539	Pneumonia Influenza 5943	HIV 6349	Septicemia 92	Liver Disease 75,837

and proliferation of underlying smooth muscle cells, vessels progressively congest with lipid-filled plaques, fibrous scar tissue, or both. This change reduces the vessels' capacity for flood flow, causing the myocardium to receive diminished oxygen (**ischemia**) from inadequate blood flow.

The roughened, hardened lining of the artery frequently causes the slowly flowing blood to clot. When a blood clot (**thrombus**) forms, it plugs one of the smaller coronary vessels, causing necrosis (death) of a portion of the myocardium. In this case, the person can suffer a heart attack or **myocardial infarction**. With only moderate

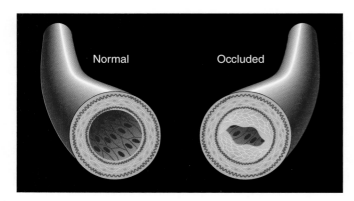

Figure 20.12
Left, Cross section of a normal coronary artery (magnification × 170). **Right,** Deterioration of a coronary artery in atherosclerosis; deposits of fatty substances roughen the vessel's center.

blockage (but with blood flow reduced below the heart's requirement), the person may experience temporary chest pain termed **angina pectoris.** The pains usually magnify during exertion because increased physical activity causes a great demand for myocardial blood flow. Anginal attacks provide vivid evidence of the importance of adequate oxygen supply to the myocardium.

Risk Factors for Coronary Heart Disease

Various personal characteristics and environmental factors identified over the past 45 years indicate a person's susceptibility to CHD. In general, the greater the number of the risk factors, the more likely coronary artery disease exists or will emerge in the near future. This does not mean that a specific risk factor causes disease, as diverse factors may act and interact in a cause-and-effect manner. However, risk factor identification and prudent modification (where possible) improve an individual's chances to avoid CHD.

The following risk factors *can* be modified:

- Cigarette smoking
- Physical inactivity
- Hypertension
- Elevated blood lipids
- Visceral-abdominal adiposity
- Diabetes mellitus
- Obesity
- ECG abnormalities
- Elevated homocysteine levels
- High-strung, nervous personality and behavior patterns
- Psychosocial charac-

teristics of work (e.g., low job control and low pay)
- High uric acid levels
- Pulmonary function abnormalities
- Tension and stress
- High-fat diet

The following risk factors are considered fixed, i.e., they *cannot* be modified.

- Age
- Gender
- Heredity
- Race
- Male-pattern baldness

Quantifying the importance of each CHD risk factor in relation to the others becomes difficult because many of the factors interrelate. For example, blood lipid abnormalities, diabetes, heredity, and obesity often go hand-in-hand. In addition, increasing daily physical activity generally lowers body weight, body fat, blood lipids, tension, stress, and risk for developing type 2 diabetes.

Five "treatable" factors (elevated serum lipids, high blood pressure, physical inactivity, cigarette smoking, and obesity) represent the **primary CHD risk factors**. Although some risk factors link closely with CHD, the associations do not necessarily infer causality. In some instances, risk factor reduction may not offer effective protection from the disease. Nonetheless, a prudent approach to CHD prevention assumes that eliminating or reducing one or more risk factors decreases the likelihood of contracting CHD.

Age, Gender, and Heredity
Figure 20.13 indicates that after age 35 in males and age 45 in females, the chances of dying from CHD increase progressively and dramatically. Consequently, age per se represents a significant CHD risk factor. From the perspective of causality, however, chronologic age symbolizes more of an associative risk because of its close link to other more likely "causal" risk factors like hypertension, elevated blood lipids, and glucose intolerance.

Between ages 55 and 65, about 13 of every 100 men and 6 of 100 women die from CHD. At most ages, women fare much better than men. For example, in middle age, a man has about a sixfold greater chance of dying from a heart attack. American women still lead women from all other countries in heart disease; the specific "gender advantage" decreases significantly after menopause. This has fueled speculation that hormonal differences between the sexes provide CHD protection for women. For some unknown reason, heart attacks that strike at an early age tend to run in families.

Blood Lipid Abnormalities
Overwhelming evidence links high blood lipid levels with increased heart disease risk.

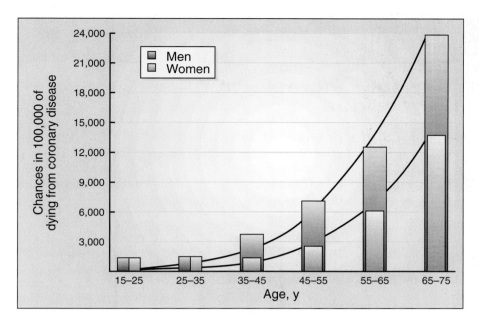

Figure 20.13
Chances of a single individual dying from coronary heart disease. (Data from the American Heart Association).

risk. In contrast, elevated cholesterol-rich, low-density lipoproteins (LDL) represent an increased risk.

LDLs transport cholesterol throughout the body for delivery to cells, including those of the arteries' smooth muscle walls. LDLs then become oxidized here and ultimately contribute to the artery-narrowing process of atherosclerosis. Whereas LDL carries cholesterol to tissues and contributes to arterial damage, HDL acts as a scavenger, gathering cholesterol from cells (including cells in arterial walls) and returning it for metabolism to the liver and excretion in bile.

Research continues to clarify HDL's protective effect and what factors raise its levels. For one thing, cigarette smoking adversely affects plasma HDL concentrations. This may account for the significant CHD risk with smoking. From an exercise perspective, endurance athletes posses relatively high HDL levels; favorable alterations also occur in sedentary people who engage in either moderate or vigorous aerobic training. Concurrently, exercise decreases LDL, which produces the net effect of considerably improved ratios of HDL-to-LDL, or HDL-to-total cholesterol. The exercise effect occurs independently of

Cholesterol and Triglycerides

The accompanying *How to Classify Values for Cholesterol, Lipoproteins, and Triglycerides* presents serum cholesterol, triglyceride, and lipoprotein levels above which young and older adults should seek advice on treatment. In general, a cholesterol value of 200 mg·dL^{-1} or lower represents a desirable level. A cholesterol of 230 mg·dL^{-1} increases heart attack risk to about twice that of a person with 180 mg·dL^{-1}, and a value of 300 mg·dL^{-1} increases the risk fourfold. The term **hyperlipidemia** refers to an increased blood plasma lipid level.

Importance of Cholesterol Forms

Cholesterol and triglycerides represent the two most common lipids associated with CHD risk. Recall from Chapter 2 that these lipids remain insoluble in water so they do not circulate freely in blood plasma. Rather, they transport combined with a carrier protein to form a **lipoprotein**. Lipoprotein varies in size depending on the quantity of protein and lipid it contains. **Hyperlipidemia** refers to a general elevation in blood lipids, whereas **hyperlipoproteinemia** more meaningfully describes elevation in the specific lipoproteins. Table 20.2 lists the four different lipoproteins, their approximate density, and percentage composition in blood. *Serum cholesterol represents a composite of the total cholesterol contained in the different lipoproteins.*

The distribution of cholesterol among various lipoproteins more powerfully predicts heart disease risk than simply total plasma lipids. This helps to explain how one person with a high total serum cholesterol may not develop CHD, while it develops in another person with a lower cholesterol level. Specifically, elevated high-density lipoproteins (HDL), which contain the largest quantity of protein and least cholesterol, relate to low heart disease

Should Children Have Cholesterol Measured?

Guidelines issued by the National Cholesterol Education Program conclude "yes" if a family history of high cholesterol or heart disease exists (particularly if a parent suffered a heart attack before age 50). Shockingly, this parental "cardiac proneness" includes up to one-fourth of the United States adult population! Research with children age 10 to 15 years indicates that lifestyle habits like regular exercise, improved cardiovascular fitness, and a prudent nutritional profile contribute to favorable lipid profiles similar to effects seen with adults.

How to Classify Values for Cholesterol, Lipoproteins, and Triglycerides

Important risk factors for development of atherosclerosis include high levels of serum cholesterol, triglyceride, and low-density lipoprotein cholesterol (LDL-C), and a low level of high-density lipoprotein cholesterol (HDL-C). The primary sites for artery-narrowing plaque formation (i.e., incorpo-ration of connective tissue, smooth muscle, cellular debris, minerals, and cholesterol) include the aorta and carotid, coronary, femoral, and iliac arteries. Specific cut-off values for total cholesterol, LDL-C and HDL-C, and triglyceride relate to varying levels of increased coronary heart disease risk.

Classification of serum total cholesterol, LDL-C and HDL-C, and triglyceride levels.

SERUM CHOLESTEROL AND LIPOPROTEIN

Total Cholesterol	Classification
<200 mg · dL^{-1} (5.2 mmol · L^{-1})	Desirable cholesterol
200–239 mg · dL^{-1} (5.3–6.2 mmol · L^{-1})	Borderline high cholesterol
>240 mg · dL^{-1} (6.2 mmol · L^{-1})	High cholesterol

LDL Cholesterol	Classification
<130 mg · dL^{-1} (3.4 mmol · L^{-1})	Desirable
130–159 mg · dL^{-1} (3.4–4.1 mmol · L^{-1})	Borderline high
>160 mg · dL^{-1} (4.1 mmol · L^{-1})	High

HDL Cholesterol	Classification
<35 mg · dL^{-1} (0.9 mmol · L^{-1})	Low

SERUM TRIGLYCERIDE

Serum Triglycerides	Classification	Comments
<200 mg · dL^{-1} (2.3 mmol · L^{-1})	Normal	
200–400 mg · dL^{-1} (2.3–4.5 mmol · L^{-1})	Borderline high	Check for accompanying primary or secondary dyslipidemias
400–1000 mg · dL^{-1} (4.5–11.3 mmol · L^{-1})	High	Check for accompanying primary or secondary dyslipidemias
>1000 mg · dL^{-1} (11.3 mmol · L^{-1})	Very high	Increased risk for acute pancreatitis

From expert panel on detection, evaluation, and treatment of high blood pressure, and cholesterol in adults. *JAMA*, 269:3015, 1993.

the diet's lipid content or the exerciser's body composition. Moderate consumption of alcohol (equivalent to about 2 oz or 30 mL of 90 proof alcohol, three 6-oz glasses of wine, or a bit less than three 12-oz cans of beer) reduces an otherwise healthy person's risk of heart attack. The cardiopro-tective mechanism may relate to alcohol's effect in raising HDL and lowering LDL, and blunting arterial smooth muscle cell proliferation. Excessive alcohol consumption offers no lipoprotein benefit; it also greatly increases risk of liver disease and cancer.

TABLE 20.2
Approximate composition of lipoproteins in the blood

	CHYLOMICRONS	VERY-LOW DENSITY LIPOPROTEINS (VLDL: PREBETA)	LOW-DENSITY LIPOPROTEINS (LDL: BETA)	HIGH-DENSITY LIPOPROTEINS (HDL: ALPHA)
Density, $g \cdot cm^{-3}$	0.95	0.95–1.006	1.006–1.019	1.063–1.210
Protein, %	0.5–1.0	5–15	25	45–55
Lipid, %	99	95	75	50
Cholesterol, %	2–5	10–20	40–45	18
Triglyceride, %	85	50–70	5–10	2
Phospholipid, %	3–6	10–20	20–25	30

Factors That Affect Cholesterol and Lipoprotein Levels. Diverse behaviors can significantly impact the blood lipid profile. Behaviors that favorably affect cholesterol and lipoprotein levels include:

- Weight loss (through food restriction and/or exercise)
- Regular aerobic exercise (independent of weight loss)
- Increased intake of water-soluble fibers (e.g., fibers in beans, legumes, and oat bran)
- Increased dietary intake of polyunsaturated to saturated fatty acid ratio and monounsaturated fatty acids
- Increased dietary intake of unique polyunsaturated fatty acids in fish oils
- Moderate alcohol consumption

Variables that adversely affect cholesterol and lipoprotein levels include:

- Cigarette smoking
- Diet high in saturated fatty acids and preformed cholesterol
- Emotionally stressful situations
- Certain oral contraceptives

Cholesterol Ratios Important

An effective way to evaluate lipoprotein status divides total cholesterol by HDL cholesterol. This ratio represents a superior index of heart disease risk than either total cholesterol or LDL:cholesterol level. A cholesterol:HDL ratio greater than 4.5 indicates high risk for heart disease, whereas an optimal ratio equals 3.5 or lower.

- Sedentary lifestyle
- Weight gain (through increased food intake and/or lack of exercise)

Homocysteine and Coronary Heart Disease

In 1969, an 8-year-old boy died of a stroke. An autopsy revealed that his arteries had the sclerotic look of the blood vessels of an elderly man, and his blood contained excess levels of the amino acid **homocysteine.** His rare genetic disorder, homocystinuria, causes premature hardening of the arteries and early death from heart attack or stroke. In the years after this observation, an impressive number of studies have shown a strong positive association between plasma homocysteine levels and heart attack and mortality risks. In the presence of other conventional CHD risks (e.g., smoking and hypertension), synergistic effects magnify the negative impact of homocysteine.

All individuals produce homocysteine, but it normally converts to other nondamaging amino acids. Three B-vitamins (folic acid, B_6, and B_{12}) facilitate the conversion. If the conversion slows due to a genetic defect or vitamin deficiency, homocysteine levels increase and promote cholesterol's damaging effects on the arterial lumen. Figure 20.14 proposes a mechanism for homocysteine damage. The homocysteine model helps to explain why some people with low to normal cholesterol levels contract heart disease.

Excessive homocysteine causes blood platelets to clump, fostering blood clots and deterioration of smooth muscle cells that line the arterial wall. Chronic homocysteine exposure can scar and thicken arteries and provide a fertile medium for circulating LDL-cholesterol to initiate damage. People with elevated homocysteine levels run a 4.5 times greater statistical risk of death from heart disease than individuals with normal levels.

It remains uncertain what causes some people to accu-

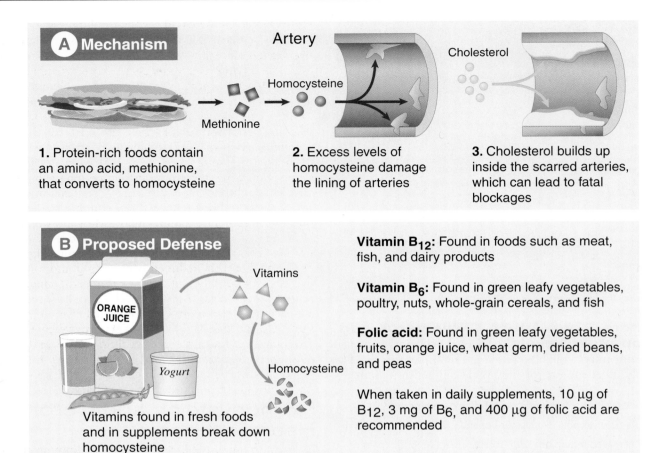

Figure 20.14

A, Proposed mechanism for how the amino acid homocysteine damages the lining of arteries and sets the stage for cholesterol infiltration into a vessel. **B,** Proposed defense against the possible harmful effects of elevated homocysteine levels.

mulate homocysteine, but the evidence points to deficiency of B-vitamins. Also, no clear standard of normal or desirable levels of homocysteine currently exists; research needs to show that normalizing homocysteine actually reduces risk of heart attack and stroke. Nevertheless, sufficient data support the practice of consuming adequate B-vitamins, particularly folic acid. Even small amounts of this vitamin (plentiful in enriched whole-grain cereals, nuts and seeds, dark green leafy vegetables, beans and peas, and orange juice) lower homocysteine levels. In 1999, all white flour, breads, pasta, grits, white rice, and cornmeal will be fortified with folic acid. Between 180 to 200 micrograms (μg) represent the current RDA for folic acid; 500 to 700 μg probably presents a better dietary target. Recent research shows that people who every day ate cereal containing 127 μg of folic acid—an amount that approximates the RDA recommendation—raised their folic acid level by 31%, but lowered homocysteine level only 3.7%, not enough to prevent vessel damage. Cereals with 499 and 665 μg of folic acid reduced homocysteine by 11% and 14%, respectively, supporting the need for increased levels of folic acid in the diet.

Apoprotein

The **apoproteins** represent a class of specific proteins embedded in the outer shell of a lipoprotein particle that (a) increase the solubility of the lipoprotein's cholesterol and triglyceride components, (b) act as ligands for specific lipoprotein receptors in cell membranes, and (c) serve as important cofactors to activate enzymes in lipoprotein metabolism. Researchers now believe that specific apoproteins more reliably predict heart disease proneness than total cholesterol level.

Physical Activity and Coronary Heart Disease

A critique of 43 studies of the relationship between physical inactivity and CHD concluded that lack of regular exercise contributes to heart disease in a cause-and-effect

Risk Factors in Children and Adolescents

Multiple CHD risk factors—obesity, elevated blood lipids, physical inactivity, cigarette smoking, and a family history of heart disease—frequently occur in young children and adolescents. In addition, the risks often interrelate as the fattest children generally have the highest cholesterol and triglyceride levels and lowest physical activity levels. Schools must initiate programs aimed at reducing risk factors in children and adolescents, but current efforts have fallen short, particularly regarding tobacco use. The 1998 Youth Risk Behavior Study from the *Centers for Disease Control and Prevention* reported that cigarette use among black, white, and Hispanic high school students jumped considerably between 1991 and 1997. Moreover, there was a precipitous 80% increase from 1991 to 1997 in percentage of black males who smoked. The tobacco industry's advertising and marketing campaign to attract new smokers (coupled with renewed glamorization of tobacco products in movies, TV, and music videos) apparently overwhelms school efforts at risk intervention at an early age.

manner, with the sedentary person at almost twice the risk as the most active individual. The strength of this protective association equaled that observed between CHD and hypertension, cigarette smoking, and high serum cholesterol. *This places physical inactivity as the greater heart disease risk, considering that more people lead sedentary lives than have one or more of the other risk factors.* Although vigorous exercise does entail a small risk of sudden death during the activity, the important longer-term health benefits of regular exercise far outweigh any potential acute risk.

Hypertension

More than 35 million Americans currently have systolic blood pressures over 140 mm Hg (**systolic hypertension**) or diastolic pressures that exceed 90 mm Hg (**diastolic hypertension**). These values form the lower limit for the classification of **borderline high blood pressure**. One of every five people experience chronic abnormally high blood pressure sometime during their lives. Uncorrected hypertension leads to heart failure, heart attack, stroke, or kidney failure.

Hypertension, often labeled the "silent killer," generally progresses unnoticed for decades before inflicting its deadly blow. The cause(s) of hypertension remains unknown in more than 90% of cases. Statistics indicate that the optimal blood pressure for longevity averages about 110 mm Hg systolic and 70 mm Hg diastolic. Anything

higher results in increased cardiovascular disease risk. For example, a man with systolic blood pressure above 150 mm Hg has more than twice the heart disease risk as someone with 120 mm Hg. Many people have a genetic predisposition toward hypertension that increases their tendency to retain salt, heightens the reactivity of their blood vessels to stress, and causes higher levels of chemicals that constrict the peripheral vasculature.

Modification of lifestyle behaviors often lower blood pressure. Important modifications include weight loss, cessation of smoking (nicotine constricts peripheral blood vessels, which elevates blood pressure), and reducing salt intake (excess sodium retains fluid, which elevates blood pressure in susceptible individuals). Men and women age 30 to 54 years with mild hypertension modestly lowered systolic (2.9 mm Hg) and diastolic (2.3 mm Hg) blood pressure when they reduced body weight and salt intake over an 18-month period. No blood pressure changes occurred for subjects who undertook only stress reduction and relaxation techniques, or consumed calcium, magnesium, phosphorus, and fish oil dietary supplements. Prescription drugs that either reduce fluid volume or decrease peripheral resistance to blood flow effectively treat high blood pressure. Experts estimate that each 2 mm Hg reduction in blood pressure decreases CHD risk by 4% and stroke by 6%.

Exercise and Hypertension

As pointed out in Chapter 14, exercise training reduces blood pressure in hypertensive patients. Prudent counsel recommends periodic blood pressure measurement and regular aerobic exercise for preventive and therapeutic management.

Cigarette Smoking

In terms of health status, the more a person smokes, the poorer his or her future health status. Cigarette smoking represents one of the strongest predictors of CHD. In fact, the probability of death from heart disease for smokers nearly doubles over that of nonsmokers. Risk for CHD (and lung cancer) increases the more one smokes, the deeper one inhales, and the stronger the cigarette's tars and noxious byproducts. In addition, smokers experience nearly five times the risk for stroke as nonsmokers, and those who smoke a pack or more a day have an 11-times greater chance of suffering a deadly stroke that strikes younger men and women.

Surprisingly, CHD risk from smoking translates to two to three times more deaths than excess mortality from lung cancer. Even exposure to second-hand smoke increases CHD risk. Three hours of second-hand smoke exposure equals smoking one pack of cigarettes. The good news: If a smoker for 40 years stops, CHD risk returns to that of a "never smoker" within 5 years, regardless of age. As for cancer, a substantial risk decline occurs but it takes longer.

Obesity

Obesity's association with many diseases makes the quantitative importance of excess body fat per se as a health risk difficult to determine. Nevertheless, the death rate for men weighing 30% in excess of ideal weight exceeds the risk for a normal-weight individuals by 70%. The overfat condition often accompanies multiple risk factors like hypertension and elevated serum lipids. In addition, an obese person usually consumes a highly atherogenic diet rich in saturated fatty acids and cholesterol. Gaining weight also increases the chance for developing impaired glucose tolerance (type 2 diabetes) and abnormal serum uric acid.

Weight loss and accompanying body fat reduction help normalize plasma cholesterol and triglycerides, and beneficially affect blood pressure and type 2 diabetes. Age-related gains in body mass partly explain the expected increase in blood pressure with age.

Personality and Behavior Patterns

A distinct personality exists that may increase susceptibility to heart disease. The coronary-prone behaviors (hard-driving, ambitious, impatient, short-tempered, hostile, and restless) typify what psychologists call the **Type A personality**. Unrelenting pressures, drives, deadlines, anxieties, depression, and a constant struggle against the limitations of time comprise the Type A stress syndrome, with its accompanying excessive stimulation of the body's "fight or flight" hormonal response, which may impair cardiovascular health.

The opposite style of behavior, exemplified by the equally capable but easy going, no pressure, "laid back" **Type B personality**, functions under no time pressure. The absence of Type A behaviors characterizes this personality type. Generally, most people classify as neither all Type A nor all Type B, but rather a blend of both types of behavior patterns.

The precise manner in which personality and behavior influence CHD development remains unknown, let alone whether one's basic personality "type" can significantly influence a disease process. One desirable strategy recognizes, manage, and effectively directs excess stress elsewhere. To this end, regular exercise blended with behavior modification can channel potentially harmful behaviors into ones that produce positive "spin-off." Interestingly, laughter may play an important role in the stress response and positively combat disease processes. Individuals who laugh easily, spontaneously, and hard on a regular basis have lower CHD incidence, recover faster from surgery, and geneally remain less susceptible to disease.

Physical Inactivity

Enough evidence exists relating sedentary habits to poor health to classify physical inactivity as a major risk factor for early death. The maintenance of physical fitness throughout life provides significant protection from CHD risk factors and occurrence of actual disease. In a nine-year study of Californians, sedentary men and women died prematurely at twice the rate compared to counterparts who exercised frequently. People who reported even mild exercise experienced better health than those who remained sedentary.

Increased physical activity exerts potent and direct effects on other risk factors. It reduces blood lipid levels, lowers blood pressure, improves pulmonary function, normalizes glucose metabolism, alleviates tension and stress, decreases body fat levels, and improves uric acid levels. All of these changes contribute to lower overall CHD risk, an encompassing effect not possible by modifying any other singular risk factor.

Research with animals and humans shows that regular exercise diminishes CHD risk in the following ways:

- Improves myocardial circulation and metabolism to protect the heart from oxygen lack; this includes possibly enhanced vascularization and modest increases in cardiac glycogen stores and anaerobic capacity
- Enhances the myocardium's contractile properties to maintain or increase contractility during a specific challenge
- Provides more favorable blood clotting characteristics
- Favorably alters heart rate and blood pressure so the work of the heart (rate-pressure product) decreases during rest and exercise
- Establishes a favorable neural-hormonal balance to reduce myocardial oxygen demands

Figure 20.15 illustrates how the American Heart Association uses risk factors to help the public identify their likelihood for heart disease. Notice that physical inactivity, body weight, smoking habits, diabetes, and blood pressure and cholesterol status (all modifiable risk factors) contribute significantly to the overall CHD risk score.

Interaction Among Risk Factors

Smoking generally acts independently of other risk factors to increase CHD risk. Other risk factors, however, interact with each other and CHD itself to accentuate disease risk. Figure 20.16 quantifies the interaction of three primary CHD risk factors elevated in the same person. With one risk factor, a 45-year-old man's chance for CHD symptoms during the year averages about twice that of a man without risks. The prospect

---

Diabetes Risk Significantly Lowered with Regular Exercise

Men who exercise five or more times a week show a 42% lower risk of type 2 diabetes than men who exercise less than once a week. The exercise benefits become most pronounced among obese participants. The risk of diabetes decreases approximately 6% for every 500 kcal of additional weekly exercise.

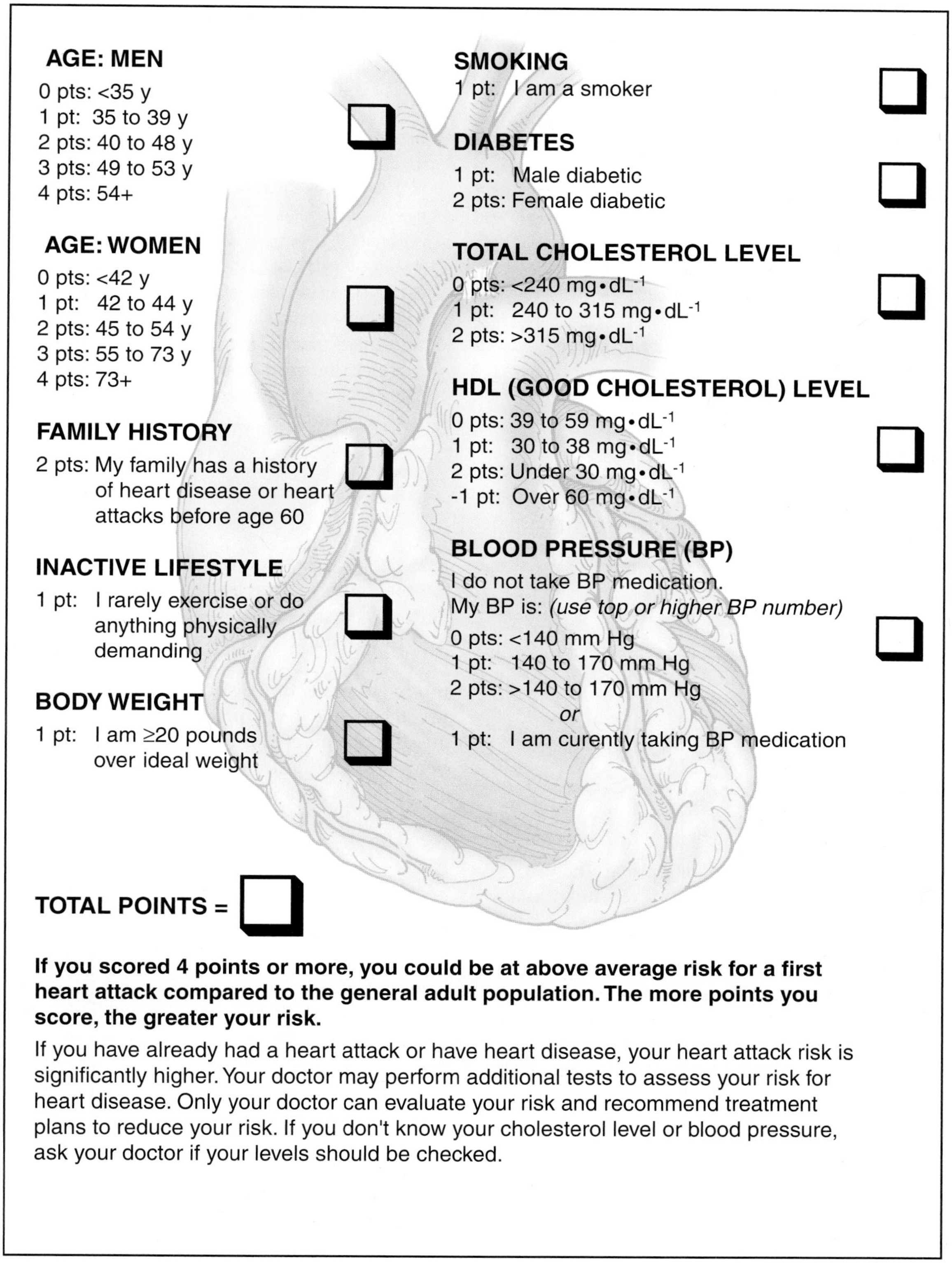

AGE: MEN

0 pts: <35 y
1 pt: 35 to 39 y
2 pts: 40 to 48 y
3 pts: 49 to 53 y
4 pts: 54+

AGE: WOMEN

0 pts: <42 y
1 pt: 42 to 44 y
2 pts: 45 to 54 y
3 pts: 55 to 73 y
4 pts: 73+

FAMILY HISTORY

2 pts: My family has a history
of heart disease or heart
attacks before age 60

INACTIVE LIFESTYLE

1 pt: I rarely exercise or do
anything physically
demanding

BODY WEIGHT

1 pt: I am ≥20 pounds
over ideal weight

SMOKING

1 pt: I am a smoker

DIABETES

1 pt: Male diabetic
2 pts: Female diabetic

TOTAL CHOLESTEROL LEVEL

0 pts: <240 mg•dL^{-1}
1 pt: 240 to 315 mg•dL^{-1}
2 pts: >315 mg•dL^{-1}

HDL (GOOD CHOLESTEROL) LEVEL

0 pts: 39 to 59 mg•dL^{-1}
1 pt: 30 to 38 mg•dL^{-1}
2 pts: Under 30 mg•dL^{-1}
-1 pt: Over 60 mg•dL^{-1}

BLOOD PRESSURE (BP)

I do not take BP medication.
My BP is: *(use top or higher BP number)*

0 pts: <140 mm Hg
1 pt: 140 to 170 mm Hg
2 pts: >140 to 170 mm Hg
or
1 pt: I am curently taking BP medication

TOTAL POINTS =

If you scored 4 points or more, you could be at above average risk for a first heart attack compared to the general adult population. The more points you score, the greater your risk.

If you have already had a heart attack or have heart disease, your heart attack risk is significantly higher. Your doctor may perform additional tests to assess your risk for heart disease. Only your doctor can evaluate your risk and recommend treatment plans to reduce your risk. If you don't know your cholesterol level or blood pressure, ask your doctor if your levels should be checked.

Figure 20.15
American Heart Association's checklist to evaluate coronary heart disease risk.

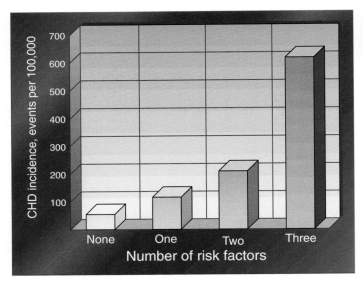

Figure 20.16
Relationship between a combination of abnormal CHD risk factors (cholesterol >250 mg · dL^{-1}; systolic blood pressure >160 mm Hg; smoking >1 pack a day), and incidence of coronary heart disease.

Exercise Is Good Medicine for the Colon

The series of studies of the health and exercise habits of Harvard alumni indicates that physically active men had about one-half the risk of colon cancer as their inactive classmates. The protection disappeared if the men stopped exercising. One mechanism proposes that exercise protects against this major killer by speeding the passage of food residues through the digestive tract. This reduces the colon's exposure to any potential carcinogens in food.

for chest pain, heart attack, or sudden death with three risk factors increases five times compared with no risk factors.

Behavioral Changes Improve Overall Health Profile

Different health-promoting habits prove effective in areas other than those related to one's heart attack risk. Table 20.3 ranks the value of several health-saving tactics that reduce risk or bolster resistance to cancer, heart attack, stroke, and diabetes.

A low-fat diet effectively protects against type 2 diabetes, heart attack, and breast and colon cancers (and provides moderate protection against other cancers). A diet rich in vegetables and fruits proves most effective against colon and throat cancers, and offers some protection against diabetes and cardiovascular disease. Smoking, the country's single deadliest habit, represents the primary cause of lung cancer and heart attack. Regular exercise and weight control offer their greatest protection in reducing risk of heart disease, stroke, and diabetes, and provide some protection against certain cancers.

TABLE 20.3
Preventing major diseases: a checklist of health-saving tactics

	NO TOBACCO	LOW-FAT DIET	HIGH-FIBER DIET	AVOID ALCOHOL	AVOID SALTED, PICKLED FOODS	DIET HIGH IN VEGETABLES AND FRUITS	EXERCISE, WEIGHT CONTROL
Cancer							
Lung	√√√	√				√	
Breast		√√√	√			√√	√
Colon		√√√	√√√			√√√	√
Liver				√√√	√	√√	
Heart Attack	√√√	√√√				√√	√√√
Stroke	√				√√√	√√	√√
Type 2 diabetes		√√√	√			√√	√√

√√√ Highly effective   √√ Moderately effective   √ Somewhat effective
Modified from American Medical Foundation.

summary

1. *The Surgeon General's Report: Physical Activity and Health* represents the first governmentally sanctioned report endorsing increased physical activity for U.S. citizens to combat the increasingly large number of physical ailments associated with sedentary living.

2. Major conclusions of the Report include: (a) people of all ages benefit from regular physical activity, (b) significant health and quality of life benefits emerge with just moderate physical activity (e.g., 30 min brisk walking or raking leaves, 15 min running, or 45 min playing volleyball) on most days, and (c) regular exercise reduces general premature mortality risk, and specific risks of coronary heart disease, hypertension, osteoporosis, colon cancer, and type 2 diabetes.

3. Exercise scientists play an important role in the emerging "new gerontology," which concentrates on successful aging (maintenance and even enhancement of physical and cognitive functions) rather than disease-related processes and physical frailty.

4. Physiologic and performance capabilities generally decline after age 30. The decline rates of various functions differ within and among individuals. Regular exercise enables older persons to retain higher levels of functional capacity, particularly cardiovascular and muscular functions.

5. Aging alters endocrine function, particularly for the pituitary, pancreas, adrenal, and thyroid glands.

6. Vigorous physical activity early in life contributes little to increased longevity or health status in later life. However, a physically active lifestyle throughout life confers significant health-related benefits.

7. Coronary heart disease (CHD) represents the single largest cause of death in the Western world. The pathogenesis of CHD involves degenerative changes in the inner lining of the arterial wall that result in progressive occlusion.

8. Numerous factors indicate an individual's susceptibility to CHD. Important risk factors include age and gender, elevated blood lipids, hypertension, cigarette smoking, obesity, physical inactivity, diet, heredity, and ECG abnormalities during rest and exercise.

9. A cholesterol value of 200 $mg \cdot dL^{-1}$ or lower represents a desirable cholesterol level. Cholesterol of 230 $mg \cdot dL^{-1}$ increases heart attack risk to about twice that of a person with 180 $mg \cdot dL^{-1}$, and a value of 300 $mg \cdot dL^{-1}$ increases CHD risk fourfold.

10. The distribution of HDL and LDL-cholesterol more powerfully predicts heart disease risk than simply the total quantity of serum cholesterol.

11. Excess levels of the amino acid homocysteine cause clumping of blood platelets, which fosters blood clots and deterioration of smooth muscle cells that line the arterial wall. Adequate folic acid and vitamin B_6 and B_{12} intake defends against elevated homocysteine levels.

12. Cigarette smoking represents the strongest predictor of CHD. The probability of death from heart disease for smokers nearly doubles that of nonsmokers. The adverse effect of cigarette smoke on lipoprotein levels represents one mechanism for increased risk.

13. The interaction of CHD risk factors significantly magnifies their individual effect in predicting one's likelihood for disease.

14. Proper nutrition, exercise, and weight control modify many CHD risk factors. Risk intervention generally improves an individual's health outlook.

thought questions

1. The following case provides general descriptive information about an individual, including personal information and results of a graded exercise stress test (GXT). Summarize the case, list and analyze the risk factors, and react to the results of the stress test. Make recommendations for the person for exercise, risk reduction, and health maintenance.

   DATA: Caucasian male stockbroker, age, 39 y.; body mass, 92 kg; stature, 179 cm; percent body fat, 29%; total cholesterol, 255 $mg \cdot dL^{-1}$, HDL cholesterol, 35 $mg \cdot dL^{-1}$; mother died of heart attack at age 46; has remained sedentary since college days, when he regularly participated in intramural sports.

   GXT test: 3 mph; 2.5% increase in treadmill grade every 2 min; SBP = systolic blood pressure, DBP = diastolic blood pressure (mm Hg)

% Grade	METs	SBP	DBP	HR	ECG	Symptoms
Rest		128	89	82	normal	none
2.5	4.3	149	89	140	normal	none
5.0	5.4	154	88	154	normal	none
7.5	6.4	162	84	165	normal	none
10	7.4	180	83	172	normal	none
12.5	8.5	186	83	184	normal	none
15	9.5	198	86	197	normal	none

2. If regular physical activity contributes little to overall life span, what other reasons exist for maintaining a physically active lifestyle throughout middle and old age?

3. Respond to the statement: "The fact that overwhelming epidemiological evidence links physical activity on the job or in leisure time to reduced CHD risk does not necessarily prove that exercise benefits cardiovascular health."

4. For children and adults with the same $\dot{V}O_{2max}$ ($mL \cdot kg^{-1} \cdot min^{-1}$), what factors explain the relatively poorer performances of children in aerobic activities like a 10-K run?

selected references

ACSM Position Stand on Exercise and Physical Activity for Older Adults. *Med. Sci. Sports Exerc.*, 30:992, 1998.

ADA/ACSM Diabetes Mellitus and Exercise Joint Position Paper. *Med. Sci. Sports Exerc.*, 29:I, 1997.

Anderson, R.E.: Effects of lifestyle activity vs structured aerobic exercise in obese women. *JAMA*, 281:335, 1999.

Åstrand, P.O., et al.: A 33-yr. follow-up of peak oxygen uptake and related variables of former physical education students. *J. Appl. Physiol.*, 82:1844, 1997.

Babb, T.G.: Mechanical ventilatory constraints in aging, lung disease and obesity: perspectives and brief review. *Med. Sci. Sports Exerc.*, 31, No. 1(Suppl.):S12, 1999.

Bailey, D.A.: The Saskatchewan Pediatric Bone Mineral Accrual Study: bone mineral acquisition during the growing years. *Int. J. Sports Med.*, 18 Suppl 3:S191, 1997.

Bailey, D.A., et al.: A Six-Year Longitudinal Study of the Relationship of Physical Activity to Bone Mineral Accrual in Growing Children: The University of Saskatchewan Bone Mineral Accrual Study. *J. Bone Miner. Res.*, 14:1672, 1999.

Beniamini, Y., et al.: High-intensity strength training of patients enrolled in an outpatient cardiac rehabilitation program. *J. Cardiopulm. Rehab.*, 19(1):8–17, 1998.

Berenson, G.S., et al.: Association between multiple cardiovascular risk factors and atherosclerosis in children and young adults. *N. Engl. J. Med.*, 338:1650, 1998.

Blair, S. N., et al.: Changes in physical fitness and all cause mortality: a prospective study of healthy and unhealthy men. *JAMA*, 273:1093, 1995.

Blair, S.N., et al.: Physical activity, nutrition, and chronic disease. *Med. Sci. Sports Exerc.*, 28:335, 1997.

Blair, S.N., and Connelly, J.C.: How much physical activity should we do? The case for moderate amounts and intensities of physical activity. *Res. Q. Exerc. Sport*, 67:193, 1996.

Both, F. W., et al.: Effect of aging on human skeletal muscle and motor function. *Med. Sci. Sports Exerc.*, 26:556, 1994.

Brönstrup, A., et al.: Effects of folic acid and combinations of folic acid and vitamin B-12 on plasma homocysteine concentrations in healthy young women. *Am. J. Clin. Nutr.*, 68:1104, 1998.

Burke, A.P., et al.: Plaque rupture and sudden death related to exertion in men with coronary artery disease. *JAMA*, 281:921, 1999.

Cartee, G.D.: Aging skeletal muscle: response to exercise. *Exerc. Sport Sci. Rev.*, 22:91, 1994.

Centers for Disease Control and Prevention. Prevalence of sedentary lifestyle. *MMWR*, 46:941, 1997.

Chodzko-Zajko, W.J.: Normal aging and human physiology. *Semin Speech Lang.*, May; 18:95, 1997.

Consensus statement. *Physical Activity, Fitness, and Health.* Bouchard, C., et al. (eds.). Champaign, IL: Human Kinetics, 1994.

Covey, M.K., et al.: Reliability of submaximal exercise tests in patients with COPD. Chronic obstructive pulmonary disease. *Med. Sci. Sports Exerc.*, 31:1257, 1999.

DeSerres S.J., and Enoka, R.M.: Older adults can maximally activate the biceps brachi muscle by voluntary command. *J. Appl. Physiol.*, 84:284, 1998.

Despres, J.P., et al.: Plasma post-heparin lipase activities in the HERITAGE Family Study: the reproducibility, gender differences, and associations with lipoprotein levels. Health, risk factors, exercise training and genetics. *Clin. Biochem.*, 32:157, 1999.

Dunn, A.L., et al.: Comparison of lifestyle and structured interventions to increase physical activity and cardiorespiratory fitness. *JAMA*, 281:327, 1999.

Durstine, J. L., and Haskell, W. L.: Effects of exercise training on plasma lipids and lipoproteins. *Exerc. Sport Sci. Rev.*, 22:477, 1994.

Enos, W.F., et al.: Coronary disease among United States soldiers killed in action in Korea. *JAMA*, 152:1090, 1953.

Ettinger, W.H., et al.: A randomized trial comparing aerobic exercise and resistance exercise with a health education program in older adults with knee osteoarthritis: The Fitness Arthritis and Seniors Trial—(FAST). *JAMA*, 277:25, 1997.

Evans, W.J.: Exercise training guidelines for the elderly. *Med. Sci. Sports Exerc.*, 31:12, 1999.

Farrell, S.W., et al.: Influence of cardiorespiratory fitness levels and other predictors on cardiovascular disease mortality in men. *Med. Sci. Sports Exerc.*, 30:899, 1998.

Feigenbaum, M.S., et al.: Prescription of resistance training for health and disease. *Med. Sci. Sports Exerc.*, 31:38, 1999.

Fiatarone, M.A., et al.: Exercise training and nutritional supplementation for physical frailty in very elderly people. *N. Engl. J. Med.*, 330:1769, 1994.

Finch, C.E., and Tanzi, R.E., Genetics of aging. *Science*, 278:407, 1997.

FigzGerald, M.D., et al.: Age-related decline in maximal aerobic capacity in regularly exercising vs. sedentary females: a meta-analysis. *J. Appl. Physiol.*, 83:160, 1997.

Fried, L.P., et al.: Risk factors for 5-year mortality in older adults. *JAMA*, 279:585, 1998.

Fried, L.P., et al.: Risk factors and 5-year mortality in older adults: the Cardiovascular Health Study, *JAMA*, 279:585, 1998.

First, R.E., et al.: Athletes have a lower lifetime occurrence of breast cancer and cancers of the reproductive system. *Adv. Exp. Med. Biol.*, 322:29, 1992.

Gallager, D., et al.: Appendicular skeletal muscle mass: effects of age, gender, and ethnicity. *J. Appl. Physiol.*, 83:229, 1997.

Goldberg, R.J., et al.: A two decades (1975 to 1995) long experience in the incidence, in-hospital and long-term—fatality rates of acute myocardial infarction: a community wide perspective. *J. Am. Coll. Cardiol.*, 33:1533, 1999.

Grabber, MD, and Eon, RCA.: Changes in movement capabilities with aging. *Exerc. Sport Sci. Rev.*, 23:65, 1995.

Graham, IM, et al., Plasma homocysteine as a risk factor for vascular disease. The European Concerted Action Project. *JAMA*, 277:1775, 1997.

Grundy, S.M.: Primary prevention of coronary heart disease: selection of patients for aggressive cholesterol management. *Am J. Med.*, 107(2A):2S, 1999.

Gudat, V., et. al.: Physical activity, fitness, and non-insulin-dependent (Type 2) diabetes mellitus. In: *Physical Activity, Fitness, and Health.* Bouchard, C., et al. (eds). Champaign, IL: Human Kinetics, 1994.

Hagerman, F.C., et al.: A 20-yr longitudinal study of Olympic oarsmen. *Med. Sci. Sports Exerc.*, 28:1150, 1996.

Hakim, A.A., et al.: Effects of walking on mortality among nonsmoking retired men. *N. Engl. J. Med.*, 338:94, 1998.

Havranek, E.P.: Primary prevention of CHD: nine ways to reduce risk. *Am Fam. Physician.*, 59:1455–63, 1999.

He, J., et al.: Passive smoking and the risk of coronary heart disease—a meta-analysis of epidemiologic studies. *N. Engl. J. Med.*, 340:920, 1999.

Heckbert, S.R., et al.: Duration of estrogen replacement therapy in relation to risk of incident of myocardial infarction in postmenopausal women. *Arch. Intern. Med.*, 157:1330, 1997.

Houmard, J.A., et al.: Fiber type and citrate synthase activity in human gastrocnemius and vastus lateralis with aging. *J. Appl. Physiol.*, 85:1337, 1998.

Howard, G., et al.: Cigarette smoking and progression of atherosclerosis: The Atherosclerosis Risk in Communities (ARIC) Study. *JAMA*, 279:119, 1998.

Huang, Y., et al.: Physical fitness, physical activity, and functional limitation in adults aged 40 and older. *Med. Sci. Sports Exerc.*, 30:1430, 1998.

Huang, Z., et al.: Body weight, weight change, and risk for hypertension in women. *Ann. Intern. Med.*, 128:81, 1998.

Hunink, M.G.M., et al.: The recent decline in mortality from coronary heart disease, 1980–1990: The effect of secular trends in risk factors and treatment. *JAMA*, 277:535, 1997.

Izquierdo, M., et al.: Maximal and explosive force production capacity and balance performance in men of different ages. *Eur. J. Appl. Physiol.*, 79:260, 1999.

Jackson, A.S., et al.: Changes in aerobic power of women, ages 20–64 yr. *Med. Sci. Sports Exerc.*, 28:884, 1996.

Jackson, A. S., et al.: Changes in aerobic power of men, ages 25–70 yr. *Med. Sci. Sports Exerc.*, 27:113, 1995.

Kasch, F. W., et al.: The effect of physical activity and inactivity on aerobic power in older men (a longitudinal study). *Phys. Sportsmed.*, 18:73, 1990.

Kujala, V.M., et al.: Relationship of leisure-time physical activity and mortality: the Finnish Twin Cohort. *JAMA*, 279:440, 1998.

Kushi, L.H., et al.: Physical activity and mortality in postmenopausal women. *JAMA*, 277:1287, 1997.

Lamberts, S.W.J., et al.: The endocrinology of aging. *Science*, 278:419, 1997.

Laughlin, M.H., et al.: Exercise training-induced adaptations in the coronary circulation. *Med. Sci. Sports Exerc.*, 30:352, 1998.

Layne, J.E., and Nelson, M.E.: The effects of progressive resistance training on bone density: a review. *Med. Sci. Sports Exerc.*, 31:25, 1999.

Lee, I-M., et al.: Exercise and risk of stroke in male physicians. *Stroke*, 30:1, 1999.

Lemaitre, R.N., et al.: Leisure-time physical activity and the risk of primary cardiac arrest. *Arch. Intern. Med.*, 159:686, 1999.

Lindahl, B., et al.: Improved fibrinolysis by intense lifestyle intervention. A randomized trial in subjects with impaired glucose tolerance. *J. Intern. Med.*, 246:105, 1999.

Lindle, R.S., et al.: Age and gender comparisons of muscle strength in 654 women and men aged 20–93 yr. *J. Appl. Physiol.*, 83:1581, 1997.

Lynch, N.A., et al.: Muscle quality. I. Age-associated differences between arm and leg muscle groups. *J. Appl. Physiol.*, 86:188, 1999.

Marrugat, J., et al.: Mortality differences between men and women following first myocardial infarction. *JAMA*, 280:1405, 1999.

Mayer-Davis, E. J., et al.: Intensity and amount of physical activity in relation to insulin sensitivity. *JAMA*, 279:669, 1998.

McCartney, N.: Role of resistance training in heart disease. *Med. Sci. Sports Exerc.*, 10 (Suppl): S396, 1998.

McMurray, R.G., et al.: Is physical activity or aerobic power more influential on reducing cardiovascular disease risk factors? *Med. Sci. Sports Exerc.*, 30:1521, 1998.

Miller, M., et al.: Normal triglyceride levels and coronary artery disease events: The Baltimore Coronary Observational Long-Term Study. *J. Am. Coll. Cardiol.*, May, 1998.

Mitchell, T.L., and Gibbons, L.W.: Controlling blood lipids. Part 1: A practical role for diet and exercise. *Phys. Sportsmed.*, 26(10):41, 1998.

Morey, M.C., et al.: Physical fitness and functional limitations in community-dwelling older adults. *Med. Sci. Sports Exerc.*, 30:715, 1998.

Morris, J. N.: Exercise in the prevention of coronary heart disease: today's best bet in public health. *Med. Sci. Sports Exerc.*, 26:807, 1994.

Morris, J.N., et al.: Coronary heart disease and physical activity of work. *Lancet*, 265:1053, 1953.

Nappo, F., et al.: Impairment of endothelial functions by acute hyperhomocysteinemia and reversal by antioxidant vitamins. *JAMA*, 281:2113, 1999.

Nygård, O., et al.: Major lifestyle determinants of plasma total homocysteine distribution: The Horland Homocysteine Study. *Am. J. Clin. Nutr.*, 67:263, 1998.

Ornish, D., et al.: Intensive lifestyle changes for reversal of coronary heart disease. *JAMA*, 280:2001, 1998.

Parish, S., et al.: Cigarette smoking, tar yields, and non-fatal myocardial infarction: 14000 cases and 32000 controls. *Br. Med. J.*, 311:471, 1995.

Pate, R.R., et al.: Physical activity and public health: a recommendation from the Centers for Disease Control and Prevention and American College of Sports Medicine. *JAMA*, 273:402, 1995.

Poehlman, E.T., et al.: Endurance exercise in aging humans: effects on energy metabolism. *Exerc. Sport Sci. Rev.*, 22:751, 1994.

Pollock, M.L., et al.: Twenty-year follow-up of aerobic power and body composition of older track athletes. *J. Appl. Physiol.*, 82:1508, 1997.

Pollock, M.L., et al.: The recommended quantity and quality of exercise for developing and maintaining cardiorespiratory fitness, strength, and flexibility in healthy adults. *Med. Sci. Sports Exerc.*, 30:975, 1998.

Powell, K.E., et al.: Injury rates from walking, gardening, weightlifting, outdoor bicycling, and aerobics. *Med. Sci. Sports Exerc.*, 30:1246, 1998.

Procter, D.N. and Joyner, M.J.: Skeletal muscle mass and the reduction of VO_{2max} in trained older subjects. *J. Appl. Physiol.*, 82:1411, 1997.

Province, M.A., et al.: Ten effects of exercise on falls in elderly patients: a preplanned meta-analysis of the FICSIT trials. *JAMA*, 273, 1995.

Ridker, P.M., et al.: Homocysteine and risk of cardiovascular disease among postmenopausal women. *JAMA*, 281:1817, 1999.

Rifici, V.A., et al.: Red wine inhibits the cell-mediated oxidation of LDL and HDL. *J. Am. Coll. Nutr.*, 18:137, 1999.

Rockhill, B., et al.: Physical activity and breast cancer risk in a cohort of young women. *J. Natl. Cancer Inst.*, 90:1155, 1998.

Rogers, M.A., and Evans, W.J.: Changes in skeletal muscle with aging: effects of exercise training. In: *Exercise and Sport Sciences Reviews, Vol. 21.* Holloszy, J. O (eds). Baltimore, MD: Williams & Wilkins, 1993.

Rosen, M.J., et al.: Predictors of age-associated decline in maximal aerobic capacity: a comparison of four statistical models. *J. Appl. Physiol.*, 84:2163, 1998.

Sacco, R.L., et al.: The protective effect of moderate alcohol consumption on ischemic stroke. *JAMA*, 28:913, 1999.

Shephard, R. J.: Exercise and sudden death: an overview. *Sport Sci. Rev.*, 4:1, 1995.

Shephard, R.J., et al.: Exercise as cardiovascular therapy. *Circulation*, 7:963, 1999.

Shephard, R.J., and Baldy, G.J.: Exercise as cardiovascular therapy. *Circulation*, 99:963, 1999.

Simonen, R.L., et al.: The effect of lifelong exercise on psychomotor reaction time: a study of 38 pairs of male monozygotic twins. *Med. Sci. Sports Exerc.*, 30:1445, 1998.

Spina, R.J.: Cardiovascular adaptations to endurance exercise training in older men and women. *Exerc. Sport Sci. Revs.* 27:317, 1999.

Stefanick, M.L., et al.: Effects of diet and exercise in men and postmenopausal women with low levels of HDL cholesterol and high levels of LDL cholesterol. *N. Engl. J. Med.*, 339:12, 1998.

Stein, J.H., and McBride, P.E.: Hyperhomocysteinemia and atherosclerotic vascular disease. *Arch. Intern. Med.*, 158:1301, 1998.

Strong, J.P., et al.: Prevalence and extent of atherosclerosis in adolescents and young adults. *JAMA*, 281:727, 1999.

Thune, I., et al.: Physical activity improves the metabolic risk profile in men and women. *Arch. Intern. Med.*, 158:1633, 1998.

Tracy, B.L., et al.: Muscle quality. II. Effects of strength training in 65 to 75-year-old men and women. *J. Appl. Physiol.*, 86:195, 1999.

Trappe. A.W., et al.: Aging among elite distance runners: a 22-yr. longitudinal study. *J. Appl. Physiol.*, 80:285, 1996.

U.S. Department of Health and Human Services. Surgeon General's Report: Physical Activity and Health. Washington, D.C., 1996.

Wescott, W.L., and Baechle, T.R.: *Strength Training Past 50*. Champaign, IL: Human Kinetics, 1998.

Wiebe, C.G., et al.: Exercise cardiac function in young through elderly endurance trained women. *Med. Sci. Sports Exerc.*, 31:684, 1999.

Williams, P.T.: Relationship of heart disease risk factors to exercise quantity and intensity. *Arch Intern. Med.*, 158:237, 1998.

Xiao-ren, P., et al.: Effects of diet and exercise in preventing NIDDM in people with impaired glucose tolerance. *Diabetes Care*, 20:537, 1997.

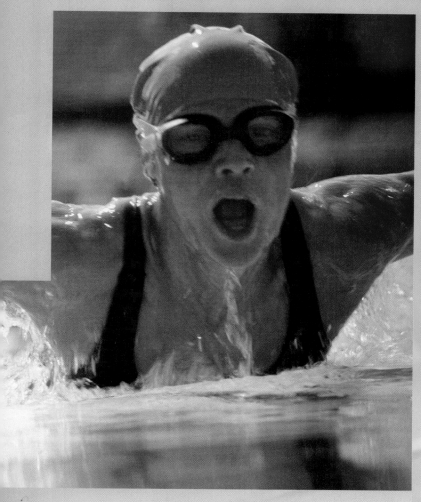

CHAPTER

21

Topics covered in this chapter

The Exercise Physiologist/Health-Fitness Professional In the Clinical Setting

Sports Medicine and Exercise Physiology: A Vital Link

Training and Certification by Professional Organizations

Exercise Programs for Special Populations

Oncology

Cardiovascular Diseases

Cardiac Disease Assessment

Stress Test Protocols

Maximal Treadmill, Cycle Ergometer, and Swimming Tests

Safety of Stress Testing

Exercise-Induced Indicators of CHD

Invasive Physiologic Tests

Patient Classification for Cardiac Rehabilitation

Phases of Cardiac Rehabilitation

Exercise Prescription

The Rehabilitation Program

Cardiac Medications

Pulmonary Diseases

Pulmonary Assessments

Pulmonary Rehabilitation and Exercise Prescription

Pulmonary Medications

Summary

Thought Questions

Selected References

Clinical Exercise Physiology for Health-Related Professionals

- Describe the role of an exercise physiologist/health-fitness professional in the clinical setting.

- Outline broad stages of the progression of HIV and give guidelines for prescribing exercise for these patients.

- List five ACSM certifications and give the qualifications required for each.

- Discuss the potential benefits of physical activity and the role of the clinical exercise physiologist in rehabilitating patients recovering from cancer.

- List at least seven goals of the clinical exercise physiologist in treating patients with deconditioning, immobility, and disuse syndromes.

- List three different diseases of the heart muscle.

- Categorize two different diseases that affect heart valves and the cardiac nervous system.

- Describe the steps in cardiac disease assessment.

- List at least four important reasons for including stress testing to evaluate for coronary heart disease.

- Identify the specifics of different exercise stress test protocols.

- List several indicators of coronary heart disease during an exercise stress test.

- Give advantages and limitations of different modes of exercise for graded exercise stress testing.

- Describe the use of the rating of perceived exertion scale for exercise stress testing and exercise training.

- Define the following terms for stress test results: true-positive, false-negative, true-negative, and false-positive.

- List four reasons for stopping a stress test.

- Outline an approach for individualizing an "exercise prescription."

- Describe phases of a cardiac rehabilitation program.

- Categorize different diseases that affect the pulmonary system.

- Discuss the roles of physical activity and exercise prescription in pulmonary rehabilitation.

The Exercise Physiologist/Health-Fitness Professional in the Clinical Setting

The strong link between regular physical activity and good health has enhanced, the exercise physiologist's role has extended beyond traditional lines. A clinical exercise physiologist becomes part of the health/fitness professional team. This team approach to preventive and rehabilitative services requires different personnel depending on program mission, population served, location, number of participants, space availability, and funding level. A comprehensive clinical program can include the following personnel, in addition to the exercise physiologist:

- Physicians
- Certified personnel (exercise leaders, health-fitness instructors, directors, exercise test technologists, preventive and rehabilitative exercise specialists, preventive and rehabilitative exercise directors)
- Dietitians
- Nurses
- Physical therapists
- Occupational therapists
- Social workers
- Respiratory therapists
- Psychologists
- Health educators

The team of health professionals work in harmony to restore a patient's mobility, functional capacity, and overall health. Issues about available funding, specific client needs, and programmatic direction dictate the extent of part-time and full-time personnel.

Figure 21.1 illustrates five categories of health-impairment status that the exercise physiologist frequently encounters in the clinical setting. Within this framework, the term **disability** refers to an individual's diminished functional capacity, whereas **handicap** refers to a physical performance frame of reference defined by society. Individuals considered handicapped no longer perform tasks expected by society. Having a functional limitation, however, does not necessarily result in disability or handicap.

Sports Medicine and Exercise Physiology: A Vital Link

The traditional view of **sports medicine** involves rehabilitating athletes from sports-related injuries. *A more*

close up

Exercise Prescription for HIV-Positive Patients

An estimated 11 to 13 million individuals worldwide carry the human immunodeficiency virus (HIV). HIV infection represents a chronic disease involving three stages:

1. *Healthy carrier:* The virus infects few CD4-bearing cells (helper T cells) without being clinically detectable except by blood testing. Individuals can remain in this stage for up to 10 years and stay free of significant symptoms despite the presence of infection.
2. *Symptomatic infections:* Mild symptoms such as fatigue, intermittent fever, and weight loss become evident with diminished CD4 count.
3. *AIDS:* Acquired immune deficiency syndrome (AIDS) depletes CD4 cells and initiates major complications resulting from opportunistic infection or malignancy. The person's health deteriorates, leading to chronic fever, fatigue, sleep loss, fluid build-up in the lungs, and eventually death.

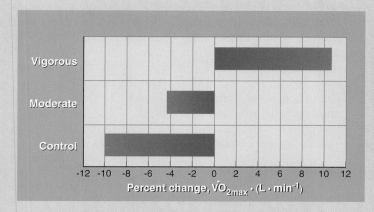

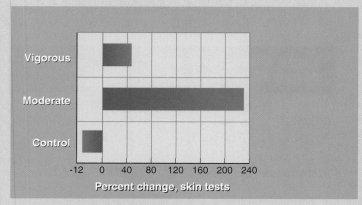

From Stringer, W. W., et al.: The effect of exercise training on aerobic fitness, immune indices, and quality of life in HIV+ patients. *Med. Sci. Sports Exerc.*, 30:11, 1998.

Treatment Modalities

Treatment modalities are rapidly changing as new information emerges about disease progression. During the early asymptomatic stages, moderate aerobic exercise training appears useful and may even delay disease progression by increasing CD4 cell number and/or upgrading the patient's general physical and psychological profiles. Some evidence suggests that even strenuous aerobic exercise can safely improve aerobic power, without acute worsening of CD4 cell count compared with nonexercise controls, or individuals engaged in only light to moderate aerobic exercise.

The figure displays results for percent change in $\dot{V}O_{2max}$ with 6 weeks of exercise training. HIV positive (HIV+) patients either (a) served as controls (no exercise), (b) trained moderately (1 h · d^{-1}, 3d · wk^{-1} for 6 wk at exercise intensity of 80% of the lactate threshold [LT] determined from a graded exercise stress test), or (c) trained vigorously (1 h · d^{-1}, 3d · wk^{-1} for 6 wk at exercise intensity equal to 50% of the difference between LT and $\dot{V}O_{2max}$). Impressive and significant increases in $\dot{V}O_{2max}$ occurred for the vigorous exercise group, whereas this measure decreased for both control and moderate training groups. Skin test scores (Candida albicans antigen, a measure of immunologic function) showed improved immune response in both exercise groups, but reached statistical significance only in the moderate exercisers. No reported episodes of immuno-compromised infections occurred during the 6-week experimental period. Quality of life measures improved for exercisers compared with nonexercisers, and exercise training did not adversely affect the level of protective CD4 cells.

Exercise Guidelines for HIV+ Individuals

Aerobic exercise training can serve as nonpharmacologic therapy within the total treatment of HIV+ patients in the intermediate stages of disease. The following guidelines are warranted for HIV+ individuals who are asymptomatic or with mild symptoms:

- Continue unrestricted physical activity.
- Follow American College of Sports Medicine guidelines for moderate exercise: minimum 3 days per week, 30 minutes a day at 50-70% HR_{max}.
- If condition worsens, the patient should continue to exercise on a symptom-limited basis.
- Reduce or curtail exercise during acute illness.

References

1. Brenner, I.K.M., et al.: Infection in athletes. *Sports Med.*, 17: 86, 1994.
2. Eichner, E.R., et al.: Immunology and exercise. Physiology, pathophysiology, and implications for HIV infection. *Med. Clin. North. Am.*, 78:377, 1994.
3. Rigsby, L. R., et al.: Effects of exercise training on men seropositive for the human immunodeficiency virus-1. *Med. Sci. Sports Exerc.*, 24:6, 1992.

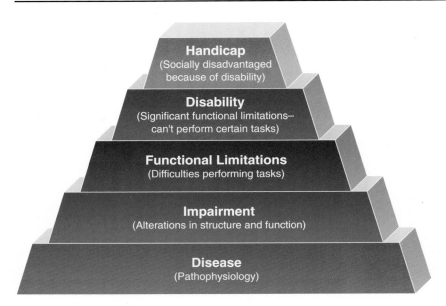

Figure 21.1
Categories of status related to physical, physiologic, and health-related impairment.

contemporary view relates sports medicine to the scientific and medical aspects of physical activity, physical fitness, and exercise/sports performance. Thus, a close link ties sports medicine to clinical exercise physiology. The sports medicine professional and exercise physiologist work hand-in-hand with similar populations. These include, at one extreme, the sedentary person who needs only a modest amount of regular exercise to reduce risk of degenerative diseases; at the other extreme, able-bodied and disabled athletes who strive to enhance sports performance. The prescription of physical activity and athletic competition for the physically challenged also plays an important role in sports medicine and exercise physiology, providing unique opportunities for research, clinical practice, and professional advancement.

Carefully prescribed physical activity significantly contributes to overall health and quality of life. Exercise physiologists assume important clinical positions alongside sports medicine professionals; their role includes testing, diagnosing, treating, and rehabilitating individuals with diverse diseases and physical disabilities.

Training and Certification by Professional Organizations

To accomplish their responsibilities in the clinical setting, the health-fitness professional must integrate unique knowledge, skills, and abilities related to exercise, physical fitness, and health. Different professional organizations provide leadership in training and certifying health-fitness professionals at different levels. Table 21.1 lists organizations offering training/certification programs with diverse emphases and specializations. The **American College of Sports Medicine (ACSM)** has emerged as the preeminent academic organization offering comprehensive programs in several areas related to the health-fitness profession. ACSM certifications encompass cognitive and practical competencies that are evaluated by written and practical examinations. The candidate must successfully complete these components (scored separately) to receive the world-recognized ACSM certification.

ACSM Qualifications and Certifications

Health-fitness professionals should be knowledgeable and competent in different areas (including first-aid and CPR certification), depending on personal interest. Table 21.2 presents content areas for different ACSM certifications. Each has general and specific learning objectives. Examples of general objectives for an **exercise leader** in exercise physiology include how to:

- Define aerobic and anaerobic metabolism.
- Describe the role of carbohydrates, fats, and proteins as fuel for aerobic and anaerobic exercise performance.
- Define the relationship of METs and kilocalories to levels of physical activity.

Less Structure and More Movement

From a public health perspective, it may be beneficial to take a less technical approach to physical fitness when recommending physical activity to individuals. People should be more active in daily life — go for a walk, garden more, watch less television, take the stairs, and do whatever practical to upgrade daily energy output.

TABLE 21.1
Organizations that offer training/certification programs related to physical activity

ORGANIZATION	AREAS OF SPECIALIZATION AND CERTIFICATION
Aerobics and Fitness Association of America (AFAA) 15250 Ventura Blvd., Suite 200 Sherman Oaks, CA 91403	AFP Fitness Practitioner, Primary Aerobics Instructor, Personal Trainer & Fitness Counselor, Step Reebok Certification, Weight Room/Resistance Training Certification, Emergency Response Certification
American College Sports Medicine (ACSM) 401 West Michigan Street Indianapolis, IN 46202	Exercise Leader, Health/Fitness Instructor, Exercise Test Technologist, Health/Fitness Director, Exercise Specialist, Program Director
American Council on Exercise (ACE) 5820 Oberlin Drive, Suite 102 San Diego, CA 92121	Group Fitness Instructor, Personal Trainer, Lifestyle & Weight Management Consultant
Canadian Aerobics Instructors Network (CAIN) 2441 Lakeshore Road West, P.O. Box 70029 Oakville, ON L6L 6M9	CIAI Instructor, Certified Personal Trainer
Canadian Personal Trainers Network (CPTN) Ontario Fitness Council (OFC) 1185 Eglington Ave. East, Suite 407 North York, ON M3C 3C6	CPTN/OFC Certified Personal Trainer, CPTN Certified Specialty Personal Trainer, CPTN/OFC Assessor of Personal Trainers, CPTN/OFC Course Conductor for Personal Trainers
Canadian Society for Exercise Physiology 1600 James Naismith Drive, Suite 311 Gloucester, ON K1B 5N4	CFC-Certified Fitness Consultant, PFLC-Professional Fitness and Lifestyle Consultant, AFAC-Accredited Fitness Appraisal Center
The Cooper Institute for Aerobics Research 12330 Preston Road Dallas, TX 75230	PFS-Physical Fitness Specialists (Personal Trainer), GEL-Group Exercise Leadership (Aerobic Instructor), ADV.PFS-Advanced Physical Fitness Specialist, Biomechanics of Strength Training, Health Promotion Director
Disabled Sports USA 451 Hungerford Drive, Suite 100 Rockville, MD 20850	Adapted Fitness Instructor
International Sports Sciences Association (ISSA) 1036 Santa Barbara Street, Suite 7 Santa Barbara, CA 93101	Certified Fitness Trainer, Specialist in Performance Nutrition, Fitness Therapist (Sports Medicine), Aerobic Fitness Trainer, Specialist in Fitness for the Physically Limited, Specialist in Martial Arts Conditioning, Specialist in Sports Management, Specialist in Water Fitness Trainer, Certified Police Fitness Instructor
International Weightlifting Association (IWA) P.O. Box 444 Hudson, OH 44236	CWT-Certified Weight Trainer
Jazzercise 2808 Roosevelt Blvd. Carlsbad, CA 92008	Certified Jazzercise Instructor
National Federation of Personal Trainers (NFPT) P.O. Box 4579 Lafayette, IN, 47903	Certified Personal Fitness Trainer
National Strength & Conditioning Association (NSCA) P.O. Box 38909 Colorado Springs, CO 80937	Certified Strength and Conditioning Specialist, Certified Personal Trainer
YMCA of the USA 101 North Wacker Drive Chicago, IL 60606	Certified Fitness Leader (Stage I-Theory, II-Applied Theory, III-Practical, Certified Specialty Leader, Trainer of Fitness Leaders, Trainer of Trainers

TABLE 21.2
Major knowledge/competency areas required for individuals interested in ACSM certifications

Functional anatomy and biomechanics
Exercise physiology
Pathophysiology and risk factors
Human development and aging
Human behavior and psychology
Health appraisal and fitness testing
ECG
Emergency procedures and safety
Exercise programming
Program administration

From *ACSM's Guidelines for Exercise Testing and Prescription*, 5th Ed. Baltimore, MD: Williams & Wilkins, 1995.

Health and Fitness Track

The **Health and Fitness Track** encompasses the Exercise Leader, Health/Fitness Instructor, and Health/Fitness Director categories.

Exercise Leader. An **Exercise Leader** must know about physical fitness (including basic motivation and counseling techniques) for healthy individuals and those with cardiovascular and pulmonary diseases. This category requires at least 250 hours of hands-on leadership experience, or an academic background in an appropriate allied health field.

Health/Fitness Instructor. A bachelors degree in exercise science, physical education, or appropriate allied health field represents the minimum education prerequisite for a **Health/Fitness Instructor**. These individuals must demonstrate competency in physical fitness testing, designing and executing an exercise program, leading exercise, and organizing and operating fitness facilities. The Health/Fitness Instructor has added responsibility for (a) training and/or supervising exercise leaders during an exercise program, and (b) serving as an exercise leader. Health/Fitness Instructors also function as health counselors to offer multiple intervention strategies for lifestyle change.

Health/Fitness Director. The minimum educational prerequisite for **Health/Fitness Director** certification requires a postgraduate degree in an appropriate allied health field. Health/Fitness Directors must acquire a Health/Fitness Instructor or exercise specialist certification. This level requires supervision by a certified program director and physician during an approved internship, or at

least 1 year of practical experience. Health/Fitness Directors require leadership qualities that ensure competency in training and supervising personnel, and proficiency in oral presentations.

ACSM Clinical Track

The title "clinical" indicates that certified personnel in these areas provide leadership in health and fitness and/or clinical programs. These professionals possess added clinical skills and knowledge that allow them to work with higher risk, symptomatic populations.

Exercise Test Technologist. **Exercise Test Technologists** administer exercise tests to individuals in good health and various states of illness. They need to demonstrate appropriate knowledge of functional anatomy, exercise physiology, pathophysiology, electrocardiography, and psychology. They must know how to recognize contraindications to testing during preliminary screening, administer tests, record data, implement emergency procedures, summarize test data, and communicate test results to other health professionals. Certification as an Exercise Test Technologist does *not* require prerequisite experience or special level of education.

Preventive/Rehabilitative Exercise Specialist. Unique competencies for the category **Preventive/Rehabilitative Exercise Specialist** include the ability to lead exercises for persons with medical limitations (particularly cardiorespiratory and related diseases) and healthy populations. The position requires a bachelors or graduate degree in an appropriate allied health field and an internship of six months or more (800 hours), largely with cardiopulmonary disease patients in a rehabilitative setting. The preventive/rehabilitative exercise specialist conducts and administers exercise tests, evaluates and interprets clinical data and formulates an exercise prescription, conducts exercise sessions, and demonstrates leadership, enthusiasm, and creativity. This person can respond appropriately to complications during exercise testing and training, and can modify exercise prescriptions for patients with specific needs.

Preventive/Rehabilitative Program Director. The **Preventive/Rehabilitative Program Director** holds an advanced degree in an appropriate allied health-related area. The certification requires an internship or practical experience of at least 2 years. This health professional works with cardiopulmonary disease patients in a rehabilitative setting, conducts and administers exercise tests, evaluates and interprets clinical data, formulates exercise prescriptions, conducts exercise sessions, responds appropriately to complications during exercise testing and training, modifies exercise prescriptions for patients with specific limitations, and makes administrative decisions regarding all aspects of a specific program.

Exercise Programs for Special Populations

The following sections present the clinical applications of exercise physiology for oncology (cancer), cardiovascular disease, and pulmonary system disabilities.

Oncology

Cancer represents a group of diseases collectively characterized by uncontrolled growth of abnormal cells. More than 100 different types of cancers exist, most occurring in adults. *Fifty percent of all cancers in adults affect the breast, lung, bowel, or uterus.* Cancer remains the second leading cause of death in the United States; approximately one-third of the population has some type of cancer. In 1997, 600,000 Americans died from cancer, and about 1.2 million new cases were diagnosed. Minorities (with different cultural backgrounds and health-nutrition beliefs) consistently had higher cancer rates, although the reasons remain unknown. Cancer represents the leading cause of death in women between ages 25 and 44 years.

The current population of more than eight million cancer survivors (many initially diagnosed in the 1970s) illustrates the need for increased rehabilitative options. The most serious outcomes for most cancer patients and survivors include loss of body mass and functional status. Depressed functional status includes difficulty walking (even a short distance) and serious fatigue that limits completion of simple household chores. Approximately 75% of cancer survivors report extreme fatigue during and following radiotherapy or chemotherapy, accompanied by weight loss and decreased muscular strength and cardiovascular endurance. Maintaining and restoring functional capacity challenges the cancer survivor, even those patients considered "cured." Sufficient rationale now justifies exercise intervention for cancer survivors.

Decreased Cancer Prevalence Associated with Increased Physical Activity

Evidence from more than 25 research studies on humans (from different continents with different diets, ways of life, environmental circumstances, race, ethnicity and socio-economic backgrounds) and laboratory animals (undergoing voluntary or forced exercise) show a reduced risk of cancer development associated with higher levels of regular physical activity.

Increased regular physical activity can assist the cancer patient in recuperating and returning to a normal, independent lifestyle. Table 21.3 lists general preventive and intervention goals for a cancer patient who faces sustained periods of inactivity and bed rest. The health-care team strives to upgrade the patient to a level of function that allows return to work and pursuit of normal recreational activities.

Exercise Effects on Cancer

Epidemiologic evidence shows that regular exercise can reduce risk for certain cancers by:

TABLE 21.3
Ten goals of clinical exercise physiologists in treating patients with deconditioning, immobility, or disuse syndromes

1. Improve overall functional status
2. Improve active motion for nonrestrictive segments and joints
3. Prevent loss of flexibility by active motion and passive movements
4. Stimulate peripheral and central circulation through active motion exercise based on current functional level
5. Increase ventilatory function by use of systematic breathing exercises
6. Prevent thrombosis through physical activities
7. Prevent loss of motor control and muscle strength and endurance with resistance exercises
8. Reduce the rate of bone loss through weight-bearing aerobic and muscle-strengthening exercises
9. Through active aerobic and resistance exercise, slow the loss of fat-free body mass and subsequent reduction of BMR that accompanies deconditioning
10. Monitor signs of increased fatigue or weakness, lethargy, dyspnea, pallor, dizziness, claudication, or cramping during or following exercise

Incidence and Types of Cancer

Type of Cancer	Incidence per 1000 people (all ages)
Lung, bronchial	125
Leukemia	58
Female breast	159
Genitourinary	173
Digestive	185
Bone	52
Skin	44

- Reducing levels of plasma glucose and insulin
- Increasing levels of corticosteroid hormones
- Increasing anti-inflammatory cytokines
- Augmenting insulin-receptor expression in cancer-fighting T cells
- Increasing interferon production
- Stimulating glycogen synthetase activity
- Augmenting leukocyte function
- Improving ascorbic acid metabolism
- Exerting beneficial effects on pro-virus or oncogene activation

Exercise Prescription and Cancer

What constitutes the proper exercise prescription for cancer patients? Unfortunately, little research exists on the timing of exercise relative to various phases of carcinogenesis. This makes it difficult to determine when to initiate exercise intervention. With such little objective information on exercise prescription and cancer rehabilitation, health-fitness professionals generally recommend a symptom-limited, progressive, and individualized exercise prescription. Prudent ambulation of any kind proves beneficial for the most sedentary and deconditioned patient.

Cancer patients can participate in an exercise stress test, which also serves as a basis for the exercise prescription. Similar testing procedures apply as with healthy individuals, except feelings of fatigue require greater attention.

The exercise prescription should encourage ambulation if the patient has no specific exercise contraindications. The prescription also should involve range of motion and flexibility exercises, and exercises to improve muscular strength and overall mobility (e.g., submaximal static exercises for antigravity muscles, deep breathing exercises, and dynamic trunk rotation movements). In most cases, preference goes to low-level exercise for short periods, performed several times daily. Exercise progression and intensity are individualized, with initial work/rest ratios of 1:1 progressing to 2:1. Eventually, continuous exercise can be prescribed, as tolerated, starting with 3 to 5 minutes, then 10 minutes, and moving up to 30 to 45 minutes whenever possible.

Breast Cancer and Exercise

Carcinoma of the breast, one of the most common forms of cancer in white females age 40 years and older represents the leading cause of death in women between ages 40 to 60 years. Approximately 184,000 new cases of breast cancer are diagnosed annually, which means that one of every nine females develops breast cancer at some time during her life, with a high rate of reoccurrence. In 1996, over 44,300 women died from breast cancer; only heart disease and lung cancer kill more women yearly. Primary breast cancer risk factors include a positive family history of breast cancer, a personal history of cancer, first menstrual period at an early age, menopause at a late age, first childbirth after age 30 or no childbirth, and a high-fat diet.

Although limited data exists on the role of exercise in breast cancer rehabilitation, available research suggests:

- Physical activity has a pronounced protective effect for postmenopausal women compared with pre-menopausal women.
- Physical activity plays an important "psychological" role in post-surgery rehabilitation.

A study from one of our laboratories tested 28 patients recovering from breast cancer surgery to evaluate the effects of a 10-week circuit resistance training program on depression, self-esteem, and anxiety (Fig. 21.2). The program, conducted 4 days per week, consisted of self-paced hydraulic resistance exercises performed in a 14-station aerobic exercise circuit.

Exercisers exhibited a 38% decrease in depression compared with a 13% increase for nonexercising controls also recovering from breast cancer surgery. Exercisers exhibited a 16% decrease in trait anxiety and a 20% decrease in

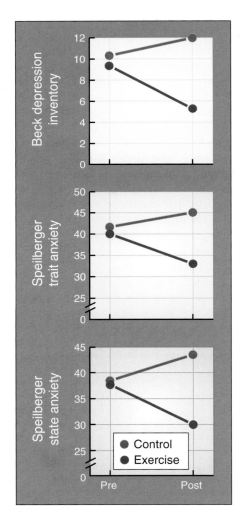

Figure 21.2
Effects of 10 weeks of moderate aerobic resistance exercise on depression (**top**), and trait (**middle**) and state (**lower**) anxiety in women recovering form breast cancer surgery. (Data courtesy of M. Segar, Applied Physiology Laboratory, University of Michigan, Ann Arbor, MI, 1996.)

Possible Mechanisms for Breast Cancer Protection with Exercise

1. Alteration in cumulative exposure to estrogen (a primary risk factor for the disease)
   - Changes in menstrual/ovulatory patterns
   - Delayed onset of menarche
   - Increased number of menstrual cycles without ovulation
   - Increased menstrual irregularity results in fewer cycles
   - Decreased levels of body fat
2. Immune system enhancement
3. Healthy lifestyle that accompanies regular exercise
   - Prevention of excess body fat
   - Consumption of low-fat diets
   - Consumption of fruits and vegetables
   - Abstinence from smoking
   - Attention to preventive health practices
   - Less depression and anxiety
   - Greater self-esteem

state anxiety compared to significant increases in both variables for controls. These results demonstrate that a planned, moderate aerobic resistance exercise program can exert positive effects on psychosocial variables during breast cancer rehabilitation.

Cardiovascular Diseases

Heart disease accounts for the greatest number of deaths among industrialized nations. More than two million deaths occur from cardiovascular diseases in the United States each year, and one in four Americans will suffer some form of cardiovascular disease in their lifetime. Fortunately, occurrence and death from cardiovascular disease have declined during the past decade, due in part to aggressive steps to reduce risk factors, and early screening and implementation of cardiac prevention and rehabilitation programs.

Cardiac patients can participate in regular aerobic exercise after consideration for specific pathophysiology, mechanisms that may limit exercise capacity, and individual differences in functional capacity. Table 21.4 lists three different categories of heart disease that lead to functional disability. By far, diseases of the myocardium become most prevalent, particularly with advancing age. The following terms frequently describe these diseases: degenerative heart disease (DHD), atherosclerotic cardiovascular disease, arteriosclerotic cardiovascular disease, coronary artery disease (CAD), or coronary heart disease (CHD).

Diseases of the Myocardium

Recent advances in molecular biology have isolated a possible genetic link to CHD. This gene (on chromosome 19 near the gene related to LDL-cholesterol receptor functioning), called the **atherosclerosis susceptibility gene (ATHS)**, accounts for almost 50% of all CHD cases. The ATHS gene causes a set of characteristics (abdominal obesity, low levels of HDL-cholesterol, and high levels of LDL-cholesterol) that triple a person's risk of myocardial infarction.

CHD pathogenesis probably progresses along the following sequence:

1. Injury to the coronary artery's endothelial cell wall
2. Fibroblastic proliferation of the artery's inner lining (intima)
3. Accumulation of lipids at the junction of the arterial intima and middle lining, further obstructing blood flow

TABLE 21.4
Three categories of heart disease that lead to functional disability

DISEASES AFFECTING THE HEART MUSCLE	DISEASES AFFECTING HEART VALVES	DISEASES AFFECTING THE CARDIAC NERVOUS SYSTEM
CHD	Rheumatic fever	Arrhythmias
Angina	Endocarditis	Tachycardia
Myocardial infarction	Mitral valve prolapse	Bradycardia
Pericarditis	Congenital deformations	
Congestive heart failure		
Aneurysms		

TABLE 21.5
Similarity of symptoms of angina and heartburn

ANGINA	HEARTBURN
• Gripping, viselike feelings of pain or pressure behind the breast bone	• Frequent feeling of heartburn
• Pain that radiates to the neck, jaw, back, shoulders, or arms (usually left)	• Frequent use of antacids to relieve pain
• Toothache	• Heartburn wakes person up at night
• Burning indigestion	• Acid or bitter taste in mouth
• Shortness of breath	• Burning chest sensation
• Nausea	• Discomfort after eating spicy food
• Frequent belching	• Difficulty in swallowing

4. Deterioration and formation of hyaline (a clear, homogeneous substance formed in degeneration) in the vessel's intima.
5. Calcium deposition at edges of hyalinated area.

The major disorders caused by reduced myocardial blood supply include angina pectoris, myocardial infarction, and congestive heart failure.

Angina Pectoris. Angina pectoris, characterized by acute chest pain, results from an imbalance between the oxygen demands of the heart and its oxygen supply. Current theory suggests that angina pain results from metabolite accumulation within an ischemic segment of heart muscle. The sensation of angina pectoris includes squeezing, burning, and pressing or "choking" in the chest region, which can often become confused with simple heartburn (Table 21.5). Angina pain usually lasts up to three minutes, but can continue for longer intervals. About one-third of individuals who suffer from angina die suddenly from myocardial infarction. Several types of angina exist, including **chronic stable angina** (often referred to as "walk-through" angina), which occur at a predictable level of physical exertion. Vasodilators like nitroglycerin reduce cardiac work-load to effectively control this uncomfortable and potentially debilitating condition.

Figure 21.3 shows the usual pattern of pain associated with an episode of acute angina pectoris. Pain occurs in the left shoulder or along the arm to the elbow. Occasionally, angina pain occurs in the back area of the left scapula along the spinal cord.

Myocardial Infarction

Myocardial infarction (MI, heart attack, or coronary occlusion) results from inadequate perfusion of blood in the coronary arteries, and/or imbalance in myocardial oxygen demand and supply during physical activity caused by significant occlusion of coronary vasculature. Sudden occlusion results from prior clot formation initiated from plaque accumulation in one or more coronary arteries. Severe fatigue for several days without specific pain usually precedes the onset of an MI. Figure 21.4 displays the diverse locations of early warning signs of the onset of an MI. Severe, unrelenting chest pain can last from 30 minutes to one hour during an MI.

Pericarditis

Pericarditis, an inflammation of the heart's outer pericardial lining or sac, classifies as either acute or chronic (recurring or constrictive). Acute pericarditis symptoms vary but usually include chest pain, dyspnea, and elevated resting heart rate and body temperature. In chronic pericarditis, inflammation creates extreme chest pain due to fluid accumulation in the pericardial sac, which prevents the heart from fully expanding during diastole. The prognosis for acute viral pericarditis is excellent, whereas

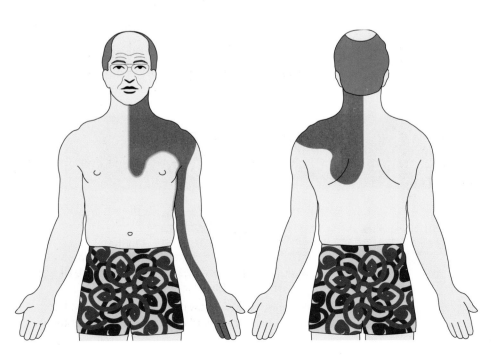

Figure 21.3
Location of pain generally associated with angina pectoris.

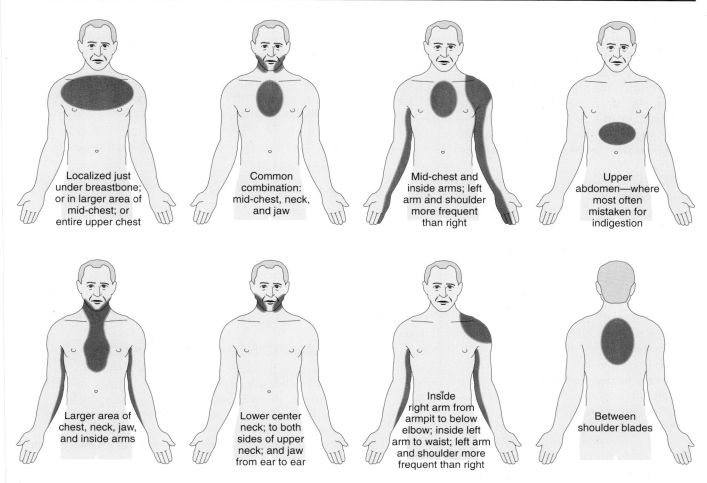

Figure 21.4
Location of early warning signs of myocardial infarction. Note diverse locations of pain.

chronic pericarditis from bacterial origin presents a more serious pathology.

Congestive Heart Failure

Congestive heart failure (CHF or chronic decompensation) occurs when cardiac output cannot keep pace with venous return. The heart fails from intrinsic myocardial disease, chronic hypertension, or structural defects that impair pump performance. When this occurs, left ventricular output diminishes and blood accumulates in the pulmonary vasculature. This causes shortness of breath and eventual flooding of the pulmonary alveoli with plasma filtrate, a condition referred to as **pulmonary congestion**. Common CHF symptoms include dyspnea, coughing with large amounts of frothy blood-tinged sputum, pulmonary edema, general fatigue, and overall muscular weakness. Heart failure can occur from the right or left heart, each with different symptomatologies and prognoses depending on initiation of treatment.

Aneurysm

An **aneurysm** is an abnormal dilatation in the wall of an artery or vein or the myocardium. Vascular aneurysms oc-

cur when a vessel's wall weakens from trauma, congenital vascular disease, infection, or atherosclerosis. These are identified as either "arterial" or "venous," and classified according to the specific vasculature area affected (e.g., thoracic aneurysm). A routine chest x-ray uncovers most aneurysms. Common symptoms include chest pain with a specific, palpable, pulsating mass in the chest, abdomen, or lower back.

Heart Valve Diseases

Diseases and abnormalities that affect heart valve structure and function include:

- **Stenosis:** Valve narrowing or constriction that prevents it from opening fully; caused by growths, scars, or abnormal mineral deposits.

- **Insufficiency** (also called regurgitation): Heart valves do not close properly, causing blood to flow back into the heart's chambers during diastole.

- **Prolapse** (only affects mitral valve): Enlarged valve leaflets bulge backward into the left atrium during the cardiac cycle.

Valvular abnormalities increase myocardial work-load, requiring the heart to generate greater force to pump blood through a constricted valve, or to maintain cardiac output if blood seeps back into a chamber. Heart valve stenosis frequently results from **rheumatic fever**, a potentially fatal infection by streptococcal bacteria that can lead to rheumatic heart disease (valvular scarring and heart valve deformity). The two most common symptoms of this valve pathology include fever and joint pain.

Endocarditis

Endocarditis, an inflammation of the endocardium usually of bacterial origin, damages the tricuspid, aortic, or mitral valves resulting from direct invasion of bacteria into the tissue. Patients initially have musculoskeletal symptoms, including arthritis, low back pain, and general weakness in one or more joints. Antibiotic drugs usually prove effective in treating this disease.

Congenital Malformations

Congenital heart defects appear in one of every 100 births; they include defects of the heart valves such as ventricular or atrial septal defects (hole between the ventricles and atria) and patent ductus arteriosus (shunt caused by an opening between the aorta and pulmonary artery). These defects require surgical repair.

Mitral Valve Prolapse

Mitral valve prolapse (MVP) occurs in about 10% of Americans; it involves variations in either the mitral valve's shape or structure. This defect has been called "floppy valve syndrome," "Barlow's syndrome," and the "click-murmur syndrome." MVP usually remains benign, but frequency of diagnosis has increased over the past decade due to its association with endocarditis, atherosclerosis, and muscular dystrophy. MVP probably results from connective tissue abnormalities in mitral valve leaflets. Sixty percent of patients with MVP have no symptoms; the remainder experience profound fatigue during exercise.

Cardiac Nervous System Diseases

Diseases that affect the heart's electrical conduction system include **dysrhythmias (arrhythmias)** that cause the heart to:

- Beat too quickly (tachycardia)
- Beat too slowly (bradycardia)
- Generate extra beats (ectopic, extrasystole, or premature ventricular contractions)
- Fibrillate (fine rapid contractions or twitching of cardiac muscle fibers)

Dysrhythmias usually change circulatory dynamics and can result in low blood pressure, heart failure, and shock. They often occur following a stroke induced by physical exertion or other stressor.

In adults, **sinus tachycardia** represents a resting heart rate greater than 100 b·min^{-1}, whereas in **sinus bradycardia** resting heart rate goes below 60 b·min^{-1}. Asymptomatic sinus bradycardia often occurs in endurance athletes and young adults. This form of bradycardia represents a benign dysrhythmia; it actually may reflect a beneficial adaptation because of a longer diastole for ventricular filling during the cardiac cycle.

Cardiac Disease Assessment

thorough cardiac disease assessment includes the following:

- Patient medical history
- Physical examination
- Laboratory tests
- Physiological tests

Patient Medical History

A carefully obtained patient history documents the most common complaints and establishes a basis for CHD risk profiling. Because most CHD symptoms include chest pain, this pain's differential diagnosis becomes a primary focus. Table 21.6 lists a limited differential diagnosis of chest pain, including possible causes and pathogenesis.

Physical Examination

A physician, nurse, or physician's assistant usually conducts the physical examination that includes the patient's vital signs (body temperature, heart rate, breathing rate, and blood pressure). Resting heart rate provides a noninvasive measure of cardiovascular efficiency. Evidence of sinus tachycardia and increased breathing rate and systolic blood pressure could alter the exercise prescription.

For purposes of prescribing exercise and identifying early warning signs of CHD, the clinical exercise physiologist must know a patient's normal heart rate and blood pressure response to incremental exercise. For example, an increase in systolic blood pressure of 20 mm Hg or more (**hypertensive response**) in low-level physical activity (2 to 4 METs) can indicate overall cardiovascular impairment and warn of an increased myocardial oxygen demand (suggestive of potential coronary ischemia). In contrast, failure for systolic blood pressure to increase (**hypotensive response**) during moderate physical activity can indicate left ventricular dysfunction; at high exercise intensities, a hypotensive response signals significant mortality risk. Individuals unable to elevate systolic blood pressures above 140 mm Hg during maximal exercise often have significant but dormant cardiac disease.

Heart Auscultation

Listening to (**auscultation**) heart sounds provides important information about cardiac function. The exercise physiologist should become familiar with different abnor-

TABLE 21.6
Chest pain diagnosis

PAIN/COMPLAINT/FINDINGS	POSSIBLE CAUSES	STIMULI	POSSIBLE PATHOLOGY
Pressure, ache, tightness or burning in midsternum, left shoulder, arm; diaphoresis; nausea; vomiting; ST-segment changes	MI	Exertion; cold; smoking; heavy meal; fluid overload	CHD
Sharp pain worsens with inspiration, improves with sitting	Inflammation	Acute MI	Pericarditis
Chest tightness with breathlessness; low-grade fever	Infection	IV drug use; microbes	Myocarditis; endocarditis
Sharp, stabbing pain, breathlessness, cough; loss of consciousness	Pulmonary	Recent surgery	Pulmonary embolism
Burning pain in stomach; indigestion relieved by antacids	Referred pain	Heavy meal, spicy food	Esophageal reflux
Angina pain; breathlessness; wide pulse pressure; ventricular hypertrophy on ECG	Ventricular outflow tract obstruction	Exertion; CHD	Aortic stenosis Mitral valve prolapse

mal heart sounds, including how to identify heart murmurs. Auscultation can readily diagnose valvular diseases (e.g., MVP diagnosed by the classic click-murmur sounds) and congenital abnormalities (regurgitation sounds in ventricular septal defects).

Laboratory Tests

The following laboratory tests provide significant information for confirming and documenting the extent of CHD:

- Chest x-ray
- Electrocardiogram (ECG)
- Blood lipid and lipoproteins
- Serum enzymes

Chest x-rays (Figure 21.5) reveal the size and shape of the heart and lungs, and resting and exercise ECG provide essential information to assess cardiac function for electrical conductivity and myocardial oxygenation.

Correctly reading and interpreting an ECG requires specialized training and considerable practice. Table 21.7 lists the six different categories of ECG interpretations. Later in this chapter, various ECG abnormalities and abnormal physiologic responses to exercise are described; how to count heart rate from ECG tracings is also detailed. Careful monitoring of ECG changes during exercise targets individuals with potential CHD for further evaluation. Table 21.8 lists common ECG changes associated with CHD.

Routine laboratory testing for CHD risk includes analysis of the blood lipid and lipoprotein profile. Alterations in serum enzymes often diagnose or exclude an acute MI. When myocardial cell death (**necrosis**) or prolonged lack of blood flow (**ischemia**) occur, enzymes from the damaged muscle leak into the blood because of the plasma membrane's increased permeability. This increases serum levels of three enzymes:

1. *Creatine phosphokinase (CPK)*. Elevated CPK reflects either skeletal or cardiac muscle necrosis

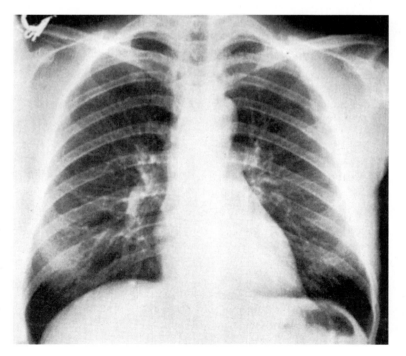

Figure 21.5
Typical chest x-ray.

TABLE 21.7
Six categories for ECG interpretation

1. **Measurements**
   - Heart rate (atrial and ventricular)
   - PR interval (0.12 to 0.20 s)
   - QRS duration (0.06 to 0.10 s)
   - QT interval (HR dependent)
   - Frontal plane QRS Axis ($-30°$ to $+90°$)
2. **Rhythm diagnosis**
3. **Conduction diagnosis**
4. **Wave form description**
   - P wave (atrial enlargement)
   - QRS complex (ventricular hypertrophy, infarction)
   - ST segment (elevated or depressed)
   - T wave (flattened or inverted)
   - U wave (prominent or inverted)
5. **ECG diagnosis**
   - Within normal limits
   - Borderline abnormal
   - Abnormal
6. **Comparison with previous ECG**

From Fardy, P., and Yanowitz, F.G.: *Cardiac Rehabilitation, Adult Fitness and Exercise Testing.* Baltimore, MD: Williams & Wilkins, 1996.

2. *Lactate dehydrogenase (LDH).* LDH, like CPK, fractionates into different isoenzyme markers, one of which increases during an MI
3. *Serum glutamic oxaloacetic transaminase (SGOT)*

Noninvasive Physiological Tests

Noninvasive physiological tests can identify specific cardiac dysfunction with minimal patient discomfort and risk.

Echocardiography

Echocardiography uses pulses of reflected **ultrasound** to evaluate heart function and morphology; it identifies the heart's structural components, and measures distances from the echo transducers. This allows estimation of various heart chamber sizes (volumes), in addition to blood vessel dimensions and thickness of various myocardial components. The echocardiogram has surpassed the ECG in recognizing chamber enlargement, myocardial hypertrophy, and other structural abnormalities. Echocardiograms can diagnose heart murmurs, evaluate valvular lesions, and determine the extent of congenital heart diseases and cardiomyopathies.

Graded Exercise Stress Test (GXT)

For many people, an important part of their medical evaluation includes a **graded exercise stress test (GXT)**. The term stress test describes the systematic use of exercise for two purposes:

1. Observe cardiac rhythm abnormalities during exercise
2. Assess physiological adjustments to increased metabolic demands

The most common modes for exercise stress testing include multistage bicycle and treadmill tests. The test, "graded" for exercise intensity, includes submaximal exercise levels of three to five minutes duration each, progressing up to a self-imposed fatigue level. The graded nature of testing allows detection of ischemic manifestations and rhythm disorders with small increments in exercise intensity. The stress test can provide a reliable, quantitative index of the person's level of functional impairment. *For most screening purposes, the test need not be maximal; instead, the person exercises to at least 85% of age-predicted maximum heart rate.*

A resting ECG usually precedes the GXT to establish that the person can engage safely in subsequent graded exercise. The resting ECG provides an important baseline measure.

TABLE 21.8
Normal and abnormal ECG changes commonly observed during exercise

NORMAL ECG CHANGES IN HEALTHY INDIVIDUALS[a]	ABNORMAL ECG CHANGES WITH CHD
1. Slight increase in P wave amplitude	1. Appearance of bundle branch block at a critical HR
2. Shortening of PR interval	2. Recurrent or multifocal PVCs during exercise and recovery
3. Shift to the right of QRS axis	3. Ventricular tachycardia
4. ST segment depression <1.0 mm	4. Appearance of bradyarrhythmias, tachyarrhythmias
5. Decreased T wave amplitude	5. ST segment depression/elevation of >1.0 mm 0.08 s after J point
6. Single or rare PVC during exercise and recovery	6. Exercise bradycardia
7. Single or rare PVC or PAC	7. Submaximal exercise tachycardia
	8. Increase in frequency or severity of any known arrhythmia

[a] PVC, premature ventricular contraction; PAC, premature atrial contraction.

Why Stress Test?

Stress testing is important in an overall CHD evaluation to:

Keeping the Cardiovascular System Young

A 30-min program of rapid walking performed by an older person 3 or 4 times a week can turn back the biologic clock by 10 years for cardiovascular function and aerobic fitness.

- *Detect heart disease.* An exercise ECG can diagnose overt heart disease, and also screen for possible "silent" coronary disease in seemingly healthy individuals. Approximately 25 to 40% of people with confirmed coronary artery disease have normal resting electrocardiograms. ECG analysis during exercise uncovers about 80% of these abnormalities.

- R*eproduce and assess exercise-related chest symptoms.* Individuals older than age 40 often suffer angina symptoms with physical exertion. ECG analysis during graded exercise provides a more objective and valid diagnosis of exercise-induced pain.

- *Screen candidates for preventive and rehabilitative exercise programs.* Stress test results help with the design of an exercise program within the person's functional capacity and health status. Repeated testing evaluates training progress and determines how to safely modify the initial exercise prescription.

- *Detect abnormal blood pressure responses.* Many individuals with normal resting blood pressure show higher than normal increases in systolic blood pressure with exercise. Exercise hypertension often signifies developing cardiovascular complications.

- *Monitor responses to various therapeutic interventions (drug, surgical, and dietary) designed to improve cardiovascular health and function.* For example, the patient's adjustment to exercise and how well he or she reaches a target heart rate without complications indicate success of coronary bypass surgery.

- *Define functional aerobic capacity and evaluate its degree of deviation from normal standards.* Metabolic measurements during the GXT allow determination of the $\dot{V}O_{2max}$ or $\dot{V}O_{2peak}$.

Who Should Be Stress-Tested? Table 21.9 shows a classification system by age and health status for screening and supervisory procedures for both stress testing and participation in a regular exercise program. These guidelines apply for healthy individuals and those at higher risk. Seemingly healthy young adults can begin moderate inten-

TABLE 21.9
Classification system by age and health status for stress testing

| | APPARENTLY HEALTHY | | HIGHER RISK[a] | | |
	≤40 Y (♂) ≤50 Y (♀)	OLDER	NO SYMPTOMS	SYMPTOMS	WITH DISEASE[b]
Medical exam and diagnostic test recommended prior to:					
Moderate exercise	No[c]	No	No	Re	Rec
Vigorous exercise	No	Rec	Rec	Rec	Rec
Physician supervision recommended during exercise test:					
Submaximal testing	No	No	No	Rec	Rec
Maximal testing	No	Rec	Rec	Rec	Rec

[a] Person with two or more primary CHD risk factors.

[b] Persons with known cardiac, pulmonary, or metabolic disease.

[c] No does not mean "not necessary"; just not recommended at this time.

Rec = recommended.

Moderate = exercise intensity of 40 to 60% $\dot{V}O_{2max}$ performed for 30–60 min.

Vigorous = exercise intensity of >60% $\dot{V}O_{2max}$ that results in fatigue within 20 min.

From *ACSM's Guidelines for Exercise Testing and Prescription.* 5th Ed. Baltimore, MD: Williams & Wilkins, 1995.

sity exercise (40-60% $\dot{V}O_{2max}$) without an exercise stress test or medical examination. Men above age 40 and women above age 50 should have a medical examination that includes a stress test before starting an exercise program. A GXT that precedes exercise training takes on added importance for higher risk individuals of any age. These include people with two or more major CHD risk factors and/or symptoms suggestive of cardiopulmonary or metabolic disease (see Chapter 20). An individual with these diseases should undergo a thorough medical evaluation before modifying their normal routine for physical activity.

Informed Consent. All testing and exercise training must be performed on "informed volunteers." *Informed consent raises awareness about all potential risks of*

participation. The informed consent must include a written statement that the person had an opportunity to ask questions about the procedures with sufficient information clearly provided so consent occurs from a knowledgeable (informed) perspective. A legal guardian or parent must sign the consent form for a minor. Individuals need assurance that test results remain confidential. They should understand that they can terminate the exercise testing or training program at any time and for any reason. Table 21.10 presents a sample informed consent statement.

Contraindications to Stress Testing. Certain conditions preclude administering a stress test while other conditions require that the GXT be administered under more closely monitored conditions.

TABLE 21.10
Informed consent for a graded exercise stress test

Name _____

1. **Explanation of the exercise test**
   You will perform an exercise test on a cycle ergometer or a motor-driven treadmill. The exercise intensity begins at a level you can easily accomplish and will advance in stages of difficulty depending on your fitness level. We may stop the test at any time because of signs of fatigue, or you may stop the test when you wish because of fatigue or discomfort that you feel, particularly at the higher exercise levels.

2. **Risks and Discomforts**
   The possibility exists that certain abnormal changes can occur during the test. These include abnormal blood pressure, fainting, disorder of heart beat, and in rare instances, heart attack, stroke, or death. Every effort will be made to minimize these risks by evaluating preliminary information related to your health and fitness, and by observations during testing. Emergency equipment and available trained personnel can deal with unusual situations that may arise.

3. **Responsibilities of the Participant**
   Information you possess about your health status or previous experiences of unusual feelings with physical effort may affect the safety and value of your exercise test you should report this information now. Your prompt reporting of how you feel during the exercise test also is important. You are responsible for fully disclosing such information when requested to do so by the testing staff.

4. **Expected Benefits from the Test**
   The results obtained from the exercise test may assist in diagnosing your illness, or evaluating what type of physical activities you might do with low risk.

5. **Inquires**
   We encourage you to ask any questions about the procedures used in the exercise test or in the estimation of your functional capacity. If you have doubts or questions, please ask us for further explanations.

6. **Freedom of Consent**
   Your permission to perform this exercise test is voluntary. You are free to deny consent or stop the test at any point.
   I have read this form and understand the test procedures. I voluntarily consent to participate in this test.

Date: _____

Signature of Patient: _____

Signature of Witness: _____

Questions: _____

_____

Responses: _____

Signature of Physician or Delegate: _____

Absolute Contraindications.   Under no circumstances should a stress test be administered without direct medical supervision if any of the following exist:

- Resting ECG suggestive of acute cardiac disease
- Recent complicated myocardial infarction
- Unstable angina pectoris
- Uncontrolled ventricular arrhythmia
- Uncontrolled atrial arrhythmia that compromises cardiac function
- Third degree AV heart block without pacemaker
- Acute congestive heart failure
- Severe aortic stenosis
- Active or suspected myocarditis or pericarditis
- Recent systemic or pulmonary embolism
- Acute infections
- Acute emotional distress

Relative Contraindications.   In the presence of any of the following conditions, a GXT can be administered with caution and with medical personal in close proximity to the test area.

- Resting diastolic blood pressure >115 mm Hg or systolic blood pressure ≥200 mm Hg
- Moderate valvular disease
- Electrolyte abnormalities
- Frequent or complex ventricular ectopy
- Ventricular aneurysm
- Uncontrolled metabolic disease (diabetes, thyrotoxicosis)
- Chronic infectious disease (hepatitis, mononucleosis, AIDS)
- Neuromuscular or musculoskeletal disorders
- Pregnancy (complicated or in the last trimester)
- Psychological distress/apprehension about taking the test

Field Tests of Cardiorespiratory Fitness

Field tests estimate cardiorespiratory fitness (primarily $\dot{V}O_{2max}$) and endurance performance. The tests require little equipment, can be administered in different locations, and usually involve walking, jogging or stationary cycling, forms of exercise familiar to most individuals. Except for stationary cycling, field testing does not lend itself to (a) ECG monitoring (except heart rate, which has limited diagnostic utility), or (b) monitoring blood pressure and metabolic responses to exercise.

Two common endurance field tests include:

1. One-mile walk test: Individuals walk as fast as possible on a measured track, with heart rate recorded after the mile. The person's body weight, sex, age, time to complete the mile, and heart rate response are used to predict $\dot{V}O_{2max}$.

2. Twelve-minute or 1.5-mile run-walk test: Individual walks, jogs, or runs as fast as possible for 12 minutes or for 1.5 miles.

Laboratory-based GXTs remain preferable to field tests because of control over test environment and exercise intensity. The most popular tests use a treadmill, stationary cycle ergometer, or bench step-up.

Maximal Versus Submaximal Tests

A *maximal GXT (GXT$_{max}$) represents the most common noninvasive method to screen for CHD and determine $\dot{V}O_{2max}$ or $\dot{V}O_{2peak}$.* Individuals exercise until they decide to stop, or develop abnormal symptoms that signal test termination (Table 21.11); the term **symptom limited** describes such tests.

GXT$_{max}$ normally progress through several stages (multistage); the duration, starting point, and increments between stages vary with the person (e.g., young active; healthy sedentary; questionable health status). The advantages of a GXT$_{max}$ include ability to directly determine $\dot{V}O_{2max}$ and maximal cardiovascular responses, screen for abnormal ECG patterns not revealed during rest or low intensity exercise, and establish more precise training levels. Disadvantages include the significant stress placed on the person; al-

---

TABLE 21.11
Criteria for stopping a GXT in apparently healthy adults

1. Onset of angina or angina-like symptoms
2. Ventricular tachycardia
3. Significant decrease in systolic blood pressure of 20 mm Hg or more
4. Failure of the systolic blood pressure and/or heart rate to rise with an increase in exercise load
5. Light-headedness, confusion, ataxia, pallor, cyanosis, nausea, or signs of severe peripheral circulatory insufficiency
6. Early onset horizontal or downsloping S-T segment depression or elevation (>4 mm)
7. Increasing ventricular ectopy, multiform PVCs
8. Excessive increase in blood pressure: systolic BP >260 mm Hg; diastolic BP >115 mm Hg
9. Increase in heart rate <25 b · min^{-1} of predicted normal value (in the absence of beta blockade medication)
10. Sustained supraventricular tachycardia
11. Subject requests to stop test for whatever reason
12. Equipment failure

From *ACSM's Guidelines for Exercises Testing and Prescription.* 5 Ed., ACSM. Baltimore, MD: Williams & Wilkins, 1995.

How To Recognize Vital Signs

Proper handling of potentially critical situations requires the ability to recognize physiological signs of injury. When evaluating the seriously ill or injured, one must be aware of nine **vital signs:**

1. Heart (pulse) rate
2. Breathing rate (respiration)
3. Blood pressure
4. Body temperature
5. Skin color
6. Pupils of the eye
7. Movement
8. Presence of pain
9. State of consciousness

Heart (Pulse) Rate

A normal pulse rate per minute for adults ranges between 60 and 80 b·min^{-1}, and in children from 80 to 100 b·min^{-1}. Any alteration from normality can indicate the presence of a pathological condition. For example, a rapid but weak pulse could indicate shock, bleeding, diabetic coma, or heat exhaustion. A rapid and strong pulse may indicate heatstroke or severe fright. A strong but slow pulse could indicate a skull fracture or stroke, whereas no pulse means cardiac arrest or death.

Breathing Rate (Respiration)

The normal breathing rate in adults approximates 12 breathes per minute, and 20 to 25 in children. Breathing cab be **shallow, irregular,** or **gasping.** Frothy blood from the mouth indicates a chest injury involving the lung. **Look, listen, and feel;** look to ascertain whether the chest is rising or falling; listen for air passing in and out of the mouth or nose or both; and feel how the chest is moving.

Blood Pressure

Normal systolic blood pressure for 15 to 20-year-old males ranges from 115 to 120 mm Hg; the diastolic pressure ranges from 75 to 80 mm Hg. Female blood pressure usually records 8 to 10 mm Hg lower for both systolic and diastolic pressures. Between the age of 15 to 20, a systolic pressure of 135 mm Hg and above may be excessive; while a pressure of 110 mm Hg or lower may be considered too low. Diastolic pressure should not exceed 60 for females and 85 mm Hg for males, respectively. A dramatically lowered blood pressure can indicate hemorrhage, shock, heart attack, or internal organ injury.

Body Temperature

Normal body temperature averages 98.6° F (37° C). Temperature can be measured under the tongue, in the armpit, or in the rectum. Changes in body temperature can also be palpated. Hot dry skin can indicate disease, infection, or overexposure to environmental heat. Cool, clammy skin can indicate trauma, shock, or heat exhaustion. Cool, dry skin can be the result of overexposure to cold. A rise or fall of the internal temperature can be caused by a variety of circumstances such as the onset of a communicable disease, cold exposure, pain, fear, or nervousness.

Skin Color

For individuals who are lightly pigmented, the skin can be a good indicator of the state of health. Three skin colors are commonly identified in medical emergencies:

1. Red: may indicate heatstroke, high blood pressure, or carbon monoxide poisoning
2. White: a pale, ashen, or white skin can mean insufficient circulation, shock, fright, hemorrhage, heat exhaustion, or insulin shock
3. Blue: usually means that circulating blood is poorly oxygenated indicating an airway obstruction or respiratory insufficiency

Assessing a dark skinned individual becomes complicated. These individuals normally have pink coloration of the nail beds and inside the lips, mouth, and tongue. Changes in these indicate a medical emergency.

Pupils

The pupils are extremely sensitive to situations affecting the nervous system. Although most persons have pupils of regular outline and equal size, some individuals have pupils that may be irregular and unequal. A constricted pupil can indicate a central nervous system response to a depressant drug. If one or both pupils are dilated, the individual may have sustained a head injury, may be experiencing shock, heatstroke, or hemorrhage, or may have ingested a stimulant drug. The pupil's response to light should also be noted. If one or both pupils fail to accommodate to light, there may be brain injury, or alcohol or drug poisoning. Pupil response is more critical in evaluation than pupil size.

State of Consciousness

Normally, individuals are alert, aware of their environment, and respond quickly to vocal stimulation. Head injury, heatstroke, and diabetic coma can vary an individual's level of consciousness awareness.

Movement

The inability to move a body part can indicate a serious central nervous system injury. An inability to move one side of the body can the result of a head injury or cerebrovascular accident. Paralysis of the upper limb can indicate a spinal injury, inability to move the lower extremities could mean an injury below the neck, and pressure on the spinal cord could lead to limited use of the limbs.

Abnormal Nerve Response

Numbness or tingling in a limb with or without movement can indicate nerve or cold damage. Blocking of a main artery can produce severe pain, loss of sensation, or lack of a pulse in a limb. A complete lack of pain or of awareness of serious but obvious injury can be caused by shock, hysteria, drug usage, or spinal cord injury. Generalized or localized pain in an injured region probably means there is no spinal cord injury.

though GXT$_{max}$ exhibits low risk, the discomfort of being pushed to maximum without prior physical conditioning may deter some persons from participating in a subsequent exercise-fitness program. For most healthy people, about the same physiologic information can be obtained from a submaximum test as from a test requiring all-out effort.

The criteria for stopping a test distinguish one GXT protocol from another; otherwise, any of the protocols are effective. In all instances, an abnormal response should result in test termination.

Important factors that influence a person's physiologic response to submaximal or maximal exercise include:

- Ambient temperature and relative humidity
- Subject's sleep state (number of sleep hours prior to testing)
- Emotional state
- Medication
- Time of day
- Caffeine intake
- Time since last meal
- Time since last exercise
- Testing environment (type and appearance of testing room; physical appearance and behavior of test personnel)

Test standardization and attention to details increase the likelihood that the level of exercise stress rather than any extraneous factor influences the person's physiologic responses to a GXT.

Stress Test Protocols

Test duration, initial exercise intensity level, and increments of intensity between stages for GXT protocols dictate which test to administer. In a national survey of 1400 exercise stress test centers, 71% used treadmills, 17% bicycle ergometers, and only 12% step tests. No statistics are available for arm-cranking or swimming stress tests.

Treadmill Tests

Treadmill tests accommodate individuals through a broad spectrum of fitness using the "natural" activities of walking and running. (Figure 7.10 outlined dif-ferent treadmill protocols.) Table 21.12 presents adaptations of the **Naughton** (best for deconditioned persons), **Balke** (best for normal, inactive persons), and **Bruce** (best for active, young persons) treadmill test protocols.

Each protocol has advantages and disadvantages. The Bruce test, for example, uses a more abrupt increase in exercise intensity between stages. Although this may benefit sensitivity to ischemic ECG responses, it also means the person must tolerate the increased exercise level. A stress test should begin at a low level, with two- to three-minute increments in exercise intensity. A warm-up should be used, either separately or incorporated into the test. Total

TABLE 21.12
Adaptations of the Naughton, Balke, and Bruce treadmill protocols for different populations

STAGE	METs	SPEED+ km · h^{-1}	GRADE %	TIME MIN
For very sedentary adults (modified Naughton test[a])				
1	2.5	3.2	0	3
2	3.5	3.2	3.5	3
3	4.5	3.2	7	3
4	5.4	3.2	10.5	3
5	6.4	3.2	14	3
6	7.3	3.2	17.5	3
7	8.5	4.8	12.5	3
8	9.5	4.8	15	3
9	10.5	4.8	17.5	3
For normal sedentary adults (modified Balke test[b])				
1	4.3	4.8	2.5	2
2	5.4	4.8	5	2
3	6.4	4.8	7.5	2
4	7.4	4.8	10	2
5	8.5	4.8	12.5	2
6	9.5	4.8	15	2
7	10.5	4.8	17.5	2
8	11.6	4.8	20	2
9	12.6	4.8	22.5	2
10	13.6	4.8	25	2
For young active adults (modified Bruce test[c])				
1	5	2.7	10	3
2	7	4	12	3
3	9.5	5.4	14	3
4	13	6.7	16	3
5	16	8	18	3

+ 1 km = 0.625 miles.

[a] Naughton, J.P.: Methods of Exercise Testing. In: *Exercise Testing and Exercise Training in Coronary Heart Disease*. New York: Academic Press, 1973.

[b] Balke, B.: *Advanced Exercise Procedures for Evaluation of the Cardiovascular System*. Monograph. Milwaukee: The Burdick Corp., 1970.

[c] Bruce, R.A.: Multi-stage treadmill test of maximal and submaximal exercise. In: *AHA: Exercise Testing and Training of Apparently Healthy Individuals: A Handbook for Physicians*. New York. 1972.

test duration should last at least eight minutes. A test longer than 20 minutes provides no additional ECG or physiologic data than shorter durations. A longer test can establish more precise end-points for setting training guidelines, however.

Bicycle Ergometer Tests

Bicycle ergometers have distinct advantages over other exercise devices. In contrast to treadmills, power output (easily calculated and regulated) on the ergometer is independent of body mass. Most ergometers are portable, safe, and relatively inexpensive. Electrically braked and weight-loaded, friction-type devices represent the two most common ergometers. For electrically braked ergometers, preselected power output remains fixed within a range of pedaling frequencies. Power output with weight-loaded ergometers relates directly to frictional resistance and pedaling rate.

The same general guidelines used for treadmill testing apply to testing on a bicycle ergometer (and arm-crank ergometer). Power output on a bicycle ergometer is usually expressed in kg–$m \cdot min^{-1}$ or watts ($1\ W = 6.12\ kg$–$m \cdot min^{-1}$). Bicycle ergometer tests generally use two- to four-minute stages of graded exercise. Initial resistance ranges between 0 and 30 W; power output generally increases 15 to 30 W per stage. Pedaling at 50 or 60 revolutions per minute represents the typical rpm for weight-loaded ergometers.

Arm-Crank Ergometer Tests

Stress testing can employ arm cranking (Fig. 21.6) as the exercise stressor, particularly when formulating the exercise prescription for upper-body exercise. Arm-crank exercise generally produces up to 30% lower $\dot{V}O_{2max}$ val-

ues, and 10 to 15 $b \cdot min^{-1}$ lower maximum heart rates compared with treadmill or bicycle exercise. Unfortunately, arm-crank exercise interferes with blood pressure measurement during exercise. Blood pressure, heart rate, and oxygen uptake values remain higher during submaximal arm-cranking compared to the same power output in leg exercise. The same graded protocols developed for leg cycling tests can evaluate a patient's response to upper-body exercise. Of course, the starting frictional resistance will be less, with incremental power output levels adjusted accordingly.

Maximal Treadmill, Cycle Ergometer, and Swimming Tests

Studies have compared the physiologic and metabolic responses to different exercise modes in CHD patients and healthy individuals. Figure 21.7 shows $\dot{V}O_{2max}$ and HR_{max} in healthy adults and CHD patients during graded exercise on a treadmill, cycle ergometer, and tethered swimming apparatus. For both groups, treadmill exercise produced the highest $\dot{V}O_{2max}$ scores followed by cycling and swimming exercise. *These differences largely relate to differences in the quantity of muscle mass activated in the activity.* In each exercise mode, healthy adults achieved on average between 67% (treadmill) and 100% (swimming) higher maximum values than CHD patients. Maximal heart rate in healthy adults followed the same trend as $\dot{V}O_{2max}$ (treadmill < bicycle < swim). In contrast, no significant heart rate differences emerged among test modes for CHD patients, although they achieved significantly lower maximum heart rates than healthy adults in each exercise mode (8% lower swimming; 17% lower walking and cycling). Some researchers suggest that equivalent maximal heart rates for CHD patients during swimming and treadmill exercise occur because patients experience less cardiac symptoms during swimming, thus enabling them to reach relatively higher exercise heart rates.

The relative constancy in maximal heart rate of CHD patients across exercise modes (and patients' equivalent submaximal HR–$\dot{V}O_2$ relationships in land and water) indicates that one can establish an exercise training heart rate for these patients from land-based exercise with equivalence for walking, cycling, and swimming. Arm-crank ergometry remains an exception because of its lack of HR–$\dot{V}O_2$ equivalence with other exercise modes, particularly at intensities above 60% of maximum. Arm-crank exercise cannot be used to generate exercise prescriptions for exercise in water. Because of skill requirements in swimming (large variations in exercise economy) and the relatively large energy cost of even slow swimming, swimming may initially be inappropriate for CHD patients with depressed functional capacities. Water aerobics and walking in water provide suitable alternatives.

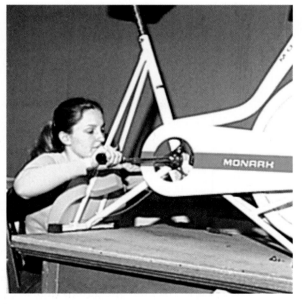

Figure 21.6
Arm-crank ergometer. (Modified from bicycle ergometer).

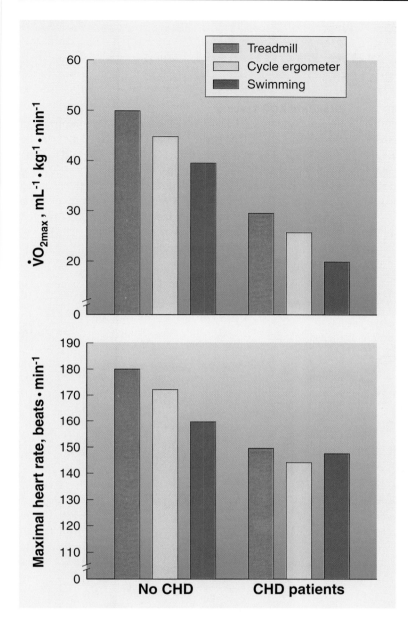

Figure 21.7
Maximal oxygen uptake ($\dot{V}O_{2max}$; **top**) and maximal heart rate (**bottom**) during treadmill, cycle ergometer, and swimming exercise for individuals with and without CHD. (Modified from Porcari, J., et al.: Aquatics programming in cardiac rehabilitation. In *Training Techniques in Cardiac Rehabilitation*. Monograph Number 3. Fardy, P.S. et al., (eds.), Champaign, IL: Human Kinetics, 1998.)

in 3000. In most middle-aged men and women test risk generally increases about 6 to 12 times higher than for young adults. For patients with documented CHD (including previous myocardial infarction or episodes of angina), risk of cardiovascular incident in stress testing increases 30 to 60 times above normal. Based on total risk analyses, many experts believe that a lower "overall risk" exists for those who take a GXT and then initiate a regular exercise program than for those who take no GXT and remain sedentary. Sedentary lifestyle directly relates to higher risk of heart disease and death than the small elevated risk of death that exists during exercise.

Stress Test Outcomes

The clinical value of a stress test depends on how well it detects heart disease, that is, its **sensitivity**. *Sensitivity of a stress test refers to the percentage of people with actual disease who have an abnormal test result.* Four possible outcomes from a graded exercise stress test include:

- **True-Positive**: Test results correctly diagnose heart disease (test successful).

- **False-Negative**: Normal test results, but heart disease present (test unsuccessful; heart disease goes undiagnosed).

- **True-Negative**: Test results normal; no heart disease (test successful).

- **False-Positive**: Test results abnormal; person does not have heart disease (test unsuccessful; healthy person diagnosed with heart disease).

False-negative results occur 25% of the time, with 15% false-positives. False-negatives and false-positives have dramatic ramifications, particularly a false-negative result. Whenever a stress test indicates presence of heart disease, subsequent thallium imaging or angiocardiography (see page 611) confirms the diagnosis. Similarly, a normal stress test does not rule out heart disease. In spite of these limitations, the predictive value of an abnormal stress test exceeds the predictive value of a normal test.

Safety of Stress Testing

The yearly death rate from stress testing ranges between 2% to 12% for men who show clinical evidence of heart disease. Such broad variation in expected mortality directly relates to the number and severity of diseased coronary arteries.

In approximately 170,000 submaximal and maximal stress tests, only 16 high-risk but apparently healthy patients suffered coronary episodes. This represents about one person per 10,000, or approximately 0.01% of the total group In more than 9000 stress tests, no cardiovascular episodes occurred for subjects with increased heart disease risk. In other reports, risk of coronary episodes for healthy, middle-aged adults during a maximum stress test equaled about 1

How to Determine Heart Rate From An Electrocardiographic Tracing

The **electrocardiogram (ECG)** depicts the pattern of electrical activity across the myocardium recorded by an **electrocardiograph**. As the wave of depolarization travels throughout the heart, electrical currents spread through the highly conductive body fluids for monitoring by electrodes placed on the skin's surface. Standard markings on the ECG paper allow time interval and voltage measurements during ECG propagation.

Standard ECG Tracing

Figure 1 shows a standard ECG tracing with time recorded on the horizontal axis. The paper normally moves at 25 mm per second. A repeating grid marks the ECG paper; major grid lines occur 5 mm apart (at 25 mm $\cdot s^{-1}$ paper speed, 5 mm = 0.20 s), minor grid lines occur 1 mm apart (at 25 mm $\cdot s^{-1}$ paper speed, 1 mm equals 0.04 s). The graph's vertical axis indicates electrical voltage. The standard calibration factor equals 0.1 mV (millivolt) per mm of vertical deflection.

Figure 1
Normal ECG tracing.

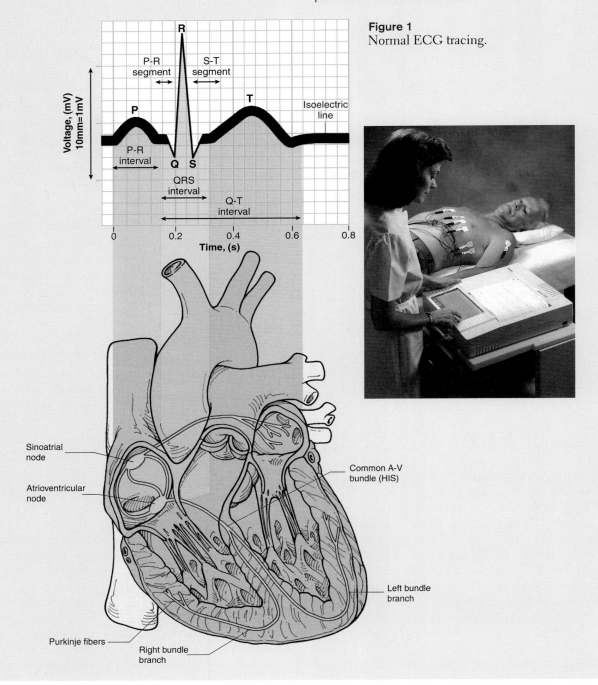

Determining Heart Rate

Three methods determine heart rate from the standard ECG tracing.

Method #1

Figure 2A shows the standard **R-R method**. The R-R interval indicates the time between successive R waves. An approximate heart rate in beats per minute (b·min^{-1}) can be determined by dividing 1500 (60 s ×25 mm·s^{-1}) by the number of mm between adjacent R waves. In the example, heart rate equals 125 b·min^{-1}, since 12 mm occurs between two successive R waves.

Method #2

A second way to determine heart rate from an ECG tracing begins with an R wave that falls on a thick blue line of the tracing (Fig. 2B). Moving to the right, the next six thick lines to represent heart rates of 300, 150, 100, 75, 60, and 50 b·min^{-1} (these numbers need to be memorized). If the next R wave (after the first one falling on the thick line) falls on either the first through sixth subsequent thick lines, the corresponding number (300 to 50) indicates heart rate in b·min^{-1}. Interpolation becomes necessary if the next R wave falls between two thick lines. In this instance the first R wave fall between points 60 and 75 at 70 b·min^{-1}.

Method #3

The third method (Fig. 2C), often used with irregular heart rates, counts the number of complete R-R intervals in a 6-second ECG strip multiplied by 10. In this example, six complete R-to-R intervals occur in six seconds; this equals a heart rate of 60 b·min^{-1} (6×10 = 60).

A

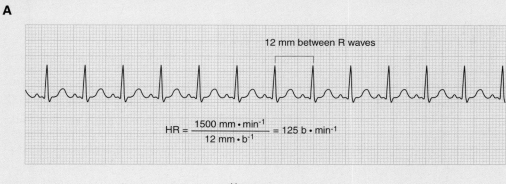

12 mm between R waves

$$HR = \frac{1500 \text{ mm} \cdot \text{min}^{-1}}{12 \text{ mm} \cdot \text{b}^{-1}} = 125 \text{ b} \cdot \text{min}^{-1}$$

B

Start 300 150 100 75 60 50

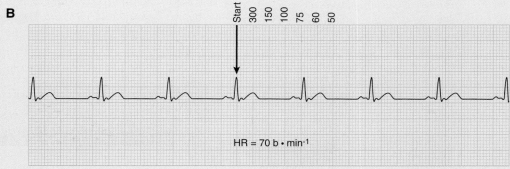

HR = 70 b · min^{-1}

C

3-second mark

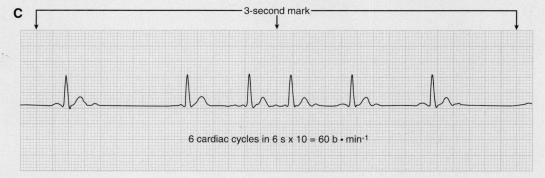

6 cardiac cycles in 6 s x 10 = 60 b · min^{-1}

Figure 2.
Three methods for determining heart rate from ECG tracings.

Exercise-Induced Indicators of CHD

Exercise reveals important clues about CHD because the stress of exercise creates the greatest demand for coronary blood flow.

Angina Pectoris

Approximately 30% of initial manifestations of CHD during exercise comes from chest-related pain (**angina pectoris**). This condition indicates insufficiency of coronary blood flow, where oxygen supply momentarily reaches critically low levels. **Myocardial ischemia** (insufficient oxygen supply caused by coronary atherosclerosis) stimulates sensory nerves in the walls of coronary arteries and myocardium. (Refer to Figure 21.3 for locations of angina pain.) After resting a few minutes, the pain usually subsides without permanent damage to the heart muscle.

ECG Disorders

Alterations in the heart's normal pattern of electrical activity may indicate:

- Extensive coronary artery obstruction.
- Insufficient myocardial oxygen supply.
- Increased death risk from CHD.

These electrical "clues" rarely show up until the heart's metabolic (and blood flow) requirements increase above resting level. The most common ECG abnormalities observed during exercise indicate myocardial ischemia (coronary artery obstruction accounts for most myocardial ischemia). Significant obstruction refers to more than 50% diameter reduction from occlusion. A 50% diameter reduction equals a 75% loss in the arterial lumen. A significantly obstructed coronary artery can still maintain adequate blood flow at rest, but cannot deliver sufficient blood (and oxygen) to meet increased myocardial needs with exercise. Ischemia does not always produce angina pectoris; its diagnosis most readily occurs through depressions of the S-T segment of the ECG. Figure 21.8 shows three types of S-T segment depression: upsloping, horizontal, and downsloping.

Cardiac Rhythm Abnormalities. Exercise can induce abnormalities in the S-T segment of the ECG; exercise also provides a way to observe normal and abnormal cardiac rhythms. Alterations in cardiac rhythm (arrhythmia) with exercise frequently appear as **premature ventricular contractions** (PVCs; Fig. 21.9). In this case, the ventricles demonstrate disorganized electrical activity. The ECG shows this as an "extra" ventricular beat (QRS complex), which occurs without a P wave normally preceding it.

PVCs in exercise generally herald the presence of severe ischemic atherosclerotic heart disease, often involving two or more major coronary vessels. Individuals who experience frequent PVCs have a high risk of sudden death from ventricular fibrillation, an electrical instability when ventricles fail to contract synchronously. This drastically disrupts myocardial function, causing cardiac output to fall dramatically.

Other Indices of CHD

Two useful non-electrocardiographic indicators of possible CHD include blood pressure and heart rate response to exercise.

Hypertensive Response. During a graded exercise test, a normal, progressive transition in systolic blood pressure occurs from about 120 mm Hg at rest to 160 to 190 mm Hg during peak exercise. Diastolic pressure generally changes less than 10 mm Hg. Strenuous exercise can elevate systolic blood pressure close to 250 mm Hg, whereas diastolic pressure can approach 150 mm Hg. Abnormal blood pressure responses to exercise often provide a significant clue to cardiovascular disease.

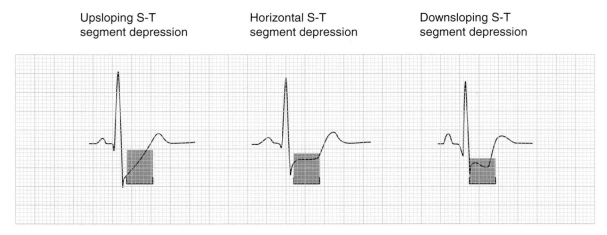

Upsloping S-T segment depression   Horizontal S-T segment depression   Downsloping S-T segment depression

Figure 21.8
Three types of S-T segment depression: upsloping, horizontal, and downsloping.

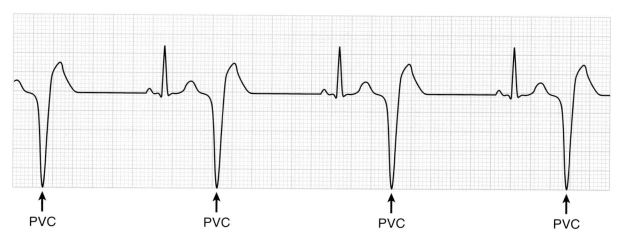

Figure 21.9
ECG tracing illustrating premature ventricular contractions (PVCs).

Hypotensive Response. Failure of blood pressure to increase with exercise can indicate cardiovascular malfunction. For example, diminished cardiac reserve may exist if systolic blood pressure does not increase by at least 20 or 30 mm Hg during graded exercise.

Heart Rate Response. An abnormally rapid heart rate (**tachycardia**) early in submaximal exercise often foretells cardiac problems. Likewise, abnormally low exercise heart rate (**bradycardia**) can reflect sinus node malfunction (**sick sinus node syndrome**). Inability of heart rate to increase during exercise, especially when accompanied by extreme fatigue, also indicates cardiac strain and heart disease.

Invasive Physiologic Tests

Invasive physiological tests provide diagnostic information unavailable through noninvasive procedures. This information includes extent, severity, and location of coronary atherosclerosis, degree of ventricular dysfunction, and specific cardiac abnormalities.

Radionucleotide Studies

Radionucleotide studies require radioactive isotope injection during rest and exercise. Two types of radionucleotide procedures are 1) **thallium imaging**, which evaluates areas of myocardial blood flow and tissue perfusion to differentiate between a true- and a false-positive S-T segment depression obtained by ECG evaluation, and 2) **ventriculography**, an imaging procedure that provides information about left ventricular functional dynamics.

Cardiac Catheterization

In **cardiac catheterization**, a small diameter, flexible tube (catheter) is guided by x-ray directly into an arm or leg vein and/or artery up into the right or left side of the heart. Sen-

sors on the catheter tip accurately measure pressure gradients at various locations within the heart's chambers or large vessels and also assess the heart's electrical patterns (to determine coronary artery blocking). The oxygen content of arterial and mixed-venous blood comes from blood sampled from the ventricles or atria. Cardiac catheterization takes place under local anesthesia, depending on the point of catheter entry (arm or leg). The patient remains awake during the procedure, and test results usually become available on the day of testing.

Coronary Angiography

Coronary angiography provides an intracardiac x-ray after a radiopaque contrast medium enters the coronary blood vessels, and its passage is viewed during a cardiac cycle. This technique accurately assesses the extent of atherosclerosis and serves as the criterion "gold standard" for viewing coronary blood flow. It also creates a baseline for other test comparisons and validations. Angiography does not show how readily blood flows within local portions of the myocardium (does not measure capillary blood flow), and it cannot be used during exercise.

Patient Classification for Cardiac Rehabilitation

Clinical symptoms show in the early stages of CHD, but they do emerge as the disease progresses and coronary arteries narrow. CHD disease often first presents as slight angina pain accompanied by decreases in functional capacity. With disease progression, ischemia produces necrosis of myocardial tissue. In severe cases, the patient experiences persistent chest pain, anxiety, nausea, vomiting, and dyspnea. If untreated, this leads to myocardial weakening and eventual heart failure when cardiac output fails to support metabolic needs. A persistent cough can reflect congestive heart failure (pulmonary congestion), with the patient sometimes coughing up blood. At this stage, the patient becomes short of breath, even when sitting at rest, and can suffer a sudden mild to massive MI.

Table 21.13 shows a system for classifying the functional and therapeutic characteristics of various stages of heart disease. It should be emphasized that substantial individual differences exist in symptoms, functional capacities, and appropriate rehabilitation requirements. Whenever patients undertake rehabilitation, their classification should result from available medical screening information and the most recent GXT.

Phases of Cardiac Rehabilitation

Most cardiac rehabilitation programs consist of three distinct phases, each with different objectives, different patient activities, and levels of supervision (Table 21.14). Patients must complete a GXT without symptoms before progressing to the next phase. These phases include inpatient, outpatient, in-home, and community (Table 21.15.)

TABLE 21.13
Functional and therapeutic classifications of heart disease

Functional Capacity Classification

Class I — No limitation of physical activity. Ordinary physical activity does not cause undue fatigue, palpitation, dyspnea, or anginal pain

Class II — Slight limitation of physical activity. Comfortable at rest, but ordinary physical activity results in fatigue, palpitation, dyspnea, or anginal pain

Class III — Marked limitation of physical activity. Comfortable at rest, but less than ordinary activity causes fatigue, palpitation, dyspnea, or anginal pain

Class IV — Unable to carry on any physical activity without discomfort. Symptoms of cardiac insufficiency or angina may be present even at rest. If any physical activity is undertaken, discomfort increases

Therapeutic Classification

Class A — Physical activity need not be restricted

Class B — Ordinary physical activity need not be restricted, but usually severe or competitive efforts should be avoided

Class C — Ordinary physical activity should be moderately restricted, and more strenuous efforts should be discontinued

Class D — Ordinary physical activity should be markedly restricted

Class E — Patient should be at complete rest and confined to bed or a chair

From New York Heart Association.

A properly prescribed and monitored rehabilitation program allows cardiac patients to safely improve functional capacity comparable to a healthy person of the same age. Clinical symptoms like angina and ECG abnormalities can improve or even disappear. Physiologic adjustments to training actually reduce the heart's work at a given exercise level. For example, reduced exercise heart rate and blood pressure (two major determinants of myocardial oxygen uptake) and improved myocardial contractility reduce myocardial effort. This delays the onset of angina pain allowing exercise of greater intensity and duration. *For individuals whose occupations predominantly require arm work, training should emphasize this musculature because many of the cardiovascular benefits of exercise training appear in activities utilizing the trained musculature.*

Patients enter a cardiac rehabilitation program based partially on their level of CHD risk. Table 21.16 shows an example of a three-level CHD risk classification system. Proper identification of CHD risk makes patient management easier and safer.

Exercise Prescription

Heart rate and oxygen uptake data obtained during the GXT form the basis for an individualized exercise prescription. Many people who start exercising do not recognize their limitations and exercise above a prudent level. Even group exercise programs that require medical clearance may not be appropriate because members often all exercise at about the *same* work level (walk, jog, or swim at a similar pace) without much attention paid to individual differences in physical fitness.

Figure 21.10 illustrates a practical approach for functional translation of treadmill or cycle ergometer exercise test responses to an exercise prescription. Heart rate (A) during the Bruce test is plotted as a function of time. Line B depicts a mathematical line of "best fit" drawn through the data points. A target zone for heart rate is 60 to 75% of maximum heart rate (167 b · min^{-1}; shaded portion represented as C). The individualized prescription includes pace (14.0 to 15.4 min per mile and/or 3.9 to 5.9 METs) (E). The acceptable range of exercise intensity in area C, based on heart rate response during the graded exercise test, includes the following recreational activities: bicycling, touch football, canoeing, alpine skiing, aerobics, volleyball, tennis and badminton, swimming, skating, and water-skiing. This quantitative method of assigning exercise improves exercise prescription specificity and precision for previously sedentary, healthy individuals and patients with diagnosed cardiovascular diseases.

Guidelines

Any exercise prescription should begin with 5 to 15 minutes of light stretching and range-of-motion activities, followed by several minutes of light to moderate preliminary, rhythmic "warm-up" movements. The aerobic conditioning phase

TABLE 21.14
Three phases of a cardiac rehabilitation program

PHASE	DURATION	TREATMENT OBJECTIVES	ROLE OF EXERCISE PHYSIOLOGIST	PATIENT ACTIVITIES	PATIENT EDUCATION	DISCHARGE
Phase I Hospital inpatient; usually follows surgery; usually coordinated with physician, physical therapist, and exercise physiologist	6 to 14 d; 1–7 d in ICU, 7–14 d in ward	1. Prevent the effects of bed rest and deconditioning 2. Reduce orthostatic hypotension 3. Maintain joint mobility	1. Supervise low level exercise 2. Monitor daily living activities 3. Evaluate heart rate and blood pressure responses	1. Range of motion activities 2. Progressive ambulation, stair climbing 3. MET activities not to exceed 1–3 METs, or $HR > 20\ b \cdot min^{-1}$ above resting 4. Includes continuous ambulatory monitoring	1. Lifestyle education 2. Identifying personal risk factors	Before discharge, patient completes low-level, symptom-limited GXT with no complications; purpose of GXT evaluates functional capacity and determines symptom-limited HR for Phase II prescription
Phase II Convalescent (outpatient) stage following hospital discharge; at a supervised cardiac rehab center (YMCA, hospital, or university center)	14-d to 12-wk post-coronary event; usually begins immediately after hospital discharge	1. Move from recuperation to improving functional capacity; promote return to normal daily activities 2. Promote positive lifestyle changes	1. Formulate exercise prescription based on GXT results 2. Monitor HR, BP, RPE, and determine energy expenditure during exercise 3. Ensure progression for discharge to Phase III	1. Individually prescribed progressive exercise using different modes (walking, cycling, arm exercise, circuit resistance training, swimming) 2. Careful monitoring (including frequent GXT) during progressive increases in exercise intensity	1. Risk factor modification programs 2. Comprehensive patient and family education	Before discharge, patient must complete a symptom-limited maximal GXT without complications
Phase III Non-hospital-based community rehab program; patients may have finished a Phase I or II program, or may enter with no prior involvement; patients stable with decreasing or no angina, controlled arrhythmias, ability to self regulate exercise; minimal functional capacity (>6 METs)	4 to 6 months or longer; some patients may be in Phase III for 1 y or more	1. Maintenance of function 2. Compliance with an exercise program 3. Risk factor modification	1. Formulate exercise prescription based on GXT results 2. Monitor HR, BP, RPE, and sometimes energy expenditure during exercise 3. Ensure compliance 4. Help patients with self selection of different activities	1. Individually prescribed progressive exercise using a variety of modes (walking, cycling, arm exercise, circuit resistance training, swimming) 2. Successfully completes maximal GXT	1. Maintenance of risk factor modification	Before discharge, patient completes symptom-limited maximal GXT without complications; patient resumes normal life

should progress in duration so individuals eventually perform 30 to 45 minutes of continuous activity at the prescribed intensity, followed by 5- to 15-minutes of low-intensity walking or other rhythmic activities.

Most cardiac rehabilitation patients can tolerate exercising three days per week with no more than a two-day lapse between exercise sessions. For elderly patients or those with poor functional capacity (< 5 METs), low-intensity exercise should be performed daily or twice daily. As a patient's functional capacity improves, exercise inten-

TABLE 21.15
Types of exercise programs related to patient symptoms

TYPE	PARTICIPANTS	ENTRY MET LEVEL	SUPERVISION
A. Unsupervised	Asymptomatic	8+	None
B. Supervised			
1. Inpatient	All symptomatics—post myocardial infarction, postoperative, pulmonary disease	3	Supervised ambulatory therapy
2. Outpatient	All symptomatics—post myocardial infarction, postoperative pulmonary disease	3+	Exercise specialist, physician on call
3. In Home	Symptomatic + asymptomatic	>3–5	Unsupervised; periodic hospital reevaluation
4. Community	Symptomatic + asymptomatic, 6–8 wk post infarct, 4–8 wk postoperative	>5	Exercise program director + exercise specialist

sity and duration can increase progressively with little fear of complications. The most recent GXT serves as the basis for updating the exercise prescription.

Along with an exercise prescription, three other important components of cardiac rehabilitation include (a) patient education, (b) appropriate drug intervention, and (c) family support counseling. A trained social worker often coordinates these aspects of the rehabilitative process.

Beneficial Effects of Resistance Exercise

Resistance exercise helps restore and maintain muscular strength and preserve fat-free body mass as part of a comprehensive cardiac rehabilitation program. Because blood pressure increases substantially with straining-type exercises, resistance training for the cardiac patient should consist of relatively light resistance (30 to 60% estimated 1-RM) with at least 15 repetitions. Progression should be slow, starting with one set and advancing to three sets, depending on the patient's fitness level. Table 21.17 provides guidelines for circuit resistance training (CRT) for cardiac patients for use with traditional programs (machines, free weights) and less expensive alternatives (sand- and cloth-filled bags). Table 21.18 summarizes the results of 12 CRT studies for male cardiac patients. Information includes training duration, mode and intensity of exercise, changes in muscular strength, aerobic capacity, percent body fat and body mass, and incidence of cardiovascular complications.

For heart transplant patients, a carefully supervised total body (including back) resistance training program (3 days weekly for 6 months) increases functional strength and muscle mass to counter the generally debilitating effects of immunosuppressive medication.

The Rehabilitation Program

The most effective preventive and rehabilitative programs emphasize individualized exercise. Some CHD patients have a reduced heart rate response to exercise with a corresponding decrease in maximum heart rate. Use of-population based target heart rates for these individuals overestimates a prudent training intensity. This argues for exercise testing of each patient to their symptom-limited maximum, and then formulating the exercise prescription based on the patient's *actual* heart rate data.

Patients should engage in endurance-type activities at least three times weekly for 20 to 40 minutes each exercise session at 50 to 75% of exercise capacity, or similar oxygen uptake capacity measured on the GXT. This "target zone" puts individuals at or above a threshold level to achieve a training effect. Ideally, the personalized exercise prescription includes recommendations for weight loss and dietary modification (if necessary), warm-up and cool-down activities, and developmental total body or muscle-specific strength improvement program.

Cardiac Rehabilitation Outcomes

Comprehensive long-term rehabilitation attempts to diminish the following adverse consequences of CHD:

TABLE 21.16
Classification of CHD risk by specific characteristics

CHD RISK LEVEL	CHARACTERISTICS
Low	1. Uncomplicated clinical symptoms 2. No evidence of MI 3. Functional capacity ≥7 METs 4. Normal left ventricular function 5. Absence of significant ventricular ectopy
Moderate	1. ST segment depression ≥2 mm, flat or downsloping 2. Reversible thallium defects 3. Moderate to good left ventricular function 4. Changing pattern, or new development of angina
High	1. Prior MI or infarct involving ≥35% of left ventricle 2. Ejection fraction ≤35% at rest 3. Fall in exercise SBP or failure of SBP to rise more than 10 mm Hg on GXT 4. Persistent or recurrent ischemic pain 24 h or more after hospital admission 5. Functional capacity ≤5 METs with hypotensive BP response, or ≥1 mm ST segment depression 6. Congestive heart failure 7. ≥2 mm ST segment depression at peak HR ≤135 b · min^{-1} 8. High-grade ventricular ectopy

From *Guidelines for Cardiac Rehabilitation Programs. American Association of Cardiovascular and Pulmonary Rehabilitation.* Champaign, IL: Human Kinetics, 1991.

- Physiologic effects of cardiac illness
- Psychologic effects of cardiac illness
- Sudden death or reinfarction
- Progression of the atherosclerotic process

Considerable scientific evidence exists about the positive outcomes in two major areas of cardiac rehabilitation: (a) exercise training, and (b) education, counseling, and behavioral interventions.

Exercise Training

Table 21.19 summarizes scientific evidence from a critical review of 400 reports concerning 16 cardiac rehabilitation outcomes from exercise training. The last column (similar to Table 21.20) rates the strength of the evidence on a three-letter scale ranging from (A) well-designed study, (B) scientific evidence with less consistent results, to (C) opinions of experts, and poorly controlled trials. The strongest outcome evidence supporting the positive effects of exercise relate to exercise tolerance, morbidity, changes in atherosclerosis, outcomes with heart failure patients, and stress reduction and improved psychological well-being.

Education, Counseling, and Behavioral Interventions

Table 21.20 summarizes the scientific basis for cardiac rehabilitation outcomes with education, counseling, and behavioral interventions. Consistent positive effects occur in areas of stress reduction and psychological well being. Behavior modification, stress management, and relaxation techniques lower levels of self-reported emotional distress and positively redirect Type-A behaviors.

Supervision Level

The American College of Sports Medicine categorizes several types of exercise programs with specific criteria for entry and supervision (refer to Table 21.15).

The classification includes unsupervised and supervised programs with four subdivisions of the supervised category. Unsupervised programs include asymptomatic participants of any age with functional capacities of at least eight METs, and no known major risk factors. People with specific needs enroll in a supervised exercise program, and include asymptomatic physically active or inactive persons of any age with CHD risk factors but without known disease (B4), and symptomatic individuals (B1-3), including those with recent CHD and others who report a change in disease status.

Program Administration

Administration of health/fitness/wellness programs requires attention to the following:

- How a program fits within the organizational unit (hospital, community center, private business, university)
- Program development
- Program planning
- Day-to-day operations
- Program evaluation
- Funding

Every program needs a **mission statement** (a clearly defined, concise statement about the reason for the program's existence [sometimes referred to as the major objective of the program], e.g., "To a provide comprehensive health/fitness program for all company employees"). A **strategic plan** outlines a strategy to achieve the mission. The plan has specific goals, objectives, and a strategy of action to create a successful program. The exercise physiolo-

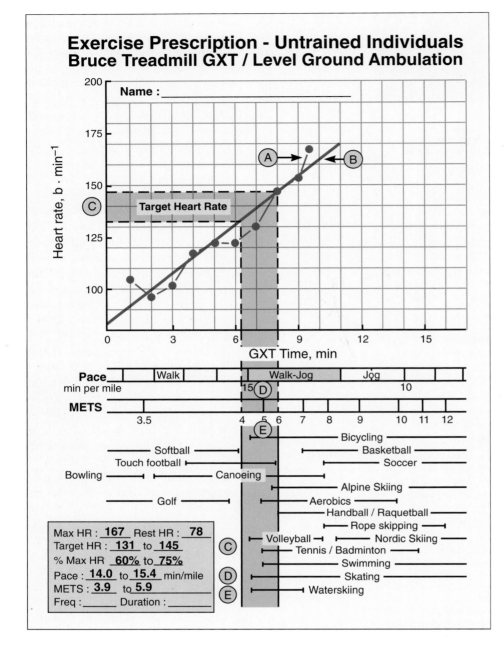

Exercise Prescription - Untrained Individuals
Bruce Treadmill GXT / Level Ground Ambulation

Max HR : **167** Rest HR : **78**
Target HR : **131** to **145**
% Max HR **60%** to **75%**
Pace : **14.0** to **15.4** min/mile
METS : **3.9** to **5.9**
Freq :_____ Duration :_____

Figure 21.10
Exercise prescription based on functional translation algorithm for level ground ambulation. (Courtesy of Dr. C. Foster, Department of Medicine, Cardiovascular Disease Section, Sinai Samaritan Center, Milwaukee, WI).

creases in drug therapy. Patients and program personnel need awareness of drugs patients take and their side effects. Table 21.21 lists six classifications of common cardiac drugs along with trade names, side effects, and possible effects on exercise response.

Pulmonary Diseases

The exercise physiologist's involvement in treating patients with pulmonary disease focuses primarily on improving ventilation, decreasing the work of breathing, and increasing overall level of functional capacity. The exercise physiologist interprets clinical information from the personal history, physical examination, pertinent laboratory data, and imaging studies. Disorders of the cardiovascular system usually impair pulmonary function. Conversely, cardiovascular complications often follow pulmonary disease onset.

Restrictive (reduced lung volume dimensions), and **obstructive** (impeded air flow) lung diseases represent two common classifications for pulmonary dysfunction. Although a convenient classification system, several pulmonary disorders combine both restrictive and obstructive impairments.

Restrictive Lung Dysfunction

Restrictive lung dysfunction (RLD), characterized by an abnormal reduction in pulmonary ventilation, includes diminished lung expansion and decreased tidal volume. The chest and lung tissues in RLD tend to stiffen and offer considerable resistance to expansion under normal pulmonary pressure differentials. This represents a reduction in **lung compliance**, that is, a change in lung volume per unit

gist plays an important role in the program's day-to-day operations, including periodic evaluation of the program's contribution to revenues, allocation of resources, cost, productivity, growth, public image, and strategic fit within the organization.

Cardiac Medications

Knowledge about physiologic effects of drug intervention allows the clinical exercise physiologist to accurately assess a patient's response during physical activity. Improvements in functional capacity often permit de-

TABLE 21.17
Guidelines for circuit resistance training (CRT) for cardiac patients

CRT PARAMETER	CARDIAC RECOMMENDATIONS
Resistance	30–60% of 1-RM or low to moderate loads
Repetitions	8–20
	10 to 15 most often recommended
Exercise duration	20 to 30 minutes
Number of stations	5 to 18
Number of circuits/sets	1 to 3
	Depends on patient's fitness level
Rest interval between stations	At least 30 seconds
	Shorter rest intervals may produce greater improvement in cardiovascular endurance
	Greater HR/BP recovery with longer rest intervals and less risk of cardiovascular complications
Speed of muscle contraction	Lift to a count of 2, lower to a count of 4
	Complete limb flexion/extension
Placement of CRT session	After the program's aerobic phase
	Assures adequate warm-up, less risk of musculoskeletal injury, and prioritizes aerobic phase
Frequency	Alternating 2 to 3 days a week
Progression	Increase resistance when 10 to 15 reps are performed comfortably (RPE 11–13)
	Increase sets depending upon time allotment for session, fitness level, and subject fatigue
Specificity	All major muscle groups

Modified from Verrill, D.E., and Ribisl, P.M.: Resistive exercise training in cardiac rehabilitation—an update. *Sports Med.*, 21:371, 1996.

change in intra-alveolar pressure. Decreased pulmonary compliance increases the energy cost of ventilation, even at rest. Eventually, RLD progresses to a point where significant decreases occur in all lung volumes and capacities.

Table 21.22 lists major RLDs, along with causes, signs and symptoms, and treatments. Other known causes of RLD include rheumatoid arthritis, immunologic impairment, massive obesity, diabetes mellitus, trauma from impact injuries, penetrating wounds, burns and other inhalation injuries, radiation trauma, poisoning, and complications from drug therapy (including negative reactions to antibiotics and anti-inflammatory drugs).

Chronic Obstructive Pulmonary Disease
Chronic obstructive pulmonary disease (COPD) , also termed **chronic airflow limitations** or CAL, includes res-

piratory diseases that produce airflow obstruction. This ultimately affects the lung's mechanical function and compromises alveolar gas exchange. In the United States, COPD ranks as the fifth leading cause of death and the second leading cause of morbidity. The natural history of COPD spans 20 to 50 years, and closely links with chronic cigarette smoking.

Changes in pulmonary function, most notably a decrease in expiratory flow rates and an increase in residual lung volume, usually diagnose COPD. Classic symptoms include spontaneous spasms of bronchial smooth muscle that produce chronic coughing, inflammation and thickening of the mucosal lining of the bronchi and bronchioles, increased mucus production, wheezing, and dyspnea upon physical exertion. Table 21.23 summarizes differences among major COPD conditions.

In all forms of COPD, airways narrow to obstruct airflow. Airway narrowing hinders alveolar ventilation by trapping air in the bronchi and alveoli; in essence, COPD increases physiologic dead space. Obstruction particularly increases resistance to airflow during expiration, impairs normal alveolar gas exchange, diminishes exercise capacity, and reduces ventilatory capacity.

The following brief discussion centers on three major COPD diseases: (a) chronic bronchitis, (b) emphysema, and (c) cystic fibrosis. Chapter 10 discusses obstructive conditions of asthma and exercise-induced bronchospasm.

Chronic Bronchitis
Acute bronchitis refers to self-limiting and short duration inflammation of the trachea and bronchi. In contrast,

Factors Predisposing to COPD
- Chronic cigarette smoking
- Air pollution
- Occupational exposure to irritating dusts or gases
- Heredity
- Infection
- Allergies
- Aging
- Drugs

TABLE 21.18
Summary of circuit resistance training (CRT) studies with male cardiac patients

N	CLINICAL STATUS	DURATION OF TRAINING	MODE/ INTENSITY OF CRT	STRENGTH GAINS	AEROBIC CAPACITY	% FAT/ WEIGHT CHANGE	CARDIOVASCULAR COMPLICATIONS
8	CABG (9–10 wk post surg.)	8 wk	3 circuits, 8–16 reps, 20 s work intervals	22% ↑ upper, 18% ↑ lower-body strength	11% ↑ $\dot{V}O_{2max}$	No changes	None
13	MI, CABG (4 pts. EF < 40%, 5–6 wk post-event)	Averaged 6 weight-lifting sessions	1 circuit, 10–14 reps of a 10-RM estimate; aerobic exercise	25% ave. ↑ upper/lower-body strength	Not measured	Not reported	None
16	PTCA, CABG, MI, CAD, "high risk"	24 wk, 3×/wk	1 circuit at 30–40% of 1-RM; aerobic exercise 70–85% HRmax	22% ave. ↑ upper/lower-body strength	Not measured	No changes	None
10	CAD, MI, CABG, angina	10 wk, 2×/wk	2 circuits at 40–80% of 1-RM; aerobic exercise 60–85% HRmax	42% ↑ upper, 23% ↑ lower-body strength	15% ↑ max cycle power output; 109% ↑ max cycle time	Not reported	None
9	MI, angina, CABG	10 wk, 3×/wk	1 circuit at 80% 1-RM; sit-ups; aerobic exercise at 45–64% HRmax	29% ave. ↑ upper/lower-body strength	Not measured	No changes	None
20	MI, CAD, CABG, angina	10 wk, 3×/wk	2 circuits of 40% 1-RM; aerobic exercise at 85% HRmax	24% ave. ↑ upper/lower-body strength	12% ↑ Bruce treadmill time	No weight change; small decrease in body fat	1 pt. hypotensive; 4 pts. PVCs with bigeminy
16	8–12 wk post-MI (EF = 40–45%)	12 wk, 3×/wk	Hydraulic CRT, 40 min/d, 3 d/wk, 20-s. work: rest intervals	29% ↑ upper, 23% ↑ lower-body strength	19% ↑ $\dot{V}O_{2max}$; 23% ↑ peak cycle erogometer workload	Not reported	None
8	≥2 wk post-MI (no anterior Q wave)	10 wk, 3×/wk	2 circuits at 40% of 1-RM; aerobic exercise	22% ↑ upper, 29% ↑ lower-body strength	15% ↑ $\dot{V}O_{2max}$	No changes	None
14	MI, CABG, PTCA, angina, valvular	12 wk, 3×/wk	3 circuits at 40–70% 1-RM; aerobic exercise at 70–85% HRmax	30% ↑ upper, 35% ↑ lower-body strength	14% ↑ $\dot{V}O_{2max}$	Not reported	None
17	MI, CAD, CABG	3 y, 3×/wk	2 circuits at 40% of 1-RM; aerobic exercise at 85% HRmax	13% ↑ upper, 40% ↑ lower-body strength	Not measured	No changes	None
9	CRP participants	10 wk	CRT (intensity not specified); aerobic exercise	19% ↑ max isometric voluntary contraction	No change in $\dot{V}O_{2max}$; 19% ↑ cycle time to exhaustion	Not reported	None
57	6–16 wk post-MI	10 wk	2 circuits at 20–60% 1-RM; aerobic exercise 70–85% HRmax	10.5–13.5% ↑ upper-body strength	4.4–13.4% ↑ $\dot{V}O_{2max}$	Not reported	None

CABG = Coronary artery bypass grafting; MI = Myocardial infarction; EF = Ejection fraction; CAD = Coronary artery disease; PTCA = Percutaneous transluminal coronary angioplasty; 1-RM = One repetition maximum; $\dot{V}O_{2max}$ = Maximal oxygen uptake; HR = Heart rate; PVC = Premature ventricular contraction; pt(s) = patient(s); incr. = increase; ave. = average; and CRP = Cardiopulmonary rehabilitation program.

Modified from Verrill, D.E., and Ribisl, P.M.: Resistive exercise training in cardiac rehabilitation—an update. *Sports Med.*, 21:371, 1996.

TABLE 21.19
Summary of evidence for positive cardiac rehabilitation outcomes: Effects of exercise training

POSITIVE OUTCOME	TOTAL NUMBER OF STUDIES	EVIDENCE BASE[a]			STRENGTH OF EVIDENCE[b]
		RANDOMIZED STUDIES	NONRANDOMIZED STUDIES	OBSERVATIONAL STUDIES	
Exercise tolerance	114	46	25	43	A
Exercise tolerance (strength training)	7	4	3	0	B
Exercise habits	15	10	2	3	B
Symptoms	26	12	7	7	B
Smoking	24	12	8	4	B
Lipids	37	18	6	13	B
Body weight	34	11	7	16	C
Blood pressure	18	9	6	3	B
Psychological well-being	20	9	8	3	B
Social adjustment and functioning	6	2	2	2	B
Return to work	28	10	9	9	A
Morbidity	42 (+2 survey reports)	15	14	13	A
Mortality	31 (+2 survey reports)	17	8	6	B
Pathophysiologic measures:					
Changes in atherosclerosis	9	5	1	3	A/B
Changes in hemodynamic measurements	5	0	0	5	B
Changes in myocardial perfusion/myocardial ischemia	11	6	2	3	B
Changes in myocardial contractility, ventricular wall motion abnormalities, and/or ventricular ejection fraction	22	9	5	8	B
Changes in cardiac arrhythmias	5	4	0	1	B
Heart failure patients	12	5	3	4	A
Cardiac transplantation patients	5	0	1	4	B
Elderly patients	7	0	1	6	B

[a] Number of studies from scientific literature by type of study design

[b] Rating for strength of evidence:

A Scientific evidence from well-designed and well-conducted controlled trials (randomized and nonrandomized) provides statistically significant results that consistently support the guideline statement.

B Scientific evidence is provided by observational studies or by controlled trials with less consistent results

C Guideline statement support by expert opinion: the available scientific evidence did not present consistent results or controlled trials were lacking.

From Wenger, N.K., et al.: *Cardiac Rehabilitation as Secondary Prevention*. Clinical Practice Guideline. Quick Reference Guide for Clinicians, No. 17. Rockville, MD: U.S. Department of Health and Human Services, Public Health Service, Agency for Health Care Policy and Research and National Heart, Lung, and Blood Institute. AHCPR Pub. No. 96-0673. October 1995.

How to Recognize Major Signs and Symptoms of Cardiopulmonary Disease

Diseases of the cardiopulmonary system are the leading cause of death. Heart diseases include afflictions affecting the heart muscle (angina, myocardial infarct, pericarditis, congestive heart failure, and aneurysms), heart valves (rheumatic fever, endocarditis, mitral valve prolapse, congenital deformations), and the cardiac nervous system (arrhythmias). Pulmonary disease includes restrictive lung dysfunction (diseases affecting compliance, volumes, capacities, and the work of breathing), and chronic obstructive pulmonary disorders (bronchitis, emphysema, asthma, cystic fibrosis).

Individuals with undiagnosed cardiopulmonary diseases exhibit specific signs and symptoms during rest and exercise (see table). Signs and symptoms of cardiopulmonary disease in the clinical context help identify individuals in need of further evaluation.

MAJOR SIGNS AND SYMPTOMS OF CARDIOPULMONARY DISEASE

- Pain, discomfort (or other angina equivalent) in the chest, neck, or arms
- Shortness of breath at rest or with mild exertion
- Dizziness or syncope (feeling of light-headedness or faintness)
- Dyspnea (shortness of breath or labored breathing) on rising from supine position or at night during sleep
- Palpitations or tachycardia (unexplained increased heart rate) during rest or mild exercise
- Ankle edema (swelling)
- Intermittent claudication (ischemic pain described as an aching, weakness, tightness or cramping sensation during physical activity) in the calf of the leg
- Known heart murmur
- Unusual fatigue accompanied by moderate to extreme dyspnea during usual activity

TABLE 21.20
Summary of evidence for positive cardiac rehabilitation outcomes: Effects of education, counseling, and behavioral interventions

POSITIVE OUTCOME	TOTAL NUMBER OF STUDIES	EVIDENCE BASE[a]			STRENGTH OF EVIDENCE[b]
		RANDOMIZED STUDIES	NONRANDOMIZED STUDIES	OBSERVATIONAL STUDIES	
Smoking	7	5	1	1	B
Lipids	18	12	3	3	B
Weight	5	3	1	1	B
Blood pressure	2	0	2	0	B
Exercise tolerance	3	1	1	1	C
Symptoms	4	2	1	1	B
Return to work	3	2	0	1	C
Stress/psychological well-being	14	7	5	2	A
Morbidity	3	3	0	0	B
Mortality	8	8	0	0	B

[a] Number of studies from scientific literature by type of study design.

[b] Rating for strength of evidence:

A Scientific evidence from well-designed and well-conducted controlled trials (randomized and nonrandomized) provides statistically significant results that consistently support the guideline statement.
B Scientific evidence is provided by observational studies or by controlled trials with less consistent results
C Guideline statement support by expert opinion: the available scientific evidence did not present consistent results or controlled trials were lacking.

From Wenger, N.K., et al.: *Cardiac Rehabilitation as Secondary Prevention.* Clinical Practice Guideline. Quick Reference Guide for Clinicians, No. 17. Rockville, MD: U.S. Department of Health and Human Services, Public Health Service, Agency for Health Care Policy and Research and National Heart, Lung, and Blood Institute. AHCPR Pub. No. 96-0673. October 1995.

TABLE 21.21
Six classifications of common cardiac drugs, along with trade names, side effects, and possible effects on exercise response

TYPE/TRADE NAME	USE	SIDE EFFECTS	EFFECTS ON EXERCISE RESPONSE
I. Anti-anginal Agents			
A. Nitroglycerin compounds [*Amyl nitrate; Isordil; Nitrostat*]	Smooth muscle relaxation; decrease cardiac output	Headache, dizziness, hypotension	Hypotension; increase exercise capacity
B. Beta blockers [*Inderal;Propranolol; Lopressor; Corgard; Biocadren*]	Block beta receptors; decrease sympathetic tone; decrease HR, contractility, and BP	Bradycardia, heart block, insomnia, nausea, fatigue, weakness, increased cholesterol and blood sugar	Decrease HR; hypotension; decrease cardiac contractility
C. Calcium Antagonists [*Verapamil; Nifedipine; Procardia*]	Block influx of calcium; dilate coronary arteries; suppress dysrhythmias	Dizziness, syncope, flushing, hypotension headache, fluid retention	Hypotension
II. Antihypertensive Agents			
A. Diuretics [*Thiazides, Lasix, Aldactone*]	Inhibit NA$^+$ and Cl$^-$ reabsorption in kidneys; increase excretion of sodium and water, and control high BP and fluid retention	Drowsiness, dehydration, electrolyte imbalance; gout, nausea, pain, hearing loss, elevated cholesterol, and lipoproteins	Hypotension
B. Vasodilators [*Hydralazine, Captopril, Apresoline, Loniten, Minoxidil*]	Dilate peripheral blood vessels; used in conjunction with diuretics; decrease BP	Increase HR and contractility; headache, drowsiness, nausea, vomiting, diarrhea	
C. Drugs interfering with sympathetic nervous system [*Reserprine, Propranolol, Aldomet, Catapres, Minipress*]	Decrease BP, HR, and cardiac output by dilating blood vessels	Drowsiness, depression, sexual dysfunction, fatigue, dry mouth, stuffy nose, fever, upset stomach, fluid retention, weight gain	Hypotension
III. Digitalis Glycosides Derviatives [*Digoxin, Lonoxin, Digitoxin*]	Strengthen heart's pumping force and decrease electrical conduction	Arrhythmias, heart block, altered ECG, fatigue, weakness, headache, nausea, vomiting	Increase exercise capacity; increase myocardial contractility
IV. Anticoagulant Agents [*Coumadin, Sodium Heparin, Aspirin, Persantine*]	Prevent blood clot formation	Easy bruising, stomach irritation, joint or abdominal pain, difficulty in swallowing, unexplained swelling, uncontrolled bleeding	
V. Antilipidemic Agents [*Cholestyramine, Lopid, Niacin, Atromid-S, Mevacor, Questran Zocor*]	Interfere with lipid metabolism and lower cholesterol and low-density lipoproteins	Nausea, vomiting, diarrhea, constipation, flatulence, abdominal discomfort, glucose intolerance	
VI. Antiarrhythmic Agents [*Cardioquin, Procaine, Quinidine Lidocaine, Dilantin, Propranolol, Bretylium tosylate, Verapamil*]	Alter conduction patterns throughout myocardium	Nausea, palpitations, vomiting, rash, insomnia, dizziness, shortness of breath, swollen ankles, coughing up blood, fever, psychosis, impotence	Hypotension; decrease HR and cardiac contractility

TABLE 21.22
Major restrictive lung diseases, their causes, signs and symptoms, and treatment

CAUSES/TYPE	ETIOLOGY	SIGNS AND SYMPTOMS	TREATMENT
I. Maturational			
a. *Abnormal fetal lung development*	Premature birth; (hypoplasia-reduced lung tissue)	Asymptomatic; pulmonary insufficiency	No specific treatment
b. *Respiratory distress syndrome* (hyaline membrane disease)	Insufficient maturation of lungs due to premature birth	↑ respiration rate; ↓ lung volumes; ↓ PaO_2; acidemia; rapid and labored respiration pressure	Treat mother prior to birth (corticosteroids); Hyperalimentation; continuous positive airway
c. *Aging*	Aging and cumulative effects of pollution, noxious gas, inhaled drug use, and cigarette smoking	↑ residual volume; ↓ vital capacity; repetitive periodic apnea	No specific treatment; increase physical activity
II. Pulmonary			
a. *Idiopathic pulmonary fibrosis* (IPF)	Unknown origin (perhaps viral or genetic)	↓ lung volumes; pulmonary hypertension; dyspnea; cough; weight loss, fatigue	Corticosteroids; maintain adequate nutrition and ventilation
b. *Coal workers' pneumoconiosis*	Repeated inhalation of coal dust over 10–12 y	↓ TLC, VC, FRC; ↓ lung compliance; dyspnea; ↓ PaO_2; pulmonary hypertension; cough	Nonreversible, no known cure
c. *Asbestosis*	Chronic exposure to asbestos	↓ lung volumes; abnormal x-ray; ↓ PaO_2; dyspnea on exertion, shortness of breath	Nonreversible, no known cure
d. *Pneumonia*	Inflammatory process caused by various bacteria, microbes, viruses	↓ lung volumes; abnormal x-ray; tachypneic dyspnea; high fever, chills, cough; pleuritic pain	Drug therapy (antibiotic)
e. *Adult respiratory distress syndrome*	Acute lung injury (fat emboli, drowning, drug induced, shock, blood transfusion, pneumonia)	Abnormal lung function tests; PaO_2 < 60 mm Hg; extreme dyspnea; cyanotic; headache; anxiety	Intubation and mechanical ventilation
f. *Bronchogenic carcinoma*	Tobacco use	Variable depending on type and location of growth	Surgery, radiation, chemotherapy
g. *Pleural effusions*	Accumulation of fluid within pleural space; heart failure; cirrhosis	Shortness of breath; pleuritic chest pain; ↓ PaO_2	Specific drainage
III. Cardiovasvular			
a. *Pulmonary edema*	↑ pulmonary capillary hydrostatic pressure secondary to left ventricular failure	↑ respiration rate; ↓ lung volumes; ↓ PaO_2; arrhythmias; feeling of suffocation, shortness of breath, cyanotic, cough	Drug therapy, diuretics; supplemental O_2
b. *Pulmonary emboli*	Complications of venous thrombosis	↓ lung volumes; ↓ PaO_2; tachycardia; acute dyspnea, shortness of breath; syncope	Heparin therapy; mechanical ventilation

TABLE 21.23
Differences among major COPD diseases

NAME	AREA AFFECTED	RESULT
Bronchitis	Membrane lining bronchial tubes	Inflammation of bronchial lining
Bronchiectasis	Bronchial tubes (bronchi or air passages)	Bronchial dilation with inflammation
Emphysema	Air spaces beyond terminal bronchioles (aleveoli)	Breakdown of alveolar walls; air spaces enlarged
Asthma	Bronchioles (small airways)	Bronchioles obstructed by muscle spasm; swelling of mucosa; thick secretions
Cystic fibrosis	Bronchioles	Bronchioles become obstructed and obliterated; plugs of mucus cling to airway walls leading to bronchitis, atelectasis, pneumonia, or pulmonary abscess

chronic bronchitis mostly occurs with chronic exposure to nonspecific irritants. Increases in mucus secretion accompany prolonged respiratory tract inflammation. Over time, the swollen mucous membranes and thick sputum obstruct airways, causing wheezing and persistent coughing. Partial or complete airway blockage from mucus secretion causes insufficient arterial saturation and edema, which produces the characteristic look known as the "Blue Bloater" (Fig. 21.11). Chronic bronchitis develops slowly and worsens over time. Patients usually have been long-term smokers. Functional exercise capacity remains low,

and fatigue occurs readily with only moderate effort. If left untreated, the disease can lead to death.

Emphysema

Abnormal, permanent enlargement of air spaces distal to the terminal bronchi characterizes **emphysema**. This disease often develops from chronic bronchitis and occurs frequently in long-term cigarette smokers. Symptoms include extreme dyspnea, hypercapnia, persistent cough, cyanosis, and digital clubbing (evidence of chronic hypoxemia; Fig. 21.12). Patients frequently appear thin; they lean forward with arms braced on the knees to support their shoulders and chest for easier breathing. The effects of trapped air and alveolar distention change the size and shape of the chest, causing the characteristic emphysemic "barrel chest" appearance (Fig. 21.13).

Although exercise cannot "cure" emphysema, it does enhance cardiovascular fitness and strengthens respiratory musculature. Regular exercise can also improve a patient's psychological state.

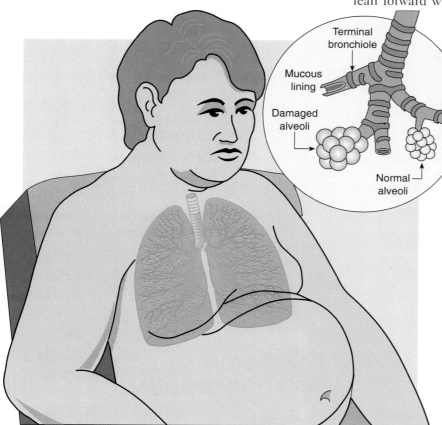

Figure 21.11
Individuals with chronic bronchitis usually develop cyanosis and pulmonary edema with the characteristic appearance known as "Blue Bloater." The effects of chronic bronchitis displayed in the insert illustrate misshapen or large alveolar sacs with reduced surface for oxygen and carbon dioxide exchange.

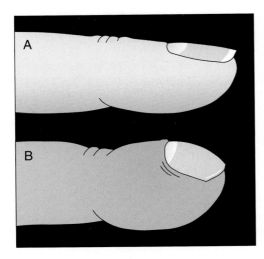

Figure 21.12
Normal digit configuration (**A**) and example of digital clubbing (**B**), indicating chronic tissue hypoxia, a common physical sign of emphysema.

Cystic Fibrosis

The term **cystic fibrosis (CF)** originated from observing cysts and scar tissue on the pancreas of autopsied patients. Although pancreatic cysts and scar tissue often exist, they are not primary characteristics of the disease (although the

TABLE 21.24
Clinical signs and symptoms of cystic fibrosis and related pulmonary involvement

Early Stages

- Persistent cough and wheezing
- Recurrent pneumonia
- Excessive appetite but poor weight gain
- Salty skin or sweat
- Bulky, foul-smelling stools (undigested lipids)

Latter Stages
(with significant pulmonary Involvement)

- Tachypnea (rapid breathing)
- Sustained chronic cough with mucus production on vomiting
- Barrel chest
- Cyanosis and digital clubbing
- Exertional dyspnea with decreased exercise capacity
- Pneumothorax
- Right heart failure secondary to pulmonary hypertension

term cystic fibrosis remains in use). Table 21.24 lists clinical signs and symptoms of CF. The disease, characterized by thickened secretions of all exocrine glands (e.g., pancreatic, pulmonic, and gastrointestinal), eventually obstructs pulmonary air flow. The most common inherited genetic disease in Caucasians, CF afflicts approximately one in 2000 white newborn infants in the United States. The disease, inherited as a recessive trait (both parents are carriers), has no current cure and remains fatal.

Pulmonary system involvement represents the most common and severe manifestation of CF. Airway obstruction leads to a chronic state of hyperinflation. Over time, RLD superimposes on the obstructive disorder, leading to chronic hypoxia, hypercapnia, and acidosis. Pneumothorax and pulmonary hypertension eventually follow and cause death.

Treatment of CF includes antibiotics, enzyme supplements, nutritional intervention, and frequent secretion removal. Many patients also benefit from regular physical activity. Twenty minutes of aerobic exercise can replace one session of secretion removal in some children. Increased minute ventilation with aerobic exercise helps clear excessive secretions from the airways. Improved fitness may play a role in delaying the crippling effects of CF.

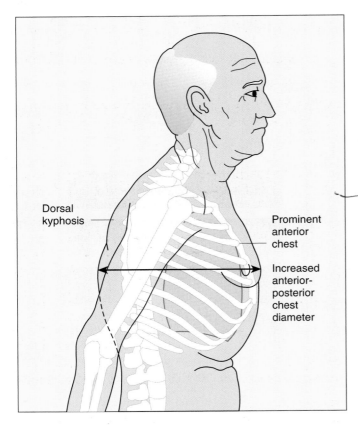

Dorsal kyphosis

Prominent anterior chest

Increased anterior-posterior chest diameter

Figure 21.13
Emphysema traps air in the lungs, making exhalation difficult. With time, changes in the patient's physical features include a "barrel chest" appearance.

Pulmonary Assessments

Chest and lung imaging provide the most common pulmonary assessment techniques. These include conventional x-ray and computed tomography (CT) scanning to (a) screen for abnormalities, (b) provide a baseline for subsequent assessments, and (c) monitor disease progression. Magnetic resonance imaging (MRI) plays a limited role because the density of large portions of the lungs cannot generate clear magnetic signals. Static and dynamic tests of lung function, pulmonary diffusing capacity, and flow-volume loops also provide diagnostic information.

Pulmonary Rehabilitation and Exercise Prescription

Despite the prevalence of COPD and RLD, pulmonary rehabilitation receives considerably less attention than programs for cardiovascular and musculoskeletal diseases. Perhaps de-emphasis has resulted from rehabilitation's failure to markedly improve pulmonary function or reverse the natural progression of these debilitating and often deadly diseases. Nevertheless, pulmonary rehabilitation can have marked, positive effects on exercise capacity, improved respiratory muscle function, improved psychological status, enhanced quality of life variables (e.g., self-esteem and self-efficacy), reduced frequency of hospitalization, and attenuated disease progression. Major goals for pulmonary rehabilitation include:

- Improve health status
- Improve respiratory symptoms (shortness of breath and cough)
- Recognize early signs requiring medical intervention
- Decrease frequency and severity of respiratory problems
- Obtain maximal arterial oxygen saturation
- Improve daily functional capacity through enhanced muscular strength, joint flexibility, and cardiorespiratory endurance
- Improve strength and power of the ventilatory musculature
- Improve body composition to enhance functional capacity
- Improve nutritional status

Pulmonary rehabilitation programs include the following five components:

1. General care
2. Pulmonary respiratory care
3. Exercise and functional training
4. Education
5. Psychosocial management

The exercise and functional training aspects of rehabilitation are particularly important to individuals with end-stage disease because the effects of weakness, fatigue, and severe dyspnea profoundly limit physical activity. Physiological monitoring during exercise rehabilitation should measure heart rate, blood pressure, respiratory rate, arterial oxygen saturation by pulse oximetry (indicates arterial oxygen desaturation), and dyspnea.

Dyspnea monitoring involves a perceived dyspnea scale (Fig. 21.14), similar to the Borg scale for rating of perceived exertion. Extreme shortness of breath, fatigue, palpitations, chest discomfort, or a decrease of 3 to 5% on pulse oximetry indicate the need to terminate the exercise test.

The pretraining GXT and spirometric analyses govern the exercise prescription. Exercise stress test interpretation includes determining: (a) whether the test terminated for cardiovascular or ventilatory endpoints, (b) the difference between pre- and postexercise pulmonary function (e.g., a decrease of 10% in $FEV_{1.0}$ indicates the need for bronchodilator therapy before exercise), and (c) the need for supplemental oxygen due to arterial oxygen desaturation (e.g., a decrease in Pa_{O_2} of more than 20 mm Hg or a Pa_{O_2} of less than 55 mm Hg) during exercise.

The exercise prescription for a patient with mild lung disease (shortness of breath with heavy exercise) mirrors that for a healthy individual. For patients with moderate lung disease (shortness of breath with normal daily activities or clinical symptoms of RLD or COPD), exercise can proceed: (a) at an intensity no greater than 75% of ventilatory reserve, (b) in the middle of the calculated training heart rate range (50 to 70% of age-predicted HR_{max}), or (c) at the point where the patient becomes noticeably dyspneic. For most individuals, dyspnea occurs between 40 to

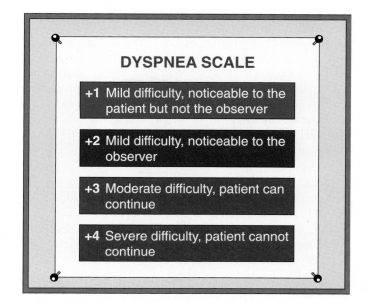

Figure 21.14
Dyspnea scale. Grading of subjective ratings of dyspnea intensity during exercise testing occurs on a scale of 1 to 4. Dyspnea usually accompanies poor exercise capacity and impaired ability to increase systolic blood pressure during graded exercise testing.

TABLE 21.25
Major pulmonary medications: Uses and side effects

DRUG/NAME	ACTION AND CLINICAL USES	SIDE EFFECTS
Sympathomimetics Isoproterenol, Ephedrine, Bronkosol, Alupent, Brethine, Proventil, Ventolin	Decrease intracellular calcium; smooth muscle relaxation; bronchodilation	Tachycardia, palpitations, GI distress, nervousness, headache, dizziness
Methylxanthines Amnodur, Elixophyllin, Theodur, Choladril	Increase cAMP; block the decrease of cAMP	Agitation, hypotension, chest pain, nausea, tachycardia, palpitations, GI distress, nervousness, headache, dizziness
Alpha Sympatholytics	Block the decrease of cAMP; bronchodilation	Agitation, hypotension, chest pain, nausea, tachycardia, palpitations, GI distress, nervousness, headache, dizziness
Parasympatholytics Atrovent, Atropine sulfate	Block parasympathetic stimulation and prevents increases in cGMP; prevents bronchoconstriction	Central nervous system stimulation with low doses and depression with high doses; delirium, hallucinations, decreased GI activity
Glucocorticoids Prednisone, Cortisol, Azmacort, Vanceril	Decrease inflammatory response; bronchodilation	Obesity, growth suppresion, hyperglycemia and diabetes, mood changes, irritability or depression, thinning of skin, muscle wasting
Cromolyn sodium Intal, Fivent	Prevents influx of calcium ions, thus blocking mast cell release of mediators responsible for bronchoconstriction; bronchodilation	Throat irritation, hoarseness, dry mouth, cough, chest tightness, bronchospasm

85% of maximum MET level on a GXT. Under these circumstances, exercise duration usually lasts 20 minutes, three times a week. If 5- to 15-minute exercise durations are more desirable, exercise frequency should increase to five to seven days weekly.

Patients with severe lung disease (shortness of breath during most daily activities, and FVC and $FEV_{1.0}$ below 55% of predicted values) require a modified approach to exercise testing and prescription. Usually low-level, discontinuous testing can begin at two to three METs with increments every several minutes. Symptom-limited walking speeds and distances provide helpful guidelines for formulating an exercise prescription. Brief bouts of interval exercise often benefit this population. Patients should exercise a minimum of once daily because of the low initial training prescription. Even small gains in exercise tolerance for these patients improves functional capacity and quality of life indices.

For all pulmonary disease patients, regular exercise contributes to improved respiratory muscle function. Two approaches can achieve this goal:

1. Provide resistance training for improved strength and power of ventilatory muscles by use of a **continuous positive airway pressure (CPAP) device.** This overloads ventilatory muscles in a manner similar to progressive resistance exercise for other skeletal muscles.

2. Increase endurance performance capacity of respiratory muscles through regular and progressive aerobic exercise training.

Pulmonary Medications

Pulmonary medications include bronchodilators, anti-inflammatory agents, decongestants, antihistamines, mucokinetic agents, respiratory stimulants, depressants, and paralyzing and antimicrobial agents. These groups of drugs promote bronchodilation, facilitate removal of lung secretions, improve alveolar ventilation and arterial oxygenation, and optimize breathing patterns. Table 21.25 lists common drugs to treat pulmonary disease.

summary

1. "Disability" represents diminished functional capacity, whereas "handicap" refers to a physical performance frame of reference defined by society. People are considered handicapped when they can no longer perform expected tasks. However, loss of functional ability does not necessarily mean disabled or handicapped.

2. In clinical settings, an exercise physiologist health/fitness profes-

sional becomes part of a team approach to comprehensive patient health care.

3. Exercise physiologists and the other health/fitness professionals work side-by-side with diverse populations including the sedentary person who needs only a modest amount of physical exercise to reduce risk of degenerative diseases, patients recovering from surgery or requiring regular exercise to combat a decline in functional capacity brought on by serious illness, and able-bodied and disabled athletes who strive to optimize sports performance.

4. Different organizations offer training/certification programs with distinct emphases and specializations.

5. Of more than 100 different types of cancers, the most prevalent include cancers of the breast, lung, bowel, and uterus.

6. The exercise prescription for cancer patients must be symptom-limited, progressive, and individualized. For most patients, the goal of exercise prescription aims to improve level of ambulation.

7. For women recovering from breast cancer surgery, a carefully planned, aerobic circuit resistance exercise program significantly decreases depression and state and trait anxieties.

8. The major cardiovascular diseases affect either the heart muscle directly, the heart valves, or the neural regulation of cardiac function. Each disease category has its specific pathogenesis and intervention strategies.

9. Aerobic exercise programs implemented for cardiac patients should consider specific disease pathophysiology, mechanisms that can limit exercise capacity, and individual differences in functional ability.

10. Reduced myocardial blood supply causes angina pectoris, congestive heart failure, and myocardial infarction.

11. Heart valve diseases include stenosis, insufficiency, and prolapse.

12. A thorough cardiac disease assessments includes medical history, physical examination, laboratory assessments, and physiological tests.

13. Laboratory tests for cardiovascular disease include chest x-ray, electrocardiogram (ECG), blood lipid and lipoprotein analyses, and serum enzyme testing.

14. The term "stress test" describes systematic exercise for two purposes: (1) ECG observations, and (2) evaluation of physiologic adjustments to metabolic demands that exceed resting requirements.

15. Multistage bicycle and treadmill tests represent the most common modes for exercise stress testing. These tests, graded for exercise intensity, include several levels of three to five minutes of exercise that bring the person to self-imposed, symptom-limited fatigue.

16. Reasons for including a stress test (and ECG observations) in an overall CHD evaluation include: (1) diagnose overt heart disease, (2) screen for possible "silent" coronary disease in seemingly healthy individuals, (3) reproduce and assess exercise-related chest symptoms, (4) screen candidates for preventive and cardiac rehabilitative exercise programs, (5) detect an abnormal blood pressure response, (6) monitor responses to various therapeutic interventions for improving cardiovascular function, and (7) evaluate functional aerobic capacity in relation to normative standards.

17. Graded exercise testing provides a relatively safe means to obtain valuable information for clearing individuals to begin exercising, and to personalize the exercise prescription.

18. No one stress test can diagnose heart disease perfectly. Four possible outcomes from a stress test are: true-positive (test a success); false-negative (heart disease not diagnosed when present); true-negative (test a success); and false-positive (healthy person diagnosed with heart disease).

19. Exercise-induced indicators of CHD include angina pectoris, ECG disorders, cardiac rhythm abnormalities, and abnormal blood pressure and heart rate responses.

20. Cardiac patients can improve functional capacity similar to healthy people of the same age.

21. Based on diagnosis, patients enter different cardiac rehabilitation phases depending on disease severity and degree of risk.

22. Restrictive lung disease (RLD) and chronic obstructive lung disease (COPD) represent two major pulmonary diseases categories. RLD relates to a variety of dysfunctions that culminate in significantly increased resistance to lung inflation. COPD includes bronchitis, emphysema, asthma, exercise-induced bronchospasm, and cystic fibrosis.

23. Assessment of pulmonary disease requires different diagnostic tools, including chest x-ray, CT scanning, MRI, and standard spirometric lung volume testing.

24. Exercise contributes to pulmonary disease management if close attention focuses on exercise intensity, patient monitoring, and exercise progression.

25. Diverse cardiac and pulmonary medications play an important role in disease management. The clinical exercise physiologist should understand the actions of these drugs and their effects on the exercise response.

thought questions

1. Give possible reasons why exercise proves more effective for coronary heart disease patients than for patients with chronic pulmonary disease.

2. A GXT on a bicycle ergometer has established 600 kg·m · min^{-1} as the desirable exercise intensity for training a CHD patient. Discuss whether this exercise intensity would also be appropriate arm-crank exercise for this patient.

3. What recommendations would you give to a middle-age man who wants to begin an aerobic training program because he feels breathless and experiences chest discomfort while walking the golf course?

4. What type of aerobic training exercise prescription would prove most beneficial for a CHD patient who experiences angina during upper-body work as a plasterer and paper hanger. Why?

selected references

Alexander, K.P., et al.: Value of exercise treadmill testing in women. *J. Am. Col. Cardiol.*, 32:1657, 1998.

American Association of Cardiovascular and Pulmonary Rehabilitation. *Guidelines For Cardiac Rehabilitation Programs*. Champaign, IL: Human Kinetics, 1995.

American Heart Association. Cardiac rehabilitation programs: a statement for health care professionals from the American Heart Association [position statement]. *Circulation*, 90 : 1602, 1994.

Asakama, S., et al.: A simple, reliable method of assessing exercise capacity in patients with chronic heart failure. *Med. Sci. Sports Exerc.*, 31:52, 1999.

ASCM's Guidelines to Exercise Testing and Prescription. 5th Ed. Baltimore, MD: Williams & Wilkins, 1995.

Belman, M.J.: Therapeutic exercise in chronic lung disease. In *Pulmonary Rehabilitation*. Fishman, A.P. (ed.). New York, Marcel Dekker, Inc., 1996.

Blair, S.N., et al: Physical activity, nutrition, and chronic disease. *Med. Sci. Sports Exerc.*, 28:335, 1996.

Braith, R.W., et al.: Neuroendocrine hyperactivity in heart failure is buffered by endurance exercise. *Circulation*, 94:1, 1996.

Braith, R.W., et al.: Exercise training in patients with CHF and heart transplant recipients. *Med. Sci. Sports Exerc.*, 30(Suppl.):S367, 1998.

Clark, C.J., et al.: Low intensity peripheral muscle conditioning improves exercise tolerance and breathlessness in COPD. *Eur. J. Respir. J.*, 9:2590, 1996.

Cole, C.R., et al.: Heart-rate recovery immediately after exercise as a predictor of mortality. *N. Engl. J. Med.*, 341:1351, 1999.

Cooper, C.B.: Determining the role of exercise in patients with chronic pulmonary disease. *Med. Sci. Sports Exerc.*, 27:147, 1995.

Daviglus, M.I., et al.: Association of nonspecific minor ST-T abnormalities with cardiovascular mortality: The Chicago Western Electric study. *JAMA*, 281:524, 1999.

Dimeo, F., et al.: Aerobic exercise as therapy for cancer fatigue. *Med. Sci. Sports Exerc.*, 30:475, 1998.

Dimeo, F.C., et al.: Effects of physical activity on the fatigue and psychologic status of cancer patients during chemotherapy. *Cancer*, 85: 2273: 1999.

Dubach, P., et al.: Effect of exercise training on myocardial remodeling in patients with reduced left ventricular function after myocardial infarction. *Circulation*, 95:2060, 1997.

Engebretson, T.O., et al.: Quality of life and anxiety in a phase II cardiac rehabilitation program. *Med. Sci. Sports Exer.*, 31:216, 1999.

Fardy, P.S., and Yanowitz, F.G.: *Cardiac Rehabilitation, Adult Fitness, and Exercise Testing.* Baltimore: Williams & Wilkins, 1996.

Fardy, P.S., et al. (eds.): *Training Techniques in Cardiac Rehabilitation*. Monograph Number 3. Champaign, IL: Human Kinetics, 1998

Fleischmann, K.E., et al.: exercise echocardiography or exercise SPECT imaging? A meta-analysis of diagnostic test performance. *JAMA*, 280:913, 1998.

Foster, C., et al.: Physiological and pathological aspects of exercise left ventricular function. *Med. Sci. Sports Exerc.*, 30(Suppl.):S379, 1998.

Franco, M.J., et al.: Comparison of dyspnea ratings during submaximal constant work exercise with incremental testing. *Med. Sci. Sports Exerc.*, 30:479, 1998.

Franklin, B. A., et al.: Additional diagnostic tests: special populations. In: *Resource Manual for Guidelines for Exercise Testing and Prescription*. Blair, S., et al. (eds.). Philadelphia: Lea & Febiger, 1988.

Franklin, B.A., et al.: Exercise and cardiac complications: do the benefits outweigh the risks? *Phys. Sportsmed.*, 22(2): 56, 1994.

Franklin, B.A., et al.: Contemporary cardiac rehabilitation services. *Am. J. Cardiol.*, 79 : 1075, 1997.

Friedenreich, C.M., et al.: Physical activity and risk of breast cancer. *Eur. J. Cancer Prev.* 4(2):145, 1995.

Gammon, M.D., et al.: Recreational physical activity and breast cancer risk among women under age 45 years. *Am. J. Epidemiol*, 147:273, 1998.

Gibbons, L., et al.: The safety of maximal exercise testing. *Circulation*, 80:846, 1989.

Heath, G.W., and Fentem, P.H.: Physical activity among persons with disabilities—a public health perspective. *Exerc. Sport Sci. Revs.*, 25:195, 1997.

Hsia, C.C.: Cardiopulmonary limitations to exercise in restrictive lung disease. *Med. Sci. Sports Exerc.*, 31(Suppl.):S28, 1999.

Hu, F.B., et al.: Walking compared with vigorous physical activity and risk of type 2 diabetes in women. *JAMA*, 282:1433, 1999.

Keteyian, S.J., et al.: Exercise testing and training of patients with heart failure due to left ventricular systolic dysfunction. *J. Cardiopulm. Rehabil.*, 17:19, 1997.

Kobashigawa, J.A., et al.: A controlled trial of exercise rehabilitation after heart transplantation. *N. Engl. J. Med.*, 340:272, 1999.

Kohl, H.W., et al.: Maximal exercise hemodynamics and risk of mortality in apparently healthy men and women. *Med. Sci. Sports Exerc.*, 28:601, 1998.

Lauer, M.S., et al.: Impaired chronotropic response to exercise stress testing as a predictor of mortality. *JAMA*, 281:524, 1999.

Marcus, P.M., et al.: Physical activity at age 12 and adult breast cancer risk. *Cancer Causes Control*, 10:293, 1999.

McCartney, N.: Acute responses to resistance training and safety. *Med. Sci. Sports Exerc.*, 31:31, 1999.

McCartney, N.: Role of resistance training in heart disease. *Med. Sci. Sports Exerc.*, 30(Suppl.):S396, 1998.

Meyer, K., et al.: Interval training in patients with severe chronic heart failure: analysis and recommendations for exercise procedures. *Med. Sci. Sports Exerc.*, 29:306, 1997.

Morris, J.N.: Exercise in the prevention of coronary heart disease: today's best bet in public health. *Med. Sci. Sports Exerc.*, 26: 807, 1994.

Oldridge, N.B., et al.: Cardiac rehabilitation after myocardial infarction: combined experience of randomized clinical trials. *JAMA*, 260:945, 1998.

Packer, M., and Cohn, J.N., (eds.). Consensus Recommendations for the Management of Chronic Heart Failure. *Am. J. Cardiol.*, 83(2A):1A, 1999.

Reiss, T.F., et al.: Mechanical efficiency in clinically stable patients with COPD. *Thorax*, 52:981, 1997.

Rockhill, B., et al.: Physical activity and breast cancer risk in a cohort of young women. *J. Natl. Cancer Inst.*, 90:1155, 1998.

Rosamond, W.D., et al.: Trends in the incidence of myocardial infarction and in mortality due to coronary heart disease, 1987 to 1994. *N. Engl. J. Med.*, 339:861, 1998.

Serres, I., et al.: Impaired skeletal muscle endurance related to physical inactivity and altered lung function in COPD patients. *Chest*, 113:900, 1998.

Sesso, H.D., et al.: Physical activity and breast cancer risk in the College Alumni Health Study (United States). *Cancer Causes Control*, 9:433, 1998.

Shephard, R.J., et al.: Physical activity and cancer: how may protection be maximized? *Crit. Rev. Oncog.*, 8(2–3):219, 1997.

Shephard, R.J., and Baldy, G.J.: Exercise as cardiovascular therapy. *Circulation*, 99:963, 1999.

Thune, L., et al.: Physical activity and the risk of breast cancer. *New Engl. J. Med.*, 336:1269, 1997.

Verrill, D.E., and Ribisl, P.M.: Resistive exercise training in cardiac rehabilitation (an update). *Sports Med.*, 21:371, 1996.

Wells, C.L.: Physical activity and cancer prevention. Focus on breast cancer. *ACSM's Health & Fitness J.*, 3(1):13, 1999.

Wells, C.L.: Physical activity and cancer prevention. *ACSM's Health Fitness J.*, 3:13, 1999.

Whittom, F., et al.: Histochemical and morphological characteristics of the vastus lateralis muscle in patients with chronic obstructive pulmonary disease. *Med. Sci. Sports Exerc.*, 30:1467, 1998.

APPENDICES

Appendix A

Reliable Information Resources and Exercise Physiology

Appendix B

The Internet and Exercise Physiology
   Part 1. Search Engines
   Part 2. Government Related Sites
   Part 3. Exercise Physiology Related
        Sites
   Part 4. General Science Sites
   Part 5. Science and Technology News
   Part 6. Useful Resources

Appendix C

The Metric System and Conversion
   Constants in Exercise Physiology

Appendix D

Metabolic Computations in Open-Circuit
   Spirometry

Appendix E

Frequently Cited Journals in Exercise
   Physiology

Appendix F

Evaluation of Body Composition
   – Girth Method

Appendix G

Evaluation of Body Composition
   – Skinfold Method

Reliable Information Resources and Exercise Physiology

American Heart Association
Inquiries Coordinator
7272 Greenville Avenue
Dallas, TX 75231-4596
(800) 242-8721; Fax: (214) 706-1341
E-mail: dstokes@amhrt. org
http://www.americanheart.org

American Institute for Cancer Research
1759 R Street NW
Washington, DC 20009
(800) 843-8114; (202) 328-7744
Fax: (202) 328-7226
E-mail: aircrweb@aicr.org
http://www.aicr.org

Anorexia Nervosa and Related Eating Disorders
PO Box 5102
Eugene, OR 97405
(541) 344-1144
http://www.anred.com

American Public Health Association
1015 18th Street NW, Washington, DC 20036
(202) 789-5600; Fax (202) 789-5661
E-mail: comments@apha.com
http://www.apha.org

American Running and Fitness Association
4405 East West Hwy, Suite 405
Bethesda, MD 20814
(800) 776-2732

American Society for Nutritional Sciences and American Society for Clinical Nutrition
9650 Rockville Pike
Bethesda, MD 20814
(301) 530-7050; Fax: (301) 571-1892
http://www.faseb.org/asns/

Canadian Association for Health, Physical, Education Recreation and Dance (CAHPERD)
1600 James Naismith Drive
Gloucester, ON KIB 5N4
(613) 748-5622; (800) 663-8708
Fax: (613) 748-5737
E-mail: cahperd@activeliving.ca
http://www.activeliving.ca/cahperd

Canadian Society for Exercise Physiology
185 Somerset St. West, Suite 202
Ottawa, Ontario CANADA K2P OJ2
(613) 234-3755; Fax: (613) 234-3565
E-mail: info@csep.ca
http://www.csep.ca

Canadian Society for Nutritional Sciences
Department of Foods and Nutrition
University of Manitoba
Winnipeg, Manitoba, CANADA R3T 2N2

Cancer Research Foundation
1600 Duke Street
Alexandria, VA 22314
(703) 836-4412
http://www.preventcancer.org/

Centers for Disease Control and Prevention
Natural Institutes of Health
1600 Clifton Road, NE
Atlanta, GA 30333
(404) 639-3311
http://www.cdc.gov/

Food and Drug Administration (FDA)
Center for Food Safety and Applied Nutrition,
Room 4405B Federal Building, 200 C Street SW
Washington, DC 20204
(202) 205-4168; Fax: (202) 205-5295
http://www/fda/gov/

Food Insight
International Food Information Council
E-mail: foodinfo@ific.health.org
http://www.ificinfo.health.org/

Food and Nutrition Information Center
National Agriculture Library
Agriculture Research Service, USDA
10301 Baltimore Ave.
Beltsville, MD 20705-2351
(301) 504-5719; Fax: (301) 504-6409
E-mail: fnic@nal.usda.gov/fnic/
http://www.nal.usda.gov/fnic/

Food Research and Action Center (FRAC)
1875 Connecticut Avenue NW #540
Washington, DC 20009
(202) 986-2200; Fax: (202) 986-2525
http://www.iglou.com/why/resource/1100.htm

Food Safety and Inspection Service
FSIS Food Safety Education and Communications Staff
U.S. Department of Agriculture
Room 1175-South Building
1400 Independence Ave., SW
Washington, DC 20250
(202) 720-7943; Fax: (202) 720-1843
E-mail: fsis.webmaster@usda.gov
http://www.fsis.usda.gov

Health and Welfare Canada
Canadian Government Publishing Center
Minister of Supply and Services
Ottawa, Ontario CANADA KIA 0S9

International Association of Eating Disorders Professionals
123 NW 13th Street #206
Boca Raton, FL 33432-1618
(800) 800-8126

International Association of Fitness Professionals
6190 Cornerstone CT. E., Suite 204
San Diego, CA 92121-3773
(800) 999-4332, Fax: (619) 535-8234
http://www.ideafit.com

International Sports Sciences Association (ISSA)
1035 Santa Barbara Street, Unit 7
Santa Barbara, CA 93101
(800) 892-4772; Fax: (805) 884-8119
E-mail: webmaster@issaonline.com
http://www.issaonline.com

Jean Mayer United States Department of Agriculture Human Nutrition Research Center on Aging
Tufts University
132 Curtis Street
Medford, MA 02155
(617) 627-628-5000
http://www.hnrc.tufts.edu/

Massachusetts Eating Disorders Association, Inc.
1162 Beacon Street
Brookline, MA 02146
(617) 738-6332

National Academy of Sciences/Institute of Medicine, Food and Nutrition Board
2101 Constitution Avenue NW
Washington, DC 20418
(202) 334-2000; Fax: (202) 334-2316
E-mail: Fnb@nas.edu
http://www.nas.edu/fnb/

National Association of Anorexia Nervosa and Associated Disorders
PO Box 7
Highland Park, IL 60035
(847) 831-3438; Fax: (847) 433-4632
http://www.medpatients.com/Health%20
    Resources/NAANAD.htm

National Cancer Institute
Office of Cancer Communications
Building 31, Room 10A-24
Bethesda, MD 20892
(800) 422-6237
E-mail: cis@icicc.nci.nih.gov
http://www.nci.nih.gov

National Center for Nutrition and Dietetics
The American Dietetic Association
216 West Jackson Boulevard
Chicago, IL 60606-6995
(312) 899-0040 ext. 4653; Fax: (312) 899-1739
http://www.eatright.org

National Center for Health Statistics (NCHS)
National Institutes of Health
6525 Belcrest Road,
Hyattsville, MD 20782
(301) 436-8500
http://www.cdc.gov/nchswww/default.htm

National Council Against Health Fraud
PO Box 1276
Loma Linda, CA 92354-9983
Fax: (909) 824-4848
http://www.ncahf.org

National Dairy Council
10255 W. Higgins Rd.
Rosemont, IL 60018-4233

National Diabetes Information Clearinghouse
1 Information Way
Bethesda, MD 20892-3560
(301) 654-3327; Fax: (301) 907-8906
E-mail: ndic@info.niddk.nih.gov
http://www.niddk.nih.gov/health/diabetes/diabetes/diabetes.htm

National Eating Disorders Organization (NEDO)
6655 South Yale Avenue
Tulsa, OK 74136
(918) 481-4044; Fax: (918) 481-4076
http://www.laureate.com

National Eating Disorders Screening Program
One Washington Street
Suite 304
Wellesley, MA 02181-1706
http://www.nmisp.org

National Heart, Lung, and Blood Institute Information Center
PO Box 30105
Bethesda, MD 20842-0105
(301) 251-1222; Fax: (301) 251-1223
E-mail: nhlbiic@dgsys.com
http://www.nhlbi.nih.gov/nhlbi/nhlbi.htm

National Institute on Aging
Information Office
Building 31, Room 5C35
Bethesda, MD 20205

National Institute of Diabetes and Digestive and Kidney Diseases
31 Center Drive, MSC-2560
Building 31, Room 9A-04
Bethesda, MD 20892-2560
(301) 496-3583; Fax: (301) 496-7422
http://www.niddk.nih.gov

National Institutes of Health (NIH)
9000 Rockville Pike,
Bethesda, MD 20892
(301) 496-4461; Fax: (301) 496-0017
http://www.nih.gov/

National Institute of Nutrition
1335 Carling Avenue
Suite 210
Ottawa, Ontario CANADA K1Z OL2

National Library of Medicine
8600 Rockville Pike
Bethesda, MD 20894
(888) 346-3656; (301) 594-5983
http://www.nlm.nih.gov

National Kidney and Urologic Diseases Information
  Clearinghouse (NIDDK)
3 Information Way
Bethesda, MD 20892-3580
(301) 654-4415; Fax: (301) 907-8906

National Mental Health Association
1201 Prince Street
Alexandria, VA 22314-2971
(703) 684-7722; Fax: (703) 684-5968
http://www.nmha.org

National Osteoporosis Foundation
1150 17th St., NW, Suite 500
Washington, DC 20036-4603
(202) 223-2226; Fax: (202) 223-2237
http://www.nof.org

National Strength and Conditioning Association (NSCA)
PO Box 38909
Colorado Springs, CO 80937-8909
(719) 632-6722; Fax: (719) 632-6367
E-mail: nsca@usa.net
http://www.nsca-lift.org

North American Association of the Study of Obesity (NAASO)
Department Endocrinology & Metabolism
Mayo Medical Center
Mayo Clinic
200 First Street, SW
Rochester, Minnesota 55905
(507) 255-6768; Fax: (507) 255-4828
http://www.naaso.org

Nutrition Programs
446 Jeanne Mance Building
Tunney's Pasture
Ottawa, Ontario CANADA K1A 1B4

Office of Disease Prevention and Health Promotion (ODPHP)
National Institutes of Health
2131 Switzer Building, 330 C Street SW
Washington, DC 20201
(202) 205-9007; Fax: 205-9478

Overeaters Anonymous
World Service Office
6075 Zenith Court, NE
Rio Rancho, NM 87124
(505) 891-4320; Fax: (505) 891-4320
E-mail: Overeattn@technet.run.org
http://www.overeatersanonymous.org

Public Health Resource Service
15 Overlea Boulevard, 5th Floor
Toronto, Ontario CANADA M4H IA9

Sports Information Resource Centre (SIRC)
107-1600 James Naismith Drive
Gloucester, Ontario CANADA K1B 5N4
(800) 664-6413; (613) 748-5658
Fax: (613) 748-5701
E-mail: moreinfo@sirc.ca
http://www.sportquest.com/sirc/facts.html

Sports, Cardiovascular and Wellness Nutritionists (SCAN)
90 S Cascade #1190
Colorado Springs, CO 80903
(719) 475-7751; Fax: (719) 475-8748
www.nutrifit.org

The Weight-Control Information Network
National Institute of Diabetes and Digestive and Kidney
  Diseases
I WIN WAY
Bethesda, MD 20892-3665
(301) 570-2177; (800) 946-8098
Fax: (301) 570-2186
http://www.niddk.nih.gov/NutritionDocs.html

U.S. Department of Health and Human Services (DHHS)
200 Independence Avenue SW,
Washington, DC 20201
(202) 619-0257; Fax: (202) 619-3363
http://www.os.dhhs.gov

U.S. Department of Agriculture (USDA)
12th and Independence Avenue SW
Washington, DC 20250
(202) 720-3631; Fax: (202) 720-5437
http://web.fie.com/web/fed/agr

Vitamin Nutrition Information Service (VNIS)
Hoffmann-LaRoche
340 Kingsland Avenue
Nutley, NJ 07110

World Health Organization (WHO)
Headquarter Offices
Avenue Appia 20
1211 Geneva 27
Switzerland
(+41 22) 791 21 11; Fax: (+41 22) 791 0746
E-mail: info@who.cho
http://www.who.int/

The Internet and Exercise Physiology

The Internet provides a phenomenal information resource about hundreds of thousands of topics covering every facet of our society. In the basic and applied sciences, the information explosion has spawned millions of web sites in a relatively short time period. No one person can ever hope to keep current with the most up-to-the minute information about a particular topic. Just five years ago when we began our own searches about the relatively new topic of exercise and molecular biology, we had no difficulty locating web sites because so few sites dealt with topics related to exercise. What a difference five years make.

On October 6, 1999, when we used the Alta Vista search engine (www.altavista.com) to locate web sites for the terms *molecular biology*, we could visit over 2 million sites for information about this topic (if we had enough time and will power!) In fact, many of the established disciplines have at least this many or more web sites associated with their field when we searched for the following terms: biology—2,774,2365; chemistry—3,915,823; physics—5,002,195; statistics—9,813,859; computers—11,193,713. A search on "exercise physiology" showed 806,580 web sites, while general areas typically associated with exercise physiology produced a huge resource of sites (health—27,536,356; fitness—3,417,734; exercise—2,329,240; human biology—3,731,595; wellness—877,350). A search on "exercise science" yielded 2,577,680 web locations, while 104,310 matches were located for "kinesiology." Obviously, this Appendix can only provide an eclectic collection of relatively few sites germane to exercise physiology, no matter how selective we identify the categories.

The web sites we highlight in this section have been placed into one of six subcategories: 1), Search Engines, 2), Government Sites, 3), Exercise Physiology Related Sites, 4), General Science Sites, 5), Science and Technology News Sites, and 6), Useful Resource Sites.

Please let us know about your favorite sites at our email address mkk@lww.com.

PART 1. SEARCH ENGINES

A2Z Online
  http:www.a2z.com
All-In-One Search Page
  http://www.albany.net/allinone/
AltaVista
  http://www.altavista.com/

Ask Jeeves
  http://askjeeves.com/
Beaucoup!
  http://www.beaucoup.com/
ComFind
  http://www.comfind.com/
Dejanews
  http://www.dejanews.com/
Directory Guide
  http://www.directoryguide.com/
Dogpile
  http://www.dogpile.com
eBLAST
  http://www.eblast.com/
Excite
  http://www.excite.com/
Galaxy
  http://galaxy.einet.net/
GoTo
  http://www.goto.com/
Hardin Meta Directory of Internet Health Sources
  http://www.lib.uiowa.edu/hardin/md/index.html
HealthFinder
  http://www.healthfinder.gov/searchoptions/topicsaz.htm
Hotbot
  http://www.hotbot.com
Inference Find
  http://www.infind.com/
Infoseek
  http://www.infoseek.com/
Internet Grateful Med
  http://igm.nlm.nih.gov/
Internet Sleuth
  http://www.isleuth.com/
Linkstar
  http://www.linkstar.com/
Lycos
  http://www.lycos.com/
Magellan
  http://www.mckinley.com/
Mayo Clinic Health Oasis
  http://www.mayohealth.org/
MedExplorer
  http://www.medexplorer.com/
MedHunt
  http://www.hon.ch/cgi-bin/find?1

Medical Matrix
    http://www.medmatrix.org/index.asp
MedSurf
    http://www.medsurf.com/
MedWeb Plus
    http://www.medwebplus.com/
MedWeb
    http://WWW.MedWeb.Emory.Edu/MedWeb/
MedWorld
    http://www-med.stanford.edu/medworld/home/
MetaCrawler
    http://www.metacrawler.com/
Multimedia Medical Reference Library
    http://www.med-library.com/medlibrary/
Northern Light
    http://www.northernlight.com/
Pathfinder
    http://www.pathfinder.com/welcome/
Savvy Search
    http://www.cs.colostate.edu/~dreiling/smartform.html
Search Tools for the Internet
    http://www.nal.usda.gov/other_internet_sites/srchtool.
    html
Searching the Internet
    http://jan.ucc.nau.edu/~bwp2/isearch.html
The New PubMed
    http://www.ncbi.nlm.nih.gov/entrez/query.fcgi
Unified Computer Science TR Index
    http://www.cs.indiana.edu:800/cstr/
Various Search Engines
    http://ic.net/~baustin/search/search.html
Webcrawler
    http://webcrawler.com/
Welcome to PubMed
    http://www.ncbi.nlm.nih.gov/PubMed/
Yahoo!
    http://search.yahoo.com/bin/search/options

PART 2. GOVERNMENT RELATED SITES

Administration for Children & Families
    www.acf.dhhs.gov/
Agency for Health Care Policy & Research
    www.ahcpr.gov/
Agency for Toxic Substances & Disease Registry
    http://atsdr1.atsdr.cdc.gov:8080
Agricultural Network Information Center
    http://www.agnic.org/
Berkeley Lab Research Review Magazine
    http://www.lbl.gov/Science-Articles/Research-
    Review/newsstand.html
Biology Information Center
    http://www.er.doe.gov/production/ober/ober_top.html
Cancer Genome Anatomy Project
    http://www.ncbi.nlm.nih.gov/ncicgap/

Center for Food Safety & Applied Nutrition
    http://vm.cfsan.fda.gov/list.html
Center for Nutrition Policy & Promotion
    http://www2.hqnet.usda.gov/cnpp/
Centers for Disease Control & Prevention
    http://www.cdc.gov/
Clinical Guidelines for Treatment of Overweight &
    Obesity in Adults
    http://www.nhlbi.nih.gov/nhlbi/cardio/obes/prof/
    guidelns/ob_home.htm
Code of Federal Regulations
    http://www.access.gpo.gov/nara/cfr/cfr-table-
    search.html
Consumer Information Center
    http://www.pueblo.gsa.gov/
Department of Health & Human Services
    http://www.os.dhhs.gov/
Dietary Guidelines for Americans
    http://www.nalusda.gov/fnic/dga/dguide95.html
Dietary Supplements
    http://www.cfsan.fda.gov/~dms/supplmnt.html
DNA From the Beginning
    http://vector.cshl.org/dnaftb/
Environmental Protection Agency
    http://www.epa.gov/
Exercise Physiology Laboratory at NASA-Johnson Space
    Center
    http://www.jsc.nasa.gov/sa/sd/sd3/exl/index.htm
FDA Consumer
    http://www.fda.gov/fdac/698_toc.html
Federal Directory: Government Information Xchange
    http://www.info.gov/
Federal Trade Commission
    http://www.ftc.gov/
FedStats
    http://www.fedstats.gov/search.html
FedWorld Network
    http://www.fedworld.gov/
Food & Agriculture Organization of the United Nations
    (FAO)
    http://www.fao.org/
Food & Drug Administration
    http://www.fda.gov/default.htm
Food & Nutrition Information Center
    http://www.nalusda.gov/fnic/
Food & Nutrition Service
    http://www2.hqnet.usda.gov/fcs/
Food & Nutrition
    http://www.gsa.gov/staff/pa/cic/food.htm
Food Guide Pyramid Information
    http://www.nalusda.gov/fnic/Fpyr/pyramid.html
Food Labeling & Nutrition
    http://vm.cfsan.fda.gov/label.html
Food Labeling Education
    http://www.nal.usda.gov/fnic/Label/label.html
Food Surveys Research Group
    http://www.barc.usda.gov/bhnrc/foodsurvey/home.htm

Gene Map of the Human Genome
  http://www.ncbi.nlm.nih.gov/SCIENCE96/
Genes & Disease
  http://www.ncbi.nlm.nih.gov/disease/
Health Care Financing Administration
  http://www.hcfa.gov
Health Finder
  http://www.healthfinder.gov/
Health Resources & Services Administration
  www.hrsa.dhhs.gov
Human Genome Project Information
  http://www.ornl.gov/TechResources/Human_
  Genome/home.html
Indian Health Service
  http://www.ihs.gov
International Space Station
  http://station.nasa.gov/
Internet Health Resources
  http://www.health-library.com/index.html
Internet Sites Related to Food & Nutrition
  http://www.barc.usda.gov/bhnrc/foodsurvey/Sites.html
Lawrence Berkeley National Laboratory Human
  Genome Sequencing
  http://www-hgc.lbl.gov/
Library of Congress Catalogs
  http://lcweb.loc.gov/catalog/
Library of Congress
  http://www.loc.gov/
Medline (PubMed)
  http://www.ncbi.nlm.nih.gov/PubMed/
Mental Health
  http://www.mentalhealth.org/cornerstone/index.cfm
Molecular Biology Desk Reference
  http://molbio.info.nih.gov/molbio/desk.html
Morbidity & Mortality Weekly Report
  http://www2.cdc.gov/mmwr/
National Academy of Sciences
  http://www.nas.edu/
National Aeronautics & Space Administration
  http://www.nasa.gov/
National Agricultural Library
  http://www.nal.usda.gov/
National Air & Space Museum
  http://www.nasm.edu/
National Center for Biotechnology Information
  http://www.ncbi.nlm.nih.gov/
National Center for Biotechnology Information
  http://www.ncbi.nlm.nih.gov/
National Centers Health Statistics Web Search
  http://www.cdc.gov/nchswww/search/search.htm
National Highway Traffic Safety Administration
  http://www.nhtsa.dot.gov
National Institute for Occupational Safety & Health
  http://www.cdc.gov/niosh/homepage.html
National Institute on Aging
  http://www.nih.gov/nia/
National Institutes of Health
  http://www.nih.gov/index.html

National Institutes of Health Food & Nutrition Board
  http://www2.nas.edu/fnb/
National Library of Medicine
  http://www4.ncbi.nlm.nih.gov/
National Science Foundation (NSF)
  http://www.nsf.gov/
NCBI Entrez Genomes List
  http://www.ncbi.nlm.nih.gov/Entrez/Genome/org.html
NIH Library Online
  http://libwww.ncrr.nih.gov/
NSF Science & Technology Centers
  http://www.cs.brown.edu/stc/allstc.html
Nutrient Data laboratory: Agricultural Research Service
  http://www.nal.usda.gov/fnic/foodcomp/
Occupational Safety & Health Administration
  http://www.osha.gov
Office of Biological & Environmental Research
  http://www.er.doe.gov/production/ober/ober_top.html
Office of Disease Prevention & Health Promotion
  http://odphp.osophs.dhhs.gov/
Office of Health Affairs: U.S. Food & Drug
  Administration
  http://www.fda.gov/oc/oha/
Office of Naval Research
  http://web.fie.com/fedix/onr.html
Office of Science & Technology Policy
  http://www.whitehouse.gov/OSTP.html
Physical Activity & Health: Surgeon General Report
  http://www.cdc.gov/nccdphp/sgr/sgr.htm
Profiles in Science
  http://www.profiles.nlm.nih.gov/
Science & Technology Web Sites
  http://www.harvardhealthpubs.org/frindex.html
State Departments of Public Health
  http://www.fsis.usda.gov/OPHS/stategov.htm
Statistical Abstract of the United States
  http://www.census.gov/prod/www/abs/cc97stab.html
Superintendent of Documents (GPOAccess)
  http://www.access.gpo.gov/su_docs/
Team Nutrition
  http://www2.hqnet.usda.gov/cnpp/team.htm
The Genome Database
  http://gdbwww.gdb.org/
U. S. Copyright Office
  http://lcweb.loc.gov/copyright/
U.S. Census Bureau
  http://www.census.gov/
U.S. Consumer Gateway
  http://www.consumer.gov/
U.S. Department of Agriculture
  http://www.usda.gov/
U.S. Department of Agriculture Center for Nutrition
  Policy & Promotion
  http://www.usda.gov/fcs/cnpp.htm
U.S. Department of Agriculture Cooperative State
  Research, Education, & Extension Service
  http://www.reeusda.gov/

U.S. Department of Agriculture Food & Nutrition Service
http://www.usda.gov/fcs/
U.S. Department of Agriculture Healthy Eating Index
http://www2.hqnet.usda.gov/cnpp/usda_healthy_eating_index.htm
U.S. Department of Agriculture Nutrient Data Laboratory
http://www.nal.usda.gov/fnic/foodcomp/
U.S. Department of Education
http://www.ed.gov/
U.S. Government Grants & Resources
http://pegasus.uthct.edu/OtherUsefulSites/Govt.html
U.S. Government Printing Office
http://www.access.gpo.gov/su_docs/
U.S. Indian Health Service
http://www.ihs.gov/
U.S. Military Network
http://www.military-network.com/MainSite.htm
U.S. Patent & Trademark Office
http://www.uspto.gov/
U.S. Pharmacopeia
http://www.usp.org/
U.S. State & Local Gateway: Federal Funding
http://www.statelocal.gov/funding.html
Visible Human Project
http://www.nlm.nih.gov/research/visible/visible_human.html
Walk Through Time
http://physics.nist.gov/GenInt/Time/time.html
Zip Code Lookup
http://www.usps.gov/ncsc/lookups/lookup_zip+4.html

PART 3. EXERCISE PHYSIOLOGY RELATED SITES

ADIPOS: Publication in Obesity
http://www.adipos.com/index.html
Aging Research Centre (ARC)
http://www.arclab.org/
American Alliance for Health, Physical Education, Recreation & Dance
http://www.aahperd.org/
American College of Sports Medicine
http://www.acsm.org/
American Dietetic Association
http://www.eatright.org/
American Heart Association
http://www.americanheart.org/
American Journal of Clinical Nutrition
http://www.faseb.org/ajcn/
American Medical Association
http://www.ama-assn.org/
American Red Cross: CPR Training
http://www.redcross.org/hss/cpraed.html
American Society for Nutritional Sciences
http://www.nutrition.org/

Ancient Medicine/Medicina Antiqua
http://web1.ea.pvt.k12.pa.us:80/medant/
Ancient Olympic Games Virtual Museum
http://devlab.dartmouth.edu/olympic/
Applied Exercise Science Websites
http://www.edb.utexas.edu/abraham/Links.html
Artificial Muscle Project
http://www.ai.mit.edu/projects/muscle/overview.html
Artigen Health News
http://www.artigen.com/newswire/health.html
Ask an Expert
http://www.askanexpert.com/askanexpert/catscitec.shtml
Ask the Dietician
http://www.dietitian.com/
Audiovisuals about Basic Nutrition
http://www.nal.usda.gov/fnic/pubs/bibs/av/basic-av.htm
Beginners Guide to Molecular Biology
http://www.tiac.net/users/pmgannon/
Biomechanics Worldwide
http://www.per.ualberta.ca/biomechanics/bwwframe.htm
Blonz Guide: Nutrition, Food & Health Resources
http://www.blonz.com/blonz/nfindex2.htm
Body Composition Tutorial
http://nuts.uvm.edu/nusc/uww/
Canadian Journal of Applied Physiology
http://www.humankinetics.com/infok/journals/cjap/intro.htm
Cell & Molecular Biology Online
http://www.cellbio.com/
Cells Alive!
http://www.cellsalive.com/
Center for Cancer Biology & Nutrition
http://www.tamu.edu/ccbn/ccbnweb/ccbn.htm
CHID Online (Combined Health Information Database)
http://chid.nih.gov/
Clinical Guidelines About Overweight & Obesity in Adults
http://www.nhlbi.nih.gov/nhlbi/cardio/obes/prof/guidelns/ob_home.htm
Coaching Science Abstracts
http://www-rohan.sdsu.edu/dept/coachsci/intro.html
Community of Science (COS)
http://www.cos.com/
Complete Home Medical Guide
http://cpmcnet.columbia.edu/texts/guide/
Comprehensive Medical Indexes
http://www.ama-assn.org/med_link/links.htm
Cycling Performance Tips
http://www.halcyon.com/gasman/
DOCINFO
http://www.docinfo.com/index.htm
Donald B. Brown Research Chair on Obesity
http://obesity.chair.ulaval.ca/welcome.html
Electric Library: Encyclopedia
http://www.Encyclopedia.com/

Exercise Physiology Digital Image Archive
http://www.abacon.com/dia/exphys/home.html

Exercise Physiology. Methods & Mechanisms Underlying Performance
http://www.krs.hia.no/~stephens/exphys.htm

Fatfree: The Low Fat Vegetarian Archive
http://www.fatfree.com/index.shtml

Federation of American Societies for Experimental Biology
http://www.faseb.org/

Fitness Links Page
http://www.general.uwa.edu.au/u/rjwood/links.htm

Food Composition Resource List for Professionals
http://www.nal.usda.gov/fnic/pubs/bibs/gen/97fdcomp.htm

Food Finder
http://www.olen.com/food/

Food Guide Pyramid
http://www2.hqnet.usda.gov/cnpp/pyramid2.htm

From Quackery to Bacteriology
http://www.cl.utoledo.edu/canaday/quackery/quack1.html

Gatorade Sports Science Institute
http://gssiweb.com/site.html

GeroWeb
http://www.iog.wayne.edu/govlinks.html

Guide to Eating Disorders
http://eatingdisorders.miningco.com/

Guide To Medical Information & Support on the Internet
http://www.geocities.com/HotSprings/1505/guide.html

Health A to Z
http://www.healthatoz.com/

Health Directory Worldwide
http://www.healthdirectory.com/

Health on the Net Foundation
http://www.hon.ch/

Healthgate
http://www.healthgate.com/

Herbal Medicine Resource List
http://www.nal.usda.gov/fnic/pubs/bibs/gen/herbbr.htm

HMS Beagle: The BioMedNet Magazine
http://biomednet.com/hmsbeagle/index.htm

Horus' Web Links to History Resources
http://www.ucr.edu/h-gig/horuslinks.html

Hosford Muscle Tables: Skeletal Muscles of the Human Body
http://www.ptcentral.com/muscles/

Human Muscle Gene Map
http://www.bio.unipd.it/~telethon/Hmgm/HMGM.html

Hypermuscle: Muscles in Action
http://www.med.umich.edu/lrc/Hypermuscle/Hyper.html

In Vivo Sarcomere Length Measurement
http://www-neuromus.ucsd.edu/surgery/surgery.html

Institute of Medicine
http://www.iom.edu/

Intelihealth
http://www.intelihealth.com/IH/ihtIH

International Food Composition Tables Directory
http://www.crop.cri.nz/foodinfo/infoods/fdtables/0fdtable.html

International Food Information Council
http://ificinfo.health.org/

International Journal of Sport Nutrition
http://www.humankinetics.com/infok/journals/ijsn/intro.htm

Internet Drug Index
http://www.rxlist.com/

Introduction to Muscle Physiology & Design
http://muscle.ucsd.edu/MusIntro/

John B. Pierce Laboratory, Inc.
http://www.jbpierce.org/jbp/default.htm

Journal of Applied Physiology
http://jap.physiology.org/

Journal of Food Composition & Analysis
http://www.academicpress.com/jfca

KEGG Metabolic
http://www.genome.ad.jp/kegg/metabolism.html

KidsHealth
http://KidsHealth.org/index2.html

Kinesiology & Health Science Links
http://www.tahperd.sfasu.edu/links3.html

Link to Electronic Journals
http://www.eurekalert.org/links/Journals_public.html

Marathoning Start to Finish
http://www.teamoregon.com/publications/marathon/

Masters Athlete Physiology & Performance
http://www.krs.hia.no/~stephens/index.html

MayoClinic
http://www.mayohealth.org/

Medfacts
http://www.medfacts.com/

MedFinder
http://www.netmedicine.com/medfinder.htm

Medical History on the Internet
http://www.anes.uab.edu/medhist.htm

Medical World Search
http://www.mwsearch.com/

Medicine & Science in Sports & Exercise
http://www.wwilkins.com/MSSE/

Medicine & Sports Related Links
http://www.mspweb.com/

MedicineNet
http://www.medicinenet.com/

Medscape
http://www.medscape.com/

Medsite
http://www.medsite.com/

MedWeb Biomedical Internet Resources
http://www.cc.emory.edu/WHSCL/medweb.html

MedWeb Physiology
http://www.gen.emory.edu/MEDWEB/keyword/physiology.html

MedWeb Sports Medicine
http://www.gen.emory.edu/medweb/
medweb.sportsmed.html

Metabolic Pathways of Biochemistry
http://www.gwu.edu/~mpb/

Multilingual Glossary of Technical & Popular Medical Terms
http://allserv.rug.ac.be/~rvdstich/eugloss/welcome.html

Muscle Physiology & Design
http://www-neuromus.ucsd.edu/MusIntro/Jump.html

Museum of Health & Medical Science
http://www.mhms.org/

National Fraud Information Center
http://www.fraud.org/

National Research Council
http://www.iom.edu/

National Sports Medicine Institute of the United Kingdom
http://www.nsmi.org.uk/publ.html

Net Doctor
http://www.net-doctor.com/

NetBiochem
http://www-medlib.med.utah.edu/NetBiochem/
NetWelco.htm

Neuromuscular Research Lab
http://nmrc.bu.edu/

New England Journal of Medicine
http://www.nejm.org/

Nutrition & Fitness Links
http://www.lifelines.com/ntnlnk.html

Nutrition Analysis Tool
http://www.ag.uiuc.edu/~food-lab/nat/

Nutrition Navigator: Rating Guide to Nutrition Websites
http://navigator.tufts.edu/

Obesity
http://www.obesity.com/

Obesity, Health, & Metabolic Fitness
http://www.mesomorphosis.com/exclusive/gaesser/
obesity01.htm

Olympic Centennial: Athletic, Sport, Recreation Bibliography Project
http://www-nutrition.ucdavis.edu/Olympics/

Pedro's Biomolecular Research Tools
http://www.biophys.uni-duesseldorf.de/bionet/
research_tools.html

Pennington Biomedical Research Center
http://www.pbrc.edu/default.htm

Perseus Project: Ancient Olympic Games
http://olympics.tufts.edu/

Physical Activity & Health Network
http://www1.pitt.edu/~pahnet/

Physician & Sportsmedicine Online
http://www.physsportsmed.com/

Physiology & Biophysics (Biosciences)
http://physiology.med.cornell.edu/WWWVL/
PhysioWeb.html

Primer on Molecular Genetics
http://www.bis.med.jhmi.edu/Dan/DOE/intro.html

Professional Resources about Eating Disorders
http://www.nal.usda.gov/fnic/pubs/bibs/gen/
anorhpbr.htm

Quackwatch: Guide to Health Fraud, Quackery, & Intelligent Decisions
http://www.quackwatch.com/

Quick'Ndex: Your Own Medical Librarian on the Internet
http://www.healthy.net/welcome/quick.htm

Reedy's Muscle Database
http://note.cellbio.duke.edu/Faculty/~Reedy
/Muscle/MuscleDB.html

Resources for Medical History Papers
http://www.usuhs.mil/meh/histres.html

Runner's World Online
http://www.runnersworld.com/

Science of Foods
http://osu.orst.edu/instruct/nfm236/head/glossary/
index.html

Science of Obesity & Weight Control
http://www.loop.com/~bkrentzman/index.html

Scientific American
http://www.sciam.com/

Shape Up America
http://www.shapeup.org/

Something Fishy Website on Eating Disorders
http://www.something-fishy.com/ed.htm

Sportscience
http://www.sportsci.org/

Swiss Food Composition Database
http://food.ethz.ch/swifd/

The Fédération Internationale de Médecine du Sport (FIMS)
http://www.fims.org/

The Heart: An Online Exploration
http://sln.fi.edu/biosci/heart.html

The Journal of the American Medical Association
http://www.ama-assn.org/public/journals/jama/

The Lancet Interactive
http://www.thelancet.com/

The New England Journal of Medicine
http://www.nejm.org/content/index.asp

The Online Medical Dictionary
http://www.graylab.ac.uk/omd/index.html

The Physiologist
http://www.faseb.org/aps/tphys.htm

The Sleep Well
http://www.stanford.edu/~dement/

United States Sports Academy
http://www.sport.ussa.edu/

USDA Food Safety & Inspection Service
http://www.fsis.usda.gov/

Useful Links for Endurance Athletes
http://www.krs.hia.no/~stephens/coolinks.htm

Vegetarian Resource Group
http://www.vrg.org/

Virtual Anatomy
http://hyperion.advanced.org/16421/

Virtual Body
http://www.medtropolis.com/vbody/
WebMedLit
http://www.webmedlit.com/
WebSearch: Health & Medicine
http://websearch.miningco.com/
Wellness Web: Nutrition & Fitness
http://www.wellweb.com/nutrition_fitness_home-page.htm
Women in Health & Medicine
http://www.netsrq.com/~dbois/health.html
World Health Organization
http://www.who.int/   http://www.who.int/

PART 4. GENERAL SCIENCE SITES

American Association for the Advancement of Science
http://www.aaas.org/
American Institute of Physics
http://www.aip.org/history/
Armchair Scientist
http://www.areacom.it/html/arte_cultura/loris/armchair.html
Bioinformatics Links
http://www.ii.uib.no/~inge/list.html
BioMedNews
http://www.biomednet.com/biomednews
Biosciences
http://golgi.harvard.edu/biopages.list
BioSites
http://www.library.ucsf.edu/biosites/
BioTech Life Sciences Resources & Reference Tools
http://biotech.icmb.utexas.edu/
Boston Museum of Science
http://www.british-museum.ac.uk/
BrainPop
http://www.brainpop.com/indexgen.asp
Cell & Molecular Biology Online
http://www.cellbio.com/
Center for Human Simulation
http://www.uchsc.edu/sm/chs/
Center of Science & Industry
http://cosi.org/
Charles Darwin Origin of Species & Voyage of the Beagle
http://www.literature.org/Works/Charles-Darwin/
Chicago Academy of Sciences
http://www.chias.org/
Discover Magazine
http://www.discover.com/
Discovery Channel Online
http://www.discovery.com/
Exploratorium
http://www.exploratorium.org/
Franklin Institute Science Museum
http://sln.fi.edu/

History of the Health Sciences World Wide Web Links
http://www2.mc.duke.edu/misc/MLA/HHSS/histlink.htm#liv
HMS Beagle
http://www.biomednet.com/hmsbeagle/current/about/index
How Things Work
http://Landau1.phys.Virginia.EDU/Education/Teaching/HowThingsWork/
Human Anatomy On_line
http://www.innerbody.com/indexbody.html
International Museum of Surgical Science
http://www.imss.org/
International Space Station
http://station.nasa.gov/
Journals, Conferences, & Current Awareness Services
http://golgi.harvard.edu/journals.html
Life Science Dictionary
http://biotech.chem.indiana.edu/pages/dictionary.html
Marching Through the Visible Man
http://www.crd.ge.com/esl/cgsp/projects/vm/
Mayo Clinic Health Oasis
http://www.mayohealth.org/
Medical Breakthroughs
http://www.ivanhoe.com/
MedWeb: History
http://www.gen.emory.edu/MEDWEB/alphakey/history.html
Monterey Bay Aquarium Online
http://www.mbayaq.org
Museum of Questionable Medical Devices
http://eatingdisorders.miningco.com/
NASA Human Spaceflight
http://station.nasa.gov/index-m.html
NASA Shuttle Web
http://shuttle.nasa.gov/
NASA Spaace Science
http://science.nasa.gov/
NASA Spacelink
http://spacelink.nasa.gov/.index.html
National Academy of Sciences
http://www.nas.edu/
National Academy Press
http://www.nap.edu/
National Geographic
http://www.nationalgeographic.com/
National Science Teachers Association
http://www.nsta.org/
Natural History on the WWW
http://www.nhm.ac.uk/info/links/general.htm#gensite
Nature
http://www.nature.com/
New Scientist
http://www.newscientist.com/
Nobel Foundation
http://www.nobel.se/
Nobel Laureates in the Sciences
http://www.lib.lsu.edu/sci/chem/guides/srs118.html

NOVA Online
http://www.pbs.org/wgbh/nova/

Paleontology Without Walls
http://www.ucmp.berkeley.edu/exhibit/exhibits.html

People & Discoveries
http://www.pbs.org/wgbh/aso/databank/

People & Discoveries
http://www.pbs.org/wgbh/aso/databank/

Periodic Table on the WWW
http://www.shef.ac.uk/~chem/web-elements/

Popular Science
http://www.popsci.com/

Questacon
http://sunsite.anu.edu.au/Questacon/

Science & Technology
http://www.artigen.com/newswire/scitech.html

Science in the Headlines
http://www.nas.edu/headlines/

Science Now
http://sciencenow.sciencemag.org/

Science Resources
http://biotech.chem.indiana.edu/pages/scitools.html

Scientific American
http://www.scientificamerican.com/

Sirs Web Guide
http://www.sirs.com/tree/science.htm

Smithsonian Institution
http://www.si.edu/start.htm

Tech Museum of Innovation
http://www.thetech.org/

The Genome Database
http://gdbwww.gdb.org/

The John Hopkins University BioInformatics Web Server
http://www.bis.med.jhmi.edu/

The Why Files
http://whyfiles.news.wisc.edu/index.html

Visible Human Viewer
http://www.npac.syr.edu/projects/vishuman/
VisibleHuman.html

Welcome to Nye Labs OnLine
http://nyelabs.kcts.org/flash_go.html

Wellcome Institute for the History of Medicine
http://www.wellcome.ac.uk/wellcomegraphic/a2/
index.html

WorldOrtho
http://worldortho.com/

PART 5. SCIENCE AND TECHNOLOGY NEWS

ABC News: Science
http://www.abcnews.com/sections/science/

American Medical News
http://www.ama-assn.org/public/journals/amnews/
amnews.htm

CBS News SciTech
http://www.wfsb.com/prd1/now/template.display?p_
who=WFSB&p_section=205

CNN Interactive Sci-Tech
http://cnn.com/TECH/

FDA News & Publications
http://www.fda.gov/opacom/hpnews.html

Fox News: Sci-Tech
http://www.foxnews.com:80/nav/stage_scitech.sml

Institute for Scientific Information
http://www.isinet.com/

Los Angeles Times: Health
http://www.latimes.com/HOME/NEWS/HEALTH/
health.htm

MSNBC Health
http://www.msnbc.com/news/HEALTH_Front.asp?a

Nando Health/Science
http://www2.nando.net/nt/health/

Nature Science Update
http://helix.nature.com/nsu/

News File Top News Stories
http://www.newsfile.com/topcwh.htm

News Scientist
http://www.newscientist.com/

NY Times on the Web: National Science
http://www.nytimes.com/yr/mo/day/national/index-
science.html

Reuters Health
http://www.reutershealth.com/

Science Daily
http://www.sciencedaily.com/

Science News Update
http://www.ama-assn.org/sci-pubs/
sci-news/1997/pres_rel.htm

SciSeek
http://www.sciseek.com/

The Chronicle of Higher Education Information
Technology
http://chronicle.com/infotech/index.htm

The Philadelphia Inquirer Health & Science
http://sln.fi.edu/inquirer/inquirer.html

UniSci
http://www.comfind.com/

Up To The Minute News
http://www.size-acceptance.org/news/

USAToday Science
http://www.usatoday.com/life/science/lsd1.htm

PART 6. USEFUL RESOURCES

4000 Years of Women in Science
http://www.astr.ua.edu/4000WS/4000WS.html

Accesses to Major English-Language Libraries On-Line
http://www.clark.net/pub/abaa-booknet/research/
librar.html

Accesses to Major English-Language Libraries On-Line
http://www.clark.net/pub/abaa-booknet/research/
librar.html

African Americans in the Sciences
http://www.lib.lsu.edu/lib/chem/display/faces.html

Albert Einstein Online
http://www.westegg.com/einstein/

All About the Internet
http://home.rmi.net/~kgr/internet/

AltaVista Translation
http://babelfish.altavista.digital.com/cgi-bin/translate?

American Cancer Society
http://www.cancer.org/

American Diabetes Association
http://www.diabetes.org/

American Lung Association
http://www.lungusa.org/

Arthritis Foundation
http://www.arthritis.org/

Aviation, Space, & Environmental Medicine
http://www.asma.org/html/journal.htm

Best Medical Resources on the Web
http://www.priory.com/other.htm

Beyond Discoery
http://www4.nas.edu/beyond/beyonddiscovery.nsf

Bio Online
http://www.bio.com/os/start/home.html

Biochemist On-line
http://www.biochemist.com/home.htm

BioLinks
http://www.biolinks.com/

Biology Labs Virtual Courseware
http://vcourseware2.calstatela.edu/

Biomechanics World Wide
http://www.per.ualberta.ca/biomechanics/

BioMedNet
http://www.biomednet.com/

BioResearch Online
http://www2.bioresearchonline.com/content/
homepage/

Brain.com
http://www.brain.com/home.cfm

Bugs in the News!
http://falcon.cc.ukans.edu/~jbrown/bugs.html

Build It Yourself
http://northshore.shore.net/~biy/

Chem4Kids
http://chem4kids.com/

Classics in the History of Psychology
http://www.yorku.ca/dept/psych/classics/

Coaching Science Abstracts
http://www-rohan.sdsu.edu/dept/coachsci/index.htm

Contributions of 20th Century Women to Physics
http://www.physics.ucla.edu/~cwp/index.html

Diabetes.com
http://www.diabetes.com/

Educational Package in Molecular Biology
http://www.bis.med.jhmi.edu/Dan/DOE/intro.html

Email List Server
http://www.tile.net/listserv/

English Weights & Measures
http://home.clara.net/brianp/index.html

Enter Evolution: Theory & History
http://www.ucmp.berkeley.edu/history/evolution.html

Ergoworld
http://www.interface-analysis.com/ergoworld/

EurekAlert!
http://www.eurekalert.org/

GeneBrowser
http://www.natx.com/

Global Medic
http://www.globalmedic.com/

Harvard Molecular & Cell Biology Links
http://mcb.harvard.edu/BioLinks.html

Health & Fitness Links: Professional Societies
http://www.tc.columbia.edu/~academic/movement/
links/societies.html

Healthgate.com
http://www.healthgate.com/

HighWire Press
http://highwire.stanford.edu/

HospitalWeb
http://neuro-www.mgh.harvard.edu/hospitalweb.shtml

HyperHistory Online
http://www.hyperhistory.com/

International Museum of Surgical Science
http://www.imss.org/

International Olympic Committee
http://www.olympic.org/map/index.html

Internet Pathology Laboratory for Medical Education
http://www-medlib.med.utah.edu/WebPath/webpath.
html

Internet@address.finder
http://iaf.net/

Journal of Medical Genetics
http://jmg.bmjjournals.com/

Liszt,, the mailing list directory
http://www.liszt.com/

Medical/Health Science Libraries on the Web
http://www.lib.uiowa.edu/hardin-www/hslibs.html

Medicine Through Time
http://www.bbc.co.uk/education/medicine/

MendelWeb
http://www.netspace.org/MendelWeb/

MolecularVision
http://www.molvis.org/molvis/

Museums Around the World
http://www.comlab.ox.ac.uk/archive/other/museums/
world.html

NASA Astrobiology
http://astrobiology.arc.nasa.gov/index.cfm

National Academy Press
http://www.nap.edu/

National Institute of Diabetes & Digestive & Kidney
Diseases
http://www.niddk.nih.gov/

National Inventors Hall of Fame
http://www.invent.org/book/

Neurosciences on the Internet
http://www.neuroguide.com/

Newspapers Online!
http://www.newspapers.com/

Newton's Apple
http://www.pbs.org/ktca/newtons/
Nobel Prize Internet Archive
http://www.almaz.com/
Oxford English Dictionary
http://www.oed.com/
People Finder: Netscape
http://database.rsnz.govt.nz/sportsci/indexnew.html
Publicly Accessible Mailing Lists
http://www.neosoft.com/internet/paml/
Quicktime VR for Macintosh & Windows
http://www.apple.com/quicktime/qtvr/index.html
Referencing Online Documents in Scientific
Publications
http://www.beadsland.com/weapas/
Referencing Online Documents in Scientific
Publications
http://www.beadsland.com/weapas/
Roget's Thesaurus
http://humanities.uchicago.edu/forms_unrest/
ROGET.html
The Aging Research Center
http://www.graylab.ac.uk/omd/index.html
The Biology Place
http://www.biology.com/
The Chemistry Place
http://www.chemplace.com/
The Educational Resources Information Center
http://www.accesseric.org:81/
The Galileo Project
http://es.rice.edu/ES/humsoc/Galileo/
The Help Web
http://www.imaginarylandscape.com/helpweb/
The Internet Index
http://www.openmarket.com/intindex/index.cfm
The Medieval Science Page
http://members.aol.com/mcnelis/medsci_index.html
The Nephron Information Center
http://www.nephron.com/

The Scout Report
http://scout.cs.wisc.edu/report/sr/current/index.html
The Tech Museum of Innovation
http://www.thetech.org/
The Ultimates
http://www.theultimates.com/
The Virtual Resource Centre for Sport Information
http://www.sportquest.com/
Three Dimensional Medical Reconstruction
http://www.crd.ge.com/esl/cgsp/projects/medical/
Top 50 Most Useful Sites
http://www.wisecat.co.uk/useful.htm
Top Ten Links
http://www.toptenlinks.com/
TransWeb
http://www.transweb.org/
Uni Academic Guide to the Internet
http://www.aldea.com/guides/ag/attframes2.html
UniGuide to United States Universities
http://www.aldea.com/guides/gu/attframes3.html
United States & Canada Medical Schools
http://www.mc.vanderbilt.edu/~aubrey/medstu/
medical_schools.html
University of Michigan Documents Center
http://www.lib.umich.edu/libhome/Documents.
center/index.html#doctop
Using the Internet
http://www.pbs.org/uti/
What is the Internet?
http://www.isoc.org/internet/
WhoWhere? People Finder
http://www.whowhere.lycos.com/
Yahoo! People Search
http://people.yahoo.com/
Yellow Pages: Netscape
http://home.netscape.com/netcenter/yellowpages.html
You Are What You Eat
http://library.advanced.org/11163/gather/
cgi-bin/wookie.cgi/

The Metric System and Conversion Constants in Exercise Physiology

Appendix C has two parts. Part 1 deals with the metric system, Part 2 discusses le Système International d'Unités (SI units)

THE METRIC SYSTEM

Most measurements in science are expressed in terms of the metric system. This system uses units that are related to one another by some power of 10. The prefix centi- means one-hundredth, milli- means one-thousandth, and the prefix kilo- is derived from a word that means one thousand. In the following sections, we show the relationship between metric units and English units of measurement that are relevant to the material presented in this book.

UNITS OF LENGTH

Metric Unit	Equivalent Metric Units	Equivalent English Units
meter (m)	100 cm; 1000 mm	39.37 in; 3.28 ft; 1.09 yd
centimeter (cm)	0.01 m; 10 mm	0.3937 in
millimeter (mm)	0.001 m; 0.1 cm	0.03937 in

UNITS OF WEIGHT

Use the following conversions for common units of mass (weight) and volume. For example, 1 ounce = 0.06 pound. Two ounces would therefore equal $2 \times 0.06 = 0.12$ pound, and 16 ounces = 0.96 pound (16×0.06).

Metric Unit	Equivalent Metric Units	Equivalent English Units
kilogram (kg)	1,000 g 1,000,000 mg	35.3 oz; 2.2046 lb
gram (g)	0.001 kg 1,000 mg	0.353 oz
milligram (mg)	0.000001 kg 0.001	0.0000353 oz

UNITS OF VOLUME

Metric Unit	Equivalent Metric Units	Equivalent English Units
liter (L)	1000 mL	1.057 qt
milliliter (mL) or cubic centimeter (cc)	0.001 L	0.001057 qt

TEMPERATURE

To convert Fahrenheit to Celsius: $°C = (°F - 32) \div 1.8$

To convert Celsius to Fahrenheit: $°F = (1.8 \div °C) + 32$

On the Fahrenheit scale, water freezes at 32°F and boils at 212°F. On the Celsius scale, water freezes at 0°C and boils at 100°C.

UNITS OF SPEED

mph	$km \cdot hr^{-1}$	$m \cdot s^{-1}$
1	1.6	0.47
2	3.2	0.94
3	4.8	1.41
4	6.4	1.88
5	8.0	2.35
6	9.6	2.82
7	11.2	3.29
8	12.8	3.76
9	14.4	4.23
10	16.0	4.70
11	17.7	5.17
12	19.3	5.64
13	20.9	6.11
14	22.5	6.58
15	24.1	7.05
16	25.8	7.52
17	27.4	7.99
18	29.0	8.46
19	30.6	8.93
20	32.2	9.40

COMMON EXPRESSIONS OF WORK, ENERGY, AND POWER

Watts	Kilocalories (kcal)	Foot-Pounds (ft · lb)
1 watt = 0.73756 ft-lb · s^{-1}	1 kcal = 3086 ft-lb	1 ft · lb = 3.2389 × 10^{-3} kcal
1 watt = 0.01433 kcal · min^{-1}	1 kcal = 426.8 kg-m	1 ft · lb = 0.13825 kg-m
1 watt = 1.341 × 10^{-3} hp or 0.0013 hp	1 kcal = 3087.4 ft-lb	1 ft · lb = 5.050 × 10^{-3} hp · h^{-1}
1 watt = 6.12 kg-m · min^{-1}	1 kcal = 1.5593 × 10^{-3} hp · h^{-1}	

TERMINOLOGY AND UNITS OF MEASUREMENT

The American College of Sports Medicine suggests that the following terminology and units of measurement be used in scientific endeavors to promote consistency and clarity of communication, and to avoid ambiguity. The terms defined below utilize the units of measurement of the Système International d'Unités (SI units).

Exercise: Any and all activity involving generation of force by the activated muscle(s) which results in disruption of a homeostatic state. In dynamic exercise, the muscle may perform shortening (concentric) contractions or be overcome by external resistance and perform lengthening (eccentric) contractions. When muscle force results in no movement, the contraction should be termed static or isometric.

Exercise intensity: A specific level of maintenance of muscular activity that can be quantified in terms of power (energy expenditure or work performed per unit of time), isometric force sustained, or velocity of progression.

Endurance: The time limit of a person's ability to maintain either a specific isometric force or a specific power level involving combinations of concentric or eccentric muscular contractions.

Mass: A quantity of matter of an object, a direct measure of the object's inertia (note: mass = weight ÷ acceleration due to gravity; unit: gram or kilogram).

Weight: The force with which a quantity of matter is attracted toward Earth by normal acceleration of gravity (traditional unit: kilogram of weight).

Energy: The capability of producing force, performing work, or generating heat (unit: joule or kilojoule).

Force: That which changes or tends to change the state of rest or motion in matter (unit: newton).

Speed: Total distance traveled per unit of time (unit: meters per second).

Velocity: Displacement per unit of time A vector quantity requiring that direction be stated or strongly implied (unit: meters per second or kilometers per hour).

Work: Force expressed through a distance but with no limitation on time (unit: joule or kilojoule). Quantities of energy and heat expressed independently of time should also be presented in joules. The term "work" should *not* be employed synonymously with muscular exercise.

Power: The rate of performing work; the derivative of work with respect to time; the product of force and velocity (unit: watt). Other related processes such as energy release and heat transfer should, when expressed per unit of time, be quantified and presented in watts.

Torque: Effectiveness of a force to produce axial rotation (unit: newton meter).

Volume: A space occupied, for example, by a quantity of fluid gas (unit: liter or milliliter). Gas volumes should be indicated as ATPS, BTPS, or STPD.

Amount of a substance: The amount of a substance is frequently expressed in moles. A mole is the quantity of a chemical substance that has a weight in mass units (e.g., grams) numerically equal to the molecular weight, or that in the case of a gas has a volume occupied by such a weight under specified conditions. One mole of a respiratory gas is equal to 22.4 liters at STPD.

SI UNITS

The uniform numerical value system is known as the Système International d'Unités, or its abbreviation, SI. SI was developed through international cooperation to create a universally acceptable system of measurement. SI ensures that units of measurement are uniform in concept and style. The SI system permits quantities in common use to be more easily compared. Many scientific organizations endorse the concept of the SI, and leading journals in nutrition, health, and exercise science now require that laboratory data be presented in SI units. The information in this appendix has been summarized from a detailed description about the SI published in the following article:

Young DS: Implementation of SI units for clinical laboratory data. Style specifications and conversion tables. *Ann. Intern. Med.,* 106:114, 1987.

DEFINITIONS OF COMMON SI UNITS

Degree Celsius (°C)	The degree Celsius (centigrade) is equivalent to K − 273.15.
Radian (rad)	The radian is the plane angle between two radii of a circle which subtend on the circumference of an arc equal in length to the radius.
Joule (J)	The joule is the work done when the point of application of a force of one newton is displaced through a distance of one meter in the direction of the force. 1 J = 1 Nm.
Kelvin (K)	The kelvin is the fraction 1/273.16 of the thermodynamic temperature of the triple point of water.
Kilogram (kg)	The kilogram is a unit of mass equal to the mass of the international prototype of the kilogram.
Meter (m)	The meter is the length equal to 1,650,763.73 wavelengths in vacuum of the radiation that corresponds to the transition between the levels $2p_{10}$ and $5d_5$ of the krypton 86 atom.
Newton (N)	The newton is that force which, when applied to a mass of one kilogram, gives it an acceleration of one meter per second squared. $1\text{ N} = 1\text{ kg} \cdot \text{m}^{-1} \cdot \text{s}^{-2}$.
Pascal (Pa)	The pascal is the pressure produced by a force of one newton applied, with uniform distribution, over an area of one square meter. $1\text{ Pa} = 1\text{ N} \cdot \text{m}^{-2}$.
Second (s)	The second is the duration of 9,192,631,770 periods of the radiation that corresponds to the transition between the two hyperfine levels of the ground state of the cesium 133 atom.
Watt (W)	The watt is the power that in one second gives rise to the energy of one joule. $1\text{ W} = 1\text{ J} \cdot \text{s}^{-1}$.

BASE UNITS OF SI NOMENCLATURE

Physical Quantity	Base Unit	SI Symbol
Length	meter	m
Mass	kilogram	kg
Time	second	s
Amount of substance	mole	mol
Thermodynamic temperature	kelvin	K
Electric current	ampere	A
Luminous intensity	candela	cd

BASE UNITS OF SI STYLE GUIDLINES

Guidelines	Example	Incorrect Style	Correct Style
Lowercase letters are used for symbols or abreviations Exceptions:	kilogram	Kg	kg
	kelvin	k	K
	ampere	a	A
	liter	l	L
Symbols are not followed by a period	meter	m.	m
Exception: end of sentence	mole	mol.	mol
Symbols are not to be pluralized	kilograms	kgs	kg
	meters	ms	m
Names and symbols are not to be combined	force	kilogram $\cdot$ meter $\cdot$ s^{-2}	kg–m $\cdot$ s^{-2} kg–m/s^2
When numbers are printed, symbols are preferred		100 meters	100 m
		2 moles	2 mol
A space should be placed between number and symbol		50ml	50 mL
The product of units is indicated by a dot above the line		kg × m/s^2	kg–m $\cdot$ s^{-2} kg–m/s^2
Only one solidus (/) should be used per expression		mmol/L/s	mmol/(L $\cdot$ s)
A zero should be placed before the decimal		.01	0.01
Decimal numbers are preferable to fractions		$^3/_4$	0.75
		75%	0.75
Spaces are used to separate long numbers		1,500,000	1 500 000
Exception: optional with four-digit number		1,000	1000 or 1 000

For SI units in exercise physiology, the term body weight is properly referred to as *mass* (kg), height should be referred to as *stature* (m), second is *s*, minute is *min*, hour is *h*, week is *wk*, month is *mo*, year is *y*, day is *d*, gram is *g*, liter is *L*, hertz is *Hz*, joule is *J*, kilocalorie is *kcal*, ohm is *Ω*, pascal is *Pa*, revolutions per minute is *rpm*, volt is *V*, and watt is *W*. These abbreviations or symbols are used for the singular or plural form.

Metabolic Computations in Open-Circuit Spirometry

STANDARDIZING GAS VOLUMES: ENVIRONMENTAL FACTORS

Gas volumes obtained during physiologic measurements are usually expressed in one of three ways: *ATPS*, *STPD*, or *BTPS*.

ATPS refers to the volume of gas at the specific conditions of measurement, which are therefore at Ambient Temperature (273°K + ambient temperature°C), ambient Pressure, and Saturated with water vapor. Gas volumes collected during open-circuit spirometry and pulmonary function tests are measured initially at ATPS.

The volume of a gas varies, however, depending on its temperature, pressure, and content of water vapor, even though the absolute number of gas molecules remains constant. These environmental influences are summarized as follows:

Temperature: The volume of a gas varies *directly* with temperature. Increasing the temperature causes the molecules to move more rapidly; the gas mixture expands, and the volume increases proportionately (*Charles' law*).

Pressure: The volume of a gas varies *inversely* with pressure. Increasing the pressure on a gas forces the molecules closer together, causing the volume to decrease in proportion to the increase in pressure (*Boyle's law*).

Water vapor: The volume of a gas varies depending on its water vapor content. The volume of a gas is greater when the gas is saturated with water vapor than it is when the same gas is dry (i.e., contains no moisture).

These three factors—temperature, pressure, and the relative degree of saturation of the gas with water vapor—must be considered, especially when gas volumes are to be compared under different environmental conditions and used subsequently in metabolic and physiologic calculations. The standards that provide the frame of reference for expressing a volume of gas are either STPD or BTPS.

STPD refers to the volume of a gas expressed under Standard conditions of Temperature (273°K or 0°C), Pressure (760 mm Hg), and Dry (no water vapor). Expressing a gas volume STPD, for example, makes it possible to evaluate and compare the volumes of expired air measured while running in the rain at high altitude, along a beach in the cold of winter, or in a hot desert environment below sea level. *In all metabolic calculations, gas volumes are always expressed at STPD.*

1. To reduce a gas volume to standard temperature (ST), the following formula is applied:

$$\text{Gas volume ST} = V_{ATPS} \times \frac{273°K}{273°K + T°C} \qquad (1)$$

where $T°C$ = temperature of the gas in the measuring device and $273°K$ = absolute temperature Kelvin, which is equivalent to 0°C.

2. The following equation is used to express a gas volume at standard pressure (SP):

$$\text{Gas volume SP} = V_{ATPS} \times \frac{P_B}{760 \text{ mmHg}} \qquad (2)$$

where P_B = ambient barometric pressure in mm Hg and 760 = standard barometric pressure at sea level, mm Hg.

3. To reduce a gas to standard dry (SD) conditions, the effects of water vapor pressure at the particular environmental temperature must be subtracted from the volume of gas. Because expired air is 100% saturated with water vapor, it is not necessary to determine its percent saturation from measures of relative humidity. The vapor pressure in moist or completely humidified air at a particular ambient temperature can be obtained in Table D.1 and is expressed in mm Hg. This vapor pressure (P_{H_2O}) is then subtracted from the ambient barometric pressure (P_B) to reduce the gas to standard pressure dry (SPD) as follows:

$$\text{Gas volume SPD} = V_{ATPS} \times \frac{P_B - P_{H_2O}}{760} \qquad (3)$$

By combining equations (1) and (3), any volume of moist air can be converted to STPD as follows:

$$\text{Gas volume STPD} = V_{ATPS}\left(\frac{273}{273 + T°C}\right)\left(\frac{P_B - P_{H_2O}}{760}\right) \qquad (4)$$

TABLE D.1
VAPOR PRESSURE (P_{H_2O}) OF WET GAS AT TEMPERATURES NORMALLY ENCOUNTERED IN THE LABORATORY

T (°C)	P_{H_2O} (mm Hg)	T (°C)	P_{H_2O} (mm Hg)
20	17.5	31	33.7
21	18.7	32	35.7
22	19.8	33	37.7
23	21.1	34	39.9
24	22.4	35	42.2
25	23.8	36	44.6
26	25.2	37	47.1
27	26.7	38	49.7
28	28.4	39	52.4
29	30.0	40	55.3
30	31.8		

TABLE D.2
FACTORS TO REDUCE MOIST GAS TO A DRY GAS VOLUME AT 0°C AND 760 mm Hg

Barometric Pressure	15	16	17	18	19	20	21	22	23	24	25	26	27	28	29	30	31	32
700	0.855	851	847	842	838	834	829	825	821	816	812	807	802	797	793	788	783	778
702	857	853	849	845	840	836	832	827	823	818	814	809	805	800	795	790	785	780
704	860	856	852	847	843	839	834	830	825	821	816	812	807	802	797	792	787	783
706	862	858	854	850	845	841	837	832	828	823	819	814	810	804	800	795	790	785
708	865	861	856	852	848	843	839	834	830	825	821	816	812	807	802	797	792	787
710	867	863	859	855	850	846	842	837	833	828	824	819	814	809	804	799	795	790
712	870	866	861	857	853	848	844	839	836	830	826	821	817	812	807	802	797	792
714	872	868	864	859	855	851	846	842	837	833	828	824	819	814	809	804	799	794
716	875	871	866	862	858	853	849	844	840	835	831	826	822	816	812	807	802	797
718	877	873	869	864	860	856	851	847	842	838	833	828	824	819	814	809	804	799
720	880	876	871	867	863	858	854	849	845	840	836	831	826	821	816	812	807	802
722	882	878	874	869	865	861	856	852	847	843	838	833	829	824	819	814	809	804
724	885	880	876	872	867	863	858	854	849	845	840	835	831	826	821	816	811	806
726	887	883	879	874	870	866	861	856	852	847	843	838	833	829	824	818	813	808
728	890	886	881	877	872	868	863	859	854	850	845	840	836	831	826	821	816	811
730	892	888	884	879	875	871	866	861	857	852	847	843	838	833	828	823	818	813
732	895	890	886	882	877	873	868	864	859	854	850	845	840	836	831	825	820	815
734	897	893	889	884	880	875	871	866	862	857	852	847	843	838	833	828	823	818
736	900	895	891	887	882	878	873	869	864	859	855	850	845	840	835	830	825	820
738	902	898	894	889	885	880	876	871	866	862	857	852	848	843	838	833	828	822
740	905	900	896	892	887	883	878	874	869	864	860	855	850	845	840	835	830	825
742	907	903	898	894	890	885	881	876	871	867	862	857	852	847	842	837	832	827
744	910	906	901	897	892	888	883	878	874	869	864	859	855	850	845	840	834	829
746	912	908	903	899	895	890	886	881	876	872	867	862	857	852	847	842	837	832
748	915	910	906	901	897	892	888	883	879	874	869	864	860	854	850	845	839	834
750	917	913	908	904	900	895	890	886	881	876	872	867	862	857	852	847	842	837
752	920	915	911	906	902	897	893	888	883	879	874	869	864	859	854	849	844	839
754	922	918	913	909	904	900	895	891	886	881	876	872	867	862	857	852	846	841
756	925	920	916	911	907	902	898	893	888	883	879	874	869	864	859	854	849	844
758	927	923	918	914	909	905	900	896	891	886	881	876	872	866	861	856	851	846
760	930	925	921	916	912	907	902	898	893	888	883	879	874	869	864	859	854	848
762	932	928	923	919	914	910	905	900	896	891	886	881	876	871	866	861	856	851
764	936	930	926	921	916	912	907	903	898	893	888	884	879	874	869	864	858	853
766	937	933	928	924	919	915	910	905	900	896	891	886	881	876	871	866	861	855
768	940	935	931	926	922	917	912	908	903	898	893	888	883	878	873	868	863	858
770	942	938	933	928	924	919	915	910	905	901	896	891	886	881	876	871	865	860

As was the case with the correction to STPD, appropriate BTPS *correction factors* are available for converting a moist gas volume at ambient conditions to a volume BTPS. These BTPS factors for a broad range of ambient temperatures are presented in Table D.3. These factors have been computed assuming a barometric pressure of 760 mm Hg, and small deviations (± 10 mm Hg) from this pressure introduce only a minimal error.

TABLE D.3
BTPS FACTORS

T (°C)	BTPS[a]	T (°C)	BTPS
20	1.102	29	1.051
21	1.096	30	1.045
22	1.091	31	1.039
23	1.085	32	1.032
24	1.080	33	1.026
25	1.075	34	1.020
26	1.068	35	1.014
27	1.063	36	1.007
28	1.057	37	1.000

[a]Body temperature, ambient pressure, and saturated with water vapor.

CALCULATION OF OXYGEN UPTAKE

In determining oxygen uptake by open-circuit spirometry, we are interested in knowing how much oxygen has been removed from the *inspired air*. Because the composition of inspired air remains relatively constant ($CO_2 = 0.03\%$, $O_2 = 20.93\%$, $N_2 = 79.04\%$), it is possible to determine how much oxygen has been removed from the inspired air by measuring the amount and composition of the expired air. When this is done, the expired air contains more carbon dioxide (usually 2.5 to 5.0%), less oxygen (usually 15.0 to 18.5%), and more nitrogen (usually 79.04 to 79.60%). It should be noted, however, that nitrogen is inert in terms of metabolism; any change in its concentration in expired air reflects the fact that the number of oxygen molecules removed from the inspired air is not replaced by the same number of carbon dioxide molecules produced in metabolism. This results in the volume of expired air (V_E, STPD) being unequal to the inspired volume (V_I, STPD). For example, if the respiratory quotient is less than 1.00 (i.e., less CO_2 produced in relation to O_2 consumed), and 3 liters of air are inspired, *less* than 3 liters of air will be expired. In this case, the nitrogen concentration is higher in the expired air than in the inspired air. This is not to say that nitrogen has been produced, only that nitrogen molecules now represent a larger percentage of V_E compared to V_I. In fact, V_E differs from V_I in direct proportion to the change in nitrogen concentration between the inspired and expired volumes. Thus, V_I can be determined from V_E using the relative change in nitrogen in an equation known as the *Haldane transformation*.

$$V_I, \text{STPD} = V_E, \text{STPD} \times \frac{\%N_{2_E}}{\%N_{2_I}} \quad (6)$$

where $\%N_{2_I} = 79.04$ and $\%N_{2_E}$ = percent nitrogen in expired air computed from gas analysis as

$$[(100 - (\%O_{2_E} + \%CO_2)].$$

The volume of O_2 in the inspired air ($\dot{V}O_{2_I}$) can then be determined as follows:

$$\dot{V}O_{2_I} = \dot{V}_I \times \%O_{2_I} \quad (7)$$

Substituting equation (6) for V_I,

$$\dot{V}O_{2_I} = \dot{V}_E \times \frac{\%N_{2_E}}{79.04\%} \times \%O_{2_I} \quad (8)$$

where $\%O_{2_I} = 20.93\%$

The amount or volume of oxygen in the expired air ($\dot{V}O_{2_E}$) is computed as

$$\dot{V}O_{2_E} = \dot{V}_E \times \%O_{2_E} \quad (9)$$

where $\%O_{2_E}$ is the fractional concentration of oxygen in expired air determined by gas analysis (chemical or electronic methods).

The amount of O_2 removed from the inspired air each minute ($\dot{V}O_2$) can then be computed as follows:

$$\dot{V}O_{2_E} = (\dot{V}_I \times \%O_{2_I}) - (\dot{V}_E \times \%O_{2_E}) \quad (10)$$

By substitution

$$\dot{V}O_2 = \left[\left(\dot{V}_E \times \frac{\%N_{2_E}}{79.04\%}\right) \times 20.93\%\right] - (\dot{V}_E \times \%O_{2_E}) \quad (11)$$

where $\dot{V}O_2$ = volume of oxygen consumed per minute, expressed in milliliters or liters, and $\dot{V}_E$ = expired air volume per minute expressed in milliliters or liters. Equation (11) can be simplified to:

$$\dot{V}O_2 = \dot{V}_E \left[\left(\frac{\%N_{2_E}}{79.04\%} \times 20.93\%\right) - \%O_{2_E}\right] \quad (12)$$

The final form of the equation is:

$$\dot{V}O_2 = \dot{V}_E[(\%N_{2_E} \times 0.265) - \%O_{2_E}] \quad (13)$$

The value obtained within the brackets in equations (12) and (13) is referred to as the *true O_2*; this represents the "oxygen extraction" or, more precisely, the percentage of oxygen consumed for any volume of air *expired*.

Although equation (13) is the equation used most widely to compute oxygen uptake from measures of expired air, it is also possible to calculate $\dot{V}O_2$ from direct measurements of both $\dot{V}_I$ and $\dot{V}_E$. In this case, the Haldane trans-formation is not used, and oxygen uptake is calculated directly as

$$\dot{V}O_2 = (\dot{V}_I \times 20.93) - (\dot{V}_E \times \%O_{2_E}) \quad (14)$$

In situations in which only $\dot{V}_I$ is measured, the $\dot{V}_E$ can be calculated from the Haldane transformation as

$$\dot{V}_E = \dot{V}_I \frac{\%N_{2_I}}{\%N_{2_E}}$$

By substitution in equation (14), the computational equation is:

$$\dot{V}O_2 = \dot{V}_I \left[\%O_{2_I} - \left(\frac{\%N_{2_I}}{\%N_{2_E}} \times \%O_{2_E} \right) \right] \quad (15)$$

CALCULATION OF CARBON DIOXIDE PRODUCTION

The carbon dioxide production per minute ($\dot{V}_{CO_2}$) is calculated as follows:

$$\dot{V}CO_2 = \dot{V}_E(\%CO_{2_E} - \%CO_{2_I}) \quad (16)$$

where $\%CO_{2_E}$ = percent carbon dioxide in expired air determined by gas analysis, and $\%CO_{2_I}$ = percent carbon dioxide in inspired air, which is essentially constant at 0.03%.

The final form of the equation is:

$$\dot{V}CO_2 = \dot{V}_E(\%CO_{2_E} - 0.03\%) \quad (17)$$

CALCULATION OF RESPIRATORY QUOTIENT

The respiratory quotient (RQ) is calculated in one of two ways:

1. $RQ = \dot{V}CO_2 / \dot{V}O_2 \quad (18)$

or

2. $RQ = \dfrac{(\%CO_{2_E} - 0.03\%)}{\text{"True" } O_2} \quad (19)$

SAMPLE METABOLIC CALCULATIONS

The following data were obtained during the last minute of a steady-rate, 10-minute treadmill run performed at 6 miles per hour at a 5% grade.

$\dot{V}_E$: 62.1 liters, ATPS
Barometric pressure: 750 mm Hg
Temperature: 26°C
%O_2 expired: 16.86 (O_2 analyzer)
%CO_2 expired: 3.60 (CO_2 analyzer)
%N_2 expired: $[100 - (16.86 + 3.60)] = 79.54$

Determine the following:

1. $\dot{V}_E$, STPD
2. $\dot{V}O_2$, STPD
3. $\dot{V}CO_2$ STPD
4. RQ
5. kcal · min^{-1}

1. $\dot{V}_E$, STPD (use equation 4 or STPD correction factor in Table D.2).

$$\dot{V}_E, \text{STPD} = \dot{V}_E, \text{ATPS} \left(\frac{273}{273 + T°C} \right) \left(\frac{P_B - P_{H_2O}}{760} \right)$$

$$= 62.1 \left(\frac{273}{299} \right) \left(\frac{750 - 25.2}{760} \right)$$

$$= 54.07 \text{ L} \cdot \text{min}^{-1}$$

2. $\dot{V}O_2$, STPD (use equation 13)

$$\dot{V}O_2, \text{STPD} = \dot{V}_E, \text{STPD} \, [(\%N_{2_E} \times 0.265) - \%O_{2_E}]$$

$$= 54.07 \, [(0.7954 \times 0.265) - 0.1686]$$

$$= 54.07 \, (0.0422)$$

$$= 2.281 \text{ L} \cdot \text{min}^{-1}$$

3. $\dot{V}CO_2$, STPD (use equation 17)

$$\dot{V}CO_2, \text{STPD} = \dot{V}_E, \text{STPD} \, (CO_{2_E} - 0.03\%)$$

$$= 54.07 \, (0.0360 - 0.0003)$$

$$= 54.07 \, (0.0357)$$

$$= 1.930 \text{ L} \cdot \text{min}^{-1}$$

4. RQ (use equation 18 or 19)

$$RQ = \dot{V}CO_2 / \dot{V}O_2$$

$$= \frac{1.930}{2.281}$$

$$= 0.846$$

or

$$RQ = \frac{(\%CO_{2_E} - 0.03\%)}{\text{"true" } O_2}$$

$$= \frac{3.60 - .03}{4.22}$$

$$= 0.846$$

Because the exercise was performed in a steady-rate of aerobic metabolism, the obtained RQ of 0.846 can be applied in Table 8.1 to obtain the appropriate caloric transformation. In this way, the exercise oxygen uptake can be transposed to kcal of energy expended per minute as follows:

5. Energy expenditure (kcal · min^{-1}) = $\dot{V}O_2$ (liters · min^{-1}) × caloric equivalent per liter O_2 at the given steady-rate RQ

Energy expenditure $= 2.281 \times 4.862$

$$= 11.09 \text{ kcal} \cdot \text{min}^{-1}$$

Assuming that the RQ value reflects the nonprotein RQ, a reasonable estimate of both the percentage and quantity of lipid and carbohydrate metabolized during each minute of the run can be obtained from Table 8.1.

Percentage kcal derived from lipid $= 50.7\%$

Percentage kcal derived from carbohydrate $= 49.3\%$

Grams of lipid utilized $= 0.267$ g per liter of oxygen or approximately 0.61 g per minute (0.267×2.281 L O_2)

Grams of carbohydrate utilized $= 0.580$ g per liter of oxygen, or approximately 1.36 g per minute (0.580×2.281 L O_2)

APPENDIX E

Frequently Cited Journals in Exercise Physiology

Journal	Abbreviation	Journal	Abbreviation
Acta Medica Scandinavica	Acta Med Scand	Journal of Clinical Endocrinology and Metabolism	J Clin Endocrinol Metab
Acta Physiologica Scandinavica	Acta Physiol Scand	Journal of Clinical Investigation	J Clin Invest
American Journal of Clinical Nutrition	Am J Clin Nutr	Journal of Gerontology	J Gerontol
American Heart Journal	Am Heart J	Journal of Human Movement Studies	J Hum Mov Stud
American Journal of Anatomy	Am J Anat	Journal of Laboratory and Clinical Medicine	J Lab Clin Med
American Journal of Cardiology	Am J Cardiol		
American Journal of Epidemiology	Am J Epidemiol	Journal of Lipid Research	J Lipid Res
American Journal of Human Biology	Am J Hum Biol	Journal of Molecular Biology	J Mole Bio
American Journal of Physical Anthropology	Am J Phys Anthropol	Journal of Neurophysiology	J Neurophysiol
		Journal of Nutrition	J Nutr
American Journal of Physiology	Am J Physiol	Journal of Parenteral and Enteral Nutrition	JPEN
American Journal of Public Health	Am J Public Health		
American Journal of Sports Medicine	Am J Sports Med	Journal of Pediatrics	J Pediatr
Annals of Human Biology	Ann Hum Biol	Journal of Physical and Medical Rehabilitation	J Phys Med Rehabil
Annals of Internal Medicine	Ann Intern Med		
Annals of Nutrition and Metabolism	Ann Nut Met	Journal of Physiology	J Physiol
Appetite	Appetite	Journal of Sport and Exercise Psychology	J Sport Exerc Psychol
Archives of Environmental Health	Arch Environ Health		
Atherosclerosis	Atherosclerosis	Journal of Sport Psychology	J Sport Psychol
Aviation and Space Environmental Medicine	Aviat Space Environ Med	Journal of Sports Medicine and Physical Fitness	J Sports Med Phys Fitness
Brain: Journal of Neurology	Brain	Journal of Sports Sciences	J Sports Sci
British Heart Journal	Br Heart J	Journal of Strength and Conditioning Research	JSCR
British Journal of Nutrition	Br J Nutr		
British Journal of Sports Medicine	Br J Sports Med	Journal of the American Dietetic Association	J Am Diet Assoc
British Medical Journal	Br Med J		
Canadian Journal of Applied Physiology	Can J Appl Physiol	Journal of the American Medical Association (JAMA)	JAMA
Canadian Journal of Applied Sports Sciences	Can J Appl Sport Sci	Journal of Sports Medicine	J Sports Med
Cellular Physiology and Biochemistry	Cell Physiol Biochem	Lancet	Lancet
Circulation Research	Circ Res	Medicine and Science in Sports and Exercise	Med Sci Sports Exerc
Circulation: Journal of the American Heart Association	Circulation	Medicine and Sport Science	Med Sport Sci
Clinical Biomechanics	Clin Biomech	Molecular Genetics and Metabolism	Mol Gen Metabol
Clinical Chemistry	Clin Chem	Muscle and Nerve	Muscle Nerve
Clinical Nutrition	Clin Nutr	Molecular Medicine Today	Mol Med Today
Clinical Science	Clin Sci	Nature	Nature
Clinical Sports Medicine	Clin Sports Med	Neuroscience Letters	Neurosci Lett
Diabetes	Diabetes	New England Journal of Medicine	N Engl J Med
Diabetologia	Diabetologia	Nutrition Abstracts and Reviews	Nutr Abstr Rev
Endocrinology	Endocrinology	Nutrition and Metabolism	Nutr Metab
Ergonomics	Ergonomics	Nutrition Reviews	Nutr Rev
European Journal of Applied Physiology	Eur J Appl Physiol	Pediatric Exercise Science	Pediatr Exerc Sci
		Pediatrics	Pediatrics
Exercise Immunology Review	Exerc Immun Rev	Physical Therapy Reviews	Phys Ther Rev
Experientia	Experientia	Physician and Sportsmedicine	Physician Sportsmed
Experimental Brain Research	Exp Brain Res	Physiological Reviews	Physiol Rev
FASEB Journal	FASEB J	Preventive Medicine	Prev Med
Fertility and Sterility	Fertil Steril	Proceedings of the Nutrition Society	Proc Nutr Soc
Geriatrics	Geriatrics		
Growth	Growth	Psychosomatic Medicine	Psychosom Med
Human Biology	Hum Biol	Public Health Reports	Public Health Rep
Human Heredity	Hum Her	Radiology	Radiology
Human Movement Science	Hum Mov Sci	Research Quarterly for Exercise and Sports	Res Q Exerc Sport
International Journal of Obesity	Int J Obes		
International Journal of Sports Medicine	Int J Sports Med	Scandinavian Journal of Sports Science	Scand J Sports Sci
International Journal of Sport Nutrition	IJSN	Science	Science
		Science in Sport	Sci Sport
International Journal for Vitamin and Nutrition Research	Int J Vitam Nutr Res	Scientific American	Sci Am
		Sports Medicine	Sports Med
Journal of Aging and Physical Activity	J Aging Phys Act	Sports Medicine, Training and Rehabilitation	Sports Med Train Rehabil
Journal of Applied Physiology	J Appl Physiol		
Journal of Biological Chemistry	J Biol Chem	Sport Science Review	Sport Sci Rev
Journal of Biomechanics	J Biomech	World Review of Nutrition and Dietetics	World Rev Nut Diet
Journal of Bone and Joint Surgery	J Bone Joint Surg		

Evaluation of Body Composition —Girth Method

This appendix contains the age- and sex-specific equations to predict body fat percentage based on three girth measurements. There are four charts, one each for young and older men and women. In our experience, it is important to calibrate the tape measure prior to its use. Use a meter stick as the standard and check the markings on the cloth tape at 10-cm increments. A cloth tape is preferred over a metal one because there is little skin compression when applying a cloth tape to the skin's surface at a relatively constant tension.

To use the charts, measure the three girths for your age and gender as follows:

Age (years)	Sex	Site A	Site B	Site C
18–26	M	Right upper arm	Abdomen	Right forearm
	F	Abdomen	Right thigh	Right forearm
27–50	M	Buttocks	Abdomen	Right forearm
	F	Abdomen	Right thigh	Right calf

A step-by-step explanation of how to compute the relative and absolute values for body fat, lean body mass, and desirable body mass from the Appendix F charts is presented in Chapter 16. The specific equation to predict percent body fat with its corresponding constant is presented at the bottom of each of the Appendix F charts.

CHART F.1
CONVERSION CONSTANTS TO PREDICT PERCENT BODY FAT FOR YOUNG MEN[a]

Upper Arm			Abdomen			Forearm		
in	cm	Constant A	in	cm	Constant B	in	cm	Constant C
7.00	17.78	25.91	21.00	53.34	27.56	7.00	17.78	38.01
7.25	18.41	26.83	21.25	53.97	27.88	7.25	18.41	39.37
7.50	19.05	27.76	21.50	54.61	28.21	7.50	19.05	40.72
7.75	19.68	28.68	21.75	55.24	28.54	7.75	19.68	42.08
8.00	20.32	29.61	22.00	55.88	28.87	8.00	20.32	43.44
8.25	20.95	30.53	22.25	56.51	29.20	8.25	20.95	44.80
8.50	21.59	31.46	22.50	57.15	29.52	8.50	21.59	46.15
8.75	22.22	32.38	22.75	57.78	29.85	8.75	22.22	47.51
9.00	22.86	33.31	23.00	58.42	30.18	9.00	22.86	48.87
9.25	23.49	34.24	23.25	59.05	30.51	9.25	23.49	50.23
9.50	24.13	35.16	23.50	59.69	30.84	9.50	24.13	51.58
9.75	24.76	36.09	23.75	60.32	31.16	9.75	24.76	52.94
10.00	25.40	37.01	24.00	60.96	31.49	10.00	25.40	54.30
10.25	26.03	37.94	24.25	61.59	31.82	10.25	26.03	55.65
10.50	26.67	38.86	24.50	62.23	32.15	10.50	26.67	57.01
10.75	27.30	39.79	24.75	62.86	32.48	10.75	27.30	58.37
11.00	27.94	40.71	25.00	63.50	32.80	11.00	27.94	59.73
11.25	28.57	41.64	25.25	64.13	33.13	11.25	28.57	61.08
11.50	29.21	42.56	25.50	64.77	33.46	11.50	29.21	62.44
11.75	29.84	43.49	25.75	65.40	33.79	11.75	29.84	63.80
12.00	30.48	44.41	26.00	66.04	34.12	12.00	30.48	65.16
12.25	31.11	45.34	26.25	66.67	34.44	12.25	31.11	66.51
12.50	31.75	46.26	26.50	67.31	34.77	12.50	31.75	67.87
12.75	32.38	47.19	26.75	67.94	35.10	12.75	32.38	69.23
13.00	33.02	48.11	27.00	68.58	35.43	13.00	33.02	70.59
13.25	33.65	49.04	27.25	69.21	35.76	13.25	33.65	71.94
13.50	34.29	49.96	27.50	69.85	36.09	13.50	34.29	73.30

Upper Arm			Abdomen			Forearm		
in	cm	Constant A	in	cm	Constant B	in	cm	Constant C
13.75	34.92	50.89	27.75	70.48	36.41	13.75	34.92	74.66
14.00	35.56	51.82	28.00	71.12	36.74	14.00	35.56	76.02
14.25	36.19	52.74	28.25	71.75	37.07	14.25	36.19	77.37
14.50	36.83	53.67	28.50	72.39	37.40	14.50	36.83	78.73
14.75	37.46	54.59	28.75	73.02	37.73	14.75	37.46	80.09
15.00	38.10	55.52	29.00	73.66	38.05	15.00	38.10	81.45
15.25	38.73	56.44	29.25	74.29	38.38	15.25	38.73	82.80
15.50	39.37	57.37	29.50	74.93	38.71	15.50	39.37	84.16
15.75	40.00	58.29	29.75	75.56	39.04	15.75	40.00	85.52
16.00	40.64	59.22	30.00	76.20	39.37	16.00	40.64	86.88
16.25	41.27	60.14	30.25	76.83	39.69	16.25	41.27	88.23
16.50	41.91	61.07	30.50	77.47	40.02	16.50	41.91	89.59
16.75	42.54	61.99	30.75	78.10	40.35	16.75	42.54	90.95
17.00	43.18	62.92	31.00	78.74	40.68	17.00	43.18	92.31
17.25	43.81	63.84	31.25	79.37	41.01	17.25	43.81	93.66
17.50	44.45	64.77	31.50	80.01	41.33	17.50	44.45	95.02
17.75	45.08	65.69	31.75	80.64	41.66	17.75	45.08	96.38
18.00	45.72	66.62	32.00	81.28	41.99	18.00	45.72	97.74
18.25	46.35	67.54	32.25	81.91	42.32	18.25	46.35	99.09
18.50	46.99	68.47	32.50	82.55	42.65	18.50	46.99	100.45
18.75	47.62	69.40	32.75	83.18	42.97	18.75	47.62	101.81
19.00	48.26	70.32	33.00	83.82	43.30	19.00	48.26	103.17
19.25	48.89	71.25	33.25	84.45	43.63	19.25	48.89	104.52
19.50	49.53	72.17	33.50	85.09	43.96	19.50	49.53	105.88
19.75	50.16	73.10	33.75	85.72	44.29	19.75	50.16	107.24
20.00	50.80	74.02	34.00	86.36	44.61	20.00	50.80	108.60
20.25	51.43	74.95	34.25	86.99	44.94	20.25	51.43	109.95
20.50	52.07	75.87	34.50	87.63	45.27	20.50	52.07	111.31
20.75	52.70	76.80	34.75	88.26	45.60	20.75	52.70	112.67
21.00	53.34	77.72	35.00	88.90	45.93	21.00	53.34	114.02
21.25	53.97	78.65	35.25	89.53	46.25	21.25	53.97	115.38
21.50	54.61	79.57	35.50	90.17	46.58	21.50	54.61	116.74
21.75	55.24	80.50	35.75	90.80	46.91	21.75	55.24	118.10
22.00	55.88	81.42	36.00	91.44	47.24	22.00	55.88	119.45
			36.25	92.07	47.57			
			36.50	92.71	47.89			
			36.75	93.34	48.22			
			37.00	93.98	48.55			
			37.25	94.61	48.88			
			37.50	95.25	49.21			
			37.75	95.88	49.54			
			38.00	96.52	49.86			
			38.25	97.15	50.19			
			38.50	97.79	50.52			
			38.75	98.42	50.85			
			39.00	99.06	51.18			
			39.25	99.69	51.50			
			39.50	100.33	51.83			
			39.75	100.96	52.16			
			40.00	101.60	52.49			
			40.25	102.23	52.82			
			40.50	102.87	53.14			
			40.75	103.50	53.47			
			41.00	104.14	53.80			
			41.25	104.77	54.13			
			41.50	105.41	54.46			
			41.75	106.04	54.78			
			42.00	106.68	55.11			

Note: Percent Fat = Constant A + Constant B − Constant C − 10.2

CHART F.2
CONVERSION CONSTANTS TO PREDICT PERCENT BODY FAT FOR OLDER MEN[a]

Buttocks			Abdomen			Forearm		
in	cm	Constant A	in	cm	Constant B	in	cm	Constant C
28.00	71.12	29.34	25.50	64.77	22.84	7.00	17.78	21.01
28.25	71.75	29.60	25.75	65.40	23.06	7.25	18.41	21.76
28.50	72.39	29.87	26.00	66.04	23.29	7.50	19.05	22.52
28.75	73.02	30.13	26.25	66.67	23.51	7.75	19.68	23.26
29.00	73.66	30.39	26.50	67.31	23.73	8.00	20.32	24.02
29.25	74.29	30.65	26.75	67.94	23.96	8.25	20.95	24.76
29.50	74.93	30.92	27.00	68.58	24.18	8.50	21.59	25.52
29.75	75.56	31.18	27.25	69.21	24.40	8.75	22.22	26.26
30.00	76.20	31.44	27.50	69.85	24.63	9.00	22.86	27.02
30.25	76.83	31.70	27.75	70.48	24.85	9.25	23.49	27.76
30.50	77.47	31.96	28.00	71.12	25.08	9.50	24.13	28.52
30.75	78.10	32.22	28.25	71.75	25.29	9.75	24.76	29.26
31.00	78.74	32.49	28.50	72.39	25.52	10.00	25.40	30.02
31.25	79.37	32.75	28.75	73.02	25.75	10.25	26.03	30.76
31.50	80.01	33.01	29.00	73.66	25.97	10.50	26.67	31.52
31.75	80.64	33.27	29.25	74.29	26.19	10.75	27.30	32.27
32.00	81.28	33.54	29.50	74.93	26.42	11.00	27.94	33.02
32.25	81.91	33.80	29.75	75.56	26.64	11.25	28.57	33.77
32.50	82.55	34.06	30.00	76.20	26.87	11.50	29.21	34.52
32.75	83.18	34.32	30.25	76.83	27.09	11.75	29.84	35.27
33.00	83.82	34.58	30.50	77.47	27.32	12.00	30.48	36.02
33.25	84.45	34.84	30.75	78.10	27.54	12.25	31.11	36.77
33.50	85.09	35.11	31.00	78.74	27.76	12.50	31.75	37.53
33.75	85.72	35.37	31.25	79.37	27.98	12.75	32.38	38.27
34.00	86.36	35.63	31.50	80.01	28.21	13.00	33.02	39.03
34.25	86.99	35.89	31.75	80.64	28.43	13.25	33.65	39.77
34.50	87.63	36.16	32.00	81.28	28.66	13.50	34.29	40.53
34.75	88.26	36.42	32.25	81.91	28.88	13.75	34.92	41.27
35.00	88.90	36.68	32.50	82.55	29.11	14.00	35.56	42.03
35.25	89.53	36.94	32.75	83.18	29.33	14.25	36.19	42.77
35.50	90.17	37.20	33.00	83.82	29.55	14.50	36.83	43.53
35.75	90.80	37.46	33.25	84.45	29.78	14.75	37.46	44.27
36.00	91.44	37.73	33.50	85.09	30.00	15.00	38.10	45.03
36.25	92.07	37.99	33.75	85.72	30.22	15.25	38.73	45.77
36.50	92.71	38.25	34.00	86.36	30.45	15.50	39.37	46.53
36.75	93.34	38.51	34.25	86.99	30.67	15.75	40.00	47.28
37.00	93.98	38.78	34.50	87.63	30.89	16.00	40.64	48.03
37.25	94.61	39.04	34.75	88.26	31.12	16.25	41.27	48.78
37.50	95.25	39.30	35.00	88.90	31.35	16.50	41.91	49.53
37.75	95.88	39.56	35.25	89.53	31.57	16.75	42.54	50.28
38.00	96.52	39.82	35.50	90.17	31.79	17.00	43.18	51.03
38.25	97.15	40.08	35.75	90.80	32.02	17.25	43.81	51.78
38.50	97.79	40.35	36.00	91.44	32.24	17.50	44.45	52.54
38.75	98.42	40.61	36.25	92.07	32.46	17.75	45.08	53.28
39.00	99.06	40.87	36.50	92.71	32.69	18.00	45.72	54.04
39.25	99.69	41.13	36.75	93.34	32.91	18.25	46.35	54.78
39.50	100.33	41.39	37.00	93.98	33.14			
39.75	100.96	41.66	37.25	94.61	33.36			
40.00	101.60	41.92	37.50	95.25	33.58			
40.25	102.23	42.18	37.75	95.88	33.81			
40.50	102.87	42.44	38.00	96.52	34.03			
40.75	103.50	42.70	38.25	97.15	34.26			
41.00	104.14	42.97	38.50	97.79	34.48			
41.25	104.77	43.23	38.75	98.42	34.70			
41.50	105.41	43.49	39.00	99.06	34.93			
41.75	106.04	43.75	39.25	99.69	35.15			
42.00	106.68	44.02	39.50	100.33	35.38			
42.25	107.31	44.28	39.75	100.96	35.59			
42.50	107.95	44.54	40.00	101.60	35.82			

Buttocks			Abdomen			Forearm		
in	**cm**	**Constant A**	**in**	**cm**	**Constant B**	**in**	**cm**	**Constant C**
42.75	108.58	44.80	40.25	102.23	36.05			
43.00	109.22	45.06	40.50	102.87	36.27			
43.25	109.85	45.32	40.75	103.50	36.49			
43.50	110.49	45.59	41.00	104.14	36.72			
43.75	111.12	45.85	41.25	104.77	36.94			
44.00	111.76	46.12	41.50	105.41	37.17			
44.25	112.39	46.37	41.75	106.04	37.39			
44.50	113.03	46.64	42.00	106.68	37.62			
44.75	113.66	46.89	42.25	107.31	37.87			
45.00	114.30	47.16	42.50	107.95	38.06			
45.25	114.93	47.42	42.75	108.58	38.28			
45.50	115.57	47.68	43.00	109.22	38.51			
45.75	116.20	47.94	43.25	109.85	38.73			
46.00	116.84	48.21	43.50	110.49	38.96			
46.25	117.47	48.47	43.75	111.12	39.18			
46.50	118.11	48.73	44.00	111.76	39.41			
46.75	118.74	48.99	44.25	112.39	39.63			
47.00	119.38	49.26	44.50	113.03	39.85			
47.25	120.01	49.52	44.75	113.66	40.08			
47.50	120.65	49.78	45.00	114.30	40.30			
47.75	121.28	50.04						
48.00	121.92	50.30						
48.25	122.55	50.56						
48.50	123.19	50.83						
48.75	123.82	51.09						
49.00	124.46	51.35						

Note: Percent Fat = Constant A + Constant B − Constant C − 15.0

[a]Copyright © 1986, 1991, 1996, 2000 by Frank I. Katch, Victor L. Katch, and William D. McArdle, and Fitness Technologies, Inc., 1132 Lincoln Ave. Ann Arbor, MI 48104. No part of this appendix may be reproduced in any manner without written permission from the copyright holders.

CHART F.3
CONVERSION CONSTANTS TO PREDICT PERCENT BODY FAT FOR YOUNG WOMEN[a]

Abdomen			Thigh			Forearm		
in	**cm**	**Constant A**	**in**	**cm**	**Constant B**	**in**	**cm**	**Constant C**
20.00	50.80	26.74	14.00	35.56	29.13	6.00	15.24	25.86
20.25	51.43	27.07	14.25	36.19	29.65	6.25	15.87	26.94
20.50	52.07	27.41	14.50	36.83	30.17	6.50	16.51	28.02
20.75	52.70	27.74	14.75	37.46	30.69	6.75	17.14	29.10
21.00	53.34	28.07	15.00	38.10	31.21	7.00	17.78	30.17
21.25	53.97	28.41	15.25	38.73	31.73	7.25	18.41	31.25
21.50	54.61	28.74	15.50	39.37	32.25	7.50	19.05	32.33
21.75	55.24	29.08	15.75	40.00	32.77	7.75	19.68	33.41
22.00	55.88	29.41	16.00	40.64	33.29	8.00	20.32	34.48
22.25	56.51	29.74	16.25	41.27	33.81	8.25	20.95	35.56
22.50	57.15	30.08	16.50	41.91	34.33	8.50	21.59	36.64
22.75	57.78	30.41	16.75	42.54	34.85	8.75	22.22	37.72
23.00	58.42	30.75	17.00	43.18	35.37	9.00	22.86	38.79
23.25	59.05	31.08	17.25	43.81	35.89	9.25	23.49	39.87
23.50	59.69	31.42	17.50	44.45	36.41	9.50	24.13	40.95
23.75	60.32	31.75	17.75	45.08	36.93	9.75	24.76	42.03
24.00	60.96	32.08	18.00	45.72	37.45	10.00	25.40	43.10
24.25	61.59	32.42	18.25	46.35	37.97	10.25	26.03	44.18
24.50	62.23	32.75	18.50	46.99	38.49	10.50	26.67	45.26
24.75	62.86	33.09	18.75	47.62	39.01	10.75	27.30	46.34
25.00	63.50	33.42	19.00	48.26	39.53	11.00	27.94	47.41
25.25	64.13	33.76	19.25	48.89	40.05	11.25	28.57	48.49
25.50	64.77	34.09	19.50	49.53	40.57	11.50	29.21	49.57

Continued

Abdomen			Thigh			Forearm		
in	cm	Constant A	in	cm	Constant B	in	cm	Constant C
25.75	65.40	34.42	19.75	50.16	41.09	11.75	29.84	50.65
26.00	66.04	34.76	20.00	50.80	41.61	12.00	30.48	51.73
26.25	66.67	35.09	20.25	51.43	42.13	12.25	31.11	52.80
26.50	67.31	35.43	20.50	52.07	42.65	12.50	31.75	53.88
26.75	67.94	35.76	20.75	52.70	43.17	12.75	32.38	54.96
27.00	68.58	36.10	21.00	53.34	43.69	13.00	33.02	56.04
27.25	69.21	36.43	21.25	53.97	44.21	13.25	33.65	57.11
27.50	69.85	36.76	21.50	54.61	44.73	13.50	34.29	58.19
27.75	70.48	37.10	21.75	55.24	45.25	13.75	34.92	59.27
28.00	71.12	37.43	22.00	55.88	45.77	14.00	35.56	60.35
28.25	71.75	37.77	22.25	56.51	46.29	14.25	36.19	61.42
28.50	72.39	38.10	22.50	57.15	46.81	14.50	36.83	62.50
28.75	73.02	38.43	22.75	57.78	47.33	14.75	37.46	63.58
29.00	73.66	38.77	23.00	58.42	47.85	15.00	38.10	64.66
29.25	74.29	39.10	23.25	59.05	48.37	15.25	38.73	65.73
29.50	74.93	39.44	23.50	59.69	48.89	15.50	39.37	66.81
29.75	75.56	39.77	23.75	60.32	49.41	15.75	40.00	67.89
30.00	76.20	40.11	24.00	60.96	49.93	16.00	40.64	68.97
30.25	76.83	40.44	24.25	61.59	50.45	16.25	41.27	70.04
30.50	77.47	40.77	24.50	62.23	50.97	16.50	41.91	71.12
30.75	78.10	41.11	24.75	62.86	51.49	16.75	42.54	72.20
31.00	78.74	41.44	25.00	63.50	52.01	17.00	43.18	73.28
31.25	79.37	41.78	25.25	64.13	52.53	17.25	43.81	74.36
31.50	80.01	42.11	25.50	64.77	53.05	17.50	44.45	75.43
31.75	80.64	42.45	25.75	65.40	53.57	17.75	45.08	76.51
32.00	81.28	42.78	26.00	66.04	54.09	18.00	45.72	77.59
32.25	81.91	43.11	26.25	66.67	54.61	18.25	46.35	78.67
32.50	82.55	43.45	26.50	67.31	55.13	18.50	46.99	79.74
32.75	83.18	43.78	26.75	67.94	55.65	18.75	47.62	80.82
33.00	83.82	44.12	27.00	68.58	56.17	19.00	48.26	81.90
33.25	84.45	44.45	27.25	69.21	56.69	19.25	48.89	82.98
33.50	85.09	44.78	27.50	69.85	57.21	19.50	49.53	84.05
33.75	85.72	45.12	27.75	70.48	57.73	19.75	50.16	85.13
34.00	86.36	45.45	28.00	71.12	58.26	20.00	50.80	86.21
34.25	86.99	45.79	28.25	71.75	58.78			
34.50	87.63	46.12	28.50	72.39	59.30			
34.75	88.26	46.46	38.75	73.02	59.82			
35.00	88.90	46.79	29.00	73.66	60.34			
35.25	89.53	47.12	29.25	74.29	60.86			
35.50	90.17	47.46	29.50	74.93	61.38			
35.75	90.80	47.79	29.75	75.56	61.90			
36.00	91.44	48.13	30.00	76.20	62.42			
36.25	92.07	48.46	30.25	76.83	62.94			
36.50	92.71	48.80	30.50	77.47	63.46			
36.75	93.34	49.13	30.75	78.10	63.98			
37.00	93.98	49.46	31.00	78.74	64.50			
37.25	94.61	49.80	31.25	79.37	65.02			
37.50	95.25	50.13	31.50	80.01	65.54			
37.75	95.88	50.47	31.75	80.64	66.06			
38.00	96.52	50.80	32.00	81.28	66.58			
38.25	97.15	51.13	32.25	81.91	67.10			
38.50	97.79	51.47	32.50	82.55	67.62			
38.75	98.42	51.80	32.75	83.18	68.14			
39.00	99.06	52.14	33.00	83.82	68.66			
39.25	99.69	52.47	33.25	84.45	69.18			
39.50	100.33	52.81	33.50	85.09	69.70			
39.75	100.96	53.14	33.75	85.72	70.22			
40.00	101.60	53.47	34.00	86.36	70.74			

Note: Percent Fat = Constant A + Constant B − Constant C − 19.6

CHART F.4
CONVERSION CONSTANTS TO PREDICT PERCENT BODY FAT FOR OLDER WOMEN[a]

Abdomen			Thigh			Forearm		
in	cm	Constant A	in	cm	Constant B	in	cm	Constant C
25.00	63.50	29.69	14.00	35.56	17.31	10.00	25.40	14.46
25.25	64.13	29.98	14.25	36.19	17.62	10.25	26.03	14.82
25.50	64.77	30.28	14.50	36.83	17.93	10.50	26.67	15.18
25.75	65.40	30.58	14.75	37.46	18.24	10.75	27.30	15.54
26.00	66.04	30.87	15.00	38.10	18.55	11.00	27.94	15.91
26.25	66.67	31.17	15.25	38.73	18.86	11.25	28.57	16.27
26.50	67.31	31.47	15.50	39.37	19.17	11.50	29.21	16.63
26.75	67.94	31.76	15.75	40.00	19.47	11.75	29.84	16.99
27.00	68.58	32.06	16.00	40.64	19.78	12.00	30.48	17.35
27.25	69.21	32.36	16.25	41.27	20.09	12.25	31.11	17.71
27.50	69.85	32.65	16.50	41.91	20.40	12.50	31.75	18.08
27.75	70.48	32.95	16.75	42.54	20.71	12.75	32.38	18.44
28.00	71.12	33.25	17.00	43.18	21.02	13.00	33.02	18.80
28.25	71.75	33.55	17.25	43.81	21.33	13.25	33.65	19.16
28.50	72.39	33.84	17.50	44.45	21.64	13.50	34.29	19.52
28.75	73.02	34.14	17.75	45.08	21.95	13.75	34.92	19.88
29.00	73.66	34.44	18.00	45.72	22.26	14.00	35.56	20.24
29.25	74.29	34.73	18.25	46.35	22.57	14.25	36.19	20.61
29.50	74.93	35.03	18.50	46.99	22.87	14.50	36.83	20.97
29.75	75.56	35.33	18.75	47.62	23.18	14.75	37.46	21.33
30.00	76.20	35.62	19.00	38.26	23.49	15.00	38.10	21.69
30.25	76.83	35.92	19.25	48.89	23.80	15.25	38.73	22.05
30.50	77.47	36.22	19.50	49.53	24.11	15.50	39.37	22.41
30.75	78.10	36.51	19.75	50.16	24.42	15.75	40.00	22.77
31.00	78.74	36.81	20.00	50.80	24.73	16.00	40.64	23.14
31.25	79.37	37.11	20.25	51.43	25.04	16.25	41.27	23.50
31.50	80.01	37.40	20.50	52.07	25.35	16.50	41.91	23.86
31.75	80.64	37.70	20.75	52.70	25.66	16.75	42.54	24.22
32.00	81.28	38.00	21.00	53.34	25.97	17.00	43.18	24.58
32.25	81.91	38.30	21.25	53.97	26.28	17.25	43.81	24.94
32.50	82.55	38.59	21.50	54.61	26.58	17.50	44.45	25.31
32.75	83.18	38.89	21.75	55.24	26.89	17.75	45.08	25.67
33.00	83.82	39.19	22.00	55.88	27.20	18.00	45.72	26.03
33.25	84.45	39.48	22.25	56.51	27.51	18.25	46.35	26.39
33.50	85.09	39.78	22.50	57.15	27.82	18.50	46.99	26.75
33.75	85.72	40.08	22.75	57.78	28.13	18.75	47.62	27.11
34.00	86.36	40.37	23.00	58.42	28.44	19.00	48.26	27.47
34.25	86.99	40.67	23.25	59.05	28.75	19.25	48.89	27.84
34.50	87.63	40.97	23.50	59.69	29.06	19.50	49.53	28.20
34.75	88.26	41.26	23.75	60.32	29.37	19.75	50.16	28.56
35.00	88.90	41.56	24.00	60.96	29.68	20.00	50.80	28.92
35.25	89.53	41.86	24.25	61.59	29.98	20.25	51.43	29.28
35.50	90.17	42.15	24.50	62.23	30.29	20.50	52.07	29.64
35.75	90.80	42.45	24.75	62.86	30.60	20.75	52.70	30.00
36.00	91.44	42.75	25.00	63.50	30.91	21.00	53.34	30.37
36.25	92.07	43.05	25.25	64.13	31.22	21.25	53.97	30.73
36.50	92.71	43.34	25.50	64.77	31.53	21.50	54.61	31.09
36.75	93.35	43.64	25.75	65.40	31.84	21.75	55.24	31.45
37.00	93.98	43.94	26.00	66.04	32.15	22.00	55.88	31.81
37.25	94.62	44.23	26.25	66.67	32.46	22.25	56.51	32.17
37.50	95.25	44.53	26.50	67.31	32.77	22.50	57.15	32.54
37.75	95.89	44.83	26.75	67.94	33.08	22.75	57.78	32.90
38.00	96.52	45.12	27.00	68.58	33.38	23.00	58.42	33.26
38.25	97.16	45.42	27.25	69.21	33.69	23.25	59.05	33.62
38.50	97.79	45.72	27.50	69.85	34.00	23.50	59.69	33.98
38.75	98.43	46.01	27.75	70.48	34.31	23.75	60.32	34.34
39.00	99.06	46.31	28.00	71.12	34.62	24.00	60.96	34.70

Continued

	Abdomen			Thigh			Forearm	
in	**cm**	**Constant A**	**in**	**cm**	**Constant B**	**in**	**cm**	**Constant C**
39.25	99.70	46.61	28.25	71.75	34.93	24.25	61.59	35.07
39.50	100.33	46.90	28.50	72.39	35.24	24.50	62.23	35.43
39.75	100.97	47.20	28.75	73.02	35.55	24.75	62.86	35.79
40.00	101.60	47.50	29.00	73.66	35.86	25.00	63.50	36.15
40.25	101.24	47.79	29.25	74.29	36.17			
40.50	102.87	48.09	29.50	74.93	36.48			
40.75	103.51	48.39	29.75	75.56	36.79			
41.00	104.14	48.69	30.00	76.20	37.09			
41.25	104.78	48.98	30.25	76.83	37.40			
41.50	105.41	49.28	30.50	77.47	37.71			
41.75	106.05	49.58	30.75	78.10	38.02			
42.00	106.68	49.87	31.00	78.74	38.33			
42.25	107.32	50.17	31.25	79.37	38.64			
42.50	107.95	50.47	31.50	80.01	38.95			
42.75	108.59	50.76	31.75	80.64	39.26			
43.00	109.22	51.06	32.00	81.28	39.57			
43.25	109.86	51.36	32.25	81.91	39.88			
43.50	110.49	51.65	32.50	82.55	40.19			
43.75	111.13	51.95	32.75	83.18	40.49			
44.00	111.76	52.25	33.00	83.82	40.80			
44.25	112.40	52.54	33.25	84.45	41.11			
44.50	113.03	52.84	33.50	85.09	41.42			
44.75	113.67	53.14	33.75	85.72	41.73			
45.00	114.30	53.44	34.00	86.36	42.04			

Note: Percent Fat = Constant A + Constant B − Constant C − 19.6

APPENDIX G

Evaluation of Body Composition – Skinfold Method

Use of skinfold equations to predict body density (Db) and/or percent body fat (%BF) use regression analyses in which scores obtained on several variables are multiplied by constants to arrive at a predicted Db or %BF. Solving these equations require extensive computations that are ill suited for field work, and are subject to error, particularly when done by hand or with calculators.

A nomogram is a pictorial method that simplifies computations by providing a simple "look-up" method to solve the equation.

THE NOMOGRAM

Figure G-1 presents the nomogram to estimate percent body fat for college-aged men and women from the sum of three skinfolds plus age using the Jackson et al. generalized equations (see below).

VARIABLES

- For men, obtain the following variables: skinfolds in mm (chest, abdomen, thigh); age in yr
- For women, obtain the following variables: skinfolds in mm (triceps, thigh, suprailiac); age in yr

USING THE NOMOGRAM

1. Sum the three skinfolds.
2. Locate on the right-scale, sum of the three skinfolds, mm.
3. Locate on the left-scale, age in years.
4. With a rule connect the two points (right-scale and left-scale); read the resulting percent body fat from the center scale (male or female).

EXAMPLE

Data for a women, age 30 yr.; triceps skinfold = 15 mm; thigh skinfold = 15 mm; suprailiac skinfold = 25 mm.

1. Sum skinfolds = 55 mm
2. Place rule on right-scale over 55 mm; connect to left-scale at age 30
3. Read percent body fat: 23%.

CAUTION

Although nomograms can save time they are subject to error, particularly interpolation error where precision and accuracy can be compromised. At best, interpolation of the %BF value for males and females in the present nomogram becomes limited to no more than one-half of a whole percent. Also, since the nomogram uses the Siri equation to convert body density to percent body fat it should not be

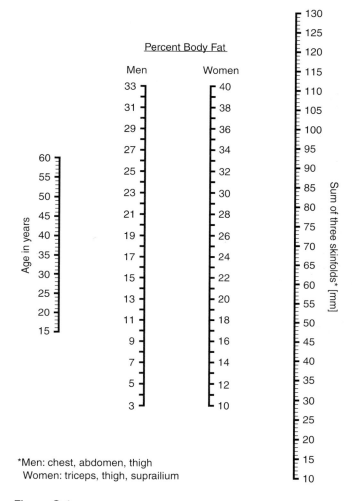

*Men: chest, abdomen, thigh
Women: triceps, thigh, suprailium

Figure G-1
Nomogram to estimate percent body fat of college-aged men and women using Jackson et al. generalized equations. *Note.* From "A Nomogram for the Estimate of Percent Body Fat From Generalized Equations" by W.B. Baun and M.R. Baun, 1981, *Research Quarterly for Exercise and Sport*, 52, p. 382. Copyright 1981 by AAHPERD. Reprinted by permission.

used with populations where other density-to-percent fat conversions are more appropriate.

EQUATIONS

Check the accuracy of using the nomogram by solving the following equations to predict body density. Convert body density to percent body fat using the Siri equations (%BF $= 495 \div$ Db $- 450$).

1. Equation for males: Σ3SKF equals sum of chest, abdomen and thigh skinfold
   Db $= 1.10938 - (0.0008267 \times \Sigma3SKF) +$
   $([0.0000016 \times \Sigma3SKF]^2) - (0.0002574 \times$ age)
2. Equation for females: Σ3SKF equals sum of triceps, thigh and suprailiac skinfold
   Db $= 1.0994921 - (0.0009929 \times \Sigma3SKF) +$
   $([0.0000023 \times \Sigma3SKF]^2) - (0.0001392 \times$ age)

References

1. Jackson, A.S., Pollock, M.L.: Generalized equations for predicting body density of men. *Br. J. Nutr.*, 40: 497, 1978.
2. Jackson, A.S., et al.: Generalized equations for predicting body density of women. *Med. Sci. Sports Exerc.*, 12: 175, 1980
3. Baun, W.B., Baun M.R.: A nomogram for the estimate of percent body fat from generalized equations. *Res. Quart. Exerc. Sport*, 52:382, 1981.

Page numbers in *italics* denote figures; those followed by a t denote tables.

A

A band, 316, *317*
Acarbose, 345
Acclimatization
 altitude, 450–453, 451t
 cold, 447
 heat, 443–444, *444*, 444t
Acetylcholine, 277, 306–307
Acetyl–coenzyme A, 108–110, *109–110*
Acid(s)
 characteristics, 118
 pH, 119
Acid-base regulation, 118–120
 altitude acclimatization, 452
 buffering systems, 119–120
Acidosis, defined, 119
Acini, 340, *340*
Acromegaly, 335
ACSM. *See* American College of Sports
 Medicine
Actin-myosin orientation. *See also* Myosin
 crossbridges
 ATP and, 320–321
 during crossbridge oscillation, 319–320, *320*
 ultrastructure, 316–318, *318*
Action potential, 307, *307*
Actomyosin
 dissociation, 321
 formation, 319
Acute mountain sickness (AMS), 455
Addictive behaviors, warning signs, 474–475
Addison's syndrome, 336
Adenosine diphosphate (ADP), 98
Adenosine monophosphate (AMP), 98
Adenosine triphosphate (ATP)
 discovery, 97
 as energy currency, 98, 100, *100*
 high-energy bonds, 98, *98*
 hydrolysis, 98
 in muscle action, 320–321
 resynthesis, 100–101, *101*
 storage, 100
Adenosine triphosphate-phosphocreatine (ATP-
 PCr) energy system. *See* ATP-PCr energy
 system
Adipocytes. *See* Fat cells
Adipose tissue, 504, 533–534
Adolescents
 CHD risk factors, 579
 physical activity patterns, 556
 steroid abuse, 464
ADP (adenosine diphosphate), 98
Adrenal cortex hormones
 aging and, 563, *564*
 described, 333t, 338–340
 endurance training response, 350
Adrenal glands, 338, *338*

Adrenal medulla hormones
 described, 333t, 338
 endurance training response, 350
Adrenergic fibers, 282, 303
Adrenocorticotropic hormone (ACTH), 332t,
 335–336, 347
Aerobic capacity (VO_{2max}). *See also*
 Cardiorespiratory fitness
 aerobic training at percentage of, 376
 age differences, 197–198, *198*, 362t, 565, *565*,
 566
 aging and, 27, *27*
 altitude and, 455, 456
 of CHD patients, 606, *607*
 classification, 362t, 363
 criteria for, 189–190, *191*
 criterion standards
 adults, 362t, 363
 children, 363, 363t
 described, *131*, 131–132
 energy sources, 132, *133*
 factors affecting, 194–198
 gender differences, 195–196, 196t, 197, *197*,
 362t, 363
 genetic influences, 194–195
 improvement
 continuous, 368, *369*
 individual differences, 363–364, *364*
 maintenance, 382
 maximum cardiac output and, 290, *290*
 maximum heart rate and, 377, *377*
 measurement, 189–190
 of Olympic wheelchair-dependent athletes,
 193
 of Olympic-caliber athletes, *190*
 prediction, 198–201
 estimation errors, 198, 200
 from heart rate, 200, 200–201
 from nonexercise data, 202, 202t–203t
 from step test performance, 199
 from walking test, 195
 stroke volume and, 286–287, 287t
 tests, 190–194. *See also* Stress testing
 continuous versus discontinuous, 191–192,
 191t
 protocol manipulations, 192–194
 treadmill protocols, 192, *192*
 ventilatory limitations, 258–260
Aerobic energy system
 described, 127, 129–*131*, 129–132
 evaluation, 188–198
 training. *See* Aerobic training
Aerobic training
 adaptations, 368–375, 370t, *375*
 body composition, 374–375
 body heat transfer, 375
 cardiovascular, 360, 370–373, *372*, 373t

 metabolic, 369, 369–370
 muscle fiber type distribution, 324, *325*
 pulmonary, 373–374, *374*
 cardiac output during, 289, *289*
 for children, 376
 continuous, 380
 duration, 366
 evaluation, 362–363, 365
 factors affecting, 366–368
 frequency, 366
 goals, 366, 367
 guidelines, 376
 intensity
 establishment, 376–380
 evaluation, 366–368, 368–369
 low, 378
 and maintenance of aerobic fitness, 382
 interval, 380–382, 381t
 at lactate threshold, 380
 at percentage of maximum heart rate, 376–378,
 377
 at percentage of VO_{2max}, 376
 at perception of effort, 378, 380
 program development, 375–380
 response, 363–364, *364*
 specificity, 359, *360*
Aerobic workout, ideal, 380
Afferent neurons, 301
Afterload, 287
Age differences
 aerobic capacity, 197–198, 362t, 363, 565, *565*,
 566
 anaerobic power, 186, 566
 basal metabolic rate, 156, *156*
 body fat, 567, *568*, 569
 coronary heart disease, 574–575, *575*
 leisure activity intensity categorization, 164,
 165t
 maximum heart rate, 567, *568*
 minute ventilation, 567, *568*
 muscle mass, 559
 oxygen pulse, 567, *568*
 resting daily energy expenditure, 158
 running economy, *167*, 167–168, 566
 thermoregulation, 445
Aging
 and aerobic capacity, 27, *27*
 and bodily function, 558, 558–568
 and body composition, 567–568, 569
 and cardiovascular function, 565, 565–566
 and endocrine function, 559, 563, *564*
 and endurance performance, 566–567, *567*
 exercise training response, 565–566
 and joint flexibility, 559
 and muscle strength, 559, *559*
 and nervous system function, 563
 and pulmonary function, 565

and resistance training, 413
  successful, 558
Air
  composition, 242, 242t
  gas movement in, 242–243
  nitrogen concentration, altitude training and, 456
Air displacement, body volume measurement by, *511*, 511–512
Air resistance, effects, 172, 174
Airway resistance, smoking and, 260
Alanine, structure, *53*
Alanine-glucose cycle, 57, 59, *59*
Alcohol
  abuse, 474, 476
  coronary heart disease and, 576–577
  and fluid replacement, 478
  level, in beverages and the body, 476
  physiological effects, 476, 478
  psychological effects, 476
  use among athletes, 476, 477t
Aldosterone
  described, 333t, 338–339
  endurance training response, 350
  exercise-induced release, 82
  in heat stress response, 434
  hypertension and, 339
Alkaline solution, 118, 119
Alkalosis
  defined, 119
  pre-exercise, ergogenic effects, 478–479, 479t
All-or-none principle, 308
All-out anaerobic endurance tests, 184, 185–186
All-out exercise duration, performance classifications based on, 359
Alpha motoneurons, 301, 306
Altitude
  acclimatization adjustments, 450–453, 451t
  exercise capacity at, 455
  extreme, nutrition and, 436t, 437, *437*
  medical problems related to, 453, 455
  oxygen loading at, 449–450
  stress of, 449–450, *450*
  training, and sea-level performance, 455–458, *457*
Alveolar air, 242, 242t
Alveolar ventilation, 237–238, 237t, *238*
Alveolus, anatomy, 232–233, *233*
Ambient air, 242, 242t
Ambient temperature
  evaporative heat loss and, 432
  extreme, nutrition and, 436t, 437, *437*
  water requirements and, 441t
Amenorrhea, athletic, 77, 78, *78*, 506
American Alliance for Health, Physical Education, Recreation and Dance (AAHPERD), 23
American Association for the Advancement of Physical Education (AAAPE), 23
American College of Sports Medicine (ACSM)
  awards, Nordic recipients, 22t
  certification programs, 590–592, 592t
  described, 23
  on use of anabolic steroids, 467
American Heart Association (AHA), CHD risk factor checklist, 580
American Journal of Physiology, 15
American Society of Exercise Physiology (ASEP), 23

Amherst College, sports science movement, 11–13, *12–14*
Amino acid supplements, as ergogenic aid, 468
Amino acids, 51–54
  branched–chain, 114
  energy release, 114–116, *116*
  essential, 52, 53
  glucogenic, 115
  ketogenic, 115–116
  nonessential, 53–54
AMP (adenosine monophosphate), 98
Amphetamines, 471
Anabolic reactions, 99
Anabolic steroids, 463–467
  ACSM position statement, 467
  cost, 464t
  dosage, 465, *465*
  ergogenic effectiveness, 464–465
  estimates of use, 463–464
  examples, 464t
  female use of, 466
  and life-threatening disease, 465–466
  and plasma lipoproteins, 466
  pyramiding, 463
  risks, 465
  side effects, 466t
  stacking, 463
  structure and action, 463
  substitutes, 468
Anabolism
  mineral contribution, 75
  protein retention, 54–55
Anaerobic endurance, 184, 185–186
Anaerobic energy, 181–188. *See also* Energy system, immediate; Energy system, short-term
  age differences, 186, 566
  energy sources, 132, *133*
  gender differences, 186–187
  individual differences, 188, *189*
  performance tests, 184, 185–186
  training effects, 188, *189*, 360–362
Anaerobic fatigue, 185
Anaerobic threshold, 258
Anatomic dead space, 237
Androgens. *See also* Anabolic steroids
  hepatic toxicity, 465–466
Androlone-D 200, 464t
Andrometer, 13, *14*
Andropause, 563, *564*
Androstenedione, 466–468
Anemia
  exercise-induced, 81–82, *82*
  iron deficiency, 80
Aneurysm, 597
Angina pectoris
  causes, 574, 596
  exercise-induced, 271, 610
  heartburn versus, 596t
  pain pattern, 596, *596*
  stable, chronic, 596
Angiography, coronary, 611
Angiotensin, 338
Animal polysaccharides, 44–45
Ankle flexion, assessment, 561
Ankle weights, walking and, 170
Anorexia athletica, 80
Anorexia nervosa, 79
Anterior motoneuron, 305–306, *306*

Anthropometric assessment, 10, 13
Antidiuretic hormone (ADH)
  described, 332t, 336–337
  endurance training response, 348
  exercise-induced release, 82
  in heat stress response, 434
Antioxidant enzymes, 73
Antioxidants
  dietary sources, 74
  exercise and, 73
  vitamins as, 72–74
Aortic bodies, in ventilatory control, 251, *251*
Apoproteins, 578
Applied research, 34, 34–35
Archimedes' principle, 507–508, *508*
Arm girth, measurement, 548
Arm-crank ergometer test, 606, *606*
Arrhythmias, 278, 280, 598, 610, *611*
Arterial blood, cardiac output and, 284
Arteries, anatomy, 265, *266*
Arteriole, 265, *266*
Arteriovenous-oxygen difference, 247
Ascending nerve tracts, 301
Ascorbic acid (vitamin C), 71t, 73, 74, 80–81
Asmussen, E., *20*, 20–21
Associations. *See* Relationships between variables
Asthma, exercise-induced, 239
Åstrand, P., 21, *21*
Astrand treadmill test, *192*
Atherosclerosis, 573–574, *574*
Atherosclerosis susceptibility gene (ATHS), 595
Athlete(s)
  aerobic capacity, *190*, 193
  alcohol use, 476, 477t
  body composition, 522–525, 523t
  body fat, 505t
  body mass index, 520
  diets, 207, 208t
  elite
    food intake, 210, *212*
    muscle fiber type distribution, 323–326, *325*
  endurance
    muscle fiber type distribution, 324, *325*
    resting cardiac output, 285
  female, eating disorders, 77, 78
  food intake model, 213, 215t
  food requirements, 214, 215t
  former, age at death, 569, *570*
  heart dimensions, 292–293, 293t
  iron requirements, 82
  longevity, 568, 570
  protein requirements, 56–57
Athletic amenorrhea, 77, 78, *78*
Athletic groups, muscle fiber type distribution, 323–326, *325*
ATP. *See* Adenosine triphosphate
ATP-PCr energy system
  described, 101, 125
  evaluation, 181–183
  oxygen deficit and, 130, *130*
  training, 101, 360–361, 368
Atrial contraction, 265
Atrial fibrillation, 278
Atrioventricular bundle, 275, *275*
Atrioventricular node, 275, *275*
Atrioventricular valves, 265
Atwater, W. O., 143
Atwater Factors, 62
Atwater-Rosa calorimeter, 143

Autonomic nervous system
  conscious modulation of, 302
  divisions, 302–303, 303t
Autonomic reflex arc, 303, *304*
Average power output, 185
Axon, 305, *306*

B

Back-lift dynamometer, 390, *392*
Bag technique, oxygen uptake measurement, 145–146, *146*
Balke treadmill test, *192*, 605, 605t
Ballet dancers, menstrual dysfunction, 506
Baroreceptors, 278, *278*, 301
"Barrel chest" appearance, 623, *624*
Basal metabolic rate (BMR), 155–159
  age differences, 156, *156*
  body size and, 156, *156*
  climate and, 159
  gender differences, 156, *156*
  measurement, 155–156
  thyroid hormones and, 337, *337*
  weight loss and, 542, *542*
Base(s), characteristics, 118–119
Basic research, 34, 34–35, *35*
Behavioral interventions
  cardiac rehabilitation, 614, 620t
  disease prevention, 582, 582t
Bench press, 1-RM test, 394–395
Bergström, J., 21, *21*
Beta blockers, 278
Beta–carotene, 73–74
Beta-endorphin, 351
Beta-hydroxy-beta-methylbutyrate (HMB), 482
Beta-lipotropohin, 351
Beta–oxidation, 113, *113*
Between-subject variability, 32
Bicarbonate, carbon dioxide as, 248–249, *249*
Bicycling. *See* Cycling
Binge-eating disorder, warning signs, 79–80
Bioelectrical impedance analysis (BIA), 517–518, *518*
Biological variation, 31–32
Biotin, 71t
Blood, components, *247*
Blood alcohol level, 476
Blood boosting
  with erythropoietin, 490
  with red blood cell reinfusion, 489–490, *490*, 491t
Blood clot, coronary, 271, 574
Blood distribution, 280–282
  aerobic training adaptations, 373
  exercise effects, 280
  hormonal factors, 282, *282*
  local factors, 280
  neural factors, 280, 282, *282*
Blood flow. *See also* Circulation
  aerobic training adaptations, 373
  redistribution, during exercise, 280–282, 289, *289*
  regulation, 280
  resistance to, factors affecting, 280
  velocity, 244
Blood pressure
  abnormalities, exercise-induced, 610–611
  aerobic training adaptations, 373, 373t
  cardiac output and, 268, *268*
  classification, 269

determinants, 267
during exercise, 268, *268*, 270, 270t, *271*
high. *See* Hypertension
maintenance, during exercise in heat, 439
measurement, 269
in recovery, 270
resting, 268
Blood sugar. *See* Glucose
Blood vessel radius, blood flow and, 280
Blood vessel walls, *266*
"Blue bloater," 623, *623*
BMI. *See* Body mass index
BOD POD, for body volume measurement, *511*, 511–512
Bodily function, aging and, 558, *558–568*
Body builders
  body composition, 523, 525
  steroid use, 463
Body composition
  aerobic training adaptations, 374–375
  aging and, 567–568, *569*
  assessment, 506–518
    by air displacement, *511*, 511–512
    by bioelectrical impedance analysis, 517–518, *518*
    direct, 507, *507*
    by dual-energy x-ray absorptiometry, 518, *519*
    by girth measurements, 515, 517, *517*, 673–679
    by hydrostatic weighing, 507–511
    indirect, 507
    model, 501, 503, *503*
    reference man and woman, 504, *504*
    by skinfold measurements, 512–515, *516*, 517, 680–681
  average values, 520–522
  of champion athletes, 522–525, 523t
  exercise effects, 547, 549
  resistance training adaptations, 419, 420t
  spot reduction and, 550
Body density
  computation, 505
  measurement, by hydrostatic weighing, 508
  residual lung volume and, 509, *510*
Body fat. *See* Fat (body)
Body inversion, blood pressure response, 270
Body mass
  energy expenditure during walking and, 169, 170t
  exercise energy cost and, 162, 162t, *163*
  fat-free. *See* Fat-free body mass
  food intake and, 539–540
  lean, 505
  maximal oxygen uptake and, 196, 196t
  minimal, 505
Body mass index (BMI)
  calculation, 518, 536
  and health risk, 536
  limitations, 520
  and mortality ratio, 519, *519*
  and overweightness, 536
Body position, circulatory dynamics and, 287, 288t
Body size
  basal metabolic rate and, 156, *156*
  resting daily energy expenditure and, 158
Body surface area, calculation, 157
Body surface area-to-mass ratio, heat dissipation and, 445

Body temperature
  during exercise, 439, *439*
  fluctuations, 429, *430*
  measurement, 430
  oxyhemoglobin dissociation curve and, *246*, 247
  regulation. *See* Thermoregulation
  ventilatory control and, 253
Body volume, measurement
  by air displacement, *511*, 511–512
  by hydrostatic weighing, 511, *511*
Body weight
  assessment, 501, 502t
  carbohydrate intake and, 211
  cycling, 542–543
  evaluation
    by body mass index, 518–520
    by height-weight tables, 501, 502t
  gain. *See* Weight gain
  goal, determination, 521–522
  loss. *See* Weight loss
  physical activity and, 212, 214
  underweight versus thin, 505
Bohr effect, *246*, 247
Bomb calorimeter, 61, *61*
Bone
  health, exercise and, 78
  mineral accrual, 567–568
  resistance training adaptations, 415, 415t
Bonking, 47, 135
Bradycardia, 277, 598
Brain
  anatomic areas, 297–298, *299*
  blood flow, during exercise, 289
  neurotransmitters, 301, 302t
  organization, 298–299, *299*
Branched–chain amino acids, 114
Breast cancer, and exercise, *594*, 594–595
Breath-holding
  dangers, 454
  effect on ventilatory control, 252
Breathing. *See* Ventilation
British Association of Sport and Exercise Sciences (BASES), 23
Bronchi, anatomy, 231–232, *232*
Bronchioles, anatomy, 232, *232*
Bronchitis
  acute, 617
  chronic, 617, 623, *623*
Bronchospasm, exercise-induced, 239
Bruce treadmill test
  described, *192*, 605, 605t
  exercise prescription based on, 612, *616*
Buffering capacity
  anaerobic energy transfer capacity and, 188
  enhancement, 189, 478–479, 479t
Buffering system(s)
  acid-base regulation, 119–120
  chemical, 120
  lactate acid, 120, 151, 255
  renal, 120
  and strenuous exercise, 120, *121*
  ventilatory, 120, 231
Bulimia nervosa, warning signs, 79
Bundle of His, 275, *275*
Buoyancy, swimming economy and, 175–176
Burnout. *See* Overtraining

C

Cable tensiometry, 390, *390*
Caffeine
  absorption, 471, 473
  effects on creatine supplementation, 487
  effects on muscle, 475
  ergogenic effects, 473, *473*
  ergogenic mechanism, 473, 475
  lipolysis stimulation, 330
  products containing, 471, 472t
  side effects, 475
Calcium, 76t
  dietary, importance, 77
  and estrogen, 77
  and exercise, 77
  functions, 75, 77
  in muscle function, 318, 321–322
Caliper, skinfold, *512*, 512–513
Calories
  calculation, from composition, 62, 62t, 65
  defined, 61
  direct measurement, *61*, 61–62
  food energy from, 65. *See also* Energy value
Calorimeter, bomb, 61, *61*
Calorimetry
  calibration methods, 147–148, *148*
  direct, 143–144, *144*, 148
  indirect, 144–148, *146–147*
Cancer
  exercise effects, 593–594
  exercise prescription, 594
  incidence and types, 593
  menstruation onset and, 506
  prevention, 582, 582t, 593
Capillary, 265, *266*
Carbamino compounds, carbon dioxide as, 248, *249*
Carbohydrate loading
  applicability, 224
  beverage, oral rehydration beverage versus, 221
  and muscle girth, 45
  negative aspects, 224
  procedure, 223
    modified, 224
Carbohydrates, 41–47. *See also* Glucose
  complex, 42
  content, common foods, 46, *46*
  conversions, 45
  depletion, and fatigue, 47
  energy distribution, 44, *44*
  energy release from, 105–111
  excess, metabolic fate, *118*
  exercise performance and, 46–47, *47*
  food sources, glycemic index of, 216, *217*
  functions, 45
  intake. *See also* Carbohydrate loading
    altitude tolerance and, 455
    body weight and, 217
    during exercise, 217–219, *218*, 222
    during intense training, 221
    overtraining and, 128, 221
    pancreatic hormones and, 341, *341*
    post-exercise, 219, 221
    precompetition, 214–216
    pre-exercise, 216–217
    during prolonged exercise, 222
    recommended, 46, 207–209, *209*
    replacement recommendations, 89–90, *91*
  metabolic mill, 116, *117*

  metabolism
    aerobic training adaptations, 369–370
    role of water-soluble vitamins, 72
    in oral rehydration beverage, 218
    respiratory quotient for, 149
    simple, 42
Carbon dioxide
  in alveolar air, 242, 242t
  in ambient air, 242, 242t
  as bicarbonate, 248–249, *249*
  calculation, by open-circuit spirometry, 670
  as carbamino compounds, 248, *249*
  chemical analysis, 147–148, *148*
  partial pressure
    effect on ventilatory control, 251–252
    during exercise, 252, 252–253
  in solution, 248, *249*
  in tissues, 249
  transport
    in blood, 248–249, *249*
    in lungs, 243, *244*, 249
  ventilatory equivalent for, 255
Carbon dioxide rebreathing method, for cardiac output measurement, 285
Carbonic acid, 248
Carbonic anhydrase, 249
Cardiac arrest, myocardial infarction versus, 571
Cardiac catheterization, 611
Cardiac conduction, *275*, 275–276
Cardiac hypertrophy
  in athletes, 292–293, 293t, 370–371
  physiological versus pathological, 415–416
Cardiac medications, 616, 621t
Cardiac nervous system disease, 598
Cardiac output
  aerobic training adaptations, 372
  blood pressure and, 268, *268*
  body position and, 287, 288t
  determinants, 284
  distribution, 288–289, *289*
  exercise, 285–286
  gender differences, 290
  in heart disease, 291
  maximum, 290, *290*
  measurement, 284–285, *285*
  oxygen transport and, 289–290
  oxygen uptake and, 284–285
  resting, 285
Cardiac rehabilitation
  CHD risk and, 612, 615t
  exercise prescription, 612–614, *616*, 617t–618t
  exercise program types, 612, 614t
  outcomes
    with education, counseling, and behavioral interventions, 614, 620t
    with exercise training, 614, 619t
    supervision level and, 614, 621t
  patient classification, 611–612, 612t
  phases, 612, 613t
  program administration, 615–616
Cardiopulmonary disease, signs and symptoms, 620
Cardiopulmonary resuscitation (CPR), 280
Cardiorespiratory fitness (CR-F). *See also* Aerobic capacity
  in children, 363, 363t
  evaluation, 362t–363t, 363–364, *364*, 365
  field tests, 603
  heart rate and, 368, *368*

  improvement
    individual differences, 363–364
    initial level and, 366
  laboratory tests, 603, 605. *See also* Stress testing
  maintenance, 382
Cardiovascular adaptations
  aerobic training, 360, 370–373, *372*, 373t
  altitude acclimatization, 451
  resistance training, 415–416, 415t
Cardiovascular center, in medulla, 277–278, *278*
Cardiovascular disease. *See also specific type, e.g.,* Coronary heart disease
  assessment, 598–605
  cardiac output in, 291
  categories, 595–598, 595t
  classifications, 611–612, 612t
  end-stage, treatment, 273
  incidence, 595
  rehabilitation. *See* Cardiac rehabilitation
Cardiovascular system
  aging and, 565, *565*–566
  components, *264*, 264–267
  in exercise
    dynamics, 284–294
    integrated response, 282–283, 283t
  functions, 263
  regulation, 275–283
Carnegie Institute, nutrition laboratory, 19
Carnitine supplementation, 480
Carotid artery palpation, 278
Carotid bodies, 251, *251*
Catabolic reactions, 99
Catalase, 73
Catecholamines
  cardiovascular effects, 276–277
  endurance training response, 350, *350*
  exercise response, 333t, 338
  training effects on, 277
Catheterization, cardiac, 611
Causality, establishing, 27–29
Cell body, 305, *306*
Cellular adaptations, altitude acclimatization, 453
Cellular oxidation, *102–103*, 102–104
Central command system, cardiovascular modulation, 277, 279
Central nervous system, 297–301, *298*. *See also* Brain; Spinal cord
Cerebellum, 298, 299
Cerebral cortex, 298, 299
Cerebral edema, high-altitude, 455
Cerebrum, 298, 299
Cervical vertebra, *300*
Cheating, defined, 391t
Chemical buffers, 120
Chemoreceptors, 301
Chest, barrel, 623, *624*
Chest pain, differential diagnosis, 599t
Chest x-rays, 599, *599*
CHF (congestive heart failure), 597
Children. *See also* Adolescents
  aerobic training, 376
  anaerobic power, 186, 566
  bone mineral accrual, 567–568
  cardiorespiratory fitness standards, 363, 363t
  CHD risk factors, 579
  cholesterol measurement, 575
  exercise physiology differences, 566
  maternal exercise effects, 383–384, 384t, 386

obese, 531, 546
physical activity patterns, 556
resistance training, 402, 402t
running performance, 363
steroid abuse, 464
thermoregulation, 445
Chloride shift, 249
Chlorine (chloride), 76t, 77–78
Cholesterol. *See also* Lipoproteins
"bad," 49. *See also* Low-density lipoproteins
blood level
classification, 576
coronary heart disease and, 575
factors affecting, 577
content, common foods, 51t
functions, 49
"good," 49. *See also* High-density lipoproteins
measurement, in children, 575
recommended intake, 51
sources, 49
terms on food labels, 64
transport, 49
Cholesterol:HDL ratio, 577
Cholinergic fibers, 282, 303
Cholinesterase, 307
Chromium, 76t, 481
alleged benefits, 481, 483, 483t
side effects, 483–484
Chronic obstructive pulmonary disease (COPD),
617, 623–624
differences among, 623t
predisposing factors, 617
ventilatory requirements, 259
Chylomicrons, 49, 577t
Circuit resistance training (CRT)
for cardiac rehabilitation, 614, 617t–618t
defined, 391t
metabolic stress, 416, 419, 419t
sequence of progression, *416*
Circulation. *See also* Blood flow
at altitude, 451, 455
coronary, 271, 272, 289
pulmonary, 264, *265*
renal, 280
systemic, 264, *265*
thermoregulatory response, 431, 434
Clenbuterol, 468
Climate, energy expenditure and, 159
Closed-circuit spirometry, 144, *144*
Clothing, thermoregulation and, 434–436
Coal miner, energy expenditure by, 160, 160t,
162
Coenzyme Q$_{10}$, 484
Coenzymes, 69
Cold stress
acclimatization, 447
evaluation, 447–448
fluid loss, 441, *442*
thermoregulation, 431
Cold-weather clothing, thermoregulation and,
434–436
Colon cancer, 582
Complex carbohydrates, 42
Compliance, exercise, 364, *366*
Computerized measurement
metabolic and cardiovascular response to
exercise, 146–147, *147*
muscle strength, 392–393
Concentric muscle action

described, 391t, 396, 396–397
for reducing muscle soreness, 420, 423, *423*
Conduction
cardiac, 275, 275–276
heat loss by, 432
Congenital heart defects, 598
Congestive heart failure (CHF), 597
Connective tissue
damage, muscle soreness and, 423
resistance training adaptations, 415
Constructs, 33
Continuous variable, 26
Control group, 28
Convection, 432
Conversational exercise, 367
Conversion constants, 664–666
Cool-down, active, 267
COPD. *See* Chronic obstructive pulmonary
disease
Copper, 76t
Cori cycle, 108, *108*
Coronary angiography, 611
Coronary arteries, 271, 272
Coronary circulation, 271, 272, 289
Coronary heart disease
age differences, 574–575, *575*
behavioral interventions, 582, 582t
deaths caused by, 571, 572–573
exercise-induced indicators, 610–611
gender differences, 571–573, 574–575
genetic influences, 575, 595
homocysteine and, 577–578, *578*
laboratory tests, 599–600
as lifelong process, 573–574, *574*
lipid abnormalities and, 575–577
obesity and, 579–580
pathogenesis, 595–596
patient medical history, 598
personality patterns and, 580
physical activity and, 578–579, 580
physical examination, 598–599
physiological tests, 600–611
rehabilitation. *See* Cardiac rehabilitation
risk factors, 574–582
AHA checklist, *580*
in children and adolescents, 579
classification, 612, 615t
interactions, 580, 582, *582*
primary, 574
smoking and, 572, 579
Coronary occlusion. *See* Myocardial infarction
Corpus striatum, 298
Corticotropin, 332t, 335–336, 347
Cortisol
described, 333t, 339–340
endurance training response, 350
release
inhibitors, 480–481
resistance training and, 481
Counseling, cardiac rehabilitation, 614, 620t
CPR (cardiopulmonary resuscitation), 280
Creatine, 484–487
caffeine effects, 487
documented benefits, 484–486, 485t
effects on body mass, 486
in energy transfer, 484
ergogenic mechanism, 486, 487
loading, 486–487, *488*
Creatine kinase, 125, 420

Creatine phosphate. *See* Phosphocreatine
Creatine phosphokinase, 599
Criticism of source material, 11
Crossed-extensor reflex, 304, *305*
CRT. *See* Circuit resistance training
Cureton, T. K., 22, *22*
Curl-up muscular endurance test, 417
Cushing's disease, 336
Cycle ergometer test
exercise prescription based on, 612, *616*
maximal, in CHD patients, 606, *607*
measurement of work, 134–135
protocols, 606
Wingate, 184–185, *186*
Cyclic 3,5-adenosine monophosphate (cyclic-
AMP), 330
Cycling. *See also* Cycle ergometer test
economy, muscle fiber type and, 167
helmet, thermoregulation and, 436
power test, 182–183
Cystic fibrosis, 624, 624t
Cytochromes, 102–103, *103*

D

De Arte Gymnastica, 9
Dead space
anatomic, 237
physiologic, 238, *238*
Deamination, protein, 54, 115
Death
age at, former athletes versus nonathletes, 569,
570
leading causes, 572–573
risk
and fitness level, 569, *570*, 571
and regular exercise, 569, *570*
Deconate, 464t
Dehydration
chronic, 90
consequences, 441
defined, 85
Dehydroepiandrosterone (DHEA), 340
aging and, 563, *564*
as ergogenic aid, 469–471
plasma levels, 469–470, *470*
safety, 470–471
Delayed-onset muscle soreness (DOMS)
after downhill running, 420, *421*
causes, 419, 422, 422–423
cell damage, 420–421, *421*
and eccentric muscle action, 419–420
reducing, 423, *423*
treatment, 420–422, *421*
Dendrite, 305, *306*
Denmark, contributions to exercise physiology,
19–21
Dependent variable, 27
Descending nerve tracts, 301
Detraining, 360, *361*
Dextrose. *See* Glucose
DHEA. *See* Dehydroepiandrosterone
Diabetes mellitus, 342–346
behavioral interventions, 582, 582t
blood tests, 343, 344
exercise and, 345–346, *346*, 350–351
and heart attacks in women, 572–573
type 1, 344, 345, 350–351
type 2
aging and, 559

described, 344–345
    exercise and, 351, 563
    oral medications, 345
    warning signs, 343
Diaphragm, 233, *234*
Diastole, 268
Diastolic blood pressure, 269
    aerobic training adaptations, 373, 373t
    during exercise, 268, 270, 270t
Diastolic filling, 287
Diencephalon, 298, 299
Diet(s). *See also* Dieting; Food intake; Nutrient
        intake
    of athletes versus nonathletes, 207, 208t
    endurance performance and, *221,* 221–222,
        224
    energy expenditure and, 159
    for increasing muscle glycogen. *See*
        Carbohydrate loading
    lactovegetarian, 55
    mixed, respiratory quotient for, 149
    quality evaluation, 208–209, 210t
    recommended, 207–208, 209
    vegetarian, 55, 80–81, 208
Diet Quality Index, 208–209, 210t
Dietary Guidelines for Americans, 211
Dietary-induced thermogenesis, 159
Dieting, 541–545
    combined with exercise, 549–550
    popular methods, 544t
    selection of diet plan, 543
    setpoint theory and, 542, *542*
    unpredictability of results, 542
    weight cycling and, 542–543
Digital clubbing, in emphysema, 623, *624*
Dill, D. B., 19, *19*
Diphosphoglycerate, *246,* 247–248
Disability, 588, *590*
Disaccharides, 42
Discrete variable, 26
Disease prevention, behavioral changes, 582,
        582t
Diuretic use, 441–442
Diving, breath-hold, 252, 454
Double product, 271–272
Double-blind procedure, 28
Down-regulation, 330
Drafting, aerodynamic effects, 174
Drag forces, during swimming, 175
Drugs. *See also* Medications
    banned, 463
    for ergogenic purposes, 463–489
Dual-energy x-ray absorptiometry (DXA), 518,
        519
Dwarfism, 335
Dynamic constant external resistance (DCER)
        training, 391t, 397, 403–404, *404*
Dynamometry, *390,* 392, 393
Dyspnea, 240
Dyspnea scale, 625, *625*
Dysrhythmias, 278, 280, 598, 610, *611*

E

Eating disorders, 77, 78, 79–80
Eccentric hypertrophy, aerobic training, 370–371
Eccentric muscle action, 391t, *396,* 397, 419–420
Echocardiography, 292, 600
Economy of movement, 166, *167*

Edema, high-altitude, 455
Education, cardiac rehabilitation, 614, 620t
Efferent neurons, 301
EKG. *See* Electrocardiogram (ECG)
Electrocardiogram (ECG)
    abnormalities
        in coronary heart disease, 599, 600t
        exercise-induced, 610, *610*
    described, 275–276
    electrode placement, 281
    during exercise, 599, 600t
    heart rate determination, 608–609
    interpretive categories, 599, 600t
    phases, 276
Electrode placement, electrocardiogram, 281
Electrolytes, 77–78, 82, 89. *See also* Chlorine;
        Potassium; Sodium
    in oral rehydration beverage, 219
    replacement, 442–443
Electromechanical devices, muscle strength
        measurement, 392–393
Electron transport
    ATP regeneration, 108–110, *109, 111*
    described, 102–103, *102–103*
    efficiency, 104
Electronic discussion groups, 22–23
*Elementary Anatomy and Physiology for Colleges,
        Academies, and Other Schools* (Hitchcock
        and Hitchcock), *13,* 18
Elite athletes
    food intake, 210, *212*
    muscle fiber type distribution, 323–326, *325*
Ellestad treadmill test, *192*
Emphysema, 623, *624*
Empirical research, *34,* 34–35
Endocarditis, 598
Endocrine function
    aging and, 559, 563, *564*
    endurance training and, 346–351, 347t
    resistance training and, 351
Endocrine glands. *See also specific gland*
    described, 329
    stimulation, 331
Endocrine system, 329–331, *330*
Endomysium, 315, *316*
Endorphins, 332t, 336, 351
Endurance
    muscle, 391t, 417–418
    muscle fibers for, 112
Endurance athletes
    body composition, 522, 523t
    muscle fiber type distribution, 324, *325*
    resting cardiac output, 285
Endurance performance
    aging and, 566–567, *567*
    at altitude, 455
    glycogen stores and, *221,* 221–222, 224
    onset of blood lactate accumulation and, 258
Endurance tests
    anaerobic, 184, 185–186
    assessment, 417–418
Endurance training, and endocrine function,
        346–351, 347t
Energy
    free, 98
    mathematical expressions, 183
Energy balance equation
    weight gain based on, 550–551
    weight loss based on, *540,* 540–541

by diet only, 541–545
by diet plus exercise, 549–550
by exercise only, 545–547, 549
Energy demands, ventilation and, 254–258
Energy expenditure. *See also* Oxygen uptake
    and body fat, 532, 546, 547
    of breathing, *250,* 259
    by coal miner, 160, 160t, 162
    daily
        average rates, 163, 163t
        components, 155
        resting, 157, 158
        total, factors affecting, 157, 159
    economy of movement and, 166, *167*
    exercise effects on, 547
    exercise intensity and, 164, 164t
    gross, 160
    heart rate as estimation of, 164–165, *165*
    maximizing, 547, 549
    measurement, 143–152. *See also* Calorimetry
    mechanical efficiency and, 167
    net, 160
    personal assessment, 541
    during physical activity, 157, 159, 160–166
    of recreational and sports activities, 162, 162t,
        163
    at rest. *See* Basal metabolic rate
    during rowing, 160
    during running, *169,* 170–174, 171t
    during swimming, 174–175, *175–176*
    during walking, 168–170, *169,* 170t
Energy intake. *See* Fluid replacement; Food
        intake; Nutrient intake
Energy metabolism
    regulation, 117–118
    role of oxygen, 104
Energy output, increasing, 546–547
Energy release
    from carbohydrates, 105–111
    from fat, 112–114, 117
    from protein, 114–116
Energy system
    and exercise intensity and duration, 132–133,
        135, 357–358, *358*
    immediate (ATP-PCr)
        described, 101, 125
        evaluation, 181–183
        oxygen deficit and, 130, *130*
        training, 101, 360–361, 368
    long-term (aerobic)
        described, 127, *129–131,* 129–132
        evaluation, 188–198
        training. *See* Aerobic training
    short-term (glycolytic; lactic acid)
        described, *126,* 126–127
        evaluation, *181,* 183–187
        training, 361–362, 368
    specificity-generality concept, 180, *181*
Energy transfer
    by chemical bonds, 101–102
    during exercise, overview, 180–181, *181*
    by oxidation-reduction reactions, 102–104,
        103–104
Energy value
    of foods, *61,* 61–62
    of meal, 62, 62t, 65
    terms on food labels, 64
Enervation ratio, 305
Environment, energy expenditure and, 159

Environmental stress
  nutrition and, 436t, 437, *437*
  thermoregulation and, 438–449
Enzymes
  aerobic training adaptations, 369
  as biologic catalysts, 98
  coronary heart disease and, 599–600
  hormonal effects, 331
  and pH, 119
Epidemiologic research, 28
Epimysium, 315, *316*
Epinephrine
  cardiovascular effects, 276–277, 282
  in cold stress, 431
  described, 333t, 338
  endurance training response, 350, *350*
Ergogenic aids, 462–495. *See also specific agent*
  banned, 463
  defined, 462
  mechanisms, 462
  pharmacologic and nutritional agents, 462–489
  physiologic agents, 489–494
Erythropoietin
  in altitude acclimatization, 452
  blood boosting with, 490
Essential fat, 504
Estradiol, aging and, 563, *564*
Estrogen, 334t, 340
Euhydration, 85
European College of Sport Science (ECSS), 23
*European Journal of Applied Physiology and
    Occupational Physiology*, 16
Evaporation
  during exercise, 433
  gender differences, 445
  heat loss by, 432, 434
Excess post-exercise oxygen consumption
    (EPOC), *136*, 136–140
Excitation, neuronal, 306–307
Excitation-contraction coupling, 321, *321*, 322
Excitatory postsynaptic potential (EPSP), 307
Exercise. *See also* Physical activity
  aerobic. *See* Aerobic training
  aging response, 565–566
  at altitude, 449–458
  anaerobic, 360–362
  anemia caused by, 81–82, *82*
  anticipatory heart rate, 277, *277*, 283t
  breast cancer and, *594*, 594–595
  bronchospasm caused by, 239
  cancer and, 593–594
  carbohydrate intake and, 216–224
  in cold, 441, *442*, 447–448
  colon cancer and, 582
  compliance, 364, *366*
  conversational, 367
  death risk and, 569, *570*
  diabetes and, 345–346, *346*, 350–351
  effects on blood distribution, 280
  effects on body composition, 547, *549*
  effects on energy expenditure, 547
  effects on food intake, 546–547
  effects on lipoprotein levels, 575–576
  endorphins and, 351
  endurance. *See* Endurance performance;
      Endurance training
  energy cost, body mass and, 162, 162t, *163*
  energy requirements, 357–358, *358*
  energy spectrum, 132–133, *133*, 135

energy transfer, 180–181, *181*
fat catabolism, 114
fluid intake and. *See* Fluid replacement
food intake and, 209–216
free radical production caused by, 73
health improvements through, 568–569, *570*
in heat, 82–83, 438–447
immune response and, 349
intensity. *See* Exercise intensity
interval. *See* Interval training
isokinetic, 405–407, *406*
life expectancy and, 568–569, *570*
menstrual dysfunction and, 505–506
perceived exertion during, 378, 380
performance. *See* Exercise performance
during pregnancy, 382–386
prescription. *See* Exercise prescription
protein sparing effects, 550
psychologic benefits, 375
resistance. *See* Progressive resistance exercise;
    Resistance training
responders and nonresponders, 363–364, *364*
rhythmic, blood pressure response, 268, *268*,
    270, *271*
static. *See* Isometric training
strenuous, buffering systems and, 120, *121*
sweating during, 439–441, *440*
thermoregulation and, 444–445
training principles, 358–360
upper-body. *See* Upper-body exercise
ventilation during, 254–260
for weight loss, 545–547, 549–550, 549t
Exercise intensity
  aerobic
      establishment, 376–380
      evaluation, 366–368, *368–369*
      low, 378
      and maintenance of aerobic fitness, 382
  defined, 391t
  energy system and, 132–133, 135, 357–358,
      358
  factors limiting, 229
  glycogen depletion and, 187, *188*
  heart rate as measure of, 367
  physical activity classification based on, 164,
      164t
Exercise Leader, 590, 592
Exercise mode, maximal oxygen uptake and,
    194–195
Exercise performance
  carbohydrates and, 46–47, *47*
  classifications, 358, *359*
  minerals and, 82–83
  smoking and, 259–260
  specificity-generality concept, 180, *181*,
      358–359
  vitamins and, 74
Exercise physiology
  as academic discipline
      components, 6, *7*
      first course of study, 17–18
      first department, 13–15
      first textbook, 18
      focus, 6
      names for departments, 16, 16t
  clinical, 587–628
      cardiovascular diseases and, 595–616
      certification program, 592
      oncology and, 593–595

pulmonary diseases and, 616–617, 623–626
setting, 588
sports medicine and, 588, 590
treatment goals, 593t
contemporary developments, 22–23
information resources, 651–653
Internet and, 654–663
Internet sites, 657–660
journals, 672
mentoring, 23
origins, 7–24
professional organizations, 23, 651–653
research
    evaluation, 30–31
    first, 15
    origins, 14, 15, 18–19
    publications, 15–16, 18
scientific development
    in ancient Greece, 8, 9
    in Nordic countries, 19–22, 22t
    in United States, 8–18
scientific method and, 25–36
training/certification programs, 590–592, 591t
Exercise prescription
  cancer, 594
  cardiac rehabilitation, 612–614, *616*,
      617t–618t. *See also* Cardiac rehabilitation
  cardiac transplantation, 273
  HIV-positive patients, 589
  pulmonary rehabilitation, 625–626
Exercise pressor reflex, 278
Exercise stress testing. *See* Stress testing
Exercise Test Technologist, 592
Exercise-to-rest (E-to-R) method, 139–140
Exocrine glands, 329
Experiment(s)
  defined, 27–28
  expectation effects, 32
  publishing results, 34
  testing effects, 29
Expiration, 234, *234*
Expiratory reserve volume, 235, *235*
External criticism, 11
Extrafusal fibers. *See* Skeletal muscle
Extrapyramidal tract, 301
Extrasystoles, 278

F

Facilitation, neuronal, 307
Facts
  finding, 25–26
  interpreting, 26, 32
Fasciculus, 315, *316*
Fast-fatigable (FF) motor unit, 308, 308t, *309*
Fast-fatigue–resistant (FR) motor unit, 308, 308t,
    309
Fast-glycolytic (FG) muscle fibers, 322
Fasting plasma glucose test (FPG), 343, *344*
Fast-oxidative-glycolytic (FOG) muscle fibers,
    322
Fast-twitch muscle fibers, 112, 132, 322, 323t
Fat (body)
  age differences, 567, 568, 569
  analysis, by dual-energy x-ray absorptiometry,
      518, *519*
  in athletes, 505t
  average values, 520–522
  computation, 508
  distribution, 515, 533–534

energy expenditure and, 532, 546, 547
essential, 504
evaluation criteria, 533–535, 538
genetic influences, 530, *530*
minimal, menstrual function and, 506
percent, 533
physical activity and, 532, 546
prediction
    by bioelectrical impedance analysis,
       517–518, *518*
    from girth measurements, 515, 517
    from skinfold measurements, 512–515, 516,
       517
spot reduction, 550
storage sites, 504
thermoregulation and, 445–446
Fat cells, 112
  location, 515, 533–534
  size and number
    after weight gain, 538
    after weight loss, 535, 538, *538*
    assessment, *534*, 534–535
    in normal and obese adults, 535, *535*
Fat mass
  computation, 508
  fat cell number and, 535, *535*
Fat patterning, 515, 533–534
Fat-free body density (FFBD), 509t
Fat-free body mass (FFM)
  computation
    from girth measurements, 515, 517
    Siri equation, 508–509
  density estimates of, 509t
  described, 505
  errors in estimation, 509, 509t
  muscle strength and, 400–401
  race and, 509
  resting daily energy expenditure and, 158
Fatigue
  anaerobic, 185
  and carbohydrate depletion, 47
  neuromuscular, 310
  nutrient-related, 135, 310
Fats. *See* Lipids (fats)
Fatty acids
  breakdown, 113, *113*
  dietary, 48, 51
  free, 51, 53, 112
  as glucose source, 113, *114*
  saturated, 48, *48*
  structure, *48*
  unsaturated, 48, *48*, 51
The Federation Internationale de Medicine
    Sportive (FIMS), 23
Female athlete triad, 77, 78
Females, steroid use by, 466
Ferritin, 80
Fiber
  content, common foods, 44t
  described, 42
  dietary, health implications, 43
  terms on food labels, 64
  water solubility, 43
Fick equation, 284
Fick method, cardiac output measurement,
    284–285, *285*
Field studies, 28–29, *29*
Field tests, cardiorespiratory fitness, 603
Finland, contributions to exercise physiology,
    21–22

First messenger, 330
Fitness
  cardiorespiratory. *See* Cardiorespiratory fitness
  defined, 58
  economic benefits, 59
  genetic contribution, 196t
  life expectancy and, 569, *570*, 571
  and wellness, 58–59
Fitz, G. W., 13–15, *15*
Five-repetition maximum (5-RM), 392, *392*
Flavin adenine dinucleotide (FAD), 102, *103*
Flavin adenine dinucleotide hydrogen (FADH$_2$),
    102, *103*
Flint, A., Jr., 9, *9*, 11
Fluid(s). *See also* Water
  gas movement in, 242–243
  loss
    in altitude acclimatization, 451
    during exercise in cold, 441, *442*
    during exercise in heat, 439–441
  replacement. *See* Fluid replacement
  volume, gastric emptying and, 218
Fluid replacement
  alcohol and, 478
  in exercise, 442
    adequacy, 90–91
    climate and, 219, 441t
    model for, 442, 443t
    recommendations, 89–90, *91*, 218–219
    with rehydration beverage, 219, 220t, 221
  during prolonged exercise, 222
Fluorine, 76t
Fluoxymesterone, 466t
Folic acid, 71t, 74
  in homocysteine conversion, 577, 578
  sources, 578
Follicle stimulating hormone (FSH)
  described, 332t, 336
  endurance training response, 347–348, *348*
Food
  antioxidant-rich, 74
  biologic value, 54
  carbohydrate content, 46, *46*, 216, *217*
  cholesterol content, 51t
  energy release from, *105*, 105–122
  energy value, *61*, 61–62
  labels, 63–64
  lipid content, 49, *50*
  protein content, 54, 54t, 55, *55*
  saturated fat content, 51t
Food Guide Pyramid, 208, *209*
Food intake. *See also* Diet(s); Dieting; Nutrient
    intake
  for athletes, 213, 214, 215t
  body mass and, 539–540
  daily average, 209, *211*
  of elite athletes, 210, *212*
  exercise and, 209–216
  exercise effects on, 546–547
  extreme, during sports activities, 210–211, *212*,
    213t
  personal assessment, 541
  physical activity and, 209–210, 212, 215t
  precompetition, 214–216
  pre-exercise, glycemic index and, 217
Football uniforms, thermoregulation and, 434
Foot-pound, defined, 183
Footwear, walking and, 169–170
Force gradation, 308

Forced expiratory volume in 2 second (FEV$_1$),
    236
Forced expiratory volume-to-forced vital capacity
    ratio (FEV$_1$/FVC), 236–237
Forced vital capacity (FVC), 235, *235*, 236
Force-power-range of motion relationship, 398,
    398–399
Force-velocity relationship, 397, 397–398
Frame size
  and body fat, 503
  evaluation, 502t
Frank-Starling's law of the heart, 287
Free energy, 98
Free fatty acids (FFA), 51, 53, 112
Free radicals, 72, 73, 421–422
Frontal lobe, 298, 299
Fructose, 42, 216–217
Functional limitation, 588, 590
Functional residual capacity (FRC), 235

G
GABA (gamma aminobutyric acid), 307
Galactose, 42
Galen, 8, 8t, 9, 263
Gamma aminobutyric acid (GABA), 307
Gamma motoneurons, 306
Gamow hypobaric chamber, 456
Gas(es)
  analysis, 147–148, *148*
  concentration, 241
  exchange, 241–245, *244*
  hyperoxic, 492–494
  movement, 242–243, *243*
  pressure, 241
  solubility, 243
  volumes, standardizing, 667–669
Gastric emptying
  factors affecting, 89–90, *90*
  fluid volume and, 218
Gender differences
  aerobic capacity, 195–196, 196t, 197, *197*,
    362t, 363
  anaerobic power, 186–187
  basal metabolic rate, 156, *156*
  cardiac output, 290
  coronary heart disease, 571–573, 574–575
  hemoglobin, 245, 290
  muscle strength, 399–402, 399t, *401*, 401t
  progressive resistance exercise, 404, *404*
  stroke volume, 285
  sweating, 445
  swimming velocity, 175
  thermoregulation, 445
Generality
  cardiac training, 360
  energy system, 180, *181*
Genetic influences
  aerobic capacity, 194–195
  body fat, 530, *530*
  coronary heart disease, 575, 595
  fitness, 196t
  maximal oxygen uptake, 194–195
  maximum heart rate, 194
  obesity, 530, 530–532, 532
  physical working capacity, 194
Gerontology, new, 557–558
Gigantism, 335
Girth measurements, 515, 517, *517*, 673–679
Glucagon, 334t, 341

endurance training response, 350
glucose interaction, 341, *341*
in glucose regulation, 44–45, 341–342, *342*
Glucocorticoids, 339–340
Glucogenesis, 44, 45
Glucolipids, 48
Gluconeogenesis, 41–42, 44, 45, 108, *108*
Glucose. *See also* Glycolysis
    blood, 44
        deficiency, 45, 216
        during exercise, 217, *218*
        regulation, 44–45, 341–342, *342*
    catabolism, energy transfer
        aerobic, 108–110, *109–110*
        anaerobic, 105–108, *106–107*
        net, 110–112, *111*
    intake, 218, 219. *See also* Carbohydrates,
        intake
    metabolism, role of insulin, 340, *340*
    production, 41
    storage, 44
    structure, 41, *42*
    synthesis. *See* Glucogenesis; Gluconeogenesis
    tolerance, aging and, 559
    uptake, in exercise, 46–47, *47*
Glucose-alanine cycle, 57, 59, *59*
Glucose-insulin interaction, 340–341, *341*
Glutamic oxaloacetic transaminase, 600
Glutamine, 480
Glutathione peroxidase (GPX), 73
Glycemic index, 216, 217, *217*
Glycerol, 113, *113*
Glycine, 307
Glycogen
    depletion
        during exercise, 135
        exercise intensity and, 187, *188*
    replenishment, 219, 221
    storage
        diet and, 45
        endurance performance and, *221*, 221–222,
            224
        resistance training and, 57
        sites, 44
    supercompensation. *See* Carbohydrate loading
Glycogen synthase, 106
Glycogenolysis, 44, 45, 105
Glycolysis
    aerobic, 107
    described, 105–108, *106–107*
    hydrogen release, 107
    lactate formation, *107*, 107–108, 126–127
    substrate-level phosphorylation, 106–107
Glycolytic power, performance tests, 185–186
Golgi, C., 311
Golgi tendon organs, *311*, 312–313, *313*
Gonadotropic hormones
    aging and, 563, *564*
    described, 332t, 336
Graded exercise stress test (GXT), 600. *See also*
    Stress testing
Greece, ancient, exercise physiology in, 8, 9
Growth hormone. *See* Human growth hormone
Guidelines for Exercise Testing and Prescription,
    23
Gymnasts, nutritional supplementation, 211, *214*
Gynecomastia, in steroid users, 465

H
H zone, 316, *317*
Haldane effect, 248
Haldane gas analyzer, 148, *148*
Haldane transformation, 161
Hand-grip dynamometer, 390, 392
Handheld weights, walking and, 170
Handicap, 588, 590
Harbor treadmill test, 192, *192*
Harpenden caliper, *512*, 513
Harvard Fatigue Laboratory, 18–19, 20
Harvard University, physical education program,
    13–15, *15*, 17–18
Harvey, W., 263
Hawthorne effect, 32
HDLs (high-density lipoproteins), 49, 575–576,
    577t
Health
    disease prevention tactics, 582, 582t
    exercise benefits, 568–569, *570*
    laws, 8, 8t
    physical activity benefits, 555–556, 557t
    Surgeon General's Report, 555–556, 557t
Health & Fitness Journal, 23
Health/Fitness Director, 592
Health/Fitness Instructor, 592
Health-fitness professional
    in clinical setting, 588
    competency areas, 592t
    training/certification programs, 590–592, 591t
Health-fitness programs, 615–616
Health-impairment categories, 588, 590
Heart
    blood supply, 271–272, *272*
    dimensions
        aerobic training adaptations, 370–371
        in athletes, 292–293, 293t
        resistance training adaptations, 415–416
    electrical impulse, 275, *275*–276
    energy supply, 272, 274
    muscle. *See* Myocardium
    as pump, 264–265, *265*
    residual volume, 287
Heart attack. *See* Myocardial infarction
Heart defects, congenital, 598
Heart disease. *See* Cardiovascular disease;
        Coronary heart disease
Heart failure, congestive, 597
Heart rate
    aerobic capacity prediction from, *200*, 200–201
    aerobic fitness and, 368, *368*
    aerobic training adaptations, 372, *372*
    anticipatory, 277, *277*, 283t
    body position and, 288t
    cardiac output and, 284
    carotid artery palpation and, 278
    catecholamine training effects, 277
    cortical influence, 277, *277*–278, *279*
    electrocardiographic determination, 608–609
    exercise, 288, *288*
    exercise-induced abnormalities, 611
    irregularities. *See* Arrhythmias
    maximum
        aerobic capacity and, 377, *377*
        aerobic training at percentage of, 376–378,
            377
        age differences, 567, *568*
        age-predicted, 377, *378*
        in CHD patients, 606, *607*
    genetic influences, 194
    for upper-body exercise, 377–378, *378*
    oxygen uptake and, 164–165, *165*, 288, *288*
    parasympathetic influence, 277, *277*
    peripheral input, 278
    reflex control, 278, *279*
    regulation, 275–281
        extrinsic, 276–280
        intrinsic, *275*, 275–276
    during step test, 363, *364*, 365
    sympathetic influence, 276–277, *277*
    training effects, 285
    training threshold, 367
    training-sensitive zone, 377, *378*
Heart rate reserve, 367
Heart sounds, auscultation, 598–599
Heart transplantation, exercise prescription, 273,
        614
Heart valve disease, 597–598
Heartburn, angina pectoris versus, 596t
Heat
    acclimatization, 443–445, *444*, 444t
    combustion, 61–62
    exercise in
        circulatory adjustments, 438–439
        mineral requirements, 82–83
        water loss, 439–443
        water requirements, 441t
    gain, factors contributing to, 429–430, *430*
    loss
        factors contributing to, 429–430, *430*
        mechanisms, 431–432
    production, measurement. *See* Calorimetry
    tolerance, factors that improve, 443–446
    transfer, aerobic training adaptations, 375
Heat cramps, 88
Heat disorders, 87–89
Heat exhaustion, 88–89
Heat stress
    evaluation, 446–447, *446–447*
    thermoregulation in, 431–432, *432*, 434
Heat Stress Index, 446–447, *447*
Heat stroke, exertional, 89
Heat syncope, 88
Height-weight tables, 501, 502t
Helmet, cycling, thermoregulation and, 436
Hematological adjustments, altitude
        acclimatization, 452, *453*
Hemoglobin
    gender differences, 245, 290
    oxygen combined with, 245
    oxygen-carrying capacity, 245–246, *246*
    saturation, 246, *246*
Hemosiderin, 80
Henderson, J., 19
Henry, F. M., 19, *19*
Henry's law, 242
Heredity. *See* Genetic influences
Hermansen, L. A., 22, *22*
Herodicus, 8
HGH-releasing hormone, 335
High-altitude cerebral edema (HACE), 455
High-altitude pulmonary edema (HAPE), 455
High-density lipoproteins (HDLs), 49, 575–576,
        577t
High-energy phosphates, 98, 101
Hill, A. V., 19, 137
Hip flexibility, assessment, 560
Historical research, validation, 10–11

Hitchcock, E., 11, 12, *12, 13*
Hitchcock, E., Jr., 11–12, *12,* 13, *13*
"Hitting the wall," 47, 135
HIV-positive patients, exercise prescription, 589
HMB (beta-hydroxy-beta-methylbutyrate), 482
Hohwü–Christensen, E., *20, 20–21*
Homocysteine, coronary heart disease and, 577–578, *578*
Hooke's law of springs, 32, *33*
Hormones. *See also* Endocrine *entries; specific hormone*
    classification, 330
    in cold stress, 431
    endurance training response, 346–351, 347t
    enzymatic effects, 331
    in heat stress, 434
    mechanism of action, 330
    nature, 330
    resistance training response, 351
    secretion
        control, 331
        resting and exercise-induced, 331–334, 332t–334t
Hultman, E., 21, *21*
The Human Body. An Account of its Structure and Activities and the Conditions of its Healthy Working (Martin), 18
Human calorimeter, 143, *144*
Human growth hormone (hGH)
    actions, 335, *336*
    aging and, 563, *564*
    described, 332t, 334–335
    endurance training and, 346–347, *348*
    as ergogenic aid, 469
    exercise and, 335
    regulation, 335, *336*
    resistance training and, 351
Humidity
    evaporative heat loss and, 432, 434
    sweating and, 87, 439, *440, 441*
Hydration, terminology, 85
Hydrochloric acid, sodium bicarbonate buffering, 120
Hydrocortisone. *See* Cortisol
Hydrodensitometry, 508
Hydrogen
    effect on ventilatory control, 252
    release, in glycolysis, 107
Hydrostatic weighing, 507–511
    body density measurement by, 508
    body fat computation and, 508–509
    body volume measurement by, 511, *511*
    limitations and errors, 509, 511
Hyperhydration, 85
Hyperlipidemia, 575
Hyperlipoproteinemia, 575
Hyperoxic gas, 492–494
    during exercise, 493, *493*
    pre-exercise, 493
    in recovery, 494, *494*
Hyperpnea, 252
Hypertension, 268
    borderline, 579
    coronary heart disease and, 572, 579
    defined, 269
    exercise and, 579
    and heart attacks in women, 572
    lifestyle and, 579
    race and, 270
    sodium-induced, 78, 80
    teenage, 339
Hypertensive response, 598, 610–611
Hyperthermia, 87–89
Hyperventilation, 240
    in altitude acclimatization, 451
    effect on ventilatory control, 252
Hypervitaminosis A, 70
Hypoglycemia, 45, 216
Hypohydration, 85
Hyponatremia, 91
Hypophyseal stalk, 334
Hypophysis, 334, *335*
Hypotensive response, 270, 598, 611
Hypothalamic releasing factor, 335
Hypothalamic-pituitary-gonadal axis, aging and, 563, *564*
Hypothalamus, 298, *299*
    as master gland, 334
    in thermoregulation, 430–431
    in ventilatory control, 250
Hypothesis testing, 33–34
Hypothetical constructs, 33

I

I band, 316, *317*
Immune response, exercise and, 349
Independent variable, 27
Indicator dilution method, 285
Individual differences, 32
    anaerobic energy transfer, 188, *189*
    exercise training, 360
    metabolic capacity, 180
    VO_{2max} improvement, 363–364, *364*
Inductive reasoning, 32
Infectious illness, immune response to, exercise and, 349
Inferior vena cava
    anatomy, 266
    collapsed, during Valsalva maneuver, 240, *240*
Information resources, exercise physiology, 651–653. *See also* Internet
Informed consent, stress testing, 602, 602t
Inhibition
    neuronal, 307
    psychological, resistance training and, 411–412
Inhibitory postsynaptic potential (IPSP), 307
Insensible water loss, 85–86, 432
Inspiration, mechanics, 233–234, *234*
Inspiratory capacity, 235
Inspiratory reserve volume, 235, *235*
Insufficiency, heart valve, 597
Insulin
    commercialization, 343, 344
    deficiency, 344
    endurance training response, 350
    functions, 340, *340*
    glucose interaction, 340–341, *341*
    in glucose regulation, 44, 341–342, *342*
    resistance, 344
Insulin-like growth factor, aging and, 563, *564*
Internal criticism, 11
International Council of Sport Science and Physical Education (ICSSPE), 23
International Olympic Committee (IOC), banned drugs, 463
International Zeitschrift für angewandte Physiologie einschliesslich Arbeitsphysiologie, 16

Internet sites, 22–23
    exercise physiology, 657–660
    general science, 660–661
    government, 655–657
    science and technology news, 661
    search engines, 654–655
    useful resources, 661–663
Interval training, 139–140, 140t, 380–382
    exercise interval, 381–382
    guidelines, 381, 381t
    rationale, 381
    relief interval, 382
Interval variable, 26
Intervertebral disc, bulging, 299
Intrafusal fibers, 310, *313*
Intraindividual variability, 31–32
Intrapulmonic pressure, 233
Iodine (iodide), 76t
Ions, 77
Iron, 76t
    absorption, 80, 81
    functions, 80
    loss, during menstrual cycle, 81
    recommended allowances, 81t
    stores, 80
Iron deficiency anemia, 80
Iron supplements, for athletes, 82
Ischemia, myocardial, 492, 574
Islets of Langerhans, 340, *340*
Isokinetic action, defined, 391t
Isokinetic dynamometer, 393
Isokinetic training, 405–407, *406*
Isometric action, 391t, 396, 397
Isometric training, 402–403, *403*, 416
Isotonic action, 397

J

Joint flexibility
    aging and, 559
    static, assessment, 560–562
Joule, 183
Journal of Applied Physiology, 16
Journals, exercise physiology, 672
Jumping test, 182

K

Karvonen, M., 22
Karvonen method, for establishment of training heart rate, 367
Katch test, 185
Ketosis
    cortisol secretion and, 339
    in diabetics, 344
Kg-m, 183
Kilocalorie (kcal), 61, 183
Kilojoule, 183
Knee-jerk reflex, 303, *304*
Komi, P., 22
Krebs cycle
    glucose catabolism, 108–110, *109–110*
    metabolic mill, 116, *117*
Krogh, A., *19,* 19–20, *20*
Krogh, M., *20, 20*

L

Lactate
    blood
        as energy source, 127
        exercise level and, *126,* 126–127, 256, 257

in maximal exercise, 187, *187*
minute ventilation and, *255*
onset of accumulation. *See* Onset of blood lactate accumulation
recovery patterns, 138, *139*
threshold. *See* Onset of blood lactate accumulation
and blood pH, during strenuous exercise, 120, *121*
formation, in glycolysis, *107*, 107–108, 126–127
paradox, 452
shuttling, 127
stacking, 362
Lactate acid buffering, 120, 151, 255
Lactate dehydrogenase, 107, 600
Lactic acid energy system. *See also* Energy system, short-term
described, *126*, 126–127
oxygen deficit and, 130, *130*
Lactic acid theory, 137
Lactose, 42
Lactovegetarian diet, 55
Lange caliper, *512*, 513
Laughter, coronary heart disease and, 580
Laws
of health, 8, 8t
scientific, 32, 33
LDLs (low-density lipoproteins), 49, 575, 577t
Leads, electrocardiogram, 281
Lean body mass (LBM), 505
Left coronary artery, 271, 272
Leg cycling power test, 182–183
Leg press, 1-RM test, 394–395
Leisure activity, intensity categorization, age and, 164, 165t
Leptin, 531, *532*
Licensing laws, early, 9
Life expectancy
for athletes, 568, *570*
current, 557–558
exercise and, 568–569, *570*
physical fitness and, 569, *570*, *571*
Lifestyle
disease prevention and, 582, 582t
hypertension and, 579
Limbic system, 299
Lindhard, J., *19*, 19–20
Ling, P. H., 21
Lipid peroxidation, 72
Lipids (fats), 47–51. *See also* Fatty acids
catabolism
and carbohydrate breakdown, 116
described, 112–114, 117
in exercise, 114
rate limit, 117
total energy transfer, 114
compound, 48–49
content, terms on food labels, 64
coronary heart disease and, 575–577
derived, 49
dietary
choosing between, 52
contribution from major food groups, 49, *50*
recommended intake, 51, 207–209, *209*
energy content, 62
energy distribution, 50, *50*
excess, metabolic fate, *118*
functions, 49–51, *50*

metabolic mill, 116, *117*
metabolism
aerobic training adaptations, 369, *369*
role of insulin, 340
role of water-soluble vitamins, 72
mobilization, 112
respiratory quotient for, 149
simple, 48, *48*
storage, 112, 504
uptake, in exercise, 51, *53*
Lipolysis, caffeine effects, 330
Lipoprotein lipase, 49, 112, 534
Lipoproteins
blood level
classification, 576
composition, 577t
coronary heart disease and, 575–577
exercise effects, 575–576
factors affecting, 577
steroid use and, 466
functions, 48
high-density, 49, 575–576, 577t
low-density, 49, 575, 577t
very-low-density, 49, 577t
Liquid meals, versus precompetition meal, 215–216
Liver function, steroid abuse and, 465–466
Liver glycogen, 44
Load-repetition relationship, 399, *400*
Long slow distance (LSD) training, 380
Longevity. *See* Life expectancy
Low back syndrome, variable resistance training and, 404–405
Low-density lipoproteins (LDLs), 49, 575, 577t
Lumbar vertebrae, *300*
Lung(s). *See also Pulmonary* entries
capacities, 235, *235*
carbon dioxide transport, 243, *244*, 249
compliance, 259, 616–617, 622t
gas exchange, 243–244, *244*
oxygen partial pressure, 246–247
surface area, 232, *232*
volume
dynamic, 235, 235–237
residual, 235, *235*, 509, 510, 511
static, 234–235, *235*
Luteinizing hormone (LH)
described, 332t, 336
endurance training response, 347–348, *348*

M

M line, 316, *317*, 318
Macronutrients, 41–59, 41–61
Magnesium, 76t
Maltose, 42
Man, reference, 504, *504*. *See also* Gender differences
Maternal exercise effects, 383–384, 384t, 386
Maximal heart rate. *See* Heart rate, maximum
Maximal oxygen uptake. *See* Aerobic capacity
Maximal voluntary muscle action (MVMA), 391t, 396
Maximum cardiac output, maximal oxygen uptake and, 290, *290*
Maximum voluntary ventilation (MVV), 236, 237
M-bridges, 318, *318*
Measurement errors, 29, 31
Measurement units, 664–666

Medications
cardiac, 616, 621t
pulmonary, 626, 626t
Medicine and Science in Sports, 16
Medicine and Science in Sports and Exercise, 16, 23
Medulla
anatomy, 298, *299*
cardiovascular center, 277–278, *279*
respiratory center, 250–251, *251*
Megavitamins, 74
Menopause, 563, *564*
Menstruation
delayed onset, and cancer risk, 506
iron loss during, 81
irregular
exercise and, 505–506
leanness and, 505–506
thermoregulation and, 445
Mentoring, 23
Mesencephalon, 298, *299*
Messenger hormones, 330
MET classification of physical activity, 164, 164t, 165t
Metabolic capacity
aerobic training adaptations, 369, 369–370
individual differences, 180
resistance training adaptations, 416, 419
specificity-generality concept, 180, *181*
Metabolic mill, 116, *117*
Metabolism, increased, free radical production and, 73
Metabolite accumulation theory of muscle soreness, 422–423
Metencephalon, 298, *299*
Metformin, 345
Methandrostenolone, 466t
Methyltestosterone, 466t
Metric system, 42, 664–666
Michigan Alcoholism Screening Test (MAST), 476, 477t
Micronutrients, 68–83
Micro-Scholander gas analyzer, 148, *148*
Midbrain, 298, *299*
Mineralocorticoids, 338–339
Minerals, 75–83. *See also* Electrolytes
and exercise performance, 82–83
functions, 75
loss, defense against, 82–83
major, 75, 76t
nature, 75
and physical activity, 75, 77–82
trace, 75, 76t
Minute ventilation, 237, 237t
age differences, 567, *568*
oxygen uptake and, 255, *255*, 258
Mission statement, health-fitness-wellness programs, 615
Mitochondria, aerobic training adaptations, 369
Mitral valve, 265
Mitral valve prolapse, 597, *598*
Mixed diet, respiratory quotient for, 149
Mixed-venous blood, cardiac output and, 284
Modified sit-and-reach test, 560
Monoamines, 301, 302t
Monosaccharides, 41–42
Monounsaturated fatty acids, 48
Mortality ratio, body mass index and, 519, *519*
Motivation, anaerobic energy transfer capacity and, 188

Motoneurons
 anterior, 305–306, *306*
 types, 306
Motor endplate, *306*, 306–307, *307*
Motor neurons, 301
Motor unit
 activation, size principle, 412
 anatomy, 305–306, *306*
 physiology, 307–310
 recruitment, 308–310, *309*
 tension-generating characteristics, 308–310, *309*
 twitch characteristics, 308, 308t, *309*
Movement
 economy, 166, *167*
 mechanical efficiency, 167
Muscle. *See also* Muscle fibers
 actions
  force-velocity relationship, 397, 397–398
  power-velocity relationship, 398, *398*
  in resistance training, 396, 396–397
 activity, in cold stress, 431
 caffeine effects, 475
 contraction
  excitation coupling, 321, *321*, 322
  relaxation after, *321*, 321–322
  sliding-filament theory, 319–321, *320*
 cross-sectional area, arm flexor strength related to, 400, *401*
 endurance, 391t, 417–418
 enervation ratio, 305
 excess, 324
 force gradation, 308
 girth, carbohydrate loading and, 45
 glycogen storage, 44
 groups
  strength curves, 408, *409*
  strength ratios, 399–400, 399t
 mass
  age differences, 559
  factors affecting, 410–411, *411*
 nerve supply, 304
 oxygen storage, 248, *248*
 relaxation, *321*, 321–322
 remodeling, 412–414
 soreness, 419–423. *See also* Delayed-onset muscle soreness
 strength. *See* Muscle strength
 types, comparison, 314–315, 315t
Muscle fibers
 for endurance, 112
 gross structure, 315, *316*
 hyperplasia, resistance training, 414–415
 hypertrophy
  aerobic training, 370–371
  male versus female, 414
  resistance training, 412
  testosterone level and, 414
 ratio of nerve fibers to, 304
 training specificity, 324
 types, 322–326
  aerobic training adaptations, 370–371
  classification, 322, 322t
  cycling economy and, 167
  distribution, by athletic group, 323–326, *325*
  measurement, 322
  resistance training adaptations, 412–415, 414t
 ultrastructure, 316–319, *317–319*

Muscle spindles, 310, *311*
Muscle strength
 age differences, 413, 559, *559*
 curves, 408, *409*
 development. *See* Resistance training
 foundations for studying, 389–390
 gender differences, 399–402, 399t, *401*, 401t
 measurement, 390, 392–393
 ratios
  by muscle group, 399–400, 399t
  for Olympic weightlifters, 400, 401t
 training zone, 399, *400*
Myelin sheath, 306, *306*
Myocardial infarction, 271
 cardiac arrest versus, 571
 causes, 574, 596
 early warning signs, 596, *597*
 illustration, *272*
Myocardium, 264
 characteristics, 314–315, 315t
 contractility, reflex control, 278, *279*
 diseases, 595–597. *See also* Coronary heart disease
 ischemia, 492, 574
 oxygen uptake, 271–272
 oxygen utilization, 271
Myofibril, ultrastructure, 316, *317*
Myofilament
 actin-myosin orientation, 316–318, *318*
 structural orientation, 316, *317*
Myoglobin
 after downhill running, 420
 muscle oxygen storage and, 248, *248*
Myosin crossbridges
 mechanical action, 319–320, *320*
 structure, 317–318, *318*
Myosin-ATPase, 321

N

Nandrolone, 464t
National Weight Control Registry (NWCR), 543–545, 545t, 546t
Naughton treadmill test, *192*, 605, 605t
Neck extension, assessment, 561
Neonates, maternal exercise effects, 383–384, 384t
Nervous system
 aging and, 563
 resistance training adaptations, *411*, 411–412
Neurilemma, 306, *306*
Neurohypophysis, 335, 336–337
Neuromotor system, 297–304, *298*
Neuromuscular fatigue, 310
Neuromuscular junction, *306*, 306–307, *307*
Neuropeptides, 301, 302t
Neurotransmitters, 301, 302t
Niacin, 71t, 74
Nicotinamide-adenine dinucleotide (NAD), 102, 103, *103*
Nicotinamide-adenine dinucleotide phosphate (NADH), 102, 103, *103*
Nicotinic acid, 71t, 74
Nielsen, M., 20, 20–21
Nitric oxide (NO)
 cardiovascular effects, 280
 as neurotransmitter, 301
Nitrogen
 altitude training and, 456
 in alveolar air, 242, 242t

 in ambient air, 242, 242t
 balance, measurement, 115
 chemical analysis, 147–148
Nodes of Ranvier, 306, *306*
Norepinephrine
 cardiovascular effects, 276–277, 282
 in cold stress, 431
 described, 333t, 338
 endurance training response, 350, *350*
Norethandrolone, 466t
Norway, contributions to exercise physiology, 21–22
Nucleoproteins, 55
Nutrient intake. *See also* Diet(s); Food intake
 recommended, 207–208, *209*
 supplementation, 211, *214*
Nutrient requirements, 207–209
Nutrition, extreme environments and, 436t, 437, *437*
Nutrition Labeling and Education Act, 64
Nutritional agents, as ergogenic aids, 462–489

O

Obesity, 529–539
 android, 534
 BMI values, 519–520
 childhood, 531, 546
 coronary heart disease and, 579–580
 creeping, 529
 fat cell size and number and, 535, *535*
 genetic influences, 530, 530–532, *532*
 gynoid, 534
 health risks, 532–533
 as long-term process, 529
 predisposing factors, 529–530
 thermogenic response, 145
 types, 533, *534*
 weight gain and, 145
Obesity gene, 530–531, *532*
Occipital lobe, 298, *299*
Occupational setting, physical testing in, 393
Older-age adults. *See* Aging
Oligomenorrhea, 77, 506
Olympic wheelchair-dependent athletes, aerobic capacity, 193
Olympic-caliber athletes, aerobic capacity, *190*
Oncology. *See* Cancer
One-mile walk test, 603
One-repetition maximum (1-RM)
 for bench and leg press, 394–395
 described, 392, *392*
 estimation, from submaximal effort, 400
Onset of blood lactate accumulation (OBLA)
 aerobic training at, 380
 causes, 258
 described, 127, 255, 256, 257, 258
 and endurance performance, 258
Open-circuit spirometry, 144–147, *146–147*, 667–671
Operational definition, 33
Opioid peptides, exercise and, 351
Oral contraceptives, coronary heart disease and, 573
Oral rehydration beverage, 219, 220t, 221
Ordinal variable, 26
Osteoporosis
 bone mineral accrual and, 567–568
 calcium deficiency and, 77
 in female athletes, 77, 78

Overload, 358, 391t, 396
Overtraining
  carbohydrates and, 128, 221
  signs and symptoms, 128, 380
  tapering versus, 128–129
Overweightness, body mass index and, 519–520, 536
Oxandrolone, 464t
Oxidation
  beta–, 113, *113*
  cellular, *102–103*, 102–104
Oxidative phosphorylation, 103–104
Oxygen
  in alveolar air, 242, 242t
  in ambient air, 242, 242t
  caloric value, 148
  chemical analysis, 147–148, *148*
  combined with hemoglobin, 245–246, *246*
  consumption. *See* Oxygen uptake
  deficit, 130, 130–131, *131*
  in energy metabolism, 104
  extraction. *See* Oxygen extraction
  loading, at altitude, 449–450
  movement, in air and fluids, 243, *243*
  myocardial utilization, 271
  partial pressure
    during exercise, 252, *252–253*
    hemoglobin saturation and, 246, *246*
    in lungs, 246–247
    plasma, 251, *251*
    in tissue, 247
  in solution, 245
  storage, in muscle, 248, *248*
  transport
    in blood, 245–248, *246*
    cardiac output and, 289–290
    in lungs, 243, *244*
  uptake. *See* Oxygen uptake
  ventilatory equivalent for, 255, 374, *374*
Oxygen extraction (a-vO$_2$ difference)
  aerobic training adaptations, 373
  cardiac output and, 284, 291, *291*
  in heart disease, 291
  during rest and exercise, 291, *291*
Oxygen pulse, age differences, 567, *568*
Oxygen uptake (VO$_2$). *See also* Energy expenditure
  and blood lactate, exercise level and, *126*, 126–127, 256, *257*
  body position and, 288t
  and body size, 132
  calculation, Haldane transformation for, 161
  cardiac output and, 284–285
  economy of movement and, 166, *167*
  exercise, 129, *129–131*
  heart rate and, 164–165, *165*, 288, *288*
  maximal. *See* Aerobic capacity
  measurement, 144–148
    by closed-circuit spirometry, 144, *144*
    by open-circuit spirometry, 144–147, *146–147*, 669–670
  myocardial, 271–272
  peak, 189, 190, 196
  during recovery, 135–140, *136*
  relative, 132
  resting, 289–290
  during upper-body exercise, 291–292, *292*
  ventilation and, 255, *255*, 258, 259, *259*
Oxyhemoglobin, 245

Oxyhemoglobin dissociation curve
  2,3-diphosphoglycerate and, *246*, 247–248
  Bohr effect, *246*, 247
  oxygen partial pressure and, 246, *246*
Oxymetholone, 464t, 466t
Oxymyoglobic curve, 248, *248*
Oxytocin
  described, 332t, 336–337
  endurance training response, 348

P

Pacinian corpuscles, 313
Pancreatic hormones
  described, 333t–334t, *340–341*, 340–342
  endurance training response, 350
Pangamic acid (vitamin B$_{15}$), 478
Pantothenic acid, 71t
Parasympathetic nervous system, 277, *277*, 302–303, 303t
Parathyroid gland, 337, *337*
Parathyroid hormone (PTH), 334t, 337
Parietal lobe, 298, *299*
Partial pressure, 241
Patella tendon reflex, 303, *304*
P[smCO[nm2. *See* Carbon dioxide, partial pressure
Peak oxygen uptake (VO$_{2peak}$), 189, 190, 196
Peak power output, 185
Peer review, 34
Peliosis hepatis, 466
Performance tests. *See* Power tests
Pericarditis, 596–597
Perimysium, 315, *316*
Periodization
  defined, 391t
  resistance training, *409*, 409–410
Periosteum, 315, *316*
Peripheral nervous system, 298, 301–304
Personality patterns, coronary heart disease and, 580
pH, 119, *119*
PH
  enzymes and, 119
  lactate and, during strenuous exercise, 120, *121*
  oxyhemoglobin dissociation curve and, *246*, 247
Pharmacologic agents, as ergogenic aids, 462–489
Phenpropionate, 464t
Phlebitis, 267, *267*
Phosphagens, 125
Phosphate bond energy, 96–104
Phosphate buffers, 120
Phosphate loading, ergogenic benefits, 480
Phosphates, high-energy, 98, 101
Phosphatidylserine (PS), 480–481
Phosphocreatine (PCr)
  creatine supplementation and, 484, 486
  as energy reservoir, 100–101, *101*, 125
Phosphofructokinase (PFK), 106
Phospholipids, 48
Phosphorus, 76t
Phosphorylation
  defined, 102
  oxidative, 103–104
  substrate-level, 106–107
Phylloquinone (vitamin K), 69, 69t
Physical activity. *See also* Exercise
  bodily function and, *558*, 558–559
  body fat and, 532, 546

  body weight and, 212, 214
  cancer and, 593
  classification, 163–164, 164t, 165t
  coronary heart disease and, 578–579, 580
  energy expenditure and, 157, 159, 160–166
  food intake and, 209–210, 212, 215t
  health benefits, 555–556, 557t
  minerals and, 75, 77–82
  of obese children, 546
  patterns and trends, 556
  protein requirements and, 56–57
  safety, 556–557
  Surgeon General's Report, 555–556, 557t
  training/certification programs, 590–592, 591t
Physical Activity and Health, 23
Physical activity ratio (PAR), 164
Physical fitness. *See* Fitness
Physical impairment, categories, 588, *590*
Physical working capacity, genetic influences, 194
Physiologic agents, as ergogenic aids, 489–494
Physiologic dead space, 238, *238*
Physiological Reviews, 15–16
The Physiology of Bodily Exercise (Lagrange), 18
Physiology of Sport (Kolb), 18
Pituitary gland
  anterior, 334, *335*
  posterior, 335, 336–337
Pituitary hormones
  anterior
    described, 332t, 334–336, *335*
    endurance training response, 346–348, 347t, *348*
  posterior
    described, 332t, 336–337
    endurance training response, 348
Placebo effect, 28
Plant polysaccharides, 42
Plasma volume, aerobic training adaptations, 371
Plyometric training, 391t, *407*, 407–408
PO$_2$. *See* Oxygen, partial pressure
Poiseuille's law, 280
Polysaccharides, 42, 44–45
Polyunsaturated fatty acids, 48
Pons, 298, *299*
Poseidon, 10
Potassium, 76t, 77–78
Power
  defined, 391t
  formula, 134, 399
Power tests, 181–183. *See also* Stress testing
  aerobic, 190–194, 191t, *192*
  anaerobic, 184, 185–186
  jumping, 182
  leg cycling, 182–183
  in occupational setting, 393
  relationships among, 183, 183t
  stair-sprinting, 182, *182*
Power-force-range of motion relationship, 398, 398–399
Power-velocity relationship, 398, *398*
Precapillary sphincter, 265
Precompetition meal, 214–216
Pregnancy
  energy expenditure and, 159
  exercise during, 382–386
    contraindications, 385
    energy cost, 382
    fetal blood supply and, 382–383

guidelines, 385
outcome, 382–384, 384t, 386
pattern, 382, 383
physiologic demands, 382
Preload, 287
Premature atrial contraction, 278
Premature ventricular contraction, 278, 610, *611*
Pressure gradients, for gas transfer, 243, *244*
Preventive/Rehabilitative Exercise Specialist, 592
Preventive/Rehabilitative Program Director, 592
PRICE acronym, 311
Primary source material, 10
The Principles of Physiology Applied to the Preservation of Health and to the Improvement of Physical and Mental Education (Combe), 18
Professional organizations, 23, 651–653
Progesterone, 334t, 340
Progressive overload, 391t
Progressive resistance exercise (PRE), 403–404, *404*
Prolactin (PRL), 332t, 336, 347
Prolapse, mitral valve, 597, 598
Pro-opiomelancortin (POMC), 336
Proprioceptors, 310–312
Protein(s), 51–59
    catabolism, 54, 114–116, *116*
    complete, 53
    deamination, 54, 115
    dietary
        contribution from major food groups, 55, 55
        precompetition, 214
        recommended intake, 55–56, 56t, 207–209, *209*
        sources, 54, 54t
        vegetarian approach, 54, 55
        for weight gain, 551
    excess, metabolic fate, 117, *118*
    functions, 54–55
    incomplete, 53–54
    metabolic mill, 116, *117*
    metabolism, role of water-soluble vitamins, 72
    predigested, 56
    requirements
        estimation, 115
        for physically active people, 56–57
    respiratory quotient for, 149
    structural, 55
    supplementation, 57
    synthesis, 54
    transamination, 53, 54, 115
Protein filaments, 317–318, *318*
Protein sparing
    carbohydrates and, 45
    exercise and, 550
Provitamins, 69
Pulmonary capillaries, 232, 233
Pulmonary circulation, 264, *265*
Pulmonary congestion, 597
Pulmonary diseases
    obstructive, 259, 617, 623–624, 623t
    restrictive, 616–617, 622t
Pulmonary edema, high-altitude, 455
Pulmonary function variables, 234–237
Pulmonary medications, 626, 626t
Pulmonary system. *See also* Lung(s)
    aerobic training adaptations, 373–374, *374*
    aging and, 565
    assessment, 624–625

illustration, 232
rehabilitation, 625–626
structure and function, 231–241
Pulmonary ventilation. *See* Ventilation
Pulse pressure, 269
Pulse rate, measurement, 199, 268, *268*
Purkinje system, 275, *275*
Push-up muscular endurance test, 418
Pyramidal tract, 301
Pyramiding, 463
Pyridoxine (vitamin B$_6$), 71t, 74
Pyruvate, glucose degradation to, 105–108, *106–107*

Q
Quebec 10-second leg cycling power test, 182–183

R
Race
    fat-free body mass and, 509
    hypertension and, 270
Radiation, heat, 431–432
Radiography, chest, 599, *599*
Radionucleotide studies, 611
Ramp test, 192
Range of motion (ROM)
    defined, 391t
    force:power and, 398, *398–399*
Rate-pressure product (RPP), 271–272
Rating of perceived exertion (RPE), 378, 380, 604
Recording error, 29, 31
Recovery
    active, 138, 267
    blood pressure in, 270
    hyperoxic gas in, 494, *494*
    optimal, 138, *139*
    oxygen uptake in, *136*, 136–140
    passive, 138
Recreational activities, energy costs, 162, 162t, *163*
Red blood cell reinfusion, 489–490, *490*, 491t
Reflex(es), 303–304, *305*
Reflex arc, autonomic, 303, *304*
Regurgitation, heart valve, 597
Rehabilitation
    cardiac. *See* Cardiac rehabilitation
    pulmonary, 625–626
Rehydration. *See also* Fluid replacement
    adequacy, 90–91
    defined, 85
    oral, 219, 220t, 221
Relationships between variables
    casual, 26–27, 27
    causal, 27–29
    factors affecting, 29, 31–32
Relaxation, after muscle contraction, *321*, 321–322
Renal buffer, 120
Renal circulation, 280
Renin, exercise-induced release, 82
Renin-angiotensin mechanism, 338
Repetition
    defined, 391t
    relationship to load, 399, *400*
Repetition maximum (RM), defined, 391t
Research continuum, in science, 34, 34–35
Research design, 30–31
Residual lung volume, 235, *235*

body density and, 509, 510
measurement errors, 511
prediction, 510
Resistance training. *See also* Muscle strength
    adaptations, 410–423, *411*, 414t
        body composition, 419, 420t
        cardiovascular, 415–416, 415t
        connective tissue and bone, 415, 415t
        metabolic, 416, 419
        muscular, 412–415, 414t
        neural, *411*, 411–412
    blood pressure response, 270, *271*
    for cardiac rehabilitation, 614, 617t–618t
    for children, 402, 402t
    circuit. *See* Circuit resistance training
    cortisol release and, 481
    definition of terms, 390, 391t
    and endocrine function, 351
    equipment, 393
    external, constant, dynamic, 391t, 397, 403–404, *404*
    factors affecting, 393
    force-power-range of motion relationship, 398, 398–399
    force-velocity relationship, 397, 397–398
    glycogen reserve requirements, 57
    isokinetic, 405–407, *406*
    isometric, 402–403, *403*
    load-repetition relationship, 399, *400*
    muscle actions, 396, 396–397
    muscle soreness after, 419–423
    objectives, 390
    for older-age adults, 413
    overload principle, 396
    periodization, *409*, 409–410
    plyometric, 407, 407–408
    power-velocity relationship, 398, *398*
    principles, 393, 396–399
    scientific foundations, 389–390
    specificity, 408, *409*
    systems, 402–410
    variable, 404–405, *405*
    for weight gain, 551
Respirations. *See* Ventilation
Respiratory center, 250–251, *251*
Respiratory chain, 102–103, *103*
Respiratory exchange ratio (R), 149–151, 255
Respiratory membrane, 232, 233
Respiratory muscles, 233–234, *234*
Respiratory quotient (RQ)
    calculation, by open-circuit spirometry, 670
    for carbohydrate, 149
    described, 148–149
    for lipid, 149
    for mixed diet, 149
    non-protein, 149, 151t
    for protein, 149
Respiratory tract, during cold-weather exercise, 448
Resting daily energy expenditure (RDEE), 157, 158
Restrictive lung dysfunction (RLD), 616–617, 622t
Reticular formation, 301
Retinol (vitamin A), 69, 69t, 70, 73, 74
Reversibility, exercise training, 360, *361*
Rheumatic fever, heart valve stenosis and, 598
Rhythmic exercise, blood pressure response, 268, *268*, 270, *271*

Riboflavin (vitamin B₂), 71t, 74
Right atrium, 266
Right coronary artery, 271, 272
Right ventricle, 266
Rigor mortis, ATP and, 321
RM (repetition maximum), defined, 391t
Rosa, E. B., 143
Rowing, energy expenditure during, 160
Running
    air resistance effects, 172, 174
    downhill, muscle soreness and, 420, *421*
    economy
        age differences, *167*, 167–168, 566
        oxygen uptake and, 166–167, *167*
        running speed and, *169*, 171
        trained versus untrained, 168
    endurance, body composition and, 522, 523t
    energy expenditure during, *169*, 170–174, 171t
    marathon, energy expenditure during, 174
    performance, in children, 363
    speed, factors affecting, 172
    treadmill
        predicted energy cost, 173
        versus track running, 174
    ultraendurance, energy intake and expenditure
        during, 210–211, 213t

S

SAID principle (specific adaptations to imposed
        demands), 358
Saltin, B., 21, *21*
Sarcolemma, 306, *307*, 315, *316*
Sarcomere, 316–319, *317–319*
Sarcoplasm, 315, *316*
Sarcoplasmic reticulum, 315, 318, *319*
Satiety hormone, 531, *532*
Saturated fat content, common foods, 51t
Saturated fatty acids, 48, *48*
Scholander, P., 22
Schwann cells, 306
Science
    certainty of, 33–34
    goals, 25
    hierarchy in, 25, *25*
    Internet sites, 660–661
    research continuum, 34, 34–35
Scientific process
    fact finding, 25–26
    hypothesis testing, 33–34
    laws, 32, 33
    levels, 25, *25*
    publishing results, 34
    theories, 32–33, 33
Second messenger, 330
Secondary source material, 10–11
Selenium, 76t
Semilunar valves, 265
Sensory neurons, 301
Sensory receptors, 301, 310–312
Septum, 265
Set, defined, 391t
Setpoint theory, 542, *542*
Sex-specific essential fat, 504
Shortness of breath. *See* Dyspnea
Shoulder elevation, assessment, 560
Shoulder rotation, assessment, 561
SI units, 665–666
Sick sinus node syndrome, 611
Simple sugars, 42

Sinoatrial (S-A) node, 275, *275*
Sinus bradycardia, 598
Sinus tachycardia, 598
Siri equation, 508–509
Sit-and-reach test, modified, 560
Size principle, 308
Skeletal muscle, *313*
    blood supply, 316
    capillarization, 316
    characteristics, 314–315, 315t
    chemical composition, 315
    fat burning adaptations, with aerobic training,
        114
    fiber type classification, 322, 322t. *See also*
        Muscle fibers, types
    gross structure, 315–316, *316*
    ultrastructure, 316–319, *317–319*
Skin friction drag, during swimming, 175
Skinfold caliper, 512, *512–513*
Skinfold equations, for prediction of body fat,
        516, 517
Skinfold measurements, 512–515, 516, 517
    calipers in, *512*, 512–513
    guidelines, 515
    nomogram, 680–681
    sites, 513–514, *514*
    timing, 513
    use of data, 514, 515t, 516, 517
Sliding-filament theory, muscle contraction,
        319–321, *320*
Slow-oxidative (SO) muscle fibers, 323, 323t
Slow-twitch (S) motor unit, 308, 308t, *309*
Slow-twitch muscle fibers, 112, 132, 323, 323t
Smoking
    coronary heart disease and, 572, 579
    effects of, 259–260
    HDL level and, 575
    and heart attacks in women, 572
Smooth muscle, characteristics, 314–315, 315t
Sodium, 76t, 77–78
    conservation, by kidneys, 82
    dietary, 78, 80
    hypertension and, 78, 80
    in oral rehydration beverage, 219
    regulation, aldosterone in, 338, 339
    terms on food labels, 64
Sodium bicarbonate
    buffering, 120
    as ergogenic aid, 478–479, 479t
Sodium citrate, as ergogenic aid, 479
Soft tissue injuries, 312
Somatic nervous system, 302
Somatopause, 563, *564*
Somatostatin, 335
Somatotropin. *See* Human growth hormone
Source material, 10–11
Spasm theory of muscle soreness, 422
Spatial summation, 307
Specific gravity, evaluation, 507–508, *508*
Specificity
    aerobic training, 359, *360*
    energy system training, 180, *181*
    exercise training, 358–359
    muscle fiber training, 324
    resistance training, 408, *409*
Sphygmograph, 11, *11*
Spinal cord
    anatomy, 299–301, *300*
    ascending nerve tracts, 301
    descending nerve tracts, 301

Spinal nerves
    compression, 299
    location and distribution, 301–302, *302*
Spindle fibers, 310, *313*
Spirometry
    closed-circuit, 144, *144*
    open-circuit, 144–147, *146–147*, 667–671
    portable, 145, *146*
Sport Science Review, 23
Sports activities, energy costs, 162, 162t, *163*
Sports anemia, 81–82, *82*
Sports medicine, and clinical exercise physiology,
        588, 590
Spot reduction, 550
Sprinting, muscle fibers for, 112
S-T segment depression, 610, *610*
Stacking, 463
Stair-sprinting test, 182, *182*
Staleness. *See* Overtraining
Stanazolol, 464t, 466t
Standard error of estimate (SEE), 198
Starch, 42
Static flexibility, assessment, 560–562
Stature, resting daily energy expenditure and, 158
Stenosis, heart valve, 597, 598
Step bench work, measurement, 135
Step test
    for cardiorespiratory fitness evaluation, 363,
        364, 365
    for maximal oxygen uptake prediction, 199
Steroids, anabolic. *See* Anabolic steroids
Sticking point, defined, 391t
Storage fat, 504
Strategic plan, health-fitness-wellness programs,
        615
Strength, 391t. *See also* Muscle strength
Stress
    coronary heart disease and, 580
    cortisol response to, 339
    immune response and, 349
Stress testing. *See also* Power tests
    contraindications, 602–603
    criteria for stopping, 603t
    ECG recordings, 281
    in evaluation of aerobic power, 190
    in evaluation of coronary heart disease
        classification system, 601–602, 601t
        purposes, 600
        rationale, 600–601
        sensitivity, 607
    graded, 600
    informed consent, 602, 602t
    maximal versus submaximal, 603, 605
    protocols, 605–606
    safety, 607
    symptom limited, 603
Stretch reflex, 310–312, *313*
Stretch-shortening cycle, 407
Stride, 172
Stroke
    heat, exertional, 89
    prevention, behavioral changes, 582, 582t
Stroke volume
    aerobic training adaptations, 371–372, *372*
    body position and, 287, 288t
    cardiac output and, 284
    exercise, *286*, 286–287
        increases, 287, 288t
        maximal oxygen uptake and, 286–287, 287t

gender differences, 285
training effects, 285
in untrained person, 285
Subcutaneous fat, 504
Sucrose, 42
Sulfonylurea, 345
Sulfur, 76t
Superior vena cava, 266
Superoxide dismutase (SOD), 73
Surgeon General's Report, on physical activity
and health, 555–556, 557t
Sweating
capacity, 85
dehydration from, 441
electrolyte concentration, 89
electrolyte loss from, 82
gender differences, 445
heat loss from, 432, 434
humidity and, 87, 439, *440*, 441
water loss from, 86–87, 439–441, *440*
Sweden, contributions to exercise physiology, 21
Swimming
breath-holding and, 252
buoyancy effects, 175–176
drag forces during, 175
energy expenditure during, 174–175, *175–176*
maximum heart rate, 377–378, *378*
oxygen uptake and, 175, *176*
tests, in CHD patients, 606, *607*
velocity
gender differences, 175
oxygen uptake and, 175, *176*
Sympathetic chain, 303
Sympathetic nervous system, 276–277, *277*,
302–303, 303t
Sympathetic outflow, vascular regulation, 282,
282
Sympathoadrenal response, 350, *350*
Sympathomimetic agents, 471
Synapse, 301
Synaptic cleft, 306, *307*
Synaptic gutter, 306, *307*
Systemic circulation, 264, *265*
Systole, 268
Systolic blood pressure, 269
aerobic training adaptations, 373, 373t
during exercise, 270, 270t
in recovery, 270
Systolic emptying, stroke volume increases and,
287

T

Tachycardia, 277, 598
Tapering, versus overtraining, 128–129
Tear theory of muscle soreness, 422
Technological error, 29
Tecumseh step test, 365
Telencephalon, 298, *299*
Television, and childhood obesity, 531
Temperature. *See* Ambient temperature; Body
temperature
Temporal lobe, 298, *299*
Temporal summation, 307
Tendon, 315, *316*
Ten-repetition maximum (10-RM), 392, *392*
Terrain, energy expenditure during walking and,
169, 170t
Testing effects, 29
Testosterone, 334t, 340

aging and, 563, *564*
endurance training response, 347–348, *348*
muscle size and, 414
resistance training response, 351
Thalamus, 298, *299*
Thallium imaging, 611
Theoretical research, *34*, 34–35
Theories, development, 32–33, *33*
Thermal balance, 429–430, *430*
Thermogenesis, dietary-induced, 159
Thermoregulation
acclimatization and, 443–445, *444*, 444t
age differences, 445
body fat and, 445–446
in children, 445
clothing and, 434–436
in cold stress, 431
exercise training and, 444–445
gender differences, 445
in heat stress, 431–432, *432*, 434
mechanisms, 429–434, 431t, *435*
role of hypothalamus, 430–431
Thiamin (vitamin B₁), 71t
Thinness, structural characteristics, 505
Thorax, compliance, 259
Thrombus, coronary, 271, 574
Thyroid function, aging and, 563
Thyroid gland, 337, *337*
Thyroid hormones
described, 333t, 337, *337*
endurance training response, 348, 350
Thyrotropin (thyroid-stimulating hormone, TSH),
332t, 335
Thyroxine (T4), 333t, 337, *337*, 431
Tidal volume (TV)
breathing rate and, 237, 237t
described, 234, *235*
distribution, 237, *238*
during exercise, 238, *239*
Tissues
carbon dioxide in, 249
gas exchange in, 244, *244*
oxygen partial pressure in, 247
Tocopherol (vitamin E), 69, 69t, 73–74, 420–422,
421
Torque, 391t
Total daily energy expenditure (TDEE), 157, 159
Total lung capacity, 235
Total strength score sum (TSSS), 401
Tour de France, energy intake and expenditure
during, 210, *212*
Trachea, anatomy, 231, *232*
Tracheal air, 242, 242t
Track running, energy expenditure, 174
Training state, maximal oxygen uptake and, 185
Training volume, 391t
Transamination, protein, *53*, 54, 115
Transferrin, 80
Treadmill running, 173, *174*
Treadmill tests
exercise prescription based on, 612, *616*
maximal, in CHD patients, 606, *607*
measurement of work, 134
protocols, 192, *192*, 605–606, 605t
Treadmill walking, 173
Triad system, 318
Triathletes, aerobic training adaptations, 371
Triceps, skinfold measurement, 548
Tricuspid valve, 265

Triglyceride level
classification, 576
coronary heart disease and, 575
Triiodothyronine (T3), 333t, 337, *337*
Troglitazone, 345
Tropomyosin, 318, *318*
Troponin, 318, *318*
Trunk extension, assessment, 561
Trunk flexibility, assessment, 560
T-tubule system, 318–319, *319*
Twelve-minute or 1.5-mile test, 603
Type A alpha motoneurons, 306
Type A personality, 580
Type B personality, 580
Type I muscle fibers, 112, 132
Type II muscle fibers, 112, 132

U

Ultrasound, 600
Underweight, versus thin, 505
University of California, Berkeley, 19
Upper-body exercise
blood pressure response, 270, 270t
cardiovascular adjustments, 291–292, *292*
maximum heart rate, 377–378, *378*
Up-regulation, 330

V

Vagus nerve, stimulation, 277
Valsalva maneuver, 240, *240*
Variability
between-subject, 32
within-subject, 31–32
Variable resistance training, 391t, 404–405, *405*
Variables
independent versus dependent, 27
types, 26
Vasoconstriction, 282, *282*, 438–439
Vasodilation, 280, 438–439
Vasomotor tone, 282
Vasopressin. *See* Antidiuretic hormone
Vegetarian diet, 55, 80–81, 208
Veins
anatomy, 266, *266*
as blood reservoirs, 266
valves in, 266, *267*
varicose, 267
Venous pooling, 267
Venous return, 266
Venous tone, 266
Ventilation
aerobic capacity limitations, 258–260
aerobic training adaptations, 373–374, *374*
alveolar, 237–238, 237t, *238*
anatomy, 231–233, *232–233*
body position and, 234
buffering function, 120, 231
depth versus rate, 238–239
disruptions in patterns, 239–240
dynamic measures, 235, 235–237
and energy demands, 254–258
during exercise, 254–260, *258*
mechanics, 233–234, *234*
minute. *See* Minute ventilation
oxygen uptake and, 255, *255*, 258, 259, *259*
rate, 237t, 238–239
regulation. *See* Ventilatory control
static measures, 234–235, *235*
voluntary, maximum, 236, 237

Ventilatory control, 250–254, *251*
  in exercise, 252–254, 253
    body temperature and, 253
    chemical, 252, 252–253
    integrated regulation, 254
    neurogenic factors, 253
    nonchemical, 253
  humoral factors, 251
  hyperventilation and breath-holding, 252
  neural factors, 250–251
  plasma $P[smCO[nm_2$ and, 251–252
  plasma Po_2 and, 251, *251*
Ventilatory equivalent
  for carbon dioxide, 255
  for oxygen, 255
Ventilatory system. *See* Pulmonary system
Ventilatory threshold, 255, 256, 257
Ventricular contraction, 265
Ventricular fibrillation, 278
Ventriculography, 611
Venule, 266, *266*
Vertebrae, 299, *300*
Very-low-density lipoproteins (VLDLs), 49, 577t
Visceral adipose tissue (V-AT), 504, 533–534
Viscous pressure drag, 175
Vitamin A (retinol), 69, 69t, 70, 73, 74
Vitamin B_1 (thiamin), 71t
Vitamin B_2 (riboflavin), 71t, 74
Vitamin B_6, 577, 578
Vitamin B_6 (pyridoxine), 71t, 74
Vitamin B_{12}, 71t, 577, 578
Vitamin B_{15} (pangamic acid), 478
Vitamin C (ascorbic acid), 71t, 73, 74, 80–81
Vitamin D, 69, 69t, 70, 74
Vitamin E (tocopherol), 69, 69t, 73–74, 420–422, *421*
Vitamin K (phylloquinone), 69, 69t
Vitamins, 68–74
  antioxidant role, 72–74
  biologic functions, 70, *71*, 72, *72*
  classification, 68–69
  exercise performance and, 74
  fat-soluble, 69, 69t, 70
  nature, 68
  toxicity, 70
  transport, 51
  water-soluble, 69–70, 71t, 72

$\dot{V}O_2$. *See* Oxygen uptake
$\dot{V}O_{2max}$. *See* Aerobic capacity

W

Waist girth, 534, 568, 569
Waist-to-hip girth ratio (WHR), 534, 537
Walking
  competition, 168, *169*
  energy expenditure during, 168–170, *169*, 170t, 173
  test
    maximal oxygen uptake prediction from, 195
    one-mile, 603
  treadmill, 173
Wallace altitude tent, 456, *457*, 458
Warm-up, 491–492
Warm-weather clothing, thermoregulation and, 436
Water (body). *See also* Fluid(s)
  absorption
    factors affecting, 89, *90*
    intestinal, 86, *87*
  compartments, 84
  functions, 84
  intake versus output, 84–86, *86*
  intoxication, 91
  loss, 84–86, *86*
    insensible, 85–86, 432
    protein breakdown and, 116
    from sweating, 86–87, 439–441, *440*
  metabolic, 84
  replacement. *See* Fluid replacement
  requirements, 84, 86
    in exercise, 86–87, 441t
  total body, distribution, 85
  uptake, glucose intake and, 219
Water vapor, in alveolar air, 242, 242t
Watt, 181
Wave drag, 175
Weight, body. *See* Body weight
Weight gain
  energy balance equation as basis for, 550–551
  fat cell size and number after, 538
  obesity and, 145
Weight loss
  calorie-counting approach, 543
  by diet only, 541–545
  by diet plus exercise, 549–550
  effects on resting metabolism, 542, *542*
  energy balance equation as basis for, *540*, 540–541
  by exercise only, 545–547, 549, 549t
  fat cell size and number after, 535, 538, *538*
  general observations, 550
  maintenance, 539, *539*, 543–545, *545*, 545t
Weightlifting
  belt, recommendations for use, 405
  body composition, 523, 525
  metabolic stress, 405
  Olympic, strength ratios, 400, 401t
Weights, energy expenditure during walking and, 170
Weir method, for calculation of energy expenditure, 150
Wellness
  economic benefits, 59
  fitness and, 58–59
Wellness programs, administration, 615–616
Wet bulb temperature (WBT), 446, *446*
Wet bulb-globe temperature (WB-GT), 446, *446*
Wind Chill Index, 448, *448*
Wind velocity, 172, 174
Wingate cycle ergometer test, 184–185, *186*
Within-subject variability, 31–32
Woman, reference, 504, *504*. *See also* Gender differences
Work
  classification, 163–164. *See also* Physical activity
  formula, 134
  mathematical expressions, 183
  measurement, 134–135
World Wide Web (www), 22–23, 654–663
Wrestlers, high school, 522–523, 523t, 524
Wrist elevation, assessment, 560

X

X-variable, 27

Y

Y-variable, 27

Z

Z line, 316, *317*
Zinc, 76t